BLACK'S
STUDENT
VETERINARY
DICTIONARY

BLACK'S STUDENT VETERINARY DICTIONARY

Edited by
Edward Boden
MBE, HonAssocRCVS, MRPharmS

A & C BLACK • LONDON

3 5 7 9 10 8 6 4 2

This edition published 2007
A & C Black Publishers Limited
36 Soho Square, London W1D 3QY
www.acblack.com

ISBN 978 0 7136 8763 7

© 2007, 2005 A & C Black Publishers Limited

A CIP catalogue record for this book is available from the British Library

Typeset in Adobe Garamond by RefineCatch Limited, Bungay, Suffolk

Printed in the UK by CPI William Clowes Beccles NR34 7TL

The publishers make no representation, express or implied,
with regard to the accuracy of the information contained in this
book and cannot accept any legal responsibility for any errors or
omissions that may take place.

This book is produced using paper made from wood grown in
managed, sustainable forests. It is natural, renewable and recyclable.
The logging and manufacturing processes conform to the environmental
regulations of the country of origin.

PREFACE

Generations of veterinary practitioners, students, farmers and pet owners have relied on *Black's Veterinary Dictionary* as a primary reference on animal health and husbandry matters. The 21st edition has been comprehensively updated; it covers the widest spectrum of veterinary data available in a single volume. The core of information on animal health, husbandry and welfare topics, and signs of diseases and their treatment, is supplemented by many new and amended entries. These reflect the numerous developments that have taken place since the 20th edition was published; they range from advances in medication to descriptions of newly identified conditions; from the resurgence of old scourges such as TB in cattle to the emerging risk of exotic diseases being imported following the relaxation of travel arrangements for dogs and cats.

A major innovation is the inclusion of entries describing the popular breeds of dog and cat, and the inheritable conditions to which they might be susceptible.

Some changes will be noticed in the spelling of certain medicines, which have been amended to conform with the recommended international non-proprietary names for medicinal substances, in accordance with EEC Directive 92/97.

Dr A.H. Andrews BVetMed, PhD, MRCVS has again acted as assistant editor. Dr Andrews, D. McK. Fraser BVM&S, CertWel. MRCVS and A.D. Malley FRCVS, MVB, BA have all made extensive suggestions and contributions. I am grateful for their input.

E.B. 2005

Note: The use of small capitals, for instance, ANTIBODY, in the text, refers the reader to the entry of that name for additional information.

Black's Veterinary Dictionary, first published in 1928, owes its existence to the late Professor William C. Miller, who was also responsible for the 1935 edition. When on the teaching staff of the Royal (Dick) Veterinary College, Edinburgh, he saw the need for such a book and modelled it on *Black's Medical Dictionary.* Professor Miller held the chair of animal husbandry at the Royal Veterinary College, London, and completed a distinguished career by becoming Director of the Animal Health Trust's equine research station at Newmarket. Editorship from the 1953 to 1995 editions was in the hands of Geoffrey P. West MRCVS, veterinary writer and journalist.

First published 1928
Second edition 1935
Third edition 1953
Fourth edition 1956
Fifth edition 1959
Sixth edition 1962
Seventh edition 1965
Eighth edition 1967
Ninth edition 1970
Tenth edition 1972
Eleventh edition 1975
Twelfth edition 1976
Thirteenth edition 1979
Fourteenth edition 1982
Fifteenth edition 1985
Sixteenth edition 1988
Seventeenth edition 1992
Eighteenth edition 1995
Nineteenth edition 1998
Twentieth edition 2001
Twenty-first edition 2005

A

Ab
(see ANTIBODY)

Abamectin
An avermectin (see AVERMECTINS) used in cattle as an ectoparasiticide and endoparasiticide.

Abbizzia spp
A group of rapidly growing African trees being exploited as a forestry crop. The seed pods have caused poisoning in goats and cattle. Clinical signs include tachycardia, anorexia, ruminal stasis, anaemia, dyspnoea and recumbency. Affected animals always show methaemglobinaemia.

Abdomen
The part of the body in front of the spine between the thorax (see CHEST) and the PELVIS. (For a description of abdominal organs, see under appropriate headings.)

Abdomen, Diseases of
(see under STOMACH, DISEASES OF; INTESTINES, DISEASES OF; DIARRHOEA; LIVER, DISEASES OF; PANCREAS, DISEASES OF; KIDNEYS, DISEASES OF; BLADDER, DISEASES OF; PERITONITIS; BLOAT; COLIC; ASCITES; HERNIA)

Abdomen, Injuries of
These include injuries to the abdominal walls, to the alimentary tract and to the organs within the abdomen. Trauma may result in damage to the liver, spleen, kidneys, or urinary bladder. Apparently small external wounds of the abdominal wall may be far more serious than their appearance suggests. Radiographs and ultrasound can be useful in diagnosis.

Diagnosis An exploratory LAPAROTOMY may be necessary to establish the internal effects of such wounds, and also the cause of internal haemorrhage, free intra-peritoneal gas, peritonitis, etc.

Obtaining a sample by PARACENTESIS may be useful, although the hollow needle may be blocked by omentum. Use of a catheter and peritoneal lavage has been effective in detecting early intra-abdominal traumatic lesions, rupture of internal organs, etc. in dogs and cats.

When a stake or other pointed object has caused a large wound in the abdominal wall, the bowels may protrude through the opening, and if the incision be extensive, evisceration may take place. When only the wall of the abdomen has been damaged, there may be severe bruising, and haemorrhage into the tissues (see HAEMATOMA).

If exposure of the abdominal contents has taken place, or if the organs have been themselves damaged, there is risk of SHOCK, haemorrhage, infection, and PERITONITIS; the latter may cause great pain and usually proves fatal. For this reason the injured animal should receive promptly the expert services of a veterinary surgeon or else be humanely destroyed. Simple WOUNDS or bruises of the abdominal walls are treated in the same way as ordinary wounds.

Abiotrophy
A degenerative condition of an organ or tissue leading to dysfunction or loss of function. Usually inherited and often involving brain or other nerve tissue. (See LYSOSOMES – Lysosomal storage disease.)

Ablation
Removal of an organ, or part of an organ, by surgery.

Ablepharia
The lack of eyelids – a normal condition in snakes.

Abnormalities, Inherited
(see GENETICS, HEREDITY AND BREEDING – Genetic defects)

Abomasum
Abomasum is the so-called 4th stomach of ruminating animals; more correctly, the 4th compartment of the ruminant stomach. It is also called the 'true' or 'rennet' stomach, and the 'reed'. It is an elongated, pear-shaped sac lying on the floor of the abdomen, on the right-hand side, and roughly between the 7th and 12th ribs.

Abomasum, Displacement of
(see STOMACH, DISEASES OF; TYMPANITIC RESONANCE IN CATTLE)

Abortifacient
A substance causing abortion.

Abortion
The termination of pregnancy. In farm animals it represents one important aspect of INFERTILITY.

A

The causes of abortion in farm animals are shown in the tables below:

Cows

Infections

Viruses
BVD/MD (bovine virus diarrhoea/mucosal disease); bovine herpesvirus 1 (infectious bovine rhinotracheitis/infectious pustular vulvovaginitis)

Chlamydia
C. psittaci

Rickettsiae
Coxiella burnetti (Q fever)
Ehrlichia phagocytophilia (tick-borne fever)

Bacteria
Salmonella dublin, S. typhimurium
Bacillus lichenformis
Brucella abortus; also B. melitensis
Actinomyces pyogenes
Listeria ivanovii, L. monocytogenes
Leptospira hardjo and other serovars
Campylobacter fetus
Besnoitia

Fungi
Aspergillus fumigatus
Mortierella wolfii

Protozoa
Neospora caninum
Toxoplasma gondii
Trichomonas fetus

Non-infectious causes

Claviceps purpurea (ergot in feed)
Stress
Recessive lethal gene
Malnutrition
Haemolytic disease
Vitamin A deficiency
Iodine deficiency

Ewes

Infections

Viruses
Border disease/Thogoto virus

Chlamydia
C. psittaci (ovis) (Enzootic abortion)

Rickettsiae
Ehrlichia phagocytophilia (tick-borne fever)
Coxiella burnetti (Q fever)

Bacteria
Bacillus licheniformis
Salmonella dublin, typhimurium, montivideo, S. abortus ovis and others
Listeria monocytogenes
Arizona spp
Actinomyces pyogenes
Brucella abortus and (not in the UK) B. ovis

Campylobacter jejuni

Fungi
Aspergillus fumigatus

Protozoa
Toxoplasma gondii

Non-infectious causes

Stress (e.g. chasing/savaging by dogs; transport)
Near-starvation
Pregnancy toxaemia
Claviceps purpurea (ergot in feed)
Iodine deficiency

Sows

Infections

Viruses
African swine fever virus
Aujeszky's disease
Smedi
Swine fever virus

Bacteria
Erysipelothrix rhusiopathiae (swine erysipelas)
Brucella abortus suis
Pasteurella multocida (occasionally)
E. coli
Leptospira pomona (not in UK) grippotyphosa, canicala, icterrhaemorrhagica

Protozoa
Toxoplasma gondii

Non-infectious causes

Malnutrition, e.g. vitamin A deficiency
(See also CARBON MONOXIDE.)

Mares

Infections

Viruses
Equine herpesvirus 1 (Equine rhinopneumonitis)
Equine viral arteritis

Bacteria
Aeromonas hydrophilia
Salmonella abortus equi
Brucella abortus (rarely)
Haempophilus equigenitalis (contagious equine metritis)
Leptospira spp (sometimes in association with equine herpesvirus 1)

Listeriosis

Non-infectious causes

Twin foals
Plant poisoning (e.g. by Locoweed)

Bitch

Neospora caninum
Brucella canis (not UK)
Streptococcus spp
Canine herpesvirus

Queen

Feline leukaemia virus, feline herpesvirus

Abortion, Contagious
(see BRUCELLOSIS)

Abortion, Enzootic, of Ewes
This disease occurs in all parts of Britain, as well as overseas.

Cause Chlamydia psittaci, which is ingested by mouth from infected material. It can remain latent for long periods in non-pregnant sheep. (See CHLAMYDIA.)

Diagnosis A competitive ELISA (cELISA) test is stated to be 100 per cent effective in testing for antibodies against abortion-causing strains of *C. psittaci*.

Signs Abortion occurs during the last 6 weeks, and usually during the last 2 or 3 weeks, of the normal period of gestation. Stillbirths and the birth of weak full-term lambs also occur. The placenta is thickened and necrotic. Most infected ewes who do not become ill have a thick, infected vaginal discharge for a week or more. Infertility is temporary, since ewes usually lamb normally the following season.

Enzootic abortion is a zoonosis (*see* ZOONOSES); **pregnant women must avoid all contact with infected sheep.**

Prevention Replacement sheep should be obtained from blood-tested disease-free flocks. Vaccines are available; antibiotics can reduce the level of abortions in an outbreak.

Abortion, Epizootic
Chlamydial abortion in cattle.

Abrasion
A superficial wound of skin or mucous membrane caused by chaffing, rubbing, etc.

Abscess
Localised pus, surrounded by inflamed tissue. A tiny abscess is known as a PUSTULE, and a diffused area that produces pus is spoken of as an area of CELLULITIS. Abscesses in cats are usually of this type and seldom 'point' (*see* below).

An acute abscess forms rapidly and as rapidly comes to a head and bursts, or else becomes reabsorbed and disappears.

Causes The direct cause of an acute abscess is either infection with bacteria, or the presence of an irritant in the tissues.

The organisms that are most often associated with the formation of abscesses include staphylococci and streptococci (see BACTERIA).

When bacteria have gained access they start to multiply, and their TOXINS may damage surrounding tissue.

White blood cells (leukocytes) – in particular, those called neutrophils – gather in the area invaded by the bacteria and engulf them. The area of invasion becomes congested with dead or dying bacteria, dead or dying leukocytes, dead tissue cells which formerly occcupied the site, and debris.

Signs Inflammation, redness, warmth, swelling, and pain; and besides these, when the abscess is of large size and is well developed, fever.

'Pointing' of an abscess means it has reached that stage when the skin covering it is dead, thin, generally glazed, and bulging. If slightly deeper, the skin over the area becomes swollen, is painful, and 'pits' on pressure. When the abscess bursts, or when it is evacuated by lancing, the pain disappears, the swelling subsides, and the temperature falls. If all the pus has been evacuated, the cavity rapidly heals; if, however, the abscess has burst into the chest or abdomen, pleurisy or peritonitis may follow. When an abscess is deeply seated so as to be out of reach of diagnosis by manipulative measures, its presence can be confirmed by blood tests.

Treatment Antibiotics may be employed as the sole means of treating multiple or deep-seated abscesses. They may be injected into a cavity following aspiration of the pus, or they may be used in addition to the lancing of an abscess. Hot fomentations, or application of a poultice, may afford relief.

After the abscess has been opened it is usually best to leave it uncovered.

A chronic abscess takes a long time to develop, seldom bursts (unless near to the surface of the body), and becomes surrounded by large amounts of fibrous tissue.

Causes Abscesses due to tuberculosis, ACTINO-MYCOSIS, staphylococci, and caseous abscess formation in the lymph nodes of sheep, are the most common types of cold or chronic abscesses. They may arise when an acute abscess, instead of bursting in the usual way, becomes surrounded by dense fibrous tissue.

Signs Swelling may be noticeable on the surface of the body (as in actinomycosis), or it may show no signs of its presence until the animal is slaughtered (as in the case of many tuberculous abscesses and in lymphadenitis of sheep). If it is present on the surface, it is found to be hard, cold, only very slightly painful, and does not rapidly increase in size.

Characteristics of the pus The contained fluid varies in its appearance and its consistency. It may be thin and watery, or it may be solid or semi-solid. To this latter type the name 'inspissated pus' is given, and the process of solidification is often spoken of as 'caseation'.

Treatment This may involve surgery, and/or the use of antibiotics, depending upon the nature of the abscess and its location.

Abyssinian
A breed of short-haired cat similar in appearance to those depicted in illustrations from ancient Egypt. It is favoured for its quiet vocalisation. Familial renal amyloidosis has been found in this breed.

Acacia Poisoning
Acacia poisoning has been recorded in cattle and goats. Signs include ataxia, excitation and prostration.

Acanthosis Nigicans
A chronic condition of the skin found mainly in dogs, especially Daschunds. The skin becomes thickened with loss of hair and excessive pigmentation, and is velvety to the touch. The condition often starts in the axillae (armpits) but the abdomen has also been seen as the primary location. The cause is unknown. It may respond to corticosteroids or radiation therapy.

Acapnia
Acapnia is a condition of diminished carbon dioxide in the blood.

Acaricide
A parasiticide effective against mites and ticks.

Acarus
A forage mite only accidentally parasitic.

Accidental Self-Injection
This has led to human infection with BRUCELLOSIS, ORF, plague, Q FEVER, and TUBERCULOSIS (TB).

Accidental self-injection with an oil-based vaccine is painful and dangerous; it requires **immediate** medical attention.

If the accident involves IMMOBILON, the effects can be reversed by an immediate self-

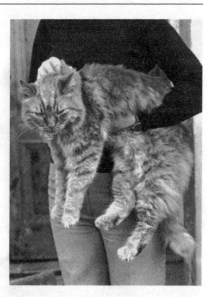

First-aid for owners: how to carry an injured cat with a suspected limb fracture. A dog may be carried similarly if not too large. An alternative for a bigger dog is to draw it gently on to a coat or rug, ready for lifting into the back of a car for transport to a veterinary surgeon. (Photo, Marc Henrie / Pedigree Petfoods.)

injection of Revivon (diprenorphine hydrochloride). A veterinary surgeon who had no Revivon with him died within 15 minutes of accidental self-injection, when a colt made a sudden violent movement. Even a scratch with a used needle can cause collapse.

Accidents
Any part of the animal may be injured in an accident. Often the damage is obvious, such as a broken limb. Serious internal injury may not be immediately apparent. Road traffic accidents are the commonest cause of accidents to dogs and cats. Care must be taken in handling injured animals, as mishandling may make the injury worse. (See also ELECTRIC SHOCK, 'STRAY VOLTAGE' AND ELECTROCUTION; FRACTURES; BLEEDING; INTERNAL HAEMORRHAGE; BURNS AND SCALDS; SHOCK; EYE, DISEASES AND INJURIES OF.)

Accommodation
(see EYE)

Acepromazine (Acetylpromazine)
Acepromazine (Acetylpromazine) is a phenothiazine-derived tranquilliser. Given by injection

before anaesthesia, it enables low doses of barbiturates to be used. 1 to 3 mg per kg bodyweight, given by mouth a quarter of an hour or more before food, may be used for the prevention of travel sickness in small animals.

Acepromazine lowers blood pressure, and so is contra-indicated in accident cases. Noradrenaline is recommended for reversing any fall in blood pressure.

Acetabulum

Acetabulum is the cup-shaped depression on the PELVIS with which the head of the femur forms the HIP-JOINT. DISLOCATION of the hip-joint sometimes occurs as the result of 'run-over' accidents, and FRACTURES of the pelvis involving the acetabulum frequently result from the same cause.

Acetaminophen

(see PARACETAMOL)

Acetic Acid

Acetic acid is used as a treatment for alkalosis, which may be caused by urea poisoning. Acetic acid may form naturally in pig mash feeds allowed to stand, or in silage and fermented hay, when it can cause illness or even death. It is one of the normal breakdown products of cellulose digesting bacteria in the rumen.

Acetonaemia

This, and ketosis, are names given to a metabolic disturbance in cattle and sheep. It may be defined as the accumulation in the blood plasma, in significant amounts, of KETONE BODIES. The disorder may occur at any time, but is commonest in winter in dairy cows kept indoors when receiving a full ration of concentrates. The condition is very rare in heifers and seldom occurs before the 3rd calving. It can be seen in cows in the 1st month after calving and is most commonly apparent at 3 weeks.

Cause The disturbance is caused by the cow's demands for carbohydrate exceeding that available from the feed. Whenever the glucose level in the blood plasma is low, as in starvation or on a low-carbohydrate diet, or when glucose is not utilisable, as in diabetes, the concentration of free fatty acids in the plasma rises. This rise is roughly paralleled by an increase in the concentration of ketone bodies, which provide a 3rd source of energy. In other words, the moderate ketosis which occurs under a variety of circumstances is to be looked upon as a normal physiological process supplying the tissues with a readily utilisable fuel when glucose is scarce.

By contrast, the severe forms of ketosis met with in the lactating cow and the diabetic cow, and characterised by high concentrations of ketone bodies in the blood and urine, are obviously harmful pathological conditions where the quantities of ketone bodies formed grossly exceed possible needs.

Signs The cow shows rapid weight loss, reduced appetite and favours roughage to concentrates. Rumen activity is reduced and faeces become harder. The animal is markedly dull, with a dull coat and reduced milk yield. The breath has a sickly sweet smell of acetone, which may also be detected in the milk and urine. Sometimes nervous signs are present, with the animal licking walls, head rope and other objects, and overexcitement. Most animals recover with treatment.

Diagnosis Rothera's test on milk; urine may be used but can cause false positives.

First-Aid Treatment consists in giving ½ a pint of glycerine or propyleneglycol, diluted in water, or a preparation containing sodium propionate.

The feeding of cut grass or flaked maize, the addition of a little molasses to feed, and exercise all aid recovery. Injections of dextrose or corticosteroids are used under veterinary control. Resistant cases are met with which defy all treatment; the cow improves up to a point but does not feed properly and dies in 10 to 20 days.

Prevention In the 2nd half of a lactation, the diet of a dairy cow should contain a greater proportion of home-grown foods with a lower digestibility than that in the diet fed during peak lactation.

At the beginning of the dry period, the cows should be fit but not fat (condition score 2.5 to 3). The cows should be kept in this condition during the dry period by a diet of relatively poor-quality forage or heavy stocking and should be given a vitamin/mineral supplement. Production rations should be introduced in the last 2 weeks of the dry period and contain both the forage and concentrate elements to be fed after calving. Cattle should not be 'steamed up' but should receive up to 3 kg (6½ lb) (dry) of the milking ration.

After calving, the quantity of production ration fed should be steadily increased as the milk production increases. For high-yielding cows the production concentrate ration should contain 16 to 18 per cent crude protein with a

A

high metolisable energy. The carbohydrate in the ration should be readily digestible. The inclusion of some ground maize may be particularly helpful in ketosis-prone herds, since some of the starch escaping rumen fermentation is digested and absorbed as sugars. Production concentrates should contain a balanced vitamin and mineral supplement.

Cows must **not** be given free access to straw. Concentrates can be fed between meals from out-of-parlour feeders, as a constituent of a complete diet, or layered in silage. High-yielding cows should not be penned for a long time in yards, but be given ample opportunity for exercise.

After the first 10 to 12 weeks of lactation, the feeding routine of the high-yielders can be modified. The home-grown forage can be slowly increased in the ration with a corresponding decrease in the more expensive highly digestible carbohydrates if the cow's performance is not affected. This change-over must be a gradual process.

Acetone

A ketone with characteristic smell found in small amounts in some samples of normal urine, and in greater quantities during the course of diabetes, acetonaemia, pneumonia, cancer, starvation, and diseases of disturbed metabolism.

Acetonuria is the excretion of ketones in the urine.

Acetylcholine

Acetylcholine is a neurotransmitter, an important link in the transmission of nerve impulses between the nerves themselves (at the synapses) and between the nerve and the muscle. Paralysis results if the body's ability to produce acetylcholine is affected by shock, injury or certain drugs, such as curare. Pharmaceutical preparations of such compounds are used in anaesthesia to produce muscle relaxation, which facilitates surgical procedures.

In the healthy animal, acetylcholine is destroyed by the enzyme cholinesterase as soon as the nerve impulse has passed. When this reaction is prevented, as in poisoning by organophosphorous insecticides, convulsions follow. Excessive salivation is an important symptom in dogs so poisoned.

Achalasia of the Oesophagus

Absence of progressive peristalsis and failure of the lower oesophageal sphincter to relax. It has been reported as an inherited condition

in Boston terriers, English springer spaniels, smooth fox terriers, wire-haired fox terriers, German shepherd dogs and Rhodesian ridgebacks.

Achondroplasia

Achondroplasia is a form of dwarfing due to disease affecting the long bones of the limbs before birth. It is noticed in some calves of certain breeds of cattle such as the Dexter, in some breeds of dogs, and in lambs. (See GENETICS, HEREDITY AND BREEDING – Genetic defects.)

Achorion
(see RINGWORM)

Acid-Fast Organisms

Acid-fast organisms are those which, when once stained with carbol-fuchsin dye, possess the power to retain their colour after immersion in strong acid solutions, which decolorise the non-acid-fast group. The important acid-fast bacteria are *Mycobacterium tuberculosis,* which causes tuberculosis in humans and other primates; *M. bovis,* which causes tuberculosis in cattle and some other mammals; *M. piscium,* which causes tuberculosis in fish; and *M. avium* var. *paratuberculosis (johnei)*, which causes Johne's disease in ruminants.

Acidosis

A condition of reduced alkaline reserve of the blood and tissues, with or without an actual fall in pH. Sudden death may occur in cattle from acidosis after gorging on grain, or following a sudden introduction of cereal-based concentrates. It is a common complication of diarrhoea, particularly in young animals. (See also BARLEY POISONING.) Sheep may similarly be affected.

Acids, Poisoning by

Strong acids are intensely destructive of animal tissue. If accidentally consumed, the effects are immediate and drastic.

Signs Excessive salivation, great pain, and destruction of the mucous membrane lining the mouth (which causes the unfortunate animal to keep its mouth open and protrude its tongue) are seen. After a short time convulsive seizures and vomiting occur, and general collapse follows; while if a large amount of acid has been taken, death from shock rapidly supervenes.

Treatment Alkaline demulcents should be given at once and in large quantities; bicarbonate of soda given in gruels or barley-water or milk is quite useful. These neutralise the acids into harmless salts, and soothe the corroded and burnt tissues. (See ACETIC ACID; HYDROCYANIC ACID (HCN).)

Acinus

Acinus is the name applied to each of the minute sacs of which secreting glands are composed.

Aciduria

Aciduria is the excretion of acid urine. It may occur as a result of feeding a specialised diet to reduce the fomation of urinary calculi (stones) in the dog and cat.

Acne

An inflammation of sebaceous glands or hair follicles, with the formation of pustules. In the horse, a contagious form of acne is sometimes due to infection with *Corynebacterium ovis*. Acne often accompanies canine distemper, and is seen on the chin of the cat.

Aconite

(*Aconitum napellus*) Also known as monkshood, it is a poisonous plant cultivated in gardens, but also growing wild in the cooler mountainous parts of both hemispheres. It is frequently cultivated in gardens in Britain for its decorative appearance. All parts of the plant are poisonous, the parts above the ground being often eaten by stock (see ACONITE POISONING). Aconite owes its poisonous properties to an alkaloid (aconitine), mainly found in the tuberous root, but present in smaller amounts in other parts of the plant. Aconitine is irritant in large doses, but smaller doses have a sedative and paralysing effect on the sensory nerves.

Aconite Poisoning

Aconite poisoning is apt to occur when herbivorous animals gain access to gardens.

In pigs poisoning sometimes occurs through eating the horseradish-like roots.

Signs The chief symptoms shown are general depression, loss of appetite, salivation, inflammation of the mucous membrane of the mouth and jaws, grinding of the teeth; pigs are nauseated and may vomit; and horses become restless and may be attacked with colic. Animals walk with an unsteady gait, and later become paralysed in their hind-limbs. The pulse becomes almost imperceptible, and unconsciousness is followed by convulsions and death.

Treatment An emetic must be given to the pig, dog and cat to induce vomiting, and a

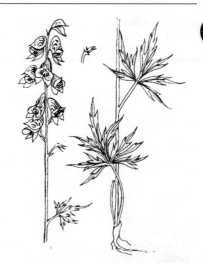

Aconite (*Aconitum napellus*). The flowers are either blue or yellow, and each has a petal which is in the shape of a helmet or hood; hence the name 'monkshood' which is often applied to the plant when growing in gardens. Height: 65 cm to 2 m (2 to 6 ft).

stomach-tube may be passed in the large herbivorous animals that do not vomit. Stimulants, such as strong black tea or coffee, should be given by mouth.

Acoprosis

Absence or scantiness of faeces.

Acorn Calves

A congenital problem most commonly seen in calves from suckler cows fed on an unsupplemented silage diet. Affected calves have domed heads and other facial deformities, and stunted limbs.

Acorn Poisoning

(see under OAK POISONING)

Acp

Acronym for ACEPROMAZINE.

Acromegaly

A condition caused by excess of the growth hormone STH, produced by the anterior lobe of the pituitary gland, leading to enlargement of the extremities and to overgrowth of connective tissue, bone and viscera. (See also SOMATOTROPHIN.)

Acropachia

Also known as hypertrophic osteopathy, or Marie's disease, it is a condition in which

A

superfluous new bone is laid down – first in the limbs and later in other parts of the skeleton. It may accompany tumours and tuberculosis in the dog.

Acrosome

A cap over the anterior part of the head of spermatozoa; it contains enzymes which aid penetration of the ovum.

ACTH

Acth is the abbreviated form of ADRENOCORTI-COTROPHIN. (See also CORTICOTROPHIN.)

Actinobacillosis

Actinobacillosis is a disease of cattle similar in some respects to ACTINOMYCOSIS, and sometimes mistaken for it.

Generally only 1 or 2 animals in a herd are affected at one time.

Swellings may be seen on lips, cheeks, jaw, and at the base of the horn. Pneumonia, infection of the liver or alimentary canal may lead to death in untreated cases. The disease occurs also in sheep and occasionally in pigs and foals.

Cause Actinobacillosis is due to infection with *Actinobacillus lignièresi*. Infection occurs through injuries, abrasions, etc. of soft tissues, and when lymph nodes are affected through invasion along the lymph vessels. Abscesses form.

Lesions may also involve the lungs, rumen, omasum, abomasum, and reticulum.

Actinobacillus seminis was discovered in a sheep in Australia. The infection, sometimes subclinical, has since been recognised in several countries including the UK, and causes polyarthritis.

Signs With *Actinobacillus lignièresi* the tongue may become infected and painful, hence its common name 'wooden tongue'. When lymph nodes in the throat are affected, the swelling and pressure caused may make swallowing and breathing difficult; if the lesion is in the skin and superficial tissues only, it may attain to a great size without causing much trouble; when the tongue is affected the animal has difficulty in mastication and swallowing and there is usually a constant dribbling of saliva from the mouth. If this is examined there may be found in it small greyish or greyish-yellow 'pus spots', in which the organism can be demonstrated by microscopic methods. Later, the saliva may become thick, purulent, and foul smelling.

Treatment Antibiotics are often effective. In intransigent cases, intravenous sodium iodide is used.

Pigs The disease has been recorded both in the UK (very rarely) and overseas, caused by *Actinobacillus equuli* (*Bacterium viscosum equi*). *Actinobacillus suis* has been recorded occasionally; it causes septicaemia in piglets and lesions in various organs. *Actinobacillus pleuropneumoniae* (formerly *Haemophilus pleuropneumoniae*) causes pleuropneumonia in pigs.

Horses *Actinobacillus equuli* causes septicaemia and internal lesions in foals (see under FOALS, DISEASES OF).

Precautions The disease can be transmitted to man. Accordingly, care must be taken over washing the hands, etc., after handling an animal with actinobacillosis.

Actinomycosis

This has been recorded in very many species of animals, including man, dogs, pigs, birds and reptiles.

The lesions produced bear a considerable resemblance to those of actinobacillosis (*see* above), and are often indistinguishable from them, but typically actinomycosis affects the cheeks, pharynx and especially the bone of the jaws (it is known as 'lumpy jaw' in cattle), while actinobacillosis is more likely to attack soft tissues only.

Cause *Actinomyces bovis*. This anaerobic bacterium is present in the digestive system of cattle, and it is probable that it can only become pathogenic by invading the tissues through a wound. It is common during the ages when the permanent cheek teeth are cutting the gums and pushing out the milk teeth.

The liver is sometimes affected, while actinomycosis and actinobacillosis have both been found in lungs and bronchi.

Yellow sulphur granules are found in the lesions.

Actinomyces (Corynebacterium) pyogenes is a major cause of abscesses and suppurative conditions.

Signs The swelling in bone and other tissue, mainly composed of dense fibrous tissue, may reach a considerable size causing interference with mastication, swallowing, or breathing, depending on the situation of the lesion. In most cases when the mouth or throat is affected, there is a constant dribbling of saliva in varying amounts from the mouth. In the earlier stages this saliva is normal in its appearance, but later becomes offensive.

Actinomycosis of the bone of the upper and lower jaws produces an increase in the size of the part and a rarefication of its bony structure, the spaces becoming filled with the proliferation of fibrous tissue which is characteristic of the disease.

When the udder is affected, hard fibrous nodules may be felt below the skin, varying in size from that of a pea to a walnut or larger, and firmly embedded in the structure of the gland itself. These swellings enclose soft centres of suppuration which, on occasions, may burst either through the covering skin, or into an adjacent milk sinus or duct. The milk from such a cow should not be used for human consumption because of the danger of the consumer contracting the disease.

Treatment Antibiotics may be effective. In intransigent cases, intravenous sodium iodide may be used.

Precautions The disease can be transmitted to man; hygienic precautions are necessary after handling infected animals.

Acuaria Uncinata
This roundworm has caused outbreaks of disease in geese, ducks, and poultry. The life-cycle of this parasite involves an intermediate host, *Daphnia pulex*, the water flea. On post-mortem examination of affected birds, worms may be found in nodules scattered over the mucous membrane of the oesophagus and proventriculus. Mortality may be high.

Acupuncture
The centuries-old Chinese technique of needle insertion at certain specified points on the surface of the body has become a part of Western veterinary medicine for treatment, analgesia, and resuscitation. Acupuncture can produce the morphine-like natural substances called ENDORPHINS which are, in effect, analgesics.

Adaptations have been made, such as the use of lasers instead of needles. Ultrasonics and heat have also been applied to the points.

Acupuncture is commonly used to relieve painful conditions; also in treating poor circulation, tissue damage, and smooth muscle dysfunction. However, it is not a panacea and must be applied by experts.

Success has been reported for the use of injections of sterile saline at acupunture points in treating intractable pain in horses. The injections were repeated at weekly intervals for upto 8 weeks.

In China, acupuncture has been used for surgical analgesia in animals and man.

Acute Disease
A disease is called acute – in contradistinction to 'chronic' – when it appears rapidly, and either causes death quickly or leads to a speedy recovery. (See also under DEATH, CAUSES OF SUDDEN.)

Ad Lib Feeding
This is a labour-saving system under which pigs or poultry help themselves to dry meal, etc., and eat as much as they wish. It is also used in dairy cattle and for intensive beef production. (See also DRY FEEDING.)

Adamantinoma
A tumour affecting the jaw and composed of cells that normally produce dental enamel.

Adder
The common viper (*Vipera berus*). About 50 cm (20 in) in length, it has dark markings on a paler ground. If disturbed, this snake may bite farm or domestic animals. The bite is dangerous; an antiserum is available.

Addison's Disease (Hypoadrenacortism)
Addison's disease (hypoadrenacortism) is caused by failure of the ADRENAL GLANDS to produce adequate amounts of corticosteroids. It may be caused by congenital defects in, injury to, or disease of the cortex of the gland, when it is known as primary hypoadrenocorticism. Secondary hypoadrenocorticism results from excessive or prolonged dosage of an animal with cortisone products, which depresses the natural production of the hormone.

Signs In the dog or cat, where it most commonly occurs, the animal may be lethargic, depressed and weak; diarrhoea and vomiting may be seen. In severe cases left untreated, death may result.

In cattle, it is associated with a high incidence of aborted, weakly or still-born calves.

Treatment The condition responds rapidly to administration of hydrocortisone or other appropriate corticoid product to restore levels of cortisol in the blood; numerous formulations are available.

A

Additives

Substances incorporated in a premix added to animals' feed, often for a purpose other than nutrition. They are mainly growth promoters, enhancers of feed conversion, or, commonly, used to provide vitami ns or minerals necessary for a healthy diet. In addition to minerals and vitamins, permitted additives include certain ANTHELMINTICS and and coccidiostats for the control of parasites in farm animals. The use of antibiotics as growth promoters, permitted to a limited extent to date, is being phased out in the EU. Specified dyes, such as the xanthins used to achieve desired coloration of farmed rainbow trout, are also permitted.

Very strict controls apply to the preparation and use of medicated feeds with the principal aim of ensuring that consumers are not put at risk from medicinal residues in food animals. The legislation is contained in the Medicines (Medicated Animal Feeding Stuffs) No. 2 Regulations 1992, the Feeding Stuffs Regulations 2000, the Feeding Stuffs (Establishments and Intermediaries) Regulations 1999 and the Feeding Stuffs (Zootechnical Products) Regulations 1999. All UK compounders, whether commercial or home mixers, must register with the Royal Pharmaceutical Society or the Department of Agriculture for Northern Ireland.

(See also under MEDICINES ACT; ANTIBIOTIC; GROWTH PROMOTERS; HORMONES IN MEAT PRODUCTION.)

Adenitis

Inflammation of a gland.

Adenofibroma

Adenofibroma is a fibrous tumour enclosing neoplastic glandular tissue.

Adenoma

A TUMOUR composed of epithelial tissue, often gland-like in appearance. It may sometimes be found in positions where glandular tissue is not normally present. A malignant form is the adenocarcinoma.

Adenomatosis

The formation of numerous adematous growths in an organ. (See PORCINE INTESTINAL ADENOMATOSIS; PULMONARY ADENOMATOSIS.)

Adenopathy

Swelling of the glands, particularly the lymph glands.

Adenosine

Adenosine is a purine which is part of the structure of certain genes controlling the formation of amino acids. Adenosine triphosphate and diphosphate are important in the contraction of muscles.

Adenovirus

This is a contraction of the original term 'adenoidal-pharyngeal conjunctival agents'. (See VIRUSES.)

ADH

(see ANTIDIURETIC HORMONE)

Adhesion Factor, Bacterial

(see BACTERIAL ADHESIVENESS)

Adhesions

Adhesions occur by the uniting or growing together of structures or organs which are normally separate and freely movable. They are generally the result of acute or chronic inflammation, and in the earlier stages the uniting material is fibrin, which later becomes resolved into fibrous tissue.

Treatment Surgical division of the obstructing bands is often necessary in the abdominal cavity and in adhesions of the walls of the vagina following injuries received at a previous parturition. (See PLEURISY; PERITONITIS.)

Adipose Tissue

Here fat is stored as an energy reserve; globules of fat form within connective tissue cells. When additional fat is stored, each cell eventually becomes spherical, its nucleus pushed to one side. (*See* illustration on page 11.)

During demanding muscular exercise, or when food is insufficient, or during a debilitating disease, the cells release the fat into the bloodstream and resume their normal shape. (See also LIPOMA.)

Adjuvant

A substance added to a vaccine, in order to stabilise the product and enhance the immune response.

Adrenal Glands (Suprarenal Glands)

These are two small organs situated at the anterior extremities of the kidneys, and are endocrine glands.

Function The cortex secretes hormones which are called steroids or corticosteroids. These include glucocorticoids, notably cortisol, concerned with the regulation of carbohydrate

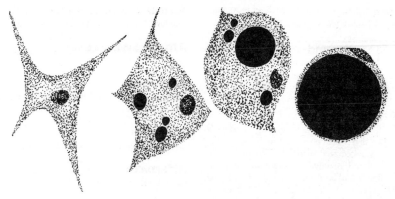

Typical fat cell formed by intake of fat globules. (Reproduced with permission from R. D. Frandson, *Anatomy and Physiology of Farm Animals*, Lea & Febiger, 1986, after Ham and Leeson, *Histology*, J. B. Lippincott Co.)

metabolism; and mineralocorticoids (which regulate sodium and potassium levels in body fluids), e.g. aldosterone. The cortex also secretes androgens; the medulla secretes adrenalin and noradrenalin.

Surgical removal of the adrenal glands (adrenalectomy) has been carried out in the treatment of CUSHING'S SYNDROME in the dog – survival being possible through hormone implants. Otherwise removal of the adrenals usually leads to death within a matter of weeks.

Atrophy The commonest cause of adrenal atrophy in the western world has been said to be corticosteroid therapy.

Adrenalin (Adrenaline)

Adrenalin (adrenaline) is the 'fight or flight' hormone from the adrenal glands (*see* above).

Its chief action is that of raising the tone of all involuntary muscle fibres, stimulating the heart, constricting the walls of the smaller arteries, and producing a rise in the blood pressure. It is used for checking capillary haemorrhage in wounds, and for warding off shock or collapse by raising the blood pressure.

Adrenocorticotrophin (Acth; Corticotrophin)

A naturally occurring hormone produced by the anterior lobe of the pituitary gland.

Aedes

(see under FLIES)

Aelurostrongylus

A lungworm of cats. (See ROUNDWORMS.)

Aerobe

A micro-organism which needs oxygen for its growth and multiplication. (See also ANAEROBE.)

Aeromonas

Aeromonas shigelloides is associated with chronic diarrhoea in cats. (See also FURUNCULOSIS.)

Aerosol

A liquid agent or solution dispersed in air in the form of a fine mist. If aerosols, for insecticidal and other purposes, are used over a long period, e.g. by a continuous evaporator, thought must be given to the effect of the chemicals used (a) on the health of the livestock; (b) on organochlorine or other residues left in the carcase to the detriment of people eating meat; (c) on the health of the stockmen.

Aerosols as a Mode of Infection Viruses excreted by animals suffering from an infectious disease may be transmitted to other animals (or man) as an aerosol. ('Coughs and sneezes spread diseases.')

Salmonella infection of veterinary surgeons through aerosols has occurred during uterine irrigation and embryotomies in cows.

Aerotropism

The tendency of micro-organisms to group themselves about a bubble of air in culture media.

Aetiology

Aetiology is the cause of a disease, or the study of such causes.

Afferent

Afferent nerve fibres carry impulses in towards the central nervous system. Efferent fibres are concerned with activities, such as movement, secretion, vascular changes, etc.

Afghan Hound
A tall breed of dog with silky coat. Inherited cataract caused by a recessive gene has been reported in the breed.

Aflatoxins
Toxins produced by fungi, e.g. *Aspergillus flavus*: they cause poisoning in animals eating contaminated feed materials. The toxins have been found mainly in groundnut meal, but sunflower and cottonseed can also be affected. The Feeding Stuffs Regulations 2000 require those products, and copra, palm kernel, maize and feeds derived from them, to be screened for the presence of toxins.

In cattle, aflatoxins may give rise to a reduced growth rate and lower milk yield. Aflatoxins are excreted in the milk. In pigs, jaundice may be seen; post mortem, the liver has a leathery appearance. Adult pigs may show bile duct carcinoma.

Aflatoxicosis in poultry is characterised by haemorrhages, anorexia, decreased efficiency in food utilisation, pathological changes in the liver, kidneys and bile ducts, and death. The problem can be prevented by storing grain with 13 per cent of moisture or less. The litter may also be a source of toxins and consequently it is important to keep the moisture in the litter to a minimum by ensuring that the ventilation of the house is adequate and that the waterers are operating correctly.

Fish are extremely susceptible to aflatoxins. As one of the precautions taken to keep animal feeds free of dangerously high levels of aflatoxins, trout have been used for testing. In young trout (as in pigs), aflatoxin poisoning is likely to result in cancer of the liver. (Mature cock fish become fully resistant.) Equally, care has to be taken with commercial dry trout feeds, to ensure that aflatoxin level is below 0.5 parts per billion; otherwise malignant tumours are apt to develop, and later liquid-filled cysts may grow to a remarkable size.

As the long-term effect is cancer of the bile ducts, animals without gall-bladders, e.g. horses and deer, are less likely to be affected. (See also MYCOTOXICOSIS; CIRRHOSIS.)

AFRC
AFRC is the abbreviation for the Agricultural and Food Research Council. This body was replaced in 1994 by the Biotechnology and Biological Sciences Research Council.

African Horse Sickness
(see HORSE-SICKNESS, AFRICAN)

African Swine Fever
(see SWINE FEVER, AFRICAN)

Africander
Cattle in origin about ¾ Brahman and ¼ British beef breed. (See also under CYTOGENETICS.)

Afrikaner
A synonym for Brahman or Zebu cattle.

Afterbirth
(see PLACENTA)

Afterbirths, Infected
Afterbirths, Infected may be a source of infection to other animals. (See SCRAPIE; BRUCELLOSIS; ABORTION, ENZOOTIC.)

Agalactia
Partial or complete absence of milk, or milk flow, from the udder. Where this is due to a failure of milk 'let down', oxytocin may be prescribed. (See SOW'S MILK, ABSENCE OF; COW'S MILK, ABSENCE OF.)

Agalactia, Contagious
This is a disease of goats especially, and sheep less commonly, characterised by inflammatory lesions in the udder, eyes, and joints. It is chiefly encountered in France, Switzerland, the Tyrol, Italy, the Pyrenees, North Africa and India.

Cause *Mycoplasma agalactiae*. The disease often occurs in the spring and the summer, and disappears with the advent of the colder weather. The infection may be carried by flies or the hands of the milkers and by the litter in a shed becoming contaminated, while the fetus may be infected before birth.

Signs Fever, mastitis, and a greatly reduced milk yield. The milk becomes yellowish-green and contains clots. In addition to the udder, both joints and eyes may be involved; a painful arthritis, and conjunctivitis followed by keratitis (with resultant temporary blindness) worsening the animal's condition.

Emaciation and death within 10 days may occur in very acute cases; otherwise recovery usually follows within a few weeks, though the former milk yield will not have been regained.

Male animals may have orchitis as well as arthritis.

Inflammation of the lymph nodes may occur, and lesions may be found also in abdominal organs and tissues, and in the chest.

Treatment Isolation of the affected animals and strict segregation of the in-contacts should be carried out.

Agar
Agar is the gelatinous substance prepared from Ceylon moss and various kinds of seaweed. It dissolves in boiling water, and, on cooling, solidifies into a gelatinous mass at a temperature slightly above that of the body. It is used extensively in preparing culture-media for use in bacteriological laboratories, and also in the treatment of chronic constipation in dog and cat.

Agar-Gel Immunodiffusion Test
A test used in diagnosis of, e.g., equine infectious anaemia. (See also COGGINS TEST.)

Agene Process
The bleaching of flour with nitrogen trichloride. The use of such flour in dog foods gave rise to HYSTERIA.

Ages of Animals

Horses By the time it has reached 17 years, which generally means about 14 years of work, a horse's powers are on the wane. Many at this age are still in possession of their full vigour, but these are generally of a class that is better looked after than the average, e.g. hunters, carriage-horses, or favourites. On an average, the feet of the horse are worn out first, not the arteries as in man, and consequently horses with good feet and legs are likely to outlast those inferior in this respect, other things being equal. After the feet come the teeth. In very many cases a horse's teeth wear out before their time. It often happens that the upper and lower rows of teeth do not wear in the normal way; the angle of their grinding surfaces becomes more and more oblique, until the chewing of the food becomes less and less effective, and the horse loses condition.

Instances are on record of horses attaining the age of 35, 45, 50, and one of a horse that was still working when 63 years old. These, however, are very exceptional. The average age at which a horse dies or is euthanased lies somewhere between 20 and 25 years.

Cattle The great majority of bullocks are killed before they reach 3 years of age, and in countries where 'prime beef' is grown they are fattened and killed between 2½ and 3 years. In the majority of herds, few cows live to be more than 8 or 10 years of age. Pedigree bulls may reach 12 or 14 years of age before being discarded. Records are in existence of cows up to 39 years old, and it is claimed that one had 30 calves.

Sheep Here again the requirements of the butcher have modified the age of the animal at death. Wether lambs are killed at ages ranging from 4 to 9 months (Christmas lambs), and older fat sheep up to 2½ years. Ewes, on the average, breed until they are from 4 to 6 or 7 years, when they too are fattened and slaughtered for mutton. Exceptionally, they reach greater ages, but unless in the case of pure breeding animals, each year over 6 reduces their ultimate value as carcases. Rams are killed after they have been used for 2 or 3 successive seasons at stud – that is, when they are 3 or 4 years of age, as a rule.

Pigs In different districts the age at which pigs are killed varies to some extent, according to the requirements of local trade. Pigs for pork production are killed at about 3½ to 4 months; bacon pigs are killed between 6 and 7½ months, and only breeding sows and boars are kept longer. Ages of up to 12 years have been recorded for sows.

Dogs and cats These are the only domesticated animals which are generally allowed to die a natural death. The average age of the dog is about 12 years, and of the cat 9 to 12, but instances are not uncommon of dogs living to 18 or 20 years of age, and of cats similarly. (See also BREEDING OF LIVESTOCK; DENTITION.)

Elephants Their normal life-span in the wild is 65 to 70; some working elephants are employed up to a similar age and then retired.

Agglutination
Agglutination is the clumping together of cells in a fluid. For example, bacteria will agglutinate when a specific antiserum is added to the suspension of bacteria. Similarly, the blood serum of one animal will cause the red blood cells of another to become agglutinated.

Agglutination is explained by the presence in the serum of an agglutinin which combines with an agglutinable substance, or agglutinogen, possessed by the organisms.

Agglutination is made use of in the Agglutination Test, which depends upon the principle that in the blood serum of an animal

A

harbouring in its body disease-producing organisms (though it may show no symptoms), there is a far greater concentration of agglutinins than in a normal animal. Minute doses (e.g. dilutions of 1 part to 100 or even 1000) of such serum will cause agglutination, while serum from a normal animal will not cause agglutination when diluted more than 1 part in 10. Incubation of the mixture at body heat usually hastens the results and enables a rapid diagnosis to be made.

Aggressiveness (Aggression)

This may be transient, as in a nursing bitch fearful for her puppies. Persistent aggressiveness can be the result of jealousy, as when the birth of a baby means a decline in status for the dog. Ill-treatment, attacks by some local pugnacious dog, being kept tied up for long periods, or being shut in an empty house are other causes. Heredity is an important factor, too, and it is unwise to breed from aggressive parents even if they look like Show winners. Brain disease – for example, encephalitis, or a brain tumour – may account for aggressiveness in any animal. So may pain. (See also ENCEPHALITIS; MENINGIOMA; RABIES; BENZOIC ACID POISONING; EQUINE VERMINOUS ARTERITIS; 'VICES'; CHLORINATED HYDROCARBONS; MUSCLES, DISEASES OF – Muscular rheumatism; OVARIES, DISEASES OF; HYPER-AESTHESIA; BOVINE SPONGIFORM ENCEPHALOPATHY; LISTERIOSIS; ANAPLASMOSIS; ACETONAEMIA; GRASS SICKNESS; HEARTWATER.)

Agonist

A type of drug which gives a positive response (e.g. contraction or relaxation of a muscle fibre, or secretion from a gland) when its molecule combines with a receptor. The latter is a specific structural component of a cell, on its membrane, and usually a protein.

Antagonist A drug which merely blocks the attachment of any other substance at the receptor, so preventing any possible active response.

Partial agonist A drug which produces a positive response at the receptor, but only a weak one. However, since it occupies the receptor it prevents any full agonist from binding so that, in the presence of agonists, partial agonists may act as antagonists.

Many drugs are now classified according to their major action, e.g. β blockers, H_1 and H_2 receptor antagonists.

β receptors are present in the heart and smooth muscle of the bronchioles, uterus, and arterioles supplying skeletal muscle. Drugs which are selective β_1 (heart) or β_2 (elsewhere) are now available. For example, CLENBUTEROL is a specific β_2 agonist; it is used as a bronchodilator to treat respiratory conditions in horses, dogs and cats.

The use of clenbuterol in cattle, where it acts as a growth promoter, is prohibited in the EU.

Air

Atmospheric air contains by volume 20.96 per cent of oxygen, 78.09 per cent of nitrogen, 0.03 per cent of carbon dioxide, 0.94 per cent of argon, and traces of a number of other elements – the most important of which are helium, hydrogen, ozone, neon, zenon, and krypton, as well as variable quantities of water vapour. (See SMOG.)

Air that has been expired from the lungs in a normal manner shows roughly a 4 per cent change in the amount of the oxygen and carbon dioxide, less of the former (16.96 per cent) and more of the latter (4.03 per cent). The nitrogen remains unaltered.

The importance of fresh air to animals is immense. (See VENTILATION; RESPIRATION; OZONE; SLURRY; CARBON MONOXIDE.)

Air Passages

(see BRONCHUS; NOSE AND NASAL PASSAGES; TRACHEA)

Air SAC

Part of the respiratory system, particularly in reference to birds.

Air Sacculitis

Inflammation of the air sacs in birds.

Airedale Terrier

A large, black-and-tan, wiry-coated breed. Entropion and cataract are inherited, probably as autosomal dominant traits.

Akabane Virus

First isolated from mosquitoes in Japan; antibodies detected in cattle, horses and sheep in Australia. A possible cause of abortion in cattle, and of birth of abnormal calves. The virus, a member of the Bunyavirus group, is teratogenic.

Some calves are born blind and walk with difficulty; some have the cerebrum virtually replaced by a water-filled cyst.

(See also Arthrogryposis under GENETICS, HEREDITY AND BREEDING – Genetic defects.)

Alanine Aminotransferase (ALT)

An enzyme involved in amino acid transfer. Liver damage results in high levels in the circulating blood. It is used as a measure of liver damage in dogs and cats.

Alaskan Malamute

A breed of dog developed from the husky. Dwarfism (chondrodysplasia) is inherited in some litters. Day blindness may also be inherited and congenital haemolytic anaemia occurs.

Albinism

Albinism is a lack of the pigment melanin in the skin – an inherited condition.

Albumins

(see PROTEINS; CONALBUMIN; ALBUMINURIA)

Albuminuria

The presence of albumin in the urine: one of the earliest signs of NEPHRITIS and cystitis (see URINARY BLADDER, DISEASES OF).

Alcohol Poisoning

Acute alcoholism is usually the result of too large doses given *bona fide*, but occasionally the larger herbivora and pigs eat fermenting windfalls in apple orchards; or are given or obtain, fresh distillers' grains, or other residue permeated with spirit, in such quantities that the animals become virtually drunk. In more serious cases they may become comatose.

Aldosterone

This is a hormone secreted by the adrenal gland. Aldosterone regulates the electrolyte balance by increasing sodium retention and potassium excretion. (See CORTICOSTEROIDS.)

Aldrin

A persistent insecticide; a chlorinated hydrocarbon used in agriculture and formerly in farm animals. Its persistence has prevented its veterinary use. Signs of toxicity include blindness, salivation, convulsions, rapid breathing. (See GAME BIRDS.)

Aleutian Disease

First described in 1956 in the USA, this disease of mink also occurs in the UK, Denmark, Sweden, New Zealand and Canada.

Mink

Signs include: failure to put on weight or even loss of weight; thirst; the presence of undigested food in the faeces – which may be tarry. Bleeding from the mouth and anaemia may also be observed. Death usually follows within a month.

Ferrets In these animals the disease is characterised by a persistent viraemia.

Signs include: loss of weight; malaise; chronic respiratory infection; and paresis or paraplegia. Bleeding from the mouth and anaemia may also be observed. Death usually follows within a month. The disease can be confused with the later stages of rabies.

Diagnosis In ferrets the counter-current electrophoresis test has been used.

Alexin

(see COMPLEMENT)

Alfadalone

(see ALFAXALONE)

Alfaxalone

Used in combination with alfadalone (in Saffan [Schering-Plough]) as a general anaesthetic in cats; it must not be used in dogs. Given by intravenous injection, It produces sedation in 9 seconds and anaesthesia after 25 seconds. It is also given by deep intramuscular injection as an induction for general anasthesia for long operations. It must not be given with other injectable anaesthetics.

Algae

Simple plant life of very varied form and size, ranging from single-cell organisms upwards to large seaweed structures. Algae can be a nuisance on farms when they block pipes or clog nipple drinkers. This happens especially in warm buildings, where either an antibiotic or sugar is being administered to poultry via the drinking water. Filters may also become blocked by algae.

The colourless *Prototheca* species are pathogenic for both animals (cattle, deer, dogs, pigs) and man. (See MASTITIS IN COWS – Algal mastitis.)

The non-toxic algae of the *Spirulina* group are used in the feed of some ornamental fish.

Algae Poisoning

Toxic freshwater algae, characteristically blue-green in colour, are found in summer on lakes in numerous locations, particularly where water has a high phosphate and nitrate content derived from farm land. Formed by the summer blooms of cyanobacteria, they can form an oily, paint-like layer several cm thick. Deaths have occurred in cattle and sheep drinking from affected water; photosensitivity is a common sign among survivors. Dogs have also been affected.

The main toxic freshwater cyanobacteria are strains of the unicellular *Microcystis aeruginosa*,

A

and the filamentous forms *Anabaena flos-aquae*, *Aphanizomenon* and *Oscillatoria agardhii*.

Signs vary according to the dominant cyanobacterium present. *Anabaena flos-aquae*, for example, can form alkaloid neuromuscular toxins which can produce symptoms within half an hour; these being muscular tremors, stupor, ataxia, prostration, convulsions, sometimes opisthotonus, and death. Dyspnoea and salivation may also be seen.

Mycrocystis strains produce a slower-acting peptide toxin, which may cause vomiting and diarrhoea, salivation, thirst, piloerection, and lachrymation. Survivors may show LIGHT SENSITISATION, with inflamed white skin and oedema of ears and eyelids.

Poisoning by algae has been recorded in dogs that have been in the sea off Denmark. In America a colourless alga is reported to have caused dysentery, blindness and deafness, and sometimes ataxia and head-tilting.

In Victoria, Australia, 17 sheep died and many others showed signs of light sensitivity after drinking from a lake affected by a thick bloom of *M. aeruginosa*. The deaths were spread over 6 months after removal from access to the lake.

Poisoning in cattle was suspected in the UK after a spell of hot weather in East Anglia caused an algal bloom in field ponds and 50 per cent of the cows in a herd suddenly showed nervous signs. BSE was ruled out as the cause.

Alimentary Canal
(see DIGESTION)

Alkali
A substance which neutralises an acid to form a salt, and turns red litmus blue. Alkalis are generally the oxides, hydroxides, carbonates, or bicarbonates of metals.

Varieties Ammonium, lithium, potassium, and sodium salts are the principal alkalis, their carbonates being weak and their bicarbonates weaker.

Uses In poisoning by acids, alkalis in dilute solution should be administered at once. (See ACIDS, POISONING BY; STOMACH, DISEASES OF; DISINFECTION; DETERGENTS.)

Alkaloids
Alkaloids constitute a large number of the active principles of plants and all possess a powerful physiological action. Like alkalis, they combine with acids to form salts, and turn red litmus blue. Many alkaloids are used in medicine, and their names almost always end in 'ine' – e.g. atropine, morphine, quinine, etc.

Aconitine } from monkshood (*Aconitum napellus*).
Aconine }
Arecoline, from areca nut (*Areca catechu*).
Atropine, from belladonna, the juice of the deadly nightshade (*Atropa belladonna*).
Caffeine, from the coffee plant (*Coffea arabica*) and from the leaves of the tea plant (*Thea sinensis*), also found in the kola nut, guarana, and species of holly, etc.
Cocaine, from coca leaves (*Coca erythroxylon*).
Digitoxin } from foxglove (*Digitalis purpurea*).
Digitalin* }
Ephedrine, from various species of *Ephedra*.
Ergotoxin* } from ergot (*Claviceps purpurea*).
Ergometrine }
Hyoscyamine, from henbane (*Hyoscyamus niger*).
Hyoscine or } also from henbane.
Scopolamine }
Morphine }
Codeine } from opium, the juice of the opium
Thebaine } poppy (*Papaver comniferans*).
Heroin }
Nicotine, from tobacco leaves (*Nicotiana tobaccum*).
Physostigmine } from Calabar beans (*Physostigma*
or *Eserine* } *venenosum*).
Pilocarpine, from jaborandi (*Pilocarpus jaborandi*).
Quinine, from cinchona or Peruvian bark (*Cinchona*, and *Cinchona rubra*).
Santonin*, from wormwood (*Artemesia pauciflora*).
Sparteine, from lupins (*Lupulinus*, sp.) and from broom (*Cytisus scoparius*).
Strychnine, from *Nux vomica* seeds (*Strychnos nux vomica*).
Veratrine, from cevadilla seeds (*Cevadilla officinale*, or *Schoenocaulon officinale*).

Those marked * are neutral principles.

A first-aid antidote for poisoning by an alkaloid is strong tea.

Allantois
A sac extending from the hind gut of the early embryo and containing urine-like fluid. The allantois fuses with the chorion to become part of the PLACENTA. (See also PERVIOUS URACHUS.)

Alleles (Allelomorphs)
Alleles (allelomorphs) are genes which influence a particular development process, processes, or character, in opposite ways, and can replace one another at a particular locus on a chromosome. They result from a previous mutation, and the original gene and its mutated form are called an 'allelomorphic pair'. Another definition is: one of a pair or series (multiple alleles) of genes occupying alternatively the same locus. (See also GENETICS, HEREDITY AND BREEDING.)

Allergic Dermatitis

Allergic dermatitis is another name for eczema caused by an allergy. For example, 'Queensland Itch' is seen in horses in Australia, where it is a result of hypersensitivity to e.g. the bites of a sandfly; in Japan it follows bites of the stable-fly. It is a disease of the hot weather, and is intensely itchy in character. Treatment involves the use of antihistamines. In the UK 'Sweet Itch' is the name for a similar or identical condition in horses. (See also ECZEMA.)

Allergy

A specific sensitivity to e.g. a plant or animal product, usually of a protein nature. In the dog and cat, sensitivity occurs most commonly from bedding, carpeting, rubber products, household cleaners, plants, and some skin dressings; in pigs, soyabean protein antigens.

The three main signs are itching, self-inflicted damage as a result, and redness; sometimes oedema of the face, ears, vulva or extremities, or skin weals.

Many foodstuffs have caused allergy in the dog, e.g. cow's milk; horse, ox, pig, sheep and chicken meat; eggs. True food allergies are less common in cats. They can, however, be distressing. All constituents of the feline diet may be involved, including colouring agents and preservatives.

Tobacco smoke was reported to be the cause of an allergy in a dog. When his owner gave up smoking, the allergy did not return.

Allergy may arise following the bites of sand-flies, stable-flies, fleas and sometimes bee or wasp stings. Pollens can produce skin changes; likewise avianised vaccines, horse serum, antibiotics, and synthetic hormone preparations. (See also ATOPIC DISEASE; ECZEMA; ANAPHYLACTIC SHOCK; ANTIHISTAMINES; LIGHT SENSITISATION; LAMINITIS; REAGINIC ANTIBODIES.)

Allograft

A piece of tissue, or a complete organ, transplanted from one animal to another of the same species. (See SKIN GRAFTING.)

Allopurinol

(1) The treatment of choice for LEISHMANIASIS in dogs. Given by mouth, it is well absorbed from the gastrointestinal tract and excreted by the kidneys. (2) It is also used in dogs to treat UROLITHIASIS.

Aloe

Cape aloes are an anthraquinone laxative with an intensely bitter taste. Aloe vera is a popular ingredient in skin preparations and the juice is reputed to be of benefit in cases of eczema.

Alopecia

Absence of hair from where it is normally present; it has to be differentiated from loss of hair due to mange, ringworm, lice infestation, and eczema.

Alopecia may be the result of a hormone imbalance, a dietary deficiency, or selenium poisoning.

A temporary alopecia is occasionally seen in newborn animals, and also in the dams of newborn animals. A deficiency of iodine or of thyroxine may produce such hair loss. In dogs, bald patches, usually symmetrical, may occur on the flanks and extend to the limbs. This type of canine alopecia usually responds to thyroid therapy. In male dogs of 5 years old and upwards, alopecia may be accompanied by an attraction for other males, and may respond to castration but not to hormone therapy. A Sertoli-cell tumour of the testicle also causes alopecia and feminisation. Symmetrical bare patches, accompanied by other symptoms, are a feature of Cushing's disease. Senile alopecia affects some cats, and a patchy loss of fur may occur from time to time in some spayed cats. Tetracyclines may occasionally cause severe hair loss in cats.

Alopecia in dogs, with symmetrical bilateral hair loss from trunk, neck and end of tail, may sometimes be due to a deficiency of the growth hormone SOMATOTROPHIN. The age group affected is 1 to 4 years. Highly pigmented skin may be a feature. Treatment with the growth hormone has proved successful.

Alphachloralose

A narcotic used for the destruction of rodents, pigeons, etc. It acts by lowering the body temperature. Accidental poisoning in dogs and cats can occur. Animals should be kept warm; emetics may be given in the early stages.

Alpaca

A type of South American camel now farmed in the UK and elsewhere for its fine wool; not reared for meat. Individuals can live for up to 20 years.

Alphavirus

Viruses of arbovirus group A and equine encephalitis viruses bear this name.

ALT

(see ALANINE AMINOTRANSFERASE)

A

Altitude

Animals unaccustomed to high altitudes can be adversely affected by them. Like humans, animals suffer hypoxia. Testicles of cats, rabbits and rats atrophy with resulting fertility problems. Hens and geese lay infertile eggs or cease laying. Ascites caused by high altitudes has been reported in all types of poultry. Acclimatisation to high altitudes results in the formation of more and smaller red blood cells so that oxygen-binding capacity is increased. (See also 'MOUNTAIN SICKNESS'.)

Altrenogest

A prostaglandin analogue used for the synchronisation of oestrus in mature sows (Regumate Porcine) and the suppression of prolonged oestrus in mares (Regumate Equine).

Aluminium Toxicity

In the rat, research in South Africa has shown that aluminium toxicity might be due to (experimental) porphyria. In Israel it has been shown that rats given aluminium salts, and then examined under ultra-violet light, show fluorescence of eyes, long bones, brain and peri-testicular fat. In rats at least, therefore, aluminium cannot be regarded as a harmless element.

Alveld

A disease of lambs in Norway, associated with the eating of bog asphodel *Narthecium ossifragum*. Signs are photosensitisation and jaundice; it is thought to be due to poisoning by microfungi present on the plant.

Alveolus

A tooth socket in the jaw. The term is also applied to the minute divisions of glands and to the air sacs of the lungs.

Alveolitis

Inflammation of an alveolus. (See EXTRINSIC ALLERGIC ALVEOLITIS.)

'Alzheimer's Disease' in Cats

A condition in geriatric cats that closely resembles the human disease. Signs include disorientation, compulsive behaviours, disturbed sleep patterns and incontinence. Histologically, changes to the brain resemble those in the human disease.

Amaurosis

Impaired vision or even loss of sight, resulting from disease of the optic nerve, brain, or spinal cord.

Amblyopia

Diminution of vision.

Amelia

An information bulletin published by the Veterinary Medicines Directorate. The title is an acronym for Animal Medicines European Legislation Information and Advice.

American Box Tortoises

A ban on the importation into the UK of tortoises from Mediterranean countries led dealers and pet shops to seek an alternative, and the choice was *Terrapene carolina*. These are terrestial, but like to take an occasional dip in water about 3 inches deep. Poor swimmers, they dislike water deeper than that. The recommended diet for them is 'earthworms, mushrooms, beans, beansprouts, cucumber, grapes, banana, and some leafy vegetables'. In winter a vitamin and mineral supplement is advisable.

American Cocker Spaniel

A breed smaller than the English spaniel and with longer hair. Cataract is an inherited trait. Other inherited conditions may include distichiasis, entropion, haemophilia, patellar luxation and prognathia.

American Quarter Horse

A breed derived mainly from dams of Spanish origin, for long bred by American Indians, and from Galloway sires brought by the early settlers. 'It was Barb blood spiced with a Celtic infusion and refined with a dash of Eastern blood that fashioned the Quarter Horse.' (R. M. Denhardt.)

Amine

An organic compound containing ammonia (NH_3).

Amino Acids

Amino acids are the 'building blocks' into which proteins can be broken down, and with which proteins can be constructed.

Amino acids contain carbon, hydrogen, and oxygen, together with an amine group (NH_2).

The quality of a protein, in terms of its value as an animal feed, depends upon its content of essential amino acids. These are lysine, methionine, tryptophane, leucine, isoleucine, phenylalanine, threonine, histidine, valine, and arginine.

LYSINE is a particularly important amino acid for growth and milk production, and is one of those prepared synthetically and added to some livestock feeds.

The pig and rat require, for rapid growth: lysine, tryptophane, leucine, isoleucine, methionine, threonine, phenylalanine, valine, and histidine. The chick needs glycine in addition to these. The cat needs TAURINE.

Aminoglycosides

A group of bactericidal antibiotics produced from *Streptomycin* species including streptomycin, neomycin, framycetin and gentamicin.

Aminonitrothiazole

A drug used against Blackhead in turkeys.

Aminotransferase

An enzyme which catalyses transfer reactions involving amino acids.

Amitraz

An ectoparasiticide for the treatment of lice and tick infestation and mange in farm animals and dogs. It must not be used on chihuahuas, nor on cats or horses. It is sold under a variety of trade names.

Ammonia (NH₃)

A few drops of ammonia on a piece of cotton-wool held a few inches from the nostrils have a good effect in reviving animals which have collapsed. (Inhalation of concentrated ammonia can prove fatal.) Ammonia fumes from litter may adversely affect poultry. (See DEEP LITTER; also QUATERNARY AMMONIUM COMPOUNDS.)

An excess of ammonia in the rumen has been cited as a cause of hypomagnesaemia in spring following massive applications of nitrogenous fertiliser. (See also UREA.)

Ammonia poisoning Hydrolysis of urea to ammonia in the rumen may occur very rapidly in cattle receiving excessive amounts of urea. If more ammonia reaches the blood and then the liver than the latter organ can detoxify, then ammonia poisoning will result. (See UREA.)

Several cows died after being fed straw which had been treated with ammonia for 5 days only and came direct from the treatment box. (It is recommended that the treatment should be for 10 days, with a 2-day interval before the product is fed to livestock.) Laryngeal oedema and emphysema of the lungs were caused. The level of ammonia in the atmosphere of animal housing must not exceed 14 ppm.

(See also LITTER, OLD.)

Amnion

The innermost of the 3 fetal envelopes. It is continuous with the skin at the umbilicus (navel), and completely encloses the fetus but is separated from actual contact with it by the amniotic fluid, or the 'liquor of the amnion', which in the mare measures about 5 or 6 litres (9 to 10H pints). (See PLACENTA.)

This 'liquor amnii' forms a kind of hydrostatic bed in which the fetus floats, and serves to protect it from injury, shocks, and extremes of temperature. It allows free though limited movements, and guards the uterus of the dam from the spasmodic fetal movements which, late in pregnancy, are often vigorous and even violent.

At birth it helps to dilate the cervical canal of the uterus and the posterior genital passages, forms part of the 'waterbag', and, on bursting, lubricates the maternal passages. (See PARTURITION.)

Amoebic Encephalitis

Amoebic encephalitis due to *Acanthamoeba castellani* was found after the euthanasia of a 4-month-old puppy. Fits and hyperkeratosis of the foot pads suggested that the cause was the distemper virus, but *A. castellani* was recovered from an area of suppurative necrosis in the brain.

(In human medicine, several species of this amoeba are recognised as an important cause of granulomatous encephalitis.) (Pearce, J. R. & others, *JAVMA* **187**, 951.)

Amoxycillin

An antibiotic resembling ampicillin, but its action is quicker and it is excreted more rapidly. Amoxycillin is often used in combination with clavulanase, which makes it more effective by blocking the effect of penicillinase, by which ampicillin is destroyed. It is used in all species.

Amphistomes

Synonym for Paramphistomes (see PARAMPHISTOMIASIS).

Ampicillin

A semi-synthetic penicillin, active against both Gram-positive and GRAM-NEGATIVE bacteria. It is not resistant to penicillinase, but can be given by mouth.

Ampoule

A small glass container having one end drawn out into a point capable of being sealed so as to preserve its contents sterile. It is used to contain solutions of drugs for hypodermic injection, while many vaccines and other biological products are also distributed in ampoules. A potential hazard of glass embolism has been recognised in human medicine, and the wisdom of allowing glass particles to settle, before filling a syringe, has been stressed.

Amprolium

A drug used for the prevention and treatment of coccidiosis in turkeys, guinea fowl and chickens.

Amputation

Removal of a limb. If a long bone of dog or cat has been shattered into several pieces, or is the site of cancer, amputation is usually the only humane course to take (other than euthanasia). It is certainly kinder than leaving the animal a permanent cripple, perhaps suffering some degree of pain for the rest of its life.

A three-legged dog or cat can be expected to revise its technique of balance and movement, and to become not merely nimble but fast as well; and to demonstrate a capacity for enjoying life.

A questionnaire was submitted to the owners of 55 dogs and 18 cats which had undergone amputation of a limb. In 26 animals the reason was cancer, and in the others it was severe injury.

All the owners stated that they were pleased the operation had been performed, although many had found it a difficult decision to make.

Amylase (Amylopsin)

A starch-splitting enzyme. (See DIGESTION.)

Amyloidosis

The deposition of an insoluble starch-like protein (amyloid) which affects the functioning of the tissues in which it is deposited. It may be associated with inflammatory conditions or chronic infections.

Anabolic

Relating to anabolism, which means tissue building, and is the opposite of catabolism or tissue breakdown.

An anabolic steroid is one derived from testosterone in which the androgenic characteristics have been reduced and the protein-building (anabolic) properties increased in proportion. Examples are nandrolone and ethylestrenol. These are used in cases of malnutrition, wasting diseases, virus diseases, and severe parasitism.

Synthetic anabolic steroids have been used as growth-promoter implants in commercial beef production, but this is prohibited in the UK and EU. They are also prohibited in competition animals. It has been found that anabolic steroids can

give rise to changes in the liver and its functioning in both animals and man; with, in some instances, tumour formation. Changes in the sexual organs may follow misuse. (See STILBENES.)

Anadromy

An anadromous fish is one that spends most of its adult life in the sea but returns to fresh water to spawn. Salmon are anadromous.

Anaemia

A reduction in the number and/or size of the red blood corpuscles or the haemoglobin in the blood. It is a sign rather than a disease, and it is important to establish the cause (obvious only in the case of acute external haemorrhage due to trauma), so that a prognosis and suitable treatment can be given.

The animal may be suffering from a chronic loss of blood due to internal bleeding, e.g. from the urinary or digestive tracts; and the owner of a cat, for instance, may fail to notice the presence of blood in the urine, and so not bring the animal for treatment until other signs of illness have become obvious.

Anticoagulants, such as Warfarin, may cause internal haemorrhage and hence anaemia.

An iron-deficient diet (and one lacking also the trace elements cobalt and copper, which aid the assimilation of iron) is another cause of anaemia; likewise a deficiency of folic acid, vitamin B_6 and vitamin B_{12}.

Both external and internal parasites (lice, fleas, ticks, liver flukes, roundworms and tapeworms) can cause anaemia.

Parasites of the bloodstream are an important cause, and include trypanosomes, piroplasms, rickettsiae. (See also FELINE INFECTIOUS ANAEMIA.)

For an incompatability between the blood of sire and dam, see haemolytic disease (under FOALS, DISEASES OF).

Aplastic anaemia means a defective, or a cessation of, regeneration of the red blood cells; it may be drug-induced. (See also RETICULOCYTES.) (In human medicine, the drugs involved have included chloramphenicol, phenylbutazone, and rarely penicillin and aspirin; deaths have resulted.)

Bracken poisoning, exposure to X-rays or other forms of irradiation are other causes; also salicylates (including aspirin).

In auto-immune haemolytic anaemia the animal forms antibodies against its own red cells.

Heinz-body haemolytic anaemia (see HEINZ BODIES) may result from kale poisoning in cattle, and from paracetamol or methylene-blue poisoning in cats; sometimes also from lead poisoning.

Signs Pallor of the mucous membranes, loss of energy and of appetite, and PICA. Dogs and cats may feel the cold more than usual, and seek warm places. In some cases fever is present, and liver enlargement. The heart rate may increase.

Treatment In the smaller animals especially, vitamin B$_{12}$ or liver extract is often a valuable method of treatment. Where cobalt or copper or iron are lacking, these must be supplied. Lice or ticks and fleas should be destroyed, and treatment against internal parasites undertaken if they are the cause. (See also PIGLET ANAEMIA; FELINE and EQUINE INFECTIOUS ANAEMIA; CANINE BABESIOSIS; HEARTWORMS; ROUNDWORMS; FLUKES.)

Anaerobe

The term applied to bacteria having the power to live without oxygen. Such organisms are found growing freely, deep in the soil, as, for example, the tetanus bacillus.

Anaesthesia, General

The use of general anaesthetics to produce loss of consciousness and sensation for operations on animals dates back to 1847, when several veterinary surgeons used ether. Chloroform was also used in 1847. Both have now been largely superseded by more effective anaesthetic agents. A wide choice is now available. The selection, dosage and means of administration will be influenced by such considerations as the species, size, and habitat of the individual as well as by the procedure to be undertaken.

Anaesthetic drugs all act by limiting the oxygen uptake of tissues. The effect on an individual tissue is proportional to its normal oxygen requirement. Since the oxygen requirement of nervous tissues is disproportionately high, these tissues are the first to be affected by anaesthetic drugs. Unconsciousness, abolition of reflexes, muscular atony, and respiratory paralysis are due to depression of the cerebral cortices, the mid-brain, the spinal cord, and the medulla respectively.

General anaesthesia is usually induced by inhalation of a volatile or gaseous anaesthetic, or by intravenous or intramuscular injection. Inhalation anaesthetics are often administered via an endotracheal tube; volatile anaesthetics such as chloroform can be simply administered by sprinkling the liquid on cotton wool and allowing the animal to inhale the vapour.

Anaesthetic agents are often used in combination with a premedicant, such as hyoscine or atropine, to reduce salivation. Two agents may be used to enhanced effect; ketamine is often used with xylazine, for example. In addition, muscle relaxants such as gallamine or suxamethonium may also be used to facilitate certain procedures. If the animal is a food animal, care must be taken to observe any precautions indicated by the drug manufacturer to avoid drug residues accumulating in meat or milk. In all cases, the manufacturers' recommendations as to dosage must be followed.

Endotracheal anaesthesia This technique depends upon the introduction into the trachea of a tube which connects with the outside. The tube is passed via the mouth under a narcotic or anaesthetic, such as pentobarbital, given intravenously, and may then be used as the route for an inhalant anaesthetic mixture. The method ensures a clear airway throughout the period of anaesthesia, and thus obviates the danger of laryngeal obstruction (e.g. by the tongue falling backwards), which sometimes causes death. The method has several other advantages, e.g. it permits an unobstructed operation field during lengthy major operations, achieves better oxygenation, facilitates an even level of anaesthesia, and permits of positive pressure ventilation of the lungs in the event of respiratory failure.

Endotracheal anaesthesia is administered in one of two ways. Insufflation anaesthesia involves the use of air/oxygen and anaesthetic vapour delivered into the tube by means of a pump or, more commonly, a mixture of gases supplied from cylinders (and sometimes bubbled through a volatile anaesthetic liquid in addition). Autoinhalation anaesthesia involves the use of a wide-bore endotracheal tube through which the animal inhales the anaesthetic mixture by its own respiratory efforts. A 'rebreathing bag' may be used.

As an alternative to general anaesthesia, EPIDURAL ANAESTHESIA (involving the injection of a local anaesthetic into the spinal canal) is used for some surgical procedures.

Cattle Many procedures are performed under local anaesthetic. Where general anaesthesia is indicated, after premedication with, for example, xylazine, halothane is administered via an endotracheal tube. Cattle take chloroform well, and recovery is rapid; however, it is little used now. Thiopental and phenobarbital, by injection, may also be used on occasion.

Endotracheal intubation is recommended in order to preserve a free airway, and to prevent inhalation of regurgitated rumen contents.

Horses By inhalation, halothane or isoflurane may be used, administered through an

A

endotracheal tube. By intravenous injection, ketamine, given after premedication with xylazine, romifidine or detomidine is effective; ketamine must not be used as sole anaesthetic in the equine. The use of thiopental, via intravenous catheter, also requires premedication. Great care must be taken that the recumbent anaesthetised horse does not suffer muscle or nerve damage, caused by the pressure of its own weight, while unconscious.

Sheep Pentobarbital, by slow intravenous injection at a dosage of 24 mg per kg bodyweight, produces anaesthesia for up to 30 minutes, with recovery over a similar period. Halothane may be given by inhalation. Alphaxolone/alphadone has been used, as well as other agents, although there are few licensed anaesthetics for sheep.

Goats Pentobarbital, by slow intravenous injection, alphaxolone/alphadolone, etorphine (Immobilon), and halothane have also been suggested for such procedures as the disbudding of kids.

Dogs and cats A wide choice is available. Pentobarbital by intravenous injection is rapid in action. Thiopental, also given intravenously, is a short-acting general anaesthetic.

Ketamine hydrochloride, given by intramuscular injection, is another choice. When given to cats, it must be used with xylazine to prevent excitability on recovery.

Alfadolone/alfaxalone (Saffan), by intramuscular or intravenous injection, is used either for the induction of anaesthesia by other drugs, or as an anaesthetic itself. It should be used with caution in dogs as it may cause a histamine reaction.

Propofol (Rapinovet), an intravenous anaesthetic for dogs and cats, is useful for minor outpatient procedures and caesarian section. Recovery is generally smooth but retching, sneezing, and pawing of the face may be seen.

Monkeys Pentobarbital sodium may be given intravenously. Ketamine hydrochloride is an alternative, given by subcutaneous, intramuscular, or intravenous injection. A mixture of ketamine and xylazine has been recommended also. Halothane is suitable.

Rabbits, rats, mice, guinea pigs
Inhalation anaesthetics such as isoflurane are safe and effective; rabbits should be sedated first. Injectable anaesthetic combinations, such as fentanyl-fluanisole and midazolam, or keta-

mine and xylazine, may be used; pentobarbital is another choice.

Birds Ether has been used but its explosive nature necessitates great care; halothane or isoflurane are more suitable. For restraint, the bird may be placed in a large, clear polythene bag, into which the tube for the anaesthetic gas is introduced.

For anaesthetic injections of ketamine or pentobarbital, the bird may be immobilised with a cylinder of paper rolled around it and secured with adhesive tape.

Reptiles Small reptiles may be anaesthetised by bathing in a weak solution of phenoxyethanol, benzocaine or tricaine mesilate. They are transferred to clean oxygenated water for recovery. Ketamine, by injection, is also used but recovery may be prolonged.

Fish Phenoxyethanol, benzocaine or tricaine mesilate, dissolved in the water, are commonly used for both exotic and farmed fish. Exotic fish species vary in their tolerance of these substances; water temperature and quality also affect their efficacy. Clean oxygenated water should be available to aid recovery.

Anaesthesia, Local and Regional

For many minor operations and diagnostic procedures, local anaesthetics are used in preference to general anaesthesia. They act by blocking conduction along the nerve fibre, producing loss of sensation and/or muscle paralysis. Drugs used include lidocaine (lignocaine) and bupivacaine. The method and site of administration can be targeted according to the specific procedure to be carried out.

Perineural anaesthesia is used when the precise location of the nerves serving the area to be anaesthetised is known. For example, when disbudding calves, the area may be anaesthetised by injecting the agent about 2.5 cm below the base of the horn bud.

Field block (nerve block) is produced when a series of injections is made along a line to remove sensation from the tissue distal to that line. Field block is typically used in the diagnosis of laminitis in horses and temporary relief of the pain it causes.

Regional anaesthesia may result from perineural or field anaesthesia. To anaesthetise a limb, a tourniquet is applied above the part of the limb to be anaesthetised and the drug given intravenously; prilocaine is the agent of choice. Loss of sensation lasts until the tourniquet is released. The precautions applying to the use of tourniquets must be observed (see under TOURNIQUET).

Surface anaesthesia is useful for facilitating certain procedures. It may be applied to a mucous surface by spray. For example, a cat's throat may be sprayed with local anaesthetic before introducing a tracheal tube. To facilitate introduction of a venous catheter, the skin of smaller species can be anasthetised by applying an anaesthetic cream, after shaving the area. The cream is protected by a waterproof dressing; the anaesthetic may take up to an hour to work. Local anaesthetics may also be used in eye drops.

Epidural (or spinal) anaesthesia results when a local anaesthetic is injected into the space surrounding the spinal cord – the epidural space. This produces a loss of sensation in the tissues served by the spinal nerves. The specific area affected depends on the site of injection. In the caudal spinal cord, anaesthesia of the perineal area results; the technique is used e.g. in difficult calvings. Epidural anaesthesia applied to the anterior part of the spinal cord may be used for operations on the recumbent animal.

Intra-articular anaesthesia, by injection into a joint, is mainly used diagnostically to identify a joint that is causing pain.

Local anaesthetics must not be used indiscriminately, since poisoning can result, and affect the brain and heart. Symptoms of poisoning include sudden collapse, or excitement, vomiting and convulsions.

Anaesthetics, Legal Requirements

The Protection of Animals (Anaesthetics) Act 1964 made it obligatory to use an anaesthetic when castrating dogs, cats, horses, asses, and mules of any age.

Castration

Only a veterinary surgeon, using an anaesthetic, is permitted to castrate any farm animal more than 2 months old; with the exception of rams for which the maximum age is 3 months.

The use of rubber rings or similar devices for castrating bulls, pigs, goats, and sheep, or for docking lambs' tails, is forbidden unless applied during the 1st week of life. The Act of 1964 also requires that an anaesthetic be used when de-horning cattle; and also for disbudding calves unless this be done by chemical cautery applied during the 1st week of life.

An anaesthetic must be used for any operation, performed with or without the use of instruments, which involves interference with the sensitive tissues or the bone structure of an animal. (See also DOCKING.)

Anaesthetics, Residues in Carcases

Dogs and cats have shown severe symptoms of poisoning after being fed on meat from animals humanely slaughtered by means of an overdose of a barbiturate anaesthetic, or chloral hydrate.

Anal

Relating to the ANUS.

Anal Glands

(see under ANUS)

Analeptics

Drugs that stimulate the central nervous system (see STIMULANTS).

Analgesics

Drugs which cause a temporary loss of the sense of pain without a loss of consciousness, i.e. analgesia.

Analgesics include non-steroidal anti-inflammatory drugs (NSAIDs) such as aspirin, paracetamol and phenylbutazone. (They are contraindicated if heart, kidney or liver disease is present.)

The most effective of the opiates is MORPHINE. (See also BUPRENORPHINE; DETOMIDINE; ACUPUNCTURE.)

Anamnesis

Anamnesis is the past history of a particular patient.

Anamnestic Response

The rapid rise in antibody level in a previously immunised animal in response to a 'booster' dose of the same vaccine. The immune system has 'remembered' what to do.

Anaphrodisia

Impairment of sexual appetite.

Anaphylactic Shock (Anaphylaxis)

The reaction to a foreign protein which sometimes follows bee or wasp stings, injections of an antibiotic or antiserum, etc., after the patient has become hypersensitised to the substance. There is often a rapid fall in blood pressure; anaphylactic shock can prove fatal. (See also ANTIHISTAMINES; HYPERSENSITIVITY; WARBLES.)

A

Anaplasmosis

This is an infectious disease of cattle, characterised by anaemia and caused by a parasite of the red blood cells, *Anaplasma marginale*.

This parasite is found in Africa, Asia, Australia, Southern Europe, South America, and the southern States of the USA. *A. centrale* (in cattle) and *A. ovis* (in sheep and goats) are other species.

Signs The disease resembles Texas fever; frequently anaplasmosis coexists with babesiosis, but pure infections may also occur. It is characterised by acute anaemia, fever, jaundice, and degeneration of the internal organs; haemoglobinuria does not occur as the rate of red-blood-cell destruction is not fast enough to produce free haemoglobin in the circulating blood. Young animals appear to be resistant, and cases in calves under 1 year old are rare. In older animals the disease may be acute or chronic, and in the former case they may die within 2 to 3 days after the appearance of the first symptoms. The disease starts with a high temperature of 40.5° to 41.5°C (105° to 107°F) and after a day or two anaemia and icterus appear. In the acute illness, aggressiveness and abortion are other symptoms.

Transmission is by ticks, e.g. *Boophilus*, *Rhipicephalus*, *Hyalomma*, *Ixodes*, *Dermacentor*, and *Haemaphysalis*. Infection is passed through the egg to the next generation of ticks. Tabanid flies and mosquitoes are carriers.

Animals which recover from anaplasmosis are in a state of premunition, and remain carriers for long periods, probably for life.

In the South African States the less serious *A. centrale* has been found to give protection against the serious *A. marginale*, and both there and in other countries successful results follow its use as an immunising agent. In other areas where Texas fever and anaplasmosis frequently occur together, cattle are often immunised by blood of a bovine infected with *A. centrale*, which produces a mild infection, and with a mild form of *Babesia bigemina*.

Anasarca

Anasarca is a condition of oedema, particularly of the tissues below the skin.

Anastomosis

The means by which the circulation is carried on when a large vessel is severed or its stream obstructed. In anatomy the term is applied to a junction between 2 or more arteries or veins which communicate with each other.

Anatoxin

A toxin rendered harmless by heat or chemical means but capable of stimulating the formation of antibodies.

Anchor Worm

(*Lernaea cyprinacea*) An exotic parasite of goldfish now to be found in some indoor ornamental pools in the UK. The worms can penetrate the fish's skin. Their removal needs to be done under anaesthesia.

Anconeal Process

Part of the elbow joint, being a projection of the ULNA. In several breeds of dog it may not develop properly.

Ancylostoma

(see HOOKWORMS)

Androgen

(see HORMONES)

Anergy

Failure or suppression of the cellular immune mechanism. This may occur in e.g. human brucellosis, and in other chronic diseases. Antianergic treatment with levamisole has been found successful in some patients. (R. D. Thorne, *Veterinary Record*, **101**, 27.) (See also IMMUNOSUPPRESSION.)

Aneuplody

The presence of an irregular number of chromosomes (not an exact multiple of the haploid number). It may arise through faulty cell division.

Aneurin

A synonym for THIAMIN.

Aneurysm

A dilatation of an artery (or sometimes of a vein) following a weakening of its walls. The result is a pulsating sac which is liable to rupture.

Aneurysms occur in the abdomen, chest, and brain, and may result from a congenital weakness of the blood vessel, from disease of its lining cells, from injury, etc.

Causes Sudden and violent muscular efforts are regarded as the chief factors in the production of aneurysms, and as would be expected, the horse is more subject to this trouble than any of the other domesticated animals.

'**Verminous aneurysm**' is a misnomer for verminous arteritis of horses caused by immature strongyle worms. (See EQUINE VER-MINOUS ARTERITIS.)

Angiogenesis

A method of treating a tumour by depriving it of its blood supply.

Angiography

A radiographic technique which enables the blood-flow to and from an organ to be visualised after injection of a contrast medium.

Angioma

A TUMOUR composed of a large number of blood vessels. They are common in the livers of cattle. (See also HAEMANGIOMA.)

Angiostrongylus

(see HEARTWORMS)

Angitis

Inflammation of a blood vessel, lymph vessel, or bile duct.

Angleberry

An old name for WARTS.

Anhidrosis

A failure of the sweat mechanism. This occurs in horses especially, but also in cattle, imported into tropical countries with humid climates.

At first, affected horses sweat excessively and their breathing is distressed after exercise. Later, sweating occurs only at the mane; the skin becomes scurfy; and breathing becomes more laboured. Heart failure may occur.

Anhydride

An oxide which can combine with water to form an acid.

Anhydrous

Containing no water.

Animal Behaviour

As a guide to animal welfare, see AGGRESSIVE-NESS; ANAESTHESIA; ANALGESICS; ETHOLOGY; ELECTRIC SHOCK; HOUSING OF ANIMALS; TRANSPORT STRESS.

Animal Boarding Establishments Act 1963

This requires that the owner of a boarding establishment shall obtain a licence from the Local Authority, and that this licence must be renewed annually. The applicant has to satisfy the licensing authority on certain personal points, and that the 'animals will at all times be kept in accommodation suitable as respects construction, size of quarters, number of occupants, exercising facilities, temperature, lighting, ventilation, and cleanliness'. The Act also requires that animals boarded 'will be adequately supplied with suitable food, drink, and bedding material, adequately exercised, and (so far as necessary) visited at suitable intervals'. Isolation facilities and fire precautions are covered by the Act, which empowers the Local Authority to inspect both the boarding establishment and the register which must be kept there.

Animal Data Centre

This is located at the National Centre for Animal Statistics, Westside, Newton, Stocksfield, Northumberland NE43 7TW.

Animal Food

(see CONCENTRATES; DIET; RATIONS; PROTEINS; POISONING; VITAMINS; ADDITIVES; PET FOODS; also DOGS' DIET; CAT FOODS, etc.)

Animal Health Act 1981

This consolidated the Diseases of Animals Acts 1950, 1953 and 1975.

Animal Health Schemes

(see under HEALTH SCHEMES)

Animal Health Trust (AHT)

A charity that is one of the world's leading centres for research into animal health. Its Equine Research Station is renowned for its studies of the physiological and anatomical factors affecting performance, and the small animal centre has particular expertise in eye problems of the dog and cat. AHT research has led to breakthroughs in anaesthesia and in the development of vaccines against equine flu and canine distemper. The address is: Animal Health Trust, PO Box 5, Newmarket, Suffolk CB8 7DW.

Animal Husbandry

(see GRAZING; PASTURE; HOUSING; WATER; DIET; DAIRY HERD; also COWS, SHEEP, PIGS, etc.)

Animal Nursing

(see VETERINARY NURSES – Lay assistants who have passed the requisite examinations under the auspices of the Royal College of Veterinary Surgeons).

Animal Transport

(see TRANSPORT)

Animal Welfare Codes

(see WELFARE CODES FOR ANIMALS)

Animals, Housing Of
(see HOUSING OF ANIMALS)

Animals (Scientific Procedures) Act 1986
This replaced the Cruelty to Animals Act 1876. The 1986 Act makes it illegal to supply animals, other than those purpose-bred in Home-Office-designated breeding establishments, for use in experimental procedures involving dogs, cats, and other animals. The Act requires all laboratories in the UK where animals are used in research to appoint a veterinary surgeon to be responsible for the care and welfare of their experimental animals.

On 1 January 1990 it became illegal to sell or supply pet or stray animals for use in scientific experiments.

The Act also represents the culmination of the efforts of three organisations – the British Veterinary Association (BVA), the Committee for the Reform of Animal Experimentation (CRAE), and the Fund for the Replacement of Animals in Medical Experiments (FRAME) – to reform animal experimentation legislation. The new Act is firmly rooted in BVA/ CRAE/ FRAME proposals sent to the Home Secretary in 1983, and represents an effective compromise between the welfare needs of animals, the legitimate demands of the public for accountability, and the equally legitimate requirements of medicine, science and commerce.

The legislation gives the Home Secretary the power and the responsibility to judge the scientific merit of the work s/he authorises and for which s/he will be answerable to Parliament.

Ankylosis
The condition of a joint in which the movement is restricted by union of the bones or adhesions. (See JOINTS, DISEASES OF.)

Anodynes
Anodynes are pain-relieving drugs.

Anoestrus
Anoestrus is the state in the female when no oestrus or 'season' is exhibited. It is a state of sexual inactivity. In most mares, for example, anoestrus occurs during the winter months, when daylight is reduced, ambient temperatures are low and, in the wild state, food is scarce. In these circumstances the pituitary gland does not release the gonadotrophins FSH and LF (see HORMONES) so that neither follicles nor *corpora lutea* develop in the ovaries.

Similar circumstances apply with cattle. Fear, hunger, cold, and pain may all result in anoestrus. (See also OESTRUS.)

Anorexia
(see APPETITE – Diminished appetite)

Anoxia
Oxygen deficiency. Cerebral anoxia, or a failure in the oxygen supply to the brain, occurs during nitrite and prussic-acid poisoning; in copper deficiency in cattle; and in the thoroughbred 'barker foal'. Anoxia is a method of slaughter allowed under the Welfare of Animals (Slaughter or Killing) Regulations 1995. (See also ANAESTHESIA.)

Ante-Mortem
Before death. An ante-mortem inspection is the name for an examination of the live animal which is used in conjunction with the findings of a post-mortem inspection, or autopsy. Under the Welfare of Animals (Slaughter or Killing) Regulations 1995, ante-mortem inspections are carried out on animals after their arrival at an abattoir and before they are stunned.

Ante-Natal Infection
Infection of the fetus before birth. Examples of this may occur with the larvae of the dog hookworm, *Ancylostoma caninum*, and with the larvae of other roundworms. (See TOXOCARA.) Toxoplasmosis is another example of an infection which may occur before birth.

Ante-Partum Paralysis
Ante-partum paralysis is a condition in which the hindquarters of the pregnant animal suddenly become paralysed. It is fairly common in the cow, has been seen in the sheep and goat, but is rare in the mare. It appears from 6 to 25 days before parturition, and is liable to affect animals in almost any condition – those that are well kept as well as others.

Signs The condition suddenly appears without any warning. The pregnant animal is found in the lying position, and is quite unable to regain her feet.

Treatment As a rule, the nearer to the day of parturition that the paralysis appears, the more favourable will be the result. Those cases that lie for 2 or more weeks are very unsatisfactory. The condition usually disappears after parturition has taken place, either almost at once or in 2 or 3 days. As a consequence, treatment should be mainly directed to ensuring that the animal is comfortable, provided with plenty of bedding, is turned over on to the opposite side 3 or 4 times a day if she does not turn herself, and receives a laxative diet so that constipation may not occur. Mashes, green food, and a variety in the food stuffs offered, are indicated. When the paralysis has occurred a considerable time before parturition is due, it is often necessary to produce artificial abortion of the fetus and so relieve the uterus of its heavy encumbrance.

Anthelmintic Resistance

Routine use of an anthelmintic tends to establish resistance to its effects. Resistance to anthelmintics in sheep has become a serious problem in Australia and is increasing in other countries where livestock are regularly dosed. The development of resistance can be discouraged by changing the class of anthelmintic used for each year's dosing programme. Worming products are labelled with the following codes that identify their chemical type.

1-BZ Benzimidazoles, probenzimodazoles
2-LM Imidazothiazoles, tetrahydropyrimidines
3-AV Avermectins, milbemycins

Products with the same codes should not be used on the same animals in successive seasons.

Anthelmintics

Anthelmintics are medicines which are given to expel parasitic worms. There is a large range of substances and formulations from which to choose. Anthelmintic drugs include abamectin, albendazole, dichlorvos, doramectin, haloxon, levamisole, moxidectin, nitroxinil, tetramisole, morantel tartrate, thiophanate. Niclosamide, dichlorophen and praziquantel preparations are used against tapeworms in the dog. (See also DRONCIT.) Fenbendazole and albendazole are broad-spectrum anthelmintics usually effective against inhibited fourth-stage ostertagia larvae in cattle.

Certain criteria apply in the selection of anthelmintics. For example, will the drug in question kill worm eggs? Is it effective against immature worms? Is it effective against adult worms of the economically important species? Does the drug discolour or taint milk? Can it be given to pregnant, or emaciated, animals? In cows, for how long must the milk be discarded after administration?

Methods of dosing include drenching; injection (e.g. in the case of tetramisole); in the feed. (See also WORMS, FARM TREATMENT AGAINST.)

Anthisan

An antihistamine.

Anthrax

An acute, usually fatal, infection found in mammals; it is commonest among the herbivora.

Cause The *Bacillus anthracis*. Under certain adverse circumstances, each rod-shaped bacillus is able to form itself into a spore. The spores of anthrax are hard to destroy. They resist drying for a period of at least 2 years. They are able to live in the soil for 10 years or more and still be capable of infecting animals. Consequently pastures that have been infected by spilled blood from a case that has died are extremely difficult to render safe for stock.

Earth-worms may carry the spores from deeper layers of the soil up to the surface. Spores have been found in bone-meal, in blood fertilisers, in wool and hides and in feeds. (See also STREAMS.)

The bacillus itself is a comparatively delicate organism and easily killed by the ordinary disinfectants.

Method of Infection In cattle, infection nearly always occurs by way of the mouth and alimentary system. Either the living organisms or else the spores are taken in on the food or with the drinking water. Flies can spread the disease. Anthrax has been caused through inoculation of vaccine contaminated by spores; sheep should not be inoculated, therefore, in a dusty shed. Unsterilised bone-meal is an important source of infection.

Signs Three forms of the disease are recognised: the peracute, the acute, and the subacute.

Cattle In most peracute cases the animal is found dead without having shown any noticeable symptoms beforehand. Acute: a temperature of 41° to 41.6° C (106° or 107°F), a thin, rapid pulse, coldness of the ears, feet, and horns, and 'blood-shot' eyes and nostrils. After a few hours this picture is followed by one of prostration, unconsciousness, and death. In either of the above types there may have been diarrhoea or dysentery.

In the subacute form the affected animal may linger for as long as 48 hours, showing nothing more than a very high temperature and laboured respirations. Occasionally cattle may be infected through the skin, when a 'carbuncle' follows, similar to that seen in man. Diffuse, painless, doughy swellings are seen in other cases, especially about the neck and the lower part of the chest.

As sudden death of an animal is often wrongly attributed to lightning strike, a farmer should consult a veterinary surgeon (who will carry out a rapid blood test) to make sure that the cause of death is not anthrax – before handling the carcase, cutting

into it, moving it, or letting farm dogs, hounds, cats, etc., feed upon it.

Sheep and goats Anthrax in these animals is almost always of the peracute type.

Horses There are two notable forms of anthrax in the horse. In one there is a marked swelling of the throat, neck, and chest. In the 2nd form of equine anthrax, a fit of shivering ushers in the fever. The pulse-rate becomes increased, the horse lies and rises again with great frequency; it shows signs of slowly increasing abdominal pain by kicking at its belly, by gazing at its flanks, or by rolling on the ground.

Pigs The disease may follow the feeding of slaughter-house refuse or the flesh of an animal that has died from an unknown disease (which has really been anthrax), or raw bone-meal intended as a fertiliser. There is sometimes swelling of the throat; the intestine may be involved. In this abdominal form the symptoms may be very vague. Otherwise the pigs are dull, lie a good deal, show a gradually increasing difficulty in respiration, and present in the early stages a swelling of the throat and head which later invades the lower parts of the neck. Recovery is not unknown.

Dogs and cats A localised form, with oedema of the head and neck (similar to that in the pig), is characteristic.

Prevention and Treatment In Great Britain, as in most developed countries, anthrax is a NOTIFIABLE DISEASE. Vaccines are not available commercially. In Brtiain, DEFRA may be contacted for information about emergency supplies of vaccine. Antibiotics, if given early enough, may be effective.

In so far as its prevention is concerned, the important points to remember are (1) disposal of the carcase by efficient and safe means (see DISPOSAL OF CARCASES) and (2) frequent observation of other animals which have been in contact with the dead one; also their isolation if showing a rise in body temperature.

Sodium hypochlorite (or bleaching powder in a hot 10 per cent solution) kills both bacilli and the spores almost instantaneously.

The milk from in-contact animals must be regarded as dangerous until such time as these are considered to be out of danger. The law forbids anyone who is not authorised to cut an anthrax carcase for any purpose whatsoever. Cases of death from this procedure are by no means unknown, and illness following the

dressing of a carcase must always be considered suspicious of anthrax until the contrary has been established. The need for reporting illness to the medical authorities by all persons whose work brings them into contact with carcases of animals cannot be too strongly stressed.

Anthrax in human patients Anthrax is now very rare in humans, only a handful of cases having been notified in recent years. It may take the form of an inflamed pustule accompanied by fever and prostration, if infection is via the skin – e.g. through a cut. In cases of internal infection, by inhaling or swallowing the spores, pneumonia or intestinal ulceration usually cause death within 2 days if not treated promptly. The infection is more often contracted by workers handling infected meat or meat and bone-meal than by farmers.

Anthrax Order 1991

This order requires the person in charge of an animal or carcase suspected of being infected with anthrax to notify the divisional veterinary manager (DVM). Investigation by a veterinary inspector will follow and the premises may be declared an infected place. The local authority has the responsibility of disposing of the carcase by incineration or other suitable method. The DVM supervises cleansing, disinfection, vaccination, etc. If the owner refuses to carry out these procedures, the DVM can have them carried out and recover the cost from the owner. The Anthrax (Amendment) Order 1996 enables the veterinary inspector to require the incineration of things that have been in contact with or used by an infected animal.

Anthroponoses

Diseases transmissible from man to lower animals. Such diseases include: tuberculosis; mumps (to dogs); scarlet fever (giving rise to mastitis in dairy cows); tonsillitis (giving rise to calf pneumonia, etc.); infestation with the beef tapeworm; influenza in pigs and birds. (Compare ZOONOSES.)

Antibiotic

A chemical compound derived from living (or synthesised) organisms which is capable, in small concentration, of inhibiting the life process of micro-organisms. To be useful in medicine, an antibiotic must (1) have powerful action in the body against 1 or more types of bacteria; (2) have specific action; (3) have low toxicity for tissues; (4) be active in the presence of body fluids; (5) not be destroyed by tissue enzymes such as trypsin; (6) be stable; (7) be not too rapidly excreted; (8) preferably not give rise to resistant strains of organisms. (Professor F. Alexander.)

Antibiotics are much used in veterinary medicine to overcome certain infections, and they have been of notable service, for instance, in the control of certain forms of mastitis in dairy cattle, in the avoidance of septicaemia following badly infected wounds, deep-seated abscesses, peritonitis, etc. Abdominal and other surgery has been rendered safer by the use of antibiotics. The prophylactic use of antibiotics has been an important factor in the intensive production of livestock and poultry. They must not, however, be used indiscriminately, be regarded as a panacea, or be given in too low a dosage. It is unwise to use antibiotics of the tetracycline group in either pregnant or very young animals owing to the adverse effects upon bone and teeth which may result.

Certain antibiotics are effective GROWTH PROMOTERS.

Selection of Antibiotic It is often necessary to begin antibiotic therapy before the results of bacteriological examinations are available, and therapy must depend on the clinical features. However, the taking of material for culture and carrying out sensitivity tests are most important procedures. Another factor in veterinary practice is the cost of the drug.

Only in a very few instances are mixtures of antibiotics superior to a single drug. In those cases in which more than 1 antibiotic is required, the full dose of each of the individual antibiotics should be given so as to exceed the MINIMUM INHIBITORY CONCENTRATION. Combined antibiotic therapy does not improve the outlook in chronic urinary infections or, indeed, many chronic infections. Mixtures of antibiotics have been most successful when used in local applications or in infections of the alimentary canal. (See ADDITIVES, and under MILK.) Ten of the most widely used antibiotics in veterinary medicine are: BENZYLPENI-CILLIN, procaine penicillin (under PROCAINE HYDROCHLORIDE), AMPICILLIN, AMOXYCILLIN, STREPTOMYCIN, NEOMYCIN, TETRACYCLINES, CHLORAMPHENICOL, ERYTHROMYCIN, GRISE-OFULVIN. (See also CEPHALOSPORIN ANTIBI-OTICS, TIAMULIN, SALINOMYCIN; and below.)

For advice on selection of antibiotics for treatment, see *The Veterinary Formulary* (RPSGB/BVA).

Antibiotic Resistance

The widespread use of antibiotics has become associated with the development of resistance to

their effects. Bacteria can become drug-resistant in 1 of 2 ways. Chromosomal resistance develops through mutation and is probably rare. Bacteria which achieve this kind of resistance are unable to transfer it to other bacteria, but pass it on to their own future generations through the ordinary process of cell division.

The 2nd method is transmissible drug resistance (TDR). This is achieved by means of PLASMIDS.

Many bacteria carry, in their cytoplasm, resistance or R factors. These are pieces of DNA which include genes coding for resistance to antibiotics and other genes which facilitate the transit of the R factor to other bacteria. Both groups of genes are carried on plasmids.

A GRAM-NEGATIVE bacterium which possesses an R factor is able to conjugate with other Gram-negative bacteria. This involves intimate contact through a protoplasmic bridge called a sex pilus. When this occurs a duplicate of the R factor is transmitted to the 2nd, recipient, cell, which thereby acquires both the drug resistance and the ability to transmit it to other bacteria.

Inside the gut of an animal being dosed with an antibiotic, these resistant bacteria survive and multiply at the expense of the antibiotic-sensitive bacteria. Cross-infection can then bring about a similar situation in other animals.

The persistence of TDR in the animal gut has been related to the pattern of antibiotic usage. Continuous low-level administration of antibiotics has been shown to increase the incidence of resistant organisms. The emergence of resistant strains of salmonella in calves receiving in-feed antibiotics has been of concern. As long ago as 1972, a MAFF study of 2166 strains of salmonella isolated from farm animals found that 90 per cent were resistant to streptomycin.

There has been concern that the use of antibiotics as growth promoters could encourage development of resistant organisms. Consequently, antibiotics used in this way should be selected from those not used therapeutically in animals or humans.

On the other hand, specific full-dose treatments for acute conditions are less likely to create persistent resistance problems. For example, administration in dairy herds of an antibiotic via the teat, over short periods of time, or as a preventive during the dry period, seems to have had little effect on drug-resistance in the herd.

Antibiotic Supplements

The use of antibiotic feed supplements is strictly regulated in the EU. (See under ADDITIVES.)

Antibiotics, Adverse Reactions to

(see PENICILLIN, SENSITIVITY TO; NEOMYCIN; CHLORAMPHENICOL; TETRACYCLINES; TYLOSIN)

Antibody (Ab)

A substance in the blood serum or other body fluids formed to exert a specific restrictive or destructive action on bacteria, their toxins, viruses, or any foreign protein.

Antibodies are not produced, like hormones, by a single organ, the blood then distributing them throughout the body. Antibody production has been shown to occur in lymph nodes close to the site of introduction of an antigen, in the skin, fat, and voluntary muscle, and locally in infected tissues.

Chemically, antibodies (belonging to a group of proteins called immunoglobulins) are protein molecules of complex structure. In the IMMUNE RESPONSE, antibody and antigen molecules combine together in what is called a complex. These complexes are removed from the body by the RETICULO-ENDOTHELIAL SYSTEM. Agglutination of bacteria and precipitation of soluble protein antigens both occur following combination of antibody and antigen molecules, and are made use of in laboratory tests.

Antibodies are not always protective; some join mast cells and eosinophils after exposure to the specific antigen resulting in the release of histamine, as happens in ALLERGY. (See also REAGINIC ANTIBODIES.)

Anticoagulants

Agents which inhibit clotting of the blood. They include WARFARIN, dicoumarol and heparin. They are used in the treatment of coronary thrombosis in humans.

Anticoagulins

Substances secreted by leeches and hookworms in order to prevent clotting of the blood, which they suck.

Anticonvulsants

Drugs used in the treatment of epilepsy to control seizures. (See also ANTISPASMODICS; PHENYTOIN SODIUM.)

Antidiuretic Hormone (ADH)

Also called vasopressin, ADH is secreted by the posterior lobe of the PITUITARY GLAND. It stimulates absorption of water by the renal tubules, thus concentrating the urine. A deficiency of ADH leads to DIABETES INSIPIDUS.

Antidotes

Antidotes neutralise the effects of poisons either (a) by changing the poisons into relatively harmless substances through some chemical action, or (b) by setting up an action in the body opposite to that of the poison.

First-aid and other antidotes are given under the various poisons – see POISONING.

Antifreeze

Garages contain a poison which claims animals as victims every year, namely ethylene glycol, or antifreeze. Cats and dogs are attracted by its sweet taste. The symptoms are depression, ataxia and coma, sometimes with vomiting and convulsions. Ethylene glycol is oxidised in the body to oxalic acid, the actual toxic agent, and crystals of calcium oxalate may be found on post-mortem examination in the kidneys and blood vessels of the brain. Treatment attempts to swamp the enzyme systems which bring about this oxidation by offering ethanol as an alternative substrate. This is achieved by the intravenous administration of 20 per cent ethanol and 5 per cent sodium bicarbonate to correct acidosis; vodka (40 per cent alcohol) is a readily available source of alcohol. An alcohol dehydrogenase inhibitor, 4-methylpyrazole, has been reported effective in cases where azotaemia (nitrogen in the blood caused by toxic kidney failure) has not occurred.

Antigen

A substance which causes the formation of antibodies. (See IMMUNE RESPONSE; VACCINE; H-Y ANTIGEN.)

Antigenetic Drift

An antigenetic change caused by mutations of genes which may change the infective and antibody characteristics of a virus.

Antiglobulin

An antiserum against the globulin part of the serum, and used in the indirect fluorescent antibody test and Coombs test.

Antihistamines

Drugs which neutralise the effects of histamine in excess in the tissues. They are used in treating allergic disorders, e.g. some cases of: laminitis, urticaria, light sensitisation, anaphylaxis, rhinitis in cats, etc. Antihistamines are often used to prevent travel sickness in dogs and cats. They include diphenhydramine hydrochloride (Benylin), mepyramine maleate (Anthisan), chlorpheniramine maleate (Piriton), and promezathine hydrochloride (Phenergan). They should not be used except under professional advice.

Antihormones
True antibodies formed consequent upon the injection of hormones.

Antiketogenic
Antiketogenic is the term applied to foods and remedies which prevent or decrease the formation of ketones.

Antimony (Hb)
Antimony (Hb) is a metallic element belonging to the class of heavy metals. Antimony salts are less used now in veterinary medicine than formerly, less toxic substitutes being preferable.

Uses Tartar emetic, the double tartrate of antimony and potassium, was used for intravenous injection against certain trypanosomes and other protozoon parasites. (See ANTIDOTES.)

Antioxidants
(see VITAMINS – Vitamin E)

Antiphlogistics
(see POULTICES AND FOMENTATIONS)

Antipyretics
Antipyretics are drugs used to reduce temperature during fevers.

Antiseptics
Agents which inhibit the growth of micro-organisms, and are suitable for application to wounds or the unbroken skin. Preparations designed to kill organisms are properly called 'disinfectants' or 'germicides'. Many substances may be either antiseptic or disinfectant according to the strength used.

Very strong antiseptic or disinfectant solutions should not be used for wounds because of the destruction of cells they cause. The dead cells may then retard healing, and in some cases are later cast off as a slough.

The following are among substances used, suitably diluted or in formulation as creams or ointments, as animal antiseptics.

Chlorine compounds in several different forms are used for cleansing wounds from the presence of organisms. Among the class may be mentioned eusol, eupad, 'TCP'*, etc. They include sodium hypochlorite and chloramines, both also used as disinfectants.

Quaternary ammonium compounds (see under this heading) are widely used in dairy hygiene. They include cetrimide and benzalkonium chloride.

Dettol*, Solution of Chloroxylenol, BP Powerful bactericide of relatively low toxicity. Useful for skin cleansing, obstetrical work, and disinfecting premises. The bactericidal action is reduced in the presence of blood or serum.

Crystal violet in 1 per cent solution forms a useful antiseptic for infected wounds, burns, fungal skin diseases, and chronic ulcers. Similarly, gentian violet.

Common salt (a teaspoonful to a pint of boiled water) is useful as a wound lotion and is usually easily obtainable when other antiseptics may be lacking.

Sulphonamides have proved of great use in wounds infected with streptococci and certain other organisms (see SULFONAMIDES).

Iodoform* is a powerful, poisonous but soothing antiseptic formerly often used for dusting on to wounds as a powder with boric acid.

Iodine* in an alcoholic solution is more penetrating and irritant, especially to delicate skins. For use on the unbroken skin **only**.

Alcohol is a very powerful antiseptic chiefly used for removing grease and septic matter from the hands of the surgeon and the skin of the patient.

Hydrogen peroxide (see under this heading).

* Their injudicious use could lead to toxicity in cats, so for them other antiseptics are preferable.

Antiserum
A serum for use against a specific condition is produced by inoculating a susceptible animal with a sub-lethal dose of the causal agent or antigen and gradually increasing the dosage until very large amounts are administered. The animal develops in its blood serum an antibody which can be made use of to confer a temporary protection in other animals against the bacterium or toxin.

The use of antiserum alone confers a temporary immunity, and in most cases this probably does not protect for longer than from 10 days to a maximum of about 21 days. Antisera are used in the treatment of existing disease, and also as a means of protecting animals exposed to infection. (See BLACK-QUARTER; TETANUS; JAUNDICE (Leptospiral) for examples of diseases where serum therapy may be useful.) (See also ANAPHYLACTIC SHOCK; IMMUNITY.)

Antisialics
Substances which reduce salivation, e.g. atropine.

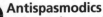

Antispasmodics

Antispasmodics are drugs which diminish spasm causing colic or 'cramp'. They mostly act upon the muscular tissues, causing them to relax, or soothing nerves which control the muscles involved. Antispasmodic drugs include ATROPINE, propantheline, cisapride and hyoscine (in Buscopan Compositum).

Antitetanic Serum (Tetanus Antitoxin, TAT)

A serum used against TETANUS. Nowadays the antitoxin is preferred.

Antitoxins (Antitoxic Sera)

Antitoxins (antitoxic sera) are substances which neutralise the harmful effects of a toxin.

Antivenin

Antivenin is a substance produced by the injection of snake venom into animals in small but increasing doses. In course of time the animal becomes immune to the particular venom injected, and the antivenin prepared from its serum is highly effective in neutralising venom injected by the bite of a snake of the same species. To be of any use it must be administered within about 1 hour of the snake bite.

Antivenom (Snake Venom Antiserum)

Antidote to the venom of adders; used for the treatment of domestic animals bitten by adders.

Antiviral

A substance used against viruses. (See also INTERFERON.)

Antizymotic

An agent which inhibits fermentation.

Antlers

Antlers are grown by stags, complete with blood supply to the velvet (the soft hairy outer layer) each year. A prime red deer stag will grow 4 kg in 3 months (May to July in the UK). Its diet must provide 600 g calcium, 300 g phosphorus and 12 g magnesium to achieve this – almost twice as much as a hind in full lactation needs.

Antrycide

A synthetic drug used in the control of trypanosomiasis.

Ants

Ants are of veterinary interest as intermediate hosts of the liver fluke *Dicroelium dendriticum*. This fluke, which is smaller than *Fasciola hepatica*, the common fluke, is found in sheep, goats, cattle, deer, hares, rabbits, pigs, dogs, donkeys, and occasionally man. In the British Isles, the fluke occurs only (it is believed) in the islands off the Scottish mainland.

The fluke's eggs are swallowed by a land-snail of the genus *Helicella*. From the snail, cercariae periodically escape and slimy clumps of them are eaten by ants (*Formica fusca* in the USA). Grazing animals, swallowing ants with the grass, then become infested.

Ants also act as the intermediate host of a tapeworm of the fowl, guinea-fowl and pigeon, *Raillietina tetragona*.

Pharaoh's ants have been shown to be of considerable medical importance. They are much smaller than the common black ant; the worker, brownish-orange in colour, measures only 2 mm in length. They are a tropical species and in a temperate climate survive where there is central heating or its equivalent.

Their nests have been found behind tiles, in light fittings, fuse-boxes, and even in hospital operating theatres! Small nests are sometimes found between the folds of sheets and towels coming from laundries.

These ants eat meat, and also sweet foods. In their quest for water they visit sinks, drains, lavatories, etc. and can therefore contaminate food. They also, apparently, feed on the discharges from infected wounds.

Pharaoh's ants constitute a public health danger since they can carry disease-producing bacteria. In the isolation unit of a school of veterinary medicine they ruined one experiment by carrying infection from known infected animals to the uninfected 'controls'.

Fire ants (*Soleropsis invicta*) have become established in the southeastern states of the USA. They are very aggressive and masses of them will attack and eat quail fledglings, for example, and unweaned rabbits. People camping out near fire-ant colonies have also been attacked; the ant 'venom' causes blurred vision, loss of consciousness and sometimes convulsions.

Antu

Alphanaphthylthiourea, used to kill rodents. One gram may prove fatal to a 9 to 11 kg (20 to 25 lb) dog. The poison gives rise to oedema of the lungs. (See also THIOUREA.) Antu is banned in the UK.

Anuran

Amphibians having no tails in the adult stage – frogs and toads. Also known as Salientia.

Anuria

Anuria is a condition in which little or no URINE is excreted or voided for some time. (See also KIDNEYS.)

Anus

The opening which terminates the alimentary canal. In health it is kept closed by the sphincter ani, a ring of muscle fibres about 2.5 cm (1 inch) thick in the horse, which is kept in a state of constant contraction by certain special nerve fibres situated in the spinal cord. If this ring fails to relax, constipation may result, while in some forms of paralysis the muscle becomes unable to retain the faeces. Imperforate anus is a defect in which an animal is born without any such opening – in effect, the absence of an anus.

Anal glands (sacs) There are two of these in the dog, situated below and to each side of the anus. They produce a malodorous fluid which possibly acts as a lubricant to aid defaecation or as a means of territorial marking. Each gland has a duct opening just inside the anus. These ducts may become blocked by a grass seed or other foreign body, so that the secretions cannot escape and the glands swell; but more commonly there is infection. Irritation or pain then results. It may be necessary to manually express the glands to relieve the blockage, or to remove them surgically.

Signs include yelping on sitting down, and tail-chasing; more commonly the dog drags itself along the ground ('scoots') or licks its hindquarters in an effort to obtain relief.

Perianal fistulae may be due to a number of causes including rupture of the anal sac, inflammation or ulceration. Except in mild cases, the condition may be difficult to treat, surgically or otherwise.

Signs include pain on defaecation and a bad smell. German shepherd dogs are said to be susceptible to the condition.

Perianal furunculosis is sometimes a recurring problem in dogs. Surgical removal of the anal sacs has been recommended to prevent recurrence.

Aorta

The principal artery of the body. It leaves the base of the left ventricle and curves upwards and backwards, giving off branches to the head and neck and forelimbs. About the level of the 8th or 9th thoracic vertebra it reaches the lower surface of the spinal column, and from there it runs back into the abdominal cavity between the lungs, piercing the diaphragm. It ends about the 5th lumbar vertebra by dividing into the two internal iliacs and the middle sacral arteries. The internal iliacs supply the 2 hind-limbs and the muscles of the pelvis. At its commencement the aorta is about 1H inches in diameter in the horse, and from there it gradually tapers as large branches leave it. It is customary to divide the aorta into thoracic aorta and abdominal aorta. (See ARTERIES; ANEURYSM.)

Aortic Rupture

This follows degenerative changes in the aorta, and is a not uncommon cause of death of male turkeys aged between 5 and 22 weeks. It was first reported in the USA and Canada. In Britain most cases occur between July and October, the birds being found dead. The condition has also been reported in ostriches.

Aortic Stenosis

A condition in which the flow of blood from the heart into the aorta is obstructed. It may result from a congenital malformation of the heart valves or an obstruction in the aorta itself. It may be an inherited condition in Boxers, German shepherd dogs and Newfoundlands. It has also been seen in cats.

Signs may include dyspnoea or congestive heart failure. (See STENOSIS.)

Aphagia

Inability, or refusal, to eat.

Aplastic

Relating to aplasia, the congenital absence of an organ. In aplastic anaemia, there is defective development or a cessation of regeneration of the red cells, etc. (See ANAEMIA.)

Apnoea

Apnoea means not breathing. Aquatic animals such as ducks and penguins display 'diving apnoea' – they hold their breath while under the water.

Apomorphine

A derivative of morphine which has a marked emetic action in the dog, and is used in that animal to induce vomiting when some poisonous or otherwise objectionable material has been taken into the stomach.

Aponeurosis

Aponeurosis is a sheet of tendinous tissue providing an insertion or attachment for muscles, which is sometimes itself attached to a bone, and sometimes is merely a method of attaching 1 muscle to another.

Apoproteins

Apoproteins are involved in the transport of LIPIDS throughout the body. Apoproteins are produced by cells in the liver or intestine. (See also LIPOPROTEIN.)

Appaloosa

The Appaloosa Horse Society of America and the British Spotted Horse Society are concerned with the breeding of this horse, which has some Arab blood and is characterised by a silky white coat with black (or chocolate-coloured) spots which can be felt with the finger.

Appetite

Pica (depraved appetite) A mineral or vitamin deficiency may account for some cases of animals eating rubbish such as coal, cinders, soil, plaster, stones, faeces, etc. Pica is often associated also with pregnancy, and is an important sign of rabies in dogs. It may result from worm infections.

In cats pica is a sign of anaemia. They will lick concrete or eat cat litter.

Excessive appetite may be a sign of dyspepsia or diabetes, of internal parasites, of tuberculosis, of listeriosis, or of the early stages of cancer.

Diminished appetite Anorexia, or a diminished appetite, is a sign usually present in most forms of dyspepsia, in gastritis and enteritis, in many fevers, and in abnormal conditions of the throat and the mouth, when the act of swallowing is difficult or painful. In other cases the appetite is in abeyance for no apparent reason. It may be merely an indication that a dog or cat or other animal has overeaten, and a rest from eating may be all that is needed. (See NURSING OF SICK ANIMALS; MINERALS; VITAMINS.)

Aquaculture

(see FISH FARMING)

Aqueduct of Sylvius (Cerebral Aqueduct)

The aqueduct of Sylvius (cerebral aqueduct) connects the 3rd and 4th ventricles of the brain, and conveys cerebrospinal fluid.

Aqueous Humour

(see EYE)

Arachnida

Arachnida is the name of the class of Arthropoda to which belong the mange mites, ticks, and spiders.

Arachidonic Acid

(see EICOSANOIDS)

Arachnoid Membrane

Arachnoid membrane is one of the membranes covering the brain and spinal cord. (See BRAIN.) Arachnoiditis is inflammation of this membrane.

Arboviruses

This is an abbreviation for arthropod-born viruses. They are responsible for diseases (such as louping-ill, equine encephalitis and yellow fever) transmitted by ticks, insects, etc. They are known as Togaviruses. (See VIRUSES table.)

ARC

The former Agricultural Research Council, under whose control a number of UK veterinary research institutes functioned, was renamed the Agricultural and Food Research Council (AFRC) and ultimately superseded by the Biotechnology and Biological Sciences Research Council (BBSRC).

Areolar Connective Tissue

Areolar connective tissue is loose in character and occurs in the body wherever a cushioning effect, with flexibility, is needed, e.g. between skin and muscle, and surrounding blood vessels.

Argulus

A crustacean parasite of freshwater fish which can cause ulceration, poor growth and transmit spring viraemia of carp. These fish lice can be removed by bathing affected fish briefly in saline.

Arizona Infection

In turkeys it was reported for the first time in the UK in 1968. The infection, mainly of birds, is caused by the Arizona group of the enterobacteriaceae – closely related to the salmonellae and the coliform group. Young birds can be infected by contact or through the egg. Nervous symptoms and eye lesions are characteristic in birds surviving the initial acute illness.

Over 300 antigenically distinct serotypes of Arizona have been identified. One at least appears to be host-adapted to sheep, and has been recovered from scouring sheep, from ewes which died in pregnancy and from aborted fetuses. Food-poisoning in man and diarrhoea in monkeys have been attributed to Arizona infection.

Arrhythmia

Arrhythmia means that the heartbeat is not occurring regularly, or that a beat is being periodically missed. It may be only temporary and of little importance; on the other hand it may be a symptom of some form of cardiac disease.

Arsanilic Acid

One of the organic compounds of arsenic which has been used as a growth supplement for pigs and poultry; now no longer used in the EU.

It should not be given within 10 days of slaughter, nor should the recommended dosage rate be exceeded, as residues – especially in the liver – may prove harmful if consumed. The permitted maximum of arsenic in liver is 1 part per million. In a random survey (1969), 4 of 93 pig livers contained from 1.2 to 3.5 ppm of arsenic.

Blindness, a staggering gait, twisting of the neck, progressive weakness and paralysis are symptoms of chronic poisoning with arsanilic acid in the pig.

Arsenic (As)

Arsenic (As) is a metal, but the term is commonly used to refer to arsenious acid. It has 2 forms: the trivalent, which is toxic; and the pentavalent (found in most organic compounds of arsenic), which is not. Arsenic is found in Scheele's green and emerald green – the two arsenites of copper; Orpiment or King's yellow, and Realgar – sulphides of arsenic; Fowler's solution (liquor arsenicalis, BP), which contains arsenic trioxide. It used to be used in older varieties of sheep-dip, rat-poisons, fly-papers, and even wall-papers.

Uses Arsenic has been used in some compound animal feeds in order to improve growth rate and to prevent histomoniasis (blackhead in turkeys). The disposal of dung containing arsenic residues causes problems: small doses over a long period may give rise to cancer. (See also ARSANILIC ACID.)

Arsenic, Poisoning By

Arsenic is an irritant poison producing in all animals gastroenteritis. The rapidity of its action depends on the amount that is taken, on the solubility of the compound, on the

presence or otherwise of food in the digestive system, and on the susceptibility of the animal.

Signs include violent purging, severe colic, straining, a staggering gait, coldness of the extremities of the body, unconsciousness, and convulsions. When the poisoning is the result of the taking of small doses for a considerable period, cumulative symptoms are observed. These include an unthrifty condition of the body generally, swelling of the joints, indigestion, constant or intermittent diarrhoea, often with a fetid odour, thirst, emaciation, and distressed breathing and heart action on moderate exercise.

Causes

Cattle have died after straying into a field of potatoes sprayed with arsenites to destroy the haulm. Others have died following the application to their backs of an arsenical dressing, and of the use of arsenic-contaminated, old bins for feeding purposes.

Sheep Probably most cases of arsenic poisoning in sheep occurred from the use of arsenical dips before other compounds were introduced. The source of this poisoning is in many cases the herbage of the pastures which becomes contaminated either from the drippings from the wool of the sheep, or from the washing of the dip out of the fleece by a shower of rain on the 2nd or 3rd day after the dipping. Absorption through wounds or laceration of the skin may result in arsenic poisoning, and when dips are made up too strong, absorption into the system may also occur. The obvious precautions, apart from care of the actual dipping, are to ensure that the sheep are kept in the draining pens long enough to ensure that their fleeces are reasonably dry (some 15 to 20 minutes) and subsequently are not allowed to remain for long thickly concentrated in small fields or paddocks. Where double dipping is carried out, the second immersion in an arsenic dip must be at half-strength.

Dogs and cats are particularly susceptible to poisoning by arsenic. The symptoms are nausea, vomiting, abdominal pain, dark fluid evacuations, and death preceded by convulsions.

Antidotes Sodium thiosulphate is a better antidote than ferric hydroxide, and a solution can be given intravenously. (See also DIPS.)

Arteries

With the exception of the pulmonary artery, which carries venous blood to the lungs, the arteries carry oxygenated blood; that is, blood which has recently been circulating in the lungs, has absorbed oxygen from the inspired air, and has become scarlet in colour. The pulmonary artery carries blood of a purple colour which has been circulating in the body and has been returned to the heart, to be sent to the lungs for oxygenation.

The arterial system begins at the left ventricle of the heart with the AORTA. This is the largest artery of the body. It divides and subdivides until the final branches end in the capillaries which ramify throughout all the body tissues except cornea, hair, horn, and teeth. The larger of these branches are called arteries, the smaller ones are arterioles, and these end in the capillaries. The capillaries pervade the tissues like the pores of a sponge, and bathe the cells of the body in arterial blood. The blood is collected by the venous system and carried back to the heart.

Structure The arteries are highly elastic tubes which are capable of great dilatation with each pulsation of the heart – a dilatation which is of considerable importance in the circulation of the blood. (See CIRCULATION OF BLOOD.) Their walls are composed of 3 coats: (1) adventitious coat, consisting of ordinary strong fibrous tissue on the outside; (2) middle coat, composed of muscle fibres and elastic fibres, in separate layers in the great arteries; (3) inner coat or intima, consisting of a layer of yellow elastic tissue on whose innermost surface rests a single continuous layer of smooth, plate-like endothelial cells, within which flows the bloodstream. The walls of the larger arteries have the muscles of their middle coat replaced to a great extent by elastic fibres so that they are capable of much distension. When an artery is cut across, its muscular coat instantly shrinks, drawing the cut end within the fibrous sheath which surrounds all arteries, and bunching it up so that only a comparatively small hole is left for the escape of blood. This in a normal case soon becomes filled up with the blood clot which is Nature's method of checking haemorrhage (see BLEEDING).

Arteries, Diseases of

These include:

(1) **Arteritis** during specific viral diseases such as African swine fever, equine viral arteritis, canine viral hepatitis, etc.

(2) **Chronic inflammation**, or **arteriosclerosis**, is a process of thickening of the arterial wall and subsequent degenerative changes, resulting in an abnormal rigidity of the tube and hindrance to the circulation.

(3) **Degenerative changes** include atheroma – thickening and degeneration of the lining of the artery. Degeneration occurs in the arteries of pigs, especially, during the course of several diseases. Examples are haemorrhagic gastritis and Herztod disease.

(4) **Thrombosis** This includes aortic-iliac THROMBOSIS, and femoral thrombosis in dogs and cats. (See also PARAPLEGIA.)

(5) **Embolism** (see main entry)

(6) **Aneurysm** (see main entry)

(7) **Equine verminous arteritis** (see main entry)

(8) **Heartworms** (see main entry)

(9) **Aortic rupture** in turkeys (see AORTIC RUPTURE)

Arthritis

Inflammation of a joint. A common disease of all farm and pet animals. (See also JOINTS, DISEASES OF.)

Causes include trauma, rheumatism, a mineral deficiency, and FLUOROSIS. Infections which cause arthritis include BRUCELLOSIS, TUBERCULOSIS, and SWINE ERYSIPELAS. (See also SYNOVITIS; BURSITIS; JOINT-ILL.)

Rheumatoid arthritis A chronic form of inflammatory arthritis, often accompanied by fever and usually with symmetrical involvement of several joints. There may be a genetic predisposition to the condition.

Open-joint injuries may lead to an acute septic arthritis following infection. Prompt treatment often leads to a full recovery.

Arthrodesis

An operation to fix a joint in a given position. By this means a pain-free, stable and strong joint can be achieved in cases of osteoarthrosis of the carpus.

Arthrogryposis

(see GENETICS – Genetic defects)

Arthroscopy

The application of endoscopic techniques to the study of joint cavities.

Arthrosis

Degenerative disease of a joint, as opposed to inflammation. (The word can also mean an articulation.)

Artifact

An apparent lesion in a histological or pathological specimen, not existing during life, but made accidentally in preparing the specimen.

Artificial Bones

In racing greyhounds, badly fractured scaphoids have been removed and replaced with plastic prostheses. (A dog called Hare Spy won a race on January 16, 1958, after such an operation.)

Artificial Induction of Parturition

(see PARTURITION, DRUG-INDUCED)

Artificial Insemination (AI)

The introduction of male germ cells (spermatozoa) into the female without actual service.

The practice is a very old one. In the 14th century Arab horse-breeders were getting mares in foal by using semen-impregnated sponges. In Italy bitches were artificially inseminated as long ago as 1780, and at the close of the 19th century the practice was applied, to a very limited extent, to mares in Britain.

It was the Russian scientist Ivanoff who saw in AI the possibilities of disease control, and in 1909, a laboratory was established in Russia for the development and improvement of existing techniques. By 1938 well over a million cattle and 15 million sheep had been inseminated in the USSR, where all the basic work was done. Denmark began to take a practical interest in AI in 1936 (and within 11 years had 100 cooperative breeding stations inseminating half a million head of cattle annually); the USA in 1937.

The UK began to practise AI on a commercial basis in 1942, and by the end of 1950 had close on a hundred centres and sub-centres in operation, serving over 60,000 farms. The introduction of prostaglandins in 1975 enabled synchronisation of oestrus in groups of cattle, greatly facilitating the use of AI. Since 1986, 'do-it-yourself' on-farm AI has been permitted after stockmen have received suitable training and the storage of semen has been adequately monitored.

Uses The use of AI in commercial cattle breeding is dependent upon the fact that, in normal mating, a bull produces up to 500 times as much semen as is required to enable 1 cow to conceive. By collecting the semen, diluting it and, if necessary, storing it in a refrigerator, the insemination of many cows from 1 ejaculate becomes possible.

AI reduces the spread of venereal disease, and hence greatly reduces the incidence of the latter. Farmers in a small way of business are able to dispense with the services of a communal bull – an animal seldom well bred and often infected with some transmissible disease. At the same time, the farmer has the advantage of the use of a healthy, pedigree bull without the considerable expense of buying, feeding, and looking after it. Owners of commercial herds are enabled to grade them up to pedigree standard, with an increase in quality and milk yield. In many of the ranching areas overseas, where stock-raising is carried out on an extensive, rather than an intensive, scale, to achieve satisfactory production of animals for trade and commercial purposes, sires have to be imported at regular intervals from the essentially sire-producing countries – of which Britain is the chief. The method of artificially inseminating a large number of females from an imported sire enables bigger generations of progeny to be raised and consequently more rapid improvement to be achieved.

Methods Various methods are employed to collect semen. Those which give best results involve the use of an artificial vagina in which to collect the semen from an ejaculation. This is used outside the female's body, being so arranged that the penis of the male enters it instead of entering the vagina. The full ejaculation is received without contamination from the female.

After the ejaculate has been collected it is either divided into fractions, each being injected by a special syringe into the cervix or uterus of another female in season, or – in commercial practice – it is diluted 20 times or more with a specially prepared 'sperm diluent', such as egg-yolk citrate buffer, and distributed into 'straws' (plastic tubes). Dilution rates of up to 1 in 100 have been successful, but it appears desirable to inseminate 12 or 13 million sperms into each cow.

The method requires skill to carry out successfully, and necessitates the employment of strict cleanliness throughout. (See CONCEPTION RATES.)

Artificial insemination has also been carried out in pigs (see FARROWING RATES), goats, dogs, turkeys and other birds, bees, etc.

A Canine AI is now practised in many parts of the world. In the UK the Kennel Club reserves the right to decide whether to accept for registration puppies obtained by means of AI rather than by normal mating. Applications are usually made by the owner of the bitch. Those concerned with a newly imported breed, and who wish to widen the genetic pool, may not be able to find a suitable male for purchase and import. However, if semen from a satisfactory dog can be obtained, and DEFRA agrees to its import under licence, AI may be a good way of increasing the available pool.

Registrations will not be accepted where AI is requested because either the prospective sire or dam is unable to mate owing to disease.

Turkey AI Farmed turkeys are now bred as male and female lines. Female lines are comparatively slender, with high egg production. Male lines are bred for meat and are much heavier. The resulting disparity between the sizes of the male and female is such that natural mating would result in injury to the female. Most turkey breeding is therefore by artificial insemination. Disposable straws, discarded after use, are used to prevent transmission of infection (notably *Mycoplasma meleagridis* and *E. coli*) but as semen is pooled from several stags, an infected stag can result in many infected hens. The technique of insemination and collection of semen requires skill.

Storage of semen Diluted semen may be stored at AI centres for a few days if kept at a temperature of 5°C. In practice, a good deal would be wasted because its fertilising power has diminished before it is all required for use. However, semen may be stored for long periods when glycerol is added to the sperm diluent. This enables the semen to be stored and transported at −196°C, using liquid nitrogen to maintain the low temperature. The advantages of this method are many. There is less wastage of semen, more can be stored, and the semen of any particular bull can be made available on any day. It is possible for several thousand cows to be got in calf by a given bull. The disadvantages of using a given bull or bulls too widely must be borne in mind, but that is a matter of policy and not of technique.

Infected semen Viruses (including that of foot-and-mouth) and mycoplasmas have, on occasion, been found in stored semen. (See also RABIES; CONTROLLED BREEDING.)

Artificial Rearing of Piglets

Cows' colostrum makes a satisfactory substitute for sows' colostrum, and may be frozen and later thawed when required. Pigs' serum as an addition enhances the value of cows' colostrum.

Artificial Respiration

This is resorted to in: (1) cessation of respiration while under general anaesthesia; (2) cases of drowning when the animal has been rescued from the water – chiefly applicable to the small animals; (3) poisoning by narcotics or paralysants; (4) cases of asphyxia from fumes, smoke, gases, etc.

Horses and cattle Release from all restraint except a loose halter or head-collar, extend the head and neck to allow a straight passage of the air into the lungs, open the mouth, and pull the tongue well out. Should the ground slope, the horse must be placed with its head downhill. While such adjustments are being carried out 1 or 2 assistants should compress the elastic posterior ribs by alternately leaning the whole weight of the body on the hands pressed on the ribs, and then releasing the pressure about once every 4 or 5 seconds, in an endeavour to stimulate the normal movements of breathing. As an alternative in a larger animal, a heavy person may sit with some vigour astride the ribs for about the same time, rise for a similar period, and then sit back again. If no response occurs, these measures should be carried out more rapidly.

The inhalation of strong solution of ammonia upon a piece of cotton-wool and held about a foot from the upper nostril often assists in inducing a gasp which is the first sign of the return to respiration, but care is needed not to allow the ammonia to come into contact with the skin or burning will occur. After 2 or 3 minutes' work the animal should be turned on to the opposite side to prevent stasis of the blood. Sometimes the mere act of turning will induce the premonitory gasp. So long as the heart continues to beat, no matter how feebly, the attempts at resuscitation should be pursued. Proprietary calf resuscitators are available to give the 'kiss of life'.

Pigs and sheep The outlines of procedure given for the larger animals are equally applicable. An ordinary domestic funnel can be used for giving pigs the 'kiss of life'.

The method of giving the 'kiss of life' to a piglet is to use a flexible polyethylene funnel, and fit this over the animal's mouth and nostrils. Air is blown into the stem of the funnel, and passes down into the piglet's lungs.

For the method to be effective, the procedure is as follows: (1) hold the piglet by its hind legs with head down in order to drain any fluid from its air passages; (2) turn the piglet with its head upwards and apply the funnel; (3) blow forcefully into the funnel; (4) remove the funnel and allow the piglet to breathe out; (5) repeat the operation. After several repetitions, the piglet should kick or show other signs of life. Lay the animal on its side or stomach and massage its chest and mouth. Piglets apparently stillborn may sometimes be revived by this method.

Piglets have been revived up to half an hour after treatment began. Of course, the heart must be beating and resuscitation started promptly to achieve success.

Dogs and cats A modification of the Schafer system is to lay the dog on its side with the head at a lower level than the rest of the body, place a hand flat over the upper side of the abdomen and the other on the rib-cage, lean heavily on the hands, and in a second or two release the pressure.

The motions of artificial respiration should in all cases be a little faster than those of normal respiration, but a slight pause should always be observed before each rhythmic movement. Use less pressure for cats.

A respiratory stimulant may be given by injection. A carbon dioxide 'Resuscitator' may be used.

Ascaridae

A class of worms belonging to the round variety or *Nemathelminthes*, which are found parasitic in the intestines of horses, pigs, dogs, and cats particularly, although they may affect other animals. They attain a size of 38 or 45 cm (15 or 18 inches) in the horse, but are small in other animals. (See ROUNDWORMS.)

Ascites

OEDEMA involving the abdomen; a very common complication of abdominal tuberculosis, of liver, kidney, or heart disease, as well as of some parasitic infestations. In poultry, ascites is sometimes associated with hypoxia ('high altitude disease') although there are other causes including toxins or, in individuals, heart defects or abdominal tumours. It is also seen in ducks with furazolidone poisoning.

Ascorbic Acid

Synthetic vitamin C.

Asepsis

The absence of pathogenic organisms. Aseptic surgery is the ideal, but among animals it may

be difficult to attain if carried out under farm conditions – despite care in sterilising instruments and the use of sterilised dressings, rubber gloves, etc. Moreover, it is an exceptionally difficult matter to prevent accidental infection in a surgical wound after the operation, for the animal cannot be put to bed, and it may object to the dressings and do all in its power to remove them. (See ANTISEPTICS; SULFONAMIDES; PENICILLIN.)

Ash Poisoning

Poisoning by *Fraxinus* species has been reported in cattle after eating the green leaves and fruits from a broken branch of a tree. Symptoms include: drowsiness, oedema involving ribs and flanks, purple discoloration of perineum.

Aspergillosis

A disease of mammals and birds produced by the growth of the fungus *Aspergillus* in the tissues of the body.

Infection probably occurs chiefly through inhalation of the fungal spores, which may be abundant in hay or straw under conditions of dampness. Entry of the spores into the body may also be by way of the mouth; in herbivorous animals from contaminated fodder or bedding; and in cat and dog from the eating of infected birds or rodents.

Once in the animal's tissues, hyphae grow out from the spores, as happens also in ringworm; and from the branching filaments more spores are produced. Local necrosis and abscess formation are caused.

Numerous organs and tissues can become infected, including the nose and nasal sinuses, the lungs, brain, uterus, and mammary glands.

Cattle and horses *Aspergillus* may cause abortion and lung sensitisation or pneumonia.

Dogs and cats Aspergillosis is a common cause of chronic nasal disease, and should be suspected when there is a discharge from one nostril.

Poultry Respiratory disease or enteritis may occur. In young turkey poults brain involvement has led to an unsteady gait, walking backwards, and turning the head to one side.

Pet parrots may die from aspergillosis, as well as wild birds.

Brain infection may occur in all species, and give rise to symptoms described under ENCEPHALITIS. Paresis and ataxia may, rarely, be caused by fungal infections of the spine.

Ketonazole, given by mouth, and irrigation of the sinuses by enilconazole in sodium chloride solution have been used in cases of canine nasal aspergillosis.

Asphodel
(see BOG ASPHODEL)

Asphyxia

Suffocation may occur during the administration of anaesthetics by inhalation, during the outbreak of fires in animal houses, where the fumes and the smoke present are responsible for oedema, and in cases of poisoning. (See also 'KITCHEN DEATHS'.)

Signs The direct cause of death from asphyxia is an insufficiency of oxygen supplied to the tissues by the blood. The first signs are a rapid and full pulse, and a quickening of the respirations. The breathing soon changes to a series of gasps, and the blood pressure rises, causing the visible membranes to become intensely injected and later blue in colour. Convulsions supervene. The convulsions are followed by quietness, when the heartbeat may be almost imperceptible and respiratory movements practically cease. The actual time of death is unnoticed as a rule, since death takes place very quietly.

During the stage of convulsions, when the amount of carbon dioxide circulating in the blood is increased, the smaller arteries vigorously contract and cause an increase in the blood pressure. This high blood pressure produces an engorgement of the right side of the heart, which cannot totally expel its contents with each beat, and becomes more and more dilated until such time as the pressure in the ventricles overcomes the strength of the muscle fibres of the heart and the organ ceases to beat. During this stage immediate relief follows bleeding from a large vein.

Treatment (see ARTIFICIAL RESPIRATION). If the breathing is shallow and the membranes livid, administration of OXYGEN is indicated.

Prevention Ensure adequate ventilation in rooms where there is a gas or solid-fuel heating system. (Many dogs and cats have been found dead in the kitchen in the morning as a result of CARBON MONOXIDE poisoning.)

Aspiration
(see PARACENTESIS)

Aspirin (Acetylsalicylic Acid)

An analgesic; also used in prevention of thrombosis. Must be used with extreme caution and under professional supervision in cats;

the dose not exceeding 10 mg/kg on alternate days.

In both cats and dogs, overdosing with aspirin may cause inflammation of the stomach, haemorrhage, some pain, and vomiting. The antidote is sodium bicarbonate which can be given in water by stomach tube; or, for first-aid purposes, by the cat-owner, in milk or water. (See SALICYLIC ACID – Salicylate poisoning.)

Aspirin has been used to lessen the effects of porcine respiratory and reproductive syndrome (PRRS/blue-eared pig disease).

Asthenia

Asthenia is another name for debility. Asthenic is applied to the exhausted state that precedes death during some fevers.

Asthma

Asthma is a term somewhat loosely applied to a number of conditions in which the main sign is breathlessness. Strictly speaking, the term should be reserved for those conditions where a true spasmodic expulsion of breath occurs without the effort of a cough. The so called 'asthma' of birds is due in nearly every case to ASPERGILLOSIS. Asthma in horses may be difficult to differentiate from 'BROKEN WIND', and in all animals from simple BRONCHITIS.

Causes These are obscure, but it is generally held that true spasmodic asthma is of nervous origin, and due to a sudden distressful contraction of the muscle fibres which lie around the smaller bronchioles. In some cases asthma may be an allergic phenomenon. In other cases a chronic inflammation of the lining mucous membrane of the small tubes is the cause.

The spores of fungi are potent allergens, and can account for many cases of asthma, especially recurrent summer asthma, in man. There are, however, a number of patients with seasonal (summer or autumn) asthma who are not sensitive to spores of any of the above nor to pollen. (See ALLERGY.)

Dog Many cases that are really chronic bronchitis are spoken of as 'bronchial asthma' owing to their similarity to asthma in man, with which many owners of animals are familiar. In true asthma the attacks of dyspnoea (i.e. distressed respiration) occur at irregular intervals, and there are periods between them when the dog is to all appearances quite normal. The attacks occur suddenly, are very distressing to witness, last for from 10 minutes to half an hour, and then suddenly cease. The dog gasps for breath, makes violent inspiratory efforts without much success, exhibits a frightened, disturbed expression, and stands till the attack passes off.

The condition appears to be hereditary in some breeds, especially the Maltese terrier. Cardiac dysfunction also gives rise to 'asthma'. (See also ATOPIC DISEASE.)

Treatment Bronchodilators, such as aminophylline, clenbuterol or ephedrine, and antihistamines or heart stimulants may be of service. The treatment used will depend on the cause of the problem. Regulation of exercise and diet is necessary. (See also CHRONIC OBSTRUCTIVE PULMONARY DISEASE; RESPIRATORY DISEASE; BRONCHITIS.)

Astragalus (Talus)

Astragalus (Talus) is the name of one of the bones of the tarsus (hock), with which the tibia forms the main joint. The articulation between these bones is sometimes referred to as the 'true hock joint', the others being more or less secondary and less freely movable joints.

Astringents

Substances which contract tissues and stop discharges; they include sulphate of zinc, alum, tannic acid, witch-hazel.

Astrocytes

Supporting cells found in the central nervous system, and each consisting of a cell body and numerous branching processes. Astrocytes are thought to be concerned with the nutrition of neighbouring nerve cells. They may also be involved in the tissue damage which ocurs in cases of stroke.

Astrovirus

Astrovirus was first detected in the faeces of children in 1975, and has since been isolated from lambs, calves, turkeys, deer, etc. It is not regarded as a serious pathogen in veterinary medicine, but studies in gnotobiotic lambs indicate that the virus multiplies in the epithelial cells of the villi of the small intestine, producing some degree of atrophy of the villi, with diarrhoea.

Asymmetric Hindquarter Syndrome (AHQS)

Outbreaks of a lop-sided condition of the hindquarters in the pig, known as asymmetric hindquarter syndrome, have been described by J. T. Done and others. This condition has been seen in Germany, Belgium, and Britain.

AHQS, which would appear to have a hereditary basis, could be of economic importance since it affects carcase conformation, and could lead to carcase condemnation.

The abnormality does not usually become obvious before pigs reach about 30 kg (66 lb) live-weight, when one thigh may be seen to be much smaller than the other though of the same length. Even in severe cases it was observed that the gait was normal.

The incidence of AHQS within litters of affected families varies from 0 to 80 per cent, and the breeds involved include Large White, Hampshire and Lacombe.

Asystole

A failure of the heart to contract, generally due to the walls having become so weak that they are unable to contract and expel the blood, with the result that the organ becomes distended – a feature found after death.

Ataxia

Ataxia means the loss of the power of governing movements, although the necessary power for these movements is still present. A staggering gait results. Ataxia is a sign which may be observed in many diverse conditions; for example, rabies, weakness or exhaustion; encephalitis; meningitis; poisoning; a brain tumour. It may be seen in all animals.

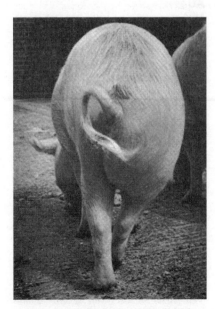

Asymmetric hindquarter syndrome (AHQS).

A

Cattle A progressive form of ataxia of unknown origin has been found in French-bred Charolais heifers, with symptoms first appearing in the 1st year: slight intermittent ataxia progresses to recumbency over 1 to 2 years. Urine is passed in a continuous but uneven squirting flow. When excited, affected heifers may show nodding of their heads.

Cats Ataxia is seen in feline infectious peritonitis poisoning by ethylene glycol (anti-freeze) and streptomycin, for example, and before eclampsia (lactation tetany). Congenital cerebellar ataxia may be seen in kittens, usually when born to mothers infected with parvovirus. There is incoordinated movement of the head, especially when feeding, and they stand with their legs apart to aid balance. The condition does not worsen and, unless very serious, kittens usually adapt well.

Atheroma

A degenerative change in the inner and middle coats of the arteries in which a deposit of lipid material is formed. (See ARTERIES, DISEASES OF.)

Atherosclerosis

A condition in which deposits of cholesterol and other material in the inner lining (intima) of arteries restricts the blood flow.

Atlas

Atlas is the name given to the 1st of the cervical vertebrae, which forms a double pivot joint with the occipital bone of the base of the skull on the one hand, and forms a single gliding pivot joint with the epistropheus – the 2nd cervical vertebra – on the other hand. The freedom of movement of the head is due almost solely to these 2 joints.

Atony

Atony means want of tone or vigour in muscles or other organs. (See also TONICS.)

Atopic Disease

A hypersensitivity to pollens and other inhaled protein particles. (See ALLERGY.) Hay-fever-like symptoms may be produced in the dog and horse; also intense itching affecting the feet, abdomen, and face. As well as sneezing, conjunctivitis, rhinitis and asthma, there may be some discoloration of the coat. In allergy tests on 208 dogs, about 40 per cent were found to be hypersensitive to human dandruff.

Atopic disease also occurs in cats and cattle (see BOVINE ATOPIC RHINITIS).

Atresia

Atresia means the absence of a natural opening, or its obliteration by membrane. Atresia of the rectum is found in newly-born pigs, lambs, calves, and foals. Atresia is sometimes met with in the vaginae of heifers, when it constitutes what is known as 'WHITE HEIFER DISEASE'.

Atrial

Relating to the atrium or AURUCLE of the heart.

Atrophic Myositis

(see under MUSCLES, DISEASES OF)

Atrophic Rhinitis

A disease of pigs affecting the nasal passages. (See under RHINITIS, ATROPHIC.)

Atrophy

Atrophy is a wasting of the tissues. Following paralysis of a motor nerve, when the muscles supplied by it are no longer able to contract, atrophy of the area takes place. This is seen in paralysis of the radial nerve. (Compare HYPERTROPHY.)

Atropine

An alkaloid contained in the leaves and root of the deadly nightshade (*Atropa belladonna*). Preparations of belladonna owe their anticholinergic actions to the presence of atropine, which blocks transmission at sensory nerve-endings and thus relieves pain and spasm in parts to which it is applied. It checks secretion in all the glands of the body when given internally; and whether given by the mouth or rubbed on the skin it causes a dilatation of the pupil of the eye and paralysis of accommodation. In large doses it induces a general stimulation of the nervous system, but this action is rapidly followed by depression, and the primary effect is not noticed in the administration of ordinary doses. The action on the heart is one of stimulation, since the inhibition fibres are paralysed, while the accelerator nerves are not interfered with, except when large doses are given and paralysis of all motor fibres occurs.

Uses Atropine is used as a premedicant to anaesthesia as it reduces secretions. It is also used to dilate the pupil in order to facilitate eye examinations. As an antidote to morphine poisoning and also to some of the organophosphorus compounds used as farm sprays, it is given as the sulphate of atropine by hypodermic injection.

Atropine Poisoning

Atropine poisoning may occur as the result of the unintentional administration of too large amounts of the alkaloid ATROPINE or of the drug BELLADONNA in one form or another, or it may be induced by feeding on the plant growing wild.

The signs of poisoning shown are restlessness, delirium, dryness of the mouth, a rapid and weak pulse, quick, short respirations, an increase in temperature, and dilatation of the pupil. In addition there is sometimes seen a loss of power in the hind-limbs.

Antidotes To those animals that vomit, an emetic should be given at once if the poison has been taken by the mouth. Horses and cattle should have their stomachs emptied by the passage of the stomach-tube, in so far as that is possible. Stimulants should be given, and pilocarpine, by injection, is the antidote.

Attenuated

A term used to describe a reduction in the virulence of a micro-organism, particularly applied to those incorporated in vaccines (see under VACCINE).

Auditory Nerve (Acoustic Nerve)

The auditory nerve (acoustic nerve) is the 8th of the cranial nerves, and is concerned with the special sense of hearing. It arises from the base of the hind-brain just behind and at the side of the pons. It is distributed to the middle and internal ears, and in addition to its acoustic function it is also concerned with the balance of the body. (See EAR.)

Aujeszky's Disease

A viral disease, primarily of pigs. It is also known as pseudorabies and infectious bulbar paralysis. It can occur in other species; the infection usually being contracted from contact with pigs or consumption of pig carcases. The disease has a very short incubation period, and is characterised by intense itching. It was first described in Hungary by Aujeszky in 1902, and has been eradicated from the UK, Denmark, Sweden and parts of other countries in the EU. It has also been found in several parts of the USA, South America, Australia, the continent of Europe, etc. In the UK the disease is NOTIFIABLE and an eradication campaign began in 1983. Monitoring continues by sampling cull animals at slaughterhouses. The infection may be windborne. Vaccines are available, but their use is prohibited in the UK except Northern

Ireland. However, gene-deleted vaccines can be used in eradication programmes as it is possible to differentiate serologically a pig which has been vaccinated from one which has been exposed to infection.

Signs

Pigs Signs include abortion, sneezing, anorexia and dullness besides some evidence of pruritus, vomiting, diarrhoea, convulsions, drooling of saliva, paralysis of the throat. Mummification of the fetuses may occur in pregnant sows affected with Aujeszky's disease. Such sows may show loss of appetite and constipation, or stiffness and muscular incoordination without itching at all. For the screening of pig serum samples, the ELISA test has been found the most sensitive, speediest and cheapest of four methods for detecting antibodies to Aujeszky's disease virus. (Central Veterinary Laboratory.)

Prevention: Intranasal vaccination with attenuated virus is more effective than parenteral vaccination with inactivated virus, as maternally derived antibodies interfere with the latter.

Dogs and cats Restlessness, loss of appetite, vomiting, salivation, signs of intense irritation (leading to biting or scratching) about the face or some other part, and occasionally moaning, groaning, or high-pitched screams are among the symptoms observed.

In one outbreak, 11 out of a pack of 51 harrier hounds died of the disease (apparently as a result of being fed raw carcase meat from a large pig unit). Infected rats may be another vector.

Cattle The first symptom to be observed is usually a persistent licking, rubbing or scratching of part of the hindquarters (or sometimes of the face) in an attempt to relieve the intense itching. The affected part soon becomes denuded of hair, and may be bitten and rubbed until it bleeds. Bellowing, salivation, and stamping with the hind-feet may be observed. Within 24 hours the animal is usually recumbent and unable to rise on account of paralysis. Death, preceded by convulsions, usually occurs within 36 to 48 hours of the onset of symptoms.

Goats Deaths have occurred in goats kept with infected pigs. Signs include restlessness, sweating, distressed bleating and convulsions; some animals may be found dead without signs being noticed.

Poultry One-day-old chicks have died after being inoculated with a Marek's disease vaccine.

A

Aujeszky's disease vaccine virus adapted to chicken cells was likely to have been the cause.

Horses The virus was isolated from the brain of a horse showing the following signs: excessive sweating, muscle tremors, and 'periods of mania'.

Public health Aujeszky's disease virus can infect people, but it seems that only laboratory workers are likely to find this a health hazard.

Aural
Relating to the ear.

Aural Cartilages
(see AURICULAR CARTILAGES)

Auricle (Atrium)
The auricles, right and left, are the chambers at the base of the heart which receive the blood from the body generally, and from the lungs respectively. Opening into the right auricle are the cranial and caudal vena cavae, which carry the venous blood that has been circulating in the head and neck and the abdomen and thorax. This blood is pumped into the right ventricle through the tricuspid valve. Opening into the left auricle are the pulmonary veins which bring the arterial blood that has been purified in the lungs; when this auricle contracts the blood is driven into the left ventricle through the mitral valve. (See HEART; CIRCULATION OF BLOOD.)

Auricular Cartilages
Auricular cartilages are the supporting structures of the ears. There are three chief cartilages in most animals, viz. the conchal, which gathers the sound waves and transmits them downwards into the cavity of the ear and gives the ear its characteristic shape; the annular, a cartilaginous ring below the former which is continuous internally with the bony acoustic canal; the scutiform, a small quadrilateral plate which lies in front of the others and serves for the attachment of muscles which move the ear.

Accidents and diseases of the cartilages of the ear are not common in animals, with the exception of dog/cat fights. Ulceration of the cartilages, chiefly the annular, occurs as a complication of ear inflammation in the dog. Laceration of the conchal cartilage is seen as the result of the application of a twitch to the ear in the horse.

Auscultation
Auscultation is a method of diagnosis by which the condition of some of the internal organs is determined by listening to the sounds they produce. Auscultation is practised by means of the stethoscope.

Autogenous
Autogenous means self-generated, and is the term applied especially to bacterial and viral vaccines manufactured from the organisms found in discharges from the body and used for the treatment of the particular individual from which the bacteria were derived.

Auto-Immune Disease
Auto-immune disease is due to a failure of the bodily defence mechanisms in which antibodies become active against some of the host's own cells. An example is spontaneous auto-immune thyroiditis which occurs in dogs, poultry, monkeys and rats, and resembles Hashimoto's thyroiditis of man. Other examples are auto-immune haemolytic disease, in which the blood's red cells are affected; and glomerulonephritis in small animals.

Immune-mediate diseases are of two kinds: (1) primary, an auto-immune reaction only against self; and (2) secondary, a similar reaction occurring when viruses, tumours, parasites, or drugs are involved.

Primary diseases are either organ-specific, e.g. auto-immune haemolytic anaemia (see under ANAEMIA), or systemic, e.g. LUPUS ERYTHEMATOSUS. (See also THROMBOCYTOPENIA; POLYARTHRITIS; PEMPHIGUS; BOVINE and CANINE AUTOIMMUNE HAEMOLYTIC ANAEMIA; DIABETES MELLITUS.)

Auto-Infection
Infection of one part of the body, hitherto healthy, from another part that already is suffering from the disease. Thus, sheep suffering from 'orf' on their feet may bite the painful areas and convey the organisms to their mouth, where the disease becomes established.

Autovaccine
A vaccine prepared from an organism isolated from from an animal and injected back into the same animal. The most common auto (or autologous) vaccine is that prepared for treatment of warts (angleberries) in cattle.

Autolysis
Self-digestion of an organism by its own enzymes. See also NECROSIS.

Autonomic Nervous System
The autonomic nervous system is that part of the nervous system which governs the automatic or

non-voluntary processes. It governs such functions as the beating of the heart, movements of the intestines, secretions from various glands, etc. It is usually regarded as composed of 2 distinct but complementary portions: the parasympathetic and the sympathetic systems.

The parasympathetic system is composed of a central portion comprising certain fibres present in the following cranial nerves: oculomotor, facial and glossopharyngeal; and the whole of the outgoing (efferent) nerves in the important vagus nerve. There is also a sacral set of autonomic nerve fibres present in the ventral roots of some of the sacral nerves.

The sympathetic system is composed of nerve fibres present in the ventral roots of the spinal nerves lying between the cervical and lumbar regions.

The 2 systems are mutually antagonistic in that stimulation of each produces opposite effects. These effects are shown in the form of the now classic table (see below).

Under normal circumstances there is a harmony preserved between the working of the 2 systems, which is flexible enough to provide for the ordinary exigencies of life. The sympathetic system is stimulated during the 'fight or flight' reaction, which comes into effect during emergency situations.

| Organ | Stimulation by chemical or other means of | |
	Parasympathetic	Sympathetic
Pupil	Contracts	Dilates
Heart	Slows	Accelerates
Salivary glands	Thin watery secretion	Thick glairy secretion
Stomach and intestines	Causes movement	Inhibits movement
Pyloric, anal, and ileocaecal	No action	Causes constriction
Bladder	Contracts	Relaxes
Bronchial muscles	Causes contraction	Causes relaxation
Gastrointestinal and bronchial glands	Produces secretion	No action
Sweat glands	No action	Causes secretion

The effect of stimulation of the parasympathetic and sympathetic nervous systems.

Autonomic Polyganglionopathy
(see FELINE DYSAUTONOMIA)

Autopsy

Autopsy (from the Greek, seeing with one's own eyes) is the examination of the internal structures of the body performed after death. From a post-mortem examination much valuable information can be learned, especially when there has been doubt about the disease condition during life. It has been said that it is 'unfair to the living animals, as well as a handicap to the progress of veterinary science, for owners to prohibit an autopsy because of sentiment'.

An autopsy is obligatory where some notifiable diseases, e.g. rabies, are involved, so that laboratory tests may be carried out to confirm or establish diagnosis. In the case of rabies, gloves and goggles must be worn, and every precaution taken, by the person carrying out the autopsy. With other communicable diseases (see ZOONOSES) similar precautions are necessary.

Valuable information can be obtained in slaughter-houses as to the extent of a disease, such as liver-fluke infestation in cattle and sheep, over a region or indeed throughout a whole country; and if suitably recorded and collated, the information can indicate the economic importance of diseases in farm animals and so lead to disease-control measures being taken as part of a regional or national campaign.

See under WOOL BALLS for an example of a layman's misinterpretation of post-mortem findings.

Autosomes

Autosomes are the chromosomes present in the nuclei of cells other than the sex-chromosomes. They are of the same type in both sexes in each species of animal, whereas the sex-chromosomes of the female are different from those of the male. (See CYTOGENETICS.)

Autumn Fly (Musca Autumnalis)

This is a non-biting fly which is a serious pest of grazing farm livestock in the UK and elsewhere. They cause cattle to huddle together and to cease feeding. Large numbers may collect on the upper part of the body, feeding on secretions from nose, mouth, eyes and on discharges from any wounds. (See FLIES – Fly control measures.)

Auxins

Plant hormones. These include oestrogens in pasture plants.

Avermectins

A group of chemical compounds derived from a fungus discovered in Japan in 1975, effective in very low dosage against nematode parasites and also against external parasites. (See IVER-MECTIN, which is the most useful of the group.) The discovery of the fungus in a soil sample was part of Merck Sharp & Dohme's international screening programme.

Technically, the avermectins are a series of macrocyclic lactone derivatives produced by fermentation of the actinomycete *Streptomyces avermitilis.*

Avian Contagious Epithelioma
(see under FOWL-POX)

Avian Infectious Encephalomyelitis

A disease of chicks and turkey poults; also known as epidemic tremor.

Cause A picornavirus. (Infection via the egg, as well as bird to bird.)

Signs If infection is egg-borne, signs are seen in the first 10 days after hatching; if infected after hatching, at 2 to 5 weeks old. There is leg weakness, followed by partial or complete paralysis of the legs. The chicks struggle to balance with the help of their wings. Trembling of the head and neck occurs in some cases.

Diagnosis An ELISA test.

Mortality A 40 per cent rate is not unusual.

Prevention Vaccination has proved very successful.

Avian Infectious Laryngotracheitis

Avian infectious laryngotracheitis of poultry is caused by a herpesvirus, prevalent in NW England. Loss of appetite, sneezing and cough-ing, a discharge from the eyes, difficulty in breathing are the main symptoms. Birds of all ages are susceptible. Mortality averages about 15 per cent. No treatment is of value. Control is best achieved by depopulation and fumiga-tion. A vaccine has been used.

Avian Influenza (Fowl Plague)

Avian influenza (fowl plague) attacks domesticat-ed fowl chiefly, but turkeys, geese, ducks, and most of the common wild birds are sometimes affected. It is not known to affect the pigeon. The disease is found in Asia, Africa, the Americas and to a lesser extent in parts of the continent of Europe, and is always liable to be introduced to countries hitherto free from it through the migrations of wild birds. An outbreak occurred among turkeys in Norfolk in 1963; this was the first recorded outbreak in Britain since 1929. An outbreak occurred in the Republic of Ireland in 1983; a slaughter policy followed. Infection may have come from Pennsylvania, where a similar policy was adopted.

Cause Myxovirus influenzae.

Signs In some cases the number attacked is small, while on the same premises the next year 80 or 90 per cent of the total inhabitants of the runs may die. The affected birds often die quite suddenly. In other instances the sick birds isolate themselves from the rest of the flock, preferring some dark out-of-the-way corner where they will be undisturbed. They are dull, disinclined to move, the tail and wings droop, the eyes are kept closed; the bird may squat on its breast with its head tucked under a wing or in amongst the shoulder feathers; food is refused, but thirst is often shown; the respira-tions are fast and laboured but not impeded by mucus; the temperature is very high at the commencement (43° to 44°C; 110° to 112°F), but falls shortly before death to below normal. (The normal temperature of birds is 41°C; 106.5°F.) The comb and wattles become purple or blue, and oedema of the head and neck is common. The illness seldom lasts more than 24 to 36 hours, and often not more than 6.

Control Vaccines are available but their use is incompatible with an eradication policy. They are used in parts of the USA and in Italy.

Avian Listeriosis

An infectious disease of poultry, occurring as an epidemic among young stock (often as an accompaniment of other diseases) or sporadically among adults.

Cause Listeria monocytogenes, a Gram-positive motile rod-shaped organism.

Signs In the epidemic type, wasting occurs over a period of days or even weeks. For 48 hours before death birds refuse all food.

The sporadic type is characterised by sudden death without much loss of condition.

Diagnosis Depends upon bacteriological methods. (See also LISTERIOSIS.)

Avian Lymphoid Leukosis

Avian lymphoid leukosis virus (LLV) infection is widespread among chickens in the UK, and causes mortality from tumours.

This disease, which has to be differentiated from Marek's disease, affects birds of 4 months upwards and is egg-transmitted, shows variable signs but, typically, the liver is enlarged.

It may be identified by the presence of neutralising antibodies in the serum or by virus detection by ELISA.

Control High standards of hygiene and flock management; no vaccines are available.

Avian Malaria
(see PLASMODIUM)

Avian Monocytosis
(see 'PULLET DISEASE')

Avian Nephritis
A viral infection first detected in the UK in 1988. In chick embryos it causes stunting, haemorrhage and oedema as well as nephritis.

Avian Sex Determination
Avian sex determination by laparoscopy has been widely used since 1976.

Avian Tuberculosis
The increase in the number of farmed poultry kept in free-range systems or with access to outdoors has led to an increase in the incidence of this disease. It is usually seen in birds over 2 years old but can occur in young birds. Ostriches are usually kept outdoors and are particularly at risk if near woodland, as wood pigeons (*Columba palamuis*) and feral pigeons are often heavily infected – as are wild birds such as starlings.

Cause Mycobacterium avium.

Signs Dullness, loss of appetite, lethargy and a tendency to squat in a sleeping position with the head tucked under one wing.

Body temperature may reach 44°C (112°F).

The comb and wattles may become almost purple, and swollen because of oedema. In young birds, there is muscle wastage and the comb may become pale in colour. The disease progresses slowly. It used to be referred to by pigeon fanciers as 'going light'.

Infection occurs following ingestion of food and water contaminated by the droppings of infected birds. Infection has been found in eagles at post-mortem examination, presumably from consumption of infected prey.

Cattle Avian tuberculosis rarely causes progressive disease, but the presence of avian TB bacteria will affect the interpretation of the tuberculin test. This infection must be differentiated from *Mycobacterium bovis* infection by using avian tuberculin as well as mammalian in the test. (See TUBERCULIN TEST.)

Sheep Avian tuberculosis can cause miliary tuberculosis in sheep.

Pigs A non-progressive infection is often found in lymph nodes at slaughter. The source of infection in housed pigs can be the use of peat as litter. *M. avium* survives in peat for a considerable period.

Post-Mortem Emaciation is usually well marked, and whitish-yellow nodules are present in the liver and spleen; also the intestines. The lungs are rarely affected in avian tuberculosis. In birds which have died suddenly, death is often found to be due to rupture of the liver, which when affected with tuberculosis is often enlarged and friable.

With valuable pedigree birds the intradermal tuberculin test may be employed, but before applying this test all birds should be examined and all thin birds destroyed, since those in the advanced stages of the disease may fail to react. Birds which pass the test should be put in clean houses on fresh ground.

(See also DISPOSAL OF CARCASES.)

Avilamycin
An antibiotic feed additive used as a growth promoter in pigs and poultry. Its use in the EU was to be phased out by 2006.

Avitaminosis
Avitaminosis is a term used to describe conditions produced by a deficiency or lack of a vitamin in the food. Thus 'avitaminosis A' means a deficiency of vitamin A. (See VITAMINS.)

Avocado Leaves
Persea americana fed to goats and sheep, during a drought in South Africa, caused death within a few days from heart disease.

Awns/Grass Seeds
A review by Kathleen E. Brennan and Peter J. Ihrke, School of Veterinary Medicine, University of California, of 182 cases in dogs and cats over a 1-year period showed that grass awns comprised 61 per cent of all foreign body cases. The most common site is the ear canal (51 per cent), and rupture of the tympanum has been an occasional sequel. Other sites are the interdigital skin conjunctiva, nose, lumbar region. Lumbar osteomyelitis has been caused. Perforation of a bronchus led to necrosis of a

lung lobe. In a cat with chronic cystitis, 2 awns were found in the bladder; and in another cat several awns were found at autopsy to have caused peritonitis. (*JAVMA*, **182**, 1201.)

Axilla

Axilla is the anatomical name for the region between the humerus and the chest wall, which corresponds to the armpit in the human being.

Axon

(see NERVES)

Azoperone

A neuroleptic drug used in pigs for reducing aggression and preventing fighting. It is used as a sedative when pigs are being transported and may be given as premedication before administering an anaesthetic or to reduce excitement when assistance at farrowing is required. Its effect may be less reliable in Vietnamese pot-bellied pigs.

It is also used for sedation in ostriches.

Azotaemia

The presence of urea and other nitrogenous products in greater concentration than normal in the blood, particularly in paralytic myoglobinuria in horses.

Azoturia

(see EQUINE MYOGLOBINURIA)

B Cells

One of the 2 types of lymphocytes. They are important in the provision of immunity, and they respond to antigens by dividing and becoming plasma cells that can produce antibody that will bind with the antigen. Their source is the bone marrow in mammals and the Bursa of Fabricius in birds. It is believed that the function of B cells is assisted by a substance provided by T CELLS. With haptens (see HAPTEN) it is apparently the B cells which recognise the protein carrier, and the T cells which recognise the hapten. (See also LYMPHOCYTE; IMMUNE RESPONSE.)

B Virus

This is a herpes virus found in monkeys which gives rise in man to an encephalitis with an almost 100 per cent mortality. It may be transmitted to man from monkeys – especially newly imported rhesus and cynomolgus monkeys. Lesions on the face and lips of monkeys should arouse suspicion of this condition.

It is believed that B virus, herpes simplex virus, and Aujeszky's disease virus have a common origin.

Babesia

Babesia is another name for piroplasm, one of the protozoan parasites belonging to the order Haemosporidia. These are generally relatively large parasites within the red blood cells and are pear-shaped, round or oval. Multiplication is by division into 2 or by budding. Infected cells frequently have 2 pyriform parasites joined at their pointed ends. Sexual multiplication takes place in the tick.

Babesiosis (Piroplasmosis) Nearly all the domestic mammals suffer from infection with some species of *Babesia*; sometimes more than 1 species may be present. The general symptoms are the appearance of fever in 8 to 10 days after infection, accompanied by haemoglobinuria, icterus; unless treated, 25 to 100 per cent of the cases are fatal. Red blood cells may be reduced in number by two-thirds. Convalescence is slow and animals may remain 'salted' for 3 to 8 years.

Transmission Development occurs in certain ticks which transmit the agent to their offspring.

The various species are similar, but are specific to their various hosts. The ticks should probably be regarded as the true or definite hosts, while the mammal is the intermediate host.

Cats *Babesia felis* is a (rare) cause of lethargy, inappetence and anaemia, and occasionally jaundice and death.

Sheep Ovine babesiosis may be due to at least 3 species of *Babesia*. There is a relatively large form, *Babesia motasi*, which is comparable to *B. bigemina* of cattle, and which produces a disease, often severe, with high temperatures, much blood-cell destruction, icterus, and haemoglobinuria. This is the 'carceag' of Eastern and Southern Europe. The 2nd parasite, of intermediate size and corresponding to *B. bovis* of cattle, is *Babesia ovis*. It produces a much milder disease with fever, jaundice, and anaemia, but recoveries generally occur. The small species is *Theileria ovis*, which appears to be similar to *T. mutans* of cattle and is relatively harmless to its host.

B. motasi, *B. ovis*, and *T. ovis* are all transmitted by *Rhipicephalus bursa*.

Animals recovered from *T. ovis* infection apparently develop a permanent immunity to it. The disease occurs in Europe, Africa, Asia, and North America.

Signs In acute cases the temperature may rise to 41.5°C (107°F), rumination ceases, there is paralysis of the hindquarters, the urine is brown, and death occurs in about a week. In benign cases there may only be a slight fever for a few days with anaemia.

A theileriosis, caused by *T. hirci*, has been described from sheep in Africa and Europe. It causes an emaciation and small haemorrhages in the conjunctiva.

Bacillary Haemoglobinurea

A disease of cattle caused by *Clostridium haemolyticum (Cl. oedematiens)* type D.

Bacillary White Diarrhoea

(see PULLORUM DISEASE)

Bacillus

This genus of Gram-positive rod-shaped organism contains many species which are not regarded as pathogenic, as well as some that are. They are found in soil, water, and on plants. Spores formed by bacilli are resistant to heat and disinfectants, and this fact is important in connection with *B. anthracis*, the cause of ANTHRAX. Another pathogenic bacillus is

B. cereus, a cause of food poisoning and also of bovine mastitis. (See BACTERIA.)

Bacitracin

An antibacterial formerly used as a feed additive; its use for this purpose has been banned in the EU.

Back-cross

Back-cross is the progeny resulting from mating a heterozygote offspring with either of its parental homozygotes. Characters in the back-crosses generally show a 1:1 ratio. Thus if a pure black bull is mated with pure red cows (all homozygous), black calves (heterozygotes) are produced. If the heifer calves are 'back-crossed' to their black father, their progeny will give 1 pure black to every 1 impure black. If a black heterozygous son of the original mating is mated to his red mother, the progeny will be 1 red to 1 black.

Back-crossing can be employed as a means of test-mating, or test-crossing to determine whether a stock of animals is homozygous, when it will never throw individuals of different type, or whether it is heterozygous, when it will give the 2 allelomorphic types. (See GENETICS, HEREDITY AND BREEDING.)

Back-Fence

(see STRIP-GRAZING)

Back Muscle Necrosis (BMN)

A disease of pigs first described in Belgium in 1960, and recognised 8 years later in West Germany (where it is colloquially known as 'banana disease'). It has been recorded in the UK, with 20 cases occurring in a single herd.

Signs A sudden and sporadic condition affecting pigs weighing over 50 kg. In the acute stage, the animal shows signs of pain, has difficulty in moving, becomes feverish, loses appetite and appears lethargic, and shows a characteristic swelling on 1 or both sides of the back. When only 1 side is affected, spinal curvature occurs with the convexity of the curve towards the swollen side.

The colloquial name 'banana disease' apparently arose from arching (as compared with lateral curvature) of the back, which is often seen in affected animals.

Some pigs die from acidosis and heart failure; some recover, apparently completely; while others are left with atrophy of the affected muscles resulting in a depression in the skin parallel to the spine. Some examples of BMN are discovered only in the slaughterhouse.

Post-Mortem examination reveals necrosis and bleeding, especially in the longissimus dorsi muscle, as well as the widely recognised condition known as PSE or pale soft exudative muscle.

Causes The disease is thought to be associated with stress; it is probable that heredity also comes into the picture.

Bacteria

Microscopic single-cell plants with important functions in nutrition and in disease processes. According to peculiarities in shape and in group formation, certain names are applied: thus a single spherical bacterium is known as 'coccus'; organisms in pairs and of the same shape (i.e. spherical) are called 'diplococci'; when in the form of a chain they are known as 'strepto-cocci'; when they are bunched together like a bunch of grapes the name 'staphylococcus' is applied. Bacteria in the form of long slender rods are known as 'bacilli'; wavy or curved forms have other names.

Reproduction The mode of multiplication of most bacteria is exceedingly simple, consisting of a splitting into 2 of a single bacterium. Since the new forms may similarly divide within half an hour, multiplication is rapid. (See illustration; see also PLASMIDS.)

Spore-Formation Some bacteria have the power to protect themselves from unfavourable conditions by changing their form to that of a 'spore'.

Size Bacteria vary in size from less than 1 MICRON (one-thousandth of a millimetre) diameter, in the case of streptococci and staphylococci, up to a length of 8 microns, in the case of the anthrax bacillus.

Mobility Not all bacteria possess the power of movement, but if a drop of fluid containing certain forms of organism which are called 'motile' be examined microscopically, it will be observed that they move actively in a definite direction. This is accomplished, in the motile organisms, by means of delicate whip-like processes which thrash backwards and forwards in the fluid and propel the body onwards. These processes are called 'flagellae'.

Methods of diagnosis

(1) *Microscopical* In order satisfactorily to examine bacteria microscopically, a drop of the

fluid containing the organisms is spread out in a thin film on a glass slide. The organisms are killed by heating the slide, and the details of their characteristics made obvious by suitable staining with appropriate dyes. (See under GRAM-NEGATIVE; also ACID-FAST.)

(2) *Cultural characteristics* By copying the conditions under which a particular bacterium grows naturally, it can be induced to grow artificially, and for this purpose various nutrient substances known as media are used. (See CULTURE MEDIUM.)

After a period of incubation on the medium on previously sterilised Petri dishes or in tubes or flasks, the bacteria form masses or colonies, visible to the naked eye.

The appearance of the colony may be sufficient in some instances for identification of the organism.

(3) (See LABORATORY TESTS)

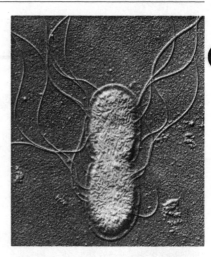

Bacterium about to divide. *Salmonella dublin* in the process of division into 2. Note also the flagellae.

(4) *Animal inoculation* This may be necessary for positive identification of the organism present in the culture. One or more labora-tory animals are inoculated and, after time allowed for lesions to develop or symptoms to appear, the animal is killed and a post-mortem examination made. The organisms recovered from the lesions may be re-examined or re-cultured.

Bacterial Adhesiveness
Some pathogenic bacteria adhere to the mucous membrane lining the intestine, and this characteristic may be an important criterion of virulence. Bacteria which possess this property include *E. coli*, *Salmonella typhimurium*, *Mycoplasma pneumoniae*, and *Moraxella bovis*.

Many strains of *E. coli* have a filamentous protein antigen called K88. This enables K88-positive *E. coli* to adhere to piglets' intestinal mucosa and to multiply there. K99 is the main adhesive antigen in cattle.

Bacterial Gill Disease
A disease of fish caused by poor water quality. The bacteria-infected gills become swollen and coated with mucus; asphyxia follows. As well as improving water quality, treatment may be attempted using copper sulphate, and zinc-free malachite green if fungal infection is also present. Dosage must be carefully calculated to avoid toxic side-effects.

Bacterial Kidney Disease
Bacterial kidney disease may affect farmed fish. Signs include pinpoint haemorrhages at the base of pectoral fins and on their sides; occasionally 'popeye' may be seen. In pacific salmon, cavernous spaces may be found in the muscles. Prolonged treatment with sulfonamides in the feed may control the disease, which may be due to infection by a coccobacillus carried by wild fish.

Bacteriophages
Bacteriophages are viruses which multiply in and destroy bacteria. Some bacteriophages have a 'tail' resembling a hypodermic syringe with which they attach themselves to bacteria and through which they 'inject' nucleic acid. 'Phages' have been photographed with the aid of the electron microscope. The growth of bacteriophages in bacteria results in the lysis of the latter, and the release of further bacteriophages. Phage-typing is a technique used for the identification of certain bacteria. Individual bacteriophages are mostly lethal only to a single bacterial species.

Bacteriostatic
An agent which inhibits the growth of micro-organisms, as opposed to killing them.

Bacteroides
Species of this anaerobic bacterium, including *B. melaninogenicus*, are frequently isolated from equine foot lesions and wounds. *B. nodosus* is one of the organisms found in foot-rot in sheep.

Baculoviruses
A group of viruses affecting insects. They are very host-specific and have been used in the

B

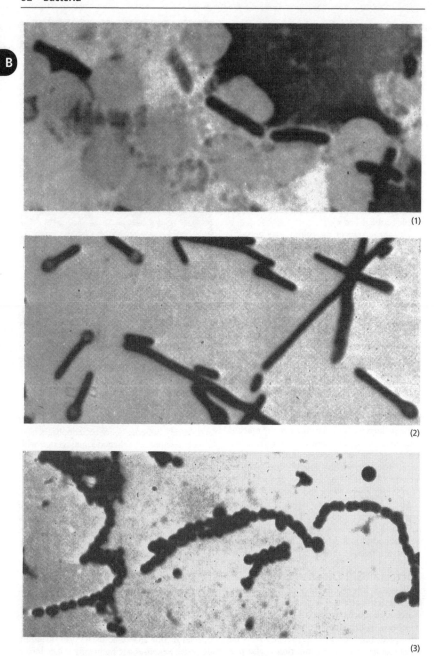

(1)

(2)

(3)

Bacteria. Photomicrographs of (1) *Bacillus anthracis* (× 4200); (2) *Clostridium tetani* (× 3250) (showing the characteristic drum-stick appearance); (3) *Streptococcus pyogenes* (× 3000).

control of specific insect pests while leaving beneficial species unharmed. Interest has also been shown in the possibility of using them as carriers of antigens in genetically engineered vaccines.

Some bacteria of veterinary importance

Name	Associated or specific diseased conditions caused
Actinobacillus lignièresi	Actinobacillosis.
A. pleuropneumoniae	Pleuropneumonia in pigs.
Actinomyces pyogenes	Abscesses in liver, kidneys, lungs or skin in sheep, cattle and pigs especially; present as a secondary organism in many suppurative conditions; causes summer mastitis in cattle.
Actinomyces bovis	Actinomycosis.
Aeromonas shigelloides	Chronic diarrhoea in cats.
Bacillus anthracis	Anthrax in all susceptible animals.
Bacillus cereus	Bovine mastitis; food poisoning.
Bacillus lichenformis	Abortion in ewes.
Baccilus piliformis	Tyzzer's disease.
Bacteroides species	Foot infections in horses.
Bacteroides nodosus	Foot-rot in sheep. Necrosis of skin or mucous membrane in rabbits after their resistance has been lowered by some other pathogen.
Bordetella bronchiseptica	Complicates distemper in the dog. Kennel cough. Atrophic rhinitis.
Brucella abortus	Brucellosis.
Brucella melitensis	Brucellosis in goats; undulant fever in man (in part).
Campylobacter fetus	Infertility, abortion.
Clostridium botulinum (*five types – A to E*)	Botulism in man and animals.
Cl. chauvoei	'Black-quarter' (and also pericarditis and meningitis in cattle) in cattle and partly in sheep.
Cl. difficile	Chronic diarrhoea in dogs and piglets.
Cl. novyi (*oedematiens*)	'Black-quarter' in cattle and pigs in part; 'black disease' in sheep; septicaemia in horses and pigs (wound infection).
Cl. septicum	Gas gangrene in man; black-quarter; braxy in sheep.
Cl. tetani	Tetanus in man and animals.
Cl. welchii (*perfringens*)	Lamb dysentery; present in many cases of gas gangrene.
Corynebacterium pseudotuberculosis	Caseous lymphadenitis in sheep; some cases of ulcerative lymphangitis and acne in horses.
C. equi	A cause of pneumonia in the horse and of tuberculosis-like lesions in the pig.
Dermatophilus congolensis	Chronic dermatitis.
Group EF-4 bacteria	Pneumonia in dogs and cats, and isolated from human dog-bite wound.
Erysipelothrix rhusiopathiae	Swine erysipelas.
Eschicheria coli (sub. types are many)	Always present in alimentary canal as commonest organism; becomes pathogenic at times, partly causing enteritis, dysentery (lambs), scour (calves and pigs), cystitis, abortion, mastitis, joint-ill, etc.
Fusiformis necrophorus	Associated with foot-rot; calf diphtheria; quittor, poll evil, and fistulous withers in horses; necrosis of the skin in dogs, pigs, and rabbits; navel-ill in calves and lambs; various other conditions in bowel and skin.
F. nodosus	Foot-rot in sheep.
Haemophilus somnus	'Sleeper syndrome' in cattle.
H. parainfluenzae *H. parasuis*	Chronic respiratory disease in pigs.
Klebsiella pneumoniae	Metritis in mares; pneumonia in dogs, etc.
Leptospira ictero-haemorrhagiae	Leptospiral jaundice, or enzootic jaundice of dogs; Weil's disease in man.
Lept. canicola	Canicola fever in man, and nephritis in dogs.
Lept. hardjo	Bovine mastitis.
Listeria monocytongens	Listeriosis.
Mycobacterium johnei	Johne's disease of cattle.

(continued)

B

Some bacteria of veterinary importance (continued from previous page)

Name	Associated or specific diseased conditions caused
Myc. tuberculosis (bovine, human, and avian types)	Tuberculosis in man and animals.
Pasteurella multocida	Fowl cholera. Haemorrhagic septicaemia in cattle.
P. haemolytica	Pneumonia.
P. tularensis	Tularaemia in rodents.
Pseudomonas mallei	Glanders in equines and man.
P. pseudomallei	Melioidosis in rats and man; occasionally in dogs and cats.
P. aeruginosa	Mastitis in cattle.
P. pyocyanea	Suppuration in wounds, otitis in the dog.
Salmonella abortus equi	Contagious abortion of mares naturally, but capable of causing abortion in pregnant ewes, cows, and sows experimentally.
S. abortus ovis	Contagious abortion of ewes occurring naturally.
S. dublin	Causes enteritis, sometimes abortion.
S. gallinarum	Klein's disease or fowl typhoid.
S. pullorum	Pullorum disease.
S. cholerae suis	Salmonellosis septicaemia in pigs.
S. typhimurium	Salmonellosis.
Serpulina (Treponema) hyodysenteriae	Swine dysentery.
Staphylococcus albus	Suppurative conditions in animals.
Staph. aureus	Suppurative conditions in animals and man, especially wound infections where other pus-producing organisms are also present. Present in various types of abscess, and in pyaemic and septi-caemic conditions. Cause of mastitis in cows.
Staph. hyicus	A primary or secondary skin pathogen causing lesions in horses, cattle, and pigs. It may also cause bone and joint lesions.
Staph. pyogenes	Often associated with the other staphylococci in above conditions; causes mastitis in cows.
Streptococcus dysgalactiae	Mastitis in cattle.
Str. equi	Strangles in horses, partly responsible for joint-ill in foals, and sterility in mares.
Str. agalactiae	Mastitis in cows.
Str. pyogenes	Many suppurative conditions, wound infections, abscesses, etc.; joint-ill in foals. (In the above conditions various other streptococci are alsofrequently present.)
Str. suis	Infects not only pigs but also horses and cats.
Str. uberis	Mastitis in cattle.
Str. zooepidemicus	Wounds in horses; mastitis in cattle and goats.
Vibrio	(*see under* CAMPYLOBACTER)
Yersinia enterocolitica	(*see under* YERSINIOSIS)
Y. pestis	Plague in man and rats. In an often subclinical form this may also occur in cats and dogs.
Y. pseudotuberculosis	(*see under* YERSINIOSIS)

For other, non-bacterial infective agents, *see* VIRUSES; RICKETTSIA; MYCOPLASMA; CHLAMYDIA.

Badgers

Several species of badger inhabit different parts of the world. The so-called true badger, *Meles meles*, can grow up to 80 cm long, excluding tail. It is an omniverous animal with greyish coat and black-and-white stripes on the face. Badgers live in extensive underground burrows called setts.

Tuberculosis in badgers caused by *Myobacterium bovis* was first described in Switzerland in 1957, and in England in 1971. Transmission of the infection to cattle led to their reinfection in the south-west of England

mainly. Badgers are now regarded as a significant reservoir of *M. bovis* infecion. However, a policy of culling badgers in TB-affected areas has been controversial.

The 2003 Krebs report on bovine tuberculosis in cattle and badgers recommended that badger culling should end in most of the UK. It would be replaced by a trial in areas repeatedly affected by TB. The trial would compare the effectiveness of culling all badgers in limited areas with the results of culling only those badgers assumed to be linked with bovine TB in other areas, and with no culling in a 3rd area.

Work on developing a vaccine to protect cattle against TB would continue.

Badgers Act 1991

This makes it an offence to damage, destroy or obstruct a sett, disturb a badger in a sett, or put a dog into a sett.

Badgers (Further Protection) Act 1991

This legalises euthanasia of a dog, and disqualification of its owner from keeping a dog, after the offending dog has killed, injured or taken a badger, or the dog's owner has ill-treated or dug a badger out of its sett.

Bakery Waste

Bakery waste has been fed to pigs. It is much safer to use than swill, provided that it contains no animal protein. Biotin deficiency may result if it is fed to excess.

Balanitis

(see PENIS, ABNORMALITIES OF)

Balance, Nutritional

The balance between what is taken in from the diet and what is excreted. For example, if an animal excretes more nitrogen than it receives from the protein in its feed, it is in negative nitrogen balance and losing protein. Similarly, reference is made to water balance, sodium balance and electrolyte balance.

Balantidium

A ciliated, protozoon parasite of pigs' intestines. As a rule, it causes no harm; but if the pig becomes debilitated from other causes, some degree of dysentery may result. The parasite is pear-shaped and about 80 microns long by 60 microns broad. The nucleus is sausage-shaped.

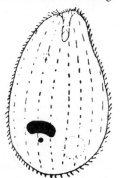

Balantidium coli.

'Baldy Calf' Syndrome

An inherited lethal disease, causing alopecia, skin cracking and ulceration with progressive loss of weight or failure to grow. It is found in the descendants of a Canadian Holstein in Australia. Inherited epidermal dysplasia has been suggested as a more appropriate name. A single autosomal recessive gene is thought to be involved.

Baling Wire

Discarded pieces of this may be swallowed by cattle and give rise to traumatic pericarditis. In Britain, it has largely been replaced by plastic baler twine. (See under HEART DISEASES.)

Ballottement

A technique of clinical examination in which the movement of any body or organ, suspended in a fluid, is detected.

'BANANA DISEASE' OF PIGS (see BACK MUSCLE NECROSIS)

Bandages and Bandaging

The application of bandages to veterinary patients is much more difficult than in human

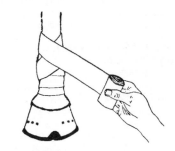

'Figure-of-eight' bandage (roller) for fetlock, also known a 'spica'.

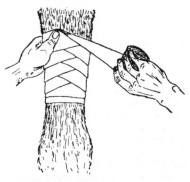

Ascending spiral-reversed bandage for fore-arm.

practice, because not only must the bandage remain in position during the movement of the patient, but it must also be comfortable, or it will be removed by the teeth or feet; and it must be so adjusted that it will not become contaminated by either urine or the faeces.

Wounds often heal more readily if left uncovered, but bandaging may be necessary to give protection against flies and the infective agents which these carry. Much will depend upon the site of the wound, its nature, and the environment of the animal.

Bandages may be needed for support, and to reduce tension on the skin. (See also illustration.)

Barbiturates

Barbiturates are derivatives of barbituric acid (malonyl-urea). They include a wide range of very valuable sedative, hypnotic or anaesthetic agents. Several are used in veterinary practice, including pentobarbitone, phenobarbitone and thiopentone. An overdose is often used to euthanase dogs and cats; and farm animals where the brain is required for examination, as in suspected BSE cases.

In case of inadvertent barbiturate poisoning, use a stomach tube and keep the animal warm. Treatment includes CNS stimulants, e.g. bemegride, doxapram, caffeine or strong coffee. (See also under EUTHANASIA; HORSE-MEAT.)

Barium-Meal Techniques in Dogs and Cats

(see under X-RAYS)

Barium Poisoning

Barium chloride is used in rat poison; the bait may be eaten by domestic pets.

The symptoms are excessive salivation, sweating (except in the dog), muscular convulsions, violent straining, palpitation of the heart, and finally general paralysis.

Treatment Induce vomiting or use a stomach pump to remove the poison. Epsom salts dissolved in water act as an antidote by converting the chloride into the insoluble sulphate of barium.

Barium Sulphate

Barium sulphate, being opaque to X-rays, is given by the mouth prior to a radiographic examination of the gastrointestinal tract for diagnostic purposes. (See X-RAYS.)

Barium Sulphide

Barium sulphide is sometimes used as a depilatory for the site of surgical operations.

Bark

A change in the tone of a dog's bark occurs in many cases of rabies.

Bark Eating

Bark eating by cattle should be regarded as a symptom of a mineral deficiency, e.g. manganese and phosphorus. The remedy is use of an appropriate mineral supplement.

Barker Foal

A maladjustment syndrome in which a violent breathing action results often in a noise like a dog barking.

Barley Poisoning

As with wheat (and to a much lesser extent, oats) an excess of barley can kill cattle and sheep not gradually accustomed to it. The main signs are severe acidosis and death. Treatment is sodium bicarbonate, by injection; gastric lavage; or rumenotomy.

It is important that barley should not be fed in a fine, powdery form. To do so is to invite severe digestive upsets, which may lead to death. Especially if ventilation is poor, dusty food also contributes to coughing and may increase the risk of pneumonia.

'Barn Itch'

The American name for sarcoptic mange in cattle.

Barrier Cream

A protective dressing for the hands and arms of veterinarians engaged in obstetrical work or rectal examinations.

Barrier, Bood-Brain

A filtering system to prevent harmful chemicals in the bloodstream from reaching the brain. The system also prevents certain medicines, such as penicillin, from treating brain infections such as bacterial meningitis. A similar barrier in the placenta protects the fetus.

Barrow

A castrated male pig.

Bars of Foot

At each of the heels of the horse's foot the wall turns inwards and forwards instead of ending abruptly. These 'reflected' portions are called the bars of the foot. They serve to strengthen the heels; they provide a gradual rather than an abrupt finish to the important wall; and they take a share in the formation of the bearing surface, on which rests the shoe.

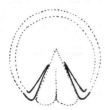

Diagram of the position of the bars of the horse's foot. The dotted line shows the outline of the wall and frog.

The bars are sometimes cut away by farriers or others, who hold the erroneous idea that by so doing they allow the heels of the foot to expand; what actually happens in such instances is that the union between the component parts of the foot is destroyed, and the resistance to contraction which they afford is lost. They should therefore be allowed to grow and maintain their natural prominence. (See also illustration.)

Bartonellosis

Infection with *Bartonella* organisms, which occasionally occurs in dogs and cattle but is of importance in laboratory rats. Symptoms are mainly those of anaemia.

Treatment Neoarsphenamine has been used.

Basic Slag

Basic slag is a by-product of the smelting industry often used as a fertiliser. It has caused poisoning in lambs, which should not be allowed access to treated fields until the slag has been well washed into the soil. Adult sheep have also been poisoned in this way, scouring badly, and so have cattle. In these animals the symptoms include: dullness, reluctance to move, inappetence, grinding of the teeth, and profuse watery black faeces.

Basenji

A small brown and white dog, originating in Africa, which is unable to bark. Inheritable congenital defects include haemolytic anaemia, inguinal hernia and persistent pupillary membrane. They may also inherit the condition intestinal lymphangiectasia, which causes loss of protein from the gut. Basenji bitches normally have only one reproductive cycle a year.

Basset Hound

A long-bodied, long-eared, short-legged breed. Ectropion, inguinal hernia and glaucoma may be inherited conditions. Back problems caused

by cervical spondylosis may occur, and failure of the anconal process (elbow) to develop properly may be seen.

Basophil

A type of white blood cell. (See under BLOOD.)

Basophilic

Blue-staining.

Baths

Bathing of animals may be undertaken for the sake of cleanliness, for the cure of a parasitic skin disease, or for the reduction of the temperature.

Cattle and sheep (see DIPS AND DIPPING)

Dogs For ordinary purposes the dog is bathed in warm water, in which it is thoroughly soaked. It is then lathered with a suitable shampoo (many proprietary brands are available) or hard soap, rinsed off and dried. A wide range of specially formulated shampoos is available for specific skin conditions.

Dish-washing detergent liquid should not be used for shampooing puppies or even adult dogs.

Cats Because cats are fastidious creatures which wash themselves nearly all over (they cannot reach the back of their necks or between their shoulder blades), the question of bathing them does not arise except in cases of a severe infestation with external parasites; very old cats which have ceased to wash themselves; entire tom cats which as a result of stress or illness have also ceased to look after themselves; as a first-aid treatment for heat stroke/stress; and in some cases where a cat has fallen into a noxious liquid.

Shampoos/flea-killers, etc. sold for use on dogs are not all safe for cats. Owners should read the small print on packets and look for 'Safe for cats' where a preparation has not been prescribed by a veterinary surgeon.

Baths are used to help the treatment of certain muscle and joint problems. Sand baths are essential for chinchillas to keep their coats in good condition. (Poultry perform dust bathing – given the opportunity.)

Bats

(see also RABIES; VAMPIRE-BATS; HISTOPLASMOSIS). Bats are mammals, and usually produce 1 offspring in late spring or early summer. Fifteen species have been identified in Britain, where they are classified as protected creatures under the Wildlife and Countryside Act 1981. They can live for up to 30 years.

Battery System

A method of intensive egg production involving keeping hens in cages with a sloping floor; 1, 2, or up to 5 birds per cage. Feeding and watering may be on the 'cafeteria' system, with food containers moving on an endless belt, electrically driven. The eggs are usually collected from racks at the front of the cages.

There have long been objections on welfare grounds to current battery systems. Benefits achieved in good examples of battery cage systems (e.g. a smaller risk from parasites, good access to food and water) may be outweighed by their deficiencies (e.g. prevention of nesting behaviour, perching, dust-bathing; bone weakness caused by lack of freedom to move about).

In the EU, battery cages are to be phased out by 2011. From January 1, 2003 the permitted cage size was increased to allow a minimum of 550 cm² per hen and since that date no new cages could be installed. 'Enriched cages', or alternative non-cage systems, were specified for new or replacement systems by January 1, 2002. The 'enriched cages' have 750 cm² space per hen and provide a nest, litter to allow pecking and scratching, and perches. The plans for alternative non-cage systems are due to be introduced by January 1, 2007.

'Cage layer fatigue', a form of leg paralysis, is sometimes encountered in battery birds. Birds let out of their cages on to a solid floor usually recover. A bone-meal supplement may help. (See also INTENSIVE LIVESTOCK PRODUCTION; EGG YIELD.)

A battery rearing system has, in a somewhat different form, been applied to pig rearing.

BCG Vaccine

BCG vaccine may be used for dogs and cats in Britain in households where a member of the household has tuberculosis. The vaccine does not cover every species of *Mycobacterium tuberculosis,* however. It cannot be used in cattle as it interfere with the tuberculin test, and has proved unsuccessful in immunising badgers. It has been used in the treatment of equine sarcoid.

Beagle

A breed of dog traditionally kept in packs. Behavioural problems may develop in solitary animals kept as pets. Inheritable conditions include cleft palate, haemolytic anaemia, glaucoma and epilepsy.

Beak

(see DE-BEAKING; SHOVEL BEAK)

Becquerel

The standard unit for measuring RADIATION.

Bedding and Bedding Materials

Whenever animals are housed in buildings, it is both necessary and economical to provide them with some form of bedding material. The reasons are as follows:

(1) All animals are able to rest more adequately in the recumbent position, and the temptation to lie is materially increased by the provision of some soft bedding upon which they may more comfortably repose than on the uncovered floor. Indeed there are some which, in the event of the bedding being inadequate, or when it becomes scraped away, will not lie down at all.

(2) The provision of a sufficiency of some non-conductor of heat (which is one of the essentials of a good bedding) minimises the risk of chills.

(3) The protection afforded to prominent bony surfaces – such as the point of the hip, the points of the elbow and hock, the stifles and knees, etc. – is important, and if neglected leads to bruises and injuries of these parts.

(4) From the point of view of cleanliness, both of the shed or loose-box and of the animal's skin, the advantages of a plentiful supply of bedding are obvious.

(5) In the case of sick animals, the supply and management of the bedding can aid recovery. (See also SLATTED FLOORS.)

Horses

Wheat straw Wheat straw undoubtedly makes the best litter for either stall or loose-box. Its main disadvantage is its inflammability.

Wheat straw should be supplied loose or in hand-tied bundles for preference. Trussed or baled straw has been pressed and has lost some of its resilience or elasticity in the process. The individual straws should be long and unbroken, and the natural resistive varnish-like coating should be still preserved in a sample. The colour should be yellowish or a golden white; it should be clean-looking and free from dustiness. Straw should be free from thistles and other weeds.

Wheat straw has a particular advantage in that horses will not eat it unless kept very short of hay.

Oat straw This straw is also very good for bedding purposes, but it possesses one or two disadvantages when compared with wheat straw. The straw is considerably softer, more easily broken and compressible than wheat, and being sweet to the taste, horses eat it.

Barley straw is inferior to either of the preceding for these reasons: it is only about half the length; it is very soft and easily compressed and therefore does not last as long as oat or wheat; more of it is required to bed the same-sized stall; and it possesses numbers of awns. The awns of barley are sharp and brittle. They irritate the softer parts of the skin, cause scratches, and sometimes penetrate the soft tissues of the udder, lips, nose, or the region about the tail.

Rye straw has the same advantages as wheat straw, but it is a little harder and rougher.

Peat-moss is quite a useful litter for horses. It is recommended for town stables and for use on board ship, or other forms of transport. A good sample should not be powdery, but should consist of a matrix of fibres in which are entangled small lumps of pressed dry moss. It is very absorbent – taking up 6 or 8 times its own weight of water. When it is used, the drains should be of the open or 'surface' variety or covered drains should be covered with old sacks, etc.

It should never be used in a loose-box in which there is an animal suffering from any respiratory disease, on account of its dusty nature.

Sand makes a fairly good bed when the sample does not contain any stones, shells, or other large particles. It is clean-looking, has a certain amount of scouring action on the coat, is cool in the summer, and comparatively easily managed. Sand should be obtained from a sand pit or the bed of a running stream; not from the sea-shore, because the latter is impregnated with salt, and likely to be licked by horses when they discover the salty taste of which they are very fond. If this habit is acquired the particles of sand that are eaten collect in the colon or caecum of the horse and may set up a condition known as 'sand colic', which is often difficult to alleviate.

Ferns and bracken make a soft bed and are easily managed, but they always look dirty and untidy, do not last as long as straws, and are rather absorbent when stamped down. With horses that eat their bedding there is a risk of bracken poisoning.

Cattle Wheat straw is the most satisfactory. Oat straw is used in parts where little or no wheat is grown. Barley straw is open to objection as a litter for cows on account of its awns, which may irritate the soft skin of the perineal region and of the udder. Sawdust has been found very convenient in cow cubicles, also shavings. Sand has been used on slippery floors below straw bedding, when it affords a good foothold for the cows and prevents accidents. (See also DEEP LITTER.) Special rubber mats have been found practicable and economic for use in cow cubicles. Shredded paper has been used for cattle (and also horses).

A disadvantage of sawdust is that its use has led to coliform mastitis (sometimes fatal) in cattle. Sand may then be preferable.

In milk-fed calves, the ingestion of peat, sawdust or wood shavings may induce hypomagnesaemia.

Pigs Many materials are used for the pig, but probably none possesses advantages over wheat straw, unless in the case of farrowing or suckling sows. These should be littered with some very short bedding which will not become entangled round the feet of the little pigs, and will not irritate the udder of the mother. For this purpose chaff, shavings, and even hay may be used according to circumstances.

Straw can make up for deficiencies in management and buildings as nothing else can. It serves the pig as a comfortable bed, as a blanket to burrow under, a plaything to avert boredom, and a source of roughage in meal-fed pigs which can help obviate digestive upsets and at least some of the scouring which reduces farmers' profits. Straw can mitigate the effects of poor floor insulation, of draughts, and of cold; and in buildings without straw, ventilation (to quote David Sainsbury) becomes a much more critical factor.

As a newborn piglet spends so much of its time lying in direct contact with the floor of its pen, much body-heat can be lost through conduction. Depending on the type of floor, this effect can be large enough to affect the piglet's growth rate and be a potential threat to its survival.' Providing straw can be equivalent to raising the ambient temperature from 10° to 18°C (50° to 64°F). Wooden and rubber floors are not as effective as straw in reducing conductive heat loss.

Dogs and cats Dogs (and pigs) have died as a result of the use for bedding of shavings of the red African hardwood (*Mansonia altissima*), which affects nose, mouth, and the feet, as well as the heart.

Fatal poisoning of cats has followed the use of sawdust, from timber treated with pentachlorophenol, used as bedding.

Hamsters Synthetic bedding materials should be avoided as they can cause injury.

Poultry (see LITTER, OLD)

Rabbits Peat-moss is recommended as it neutralises ammonia formed from urine; rabbits are particularly susceptible to ammonia in the atmosphere.

Bedlington Terrier
A small, soft-coated terrier with distinctive arched-back appearance. Together with some West Highland white terriers, they are prone to inherited copper toxicosis. The breed is relatively intolerant of high copper levels in the diet and may develop cirrhosis of the liver as a result. Zinc acetate has been used for treatment. Other inheritable conditions include brittle bones (osteogenesis imperfecta) and retinal dyspasia.

Bedsonia
(see CHLAMYDIA)

Beef Breeds and Crosses
The native British beef breeds are the Aberdeen Angus, Shorthorn Hereford, Devon, South Devon, Sussex, Galloway, Highland and Lincoln Red. Continental breeds including the Charolais, Chianinas, Simmental, Limousin, Blonde d'Aquitaine, Gebvieh, Belgian Blue and Piedmontese have been imported for use in the United Kingdom. The continental breeds are more muscular, have higher mature weights and better performance than native beef breeds, the Meat and Livestock Commission has commented.

The beef breeds are generally used as terminal sires on cows not required for breeding dairy herd replacements, and some beef cross heifers are used for suckler herd replacements. The cross-bred calves exhibit hybrid vigour and fetch a premium in the market over pure-bred dairy calves.

(See also CATTLE, BREEDS OF)

Beef Cattle Husbandry in Britain
Around 58 per cent of home-produced beef is derived from the dairy herd, partly from dairy-bred calves reared for beef and partly from culled dairy cows. A further 34 per cent comes from the beef suckler herd.

Store systems Cattle are usually on 1 farm for less than a year, typically a winter (yard finished) or summer period (grass finished),

but sometimes as short a period as 3 months. Because only part of the production cycle takes place on a single farm, the possibility for using a wide range of technical inputs is limited. The profitability is dominated by the relationship between buying and selling prices, and these systems are characterised by large year-to-year fluctuations in margins. As a generalisation, the longer the cattle are on the farm, the higher the margin.

Bees
Honey bees (*Apis* spp) represent one of the oldest forms of animal husbandry. Modern beehives are designed so that the honey-filled combs can be removed and replaced without disturbing the main chamber. This also minimises swarming. Bees are subject to several diseases of which VARROASIS is the most prevalent. The National Bee Unit, run by MAAF, provides advice on bee health issues (National Bee Unit, Sand Hutton, York YO4 1LZ). (See also under BITES, STINGS.)

Beet Tops
(see POISONING – Fodder poisoning)

Beevbilde Cattle
Breeding is based on 54 per cent polled Lincoln Red Blood, 40 per cent polled Beef Shorthorn, and 6 per cent Aberdeen Angus.

Behaviour Problems
Antisocial, or inappropriate, behaviour in dogs and cats is an increasingly common problem. There are a number of possible causes, including genetic traits in particular breeds, hormonally triggered behaviour and intentional or unintentional mistreatment. The fact that many animals are left alone for long periods while their owners are at work can encourage misbehaviour. The animal becomes distressed during the periods of absence and may resort to urinating or defecating; or in the case of dogs, chewing furniture. Then over-excitement, with uncontrolled barking and jumping, results on the owner's return. Aggressive behaviour to people or other animals is another common problem. Conversely, a pet may become obsessively attached to a single person, resenting any show of affection to that individual by another. While veterinary surgeons and 'pet counsellors' can can offer advice on correcting unacceptable behaviour, it is greatly to be preferred that the problem is avoided in the first place.

When choosing a dog or cat, it is always advisable to see the puppy or kitten in its home environment. A pup from a litter born to a well-behaved bitch in a caring home is much more likely to develop into a good companion than a dog reared on a puppy farm with little opportunity to socialise with people. And one removed too early from its litter mates may later show aggression towards, or fear of, other dogs or cats. It also helps to avoid problems if a pet is selected that the owner can cope with easily. Big dogs need lots of space and lots of exercise; long haired breeds take a lot of grooming.

Punishment for 'bad' behaviour is rarely beneficial. Removing the cause, if possible, can help; rewarding for 'good' (correct) behaviour as part of a retraining process is more effective. Retraining requires patience and perseverance. The process may be assisted by the short-term use of medication. Megestrol (Ovarid) may be useful where the behavioural problem is hormonally triggered (spraying, aggression); or tranquillising drugs may be prescribed.

Belgian Blue Cattle

A beef breed noted for exceptional hindquarter muscling. The British name is a misnomer, and 'White-blue' is said to be a better translation. Dystokia may be a problem, in breeds other than those of extreme dairy type, e.g. Holsteins. Maiden heifers should **not** be got in calf by a Belgian Blue bull.

Belladonna

Belladonna is another name for the deadly nightshade flower (*Atropa belladonna*). (See ATROPINE.)

Bemigride

A central nervous system stimulant; may be used to counter barbiturate poisoning.

Benadryl

Benadryl is the proprietary name of beta-dimethylamino-ethylbenz-hydryl ether hydrochloride, which is of use as an antihistamine in treating certain allergic conditions. (See ANTIHISTAMINES.)

Bengal

A breed of cat developed from crossing the domesic cat (*Felis cattus*) with the Asian wild cat (*F. ornata*). It is not considered as a hybrid between a wild animal and a domestic animal under the Dangerous Wild Animals Act 1976.

Benzalkonium Chloride

One of the quaternary ammonia compounds; it

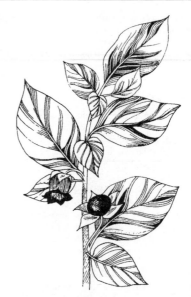

Belladonna (*Atropa belladonna*), also known as deadly nightshade, has thick, fleshy roots, dark green leaves, and purplish flowers. The berries change in colour from green to red, and then to black. The plant grows to a height of about 1.6 m (5 ft). All parts of the plant are poisonous.

is used as an antiseptic and detergent. (See under QUATERNARY.)

Benzene Hexachloride

The gamma isomer of this (lindane) is a highly effective and persistent ectoparasiticide, which was formerly the main ingredient of several proprietary preparations, designed for use as dusting powder, spray, dip, etc. Its use in animals is now banned in many countries, including the UK. It is highly toxic for fish.

BHC is the common abbreviation for the gamma isomer. (See BHC POISONING.)

Benzocaine

Benzocaine is a white powder, with local anaesthetic properties, used as a sedative for inflamed and painful surfaces and for anaesthesia in fish.

Benzocaine poisoning This has occurred in cats following use of either a benzocaine spray or ointment, and results in methaemoglobin appearing in the blood.

Signs In one case a cat showed signs of poisoning following an application of the cream to itchy areas. Cyanosis, open-mouthed breathing and vomiting occurred. Collapse followed within 15 minutes.

Improvement was noticed within 10 minutes of giving methylene blue intravenously; and within 2 hours breathing had become normal again. The cat recovered.

Benzoic Acid

Benzoic acid is an antiseptic substance formerly used for inflammatory conditions of the urinary system. It is excreted as hippuric acid, and renders the urine acid. It is used in the treatment of ringworm, and as a food preservative.

Benzoic acid poisoning Cases of this have been reported in the cat, giving rise to extreme aggressiveness, salivation, convulsions, and death. A curious symptom sometimes observed is jumping backwards and striking out with the fore-limbs 'as though catching imaginary mice'.

Benzyl Benzoate

Benzyl benzoate is a drug formerly used for treating mange in dogs and sweet itch in horses. A 25 per cent preparation may be applied to mite, etc., bites in pigeons.
Benzyl benzoate is usually employed as an emulsion. It should not be used over the whole body surface at once.

Benzylpenicillin

This antibiotic is a bactericide, active against Gram-positive bacteria, and given by parenteral or intramammary infusion. It is inactivated by penicillinase.

Bephenium Embonate

A drug which is used in sheep to kill nematodirus worms.

Bernese Mountain Dog

A large, long-haired breed, mainly black with white and brown markings. It has few inherited defects, although cleft palate may occur. Also known as Swiss mountain dog.

Berrichon Du Cher

A French breed of heavy milking sheep. The breed contains some merino blood.

Besnoitiosis

A protozoan disease usually affecting the skin and mucous membranes; other effects may include sterility. Not normally found in temperate countries.

Beta-Blocker

(see AGONIST)

Betahydroxybutyrate (BOHB)

A ketone body which can be measured in blood to determine the energy status. The higher the level, the poorer the energy intake.

Betamethasone

A corticosteroid.

BHC

BHC is an abbreviation for BENZENE HEXA-CHLORIDE.

BHC Poisoning

This may arise, especially in kittens and puppies, from a single dose (e.g. licking of BHC-containing dusting powder). Symptoms include: twitching, muscular incoordination, anxiety, convulsions.

A farmer's wife became ill (she had a convulsion) after helping to dip calves, but recovered after treatment. Two of the calves died.

BHC is highly poisonous for fish; it must be used with great care on cats, for which other insecticides such as selenium preparations are to be preferred.

The use of BHC sheep dips is no longer permitted in the UK.

BHS

Beta haemolytic streptococcus.

Bicarbonate

A salt containing HCO_3; the amount in blood determines the acid/base balance. Sodium bicarbonate is used as an antacid in ruminal acidosis.

'Big Head'

A condition associated with *Clostridium novyi* (type A) infection in rams which have slightly injured their heads as a result of fighting. It occurs in Australia and South Africa. (See also HYDROCEPHALUS.)

Bighead

Term used to describe osteodystrophia fibrosa in horses and goats.

Bile

Bile is a thick, bitter, golden-brown or greenish-yellow fluid secreted by the liver, and stored in the gall-bladder. It has digestive functions, assisting the emulsification of the fat contents of the food. It has in addition some laxative action, stimulating peristalsis, and it aids absorption not only of fats but also of fat-soluble vitamins. (See CHOLECYSTOKININ.)

Jaundice is a symptom rather than a disease; it may be caused when the flow of the bile is obstructed and does not reach the intestines, but remains circulating in the blood. As a result the pigments are deposited in the tissues and discolour them, while the visible mucous membranes are yellowish.

Vomiting of bile usually occurs when the normal passage through the intestines is obstructed, and during the course of certain digestive disorders. (See also GALLSTONES.)

Bile Acids

Steroid acids produced from the liver.

Bilharziosis

Bilharziosis is a disease caused by bilharziae or schistosomes; these are parasites of about 0.25 to 1 centimetre in length which are sometimes found in the bloodstream of cattle and sheep in Europe, and of horses, camels, cattle, sheep, and donkeys in India, Japan, and the northern seaboard countries of Africa. (See SCHISTOMIASIS.) Dogs may also suffer from these flukes.

Biliary Fever

(see CANINE BABESIOSIS; EQUINE BILIARY FEVER)

Bilirubin

A bile pigment circulating in blood; it is a breakdown product of the blood pigment haem.

Binovular Twins

Binovular Twins result from the fertilisation of 2 ova, as distinct from 'monovular twins' which arise from a single ovum.

Biocide

A biocide destroys living organisms; sodium hypochlorite (bleach) is an example.

Bioluminescence

The emission of light by an organism, such as is seen in fireflies and some fish. It results from a chemical reaction which produces light with virtually no heat.

Biomass

All the living organisms in a given area. In veterinary practice, the term is used to express stocking density as kilograms of live animals per square metre of floor space.

Biopsy

Biopsy is a diagnostic method in which a small portion of living tissue is removed from an animal and examined by special means in the laboratory so that a diagnosis may be made.

Biotechnology

The application of biological knowledge, of micro-organisms, systems or processes to a wide range of activities, such as cheese-making, animal production, waste recycling, pollution control, and human and veterinary medicine. For the manipulation of genes, see GENETIC ENGINEERING.

Biotechnology and Biological Sciences Research Council

The body established in 1994 which incorporates the work of the Agriculture and Food Research Council, and the Biotechnology Directorate and Biological Sciences Committee of the former Science and Engineering Research Council.

Biotin

A water soluble vitamin of the B group; also known as vitamin H.

A deficiency of biotin is linked to foot problems, mainly associated with the hoof. The hoof horn in horses is believed to be strengthened by a biotin-rich diet; foot lesions in pigs (see illustration) may similarly benefit, as may 'soft' or diseased claws of dogs.

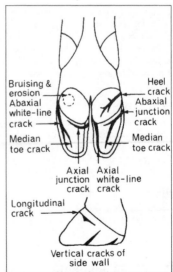

The position of foot lesions in pigs suffering from a biotin deficiency. (With acknowledgements to Dr Peter Brooks.)

Biotype

A group or strain of a micro-organism or species that has distinguishable physiological characteristics.

B

Bird-Fancier's Lung

Patients may be regarded as having bird-fancier's lung if they satisfy all the following criteria: recent history of avian exposure; serum avian precipitins; diffuse shadowing on chest radiograph; a significant reduction (less than 70 per cent predicted value) of carbon-monoxide transfer factor (single breath); and improvement or no deterioration when exposure to birds and their excreta is ceased.

In some cases there have been changes in the intestine (villous atrophy).

In the acute form, most often seen in pigeon-fanciers after cleaning the loft, influenza-like symptoms, a shortness of breath and a cough occur after 4 to 6 hours. The disease in elderly patients has to be differentiated from bronchitis and emphysema.

Bird Import Controls

Bird import controls were imposed in Great Britain in 1976, and a licence is required for all imports of captive birds and hatching eggs. All birds except those from Belgium are subject to a quarantine of 35 days. Birds imported into the EU are subject to quarantine. (See also PIGEONS.)

Bird Louse

Bird louse is a parasitic insect belonging to the order Mallophaga, which attacks most domesticated and many wild birds. The lice eat feathers and the cells shed from the surface of the skin, but they do not suck blood. Dusting with parasiticide powder is an efficient remedy. (See LICE.)

Bird Malaria

A tropical disease of fowls and turkeys caused by *Plasmodium gallinaceum, P. durae* and other species, transmitted by mosquitoes.

It may run a rapidly fatal course, or a chronic one with anaemia and greenish diarrhoea.

Birds

(see under AVIAN; also CAGE BIRDS; GAME BIRDS; TURKEYS; POULTRY; ORNITHOSIS; BOTULISM; DUCK; FALCONS; PETS; RABIES; OSTRICH; RHEA.)

Birds, Blood Sampling

The toenail-clip method enables blood to be collected into a micro-haematocrit tube or pipette. The bird can be held with its back against the palm of the hand, head between thumb and forefinger.

Larger cage birds have easily accessible jugular veins. In raptors, fowl and pigeons, the brachial vein is favoured; the tarsal vein is preferred for blood sampling in water fowl.

Birds, Humane Destruction of

For poultry and other birds, a lidless wooden box or chamber (of a size to take a polypropylene poultry crate) and a cylinder of carbon dioxide with regulating valve are useful. The box has a 1.3-cm (½-in) copper pipe drilled with 0.35-cm (⁹⁄₆₄-in) holes at 10-cm (4-in) centres fitted at levels 5 cm (2 in) and 66 cm (2 ft 2 in) from the bottom and connected by plastic tubing to the regulator valve of the cylinder.

Birdsville Disease

Birdsville disease occurs in parts of Australia, is due to a poisonous plant *Indigofera enneaphylla*, and has to be differentiated from Kimberley horse disease.

Sings Sleepiness and abnormal gait with front legs lifted high. Chronic cases drag the hind limbs.

Birth

(see PARTURITION)

Bismuth (Bi)

Bismuth (Bi) is one of the heavy metals.

Uses The carbonate, subnitrate, and the salicylate may be used in irritable and painful conditions of the stomach and intestines; also to relieve diarrhoea and vomiting.

The oxychloride and the subnitrate are used like barium, in bismuth meals prior to taking X-ray photographs of the abdominal organs for purposes of diagnosis.

Bistoury

A surgical knife used to open up stenosed (closed up) teats, fistulae, sinuses; and abscesses.

Bites, Stings and Poisoned Wounds

The bites of animals, whether domesticated or otherwise, should always be looked upon as infected WOUNDS. In countries where RABIES is present, the spread of this disease is generally by means of a bite.

TETANUS is always a hazard from bites.

Bees, wasps and hornets cause great irritation by the stings with which the females are provided. Death has been reported in pigs eating windfall apples in which wasps were feeding. The wasps stung the mucous membrane of the throat, causing great swelling and death from suffocation some hours later.

Antihistamine preparations may be used in treatment if numerous stings make this necessary.

Cat-bites are usually followed by some degree of suppuration. *Pasteurella multocida* infection of the bite wound is common. (See also RABIES; CAT-SCRATCH FEVER.)

Dog-bites are usually inflicted upon other dogs, defenceless sheep or goats, and sometimes pigs; cattle may be bitten by the herd's dog and serious wounds result. The bite is generally a punctured wound, or large tear, depending upon the part that is bitten. Where an animal is bitten in numerous places, even though no individual bite is large, there is always a considerable degree of danger. Antibiotics should be given by injection. The wounds should be dressed with some suitable antiseptic, the hair or wool being first clipped from the area; and left open. (See WOUNDS; RABIES.)

In the USA about a million dog-bites a year require medical treatment of people; and in the UK the figure has been estimated as about 99,000. Dog-bite wounds are often infected by *Pseudomonas* species, *Staphylococcus aureus*, *Streptococcus viridans*, *Pasteurella multocida*, and Group EF-4 bacteria.

Horse-bites Actinobacillosis has been transmitted to a bitten person.

Monkey-bites can transmit encephalitis caused by *Herpes simiae*; human infectious hepatitis; also TB. (*Lancet*, **2**, 553.)

Snake-bites (see SNAKES)

Spider-bites (see SPIDERS)

Bittersweet Poisoning

The common 'bittersweet' – *Solanum dulcamara* – is a frequent denizen of hedgerows and waste lands, and, although not likely to be eaten to a great extent by domesticated animals, cases of poisoning due to its ingestion have been recorded. All parts of the plant – stem, leaves, and berries – contain the toxic principle, which is an alkaloid similar to *Solanine* found in the potato.

Signs In cattle and sheep the symptoms are giddiness, quickening of the respiration, staggering gait, dilated pupil, greenish diarrhoea, and raised temperature.

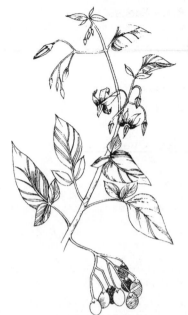

Bittersweet (*Solanum dulcamara*) has purple flowers with bright yellow anthers. The berries are first green, then yellow, finally turning to a brilliant red. This is a climbing plant and may reach a height of 2 m (6 ft) or so. Bittersweet is also known as woody nightshade.

Black Disease

Black disease is the name given to infectious necrotic hepatitis of sheep and occasionally of cattle in Australia, New Zealand, Scotland, Wales, and NW England. It is typically caused by a combined attack of immature liver flukes and bacteria, e.g. *Clostridium oedematiens*, which is one of the so-called 'gas gangrene' group, and is capable of forming resistant spores.

On post-mortem examination the most striking feature is the rapidity with which sheep dead from this disease have undergone decomposition. In carcases of sheep recently dead or killed in the later stages, the skin is a dark bluish-black colour, and the underlying tissues are congested and oedematous. In the liver, where the most constant lesions are found, there are one or more necrotic areas about 2.5 cm (1 in) in diameter.

In cattle, black disease caused by *Clostridium noyvi* (*Cl. oedematiens* type B) may not be associated with liver fluke.

Prevention An antiserum and a vaccine are available.

Black Faeces

Black faeces are passed when either iron or bismuth salts are given to dogs and pigs. The most serious cause of black motions is haemorrhage into the early part of the digestive system. A dark-coloured diarrhoea may be seen in the dog suffering from deficiency of the B vitamin.

Black-Leg

(see BLACK-QUARTER)

Black-Quarter

Black-quarter, also called black-leg, quarter-ill, etc., is an acute specific infectious disease of cattle, sometimes of sheep, and likewise of pigs, characterised by the presence of rapidly increasing swellings containing gas, and occurring in the region of the shoulder, neck, thigh, quarter, and sometimes in the diaphragm. Young cattle between the ages of 3 months and 2 years are most susceptible.

The disease has been seen in the reindeer, camel, and the buffalo.

Causes *Clostridium chauvoei*, which lives in the soil until such time as it gains entry into the animal body either along with the food or else by abrasions of the skin (see TATTOOING).

On exposure to the air, the organisms form spores which are resistant to extreme cold, or heat.

Signs The finding of a dead animal may be the first indication of the disease; though sometimes lameness is observed, and part of the udder swollen and very painful. If seen in the early stages, the swelling is hot and pits on pressure, but, increasing rapidly, it becomes puffed up with gas (emphysematous), and if pressed it crackles as if filled with screwed-up tissue-paper. Death usually occurs within 24 hours. Sheep show somewhat similar symptoms, but they may be attacked at almost any age. There are often blood-stained discharges from both the nostrils and the rectum.

Prevention Marshy ground that has been responsible for the loss of numerous animals in the past has often been rendered safe by the draining of the land and heavy liming.

Vaccine A vaccine gives very good results.

Curative There is generally no opportunity to treat cases, since death occurs after only a few hours' illness; otherwise penicillin and antiserum may be tried.

'Black Tongue'

The counterpart of human pellagra. It is shown in the dog fed a diet deficient in nicotinic acid.

(See also SHEEPDOGS *and* 'BROWN MOUTH'.) Symptoms include discoloration of the tongue, a foul odour from the mouth, ulceration, loss of appetite, and sometimes blood-stained saliva and faeces. Death will occur in the absence of treatment.

Black Vomit

Black vomit is due to the presence of blood in the stomach. Either the appearance of the vomit may be that of black masses of clotted blood, or it may resemble coffee-grounds.

Black-Water Fever

A form of babesiosis (see under BABESIA); also known as TEXAS FEVER.

Blackhead of Turkeys (Histomoniasis)

Blackhead of turkeys (histomoniasis) is a very common and fatal disease of young turkeys (from 3 weeks to 4 months old), which is caused by a small protozoon parasite, *Histomonas meleagridis*, which passes part of its life in a worm (*Heterakis gallinae*); this acts as an intermediate host. The histomonas is found in adult worms and eggs; ingestion of the latter is the chief means of spread.

Though turkeys are chiefly affected, the disease may be seen in chickens, partridges, pheasants, grouse, quail and pea-fowl.

Signs Loss of appetite and of condition. The droppings may be semi-liquid and bright yellow. Death, in 5 to 8 days, may occur in 70 to 90 per cent of turkeys, in which the disease is very acute and prevalent in summer and autumn.

Treatment Dinitridazole or nifursol, administered in the feed, may be used for prevention and treatment.

Blad

Abbreviation for BOVINE LEUKOCYTE ADHESION DEFICIENCY.

Bladder, Diseases of

(see under URINARY BLADDER, DISEASES OF; also GALL-BLADDER)

Blastocyst

Blastocyst is the name given to a very early stage in the development of the fetus.

Blastomycosis of Dogs

Infection with *Blastomyces dermatitidis*.

The disease is fairly common in both man and dogs in North America. Diagnosis depends

B

upon a laboratory demonstration of the fungus, which typically causes chronic debility often with a fatal outcome.

Infection is usually through inhalation. Bone lesions, resulting in lameness, often occur; sometimes the brain, nose, eyes, and prostate gland show lesions.

'Bleeder Horses'

Those which show blood at their nostrils after hard exercise. (See also RACEHORSES – Pulmonary haemorrhage.)

Bleeding (Haemorrhage)

Bleeding (haemorrhage) may be classified according to the vessel or vessels from which it escapes: e.g. (a) arterial, in which the blood is of a bright scarlet colour and issues in jets or spurts corresponding in rate and rhythm to the heart-beats; (b) venous, when it comes from veins, is of a dark colour, and wells up from the depth of a wound in a steady stream; and (c) capillary, when it gradually oozes from a slight injury to the network of capillaries of an area. (See also under CANINE HAEMOPHILIA; HAEMOR-RHAGIC DIATHESIS; INTERNAL HAEMORRHAGE.)

Natural arrest When an artery with a small calibre is cut, the muscular fibres in its middle coat shrink, and the cut end is slightly retracted within the stiffer fibrous covering. This results in a diminution in the size of the cut end and in a lessened capacity for output of blood. In the space between the end of the muscular coat and at the end of the fibrous coat a tiny clot commences to form, which, later, is continued into the lumen of the vessel. This is added to by further coagulation of blood, until the whole of the open end of the vessel and of the cavity of the wound is sealed by a clot. A fall in blood-pressure, due to shock and loss of blood, contributes to the natural arrest of bleeding. (See CLOTTING.)

Bleeding, external: first aid for

When a vein is cut, crimson blood will flow. From a cut artery, scarlet blood will spurt, issuing in jets corresponding with the heartbeats.

When a large vessel is cut, pressure should be applied above the wound if the bleeding is from an artery, below it if bleeding is from a vein; but the first-aider should take precautions (see RESTRAINT).

Pressure with the fingers is a helpful preliminary while someone else is finding material to use as a pressure pad. For large animals a clean pillowslip, small towel, or piece of sheet will serve; for small animals a clean handkerchief

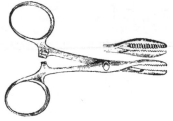

Artery forceps, with jaws shown enlarged.

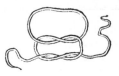

Surgeon's knot, or reef knot, used for ligaturing cut vessels.

may suffice. The pad is then placed over the wound, and held there; pressure being applied and maintained for a quarter of an hour.

Tourniquet Only if these measures fail to stop serious haemorrhage should a tourniquet be used. A tourniquet can be improvised from a rolled handkerchief, its two ends knotted, slipped around the limb, and tightened with a pencil. Tightening must be just sufficient to stop the bleeding, no more. For large animals a piece of rubber tubing or a soft rope may be used. **A tourniquet must never be left on for more than 20 minutes, or permanent damage to the limb will result.** When releasing the tourniquet, do so gradually. A tourniquet should not be used on cats, in which a pressure pad will suffice to control bleeding.

Professional help should be obtained as soon as possible.

Sometimes the actual point or points of bleeding cannot be located, especially when the wound is deep or ragged, and the blood issues in a more or less continuous stream showing no tendency to clot. In such cases it is necessary to resort to packing the wound with GELATIN SPONGE.

Professional help will also be needed to counter SHOCK. (See also BLOOD TRANSFUSIONS; DEXTRAN.)

Bleeding from special parts

(1) *The Horns* The horns of cattle are sometimes broken by falls or blows, and severe bleeding follows. If the horn is broken completely off, the haemorrhage is to the outside

from the stump, but it often happens that while the bony horn-core is fractured the horn itself holds the broken end in position, and the escaping blood finds its way down into the frontal sinus and out by the nostril. Haemorrhage from a stump may be controlled by the application of a pad and a bandage. Thermocautery, using a disbudding iron, may assist.

(2) *Legs and Feet* The tourniquet described above may be applied, to the lower side of the injury if the bleeding is venous, and above if it be arterial. When the upper parts of the limbs are injured and the haemorrhage is considerable, one of the methods of pressure is adopted until professional veterinary aid can be obtained.

(3) *Stomach* The vomiting of blood by dogs, cats, and pigs in considerable amounts is a very serious symptom of severe injury or disease in the stomach.

A dog may be offered ice cubes to lick. The animal should be kept as still as possible, and veterinary assistance obtained. Alcohol is not advisable, as it causes a dilatation of the vessels of the stomach wall and tends to promote the bleeding.

(4) *Uterus and Vagina* After parturition in all animals there is a certain risk of haemorrhage, especially in those which have a diffuse placenta, such as the mare and ass, and when the fetal membranes have been forcibly removed. If it is copious, it may prove fatal. Prompt veterinary attention is necessary. (See also under WOUNDS; INTERNAL HAEMORRHAGE.)

(5) *Navel* in piglets. See under VITAMINS – Vitamin deficiencies for prevention.

Bleeding, internal (see INTERNAL HAEMORRHAGE).

Blepharitis
Inflammation of the eyelids. It is usually associated with conjunctivitis.

Blepharospasm
Blepharospasm is a spasm of the eyelids.

Blindness
(see under EYE, DISEASES OF; also VISION)

Bloat
Also known as ruminal tympany, it occurs in cattle, sheep, and goats. With the increased use of lucerne and clovers, bloat has become of more common occurrence among cattle and is now a matter of serious economic importance. It may be of two types: free gas bloat or frothy bloat.

Free gas bloat The rumen becomes distended with gas, and pressure is exerted upon the diaphragm.

The medium-sized cow's rumen has a capacity of some 160 litres (35 gallons), and fermentation within it gives rise to bubbles of gas. This comprises carbon dioxide (CO_2) and methane (CH_4) in surprisingly large quantities; cattle producing as much as 800 litres of CO_2 in 24 hours, and as much as 500 litres of CH_4. Some of this gas, perhaps a quarter, escapes via the bloodstream to the lungs and is breathed out, but that still leaves a great deal which can be expelled only by belching. If something makes that impossible, then gas pressure builds up and is exerted on the diaphragm, heart and lungs, so that the cow is soon in considerable distress.

The cow's ability to belch may be affected by physical obstruction of the oesophagus; paralysis of the muscular wall of the rumen; and foaming of the rumen contents.

The first diagram shows a healthy state of affairs in the rumen, with the cardia – a muscular valve at the junction of oesophagus and rumen – temporarily open so that gas can escape up the oesophagus. But when this tube is obstructed by a piece of turnip or a tumour or an abscess, the gas cannot get away (or not in sufficient quantity), and 'gassy bloat' results. Paralysis of the muscular wall of the rumen has a similar effect, since expulsion of gas is aided by contraction of these muscles.

The most common cause of gassy bloat is ruminal acidosis following a barley diet, or in cases of obstruction or dysfunction of the oesophageal or cardiac sphincter.

In such cases an antacid drench may be effective, but passing a stomach tube, where this is practicable, can provide immediate relief by the release of trapped gas. Veterinary advice should be sought.

In an emergency a RUMENOTOMY may be performed or a trochar and cannula used.

Frothy bloat With the frothy type of bloat, puncturing the rumen with a trocar and cannula in an emergency may do more harm than good – not releasing gas and perhaps causing leakage of some solids into the abdominal cavity.

This frothy type of bloat is the more important from an economic point of view, as it can occur simultaneously in a number of animals, with a fatal outcome. The second

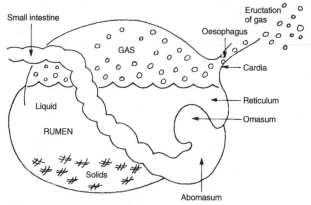

The normal rumen with gas able to escape

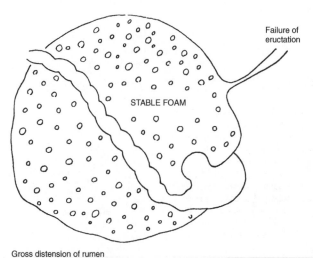

Gross distension of rumen

Acute frothy bloat – stable foam fills the rumen.

diagram shows the rumen distended by foam, with bubbles of gas trapped and unable to escape.

Signs The left side of the body, between the last rib and the hip bone, is seen to be swollen; the whole abdomen gradually becoming tense and drum-like. There is obvious distress on the part of the animal which appears restless. Breathing is rapid. (See TYMPANITIC RESONANCE.)

Prevention Frothy bloat may be prevented by limiting access to pasture, avoiding fine milled feeds and/or including an anti-foaming agent

such as poloxalene ('Bloatguard'). Dimethicone ('Birp') may also be used in the treatment of frothy bloat. A solution of sodium bicarbonate, 150 g in 1 litre (5 oz in 2 pints) of water, administered by stomach tube, is also useful.

Low-protein, low-energy supplements decreased the incidence of bloat in cattle on a high clover sward, compared with a control group in a 1996 study by C. J. C. Phillips, of Cambridge, and colleagues.

Bloat in Pigs

Bloat in Pigs affects not the stomach but the small intestine, excluding the duodenum. It is sometimes referred to as 'colonic bloat' or 'whey bloat'. (See HAEMORRHAGIC GASTROENTERITIS.)

B Block, Nerve

Applying local anaesthesia to the nerve(s) supplying a specific area to remove sensation in that part of an animal.

Blonde D'aquitaine

A French breed of cattle, for which an English breed society has been formed. (See BEEF BREEDS.)

Blood

Blood is a slightly alkaline fluid which serves as a carrier of nutrients from the digestive system to the various tissues, transports oxygen from the lungs and carbon dioxide to the lungs, carries hormones from the endocrine glands, maintains a correct water balance in the body and assists with temperature control, carries waste products to the kidneys, and has an important role in the defence of the body against bacteria, viruses, etc. By its ability to clot (see CLOTTING), blood has its own built-in safety factor for use in the event of damage to the blood vessels. Blood also assists in the maintenance of the correct pH of tissues.

Composition Blood consists of a fluid portion, or plasma, in which blood-cells are suspended. They are of three chief varieties: red blood-cells (or corpuscles), white blood-cells, and platelets.

Plasma forms about 66 per cent of the total amount of the blood and contains three protein groups – fibrinogen, serum globulin, and serum albumin. Fibrinogen is of great interest and importance, owing to its role in the coagulation of the blood.

When shed, plasma separates into two parts: a liquid, which is called serum, and a solid, which is the fibrin clot. Blood serum is therefore plasma which has lost its fibrinogen, the latter having gone to form the fibrin of the clot; but it contains two newly-formed proteins – fibrino-globulin and nucleo-protein. These are derivatives of fibrinogen which are split off from the fibrinogen when it forms the fibrin clot. (See GAMMA GLOBULIN.)

Besides the proteins mentioned above, the plasma contains non-protein nitrogenous material such as amino acids; waste products such as urea; glucose; fats; inorganic salts of sodium, potassium, calcium, magnesium, etc.

Red blood-cells constitute about 32 per cent of the total amount of the blood. Seen under the microscope they appear as biconcave discs, circular in shape, and they possess no nucleus – having lost it before entering the circulation. (*Note.* The red blood-cells of birds, fish and reptiles possess a nucleus.)

Red cells are soft, flexible, elastic envelopes containing the red blood-pigment known as haemoglobin, which is held in position by a spongy lacework of threads called stroma. They are present in large numbers in the blood. In the horse they number about 7 to 9 million per cubic millimetre, and about 6 million in the ox, on an average.

The red blood-cells are destroyed after 3 or 4 months in the circulation. New red blood-cells are formed in the red marrow of the bones, and appear first of all as nucleated red cells, called erythroblasts.

Packed cell volume The height of the column of red cells, as a percentage of total height, of a sample of centrifuged blood in the tube. The red cells lie at the bottom; the middle layer consists of the white blood-cells and platelets; and the top layer is the serum.

Blood platelets, or thrombocytes, reduce loss of blood from injured vessels by the formation of a white clot. (For a deficiency of platelets, see under THROMBOCYTOPENIA.)

Haemoglobin – a complex substance – has the power of absorbing oxygen in the lungs, parting with it to the tissues, receiving carbon dioxide in exchange, and finally, of yielding up this carbon dioxide in the lungs. When haemoglobin carries oxygen it is temporarily changed into oxyhaemoglobin, and when it is carrying carbon dioxide it is known as carboxyhaemoglobin. The process of oxidation and reduction proceeds with every respiratory cycle.

'Haemolysis' is a process by which the haemoglobin of the red blood-cells becomes dissolved and liberated from the cell-envelope. Anything which kills the cell or destroys the envelope can result in this. Natural serum of one animal can act as a haemolytic agent when injected into the body of another animal of a different species. The serum from a dog is haemolytic to the red blood-cells of a rabbit, but if this serum be heated to 57°C (135°F) it loses its haemolytic powers. The heat has destroyed the agent which caused the haemolysis.

'Agglutination' is the process by which the red cells of the blood are collected together into clumps, under the action of an agent in the blood called an 'agglutinin'. It sometimes precedes haemolysis.

White blood-cells (leukocytes) can be seen in among the red cells when blood is examined under the microscope. They are larger and fewer than the red cells, and nucleated, and possess the power of amoeboid movement. They exist in a varying proportion to the red cells, from 1 to 300, to as few as 1 to 700, and their numbers are liable to great fluctuation in the same animal at different times.

White blood-cells comprise the following:

Neutrophils, in which the cytoplasm contains granules which – with stains containing eosin and methylene blue – are not coloured markedly red or blue. The nuclei are of many shapes, and the term polymorphonuclear leukocytes is applied to neutrophils. They can migrate from the blood-vessels into the tissues and engulf bacteria (phagocytosis); are found in pus; and are very important in defence against infection.

Eosinophils have red-staining granules, contain hydrolytic enzymes, and have been observed to increase in numbers during the course of certain chronic diseases.

Basophils have blue-staining granules, containing histamine which is secreted during allergy. Basophils and mast cells have receptors for IgE antibodies, and when basophils with IgE antibodies on their surfaces are stimulated by antigen (usually of parasitic origin) they release histamine. In severe reactions the animal may die.

Monocytes have very few granules, engulf bacteria, and are important in less acute infections than those dealt with by neutrophils. When they migrate from blood-vessels into surrounding tissues, they increase in size and are called macrophages.

Lymphocytes also have few granules and are likewise formed in lymphoid tissue, e.g. lymph nodes, spleen, tonsils. B and T cells are concerned with antibody formation and form barriers against local disease. (See B CELLS.)

Coagulation (see under CLOTTING)

Temperature The temperature of the blood is not uniform throughout the body. It is coolest near the surface, and hottest in the hepatic veins. It varies from 38° to 40°C (100° to 105°F).

Blood, Diseases of

(see ANAEMIA, and the blood disorders given under that heading; also LEUKAEMIA; THROMBOCYTOPENIA; FOALS, DISEASES OF – Haemolytic disease; THROM-

BASTHENIA; CANINE HAEMOPHILIA; LEUKOPENIA; HAEMOLYSIS; VIRAEMIA; PYAEMIA; TOXAEMIA; SEPTICAEMIA)

Blood Enzymes

See creatine kinase, under CREATINE for a reference to diagnosis. Other blood enzymes, now routinely used in diagnosis, include: aldolase, alkaline phosphatase, alanine aminotransferase, aspartate aminotransferase, acetycholinesterase, gamma glutamyltransferase, glutathione peroxidase, α-hydroxybutyrate dehydrogenase, lactate dehydrogenase and superoxide dismutase.

For information on their activities in fresh serum, as compared with those in plasma containing anticoagulants and preservatives, see Jones, D. G. *Research in Veterinary Science*, **38**, 301.

Blood Parasites of British Cattle

Piroplasms	Babesia divergens (Redwater agent)
	B. major
	Theileria mutans
	T. sergenti
Rickettsiae	Cytoectes (=Ehrlichia) phago-cytophilia (Tick-borne fever agent)
	Haemobartonella bovis
	Eperythrozoon wenyoni
	E. tuomi
	E. teganodes
Flagellate	Trypanosoma theileri

Blood Poisoning

Commonly used term for bacteraemia (bacteria or toxins in the blood) or septicaemia, the same with signs of illness.

Blood Spots in Eggs

A vitamin A supplement for hens has been suggested as a means of ridding eggs of this unappetising but harmless defect.

Blood Transfusions

Blood transfusions may be used in veterinary practice in cases of anaemia and certain other blood disorders. Transfusions may also be life-saving where it is necessary to replace blood loss caused by accident, haemorrhage and shock. Plasma-substitute fluids and modified gelatin solutions, however, are often more convenient where rapid restoration of normal fluid volume is the main concern.

Blood donors must be healthy animals of the same species. Up to 10 per cent of the blood volume can usually be taken without ill effect. As a rough guide, 1 per cent of the donor's body

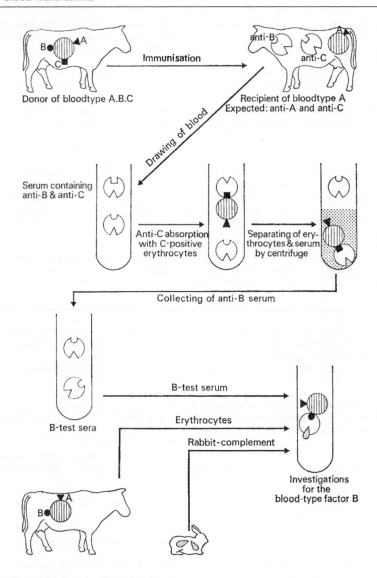

The principles of producing a test serum and its use in blood grouping. (With acknowledgements to Dr J. Moustgaard, Royal Veterinary and Agricultural College, Copenhagen.)

weight (300 ml for a 30 kg dog) may be taken. In dogs, which have 8 blood groups, adverse reactions due to incompatible blood types are rarely seen. Cats have 3 blood types: A and B, in the ratio 3:1, and AB (less than 1 per cent). Matching of donor and recipient blood should be done before transfusion, if possible.

Blood is conveniently collected from the jugular vein. Donors should be sedated and the skin in the area shaved and cleaned. A hypodermic needle or catheter is inserted and blood collected into a blood bag (dog) or 50 ml syringe (cat) containing an anticoagulant such as sodium citrate or acid citrate dextrose.

Collected blood may be stored for up to 4 weeks if refrigerated; it should be warmed to body heat before administration. This should be via a jugular or cephalic vein.

In cattle, donor and recipient are usually in the same herd, a fact which lessens the risk of introducing infection. Blood is collected from the jugular or other vein (after the skin has been cleaned and precautions taken to ensure asepsis) by means of a suitable needle (e.g.13 swg) and allowed to flow into a blood bag or sterilised bottle containing anticoagulant. This may be made by dissolving 60 mg of sodium citrate in a little water, for every 100 ml blood collected. The bottle should be shaken gently during collection. The donor's blood is then transferred to the recipient's vein. Transfusion reactions rarely occur during a first transfusion.

In the new-born foal suffering from haemolytic disease, exchange transfusion has been the means of saving life. Up to 5500 ml of the foal's blood is removed and replaced by up to 7000 ml of compatible donor's blood. The process takes up to 3 hours and requires special apparatus. See also DEXTRAN; GELATIN, SUCCINYLATED; also under FELINE INFECTIOUS ENTERITIS; DEHYDRATION.

Blood Typing, Cattle

In Canada extensive use is made of blood typing in respect of cattle, and results of a blood test have been accepted as evidence in court in a case where a man was convicted of falsifying a pedigree. The basis of this evidence was that to prove parentage of an animal, all the factors found in the blood of a calf must be present in the blood of either the sire or the dam. If certain factors found in the blood of the calf could not be found in the blood of either the sire or the dam, then that calf could not have been of that particular mating – as was proved in this case.

Blood typing is also used in the diagnosis of freemartins. In one series 228 freemartins were found out of 242 sets of twins.

Blood typing has been used to decide the paternity issue in a heifer calf born to a cow inseminated twice in the same heat period with semen from two different bulls; to reveal discrepancies in pedigrees; and to allay or confirm suspicion on the part of a Breed Society asked to register a calf born following a very short or a very long gestation period.

The work falls into two categories: commercial and research. In the former category there are routine pedigree parentage cases involving one bull, one cow, and one calf. In a series of 403 such cases, 26 (or 6.5 per cent) were found to be incorrect. Checking the parentage of bulls to be used in AI (see ARTIFICIAL INSEMINATION) as well as typing bulls being used in AI is carried out. Other applications include the diagnosis of freemartins, and the control of egg transplantation – i.e. checking that the offspring is from the egg put in and not from the host cow's own egg.

Blood typing is of service in the policing of screening tests, e.g. for brucellosis. It is not unknown for lazy or unscrupulous people to fill several sample tubes with blood from the same animal and label them as coming from several animals. If several tubes are found to have identical types, fraud is virtually certain to have occurred, since the likelihood of two samples, other than from identical twins, having the same blood type is negligible.

Thoroughbred horses must all be blood-typed as an aid to identification. (See also EQUINE BLOOD TYPING.)

The Preparation of Test Sera containing antibodies, or blood-group reagents, is based on the injection of blood corpuscles from one animal into another of the same species, or into one of a different species. The first procedure is called iso-immunisation, the second hetero-immunisation. As a result of both procedures, the recipient animal produces antibodies to the antigenic factors associated with the donor blood corpuscles, provided that these factors are not already present in the recipient animal. (No animal can produce both an antigen and its antibody.) The diagram demonstrates the principle of iso-immunisation in cattle.

It shows that the donor possesses blood-group factors A, B, and C while the recipient has only blood-group factor A. On immunisation, the recipient will therefore form antibodies to blood group factors B and C. The antibodies thus formed are called anti-B and anti-C. A serum containing several blood group antibodies is known as a crude serum. This serum will react with red corpuscles not only from the donor, but also from all cattle with the blood group factor B or C.

To obtain a blood group reagent which reacts with only one blood group factor – for example B – the anti-C antibody must be removed. To do this, the prepared crude serum is mixed with blood corpuscles which are C-positive but B-negative. The anti-C is then bound to the blood corpuscles and can be removed by centrifuging, as illustrated. This procedure is called antibody absorption. As the figure indicates, a specific B-reagent prepared in this way can be used to decide whether the blood group factor B is or is not present in a cow or bull, provided that rabbit complement is also present.

To obtain sufficiently high concentration of antibodies, donor blood corpuscles are injected into the recipient once a week for 4 to 6 weeks. The antibody concentration of the recipient's blood serum, or its titre, is estimated by determining the power of the serum to react with donor blood corpuscles, or with blood corpuscles possessing a similar antigenic structure. In some cases, one single period of immunisation is inadequate to achieve a satisfactorily high antibody concentration in the recipient's blood. This can often be achieved, however, by repeating the immunisation a few months later (reimmunisation). (See also TRANSFERRIN; EQUINE BLOOD TYPING; monoclonal antibodies under GENETIC ENGINEERING; ELECTROPHORESIS.)

Blood Urea Nitrogen (BUN)

Used as a measure of urea in the blood.

Bloodhound

A large breed of dog with pendulous ears and a lugubrious expression, possessed of an acute sense of smell; have been much used as police tracker dogs in consequence. The amount of loose skin on the face leads to both entropion and ectropion. May inherit elbow joint problems (ununited anconeal process) and posterior paralysis (Stockard's disease). Gastric torsion is not uncommon.

Blouwildebeesoog

A disease of sheep, cattle and horses, characterised by enlargement of the eyes leading to blindness. It occurs in Africa, and is apparently spread by blue-wildebeest.

Blowfly

Insects of the family Calliphoridae.

Blowfly Eradication

Sterile genetically engineered blowfly maggots have been used in attempts to eradicate blowfly infestation.

Blowfly Strike

Infestation of the skin with the maggots of blowfly; cutaneous myiasis.

Blowpipe Darts

(see PROJECTILE SYRINGE)

'Blows'

Distension of the caecum in the rabbit as a result of excessive gas formation. The rabbit assumes a huddled posture.

Bluebottle

Blowfly.

Blue Comb

Another name for 'PULLET DISEASE'.

'Blue-Ear' Disease of Pigs

Also known as porcine reproductive respiratory disease (PRRS). This devastating disease was first recognised in Europe and the USA in the late 1980s.

Cause A virus of the arterivirus genus. The infection can be wind-borne.

Signs Cyanosis of the extremities (hence the name 'blue-ear' disease) affected up to 2 per cent only of dry sows in the UK. An increase in abortions occurred in up to 3.3 per cent of sows. Premature farrowings in up to 20.6 per cent were recorded; mortality in neonatal and pre-weaning piglets was as high as 88 per cent, with a low mortality in fattening pigs. It often results in an upsurge of other latent infections in the herd, with respiratory problems being common.

Once the disease is established in a herd, little can be done. Immunity tends to build up but susceptibility may recur. As with other infectious diseases, 'All in, all out' management is advisable to control PRRS.

Diagnosis Confirmation of the disease is by serological tests.

Blue-Green Algae

(see CYANOBACTERIA)

Blue-Gray

The offspring of a Galloway or of an Aberdeen Angus crossed with a Beef Shorthorn bull. Often used as suckler cows in bleaker areas of Britain.

'Blue-Nose' Disease

'Blue-nose' disease is a form of LIGHT SENSITISATION occurring in the horse, following the eating of some particular meadow plant. The name arises from the blue discoloration observed in some cases on the muzzle (but not, for example, on the same animal's white socks). Sloughing of the non-pigmented skin occurs, and there is often intense excitement amounting to frenzy – during which the horse may injure itself. (See also ANTIHISTAMINES.)

Bluetongue

A viral disease of ruminants confined mainly to Africa but which has spread to North America and Australia, Portugal, Spain, and Cyprus and, more recently, Italy and France. Bluetongue is a NOTIFIABLE DISEASE throughout the EU.

Infection is carried by biting midges and probably the mosquito, and consequently outbreaks are commonest near the breeding haunts of such insects – damp, marshy regions.

Cattle may be symptomless carriers. A survey of 6250 sera from cattle, sheep and goats in seven Caribbean and two South American countries showed that antibody to bluetongue virus was widely distributed. Overall prevalences of antibody were 70 per cent in cattle, 67 per cent in sheep, and 76 per cent in goats. Yet, no clinical cases had been confirmed in the area; no virus isolates were available to indicate which serotype(s) was/were causing the infection.

To prevent entry of bluetongue to the EU from Canada, cattle must have a negative blood test in January; they can then be exported to the EU if they leave Canada between February 1 and April 15. This procedure ensures that they were not infected the previous summer and move out of the country before the midges carrying the infection become active.

Cause An orbivirus.

Signs In sheep, a rise in temperature up to 41.5° C (107°F), and after a week or 10 days, eruptions on the tongue, lips, and dental pads – with a swelling and blueness of these parts – mark the typical appearance of an attack. Both the mouth and nose show a discharge, and there is an accompanying smacking of the lips. In spite of the soreness of the mouth the sheep are inclined to feed, but loss of flesh is very rapid, particularly when diarrhoea sets in. In 3 to 5 days, the mouth lesions begin to heal, and the disease is seen in the feet. These become sore; sheep are stiff, and feed from the kneeling or recumbent positions. Diagnosis may be confirmed by viral isolation.

In both cattle and sheep the disease may be subclinical.

Treatment Isolation of the affected animals into shady paddocks, sheds, or orchards, where they are immune from disturbance, antiseptic mouth washes, good feeding of a soft,

succulent quality, the provision of a clean water-supply and salt-licks. Dipping has given good results.

Prevention A stockpile of quadrivalent vaccine is stored at various sites in the EU.

Boarding Kennels
(see ANIMAL BOARDING ESTABLISHMENTS ACT)

Body-Scanner
(see under X-RAYS)

Bog Asphodel

(*Narthecium ossifragum*) A cause of light sensitisation in sheep. Ears, face, and legs of white lambs may all be affected. Skin necrosis may follow the inflammation. In severe cases, jaundice may be a complication.

Cows have been fatally poisoned by the plant as a result of necrosis of kidney tissue.

In one case, cattle forced by drought to graze swampy ground where bog asphodel grew suffered 137 deaths out of 232 cattle affected. The clinical signs included depression, anorexia and diarrhoea. Extensive kidney damage was caused.

Bog Spavin

An old name for chronic synovitis of the hock (*tarsus*) of horses. It often shows as a swelling of the front of the hock joint caused by fluid. It seldom causes lameness. (See also BONE SPAVIN.)

BOHB
(see BETAHYDROXYBUTYRATE)

Bollinger, Bodies
(see FOWL POX)

Bolus

A roughly spherical mass of food, which has been chewed and mixed with saliva, ready for swallowing. Bolus also means a cylindrical mass, 3.8 to 7.5 cm (1½ to 3 in) long, and up to 1.3 cm (½ in) in diameter, of a medicine in paste or solid form for administration to horses and cattle. It is also known as a 'ball' – hence 'balling gun'. Slow-release boluses which are retained in the rumen for the administration of anthelmintics or trace elements over a period are available in a variety of forms.

A bolus of slow dissolving soluble glass containing copper, selenium and cobalt for trace element supplementation in cattle and sheep is also available.

(See WORMS, FARM TREATMENT AGAINST – Administration.)

Bombay

A breed of cat developed in the USA by crossing black American shorthairs with Burmese cats. The breed has totally black, silky fur that is difficult to keep in good condition.

Bonamiasis

A NOTIFIABLE DISEASE in the UK and other parts of the EU; it affects shellfish, notably oysters, and is caused by *Bonamia ostreae*. It is controlled in the UK by the Fish Health Regulations 1997.

Bone

Bone is composed partly of fibrous tissue, partly of phosphate and carbonate of lime. Since the bones of a young animal are composed of about 60 per cent fibrous tissue, and those of an old animal of more than 60 per cent of lime salts, one readily understands the toughness of the former and the brittleness of the latter. Two kinds of bone are noteworthy: dense bone, such as forms the shafts of the long bones of the limbs, and cancellous or spongy bone, such as is found in the short bones and at the ends of the long bones. Dense bone is found in a tube-like form, with a central cavity in which normally yellow marrow is found, composed mainly of fatty substances; the walls of the tube are stout and strong, and the outer surface is covered by 'bone membrane' or periosteum. Cancellous bone has a more open framework, is irregular in shape, and, instead of possessing a cavity, its centre is divided into innumerable tiny spaces by a fine network of bony threads, which support the important red marrow. (See MARROW.)

All bone is penetrated by a series of fine canals (Haversian canals), in which run bloodvessels, nerves, lymph-vessels, etc., for the growth, maintenance, and repair of the bone.

Varieties of Bone Apart from their structural classification, bones are arranged according to their external shape into: (a) long bones, like those of the limbs; (b) short bones, such as those of the 'knee' and hock; (c) flat bones, such as those of the skull and the shoulder-blade; (d) irregular bones, such as those of the vertebral column; and (e) the 'spongy' bones of the feet

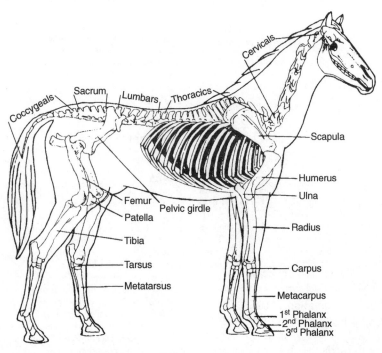

Skeleton of horse.

of horses and cattle and the claws of other animals.

The Skeleton has: (1) an axial part, consisting of the skull, the vertebrae, the ribs with their cartilages, and the sternum or breast-bone; and (2) an appendicular portion, consisting of the four limbs. In addition to these divisions, certain parts of the skeleton are embedded in the substance of organs, and are described as the visceral skeleton, e.g. the bones in the heart of the ox, the snout of the pig, the penis of the dog, etc.

Bone, Diseases of

Growth-plate disorders The growth-plate is a layer of cartilage between the diaphysis and the epiphysis of a long bone. Failure of chondrogenesis leading to cessation of growth is commonly the result of trauma to the plate, occasioned by a fracture or crush injury, or of the interruption of the vascular supply to the germinal cells. Diseases such as scurvy, rickets, osteomyelitis and endocrine disorders make the plate more vulnerable to injury and predispose to epiphyseal separation.

Epiphyseal injury in the foal, for example, may be of two types:
Type 1 Separation without fracture. After realignment healing is rapid and the prognosis is good. Femoral head detachment is the exception because if the epiphyseal vessels are damaged, avascular necrosis of the head follows.
Type 2 The most common, involving fracture of a triangular piece of metaphysis. With accurate reduction the prognosis is good.

Such injuries usually involve the epiphyses in the distal radius, distal metacarpus and proximal first phalanx. These cases often have the appearance of acute joint sprains but epiphyseal damage should always be suspected because at this age growth-plates are weaker than collateral ligaments. Radiography is essential to identify the type of defect present.

Prompt and accurate replacement of the epiphysis is required followed by external support with a cast or splint to maintain alignment. In certain instances fixation of the fragments with a compression screw may offer greater security. (Professor L. C. Vaughan.) (See VALGUS for picture.)

Acute inflammation of bone is divided into acute periostitis, or inflammation of the surface of the bone and its covering membrane, the periosteum; acute osteitis or ostitis, inflammation of the bone substance itself; and acute osteomyelitis, inflammation in the bone and the central marrow cavity.

Acute inflammation of the bone surface almost always results from external violence. Osteomyelitis is usually due to bacteria gaining access either through the blood- or lymphstreams, or through the broken tissues resulting from a deep wound. The mildest types are often due to an inflammation in a ligament or tendon spreading to the periosteum in the near vicinity and causing it to become inflamed as a consequence. (See also RHEUMATISM.)

Complete rest is essential: in fact work, or even walking, is often impossible. Hot fomentations, poultices, soothing and cooling liniments or applications are usually sufficient treatment for mild cases. The severer cases, in which infection has reached the bone, call in the first place for antibiotics, or immediate opening up of the area and the elimination of any pus that has collected. After that, any pieces of dead bone that are present are removed, and the wound treated as an infected open wound.

Chronic inflammation may result from several conditions, e.g. tuberculosis, actinomycosis, etc. Generally speaking, when a chronic suppurative inflammation affects a bone, sooner or later the pus and debris of a liquid nature will burrow through the surrounding tissues and burst on to the surface of the skin. A discharging sinus results which proves intractable to treatment. At the bottom of this sinus lies the dead piece of bone, and until it has been removed or absorbed the leakage of purulent material will continue in spite of antiseptic injections and other surface treatment.

The offending dead portion of bone must be removed in the first instance, and the whole sinus tract must be laid open. This is not always an easy matter, and much depends upon the situation of the pieces of dead bone (sequestrum), as well as of the mouth of the sinus. The area afterwards is treated as an open wound, and if all the necrotic parts have been removed, recovery generally takes place.

Exostosis is an outgrowth of rarefied bone tissue upon the surface of a bone. Among the commonest forms of exostoses are the following: certain forms of splints, ring-bones, bone spavins, some side-bones. (See also ACROPACHIA.)

Tumours of bone are sometimes met with. The commonest of these is the osteosarcoma of the limb-bones of dogs. The bony tissue is invaded by the cells that are characteristic of the tumour, and there is swelling and pain.

Rickets is a disease of young animals in which the bones of the limbs are affected, and often small pealike swellings are found at the junction of each of the ribs with its cartilage. (See also main entry for RICKETS.)

Osteomalacia is the equivalent of rickets occurring in the adult animal, especially during pregnancy. (See also main entry for OSTEOMALACIA.)

Osteodystrophic diseases are due to an incorrect calcium: phosphorus ratio in the diet, or to lack of one or more of the minerals – calcium, phosphorus, magnesium, and sometimes manganese; also, if vitamin D has been inadequate in amount in the food eaten for some considerable time (e.g. see FELINE JUVENILE OSTEODYSTROPHY). (See also OSTEODYSTROPHIC DISEASES.)

Porphyria is a rare disease, hereditary in origin, occurring in man, cattle, and pigs. It is characterised by brown or pinkish discoloration of the bones and teeth, and by changes in the urine. In cattle a hairless, scabby condition of the skin is also a symptom. (See also under HEXACHLOROBENZENE.)

Bone Grafts
(see – FRACTURES)

Bone Marrow
(see MARROW; ANAEMIA; BLOOD – Red blood-cells)

Bone-Pinning
A method of treating FRACTURES. In medullary pinning, a pointed stainless steel 'pin' is driven down the marrow cavity of the bone concerned; in ordinary pinning, transverse 'pins' are used, driven through the bone at right-angles to its length, and the pins held in position by a special adjustable metal splint. These methods obviate the use of cumbersome plaster casts, and they also enable cases of serious and multiple fracture (e.g. as caused in a dog or cat knocked down by a car) to be successfully treated – a result often impossible of achievement by older methods. These techniques require a high degree of specialised skill and strict asepsis and, of course, the use of a general anaesthetic. (See also bone-plating in the illustration; and EXTERNAL FIXATORS.)

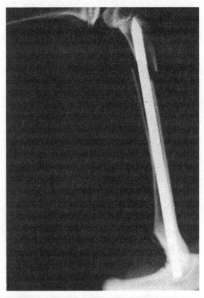

The insertion of a metal pin down the marrow cavity of the bone.

Bone Spavin
Osteitis or arthritis of the lower hock- joints of the horse. The animal is often lame; there may or may not be a hard, bony swelling.

Bonham
An Irish piglet.

Boran
An East African type of Zebu cattle.

Border Collie
A medium-sized, longish-haired dog originally bred for herding sheep. It is said that one well-trained sheepdog can do the work of 7 men. The breed is susceptible to COLLIE EYE ANOMALY (choroidal hypoplasia). Inherited deafness may be linked to coat colour. Osteochondritis dissecans may also be inherited.

'Border Disease' of Sheep
A disease occurring on the English–Welsh border, and first described in 1959. Affected lambs are known as 'hairy shakers'.

Cause The virus which causes the disease in lambs is classified as belonging to the family Togaviridae, genus *Pestivirus*.

Signs The birth-coat is altered; the amount of hair in the fleece being increased. Lambs are

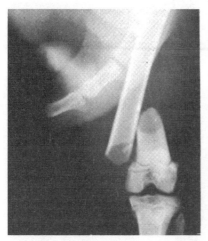
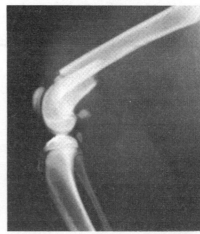

Intramedullary pinning. Two views of the fracture of the femur in a dog. (Beaumont Animals' Hospital.)

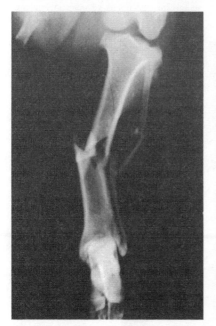
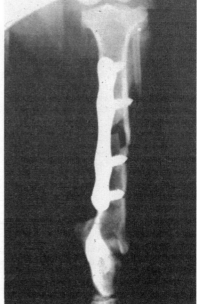

Bone-pinning – Plating. This is another technique used in veterinary practice. The radiographs show a fracture of the tibia of a dog and the use of a metal plate screwed into the bone. (Beaumont Animals' Hospital.)

smaller than normal, and grow more slowly. The shape of the head is slightly abnormal – likewise the gait which, however, shows only a slight swaying motion. Mortality is very high; most lambs die during their first few weeks.

The disease has been recognised in New Zealand, the USA, Switzerland.

A feature of the disease is acute necrosis of the placenta associated with abortion.

It appears that there is an immunological relationship between Border disease, mucosal disease, and swine fever. Possibly all three are caused by closely related viruses. In-contact piglets may be infected by sheep with Border disease.

Border Inspection Posts

The only authorised entry points for animals entering the UK from outside the EU. Animals imported into any EU member state through one of its Border Inspection Posts and found to be free from infectious or contagious disease may move on to the UK, or from the UK to another EU member state, without hindrance. Quarantine may be imposed in some cases; for example, alpacas from South America. Not every Border Inspection Post can handle all types of animal. British Border Inspection Posts, and what they can import, are as follows:

East Midlands Airport	Tropical fish
Gatwick Airport	All animals except ungulates
Glasgow Airport	All animals except ungulates
Heathrow Airport	All animals
Immingham Port	Registered equidae
Luton Airport	Ungulates including registered equidae
Manchester Airport	Cats, dogs, rodents, lagomorphs, live fish, reptiles, and birds other than ratites
Bristol Port	Ungulates other than registered equidae
Stansted Airport	Ungulates including registered equidae
Tilbury Port	Ungulates and zoo animals but not equipped to handle any species of mammal specified in the Rabies (Importation of Dogs, Cats and Other Mammals) Order 1974

Bordetella

(see under BACTERIA). *B. bronchiseptica* is a secondary invader complicating cases of canine distemper, and may also produce respiratory disease (see KENNEL COUGH) in the dog independently of viruses. This bacterium is also the cause of chronic respiratory disease in many other animals. It is an important factor in atrophic rhinitis. (See RHINITIS, ATROPHIC.)

Borna Disease

Mainly a disease of horses, but occurs also in sheep and llamas, cats and humans.

Cause A virus which is closely related to those causing EQUINE ENCEPHALITIS occurring in various tropical, subtropical and temperate regions; the diseases bearing such names as Near Eastern encephalitis, Venezuelan, Eastern, Western, and Japanese B. encephalitis.

Transmission Mosquitoes, midges, and ticks can transmit the virus, of which birds are also hosts.

Signs Depression and fever. Recovery may follow without involvement of the central nervous system, but probably in most cases such involvement does occur. Signs then include walking in circles, or pressing the head against a fixed object, a facial twitch, hanging of the head, ataxia, and paralysis.

Diagnosis depends upon a fluorescent antibody test or the detection of Joest-Degen antibodies. A differential diagnosis of Borna disease in sheep must take into account louping-ill, maedi-visna, rabies, listeriosis, scrapie, cerebro-cortical necrosis, poisons, etc.

Borogluconate

The salt of calcium used in solution for intravenous or subcutaneous injection in cases of hypocalcaemia (milk fever). It should not be given to small animals as a treatment for calcium deficiency as boron poisoning may result.

Borrelia

A species of SPIROCHAETE, causing disease in fowls in the tropics, and also human tickborne relapsing fever. The distribution of the latter is, with the exception of Australia, almost worldwide. The signs include fever, erythema, sometimes jaundice. *B. burgdorfei* causes LYME DISEASE, a disease of dog and humans characterised by arthritis, headache, lethargy, and sometimes meningitis or encephalitis. It is endemic in certain parts of the USA.

Borreliosis

A disease of dogs characterised by lameness, swollen joints and fever.

Cause Borrelia burgdorferi.

Boss Cows

(see BUNT ORDER)

Boston Terrier

Originating in the USA, this small short-haired dog has erect ears and prominent eyes. It is prone to a number of inherited conditions includng achalasia of the oesophagus, cleft palate, cataract, incomplete development of the vertebrae (hemivertebrae) and patellar luxation. The shape of the pelvis makes whelping difficult and assistance may be required.

Bot-Flies
(see under FLIES)

Bothriocephalus
Bothriocephalus is one of the parasitic tape-worms.

Botryomycosis
A suppurating granulomatous infection usually caused by *Staphylococcus aureus* (see GRANULOMA).

'Bottle-Jaw'
Oedema of the lower jaw (see illustration). Also found with liver-fluke infestations in sheep and, occasionally, cattle; and with JOHNE'S DISEASE in cattle.

Botulism
A form of food poisoning, often fatal, caused by *Clostridium botulinum* toxins, types A to G, which produce paralysis. Botulism occurs worldwide, but is especially common in the tropics. Toxin types C and D are most commonly found in birds and most mammals including cattle; A, B, E and F in people.

Cattle and sheep Large numbers may die in regions where they suffer from mineral deficiencies (especially of phosphorus) and are driven to eating the bones of dead animals to obtain the minerals they need.

Cl. botulinum may inhabit the alimentary tract of a healthy animal without ill effect. However, in a decaying carcass, rapid multiplication of the bacterium, with toxin production, occurs. Carrion is therefore the main source of

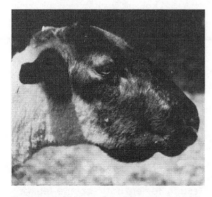

'Bottle-jaw'. Oedema of the lower jaw caused by *Haemonchus contortus*, a parasitic worm found in the abomasum of sheep and goats. It is also a cause of severe anaemia. (Reproduced by permission of Dr M. A. Taylor, Central Veterinary Laboratory, Weybridge; Crown copyright reserved.)

botulism in animals, but proliferation can also occur in decaying vegetable matter. Carcases may pollute well-water or forage, and in Britain botulism in cattle has been associated with the use of broiler litter on grazing land – such waste containing a few carcases. The worst outbreak was probably that in Queensland, Australia, where more than 5500 steers died, as a result of infection from poultry litter.

Signs Large doses of toxin may result in sudden death, but often the illness lasts a few days; the animal becoming first stiff and dejected, and then recumbent, lying on the sternum with the cow's head turned to one side. Salivation may be profuse, swallowing difficult or impossible, so that botulism has to be differentiated from rabies when making a diagnosis.

Control The use of mineral supplements where osteophagia occurs (see LAMZIEKTE), or of vaccines.

Horses The signs are ataxia, difficulty in swallowing, and posterior paralysis; or sudden death. In the UK cases have occurred in horses fed big-bale silage. Contamination of the silage by soil (which may contain *Cl. botulinum* B), or by rodent carcases, has been suggested as the source of botulism in horses. In the USA, contaminated alfalfa caused deaths of 7 out of 8 horses which showed signs of progressive muscular weakness.

Signs Difficulty in chewing and swallowing; in some outbreaks tongue paralysis has been seen; dilated pupils. Sudden death.

Dogs Botulism has occurred in packs of fox-hounds fed infected meat such as farm animals found dead.

Birds Type C botulism has been reported in Britain among both chickens and waterfowl; also pheasants. It is not uncommon in hot dry summers as water levels reduce, allowing access to mud. (See also MAGGOTS.)

Symptoms of botulism in an outbreak among captive birds included a characteristic statuesque behaviour; some individuals stood motionless for over one hour despite activity of other birds around them; paralysis, ranging from a single dropped wing to bilateral leg paralysis; inability to swallow; and terminal gasping.

Fish Botulism in fish causes high mortality. It is usually due to feeding wet trash fish to farmed fish without cleaning out the machinery between batches. The Danish name for the disease translates as 'bankruptcy disease'.

For botulism in mink, see MINK, DISEASES OF. For botulism in South African cattle, see LAMZIEKTE.

Public health Human (and also animal) botulism may occur as the result of imperfectly preserved food or when cooked food is allowed to stand and later re-heated. Although there have been very few cases of human botulism in Britain, a high proportion of trout in fish farms may be contaminated with *Cl. botulinum* type E, which can multiply at temperatures as low as 5°C, whereas the more common types A and B will not normally multiply at temperatures below 10°C.

Boutonneuse Fever

A zoonosis (see ZOONOSES) which is transmissible from dogs to people. The cause is *Rickettsia conori*. There is a rash. Wrists, ankles, and then other parts of the body may be affected. The dog tick *Rhipicephalus sanguineus* is the vector.

Bouvier Des Flanders

A medium-sized, short-tailed dog with grey or fawn coat. It has few defects; laryngeal paralysis may be inherited.

Bovine Atopic Rhinitis

A discharge from eyes and nose, with some ulceration of nasal mucosa (and formation of granuloma), are symptoms in common with those of bovine infectious rhinitis. It is often the result of an acute hypersensitivity reaction, particularly in Channel Island breeds. Recovery usually follows housing.

Bovine Atypical Interstitial Pneumonia

(see FOG FEVER)

Bovine Autoimmune Haemolytic Anaemia

A heifer died within 2 days of showing anaemia and dyspnoea, and the diagnosis was bovine auto-immune haemolytic anaemia, based on auto-agglutination (which increased on Coombs' testing) and the presence of antibovine IgG on red blood cell surfaces.

Acute haemolytic anaemia may be due to many other causes, including water intoxication, delayed copper toxicity, brassica poisoning, babesiosis, leptospirosis, and bacillary haemoglobinuria.

Bovine Embryo Collection And Transfer Regulations 1993

These apply within the UK and other member states of the EU.

Bovine Encephalomyelitis (Buss Disease)

Bovine encephalomyelitis (Buss disease) occurs in the USA, Australia, and Japan. In the USA it is a disease mainly of the summer and autumn months, and cattle under 2 years old are mainly susceptible.

Cause Chlamydia psittaci.

Signs A fever, which lasts a week or more. With loss of appetite, the animal loses condition and becomes weak. A nasal discharge or diarrhoea may be seen. Pushing the head against a wall, walking in a circle, hyperaesthesia, and convulsions are symptoms of which one or two may be seen. Economically the disease has a low incidence and generally a low mortality, but in some herds losses may be serious.

Autopsy findings include pleurisy, pericarditis and peritonitis, apart from any brain lesions.

Public health Man is susceptible.

Bovine Enzootic Leukosis

A virus-produced form of cancer, characterised by multiple malignant growths as well as, in some cases, leukaemia. The disease was first recorded in Britain in 1978, is fairly common on the European mainland, and is a NOTIFIABLE DISEASE. Occasionally cattle show symptoms before they are 2 years old, but 4 to 8 years is a more common age. Digestive disturbance, anaemia and loss of condition result.

The virus is a type C oncornavirus of the retrovirus family.

In Britain the enzootic bovine leukosis (EBL) attested herds scheme was introduced by MAFF in January 1982 to encourage the establishment of EBL-free herds, as a first step towards eradication of the disease.

Great Britain was recognised as being free of the disease in July 1999; the last case was detected in December 1996.

Testing for enzootic bovine leukosis

Breeding cattle may only be moved from one member state of the EU to another if they originate from herds which are recognised as free from EBL in accordance with the terms of the EU directive.

Bovine Ephemeral Fever
(see EPHEMERAL FEVER)

Bovine Herpes Mammillitis
An ulcerative disease of the cow's teats and udder, caused by a herpes virus. (See also VIRUS INFECTIONS OF COW'S TEATS.)

Bovine Immunodeficiency-Like Virus (BIV)
This causes a progressive wasting condition of cattle, with intercurrent diseases, poor milk yield and enlarged lymph nodes. Infection is stated to be present in North America and Europe. There is limited evidence of the degree to which BIV is present in Britain, but antibody has been found in the majority of at least one herd.

Bovine Infectious Petechial Fever
Also known as Ondiri disease, this affects cattle in Kenya, and is characterised by haemorrhages of the visible mucous membranes, fever, and diarrhoea. There may be severe conjunctivitis and protrusion of the eyeball. Death within 1 to 3 days is not uncommon, though some animals survive for longer, a few recovering. The cause is a rickettsia, believed to be spread by a biting insect, or a tick, and known as *Ehrlichia ondiri*. The bushbuck provides a reservoir of infection.

Bovine Leukocyte Adhesion Deficiency (BLAD)
An inherited problem of cattle resulting in inability to resist disease. Affected cattle usually die by 1 year old. It was discovered in the USA in 1989, and has since been found in many European countries, including the UK.

Bovine Malignant Catarrhal Fever
This infection, also known as malignant catarrh, may occur not only in cattle but also in sheep, farmed deer, and antelopes. It is most common in Africa, but cases have been recorded in the UK, other EU countries, Australasia, and North America.

Cause A herpes virus.

Signs Enlarged lymph glands, inflammation of the mucous membrane of the mouth, drooling of saliva, gastro-enteritis, keratitis (followed in some cases by blindness, and sometimes ENCEPHALITIS). Most affected animals die.

Bovine Papular Stomatitis
This pox was first described in Germany and during recent years has been reported in the UK, Australia, East Africa, etc. The disease is not accompanied by fever or systemic upset.

Characteristically, papules form in the mouth on the mucous membrane lining the cheek. Early lesions are rounded areas of intensive congestion up to 1.5 cm in diameter, which in pigmented mucous membrane are visible as roughened areas with greyish discoloration. The centre of such areas becomes necrotic and in a later stage shows a depressed centre. Removal of the caseous material leaves a raw granulating ulcer but normally epithelial regeneration occurs in 3 to 4 days. A feature of the disease is the occurrence of concentric rings of necrosis and congestion. Secondary lesions of mouth, muzzle or nostril may prolong the disease over a period of months. However, it is unusual for the animals to show signs of illness.

Cause The virus involved is the same as, or is related to, that causing pseudo-cowpox. (See also VIRUS INFECTIONS OF COW'S TEATS.)

Bovine Parvovirus
A cause of diarrhoea in calves.

Bovine Pleuropneumonia, Contagious
A NOTIFIABLE DISEASE in the UK. Affected animals have a high temperature (41.5°C/107°F), difficulty in breathing and are anorexic.

Cause *Mycoplasma pleuropneumoniae.*

Bovine Pulmonary Emphysema
(see FOG FEVER)

Bovine Quintuplets
Bovine quintuplets, all dead, were produced by a Charolais cow, which went on to conceive again within a normal period of time at the Galemire Veterinary Hospital, Cleator Moor, UK.

Bovine Respiratory Disease Complex
(see 'SHIPPING FEVER')

Bovine Rhinotracheitis, Infectious
(see RHINOTRACHEITIS)

Bovine Spongiform Encephalopathy (BSE)

'Mad cow disease'. A NOTIFIABLE DISEASE in which spaces (vacuoles) develop in the brain tissue, in the manner of a sponge.

Signs Cattle become nervous and hypersensitive to noise, and when approached or touched. They appear frightened and may be aggressive. Dairy cattle show a reluctance to enter milking parlours and may resent attempts to apply milking clusters. The gait becomes abnormal, with hind limb swaying. The head is lowered. When the animal is at rest, regular or spasmodic muscle twitching may be seen.

BSE was first recognised in 1986 although individual cattle were probably infected in the 1970s. A policy of slaughter and incineration of carcases was introduced. The heads were removed to confirm diagnosis.

Its origin is unknown but it is possible that the disease developed in a single cow following genetic mutation.

Fortuitously, a link between BSE and the use of meat and bone meal in bovine diets was established in 1987. It was at first thought that the meal responsible contained material from scrapie-infected sheep. However, the Phillips inquiry into BSE concluded that this was not the case. Current opinion favours the probability that a BSE-infected cow entered the rendering process that produces meat and bone meal, infecting cattle which spread the disease when their carcases were in turn processed into meat and bone meal. Meat and bone meal was banned from bovine diets in 1988 but could still be used in diets for other species. However, this created the potential for meal intended for cattle to be infected by contamination with that prepared for other species in the same mill. Meat and bone meal is now banned from use in all animal feeds; its possession in an animal feed plant is a criminal offence.

Specified bovine offals were prohibited from human consumption; they include brain, spinal cord, spleen, thymus, small intestine lining. All British beef exports were banned, with catastrophic effects for the farming economy. The ban could not be lifted until the UK adopted measures to lessen any risk to humans.

A new form of Creutzfeldt-Jakob disease in (mainly) young persons (new variant CJD) has been confirmed as being linked to BSE. The UK government has introduced a scheme to aid victims and their families.

Incidence At its peak in 1992, 36,681 cases had been confirmed representing about 0.3 per cent of the national herd; the disease has been declining since then. By 1996, the number had fallen to about 8000, about 0.07 per cent of the national herd. In 1997, a cull of cattle, instigated by the EU, removed those cows which could have eaten the same contaminated feed as the proved cases in the same herd. A second cull, in 1998, removed female calves born to cows around the time they showed clinical signs of the disease.

Eradication As a further precaution against the possibility of endangering public health, the carcases of animals over 30 months of age were incinerated and not used for human consumption.

Cause It is generally accepted that the cause of BSE is a prion (see PRIONS), a self-replicating infectious protein (PrP). However, it is not known how this produces the disease. Theories that BSE resulted from a change in the rendering process used to produce meat and bone meal, that it is a bovine form of scrapie or that it is an autoimmune disease have been discounted. The Phillips inquiry also discounted claims that BSE was caused by exposure to organophosphorus pesticides although it acknowledged the possibility that this might increase susceptibility to the disease.

Differential diagnosis BSE has to be differentiated from other disorders such as acetonaemia (in which short periods of delirium may occur); from listeriosis (in which cattle may become violent in the terminal stages); and from hypomagnesaemia and hypocalcaemia.

Prevention The feeding of protein or other material derived from the same species as will consume the feed should be prohibited.

Other species BSE has been recorded in several species of antelope in zoos and there is some evidence of infection in sheep. Pigs have developed BSE only after infective material was injected into the brain; they did not develop the disease when fed contaminated feed. There may be a link with FELINE SPONGIFORM ENCEPHALOPATHY as some big cats in zoos had developed a spongiform encephalopathy after having eaten bovine heads, before BSE was recognised as a disease. BSE is experimentally transmissible to mice and monkeys. (See also SCRAPIE.)

Bovine Syncytial Virus

A retrovirus which may have an involvement with bovine and bovine enzootic leukosis as well as immunodeficiency-like virus respiratory diseases. (See PNEUMONIA.)

Bovine Tuberculosis
(See TUBERCULOSIS)

Bovine Viral Diarrhoea/Mucosal Disease (BVD/MD)

Bovine viral diarrhoea (BVD) and mucosal disease (MD) are two clinically dissimilar conditions caused by the same virus.

BVD is the result of an acute infection in susceptible cattle which may occur at any age in post-natal life, and is usually a trivial illness of a few days' duration and negligible mortality. Infection in cows in early pregnancy may result in abortion, resorption of the fetus, or the birth of more persistently viraemic calves.

By contrast, MD is almost invariably fatal. It occurs in cattle which have a persistent BVD/MD viral infection acquired as fetuses. Susceptible animals are unable to produce antibody to the infecting virus. The disease develop0s, after the loss of passive immunity given by colostrum, when the animals are 6 to 9 months old.

In Britain BVD/MD virus is widespread. More than 60 per cent of adult cattle have significant levels of serum neutralising antibody.

Pigs can become infected with bovine virus diarrhoea and show signs very similar to those of SWINE FEVER.

Cause The BVD/MD virus belongs to the *Pestivirus* genus, and is a small RNA virus of the Togavirus family. There are at least 13 strains, some more pathogenic than others. The strains may show ANTIGENETIC DRIFT. The virus can survive storage at 4°C for at least 16 months; also repeated freezing and thawing.

Signs In affected animals in the very mildest cases, there may be a few ulcers in the mouth, perhaps also in the nostrils, but little else. More often, however, the animal runs a temperature of 40° or 40.5°C (104° or 105°F) with loss of appetite, scouring, and a drop in milk yield. There may be ulcers in the cleft of the foot, and lameness can be a prominent feature of the disease. With mucosal disease, signs are of severe disease with mucosal sloughing in the mouth, oesophagus and possible other parts of the alimentary tract.

Infection in early pregnancy may cause abortion, embryonic death or congenital deformities. Mid-pregnancy infection may result in apparently normal calves which may succumb to mucosal disease. Animals infected in late pregnancy produce calves born with antibodies to the disease produced by the fetus.

Diagnosis BVD/MD has to be differentiated from foot-and-mouth disease, Johne's disease,

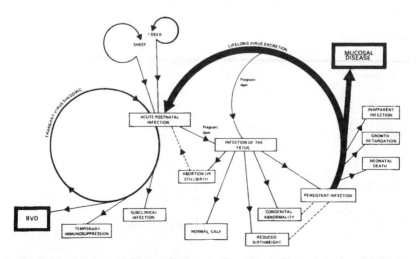

Bovine viral diarrhoea/mucosal disease: Infection cycles. (Reproduced with permission from *Veterinary Record*, **117**, 245, MAFF/HMSO. Crown copyright.)

cattle plague, and other conditions. An ELISA test is available.

B *Prevention* Various vaccines, live and inactivated, have been used in North America, with mixed results. In 1995, an inactivated vaccine was developed from a prototype created at the Institute for Animal Health, Compton, which was demonstrated as being effective by Professor Joe Brownlie and his colleagues.

Bow-Legs

Legs curved outwards from the knee occur normally in some breeds of dogs, such as the pug and bulldog, but in other breeds they are usually the sign of RICKETS. The shafts of the long bones become softened and bend outwards under the weight of the body, so that the fore-limbs especially become curved outwards. The condition is also seen in poultry and farm animals.

Bowel, Oedema of the

This disease affects mainly piglets of 8 to 14 weeks old, though occasionally it is seen in the new-born and in pigs of up to 5 months. It is usually associated with a change in management such as moving or mixing with others, but especially with a change in diet. In most cases a gelatinous fluid is found in the thickness of the stomach wall and other parts. The disease can be experimentally transmitted by inoculation of this fluid.

Cause E. COLI, mainly seroptypes 0138, 0139 or 0141.

Signs The finding of a dead pig – often the best in the litter – is usually the first indication. Puffy eyelids, from which there may be a discharge, and puffiness of snout and throat may be observed; together with leg weakness and convulsions.

Treatment Administer antibiotics by injection to affected pigs, and by injection or in feed or water to others in the group. Feed should be reduced and, if provided from hoppers, roughage should be added. Return to normal feed should be gradual.

Prevention After weaning, keep on same feed for at least 2 weeks. Change of diet should be gradual over 3 to 5 days.

Bowels

(see INTESTINES)

'Bowie'

A disease of unweaned lambs, resembling rickets, in New Zealand. A supplement of phosphates appears to be effective.

Bowman's Capsule

A part of the nephron – the unit of structure of the kidney. Fluid passes from the glomerulus into the capsule as the first stage of filtration and urine formation.

Boxer

A medium-sized, short-coated, short-nosed (brachycephalic) dog; usually brown in colour with white and black markings; a few are all white. The skull structure leads occasionally to breathing difficulties. Achalasia, cleft palate, corneal erosion, hyperplastic gingivitis and spondylitis may be inherited. The breed shows a higher than usual incidence of skin cancer. White boxers tend to be deaf.

Boxwood Poisoning

Boxwood poisoning may sometimes occur through farm animals gaining access to gardens where the plant grows, or by eating the trimmings from box hedges along with other green food taken from the garden. The plant, known botanically as *Buxus sempervirens*, contains several toxic alkaloids, the chief of which is buxine. When large quantities have been taken, or if the beast is not able to vomit, nervous symptoms, lameness, muscular twitching, dizziness, diarrhoea, and acute abdominal pains are seen. In very severe cases there is the passage of blood-stained motions, great straining, convulsions, delirium, unconsciousness, and death. Pigs are the most susceptible of the farm animals.

Brachial

Brachial is a word describing an association with the forelimb. The brachial plexus is an important group of nerves supplying the shoulder and forelimb. Tumours arising here are usually malignant. They are seen most often in dogs and cause a progressive lameness of one forelimb together with atrophy of the muscles; also signs of pain which cannot be localised. Injury to the brachial plexus involving damage to NERVES results in paralysis of the affected forelimb.

Brachycephalic

The word is applied to the short skulls of such dogs as the bulldog, toy spaniel, or pug. In such the forehead is high, the skull broad, and the face foreshortened.

Bracken Poisoning

The eating of bracken (*Pteris aquilina*) by horses, cattle or sheep may lead to serious illness and death; symptoms appearing a month or two after the first meal of the plant.

Cause Bracken contains an enzyme, thiaminase, which in the horse and pig causes a thiamine deficiency. In cattle and sheep this vitamin is produced in abundance in the rumen, and bracken poisoning is due not to thiaminase but to the 'radiomimetic-factor' also present in bracken which depresses bone-marrow function. There are complex changes in the blood and bone marrow. Poisoning is more prevalent in dry seasons than in wet weather, and young store stock are more often affected than adult cattle. The rhizomes are said to be 5 times as poisonous as the fronds – a fact of importance where reclaimed land has been ploughed.

Signs In the horse these take the form of a general loss of condition and an unsteady gait; later on, loss of appetite (but no rise in temperature), nervous spasms, and death.

Affected cattle, on the other hand, run a high temperature. They segregate themselves from the rest of the herd and cease grazing. The visible mucous membranes are pale in colour, and numerous petechial haemorrhages are found scattered over the lining of the nose, eyes, and vagina. Bracken is also associated with enzootic haematuria and upper alimentary squamous cell carcinoma.

Faeces, passed without straining, are usually blood-stained. Respirations are accelerated, and on the slightest exertion the animals fall and have some difficulty in rising. In many cases a knuckling of the fetlocks, especially of the hind-limbs, is noticeable. In some cases the throat becomes swollen, so that there is difficulty in breathing. The illness lasts from 1 to 6 days. In other cases, death may occur much sooner, and be accompanied by bleeding from nose and anus, when the carcases have some similarity to deaths from anthrax. Onset of symptoms may be delayed for up to 2 months.

In sheep, ingestion of bracken can also cause bright blindness and mandibular neoplasia.

Treatment DL-Butyl alcohol injections have been recommended for cattle in the early stages of bracken poisoning. For the horse, injections of thiamine are usually successful if the illness is tackled in time.

Prevention Bracken is usually eaten only when no other food is available; avoid the situation in which animals turn to bracken out of sheer hunger or thirst – semi-starvation of livestock is ever a false economy. Especially where the grazing is poor, it is essential to move animals to bracken-free land every 3 weeks. Avoid the use of green bracken as bedding.

Bracken and cancer During the investigation of acute bracken poisoning in cattle, it was found that certain constituents of the plant were carcinogenic in rats and mice. In 1975 one of at least two bracken carcinogens was identified as shikimic acid, a constituent of many other plants also, and it has been shown to cause lethal mutations and to be a very potent cancer-producer in mice.

Both in the UK and in Japan young bracken shoots have been eaten by people as a vegetable. A link has been established in Japan between long-term bracken fern ingestion and stomach cancer.

In some parts of the world, cancer of the bladder is an endemic condition in cattle, and in most places – states the World Health Organisation – it is associated with bracken. (See also BRIGHT BLINDNESS)

Bradshot

Another name for BRAXY.

Bradycardia

Bradycardia means slowness in the beating of the heart, with corresponding slowness of the pulse-rate. (See also HEART DISEASES – Functional disorders; PULSE.)

Bradykinin

Damaged tissue releases the polypeptide bradykinin, a powerful vasodilator and stimulator of smooth muscle and of pain receptors, possibly as part of the inflammatory response to injury.

Braford

A breed of cattle formed by crossing the Brahman and the Hereford.

Brahman

Cattle of this name in the south of the USA were developed from a mixture of several zebu breeds (*Bos indicus*) plus some Shorthorn or Hereford content.

Brailing

A means of temporarily preventing flight in pheasant poults, etc., by means of leather straps.

Brain

The brain and the spinal cord together form what is called the CENTRAL NERVOUS SYSTEM.

Parts of the brain In the domestic animals, as in man, the principal parts of the brain (front to back) are as follows:

(1) The cerebrum. This is by far the largest part, and consists of two hemispheres separated by a deep cleft. The surface of the cerebrum is increased by numerous ridges or gyri and by furrows called sulci. The hemispheres are joined by the fibres of the corpus callosum.

Each hemisphere is divided into sections or lobes, and its surface has a layer of grey matter – the cortex. At the front of each hemisphere is the olfactory bulb, which relays impulses from the olfactory nerves of the nose to the brain, and is concerned with the sense of smell.

Within the cerebral hemispheres lie the basal ganglia. At the base of the cerebrum is the thalamus. Below is the hypothalamus, containing nerve centres for the control of body temperature, and connected by a stalk or pedicle with the pituitary gland.

The lateral ventricles are located within the corresponding hemispheres and are spaces filled with cerebro-spinal fluid, and communicating with the third and fourth ventricles.

(2) The brain-stem consists of nerve tissue at the base of the brain and includes the mid-brain (of which the largest structures are the 2 cerebral peduncles and 4 quadrigeminal bodies), the pons, and the medulla oblongata.

(3) The cerebellum, which has 2 hemispheres and a middle ridge – the vermis. The cerebellum, with the pons, and the medulla oblongata are often spoken of as the hind-brain. The pons is a bridge of nerve fibres from one hemisphere

Brain of dog.

of the cerebellum to the other. The medulla continues backwards as the spinal cord.

Structure The brain is composed of white and grey matter. In the cerebrum and cerebellum the grey matter is arranged mainly as a layer on the surface, though both have grey areas imbedded in the white matter. In other parts the grey matter is found in definite masses called 'nuclei'.

The cells vary in size and shape in different parts of the brain, but all of them give off a number of processes, some of which form nerve-fibres. The cells on the surface of the cerebral hemispheres, for instance, are roughly pyramidal in shape, and each one gives off numbers of nerve-cell projections, called 'dendrites', from one end, and a single long process, called an 'axon', from the other. The white matter is made up of a large number of nerve-fibres, each of which is connected to a cell in the grey matter.

In both the grey and the white matter there is a framework of fibrous tissue cells, extremely fine and delicate, which acts as a supportive structure for the fibres and nerve cells, to which the name 'neuroglia' is applied. Permeating the grey matter is a complex system of blood-vessels, and in the white matter there are also vessels but to a lesser extent.

Meninges The brain proper is covered over by a thin membrane called the 'pia mater', the bones of the cranium are lined by a thick membrane called the 'dura mater', and between these is an irregular network called 'the arachnoid'. Between the arachnoid and the pia mater is a small amount of fluid, which serves as a kind of water-bed in which the brain floats.

Size The brain varies very much in different animals and in different breeds, but the following table gives the average relation of the weight of the brain to the weight of the body:

Cat	1 to 99
Dog	1 to 235
Sheep	1 to 317
Pig	1 to 369
Horse	1 to 593
Ox	1 to 682

From this it will be seen that the cat has proportionately to the size of its body the largest brain.

Nerves There are 12 pairs of nerves coming from the surface of the brain. They are known as cranial nerves:

1. Olfactory, to the nose (smell).
2. Optic, to the eye (sight).
3. Oculomotor ⎤
4. Trochlear   ⎦ to the muscles of the eyes.
5. Trigeminal, to the skin of the face, etc.
6. Abducens, to the muscles of the eye.
7. Facial, to the muscles of the face.
8. Auditory, to the ear (hearing).
9. Glossopharyngeal, to the tongue (taste).
10. Vagus, to heart, larynx, lungs, and stomach.
11. Spinal accessory, to muscles in the neck.
12. Hypoglossal, to the muscles of the tongue.

Blood-vessels The brain obtains its blood-supply from four main sources: two internal carotids and two occipital arteries. These branch and unite to form an irregular circle under the brain within the skull, called the 'circle of Willis'. From this, numerous smaller branches leave to supply the whole of the brain substance. By such an arrangement any possibility of deficiency of blood is obviated, for should one of the main branches become cut or occluded, the others enlarge and the same amount of blood is still supplied. The blood leaves the organ by means of large venous sinuses situated in the membranes covering the brain, and finally finds its way into the jugular veins of the neck.

Functions The cerebrum is concerned with memory, initiative, volition, intelligence, and, as well as these, it is the receiving station of the impulses that originate from the organs of sight, smell, taste, hearing, and touch. Fear, anger, and other emotions originate in the grey nerve cells of the cerebrum, which is also concerned with voluntary control of the skeletal muscles.

Sensations on the right side of the body, and muscular control in the right side, are dealt with by the left cerebral hemisphere; the right hemisphere being concerned with the left side of the body.

The cerebellum is concerned with unconscious control, with balance, and with co-ordination of complex muscular movements. Each half of the cerebellum controls the muscular system of its own side of the body, and is in communication with the opposite side of the cerebrum. It closely communicates with the nerves, internal ear, and with certain nerves of muscle-sense, monitoring the state of muscle contraction.

The hypothalamus controls many body functions including hunger, thirst, body temperature and sleep.

The thalamus acts as a vital relay station between the sensory nerves (except the olfactory nerves) and the cerebral cortex.

The basal ganglia help to control much muscular activity.

The medulla contains nerve centres for the control of involuntary, or reflex, actions such as respiration and heart-beat rates, coughing, vomiting, and the reflex part of swallowing.

Brain Diseases
Brain diseases include the following:

Abscess Infective micro-organisms may enter through an injury to the bone, through the medium of the ear (especially in the pig and dog), or may arrive by the bloodstream. Sometimes a foreign body, such as a needle that has become lodged in the throat, may pass upwards into the brain and set up an abscess. The condition may be produced during the course of pneumonia, metritis, endocarditis, etc., when the bacteria invade the bloodstream and get carried to the brain among other tissues.

For symptoms and first-aid, see under MENINGITIS; ENCEPHALITIS.

Cerebral haemorrhage Bleeding into the cranial cavity, usually as a result of trauma or a vascular problem. It may result in loss of consciousness and death. Residual signs on recovery may include hind limb instability or convulsions.

Concussion The temporary loss of consciousness resulting from a head injury. Temporary blindness may occur after the animal has regained consciousness.

In domestic animals long-term effects include changes in behaviour, such as aggressiveness and excessive libido. Fits (epileptiform convulsions) may be a sequel to a head injury in dogs. (See EPILEPSY.)

Encephalopathy Any disease of the brain, particularly one involving structural changes.

Inflammation (see ENCEPHALITIS; MENINGITIS)

Oedema of the brain is seen in salt poisoning in pigs, and in polioencephalomalacia (see CEREBROCORTICAL NECROSIS). Blindness and convulsions are produced.

(See also 'DAFT LAMBS'; HYDROCEPHALUS; CHOREA; RABIES; EQUINE ENCEPHALITIS; 'SLEEPER' SYNDROME of cattle.)

Parasites of the human brain, of animal origin, include nematodes, such as larval hookworms, *Strongyloides*, ascarid worms (*Toxocara*), filarial worms, rat lungworm (*Angiostrongylus cantonensis*), and *Gnathostoma* spp.; trematodes, such as *Fasciola hepatica* (liver fluke), *Schistosoma japonicum*, and *Paragonimus* spp. (lung fluke); the cestodes of hydatid disease, cysticercosis, and sparganosis; and fly maggots such as Tumbu fly of East and Central Africa (*Cordylobia anthropophaga*), tropical warble fly of South America (*Dermatobia hominis*), sheep botfly of parts of Russia and the region and the Mediterranean (*Rhino-oestrus purpureus*), and cattle bots and warble fly in Europe (*Hypoderma bovis* and *lineata* of cattle and *H. diana* of deer) (*Lancet*). Such parasites may similarly occur in the brains of farm and domestic animals. (See COENURIASIS and HEARTWORMS; the latter being especially important in cats.)

Transmissible encephalopathies such as scrapie and BSE.

Tuberculosis of the brain (see TUBERCU-LOSIS)

Tumours of the brain may cause a variety of signs, according to the part affected. For example, changes in character, loss of house training, seizures (cerebrum), circling movements, nystagmus (vestibular system), loss of coordination (cerebellum), a staggering gait (medulla), metabolic problems (hypothalamus). Decreased activity, drowsiness, and blindness in cats are seen as a result of a meningioma. Of the 11 per cent suspected of having bovine spongiform encephalitis (BSE) in which the disease was not confirmed, brain tumour was the commonest explanation for the signs.

Brain Surgery

In veterinary practice this is performed to treat COENURIASIS. (See under TAPEWORMS for the technique of the operation in sheep, and for the signs suggestive of this disease.) It may be necessary in small animals following a road traffic accident or to remove brain tumours.

For example, a 12-year-old cat referred to the Ohio State University's teaching hospital, had been walking in circles, aimlessly pacing, and, purring almost continuously; however, the cat was only intermittently responsive to human attention, and kept his tongue protruded from his mouth.

Under a general anaesthetic, after computerised tomography of the skull to indicate the exact site of the lesion, a hole was drilled

and through it the tumour (a meningioma) gradually removed. The cat made a perfect recovery.

Bran

A bran diet is deficient in calcium and high in phosphorus. *Osteodystrophia fibrosa* is seen in horses fed predominantly on bran (see HORSES, FEEDING OF; OSTEODYSTROPHIC DISEASES; BRAN DISEASE).

Bran Disease

Osteodystrophia fibrosa; it is seen in horses predominantly fed bran. Such a diet is deficient in calcium and contains excessive phosphorus. Bone deformities are seen, particularly swelling of the upper and lower jaws, with loosening of the teeth, and lameness. It may also occur in other animals fed a diet too high in phosphorus.

Bran Mash

Made by adding boiling water to a tablespoonful of salt and two double handfuls of bran and stirring to a porridge-like consistency; cool for 15 to 30 minutes, then give feed. Traditionally given to sick horses.

Branding

The application of an identifying mark to, usually, horses and cattle. Traditionally, a hot iron was used to sear the hide, leaving a permanent mark. A less painful method is freeze-branding. In this technique, a copper branding 'iron', cooled to −70°C with dry ice and alcohol, is applied to a clipped or shaved area for about 27 seconds.

When the branded area thaws, the hair falls out. The new hair which grows in 2 or 3 weeks is white, and therefore shows up well on a darkish animal. For a white animal, the brand has to be left on longer to kill the hair roots. The brandmark then resembles a hot-iron brand, but the hide damage may be less. (Early claims that 'there is no damage to the hide' have been disproved.)

Laser beams have been used for branding cattle in the USA. It is claimed that 'with the 5000°C temperature of the branding beam, the speed of branding is faster than the pain reflex of an animal'.

Where a permanent brand is not necessary, it is a simple matter to apply black hair dye or hair bleach, according to whether the animal is light or dark in colour.

Brassicae Species

Plants of the *Cruciferae* family – kale, cabbage, Brussels sprouts and rape. Excessive consumption can lead to haemolytic anaemia, with haemoglobinuria, especially if other foods are not available or if the kale is frosted. Certain species of brassica contain thiocyanates and produce iodine deficiencies and goitre. (See under KALE.)

Braxy

Also known as bradshot – a disease of sheep characterised by a very short period of illness, by a seasonal and regional incidence, and, in the natural state, by a high mortality. It occurs in various parts of Scotland, Ireland, the north of England, Scandinavia, etc., chiefly on hilly land. It attacks young sheep under the age of 2 years, weaned lambs being very susceptible; the best members of the flock are more liable to become attacked than poorly nourished sheep, and it is most frequently seen during a spell of cold, severe weather with hoar frosts at night.

Causes *Clostridium septicum.* It affects the mucous membrane of the 4th stomach of sheep and from there invades the tissues. It gains entrance to the alimentary canal by way of the mouth along with the grass from a 'braxy pasture'.

Infection with *Cl. septicum* is characterised by gas gangrene, and may occur in animals other than sheep – including man.

Signs These – loss of appetite, abdominal pain, diarrhoea, with a high temperature and laboured breathing – are seldom in evidence for more than 5 or 6 hours; death being sudden. A characteristic odour is perceptible from the breath and body fluids. Decomposition is very rapid. The lesions are those of a gastritis in the 4th stomach (abomasum).

Prevention Vaccination at the beginning of September, so that the animals have time to establish an immunity before the frosts begin, has given good results. On farms where the losses have been very heavy a second vaccination 14 days later may be needed. (See also under VACCINATION.)

Breathing
(see RESPIRATION)

Breathlessness

Breathlessness may be due to any condition that hinders the thorough oxygenation of the blood.

Hyperpnoea is increased depth of breathing.

Tachypnoea is the name for an increase in the rate of respiration. This may arise from such

diverse causes as anaemia, heat stress, heart disease, pneumonia, bronchitis, and paraquat poisoning.

Dyspnoea means laboured breathing, or breathing accompanied by pain or distress, such as may occur with oedema of the lungs, pneumonia, bronchitis, pleurisy, emphysema, and paraquat poisoning.

Breda Virus

A cause of diarrhoea in calves in the USA, and of respiratory disease in 2-day-old calves which very soon died.

Breech Presentation
(see PARTURITION)

Breeding, Controlled
(see CONTROLLED BREEDING)

Breeding of Dogs Act 1973

The Breeding of Dogs Act 1973 makes it unlawful for anyone to keep a dog-breeding establishment unless it has been licensed by the local authority. A breeding establishment is defined as 'any premises (including a private dwelling) where more than two bitches are kept for the purpose of breeding for sale'.

Breeding of Dogs Act 1991

This extended powers under the 1973 legislation, which permitted local authorities to inspect only those premises already licensed, or those for which a licence application had been made. Under the 1991 Act the local authority or a veterinary surgeon could apply to a magistrate for a warrant to enter and inspect the premises. Obstruction is a criminal offence.

Breeding and Sale of Dogs (Welfare) Act 1999

This amended the above two Acts. Bitches must not be mated if they are less than 1 year old; and a bitch can have not more than 6 litters in her lifetime. Records of breeding have to be kept and dogs must be identified by a tag bearing a code identifying the premises of birth.

Breeding of Livestock

Information about animals coming 'on heat' or being 'in season' is given under OESTRUS. Other information is given under PREGNANCY and PARTURITION.

Number of females per male varies. The stallion when he is 4 years old and upwards and in good condition will serve from 80 to

120 mares during a season. A 3 year old can take up to about 50 or 60, and from 15 to 20 are enough for a 2 year old. From 60 to 80 cows are sufficient for an average adult bull, but he should not serve more than 35 or 40 between 1 and 2 years of age. Twenty to 30 ewes are as many as the ram lamb will successfully serve, but shearlings may have as many as 40 to 50. Adult rams may successfully impregnate 80 ewes or more. The year-old boar should not be allowed more than 20 sows during a season, but when he is older he may have up to 30 or 35. In this connection it must be remembered that when a large number of females are served by a male, those served at the later stages are not so likely to prove fruitful as those served earlier.

When synchronisation of oestrus (heat) is practised, more males are required; for instance, 1 ram for 10 ewes.

In old age There is little reliable data, but mares have bred foals when over 30 years, cattle and sheep up to 20 years and cats till 14 years old. These, however, were all animals that had bred regularly in their younger days. It is difficult to breed from an aged female that has not previously been used for stud purposes. (See also under REPRODUCTION; ARTIFICIAL INSEMINATION.)

Brewer's Grains

Brewer's grains are a by-product of brewing used as animal feed. They consist of the malted barley after it has been exhausted. In both wet and dry forms they are used for feeding cattle, while dry grains are sometimes fed to folded sheep. If fed wet they must be fresh or they become fermented; acidosis may then result when fed. Mould can occur if stored. In the dry they can be kept for a considerable length of time without harm. They are rich in proteins and carbohydrates, but must not be fed to excess.

Some samples become infected with *Bacillus cereus*. (See BACILLUS.)

Briard

A large, long-haired dog, black, fawn or grey in colour. Many heritable defects have been eliminated by selective breeding but progressive retinal atrophy is a trait. Hip dysplasia may be due to a variety of factors.

Bridle Injuries

They take the form of: (1) injuries to the poll; (2) injuries to the chin, caused by the curb-chain; and (3) injuries of the mouth from the bit. Damage is generally only superficial but in a few cases infection sets in, and pus forms. This may burrow down into the ligamentous tissue of the poll and produce 'POLL EVIL'. In ordinary cases it suffices to protect the damaged skin by winding a piece of sheep-skin round the strap that is causing the injury, and dressing the abraded areas with an antiseptic powder each night. Those injuries to the chin that are caused by the curb-chain are usually only slight, and mainly affect young horses when they are being broken in. When they learn to answer the reins and acquire what is called a 'soft mouth', the chafed skin is allowed to heal and the condition passes off. In older horses that have 'hard mouths' and that constantly require the use of the curb-chain, the skin becomes thickened and calloused, and the surface of the bone may become irritated with a resulting deposition of new bone in the groove of the chin. Injury may be obviated by using a leather curb for young horses that have very tender skins, and by changing the bit for older animals. Care in driving of the horse, avoiding all sudden or severe pulls on the reins, will often do more to 'soften' a horse's mouth than the use of more drastic measures. Bit injuries consist of the abrasion of the mucous membrane of the lower jaw, just opposite the corners of the lips, where the bit crosses. Sometimes the membrane becomes actually ulcerated and a foul-smelling discharge escapes, but in the majority of cases the injuries are slight and heal in a few days.

Bright Blindness

This, a prevalent condition in Yorkshire hill sheep, was first described in 1965, and is characterised by progressive degeneration of the retina. The disease is of considerable economic importance in some flocks.

Cause Consumption of bracken over a period. Bright blindness has been found in several breeds of sheep, in Scotland and Wales as well as in Northern England. In some flocks the incidence may be 5 to 8 per cent among the ewes, with a peak incidence in those 2 to 4 years old. The blindness is permanent.

In ewes moved to bracken-free grazing before the disease is well advanced, the condition will not progress further.

Brisket Disease

Another name for MOUNTAIN SICKNESS.

British

The term applied to any breed of cat indicates that the animals are stockily built with round heads. For example, the British blue is stocky and round faced; the Russian blue has a bony structure more similar to the Siamese.

British Alpine

A black and white breed of goat.

British Cattle Movement Service (BCMS)

Curwen Road, Workington, Cumbria CA14 2DD. The organisation set up by the UK government to maintain a register of births, deaths and imports of cattle, issue cattle passports and process cattle movement information from farmers.

British Dane

A breed established by the Red Poll Cattle Society in the UK following the import of Danish Red cattle.

British Veterinary Association (BVA)

7 Mansfield Street, London W1G 9NQ. The veterinary surgeons' professional representative body. Its principal objects are the advancement of veterinary science in all its branches, the publication of scientific and clinical material, and the promotion of the welfare of the profession. It is intimately concerned with all matters of professional policy, and maintains contact with many outside bodies and government departments. It publishes the weekly journal *The Veterinary Record*, which has an international circulation.

The BVA Animal Welfare Foundation is a charity devoted to the promotion and protection of animal welfare; address as above.

British Veterinary Profession

(see VETERINARY PROFESSION)

Broilers

Good quality table chickens of either sex, about 5 to 8 weeks old, and weighing about 1.5 kg (3½ lbs) (liveweight).

Mortality If the chicks and their management are good, the total mortality for a broiler crop should be less than 5 per cent, frequently only 3 per cent. Most of these deaths will take place during the first fortnight. In fact, a 1.5 per cent mortality is normal and to be expected during the early period.

For commercial reasons there is often the temptation to overcrowd broilers in their houses, and this practice will inevitably increase stress and hence the liability of disease – the effects of which may be the more severe. (See also under BATTERY SYSTEM; NEWCASTLE DISEASE; POULTRY AND POULTRY KEEPING.)

Broiler ascites, and colisepticaemia lesions in the pericardium and liver, are causes of carcase rejection at processing plants; as is 'swollen head syndrome' (subcutaneous oedema). Both are caused by *E. coli*.

'Broken Mouth'

'Broken mouth' is the name given to the mouths of old sheep that have lost some of their teeth. Loss of incisor teeth is not uncommon in hill sheep and is of economic importance because a ewe needs her incisors if she is to support herself and a lamb on the hill.

The condition involves resorption of bone from the jaw following premature loss of the incisor teeth. It is already known that, in the rat, demineralisation of the skeleton can result from protein or mineral deficiency.

Broken incisors were seen in 6- to 8-month-old sheep wintered for 6 to 12 weeks on swedes or turnips. Towards the end of this period up to two-thirds of the hoggets were in poor condition. The crowns of several incisors had fractured leaving short irregular brown stumps. The enamel was normal but there was softening and loss of dentine between the apical end of the enamel and the gum margin. It was suggested that this resulted from the effects of acids produced by bacterial action on the carbohydrates in the turnips and swedes.

Signs Difficulty in feeding, dropping some of the food back into the trough, and 'quidding'.

'Broken Wind' ('Heaves')

Both are outdated expressions applied to horses with long-standing respiratory diseases, usually referred to as chronic obstructive pulmonary disease (COPD). 'Heaves' is the colloquial name for a condition in which double expiratory effort is a feature. This particular symptom may arise from several different pathological processes in the lungs, not all of which are chronic or irreversible; e.g. allergic reactions, such as immediate-type hypersensitivity (as in bronchial asthma) and extrinsic allergic alveolitis (as in 'farmer's lung'), chronic bronchiolitis following bacterial or viral infections and, very rarely, lung tumours. In every case there is widespread bronchiolitis which initially gives rise to generalised over-inflation of alveoli (so-called 'functional emphysema'). This lesion is reversible but eventually there is destructive emphysema in which there is an increase beyond normal in the size of the air-spaces with destructive changes in the alveolar walls. These changes are irreversible and lead to progressive respiratory disability and eventual failure.

Signs The clinical sign of double expiratory effort consists of an initial passive normal expiratory movement followed by an active contraction of the chest and abdominal muscles to expel the remaining air. In advanced cases this leads to hypertrophy of the rectus abdominis muscles, and the formation of a 'heaves line' beneath the posterior aspect of the rib cage – a feature characteristic of long-standing obstructive pulmonary disease in the horse.

A cough – typically dry, short, hollow and low-pitched – sometimes becomes paroxysmal after stabling or exercise; also faster breathing, audible wheezing, nasal discharge, and intolerance of exercise.

Differential diagnosis of these chronic respiratory disorders with a double expiratory effort depends upon detailed clinical evaluation, responses to corticosteroids and other drugs, the results of serological tests with appropriate antigens and, ultimately, autopsy. Infestation with the equine lungworm *Dictyocaulus arnfieldii* tuberculosis, and hydatid cysts should also be considered.

Control Vaccination against equine influenza, since many cases appear to originate from an episode of acute respiratory disease.

(See also CHRONIC OBSTRUCTIVE PULMONARY DISEASE; EMPHYSEMA.)

Bromhexine Hydrochloride

A mucolytic and expectorant; used in most animal species.

Bromocriptin

An ergot alkaloid. (See PSEUEDOPREGNANCY.)

Bronchiectasis

A condition in which there is dilatation of the walls of the bronchioles due to weakening through excessive coughing. The condition is often met with in chronic bronchitis, and the cavities produced are often filled with pus.

Bronchiolitis

Inflammation of very small bronchial tubes (bronchioles).

Bronchitis

Bronchitis is inflammation of the mucous membrane lining of the bronchi. It is a very common disease of all animals in temperate or cold climates. It may occur as an extension of inflammation of the trachea (tracheitis), and it may be followed by pneumonia or pleurisy, or both.

(a) **Acute bronchitis** This may follow exposure to smoke from a burning building, or be the result of careless administration of liquid medicines which then 'go the wrong way'. More commonly acute bronchitis may occur during the course of some virus infections, following colds and chills, and may affect farm animals housed in badly ventilated buildings. In the dog, bronchitis often occurs during the course of distemper, and in the horse it may be associated with influenza or strangles. Acute bronchitis in cattle and sheep may be parasitic. (See PARASITIC BRONCHITIS; WORMS, FARM TREATMENT AGAINST.) In pigs, too, parasitic worms may cause bronchitis. (See also under COUGHING.)

Signs A rise in temperature, accompanied by faster respiration, loss of appetite, a cough, and nasal discharge, are seen. The cough is at first hard and dry, but becomes softer and easier in the later stages. The breathing may often be heard to be wheezing and bubbling in the later stages.

Treatment Attention to hygienic conditions is of first importance. The bronchitic horse should be removed to a loose-box, provided with a plentiful supply of bedding, rugged if the weather demands, given plenty of clean water to drink, and fed on soft foods. It must on no account be drenched, for there is nearly always difficulty in swallowing, and a great risk of some of the medicine entering the trachea and complicating an already serious case. In animals suffering from bronchitis due to parasitic worms, suitable anthelmintics must be used. Where the cause is bacterial – secondary, very often, to a virus infection – the use of appropriate antibiotics is indicated. Liquid medicines should not be given. In housed livestock, attention must be paid to the ventilation. For the dog, a jacket of flannel or similar material may be made. (See NURSING OF SICK ANIMALS; KENNEL COUGH.)

(b) **Chronic bronchitis** This may follow the acute form, or it may arise as a primary condition. The smaller capillary bronchial tubes are affected and not the larger passages.

Chronic bronchitis is often seen in the old dog, very occasionally in association with tuberculosis. The latter may also cause chronic bronchitis in cattle and other animals. In the horse, chronic bronchitis may lead to EMPHYSEMA. (See also 'BROKEN WIND'.) Parasitic worms may be associated with some long-standing cases of bronchitis in animals.

Signs A loud, hard cough, often appearing in spasms, respiratory distress on the least exertion, an intermittent, white, clotted, or pus-containing nasal discharge, which is most in evidence after coughing or exercise, and a gradual loss of condition, characterises this form of bronchitis.

(c) **Bronchitis in chickens** (see under INFECTIOUS BRONCHITIS)

Bronchopneumonia
Inflammation of the bronchi and lungs.

Bronchoscopy
Examination of the bronchi by means of a bronchoscope, a tubular optical instrument with a small lamp attached which is passed through the trachea. The technique is used in cases in which clinical and radiological examinations fail to provide a diagnosis.

Bronchus, or Bronchial Tube
Bronchus, or bronchial tube, is the name applied to tubes into which the windpipe (trachea) divides, one going to either lung. The name is also applied to the later divisions of these tubes distributed throughout the lungs. Bronchioles are very small bronchial tubes.

'Brown Mouth'
A syndrome characterised mainly by gum necrosis and dysentery, occurring as a complication of virus diseases in the dog.

'Brown Nose'
A form of LIGHT SENSITISATION in cattle.

Brown Swiss
A breed of dairy cattle producing milk with a high protein level.

Brucellosis
A NOTIFIABLE DISEASE, this is an infection with *Brucella*. Five species of this genus of bacteria are important, namely: *B. abortus* (the main cause of abortion in cattle but now eradicated in Britain); *B. melitensis*, *B. suis*, *B. ovis* and *B. canis*.

Public health Human brucellosis may be caused by any of the five species of *Brucella*, as mentioned above. Infections with *Brucella* species are reportable diseases under the Zoonosis Order 1989. It often takes the form of 'undulant fever', with characteristic undulating fluctuations of the temperature. Human infection with *B. abortus* may follow the drinking of raw milk or the handling of infected fetal membranes. Infected uterine discharge drying on the cow's skin may be inhaled. It was formerly not uncommon in farm and abattoir workers, and veterinary surgeons.

For symptoms, see UNDULANT FEVER.

What was formerly known as Malta Fever in man is due to *B. melitensis*, an infection of goats and sheep, occasionally cattle. Its occurrence in the UK was limited to one outbreak resulting from imported infected cheese.

The American strain of *B. suis* (found in pigs and hares) is also pathogenic for man, causing undulant fever and arthritis.

B. canis, which infects dogs, can also cause illness in people.

B. ovis, which infects sheep, rarely causes human illness.

Horses *B. abortus* may cause fistulous withers and lameness due to infection of other ligaments. In the mare, abortion may (rarely) occur.

Cattle (see BRUCELLOSIS IN CATTLE)

Dogs In the UK, *B. abortus* was isolated from the urine of a dog which had shown symptoms of stiffness and orchitis. At autopsy, cystitis and an abscess of the prostate were found. Such a dog would be a public health risk, and a danger to cattle. Abortion is another symptom. The infection has been found in kennels, following the feeding of meat from stillborn calves. Brucellosis in dogs is probably more common than generally realised. In Chile a survey showed that 40 per cent of dogs, on farms where the dairy herds were infected with *B. abortus*, were infected.

B. canis was first isolated in 1966. In the USA it has caused outbreaks of severe illness in laboratory beagles; it causes also illness in man.

A unique feature of *B. canis* infection is lack of fever. Another feature is the duration of bacteraemia, which usually lasts for several months, but can last 3 or 4 years.

In males, epididymitis, scrotal dermatitis, and testicular degeneration may occur, although it is not uncommon for male dogs to be 'silent' carriers.

Sheep Formerly, brucellosis was an important disease of sheep in the UK.

B. ovis gives rise (in Australasia, the USA, and Europe) to infertility and scrotal oedema in rams. Abortion may occur in infected ewes. (See also RAM EPIDIDYMITIS.)

Goats In Britain, brucellosis is not a serious problem in goats.

A survey of sheep flocks and goat herds is carried out yearly to determine whether Britain remains free from brucellosis in those species. The results are sent to the EU Veterinary Directorate.

Pigs In Britain, brucellosis is not found. Overseas, abortion in pigs is caused by *B. abortus suis.*

Deer There is no evidence that deer, infected with *B. abortus*, have infected cattle grazing the same pasture.

Poultry Chickens are susceptible to *B. abortus* infection, which they have transmitted to cattle.

Wild animals The harbour porpoise around Britain may carry *Brucella maris*, which reacts with *B. abortus*. Cattle by the shore coming into contact with porpoise material may then show a positive reaction to the brucella test. *B. suis* has caused orchitis in hares abroad and, in Africa, *B. abortus* has been isolated from a waterbuck, and from rodents.

In Argentina foxes are commonly infected with *B. abortus.*

(See also FISTULOUS WITHERS; 'POLL EVIL'; BUMBLE-FOOT; RAM EPIDIDIMYTIS.)

Brucellosis in Cattle

(*Brucella melitensis* causes disease in some countries.) 'Contagious bovine abortion', also known as Bang's disease, is a specific contagious disease due to *B. abortus*. Since the infection may exist and persist in the genital system of the bull, *Brucellosis* is to be preferred as a name for the disease. In females it is characterised by a chronic inflammation of the uterus (especially of the mucous membrane); usually, but not invariably, followed by abortion between the 5th and 8th months of pregnancy.

It is important to note that not all infected animals abort. Indeed, in over half of them pregnancy runs to full term. However, any animal that has aborted once may be almost as infectious at its next and subsequent calvings as on the occasion it aborted.

Infection may occur by the mouth or through the vagina during service, when a bull which has served an infected cow is called upon to serve a clean one afterwards, or when the bull is a 'carrier'. Contamination of litter with discharges from a previous case is an important factor in the spread of the disease in a herd. The hand and arm of the man who handles an aborted fetus may also transmit infection.

In the pregnant cow a low-grade chronic inflammatory reaction is set up in the uterus with the result that an exudate accumulates between the fetal membranes and the uterine mucous membranes, especially around the cotyledons. The cotyledons may appear necrotic, owing to the presence of fibrinous adherent masses upon their surfaces, and the fetal membranes may show similar areas after they have been expelled. Quite commonly in cattle the membranes are thickened and tough. The fetus may be normal or may show a dropsical condition of the muscles and the subcutaneous tissues, and there may be fluid present in the cavities of chest, abdomen, and cranium. In some cases the fetus undergoes a process of mummification, and when it is discharged it is almost unrecognisable as a fetus.

Cows at pasture may become infected by older 'carrier' cows (which are liable to harbour the organisms in their udders) or by wild animals (e.g. foxes), dogs or birds, which have eaten or been in contact with infected membranes or discharges upon other farms near by where the disease already exists.

Signs Abortion may occur without any preliminary symptoms, and except that the calf is not a full-term one, may be practically the same as normal calving. Most cows which have aborted once will carry their next calf to full term, or practically to full term; while only very few cows will abort a calf three times. Some calves born to infected cows will be persistently infected.

As a rule, if abortion occurs early in pregnancy the fetal membranes are expelled along with the fetus, but if towards the end of the period there is almost always retention of these. A continuous reddish-brown or brownish-grey discharge follows, and persists for about 10 to 20 days (often for about 2 weeks). In some instances it slowly collects in the cavity of the uterus, little or nothing being seen at the vulva, and then it is discharged periodically, often in large amounts at a time. In the bull symptoms of infection may be very slight or absent, and laboratory methods are usually necessary to establish a diagnosis.

Brucellosis is not the only cause of abortion in cattle due to an infective agent, and in arriving at a diagnosis it must be differentiated from infections listed under ABORTION.

Immunity Infected animals gradually produce an immunity in themselves against further abortions. The organisms may persist in the system for long periods, and a cow which does not herself subsequently abort may spread infection to other cows in the herd. This natural immunity, however, is wasteful, both in the matter of calves and milk supply, so that methods have been adopted in which an effort is made to provide animals with an artificial immunity.

Testing Bulked milk from herds is routinely tested by the MILK RING TEST or an ELISA. Periodic biennial blood tests are made of suckler herds; formerly the ROSE BENGAL TEST was used but this has been replaced by an ELISA. All cows calving at 270 days' gestation or less must be reported and are investigated by blood and milk samples from the dam, examination of placenta, abomasal contents and sera of the fetus. (See also COOMBS TEST.)

Eradication In October 1985 Britain was declared officially brucellosis-free. Occasional cases have occurred following the importation of cattle. Brucellosis has been successfully eradicated from many overseas countries, including Denmark, Sweden, Norway, Finland, the Czech Republic, Slovakia and Eire. Farmers' cooperation and discipline played an important part.

Precautions All calvings under 270 days' gestation must be reported to DEFRA and investigated. The greatest care must be taken in handling and disposing of an aborted fetus, fetal membranes, discharges, etc., both in the interests of human health and in order to prevent the spread of the disease among cattle. It is worth having a veterinary surgeon examine the cause of any abortion. There can be danger from the infected cow that has carried a calf to full term. Avoid buying in replacements from non-Accredited herds. Infected farm dogs can spread infection.

Brucellosis in Sheep
(see RAM EPIDIDYMITIS)

Bruised Sole
Bruised sole is a condition of bruising of the sensitive sole of the foot, due to a badly fitting shoe, or the result of the horse having stood upon a projection, such as a stone, etc. Its character and its treatment do not differ from what is given under CORNS, except that while the corn has a more or less definite position in the foot, bruising of the sole may occur anywhere.

Bruises
The discoloration caused by bleeding under unbroken skin following a blow or other trauma (see also HAEMATOMA).

Bruit and Murmur
Bruit and murmur are words used to describe several abnormal sounds heard in connection with the heart and arteries on auscultation.

Brush Border
On the free surface of some cells, the wall may be modified to provide finger-like projections: the brush border. This is seen, for example, in the convoluted tubule of the kidney and in the alimentary canal.

Brushing and Cutting
Brushing and cutting are injuries to the horse caused by the inside of the fetlock joint or coronet being struck by the hoof or shoe of the opposite limb; although bad shoeing may be responsible in a few instances, the cause is usually faulty conformation.

A brushing boot should be fitted, and an attempt made to avoid the future occurrence of brushing by skilful shoeing. (See also SPEEDY-CUT.)

Brussels Sprouts
Cattle strip-grazing these for 6 weeks, without other food, became ill with anaemia and haemoglobinuria. The illness caused by members of the *Brassicae* species is said to be more serious near to the time of calving.

Bruxism
Grinding, gnawing or clenching of the teeth; seen mainly in cattle.

BSE
(see BOVINE SPONGIFORM ENCEPHALOPATHY)

Bubonic Plague
Bubonic plague is an infectious disease of man, rats and mice and rabbits caused by *Yersinia pestis*. Foci of infection exist in several parts of the world, including the western United States. Rats, rabbits and cats and dogs may be involved in transmitting the infection to man, usually by means of fleas.

In man bubonic plague takes one of two forms: (1) After an incubation period of 2 to

7 days, the usual symptoms include the sudden onset of fever, rigors, muscular pain, headache and prostration. Within a few days the characteristic buboes (swelling of the lymph nodes in the groin and armpits) usually appear. These are accompanied by oedema, erythema, and great pain. (2) Pulmonary plague has an incubation period of 2 or 3 days. Besides the sudden onset of fever there is a cough (usually with bloody sputum), headache, rigors, and prostration. When untreated this form of plague usually results in death within 2 to 5 days.

Various antibiotics are effective in treatment if given early enough.

The intermediate link between the infected rat and man is the rat flea.

Buccal
Related to the cheek.

Buccal Cavity
The mouth.

Buccostomy
An operation for the creation of buccal fistulae to prevent wind-sucking.

Buck
Term for the male of many species, e.g. deer, ferret, goat, hare, kangaroo.

Budgerigars
(see CAGE (AVIARY) BIRDS, DISEASES OF)

Buffalo
The Asiatic water buffalo *Bubalus bubalis* is farmed in Britain for the production of mozzarella cheese. The American 'buffalo' is the bison (*Bison bison*) and is farmed in the UK for meat. (See WATER BUFFALOES.)

Buffalo Fly
This is *Lyperosia exigua*, a parasite of importance in Australia and in India and Malaysia. It causes great irritation and even anaemia. (See FLIES.)

Buffalo Gnat
Swarms of these, which breed in running water, attack cattle, often causing them to stampede, and producing serious bites which may lead to death. Man is also attacked by these black flies (*Simulium* species).

Buffalo-Pox
A contagious disease of buffaloes which is of considerable economic importance. The infective agent is distinct from cowpox virus. (See also under POX.)

Buffer
A substance which, when added to a solution, causes resistance to any change of hydrogen ion concentration when either acid or alkali is added.

Buffing
Buffing is a term applied to the striking of the inside of one hoof at the quarter with some part of the opposite one. It is due to the same causes as BRUSHING, but it occurs in horses that do not lift their feet very high. Less damage is done than in brushing, and it is not so likely to cause stumbling or lameness.

Bufotalin
The principal poisonous substance present in the skin and saliva of the common European toad, *Bufo vulgaris*. Very small quantities will cause vomiting in dogs and cats, and 0.00917 mg per kg bodyweight has caused death from heart-failure in the cat. (See TOADS.)

Buiatrics
The study of cattle and their diseases.

Buildings
(see HOUSING OF ANIMALS)

Bulbar Paralysis, Infectious
(see AUJESZKY'S DISEASE). The term 'bulbar' relates to the medulla oblongata or the prolongation of the spinal cord into the brain.

Bull Beef
This is beef from the entire animal as opposed to the castrate. (See under ASTRATION.)

There is no question that bull beef is a more economic proposition. Feed conversion efficiency is improved, daily weight gain increased and fat deposit reduced compared with steers or heifers. Bull beef is more popular than that from steers in many parts of Europe.

Bulldog
A breed of medium-sized, smooth haired, short nosed (brachycephalic) dog which has breathing difficulties. A show of the breed that took place in very hot weather resulted in the deaths of several dogs because the abnormally large soft palate interfered with their breathing in such conditions. Bulldogs are subject to a number of inheritable conditions including cleft palate, underdevelolped (hypoplastic) trachea, and narrowing (stenosis) of the aorta and pulmonary system. Ingrowing or double eyelashes (entropion and distichiasis) are also found.The breed has changed considerably in

appearance since the beginning of the 20th century; those changes have largely contributed to the problems the bulldog suffers from today.

Bull-Dog Calves

In Dexter cattle commonly, and in other breeds occasionally, a hereditary condition, which is scientifically known as achondroplasia, occurs. Calves are born in a deformed condition in which the short limbs, dropsical swollen abdominal and thoracic cavities, and a marked foreshortening of the upper and lower jaws give the calf an appearance resembling a bull-dog. Such calves are usually dead when born.

'Bull-Dogs'

A small metal appliance used temporarily for the restraint of cattle. They are applied to the inside of the nose for holding an animal steady.

Bull Housing

Any bull housing must be secure and designed to prevent injury to the animal or stockman. The pen should be sited so that the bull can see what is happening around him; ideally, he should be able to see other cattle at times. All accommodation should have sufficient escape points to ensure the safety of those attending the bull. There should be a means of capturing and restraining the animal without having to enter the pen. Adequate space for exercise should be provided as well as sleeping accommodation, which could be a loose box. If service is to be carried out in the pen there must be a means for allowing the cow to be introduced to a service area without risk to either cow or stockmen.

The codes for the welfare of farm livestock recommend that for an adult bull of average size, the sleeping area should be not less than 16 m² (180 ft²). For very large bulls the sleeping area should not be less than 1 m² for each 60 kg liveweight (9 ft² per cwt). The exercise and service area should be at least twice the size of the sleeping accommodation.

The walls of the pen should be built up to a height of 1 m (3 ft 3 in) and extended to 2 m (6 ft 6 in) high with stout tubular steel rails. There should be a fodder rack and feeding trough at the end away from the shelter, provided with sufficient cover to protect the fodder and concentrates, and the animal while feeding, during bad weather. This arrangement encourages the bull to stay out in the open rather than in the box or shelter and is considered beneficial. The entrance to the pen should be convenient to the feeding area.

The feeding trough should be about 60 cm (2 ft) above ground level and should be fitted with a tubular tying arrangement which can be closed on the bull's neck when he puts his head through to the trough, if it is required to catch him. This equipment is very desirable as an added safety measure, as it permits the bull to be securely held before the attendant enters the pen.

An arrangement which is very useful for dealing with vicious bulls is the provision of a strong overhead wire cable running from inside the house or shelter to the opposite end of the pen. This cable is threaded through a strong ring, about 3 cm (1¼ in) in diameter. This ring, which slides along the cable, is attached to a chain which passes up through the bull's nose ring, then around the back of the horns and is hooked to the upright chain in front of the forehead. In this way, the weight of the chain is carried by the head instead of by the nose ring and considerable discomfort to the animal thereby avoided. The chain should be just sufficiently long to allow the animal to lie down comfortably. The advantage of this arrangement is that a cow can be brought into the pen for service without the necessity of having to release the bull from his tying.

Another safety device which should be provided, where possible, in the walls or railings surrounding the pen, is escape slits. These are upright openings about 38 to 45 cm (15 to 18 in) wide, sufficient to allow the attendant to pass through in case of emergency, but through which a bull could not pass. If, due to the location of the pen, it is not possible to provide these escape slits, the blind corners of the pen should be fenced off by means of sturdy upright steel rails set 38 to 45 cm (15 to 18 in) apart, behind which an attendant could seek refuge.

Bull Management

All bulls should be handled from an early age and become accustomed to being restrained by means of the bull ring. The animals should be routinely groomed and have their feet regularly handled and trimmed. There should always be two people present when the bull is handled or the pen is entered. A bull can be used for service from about a year old, but only sparingly; once a week, or 3 services in 2 weeks, until at least about 16 months old. When first using a young bull, he should be used to serve older, experienced cows.

While a bull is often turned out with cows to act as a 'sweeper' after artificial insemination, or where oestrus detection is poor, this makes it impossible to keep accurate records of service.

Because of the work involved and the lack of suitable accommodation, there has been a tendency not to keep bulls on dairy farms. Bulls should be selected to provide genetic improvement to a herd and their choice requires considerable care. (See BULL HOUSING; also PROGENY TESTING.)

Bull Mastiff

A short-coated muscular dog, somewhat resembling the original bulldog in appearance but much larger. Has fewer inherited defects than the bulldog. Cleft palate may occur, and ununited anconal process (elbow dysplasia) may be found.

Bull Terrier

A medium-sized dog, smooth coated, commonly white, with a distinctive flat profile. Originally bred for bull-fighting. Renal disease may be congenital and deafness is linked to the white colour. Cleft palate and umbilical hernia are also heritable conditions.

Bulla

A blister; plural, bullae.

'Bullets'

A form of BOLUS. They are administered to cattle and sheep by means of a special dosing 'gun', and are used as a means of supplying the animal with a long-lasting supply of magnesium, cobalt, or selenium. Bullets can be somewhat costly and not always retained, but they are widely used and have proved successful in preventing deficiency disease in sheep. (See also under COBALT.)

Bulling

A cow mounting another when in heat is said to be 'bulling'. (See also OESTRUS, DETECTION OF, IN COWS.)

Bulls, Diseases of

(see CATTLE, DISEASES OF; diseases listed under the word BOVINE; PENIS AND PREPUCE)

Bumble-Foot

Bumble-foot is a condition of the feet of poultry, waterfowl, wading birds, birds of prey and sometimes cage birds in which an abscess forms in the softer parts of the foot between the toes. It may be caused by the penetration of some sharp object, such as a piece of glass, thorn, stone, etc., or even by penetration of the skin by the bird's own talons. An abscess slowly forms, accompanied by distinct lameness. Usually a *Staphylococcus* species is involved but many other micro-organisms may be implicated. *Brucella abortus* has been isolated from a case of bumble-foot in Germany.

Treatment It is necessary to open the pus-containing cavity and evacuate the cheese-like contents.

Bun

Blood urea nitrogen. (See KIDNEYS, DISEASES OF.)

Bunostomiasis

Infestation with hookworms of the genus *Bunostomum.*

Bunt Order

Equivalent to the 'peck order' among poultry, this is the order of precedence established by cattle and pigs. With a newly mixed group of these animals there will be aggressiveness or actual fighting, until the dominant ones (usually the largest) establish their position in the social order. Once this is established, fighting will cease and the group will settle down, with the top animal being accorded precedence without having to fight for it. The second animal will be submissive to the first, but will take precedence over the rest; and so on down through the herd, with the bottom animal submissive to all. Occasionally two animals will be of equal rank, or there may be a somewhat complicated relationship between a small group as in the 'dominance circle'.

The bunt order can be important from a health point of view, and it can affect the farmer's profits. If, in large units, the batching of animals to ease management means frequent mixing or addition to established groups, stress will arise, and productive performance will decline. Stress will be reduced in the system whereby pigs occupy the same pen from birth to slaughter time. The health factor – as well as daily liveweight gains and feed conversion ratios – will be involved when there is, for example, insufficient trough space, and those animals at the bottom of the social scale may go hungry or thirsty. Similarly, the dominant animals will be able to choose more sheltered, less draughty places, while their inferiors may be cold and wet. (See also STRESS.)

Bunyaviridae

This group of viruses includes the HANTAVIRUS. Individual species may be zoonotic.

Buprenorphine Hydrochloride

An analgesic used for dogs, cats, birds, rodents and rabbits, and as a premedicant for surgery, radiography, etc.

Burial of Pet Animals

In 1992 the Environment Minister ruled that dead pets could be returned to their owners for burial, despite the 'Duty of Care' Regulations 1991.

Burns and Scalds

Though the former are caused by dry heat and the latter by moist heat, their lesions and the treatment of these are similar.

In animals a burn is usually easily recognised by singeing of the hair, or its destruction, but with a scald there may be little to be seen for several hours or even days. Moreover, a scalded area may remain concealed by a scab.

Burns and scalds are extremely painful and will give rise to shock unless they are slight. After a few hours the absorption of poisonous breakdown products from the damaged tissues may give rise to toxaemia; while destruction of skin affords means of entry for pathogenic bacteria, against which the burned tissues can offer little or no resistance. Death is a frequent sequel to extensive burns – the result of shock, toxaemia, or secondary infection.

First aid Scalds are mainly suffered by dogs, cats, and other domestic pets as a result of mishaps in the home. Placing dogs, cats and reptiles **immediately** under cold, running water will reduce the temperature of the affected area, and is likely to reduce also the pain and subsequent skin damage. This applies to burns also. Scalds from hot oil are best treated with other (cool) oily substances or emulsions such as milk. Fur-covered mammals such as chinchillas and rabbits, and birds, should not be treated with oils. Emulsions are best for such species.

Treatment Where the burn or scald is at all extensive, no time should be lost in calling in the veterinary surgeon, who will have to administer an analgesic or anaesthetic and perhaps fluid therapy before local treatment can be attempted (and in order to relieve pain, and lessen shock). This also facilitates clipping the hair to expose the affected area.

In an emergency occurring where no first-aid kit is available, a clean handkerchief (or piece of linen) either dry or soaked in strong tea may be applied as a first-aid dressing to a burn. The part should be covered, the animal kept warm and offered water to drink.

The object of treatment, besides reducing pain, is to form rapidly a coagulum of protein on the surface of the burned area and diminish absorption of those altered proteins, from the damaged tissue, which give rise to toxaemia; and also to prevent infection – to which the damaged tissue is very susceptible. Tannic acid (the useful constituent of the strong tea mentioned above) helps to form the desired coagulum. A tube or two of tannic acid jelly or bottle of Proflavine emulsion should be included in every first-aid kit for dealing with small burns. It should not be applied over large areas.

Where the animal-owner cannot obtain professional assistance, subsequent treatment must aim at avoiding sepsis, the damaged tissues being very prone to infection. Sulfathiazole or sulfanilamide powder may be dusted lightly on to the area before a first or second application of tannic acid jelly. Subsequent irrigation of the part may be carried out with a weak hypochlorite or bicarbonate solution.

For burns caused by caustic alkalis use vinegar or dilute acids; for phenol and cresol burns, swab with cotton-wool soaked in alcohol and then smear with Vaseline, oil, or fat.

Burnt Sole

Burnt sole is a condition which results from the fitting of a hot shoe to the horse's foot when the horn has been reduced to too great an extent, or when the hot shoe has been held to the foot for too long a time. It is most likely to occur when the horn is naturally thin, and when the sole is flat or convex. The heat penetrates through the thickness of the horn, and burns or blisters the sensitive structures below. It causes great pain and lameness. Professional advice should be sought.

Bursa of Fabricius

A lymphoid organ in birds, located dorsal to the cloaca, and having a similar role in immunity to that of the thymus of mammals. (See T-LYMPHOCYTES.)

Bursae

Bursae are natural small cavities interposed between soft parts of the structure of the body where unusual pressure is likely to occur. They are found between a tendon or muscle, and some underlying harder structure, often a bony prominence, between fascia and harder tissue, and some are interposed between the skin and the underlying fascia. They are lined by smooth cells which secrete a small quantity of lubricating fluid. (See BURSITIS.)

Bursal Disease

(see INFECTIOUS BURSAL DISEASE of poultry)

'Bursati'

(see ROUNDWORMS – Horses)

Bursitis

Inflammation within a bursa.

Acute bursitis is generally due to external violence. In horses, it commonly occurs after runaway accidents, falls, continued slipping when driven at fast paces, and after kicks in the shoulder, where the bursa of the biceps tendon is involved.

Chronic bursitis The blemishes resulting are very commonly seen in all the domestic and many wild animals. The walls of the bursa increase in thickness, more fluid than usual is poured out, leading to a soft, almost painless swelling. Later this becomes hard, and fibrous tissue invades the clotted material. 'Capped elbow' and 'capped hock' in the horse are instances of the condition due to lying on hard floors for a long period, or in the case of the elbow to the calkins of the shoe; 'lumpy withers' are of the same nature, due to the pressure of a badly fitting saddle, and often lead to fistulous withers; hygromata or 'big knees' in cattle result either from a shortage of bedding at the front of the stall, or from the animals continually striking their knees on a too high feeding trough when rising; in dogs the same conditions are often seen on the knees, hocks, sternum, and stifles, particularly in old and very lean individuals which lie a lot; monkeys, both in captivity and in a free state, develop similar lumps on the points of their buttocks.

'Bush Foot'

'Bush foot' is a severe lesion associated with foot-rot in pigs in New Zealand, Australia, the UK, etc. The infection involves *Fusiformis necrophorus* and spirochaetes in the UK. (See FOOT-ROT OF PIGS.)

Bush Sickness

A cobalt deficiency disease occurring in certain sheep-rearing districts of North Island, New Zealand. It is characterised by inability to thrive, emaciation, anaemia, and ultimate prostration, and affects probably all herbivorous animals, although sheep and cattle suffer most. One of the greatest sources of loss is the difficulty experienced in getting females to breed in a bush sick area.

The type of soil is usually blown coarse sand, coarse-textured gravelly sand, or 'sandy silt', and the disease is always worst on land that has been recently cleared and burnt.

The cause is a deficiency in the soil, and consequently in the herbage, of the small amounts of cobalt, which is the trace element needed to enable the body to utilise iron needed for the formation of the haemoglobin of the red blood cells. In this respect, bush sickness is very similar to conditions which are called by other names in various parts of the world such as 'Pining', 'Vanquish' or 'Vinquish' in Scotland; 'Nakuruitis' in Kenya; 'Coast disease' in Tasmania; and 'Salt sickness' in Florida.

Earlier it was shown in New Zealand that the oxide of iron deposit known as 'limonite' may – with advantage – be used on bush sick holdings as a lick. It contains very small amounts of copper and cobalt as impurities. Cobalt pellets which disintegrate slowly in the (usually 4th) stomach, giving protection for 9 months or so. (See 'BULLETS'.)

Buss Disease

(see BOVINE ENCEPHALOMYELITIS)

'Butcher's Jelly'

(see 'LICKED BEEF')

Butenolide

A fungal toxin which can cause gangrene of the feet in cattle. (See FESCUE.)

Butorphanol

A sedative and analgesic given by injection in dogs, cats and horses. It may be combined with detomidine in the horse and with medetomidine in dogs and cats. Given orally in dogs, it is used to relieve cough.

Buttercup Poisoning

The common buttercups seldom cause poisoning, although all contain a poisonous oil, protoanemonin, to a greater or lesser degree. Species most likely to cause poisoning include *Ranunculus scleratus* and *R. acris.*

Signs Stomatitis, gastroenteritis, abdominal pain; faeces are blackish. Eyelids, lips and ears may show tremors; with convulsions (and rarely death) following. (See also WEEDKILLERS.)

Butterfat

(see DIET – Fibre; also MILK)

Butyric Acid

This is a fatty acid and a product of digestion in the rumen by micro-organisms. Butyric acid is also a fermentation product in silage making. (See SILAGE.)

BVA

(see BRITISH VETERINARY ASSOCIATION)

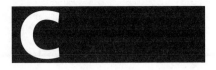

Cabbage

Excessive quantities of cabbage (*Brassica oleracea capitata*) should not be fed to livestock. It contains a goitrogenic factor and may cause goitre if it forms too large a proportion of the diet over a period. In cattle, it may lead to anaemia, haemoglobinuria and death.

Caderas, Mal De

(see MAL DE CADERAS)

Cadmium (Cd)

A metallic element whose salts are poisonous. Aerial pollution or accidental contamination of feed with fungicides, etc., containing cadmium leads to signs including hair loss, bone weakening and kidney damage. As little as 3 parts per million of cadmium in the diet of young lambs causes an 80 per cent reduction in the copper stored in the liver within 2 months.

Cadmium Anthranilate

Cadmium anthranilate has been used as a treatment for ascarid worms in the pig. It has been replaced by less toxic preparations.

Caecum

Caecum is the pouch-like blind end of the large intestine. (See INTESTINES.) Its relative size varies greatly between the species. Dilatation of the caecum is usually an acute illness. Dilatation or displacement of the caecum may often be identified by rectal examination.

Caesarean Section

An operation in which the fetus is delivered by means of an incision through the wall of the abdomen and uterus. It is chiefly performed in bitches, sows, cows, and ewes; occasionally in the mare, when the pelvic passage is for some reason unable to accommodate and discharge the fetus; when the fetus has become jammed in such a position that it cannot pass through the pelvis, and its delivery cannot be effected; when the value of the progeny is greater than the value of the dam; and when the dam is *in extremis* and it is believed that the young is or are still alive. (In this latter case the dam is usually killed and the abdomen and uterus are opened at once. There is a possibility of saving the fetus in the mare and the cow by this method, provided that not more than 2 minutes elapse between the time when the dam ceases to breathe and when the young animal commences. The foal or calf will die from lack of oxygen if this period be exceeded.)

Other indications for Caesarean section are: cases of physical immaturity of the dam, failure of the cervix to dilate, torsion of the uterus, the presence of a teratoma and, perhaps, pregnancy toxaemia.

Caesium

(see RADIOACTIVE CAESIUM)

Caffeine

Caffeine is a white crystalline alkaloid obtained from the coffee plant. It is almost identical with theine, the alkaloid of tea. Caffeine has been used as a central nervous system stimulant and a diuretic. It can be given either hypodermically or by mouth. The use of caffeine as a stimulant in greyhound or equine competitions is an offence.

Cage and Aviary Birds, Diseases of

The most common diseases of budgerigars, canaries, parrots and other birds kept in cages and aviaries are very often a consequence of nutritional deficiencies. Lack of vitamin A makes the bird more susceptible to infections such as PSITTACOSIS, BUMBLE-FOOT, respiratory and sinus infections and impaction. Calcium deficiency can lead to bone diseases such as rickets or osteomalachia in intensively bred species, especially cockatiels and African grey parrots.

Congenital and inherited conditions are also quite common. They include feather cysts (hard yellow swellings under the skin of the back). Fatty tumours and malignant growths may also occur, especially in budgerigars.

The difference in life-style between the wild, gregarious parrot, and the singly caged pet parrot accounts for behavioural problems including feather-picking.

Other causes of feather-picking include infestation with mites or lice. These are rare in caged birds but are seen in aviary birds.

Conditions affecting the crop include impaction (which may require surgical treatment) and regurgitation. Injuries to the crop may be sustained during over-enthusiastic courting rituals. In the budgerigar, regurgitation is common. There are many causes; they include inflammation of the crop caused by bacterial or fungal infection (often candidiasis), or trichomoniasis. Lack of vitamin A may cause the formation of crop crystals. A budgerigar showing the so-called randy budgie syndrome will regurgitate (chronic sexual regurgitation). Laboratory examination of the crop contents, obtained by a saline wash, is often needed to establish a diagnosis.

Prolapse of the cloaca is fairly common, especially in egg-laying hens, and can also occur in other species, especially cockatoos.

Laboured breathing, associated with rhythmical dipping of the tail, and closing of the eyes while on the perch, suggests systemic infections (e.g. chlamydiosis), heart disease, internal abscesses or enlarged liver. Gape-worms, mucus, or aspirated food material may block the upper air passages. Air-sacs may be punctured by the claws of cats, or other traumatic injury and if infected, can fill with pus or exudate. Birds with ruptured air sacs develop balloon-like swellings under the skin, especially of the base of the neck. Deflation with a needle, or more sophisticated surgery, may be needed.

So-called 'going light' in show budgerigars is a chronic and eventually fatal disease; the precise cause, which may be multifactorial, has yet to be determined. (See also TRICHOMONAS – Avian trichomoniasis.) The birds lose weight, though eating well, over a period of weeks or months. Diarrhoea is seen in a few birds; vomiting may also occur. At autopsy, enteritis is found.

Ascarids are frequently encountered nematodes in birds of the parrot family. They are seen most commonly in South Australian parakeets, especially if kept in a aviary with gallinaceous birds such as quail. Generally, nematodes are uncommon in cage birds, unless they have recently been kept in an aviary. Treatment consists of the application of a topical ivermectin preparation to the skin.

Capillaria worms may cause anaemia and diarrhoea.

Worms in the gizzard and proventriculus may cause peritonitis, air sacculitis and sudden death from visceral perforation.

Tapeworms are sometimes seen in aviary finches and in recently imported large psittacines.

Fluke may be found in ornamental water fowl and occasionally in imported psittacines.

'Scaly face' of budgerigars and cockatiels and 'tassle foot' in canaries are both caused by infestation with Knemidocuptes mites. Topical ivermectin is an appropriate treatment.

Eyeworms can be manually removed.

Fancy pigeons (Columbiforms) are affected by the same conditions as racing or feral pigeons: ascaridiasis, capillariasis, and trichomoniasis.

Some treatments for those conditions are sold by specialist suppliers to the racing pigeon fraternity.

Faulty diet, infestation by mites, and injury are among the causes of beak abnormalities, which need correcting at an early stage with scissors. In the female budgerigar especially, the nostrils may become blocked by sebaceous or other material. Horn-like excrescences near the eyes may be associated with mite infestation. Congenital beak malformations include 'scissors beak' which, in large psittacines, requires expert attention.

The feet are subject to conditions including bumblefoot, dry gangrene of the feet which may follow a fracture of the limb, unsuitable synthetic bedding material forming a tourniquet round the leg, or poisoning by ergot in the seed. Fractures of the legs result from their being caught in the wires of the cage. Dislocation of the hip is not rare. Overgrown and twisted claws are common and may be associated with mite infestation. (See also PSITTACOSIS; TUBERCULOSIS.) A perch made from abrasive material helps to keep the claws trim.

Coccidiosis, giardiasis and trichomoniasis are protozoan diseases frequently seen in small psittacines. Giardiasis may be associated with feather-plucking in cockatiels.

Viral diseases of cage birds include pox (in canaries, lovebirds, Amazon parrots); papilloma (warts) (dermal in African grey parrots, mucosal in Amazons); Pacheco's disease in Amazons; psittacine beak and feather disease (large psittacines, lovebirds, budgerigars). New viral diseases are discovered regularly.

Poisoning in budgerigars, canaries and other psittacine birds often results from their inquisitive nature. Zinc poisoning from galvanised wire used in cages and lead poisoning from paint or certain plastics are not uncommon. Washing galvanised wire with strong vinegar is a useful preventive. Waterfowl, especially ducks and swans, are liable to suffer lead poisoning from consuming lead weights discarded by anglers.

The over-heating of 'non-stick' frying pans in kitchens gives rise to vapour which can kill budgerigars and other small birds within half an hour. The substance involved is polytetrafluorethylene.

Over-heated fat in an ordinary frying pan may also prove lethal (see 'FRYING PAN' DEATHS). Birds have died after being taken into a newly painted room.

(See also under ORNITHOSIS; BIRD-FANCIER'S LUNG; *and* PETS.)

Bacterial diseases of cage birds are rare. Contact with other birds may lead to infection with staphylococci (surprisingly lethal in small birds), salmonella, mycobacteria, chlamydia and pseudotuberculosis. This latter (caused by *Yersinia pseudotuberculosis*) causes sporadic deaths of birds in aviaries – sometimes an acute outbreak, especially in overcrowded conditions. Death may occur from a bacteraemia, or follow chronic caseous lesions in lungs, air sacs, spleen, and pectoral muscles.

In exhibition budgerigars, megabacteriosis was the most common disease in 1525 birds examined at Liverpool veterinary school. Trichomoniasis, enteritis, pneumonia, hepatitis and a degenerative disease of the gizzard were also common.

'Cage Layer Fatigue'
A form of leg paralysis in poultry attributed to insufficient exercise during the rearing period. (See BATTERY SYSTEM.) Most birds recover within a week if removed from the cage or if a piece of cardboard is placed over the floor of the cage.

The long bones are found to be very fragile. The precise cause is obscure. A bone-meal supplement may prove helpful.

Cage Rearing of Piglets
This system of pig management is briefly described under WEANING.

Cairn Terrier
A small, shaggy-coated dog with erect ears; originating in Scotland. The breed is liable to inherit craniomandibular osteopathy, which causes enlargement of bones of the face and cranium, and inguinal hernia. Globoid cell leukodystrophy, causing weakness and eventual paralysis, and haemophilia are other heritable diseases.

Cake Poisoning
(see ACIDOSIS; also BARLEY, LINSEED, GOSSYPOL *and* CASTOR SEED POISONING)

Calamine, or Carbonate of Zinc
Calamine, or carbonate of zinc, is a mild astringent used to protect and soothe the irritated skin in cases of wet or weeping eczema, and is used in the form of calamine lotion. It has been used in cases of sunburn in pigs.

Calciferol
Calciferol is one of the vitamin D group of steroidal vitamins. (See VITAMIN D *and* RODENTS – Rodenticides.)

Calcification
Calcification of a tissue is said to occur when there is a deposit of calcium carbonate laid down. It is a natural process in bones and teeth. Calcification may also occur as a sequel to an inflammatory reaction (e.g. following caseation in chronic tuberculosis). Calcification in the lungs of puppies has led to death at 10 to 20 days old.

Calcined Magnesite
Calcined magnesite contains 87 to 90 per cent magnesium oxide, and being cheaper than pure magnesium oxide is used for top-dressing pastures (1250 kg per hectare; 10 cwt per acre), and for supplementary feeding of cattle in the prevention of hypomagnesaemia. In the powder form, much is apt to get wasted, but if the granular kind is well mixed with damp sugar-beet pulp or cake, the manger is usually licked clean.

Calcinosis
(see under GOUT)

Calcinosis Circumscripta
Localised deposits of calcium in nodules in subcutaneous tissues, etc. An inherited condition in dog breeds including German shepherds, Irish wolfhounds and pointers.

Calcitonin
A hormone produced by the thyroid gland. (See also CALCIUM; BLOOD.)

Calcium, Blood
Levels of calcium (Ca) in the blood are controlled by the parathyroid hormone and by the hormone calcitonin (see table under PARATHYROID GLANDS). Low blood calcium, resulting in milk fever, is frequent in cows at calving; it is also seen in horses and dogs. About half the blood calcium is bound to protein and another half is in ionised form. For an insufficiency of blood calcium, see HYPOCALCAEMIA. The calcium/phosphorus ratio is extremely important for health (e.g. see CANINE *and* FELINE JUVENILE OSTEODYSTROPHY). Resistance to infection is reduced if calcium levels are inadequate.

Calcium Borogluconate
A solution of this, given by subcutaneous or intravenous injection, is the most frequent method of treating milk fever and other acute calcium deficiencies in cattle.

Calcium Supplements
These may consist of bone meal, bone flour, ground limestone, or chalk. **Under BSE**

controls the feeding of bone meal or bone flour to ruminants is banned (see BOVINE SPONGIFORM ENCEPHALOPATHY).

Such supplements must be used with care, for an excess of calcium in the diet may interfere with the body's absorption or employment of other elements. A high calcium to phosphorous ratio will depress the growth rate in heifers.

In pigs, there is an inter-relationship of zinc and calcium in the development of PARAKERATOSIS and a calcium carbonate supplement in excess can increase the risk of PIGLET ANAEMIA.

Calcium supplements are important in the nutrition of birds and reptiles.

Calcium without phosphorus will not prevent rickets; both minerals being required for healthy bone.

The calcium:phosphorus ratio is also of great importance in dogs and cats. (See CANINE *and* FELINE JUVENILE OSTEODYSTROPHY.)

Calcium alginate, derived from seaweed, has been used as a wound dressing.

Calculi

Calculi are stones or concretions containing salts found in various parts of the body, such as the bowels, kidneys, bladder, gall-bladder, urethra, bile and pancreatic ducts. Either they are the result of the ingestion of a piece of foreign material, such as a small piece of metal or a stone (in the case of the bowels), or they originate through one or other of the body secretions being too rich in salts of potassium, calcium, sodium, or magnesium.

Urinary calculi, found in the pelvis of the kidney, in the ureters, urinary bladder, and often in the male urethra, are collections of urates, oxalates, carbonates, or phosphates, of calcium and magnesium. (See under FELINE UROLOGICAL SYNDROME.)

Urinary calculi associated with high grain rations, and the use of oestrogen implants, produce heavy losses among fattening cattle and sheep in the feed-lots of the United States and Canada. However, this condition does not seem to present the same problem in the barley beef units in this country, although outbreaks do occur in sheep fed high grain rations. The inclusion of 4 per cent salt (sodium chloride) in the ration may decrease the incidence of calculi. (See also UROLITHIASIS.)

In horses, one study found that calcium carbonate in the form of calcite plus substituted vaterite was the major component of 18 urinary calculi examined by X-ray diffraction crystallography from 14 geldings, 2 stallions, and

1 mare. In 14 of the cases the calculi were in the bladder. Calcium carbonate crystals were also demonstrated in the urine of 2 normal horses.

Intestinal calculi (enteroliths) are found in the large intestines of horses particularly. They are usually formed of phosphates and may reach enormous sizes, weighing as much as 10 kg (22 lb) in some instances. In many cases they are formed around a nucleus of metal or stone which has been accidentally taken in with the food, and in other instances they are deposited upon the surfaces of already existing coat-hair balls. (See WOOL BALLS.)

Salivary calculi are found in the duct of the parotid gland (Stenson's duct), along the side of the face of the horse. A hard swelling can usually be both seen and felt, and the horse resents handling of this part. They are rarely seen in cattle and dogs.

Biliary calculi are found either in the bile-ducts of the liver or in the gall-bladder. (*Note*. There is no gall-bladder in equines.) They may form around a minute foreign body such as a dead parasite or they may be made up of salts deposited from the bile. They are combinations of carbonates, calcium, and phosphates, along with the bile pigments, and have, accordingly, many colours; they may be yellow, brown, red, green, or chalk-white.

Pancreatic calculi in the ducts of the pancreas have been observed, but are rare.

Lacteal calculi, either in the milk sinus of the cow's udder or in the teat canal, are formed from calcium phosphate from the milk deposited around a piece of shed epithelial tissue. They may give rise to obstruction in milking.

Calf Diphtheria

Cause Fusiformis (Bacteroides) necrophorus.

Signs These may vary in severity and may merely involve a swelling of the cheek. Affected calves cease to suck or feed, salivate profusely, have difficulty in swallowing, become feverish, and may be affected with diarrhoea. The mouth is painful, the tongue swollen, and yellowish or greyish patches are seen on the surface of the mucous membrane of the cheeks, gums, tongue, and throat. On removal of one of these thickish, easily detached, membranous deposits, the underlying tissues are seen reddened and inflamed, and are very painful to the touch. In the course of 3 or 4 days the weaker or more seriously affected calves die, and others may die after 2 or 3 weeks. Some recover.

Control Isolate affected calves. Antibiotics are helpful if used early in an outbreak.

Calf Housing
Housing for calves must be warm but not stuffy (well ventilated), dry, well lit by windows, and easy to clean and disinfect. Individual pens prevent navel-sucking. Bought-in calves, in particular, are at risk of infection when placed in close contact with each other in cramped accommodation; this is exacerbated by the stress of separation from the cow, and often by transportation. (See also under COLOSTRUM.)

In the UK, standards for calf housing must meet the minimum set by the Welfare of Farmed Animals Regulations (England) 2000 (and similar legislation for Scotland and Wales). This requires that in new accommodation, a calf less than 150 kg is given 1.5 sq m of unobstructed floor space; for a calf 150 to 200 kg the space is 2 sq m and for calves more than 200 kg the space is 3 sq m. A calf must be able to stand up, turn around, lie down, rest and groom itself without hindrance and must be able to see at least one other calf unless in isolation for veterinary reasons. The width of any stall must be at least equal to the height of the calf at the withers and the length must be at least 1.1 times the length of the calf measured from the tip of the nose to the caudal edge of the pin bones (tuber ischia). The pen must be built of materials that will not harm the calves and must be able to be cleaned and disinfected. Air circulation, dust level, temperature, humidity and gas concentrations must be within limits that are not harmful to the calves. Ventilation systems must be alarmed, with a back-up system in case of failure; all automatic equipment must be serviced regularly. Calves must not be kept permanently in the dark and the light must be strong enough for them to be inspected and fed at least twice daily. All calves must be supplied with bedding and floors must be smooth but not slippery.

Calf Hutches
Individual portable pens are widely marketed. Among their advantages are the control of transmissible infections such as enteritis by preventing contact between calves. Hutches must be moved to another location and cleaned thoroughly after each occupation.

Calf Joint Laxity and Deformity Syndrome (CJLD)
A condition, apparently nutritional in origin, very similar to acorn disease (see ACORN CALVES) seen in dairy or suckler calves in herds fed predominantly silage.

Calf Pneumonia
Formerly called virus pneumonia, enzootic pneumonia of calves occurs in Britain, the rest of Europe, and North America. It is multifactorial in origin, with the environment and management often being precipitating causes. Good hygiene and the avoidance of damp, dark, cold surroundings will go a long way towards preventing it. Scours are often associated, probably the result of secondary bacterial infections. Usually, one or more bacteria, mycoplasmas or viruses are involved.

Viral infections include the following:

Parainfluenza 3 – myxovirus
Bovine adenovirus 1
Bovine adenovirus 2
Bovine adenovirus 3
Infectious bovine rhinotracheitis – a herpesvirus
Mucosal disease virus – a pestivirus
Bovine reovirus(es)
Bovine respiratory syncytial virus
Herpesvirus

Mycoplasma, including *M. bovis, M. dispar*, and ureaplasma sp. and bacteria, including *Pasteurella haemolytica, P. multocida, Haemophilus somnus*, and chlamydia, are other infective agents which may cause calf pneumonia. There is a synergism between *M. bovis* and *P. haemolytica* (an important bacterial cause of calf pneumonia). In calves housed in groups, an almost subclinical pneumonia may persist; a harsh cough being the only obvious symptom, and although growth rate is reduced there may be little or no loss of appetite, or dullness.

Often problems result from a chronic or CUFFING PNEUMONIA which is usually mycoplasmal in origin. This may be exacerbated into an acute pneumonia by other bacteria or viruses. The change for the worse often occurs following stress resulting from sale, transport, and mixing with other calves. Mortality varies; it may reach 10 per cent.

In very young calves, abscesses may form in the lungs during the course of a septicaemia arising from infection at the navel ('navel-ill'). Also in individual calves, an acute exudative, lobular pneumonia may affect calves under a month old; with, in the worst cases, areas of consolidation. (See also PNEUMONIA.)

Treatment A wide range of antibiotics may be effective, depending on the causative organism. Anti-inflammatory agents are also useful, and occasionally expectorants and diuretics. Affected calves should be moved to prevent spread of infection; good ventilation is essential.

Prevention Allow calves adequate airspace, ensure good ventilation and never house more than 30 together; do not mix age groups. Vaccines, live and inactivated, are available against specific infections.

Calf-Rearing

Calves from dairy herds are usually removed from their dams at a few hours or a few days old. They are then reared in single or group pens, being fed from buckets or feeders. Colostrum may be all or part of their diet, particularly in the calves removed early. After colostrum, they are given milk (from healthy cows) or a proprietary milk substitute, at about 2 litres twice daily when bucket fed. Proprietary milk substitutes must be given in accordance with the manufacturer's instructions. Clean water should be freely available and some form of roughage, which may be straw bedding and concentrates. Weaning usually occurs when a calf is taking 0.7 kg concentrate daily, if single penned, or 1 kg daily if in groups; this is usually at about 6 weeks of age.

The use of skim milk or whey may, where convenient, be introduced as variants of the systems given above. Under the Welfare of Livestock Regulations 1994 a minimum of 100 g of roughage should be given daily at 2 weeks of age working up to a minimum of 250 g at 20 weeks old. Concentrates providing an adequate intake of iron should also be given.

Beef calves from the suckler herd are kept with their dams for a period that depends on whether they are to be sold on or reared further. Spring-born calves are usually weaned at 5 to 8 months, the autumn-born at 8 to 10 months. Single suckling is the rule in typical beef herds but multiple suckling on nurse cows is also common practice. Under this system a cow from a dairy herd suckles 2 or more calves at a time for at least 9 to 10 weeks. Thus, a cow, according to her milk-yielding capacity, may suckle from 3 to 10 calves provided she is fed adequately and is prepared to accept different calves.

Bought-in calves may come from known farms or, more likely, from dealers via markets. Calves under a week old must not be sold at markets unless with the cow; their navels must also have healed and dried. It should be remembered that antibodies received from the dam in the colostrum protect only against infections current in the original environment – not necessarily against infections present on another farm. An early-weaning concentrate should be on offer *ad lib.*

Calf Scours
(see under DIARRHOEA)

Caliciviruses

Caliciviruses are members of the picorna virus group, and have been isolated from cats, dogs, pigs, and man. (See also FELINE CALCIVIRUS.)

California Mastitis Test (CMT)

Using Teepol as a reagent, this test may be carried out in the cowshed for the detection of cows with subclinical mastitis. The test can also be used as a rough screening test of bulk milk; slime is produced if many cells are present.

Calkins

Calkins are the portions of the heels of horses' shoes which are turned down to form projections on the ground surface of the shoe, which will obtain a grip upon the surface of paved or cobbled streets. Upon modern roads and on the land, they serve no useful purpose and may do harm. If they are too high they lead to atrophy of the frog and induce contracted heels unless the shoe possesses a bar.

Callosity

Callosity means thickening of the skin, usually accompanied by loss of hair and a dulling of sensation. Callosities are generally found on those parts of the bodies of old animals that are exposed to continued contact with the ground, such as the elbows, hocks, stifles, and the knees of cattle and dogs. (See HYGROMA.)

Callus

Callus is the lump of new bone that is laid down during the first 2 or 3 weeks after fracture, around the broken ends of the bone, and which holds these in position. (See FRACTURES.)

Calomel, or Mercurous Chloride

Calomel, or mercurous chloride, should not be confused with the much more active and poisonous mercuric chloride. Calomel is a laxative having a special action on the bile-mechanism of the liver. (See also MERCURY.)

Calorie

A unit of measurement, used for calculating the amount of energy produced by various foods. A calorie is defined as the amount of heat needed to raise the temperature of 1 g of water by 1°C. A kilo-calorie, or Calorie, equals 1000 calories. (See also CARBOHYDRATE; JOULE; METABOLISABLE ENERGY.)

Calves, Diseases of

These include CALF JOINT LAXITY AND DEFORMITY SYNDROME; DIARRHOEA; JOINT-ILL; CALF DIPHTHERIA; TUBERCULOSIS; JOHNE'S DISEASE; NECROTIC ENTERITIS; PARASITIC GASTROENTERITIS; PNEUMONIA; RINGWORM; muscular dystrophy (see under MUSCLES, DISEASES OF); GASTRIC ULCERS; RICKETS; SALMONELLOSIS; HYPOMAGNESAEMIA; PARASITIC BRONCHITIS. (See also CATTLE, DISEASES OF.)

Calves of Predetermined Sex

(see PREDETERMINED SEX OF CALVES)

Calving

(see PARTURITION *and under* TEMPERATURE)

Calving, Difficult (Dystocia)

Safety rules for the stockman are: (1) never interfere so long as progress is being achieved by the cow; (2) do not apply traction until the passage is fully open and it has been established that the calf is in a normal presentation; (3) time the traction carefully to coincide with maternal efforts; and (4) never apply that long, steady pull often favoured by the inexperienced.

The force exerted by the cow herself through her abdominal muscles and those of her uterus, in a normal calving, and the forces exerted by mechanical traction in cases of assisted calving, were evaluated by veterinarian J. C. Hindson, who used a dynamometer to measure these forces. He gave a figure of 68 kg (150 lb) for bovine maternal effort in a natural calving. Manual traction by one man was found to exert a force not much greater.

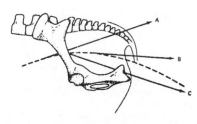

The cow's pelvis and various directions of traction.

The danger to the cow and calf of excessive force are therefore very real. Obvious risks include tearing of the soft tissues, causing paralysis in the cow, and damaging the joints and muscles of the calf. The latter's brain may also be damaged, so that what appears to be a healthy calf will never breathe.

The diagram shows the cow's pelvis and various directions of traction with the cow in a standing position. (Her failure to lie down may be due to stress, and in itself complicates delivery. Other causes of difficulty in calving include not only a large calf, an abnormal calf (monster), and an awkward presentation, but also a lack of lubrication due to loss of fluid or to death of the fetus, and inertia of the uterine and abdominal muscles – due to stress, subclinical 'milk fever', or exhaustion.)

In the diagram, line A indicates the direction of pull which would be the ideal were it not impossible because of the sacrum and vertebrae closing the roof of the pelvis. Line B is a good direction but again one usually impossible to achieve. Line C indicates the actual direction of pull, which will vary a little according to the height of the person doing the pulling, and also according to the space available in the calving area. The broken curved line indicates the direction taken by the calf.

The veterinary surgeon attending a delivery will not, of course, rely on traction alone. He or she will correct, if practicable, not only any malpresentation, but will endeavour to make good any fluid loss, treat any suspected subclinical 'milk fever', and endeavour to overcome the inertia if such be present. S/he will also form an opinion as to whether it is physically possible for that calf to pass through that pelvis; if it is not, a Caesarean operation is the likely solution.

Prevention of dystocia To minimise risks, heifers should be at a suitable weight when served; this varies with the breed. For Jerseys, the weight for serving at 15 months for calving at 2 years old is 215 kg; for Ayrshire, 290 kg; for Friesian, 310 kg; and for Holstein, 330 kg. The respective weights at calving should be: Jersey, 350 kg; Ayrshire, 490 kg; Friesian, 510 kg; and Holstein, 540 kg. Bulls should only be selected if their records revealed less than 2.5 per cent dystocia, their offspring had a below average gestation length and they were the sons of an 'easy calving' bull.

Frequent observation around calving, at least 5 checks a day, and the provision of exercise facilities should be considered as the incidence of dystocia is lower for cows kept in yards and paddocks than in pens.

Calving Earlier

Over the years, the tendency has been for heifers to calve at a younger age, usually at about 2 years old. In a herd with an average age at calving of 2 years, heifers will in practice be calving at between 22 and 26 months. The timing will depend on the maturity of the heifer as well as the time of year at which calving is required.

The Institute of Animal Science in Copenhagen has carried out experiments with groups of Danish Red identical twins, one reared on a special diet designed to give optimum growth rate and inseminated to calve when 18 months old, and the other group at an age of 30 months, and fed at a standard level.

These experiments showed that a heifer's breeding ability depends on her weight rather than on her age. The two groups came into heat for the first time when they reached a weight of between 258 and 270 kg (570 and 595 lb). In the case of the more generously reared twins, this corresponded to an age of 275 days; and with the standard-fed twins, 305 days. More than 50 per cent of the heifers conceived at the first service.

Calving Index (Calving Interval)

The ideal is to achieve an interval of 365 days between calvings. This is rarely achieved. As the gestation period is about 284 days, the cow would have to become pregnant again within about 80 days (less than 12 weeks) of calving. To ensure that cows become pregnant in the required time, services should begin shortly after 42 days (6 weeks) after calving so that there are at least two oestrous periods before 12 weeks.

The period up to 7 or 8 weeks after calving can be regarded as the acclimatisation period when the cow is adapting her feed intake to her milk production. During this time all heat periods should be recorded even though no attempt is made to serve the cow. This allows future heats to be predicted and entered on a wall chart or breeding calendar so that they can be confirmed as they occur. Cows not coming into oestrus regularly can thus be identified and treated so that they will resume normal oestrous cycles by the time breeding commences.

In very high yielding cows, it may not always be advantageous to aim at a 365-day calving interval. In such cases, return to service may be delayed for a time.

Cows that do not come into season regularly generally have cysts or other infertility disorders which, when spotted at an early stage, can be treated by the veterinary surgeon so that they are cycling regularly again before they have been calved more than 8 weeks, thus improving their chances of holding to the first service to calve within the year.

Camborough

A hybrid female developed from Large White and Landrace pigs. Litter size consistently averages 10 or more.

Cambridgeshire

A prolific breed of sheep.

Camelidae

This genus includes the llama, alpaca, vicuna, guanaco, and camel. South American camelids comprise four closely related species; all of which can interbreed and produce fertile offspring.

Drug contraindications Camels do not tolerate the trypanocidal drugs diminazine aceturate and isometamidium chloride, at doses harmless to other ruminants.

Anatomy For camel anatomy, see *The Anatomy of the Dromedary* by N. M. S. Shuts and A. J. Bezuidenhout, Oxford University Press, 1987.

Anaesthesia A mixture of xylazine and ketamine has been recommended as superior to either drug used separately: administered by intra-muscular injection in the neck.

Camels

There are two species: the one-humped Dromedary (Arabian), and the two-humped Bactrian (its head carried low). The former are found mainly in the deserts of North Africa, the Middle East, Asia, and Australia. Bactrian camels inhabit rocky, mountainous regions, including those of Turkey, parts of the former USSR, and China.

Cross breeding occurs, and mating the Dromedary to the Bactrian male produces a superior animal.

Dromedaries Body temperature varies in summer between 36° and 39°C, according to time of day. Gestation period: about 13 months. Birthweight: 26 to 52 kg. Puberty occurs in males at 4 or 5 years; in females when 3 or 4 years old. Life span: up to 40 years (but usually slaughtered for food long before such an age is reached).

In the Sahara camels often go without drinking for a week; and in the cooler months for much longer periods if grazing freely plants with a high water content.

Diseases Camel pox is the commonest viral disease diagnosed. The camel is also important as a carrier of rinderpest, foot-and-mouth disease and Rift Valley fever, although cases of the clinical diseases are rare. Among the bacterial diseases anthrax, brucellosis, salmonellosis, pasteurellosis and tetanus are not uncommon. Tuberculosis is an important disease of Bactrian camels farmed for milk production. Ringworm is the only fungal agent believed to be important and it is widely diagnosed in young animals.

Ectoparasite infections include sarcoptic mange, an important and debilitating disease of camels. The cause is *Sarcoptes scabiei* var. *cameli*. Other external parasites include fleas, lice, and ticks. (See also POX; SURRA; HAEMORRHAGIC SEPTICAEMIA; RABIES; BLACK-QUARTER; BILHARZIOSIS; SPEEDS OF ANIMALS.)

Campylobacter Infections

Campylobacter (formerly known as vibrio) are Gram-negative, non-spore forming bacteria, shaped like a comma, and motile. They are microaerophilic; that is, require little oxygen for growth. They are responsible for a variety of diseases, from dysentery to abortion, across a wide range of animal species.

C. fetus fetus can cause acute disease in animals, including sporadic abortion in cattle, abortion in sheep and bacteraemia in man.

C. fetus veneralis is an important cause of infertility in cattle (see below).

C. coli is routinely found in the intestines of healthy animals and birds; it was believed to be a cause of winter dysentery in cattle.

C. fetus jejuni is also found in mammalian and avian intestines and has been implicated in winter dysentery in cattle.

Cattle Infertility caused by *C. fetus veneralis* is due to a venereal disease, transmitted either at natural service or by artificial insemination. It should be suspected when many cows served by a particular bull fail to conceive, although usually a few become pregnant at the first mating. The genital organs of the bull, and his semen, appear normal.

One infected bull was brought into an AI centre in the Netherlands, and of 49 animals inseminated with his semen only three became pregnant. Of these three, two aborted and *C. fetus* infection was diagnosed in them. Of the remaining 46 cows, 44 were inseminated with semen from a healthy, fertile bull; and it required six or seven inseminations per cow

before pregnancy was achieved. These and many other similar experiences have led to the conclusion that infertility from this cause is temporary – cows developing an immunity some three months after the initial infection. Bulls, on the other hand, do not appear to develop any immunity and may remain 'carriers' for years.

On average, abortion due to *C. fetus* seems to occur earlier than that due to brucellosis, but later than that due to *Trichomonas*.

In an infected herd investigated in England, infertility was associated with retained afterbirth, vaginal discharges after calving, still-births, weak calves which later died, and a low conception rate. It was also found that abortions occurred between the 5th and 8th month of pregnancy – and not during the initial months of pregnancy as noted above.

Confirmation of diagnosis is dependent upon laboratory methods. A mucus agglutination test devised at the Central Veterinary Laboratory, Weybridge, is of service except when the animal is on heat.

Control A period of sexual rest, use of AI, and treatment of infected bulls by means of repeated irrigations of the prepuce with antibiotic suspensions.

C. fecalis may also cause enteritis in calves.

Ewes C. fetus intestinalis and *C. fetus jejuni* may cause infertility and abortion.

Dogs Species of campylobacter have been isolated from dogs suffering from diarrhoea or dysentery, and in some instances people in contact with those dogs were also ill with acute enteritis.

One of the species involved is *C. fetus jejuni*, iso- lated in one survey from almost 54 per cent of dogs with diarrhoea, but only from 8 per cent without diarrhoea.

Pigs *C. sputorum*, subspecies *mucosalis*, has been linked with PORCINE INTESTINAL ADENOMATOSIS, and *C. coli* with diarrhoea in piglets.

Poultry *C. fetus jejuni* is widespread in the intestines of healthy domestic fowl, including ducks and turkeys. Its importance lies in the fact that contamination of the edible parts of the bird at slaughter can cause food poisoning in consumers if the poultry meat is insufficiently cooked.

Public health Farm animals constitute a potential source of campylobacter infection for man. Campylobacters were isolated from 259 (31 per cent) of 846 faecal specimens collected from domestic animals. The highest isolation rate was found in pigs (66 per cent); lower rates were recorded for cattle (24 per cent) and sheep (22 per cent). All porcine isolates were *C. coli* while about 75 per cent of isolates from ruminants were *C. jejuni.* Cases of enteritis in people have been linked to the consumption of milk from bottle-tops that had been pecked by birds. Campylobacters were isolated from 29 out of 37 magpies which had been shot, trapped, or killed on the roads in rural areas around Truro, between June 1990 and February 1991. *Campylobacter jejuni* biotype was isolated from 25 of the birds, *C. coli* from three, *C. jejuni* biotype 2 from two and *C. lari* from one.

Canaliculus

A small channel, e.g. the minute passage leading from the lacrimal pore on each eyelid to the lacrimal sac in the nostril.

Canary

The canary, *Serinus canaria*, is a small seed-eating bird usually yellow in colour. (See under CAGE (AVIARY) BIRDS, DISEASES OF.)

Cancellous

(see BONE)

Cancer (Neoplasia)

Cancer (neoplasia) is perhaps best thought of as a group of diseases rather than as a single disease entity. All types are characterised by uncontrolled multiplication of abnormal cells. Cancer can be malignant (progressive and invasive) and will often regrow after removal; or non-malignant (benign) and will not return if removed. Malignant cancer cells usually have a primary location. If untreated, secondary growths, called metastases, may develop in other parts of the body by a process called metastasis. Two important types of malignant growth are sarcomas and carcinomas. There are several subtypes of each, classified according to the nature of their cells or the tissues affected.

Sarcomas are, as primary growths, often found in bones, cartilage, and in the connective tissue supporting various organs. Common sarcomas include osteosarcoma, fibrosarcoma, and lymphosarcoma.

Carcinomas are composed of modified epithelial tissue, and are often associated with advancing age. Primary carcinomas affect the skin and mucous membranes, for example, and

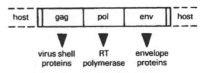

Leukaemia virus genes in cell DNA.

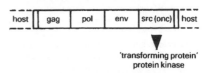

Rous sarcoma virus genes in cell DNA.

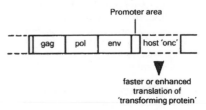

Leukaemia virus and cell oncogene.

the junction between the two, such as lips, conjunctiva, etc.

Cancer can take many forms and the names applied relate to the type, e.g. tumour; the disease caused, e.g. enzootic bovine leukosis, feline leukaemia; the tissue or organ affected, e.g. melanoma is cancer of the pigmented skin cells, osteosarcoma is cancer of the bones.

Cancer is far from rare in domestic animals and farm livestock. In the latter, however, the incidence of cancer tends to be less, because cattle, sheep, and pigs are mostly slaughtered when comparatively young. Nevertheless, sporadic bovine enzootic leukosis may appear in a clinical form in cattle under 2 years old and cancer of the liver is seen in piglets – to give but two examples.

In the old grey horse a melanoma is a common tumour. In dogs the incidence of tumours generally (including non-malignant ones) is said to be higher than in any other animal species, including the human. (See CANINE TUMOURS.) An osteosarcoma is a not uncommon form of cancer affecting a limb bone in young dogs. LEUKAEMIA provides another example of cancer. In cats, a survey of 132 with mammary gland tumours showed the ratio of malignant to benign growths to be 9:1. (See FELINE CANCER.) The relative risk in spayed cats is said to be significantly less than in intact females.

A 'rodent ulcer' is a carcinoma of the skin; less malignant than most in that, while it tends to spread and destroy much surface tissue, it does not as a rule form metastases.

The structure of some carcinomas resembles that of glands, the growth being named an adenocarcinoma. This may occur in the liver, for example.

Causes of Cancer Several different factors can lead to the production of cancer. They include: repeated irritation, by mechanical friction or radiation (e.g. X-rays, ultra-violet rays); chemical carcinogens; hormones; or viruses.

The idea that physical irritation could cause cancer was was propounded by the great 19th century pathologist Virchow. His theory was supported by the fact that cancer of the scrotum was common in chimney sweeps, cancer of the horns common in bullocks yoked for draught purposes. Cancer of the lips was common in clay-pipe smokers, and in users of early X-ray apparatus there was a high incidence of cancer, too.

Soot was probably the earliest recognised carcinogen. Japanese research workers later showed that by repeatedly painting the skin of the mouse with tar or paraffin oil, cancer often resulted. Carcinogenic compounds were isolated from tar and paraffin.

It was found too that there is a chemical relationship between one of the carcinogens in tar and the hormone oestrin. The fact that hormones were associated with the production of some tumours was confirmed. (See CANINE TUMOURS.) (For other carcinogens, see AFLA-TOXINS; BRACKEN POISONING; HORMONES IN MEAT PRODUCTION; NITROSAMINES.)

Oncogenic Viruses A wide variety of animal tumours are caused by viruses. Several oncogenic RNA viruses have been isolated: the Rous chicken sarcoma virus, the Bittner mouse mammary carcinoma virus, the Gosse mouse leukaemia virus, the Jarrett cat lymphosarcoma virus and possibly the Northern European bovine leukosis virus. Of the DNA viruses, several oncogenic viruses have been isolated, but of special importance are the herpes viruses causing Marek's disease in chickens and, recently, a fatal lymphoreticular tumour in monkeys.

Whatever their nature, all carcinogens have a common factor: they act upon DNA. W. F. Jarret, whose team at Glasgow veterinary school did pioneering work on the role of viruses in cancer, commented: 'Radiation may break it or cause adjacent units to fuse; chemicals bind tightly to it and alter its functions; viruses join into it.'

When most tumour viruses infect and enter a cell, they have mechanisms for inserting their genes into the DNA of the host cell. In effect, the host has acquired a new set of genes, and when the host cell divides and all of its genes are replicated, so are those of the virus. In this way the virus can produce copies of itself without destroying the host cell, and this is the main difference between a tumour virus and a destructive or lytic virus such as canine distemper or foot-and-mouth disease virus. One of the virus genes transferred in this way is the oncogene or tumour-producing gene responsible for producing cancerous cells.

Further research led to the discovery of a 'transforming protein' – the presence of which in a cell leads to malignancy.

Diagnosis The type and location of the cancer and the nature of the presenting signs are all factors in diagnosis. The use of endoscopes, scintigraphy and computed tomography, as well as magnetic resonance imaging, may be of considerable assistance.

Treatment Surgical removal of a malignant growth is more difficult than removal of a benign tumour, which normally has a line of demarcation to guide the surgeon. Moreover, incomplete removal of a primary cancer may be followed by cancer elsewhere, as a result of metastases.

Radium treatment is seldom used in veterinary medicine, not only because of the cost but also on the grounds that euthanasia will be preferable on humane grounds.

The localised heat treatment of skin cancer in the dog and cat has been tried in superficial skin tumours.

The most common cancer, the papilloma or wart, is treated by surgical excision or possibly by AUTOGENOUS vaccines.

Chemotherapy is used, under strict control, in dogs and cats. The drugs used are toxic and must be handled with great care; their prescribing and administration should be left to specialist veterinarians.

Control The development of vaccines against MAREKS DISEASE and FELINE LEUKAEMIA virus was a pioneering step towards the control of other virus-induced cancerous diseases.

(See also CYTOKINES.)

Candida Albicans
Candida albicans is a fungus which gives rise to the disease MONILIASIS or candidiasis; both in humans and in farm livestock.

Canicola Fever

The disease in man caused by the parasite *Leptospira canicola*, which is excreted in the urine of infected dogs. Paresis may occur and some few cases of this disease may resemble poliomyelitis. Mild conjunctivitis and nephritis accompanying symptoms of meningitis are suggestive of canicola fever. The parasite may be harboured by pigs and the disease has been recorded among workers on pig farms and milkers in dairy units. (See LEPTOSPIROSIS.)

Canine Adenovirus Infection
(see CANINE VIRAL HEPATITIS)

Canine Autoimmune Haemolytic Anaemia

A progressive disease caused by a dog forming antibodies which destroy its own red blood cells. A deficiency of platelets may occur simultaneously. This disease is a clotting disorder caused by a deficiency of blood factor VIII, and is usually fatal in males at an early age.

Signs Pale mucous membranes, lethargy, weakness, and collapse.

Diagnosis A Coombs' antiglobulin test.

Canine Babesiosis (Piroplasmosis)

Canine babesiosis (piroplasmosis), which is also called tick fever, malignant jaundice, and biliary fever, is a tick-transmitted protozoan parasitic infection increasingly common in the UK since the advent of the Pet Travel Scheme. Up to 30 per cent of dogs returning with their owners from Europe may be infected. Signs of infection are fever, weakness and malaise. Haemolytic anaemia is followed by haemoglobinurea and thrombocytopaenia. Chronic infection must be confirmed by laboratory tests. Imidocarb dipropionate is effective but must be continued after symptoms are relieved (in 24 to 48 hours) to ensure that the parasite is all destroyed. *Babesia canis* is the most common cause but *B. gibsoni* is also a possibility; this is more resistant to treatment. Tick-repellent preparations help prevent infection.

Canine Brucellosis
(see BRUCELLOSIS)

Canine Distemper
(see DISTEMPER)

Canine Dysautonomia

A syndrome resembling the Key-Gaskell syndrome in cats has been reported in dogs, and has been tentatively linked with canine parvovirus. (See FELINE DYSAUTONOMIA.)

Canine Ehrlichiosis

A rickettsial infection, formerly confined to the tropics but increasingly seen in Britain since the introduction of the Pet Travel Scheme. Infected dogs show fever, lethargy, anorexia, lymphadenopathy and thrombocytopenia; urine may be dark in colour. In the chronic form, there may be uveitis and retinal haemorrhage, with gammaglobulinaemia. Diagnosis is confirmed by serological tests. Prompt treatment with doxycycline or tetracycline is usually effective, except in German shepherd dogs, in which pancytopenia is usually irreversible. The disease is transmitted by the ticks *Rhipicephalus* and *Dermacentor* spp. Tick-control preparations help prevent infection.

Canine Fertility

It has been suggeseed that a total output of 200 million sperms per ejaculate is necessary if a dog is to be regarded as sound for breeding. Individual progressive motility of less than 70 per cent of sperms, and sperm head and midpiece abnormalities in more than 40 per cent of sperms, are associated with infertility.

Canine Filariasis
(see HEARTWORMS *and* TRACHEAL WORMS)

Canine Haemophilia

This is an uncommon disease of male dogs of virtually all breeds, characterised by an inherited defect causing abnormally slow clotting of the blood, so that bleeding may occur and continue following only a minor injury.

Cause A sex-linked recessive gene (see GENETICS). Should the dam carry this, then 50 per cent of her dog pups are likely to be affected and show symptoms. Bitches, though carriers of the gene, seldom show symptoms themselves.

Signs These may sometimes be vague and misleading, in that a temporary swelling on the forehead, for example, or transient lameness, may be attributed solely to violence of some kind. The first time that a haematoma is found in the animal, violence may again be thought to be the only cause of the bleeding, and even after repeated episodes it may be thought that the animal is suffering from warfarin poisoning. In some cases the abnormally slow clotting of the blood gives rise to excessive bleeding at teething, or if the toe-nails are inadvertently trimmed too close.

Diagnosis Confirmation depends upon laboratory tests.

Precautions Affected dogs cannot lead a rough-and-tumble life without bleeding occurring, so the owner must try to prevent knocks and bumps occurring; or agree to euthanasia. A bitch which is known to be a carrier should not, of course, be bred from.

Canine Herpesvirus

A virus isolated from vesicles affecting the genital system of the bitch and associated with infertility, abortion, and stillbirths. Infected pups usually die soon after birth. Those that recover may remain carriers of the virus.

Canine Juvenile Osteodystrophy

This is known also by other names, e.g. nutritional secondary parathyroidism. It is also found in cats, when it is referred to as FELINE JUVENILE OSTEODYSTROPHY. It arises from a calcium deficiency which, in conjunction with excess vitamin D, stimulates the release of parathyroid hormone (see the table under PARATHYROID GLANDS). Resorption of bone follows. An excess of phosphorus in the diet will also cause the condition.

Cause The main cause of this disease is feeding the dog a (muscle) meat-rich diet containing little calcium but much phosphorus. (See DOGS' DIET.)

Signs Affected animals are often in good bodily condition but are usually reluctant to move and may cry out in anticipation of being forced to do so. The usual cause of pain is fractures of the thinned bone after a minor injury or even no apparent injury. Short, hesitant steps may be taken. Splaying of the toes is sometimes seen; also swelling at the elbow or carpi.

On radiography, the skeleton appears less dense than normal, indicating demineralisation of the bones.

The bones return to normal when a balanced diet is fed but deformities left by fractures may remain.

Canine Leishmaniasis

(see LEISHMANIA; LEISHMANIASIS)

Canine Myasthenia Gravis

(see MYASTHENIA GRAVIS)

Canine Nasal Mites

A white mite, *Pneumonyssoides caninum*, is an uncommon inhabitant of the nose and nasal sinuses of dogs; and has also been found in the bronchi, and in the fat near the pelvis of the kidney.

Rubbing the nose on the ground and shaking the head are symptoms of this infestation, which has been reported from Scandinavia, America, Australia, and South Africa.

Breathing dichlorvos vapour from a polythene bag has been stated to be effective in killing the mites (but dichlorvos is also toxic to dogs).

Canine Parvovirus (CPV)

This infection appeared as a new disease entity in 1978–9 in Europe, Australia, and America. Dogs proved highly susceptible, and serious outbreaks of the illness occurred with numerous deaths. By 1981 many dogs had acquired a useful degree of immunity against the virus, following either recovery from a naturally occurring attack or vaccination; with puppies protected for up to 16 weeks by the antibodies received in the colostrum of their dams, assuming that the latter were themselves resistant.

Cause A parvovirus, possibly a mutation of the feline enteritis or the mink enteritis virus.

Canine parvovirus (CPV-2), feline panleucopenia virus (FPV), and mink enteritis virus share common antigens; however, CPV-2 has at least one specific antigen which is not present in the other viruses.

Signs The illness takes the form of a severe gastroenteritis, and diarrhoea is the main symptom. In the early outbreaks many dogs died within 48 hours. Puppies may die suddenly, within minutes of eating or playing, as a result of the virus having infected the heart muscle and caused myocarditis.

Treatment A combined antiserum preparation is available. Symptomatic treatment must include measures to overcome the severe DEHYDRATION resulting from the diarrhoea. Treatment of the myocarditis is seldom effective.

Prevention Vaccination is widely practised and has greatly reduced the incidence of the disease. Live vaccines, often combined with vaccines against distemper and other viral diseases, are available. It is essential to follow the manufacturers' directions if protection is to be effective. Annual booster doses are recommended to maintain immunity. It should be noted that apart from the effect of persisting MATERNAL ANTIBODIES, vaccination may fail in some individuals which have a defective immune system and cannot produce adequate antibodies. This occurs with all vaccines.

Canine Pasteurellosis

(see under BITES)

Canine Respiratory Disease

(see DISTEMPER; KENNEL COUGH; KLEBSIELLA)

Canine Rickettsiosis

(see ROCKY MOUNTAIN FEVER)

Canine Staphylococcal Dermatitis

This may be seen in Irish setters, collies and shelties. The lesions appear on the fine skin with few hairs on the abdomen or between the thighs. The condition is itchy, and causes the dog to scratch or lick the part. The lesions consist of roughly circular areas of reddened skin, some with a ring of blackish or greyish crust, having papules or pustules at the edge. The appearance may suggest ringworm at first glance.

The *Staphylococcus aureus* involved is resistant to penicillin, so other antibiotics must be used. An autogenous vaccine may be needed if antibiotics are not effective.

Canine Teeth

Canine teeth are the so-called 'eye-teeth', which are such prominent features of the mouths of carnivorous animals. In different animals they are known by different names, e.g.'tusks' in the pig, and 'tushes' in the horse and ass. (See DENTITION; TEETH.)

Canine Transmissible Venereal Tumours

Canine transmissible venereal tumours affect mainly the mucous membrane of the vagina or that of the prepuce; occasionally the lips of both sexes. The lesions resemble warts, and can result in infertility.

Canine Tumours

These are common. It has been suggested that the incidence of neoplasia in the dog is higher than in any other animal species including man. In fact, the age-adjusted incidence rate for mammary neoplasia is three times larger in the bitch than in women. Tumours arising in the mammary glands of the bitch and the perianal glands of the dog together may account for almost 30 per cent of all canine neoplasms. The predilection of these tumours for one sex or the other and their responsiveness, in some cases, to endocrine gland ablation or hormone therapy has promoted their designation as hormone-dependent. (See also TUMOUR; CANCER.)

Canine Viral Hepatitis (CVH)

Canine viral hepatitis (CVH) is also known as Rubarth's disease, *Hepatitis contagiosa canis,* or infectious canine hepatitis (ICH).

Dogs of all ages may be affected – even puppies a few days old – but perhaps the disease occurs most frequently in young dogs of 3 to 9 months. CVH may occur simultaneously with DISTEMPER.

Cause A canine adenovirus (CAV). CAV-1 is associated with liver, eye, kidney, and respiratory disease. (CAV-2 is implicated only in respiratory disease.)

Signs Infection may exist without symptoms, and in such cases it can be recognised only by laboratory tests. In the very acute form of the disease a dog, apparently well the night before, may be found dead in the morning. In less acute cases the dog may behave strangely and have convulsions. A high temperature, wasting, anaemia, lethargy, and coma are other symptoms observed in some cases. A thin, thready pulse is characteristic.

Vomiting, diarrhoea, and dullness may persist for 5 or 6 days, and be followed by jaundice. Such cases may be thought to be leptospiral jaundice.

Puppies may show symptoms of severe internal haemorrhage, and have blood or blood-stained fluid in the peritoneal cavity, with petechial haemorrhages from several organs. Haemorrhages, including subcutaneous ones, may also occur in older dogs. More commonly, there is fever, dullness, some vomiting, tenderness of the abdomen. Of those that survive 5 days or so, many recover. Keratitis ('blue-eye') occurs a week or two after the beginning of the illness in some cases. In older dogs, restlessness, convulsions, and coma are common.

Antiserum is useful in treatment. Glucose and vitamin K are also recommended.

Dogs which have recovered may continue to harbour the virus and act as carriers, spreading the disease to other dogs via the urine.

Diagnosis A gel diffusion test is useful at postmortem examination, especially where decomposition of the animal's body has involved cell disintegration.

Prevention Vaccines are available, both live and inactivated. Hepatitis vaccine is usually presented as a multiple vaccine in combination with distemper and parvovirus; some preparations also include protection against leptospirosis and parainfluenza. Dosage instructions vary with different brands of vaccine; normally, puppies are given two doses at an interval of 2 to 6 weeks followed by annual booster inoculations. (See under DISTEMPER.)

Cannabis Poisoning
(see MARIJUANA)

Cannibalism

Poultry Cannibalism may follow feather-picking – especially if blood is drawn – or a case of prolapse. The crowding together of housed birds is a common cause; and boredom (no scratching for insects as out-of-doors) is a factor, too. Occasionally a nutritional deficiency may be involved. In broiler plants, beak-trimming or subdued red lighting, making everything appear pink, has been resorted to. (See also SPECTACLES.)

In free range hens, cannibalism can be stimulated by the appearance of the pink of the inside of the cloaca at egg-laying. The wall of the cloaca may be penetrated, the intestine grasped and ripped out.

Pigs TAIL-BITING is a complex problem, and tail sores can lead to death. In some cases, the runt of the litter starts the vice, possibly because it is prevented by litter mates from access to the teats or trough and has nothing but tails presented to it. Cannibalism, where sows eat piglets mainly at birth or shortly afterwards, has been seen increasingly among farrowing sows kept on free range, chiefly on arable farms. The cannibal sow does not eat her own litter but guards it fiercely against other predatory sows. Thus this vice is entirely different from the occasional savaging of a litter by a hysterical sow or (more commonly) gilt in intensively kept pig herds.

Wild boar Wild boar sows must be allowed to leave the herd to give birth, returning to it later. If piglets are born near other sows they are at risk of being eaten while still in the membrane. The risk lessens when the piglets are running about.

Cannon Bone
(see METACARPAL)

Cantharides

Cantharides is a powder made from the dried bodies and wings of the Spanish fly *Cantharis vesicatoria*, or *Lytta vesicatoria*. It contains cantharidin, an irritant poison, which has been used in rubefacient and blistering applications. It can be fatal if taken internally: a young woman died after being given a drink spiked with cantharides by a would-be suitor.

Cantharidin poisoning has been reported in a horse and a mule, which died after eating hay contaminated with beetles (*Epicanta vittata*) which contain cantharidin.

Actions Cantharadin has an irritant action on the genital and urinary organs by which it is eliminated from the body. This action is responsible for its reputation as an aphrodisiac.

Canthus
Canthus is the angle at either end of the aperture between the eyelids.

Capillariasis
Infestation with *Capillaria* worms; it causes loss of condition and gastroenteritis in birds. In mammals, diarrhorea, cystitis, hepatitis or bronchial disease may be seen. *C. obsignata* has been recognised as of economic importance in intensely reared poultry in Britain.

Treatment is with flubendazole in poultry and game birds and with cambendazole and levamisole in pigeons. (See also URINARY BLADDER, DISEASES OF.)

Capillaries
Capillaries are the very minute vessels that join the ultimate arteries (or arterioles) to the commencement of the veins. Their walls consist of a single layer of fine, flat, transparent cells, joined together at their edges, and the vessels form an intricate mesh-work throughout the tissues of the body, bathing them in blood, with only the thin walls interposed, and allowing free exchange of gases and fluids. These vessels are less than 0.25 mm (1/1000th of an inch) in diameter.

Capillary Refill Time
A means of obtaining a rough assessment of the state of the peripheral circulation. It is the time taken for mucosa (e.g. in the mouth) to return to its normal colour after application of pressure. The time should normally be less than 2 seconds.

Caponisation
The castration of cockerels, carried out in order to provide a more tender carcase, and also to obviate crowing and fighting. The castrated bird is called a capon. Stilboestrol or hexoestrol, used as pellets implanted under the skin high up the neck, were used to achieve a similar effect but such hormonal treatments are now banned.

Capped Elbow
(see under BURSITIS)

Capped Hock
Capped hock is a term loosely applied to any swelling over the point of the hock. At this point

there are two bursae: the first – a false bursa, distension of which constitutes true 'capped hock' – lies between the skin and the tendon which plays over the bone; and the second, the true bursa, separates the tendon from the bone.

The lesion is virtually identical with that of capped elbow (see under BURSITIS), and treatment is practically the same.

Since the condition may be brought about in the mare by continual kicking at the heel posts of the stall (e.g. in cases of nymphomania), it is necessary to pad the heel posts or to house the horse in a loose-box.

'Cappie'

'Cappie' is a disease of sheep. (See also 'DOUBLE SCALP'.)

Caprine Arthritis-Encephalitis

A disease of goats caused by a lentivirus. It is present in Britain, Switzerland, France, Norway, the USA and Canada. It was following import of goats from Switzerland and the USA into Kenya that the disease reached Africa in 1983. In Australia a retrovirus was isolated from goats which caused a clinical disease similar to caprine arthritis-encephalitis, and produced antibodies in goats similar to those caused by maedi-visna virus, which has never been recorded in that continent.

Signs A lowered milk yield, due to mastitis, is sometimes the first sign noticed; and transmission of the virus is thought to be mainly via colostrum and milk.

The main sign, however, is arthritis. Lameness does not always accompany swelling of the joints.

Encephalitis, caused by the virus affecting the brain, affects mainly kids 2 to 4 months old. Lesions may occur in the spinal cord also. Head-tilting and trembling may be seen, together with an unsteady gait. Opisthotonus may occur. Partial paralysis may lead to recumbency and often death. A chronic interstitial pneumonia occurs in some goats and subclinical infections may occur.

Capripox Viruses

(see 'LUMPY SKIN DISEASE'; POX)

Capsule

Capsule is a term used in several senses. The term is applied to a soluble case, either of gelatine which dissolves in the stomach, or of keratin which only dissolves in the small intestine, for enclosing small doses of medicine. The term is also applied to the fibrous or membranous envelope of various organs, as of the spleen, liver, or kidney. It is also applied to a 'joint capsule'.

Car Exhaust Fumes

Car exhaust fumes from a specially adapted car engine may be used for the humane destruction of mink. The Welfare of Animals (Slaughter or Killing) Regulations 1995 state that the exhaust gas must be cooled and filtered free of any irritant material. The carbon monoxide level must reach at least 1 per cent of the volume of the chamber used before mink are placed in it and the animals must remain there until dead. Car exhaust is no longer recognised as a legal means of killing birds. (See under BIRDS, HUMANE DESTRUCTION OF.)

Car, Parked in the Sun

The temperature inside a car parked in the sun, even with two windows opened to the extent of 2.5 cm (1 in), can within 3 hours reach 33°C (92°F), when the shade temperature outside the car is only 18°C (65°F). With only one window opened 2.5 cm (1 in), or all windows closed, a dangerously high temperature would obviously be reached much sooner. A dog left in a car parked not in the shade is in danger of HEAT-STROKE; a cat similarly. (See also HYPERTHERMIA.) Owners causing suffering to their pets by leaving them in cars may face prosecution under the Protection of Animals Act 1911.

Car Sickness

(see TRAVEL SICKNESS)

Carapace

The shell of tortoises, other chelonians, and crustaceans. When assessing the health of a chelonian, it is important to relate the length of the carapace in relation to the body weight, especially as to ability to withstand a period of hibernation. The landing of crabs and lobsters in Britain is subject to the carapace being of a specified minimum length.

Carbachol

Carbachol is a potent parasympathomimetic agent which is used in the treatment of glaucoma in dogs.

Carbamates

These compounds are used as agricultural insecticides and sometimes cause accidental poisoning in animals. Carbamates inhibit cholinesterase. Symptoms of poisoning include profuse salivation, muscular tremors. Atropine is used in treatment. (See ORGANOPHOSPHORUS POISONING.)

Carbohydrate

Carbohydrate is a term used to include organic compounds containing carbon, hydrogen, and oxygen, the two latter being in the same proportions as they are present in water, viz. two parts of hydrogen to every one part of oxygen. The simplest carbohydrates are the monosaccharide sugars (e.g. glucose), then come disaccharides (e.g. cane sugar, lactose) and polysaccharides. These are complex carbohydrates, such as the starches, celluloses, and lignified compounds in hay, which must be broken down into simpler sugars by both bacterial and protozoal action and by the processes of digestion before they can be absorbed and used in the body.

Carbolic Acid

(see PHENOL)

Carbolic Acid Poisoning

Carbolic acid poisoning may occur from the application to the skin of dressings medicated with PHENOL; from the internal administration of the drug by mistake; and cases have been recorded from the use of strong carbolic disinfecting powders sprinkled on to the floors of animal buildings.

Carbon Dioxide (CO₂)

Carbon dioxide (CO_2) is a colourless gas. It is formed in the tissues during the metabolic process, taken up by the blood, exchanged for oxygen in the lungs, and expired from them with each breath. In a building, the VENTILATION must be such as will get rid of it rapidly so that it does not accumulate in the atmosphere. In the air it is present to the extent of about 0.03 per cent by volume, although this amount varies. CO_2 is used as a respiratory stimulant by anaesthetists.

Carbon Dioxide Anaesthesia

CO_2 has been widely used for anaesthetising pigs and poultry prior to slaughter. For pigs, it is necessary to have a concentration of 70 per cent CO_2 by volume. An alarm must be fitted which goes off if the level in the gassing tunnel drops below this. The pigs are driven in single file through a tunnel and inhale the CO_2 for less than a minute, after which a very brief period of unconsciousness follows – long enough, however, for hackling and 'sticking' to be accomplished without causing pain. There is no adverse effect upon the carcase. CO_2 has also been used, instead of chloroform, in lethal chambers or cabinets for the euthanasia of cats, but if it is to be humane the technique must be correct. A mixture of argon with carbon dioxide has been shown to be preferable on humane grounds to CO_2 alone.

Carbon Dioxide Snow

Carbon dioxide snow is formed when CO_2 is first compressed in a cylinder to a liquid and then released through a small nozzle. The temperature falls to about $-70°C$ and the CO_2 solidifies as a snow. This is then compressed into solid blocks, which are used for a variety of purposes where a low temperature is required for a considerable time, such as to cool meat, milk, or fish in transit by rail, to preserve tissues, bacteria, or foods, so that normal enzyme action is arrested, and sometimes to produce local anaesthesia by freezing or to cauterise a surface growth on the skin.

A piece of 'dry ice' or carbon dioxide 'snow' placed on the floor of an infested building will act as a bait for ticks which will gather round it and can then be collected and destroyed.

Carbon Fibre Implants

These have been used in the surgical repair of tendons in racehorses, and dogs, and have generally given good results.

Carbon Monoxide

Carbon monoxide poisoning may result from gas and solid-fuel heating systems in the home when there is an inadequate supply of air. Many dogs and cats have been found dead in the kitchen in the morning.

In Britain, until the late 1960s, town gas (derived from coal) contained 10 to 20 per cent of carbon monoxide. Natural and oil-based gas contain less than 1 per cent. However, where there is inadequate VENTILATION, incomplete combustion may occur leaving not carbon dioxide and water but carbon monoxide.

Stillbirths in sows have been 'associated with incomplete combustion in propane gas heaters and inadequate ventilation. In one herd when poor ventilation and faulty heaters were corrected, the stillbirth rate dropped from 28 per cent to 6.7 per cent. The pig fetus is very susceptible to carbon monoxide poisoning, and may die in the uterus or at farrowing, without clinical signs of ill health being shown by the sow.

Exhaust fumes from an ordinary motor car have been used as a source of carbon monoxide for the destruction of mink and turkeys, but this is no longer legal. (see CAR EXHAUST FUMES.)

Diagnosis Cherry-red tissues and body fluids are suggestive of poisoning. Analysis of blood samples for carboxy-haemaglobin can be used for confirmation.

Abortion may be caused by carbon monoxide even at levels too low to cause signs in adult pigs.

Carcases, Disposal of
(see under DISPOSAL)

Carcinogens
Carcinogens are oncogenic viruses or substances which give rise to CANCER. (See NITROSAMINES; BRACKEN; AFLATOXINS; HORMONES IN MEAT; *and substances mentioned under* CANCER.)

Carcinoma
(see CANCER)

Cardia
Cardia is the upper opening of the stomach at which the oesophagus terminates. It lies close behind the heart.

Cardiac Disease
(see HEART DISEASES)

Cardiac Pacemakers
(see PACEMAKER)

Cardiography
Cardiography is the process by which graphic records can be made of the heart's action. Auricular and ventricular pressures can be recorded, the sounds of the heartbeat can be converted into waves of movement and recorded on paper, and the changes in electric potential that occur can be similarly recorded. (See also under ELECTROCARDIOGRAM.)

Cardiology
Study of the heart and heart diseases.

Caries
(see TEETH, DISEASES OF)

Carminatives
Carminatives are substances which help to relieve TYMPANY or flatulence. Almost all the aromatic oils are carminatives.

Carnassial Tooth
(see under SKULL)

Carotene
A yellow pigment found in many feeds, carrots, egg yolks, etc. which can be converted into vitamin A (see VITAMINS).

Carpitis
Arthritis affecting the carpus.

Carprofen
A non-steroidal anti-inflammatory drug (NSAID) used in companion animals, farm animals and horses.

Carpus
Carpus is the wrist in man, or the 'knee' of the fore-limbs of animals.

'Carrier'
'Carrier' is an animal recovered from an infectious disease, or not showing symptoms, but capable of passing on the infection to another animal. For example, cattle may carry infectious bovine rhinotracheitis; dogs may be carriers of *leptospirae*.

Carrying Injured Dogs and Cats
(see illustration under ACCIDENTS)

Cartilage
Cartilage is a hard but pliant tissue forming parts of the skeleton, e.g. the rib cartilages, the cartilages of the larynx and ears, and the lateral cartilages of the foot, as well as the cartilages of the trachea. Microscopically it consists of cells arranged in pairs or in rows, embedded in a clear homogeneous tissue devoid of blood-vessels and nerves. The surfaces of the bones that form a joint are covered with articular cartilages, which provide smooth surfaces of contact and minimise shock and friction. In some parts of the body there are discs of cartilage interposed between bones forming a joint, e.g. between the femur and tibia and fibula there are the cartilages of the stifle joint, and between most of the adjacent vertebrae there are similar discs. When a bone is still growing, there are layers of cartilage interposed between the shaft and its extremities; these are called epiphyseal cartilages.

Diseases of cartilage Two chief diseases affect cartilages in animals. Necrosis, or death of the cells of the cartilage, results from accident, injury, or in some cases from pressure. The treatment is wholly surgical, and consists in the removal of the dead piece or pieces and the provision of drainage for discharges. Ossification: many of the cartilaginous structures of the body become ossified into bone in the normal course, especially in old age; but as the result of a single mild or many slight injuries to a cartilage, the formation of bone may take place prematurely, and interference with function results.

Caruncle
A small fleshy protuberance, which may be a normal anatomical part. In the uterus of ruminants,

for example, mushroom-shaped caruncles project from the inner surface to give attachment to the cotyledons of the fetal membranes.

Cascara

A purgative occasionally used for the relief of constipation in dogs and cats, and for the treatment of furballs in cats.

Caseation

Caseation is the drying up and necrosis of a tissue. For example, a tuberculous abscess changes into a firm, cheese-like mass, which may later calcify. (See CALCIFICATION.)

Casein

A protein of milk and an important constituent of 'solids-not-fat'.

Caseous Lymphadenitis

Caseous lymphadenitis is a chronic disease of the sheep and goat, characterised by the formation of nodules containing a cheesy pus occurring in the lymph nodes, lungs, skin, or other organs; exhibiting a tendency to produce a chronic pneumonia or pleurisy.

The disease is believed to have been introduced to the UK in a consignment of 20 goats imported from Germany in 1987. It leads to production losses and condemnation of carcases at slaughter.

Cause Corynebacterium pseudotuberculosis. Introduction of infected animals to a herd is the most important means of spreading infection. Wound infection is a common source. The organism can survive outside the animal on straw, etc. for months and in sheep dips for 24 hours. Contaminated shearing or ear-tagging tools have also been implicated.

Treatment This is difficult as the lesions become encapsulated and so inaccessible to antibiotics. Vaccines are available overseas.

Diagnosis Culture of *C. pseudotuberculosis* from pus from lesions confirms the diagnosis. ELISA tests are being developed.

Cassava

(*Manihot esculenta*) A widely grown crop for human and animal food in the tropics, and the source of tapioca. The potato-like tubers, however, if eaten raw can cause cyanide poisoning. Livestock in the tropics have died from cyanide poisoning caused by this crop. It must not be used in turkey feeds as it is not digested in the upper digestive tract but ferments in the caecum causing inflammation (typhilitis). The liquid faeces make wet litter and leg problems may follow.

Castor Seed Poisoning

Castor seed poisoning has occurred overseas through animals being accidentally fed either with the seeds themselves or with some residue from them. The seeds of the castor plant (*Ricinus communis*) contain an oil which is used not only as a medicinal agent, but also for lubricating. Processing leaves behind in the press-cakes the toxin ricine, and renders these 'castor-cakes' unsuitable as a food-stuff for all live-stock. Overseas, however, unscrupulous cattle-cake merchants sometimes sell them for feeding cattle after treating the residual press-cakes with steam, but with the result that the ricine is not all destroyed and poisoning may occur.

Signs These consist of dullness, loss of appetite, elevation of the temperature, severe abdominal pain, and usually constipation but sometimes diarrhoea. The heart's action is tumultuous, the surface of the body is cold; there may be a watery cold sweat, and the respiration is distressed. Where large amounts have been eaten the faeces are usually hard, dry, and brown in colour. Upon post-mortem examination there is an intense inflammation of the stomach and intestines, with 'false membrane' formation in the small bowel particularly.

First-Aid Give milk or oatmeal gruel pending veterinary advice.

Castration

In Britain, it is illegal to castrate horse, ass, mule, dog, or cat without the use of an anaesthetic. For other animals, an age limit is in force. (See ANAESTHETICS, LEGAL REQUIREMENTS.)

Reasons for castration To the humanitarian who has not an extensive acquaintance with animals the necessity for this operation may not be obvious, and it is advisable at the outset that the reasons for castration should be given.

Bullocks are able to be housed along with heifers without the disturbance which would otherwise occur during the oestral periods of the female, and they live together without fighting, and without becoming a risk to man. The uncertainty of the temper of an entire male animal, especially of the larger species, and the risk of injury to attendants, are well known. The same remarks apply to horses, asses and mules.

Another reason for castration of domesticated animals living under artificial conditions is that breeds and strains can be more easily kept 'pure', desirable types can be encouraged and retained, and undesirable types eliminated.

It used to be held that meat from uncastrated animals was greatly inferior to that from castrated ones. In fact, apart from such considerations as obtaining docility and avoiding promiscuous breeding, meat-quality was the main reason advanced for doing the operation. Nowadays that phrase 'greatly inferior' has tended to become 'slightly inferior'; feed conversion efficiency is better in the entire animal.

Some disadvantages of castration

The growing practice of early slaughter of meat-producing animals, so that the majority never fully mature, has posed the question: is castration still necessary or, for efficient meat production, even advisable?

In all species, the entire male grows more quickly and produces a leaner carcase than that of the castrate. Since rapid and economic production of lean flesh is essential in modern meat production, the principle of male castration may seem to be becoming out of date.

The problem differs from one species of farm animal to another. Veal calves are not castrated. They have a better food conversion ratio than castrated calves.

With pigs, boars are not castrated if going for pork and, often, for bacon. In trials, the average boar took only 151 days to reach bacon weight (90 kg; 200 lb), and had a food conversion ratio of 2.87 between 32 and 90 kg (70 and 200 lb) liveweight. If the animals in the test had been castrated they would each have required about 50 kg (1 cwt) more food to reach 90 kg (200 lb) liveweight. (See also under STRESS; BULL BEEF.)

Methods The operation consists of opening the scrotum and coverings of the testicle by a linear incision, separating the organ itself from these structures, and dividing the spermatic cord well above the epididymis which lies on the testicle, in such a way that haemorrhage from the spermatic artery does not occur.

In the interests of animal welfare, various methods of immunocastration have been tried. The aim is to 'immunise' the animal against the hormones involved in testosterone production. A series of injections is needed but the duration of effect is limited and they need repeating at ever shorter intervals.

Horses Entire colts are usually castrated when 1 year old, i.e. in early spring of the year following their birth, but they may preferably be castrated as foals, at an age of 5 months or younger. The colt may be caught with a long neck rope, and usually sedated and/or anaesthetised using detomidine, xylazine or romifidine in combination

with ketamine. When the foal can no longer stand as a result of the anaesthetic, a hind-leg is pulled forwards to expose the operation site, and castration performed with the foal lying on its side. This method has been recommended as quick, requiring less assistance, less likely to traumatise the gelding, and more humane.

After castration the colt is either turned out into a well-strawed yard or put into a roomy loose-box and given a feed; or, if climatic conditions are favourable, it may be turned out to grass again. It is always advisable to see the colt at intervals during the 24 hours after castration, to ensure that there is no bleeding, that hernia has not developed, or that no other untoward accident has happened. Cryptorchid castration is briefly mentioned under RIG.

Cattle Various methods are used, including surgical castration by removal of the testes. In the United Kingdom, the law requires that calves over 2 months old must be anaesthetised and the operation performed by a veterinary surgeon. In very young calves – i.e. those between a month and 6 weeks old – castration may be carried out by merely opening the scrotum and scraping the spermatic cord through with the edge of the knife. However, complete removal of the testicle is preferable. In larger animals the spermatic artery should be ligated to prevent haemorrhage. Alternatively, a type of emasculator may be used which has two parts to the cutting arm so that the spermatic artery is cut and crushed at the same time to prevent haemorrhage.

Another method which does not involve removal of the testes is the Burdizzo or bloodless castration method. The instrument is placed with the jaws over the neck of the scrotum in such a way that when closed they will crush the spermatic cord through the skin of the scrotum, thus preventing maturation of the testes. Ideally, an assistant presses the handles together while the operator holds the cord to prevent it moving away from the closing jaws. The method has attracted objections on welfare grounds.

Sheep The most convenient age at which lambs are castrated is when they are between a week and a month old, the operation usually being carried out at the same time as docking. The point of the scrotum is cut off transversely and each testicle exposed by the one incision. They are then held alternately by a pair of rubber-jawed forceps, turned round and round so as to twist the cord, and then pulled off, or the cord may be scraped through with a knife. Special small emasculators are also used.

The rubber-ring method (see ELASTRATOR) is also used, and the Department of Agriculture, New Zealand, has stated that there was no significant difference in the fat quality of lambs castrated at 3 weeks of age by (a) rubber ring, (b) knife, and (c) emasculator. Lambs castrated at birth by the rubber-ring method were, however, lighter and smaller.

This method is not ideal. Pain immediately following application may be severe, and subsequent ulceration of the skin may also be painful and conducive to tetanus infection.

For the castration of adult rams the Burdizzo emasculator has been used (see above). Any method of castration of adult rams which involves opening the scrotum is usually attended by a percentage of deaths, no matter with how much care and asepsis the operation is performed.

Pigs Young male pigs are usually castrated at the time they are weaned, usually 3 to 4 weeks, and in any case before they are 2 months old. Castration before weaning entails placing the newly castrated pigs back with the sow; with a fractious gilt, or with an irritable old sow, the small amount of bleeding which may occur is apt to induce the mother to attack and perhaps kill her unfortunate offspring. Some owners prefer to have the pigs castrated before they are weaned, so that the check to their growth which always follows weaning does not coincide with the check they receive from the operation. In the United States it is often the practice for piglets to be castrated when they are between 4 and 7 days old. Instead of the conventional incising of the scrotum, small incisions are made at different sites and, by means of a surgical hook, the spermatic cords are withdrawn and severed. The testicles may be left in position. It is claimed that this method reduces the danger of subsequent wound infection.

Dogs and cats A study of male cats following castration showed that there was 'a postoperative decline in fighting, roaming and urine-spraying in 88 per cent, 94 per cent, and 88 per cent, respectively'. Improvement – especially as regards urine-spraying – was obtained in most cases within a fortnight.

Castration of dogs seems to produce no reliable effect on either aggressive or scent-marking behaviour.

There are significant species differences between cats and dogs as regards the effects of castration, but 'the major effect of castration in either species is reflected by an overall reduction in the frequency of intromissions sometimes followed by a decrease in mounting behaviour. Nevertheless, some individuals retain the ability to copulate for a substantial period of time. Castration is likely to have a more pronounced effect on the mating behaviour of male cats than on that of male dogs.' (See also SPAYING *and* VASECTOMISED.)

Castration accidents or complications following the operation. Haemorrhage may occur either immediately following the operation or at any time afterwards up to the 6th or 7th day (usually within the first 24 hours). As a rule the small amount of haemorrhage which nearly always occurs immediately after the operation can be disregarded, since it comes from the vessels in the skin of the scrotum. When bleeding is alarming it is necessary to pack the scrotum with sterilised cotton wool or gauze or to search for the cut end of the cord, and apply a ligature. This is a task for a veterinary surgeon. (See under BLEEDING.)

Hernia of bowel or of omentum may occur where there is a very wide inguinal ring. The replacement or amputation of any tissue that has been protruded from the abdomen requires the services of a veterinary surgeon. All that the owner should do until s/he arrives is to secure the animal, pass underneath its abdomen a clean sheet that has been soaked in a weak solution of an antiseptic, and fix this sheet over the loins in such a way that it will support the protruded portions and prevent further prolapse.

Peritonitis, which is almost always fatal in the horse, may follow the use of unclean instruments, or may be contracted through contamination from the bedding, or by attack by flies subsequent to the operation.

TETANUS may arise as a complication following castration in horses and lambs particularly. Sometimes there is a considerable loss among lambs from this cause. In districts where tetanus is common, colts should be given a dose of tetanus anti-toxin before castration, which will protect them until the wounds have healed.

Severance of a calf's urethra by a farm worker using a Burdizzo castrator has been reported rarely.

Casualty Animals
Slaughter of an animal which is injured or sick. On a farm, slaughter is permissible with appropriate veterinary certification (see under TRANSPORT STRESS).

'Cat, Angry' Posture
This is assumed by a cat partially crippled as a result of exostoses of neck bones due to an excess

of vitamin A. The symptom may appear within 1 to 5 years of being on a virtually all-liver diet.

Cat Bites/Scratches

These may sometimes give rise in man to CAT-SCRATCH FEVER and also yersiniosis, rabies, etc., should the cat be infected with organisms causing these diseases.

'Cat Flu'

An inaccurate but convenient term widely used by owners for illness caused by FELINE VIRAL RHINOTRACHEITIS and FELINE CALCIVIRUS infection.

Cat Foods

Cats are by nature carnivorous and need a higher proportion of protein in their diet than do dogs. They have specific requirements for vitamin A, and for certain other substances, such as taurine and arachidonic acid, that they cannot make for themselves. Thus a diet based too heavily on a particular meat deficient in those substances, such as heart or liver, can cause health problems. They are also fussy eaters, which means that they may acquire a taste for a diet that is not suitable.

Reputable pet food manufacturers have studied the cat's dietary needs in great detail; they produce a range of prepared prepacked foods that are formulated to provide a palatable and nutritious diet. Such prepared foods, fed according to the manufacturer's directions, provide the necessary elements for a complete diet. However, it is often thought wise to alternate them with fresh food.

Cats with certain medical conditions, or which are obese, may require special diets; a wide range is available, which are prescribed on veterinary advice. (See also DIET; FELINE JUVENILE OSTEODYSTROPHY; 'CHASTEK PARALYSIS'; STEATITIS; TAURINE.)

Cat Leprosy

A skin disease in which granuloma formation occurs and ulcers may appear on the head and legs. The condition is a non-tuberculosis granulomatous skin disease associated with acid-fast bacilli. The main differences between the human and feline condition, on histological grounds, are the areas of caseous necrosis and the consistent lack of nerve involvement observed in cats.

Cause *Mycobacterium lepraemurium*, which is believed to be transmitted by mice and rats.

Differential Diagnosis Cat leprosy needs to be distinguished from tuberculosis, neoplasia,

foreign body granuloma, mycotic infection, nodular panniculitis, pansteatitis, and chronic abscesses secondary to feline leukaemia virus infection.

Cat Lungworm

Aleurostrongylus abstrusus can give rise to symptoms such as coughing, sneezing, and a discharge from the nostrils. Research has disclosed a relationship between infestation with this lungworm and abnormality of the pulmonary arteries. Often it is only when the cat is subjected to stress or to some other infection that lungworms cause serious illness.

Cat-Scratch Fever

Cat-scratch fever is a disease of man. The main symptom is a swelling of the lymph nodes nearest the scratch, sometimes fever, and a rash; occasionally encephalitis. The cause is a bacillus, for the identification of which the Warthin-Starry stain is used.

Catadromy

A catadromous fish is one that spends most of its adult life in fresh water but returns to the sea to spawn. Eels are catadromous.

Cataphoresis

Cataphoresis is a method of treatment by introduction of medicine through the unbroken skin by means of electric current. (See also IONIC MEDICATION, IONTOPHORESIS.)

Cataplasm

Cataplasm is another name for a poultice.

Cataplexy

Sudden onset of paralysis or collapse of short duration. Human patients suffering from NARCOLEPSY may also have attacks of cataleplexy; this is true also of the dog. A case in a bull was reported in which the animal would periodically, for no apparent reason, collapse on to its knees; getting to its feet again very soon afterwards. Apart from a 'sleepy demeanour', the bull seemed otherwise normal. There was a sudden snatch of a foreleg before attacks, which could be provoked by loud noise.

Cataract

Cataract is an opacity of the crystalline lens of the eye. (See under EYE, DISEASES AND INJURIES OF.)

Caterpillars

Several species of caterpillar have setae (hairs) which can cause an urticarial rash. Caterpillars of the brown-tailed moth (*Euproctis chrysorrhoea*) were extremely numerous in the Portsmouth area in 2 successive years, and 30 cats and a dog had lesions attributed to the caterpillars' setae which are barbed and also contain an enzyme. Loss of appetite, excessive salivation, wet patches on their flanks (probably the result of persistent licking) and redness of the underlying skin were observed. The dog developed a red rash under one eye, and later an excoriated area there which took 3 weeks to heal.

Cathartics

Another name for LAXATIVES.

Catheters

Long, slender, flexible tubes for insertion into veins, the heart, the bladder and other body cavities. They are used to remove fluids from, or introduce them into, those cavities.

The range of catheters includes cardiac, endotracheal, eustachian, and urethral instruments.

Catheter embolus During the catheterisation of a dog's vein, part of the 18-gauge catheter was accidentally severed. Radiographs showed this unusual foreign body embolism lodged in the right atrium and ventricle of the heart.

The operating veterinary surgeons had ready a cobra-shaped polyethylene end-hole catheter, which they turned into a loop snare by passing through it wire folded in half – forming a loop extending from the hole at the end of the catheter. With the guidance of a fluoroscope, they introduced the catheter with its loop snare into the right ventricle.

'The loop was enlarged by feeding one end of the doubled guide wire through the catheter loop, and the loop then passed over the foreign body, and tightened. It was safely removed, and the dog showed no ill-effects.'

Of 42 human patients in whom catheter emboli were not removed, 14 had potentially life-threatening complications; 16 died.

Cationic Proteins

(see ORIFICES, IMMUNITY AT)

Cats, Breeding Difficulties of

For the novice breeder and others, the following facts and figures may be of interest.

Dystocia In a survey of 4007 cats, dystocia occurred in only 134, i.e. 3.3 per cent. An oversize kitten is seldom a cause, unless the queen has had a fracture of the pelvis. Occasionally a malpresentation such as a turning of the fetal head may render normal birth impossible and necessitate a Caesarean operation.

Prolapse of the uterus is rare.

Ectopic pregnancy This occurs when a fertilised egg, instead of passing down one of the Fallopian tubes towards the uterus, is released from the hind end of the tube, and develops outside the uterus. Another cause is violence of some sort leading to rupture of the uterus. Mummified fetuses have been found alongside the stomach, for example.

Uterine inertia is rare. So is torsion of the uterus. In a case of the former, veterinary advice was sought concerning a 9-month-old queen in her 70th day of gestation. Following veterinary intervention, a dead kitten was born. Ninety minutes later, 3 live ones followed.

Pyometra In 183 queens the signs were distension of the abdomen, feverishness, and – in some cases – a vaginal discharge. A complete recovery followed surgery in 168 cats. Any post-operative complications in 20 per cent of the patients cleared up within a fortnight after being returned home. Euthanasia or natural death accounted for 15.

Cats, Diseases of

(see diseases beginning with the words CAT *and* FELINE. *For other diseases, see* ALOPECIA; ASPERGILLOSIS; AUJESZKY'S DISEASE; BUBONIC PLAGUE; CANCER; CHLAMYDIA infection; POX; CRYPTOCOCCOSIS; DIABETES; DIARRHOEA; ECLAMPSIA; EOSINOPHILIC GRANULOMA; GINGIVITIS; NOCARDIOSIS; PYOTHORAX; RABIES; SALMONELLOSIS; STEATITIS; toxocariasis *under* TEXOCARA; TUBERCULOSIS; TYZZER'S DISEASE; YERSINIOSIS; SPOROTRICHOSIS; POTOMAC HORSE FEVER; THROMBOSIS of femoral arteries. See also FOREIGN BODY in the trachea; NEOSPORA; PEMPHIGUS.)

Cats, Worms in

In a survey of 110 cats autopsied in the University of Sheffield, *Toxocara cati* were found in 35.4 per cent, the tapeworm *Dipylidium caninum* in 44.5 per cent, *Taenia taeniaeformis* in 4.5 per cent. In another survey made in the London area, and based on the microscopic examination of faecal samples over an 18-month period, it was found that of the 947 cats, 11.5 per cent were infected with *Toxocara cati*, 1.9 per cent with *Isospora felis*, 1.2 per cent with *D. caninum*, 1.2 per cent with *Taenia taeniaeformis*, 0.8 per cent with

I. rivolta, and 0.2 per cent with *Toxascaris leonina.* (See also 'LIZARD POISONING'; WORMS.)

Cattle, Breeds of

There are now in the world nearly 1000 breeds of cattle, including 250 major breeds. In addition, there are very many crossbreeds.

European breeds stem from *Bos taurus,* thought to have originated in temperate or western Asia. *B. indicus* (literally, Indian cattle), or zebus, have spread to SE Asia, China, Africa, the USA, and Australia. In Africa there have been many crosses between *B. indicus* and *B. taurus* groups, e.g. Africander.

(See also COWS; BULL MANAGEMENT; BEEF BREEDS AND CROSSES; CALF-REARING; HOUSING OF ANIMALS; MILK YIELDS; CATTLE HUSBANDRY.)

Cattle Crush

(see CRUSH)

Cattle, Dairy Herd Management

(see under DAIRY HERD)

Cattle, Diseases of

Many cattle diseases are multifactorial in origin. Although they may be triggered by infection with a particular bacterium or virus, an animal's susceptibility to disease is affected by its environment, management, feeding, immune status or genetic predisposition.

Surgical conditions include left or right displacement of the abomasum, abomasal torsion, abomasal ulceration, caecal dilatation and torsion, intussusception, mesenteric torsion, traumatic reticulitis, traumatic pericarditis, bloat, lameness, including sole ulceration, white line disease, foot abscesses and septic arthritis.

Other diseases include: ACTINOBACILLOSIS; ACTINOMYCOSIS; ANTHRAX; BLACK-QUARTER; BLUETONGUE; BOVINE ENCEPHALOMYELITIS; BOVINE SPONGIFORM ENCEPHALITIS; BRUCELLOSIS; CAMPYLOBACTER (VIBRIO) INFECTIONS; CATTLE PLAGUE; CEREBROCORTICAL NECROSIS; CLOSTRIDIAL ENTERITIS; COCCIDIOSIS; CONTAGIOUS BOVINE DIGITAL DERMATITIS; CONTAGIOUS BOVINE PLEURO-PNEUMONIA; ENTEQUE SECO; FOOT-AND-MOUTH DISEASE; HUSK; HYPOCUPRAEMIA; HYPOMAGNESAEMIA; JOHNE'S DISEASE; LEPTOSPIROSIS; BOVINE MALIGNANT CATARRHAL FEVER; MASTITIS; MILK FEVER; BOVINE VIRAL DIARRHOEA; MUCORMYCOSIS; PARASITIC GASTROENTERITIS; PASTEURELLOSIS; POST-PARTURIENT HAEMOGLOBINURIA; PYELONEPHRITIS; RABIES; RED-WATER FEVER; RHINOSPORIDIOSIS; RHINOTRACHEITIS; RINDERPEST; SALMONELLOSIS; 'SKIN TUBERCULOSIS'; TICK-BORNE FEVER; trichomoniasis *under* TRICHOMONAS; TUBERCULOSIS; SOOG; VIRUS INFECTIONS OF COW'S TEATS; VULVOVAGINITIS. (See also CALVES, DISEASES OF; BOVINE ENZOOTIC LEUKOSIS; 'SLEEPER SYNDROME'; EYE, DISEASES OF.)

Cattle Handling

(see COWS; CRUSH; VETERINARY FACILITIES ON THE FARM)

Cattle Husbandry

The management of cattle. It has a fundamental impact on the profitability of a dairy or beef farm and on the welfare and health of the animals.

For information on this and related health and disease problems which can cause economic loss to farmers, and for preventive measures, see under the following headings: ABORTION; ARTIFICIAL INSEMINATION; BARLEY POISONING; BEDDING; BEEF CATTLE HUSBANDRY; BEEF BREEDS AND CROSSES; BRACKEN POISONING; BULL BEEF; BULL HOUSING; BULL MANAGEMENT; BUNT ORDER; CALF HOUSING; CALF-REARING; CALVING, DIFFICULT (DYSTOCIA); CASTRATION; CLOTHING; COBALT; COLOSTRUM; COW KENNELS; COWS – Gentle treatment of; 'CONTROLLED BREEDING'; CREEP FEEDING; DAIRY HERD MANAGEMENT; DIARRHOEA; DIET; DISINFECTANTS; DRIED GRASS; ELECTRIC SHOCK; EXPOSURE; FLIES – Fly control; FOOT-BATHS; GENETICS; GRAZING BEHAVIOUR; HORMONES IN MEAT PRODUCTION; HOUSING OF ANIMALS; INFECTION; INFERTILITY; INTENSIVE LIVESTOCK PRODUCTION; ISOLATION; LAMENESS; 'LICKING SYNDROME'; LIGHTING; MILK YIELD; MILKING; MILKING MACHINES; NOTIFIABLE DISEASES; OESTRUS; OESTRUS DETECTION; PARASITES; PREGNANCY; PARTURITION; PARTURITION, DRUG-INDUCED; PASTURE, CONTAMINATION OF; PASTURE MANAGEMENT; POISONING; PROGENY TESTING; RATIONS; SEAWEED; SILAGE; SLATTED FLOORS; SLURRY; 'STEAMING UP'; STOCKING RATES; STRAW; STRIP-GRAZING; TRACE ELEMENTS; TROPICS; UREA; VENTILATION; VETERINARY FACILITIES ON THE FARM; VITAMINS; WATER; WEANING; WORMS, FARM TREATMENT AGAINST; YARDED CATTLE.

Cattle, Import Controls

Cattle may be imported into the UK through one of the following Border Inspection Posts: Bristol Port, Luton Airport, Heathrow Airport or Tilbury Docks. All animals must be accompanied by a health certificate which satisfies the 16 points laid down by the EU. Once cattle are examined and found clinically free from infectious or contagious disease at the port of entry, they may be moved around the 15 member states of the EU. Special requirements apply to cattle imported from British Columbia.

Cattle, Names Given According to Age, Sex, Etc.

Different localities have their own names for particular cattle at particular ages, periods of life, etc., and these names vary somewhat. The following is a list of the most usual names:

Bobby or slink calves Immature or unborn calves used for human food, and often removed from the uteri of cows when the latter are killed. The flesh of slink calves is often called slink veal.

Freemartin (See this heading)

Calf A young ox from birth to 6 or 9 months old; if a male, a bull calf; if a female, a cow or heifer calf.

Stag A male castrated late in life.

Steer or stot A young male ox, usually castrated, and between the ages of 6 and 24 months.

Stirk A young female of 6 to 12 months old, sometimes a male of the same age, especially in Scotland.

Bullock A 2-year-old (or more) castrated ox.

Heifer or quey A year-old female up to the 1st calving.

Malden heifer An adult female that has not been allowed to breed.

Cow-heifer A female that has calved once only.

Bull An uncastrated male.

Cow A female having had more than one calf.

Cattle Plague
(see RINDERPEST)

Cattle, Reasons for Emergency Slaughter

A Swiss survey covered 44,704 cattle slaughtered. Major causes were dystocia (8.84 per cent, 3950 cattle), BLOAT (8.44 per cent; 62 per cent of this group were aged 2 months to 3 years), respiratory diseases (6.49 per cent; 72 per cent were 2 months to 3 years old), joint disease (5.78 per cent), reticular foreign bodies (5.16 per cent), circulatory disease (5.14 per cent), enteritis (4.65 per cent), fractures unrelated to parturition (4.43 per cent; 60 per cent were 2 months to 3 years old), recumbency (4.10 per cent), claw disease (3.46 per cent; 35 per cent were aged 6 to 9 years, 27 per cent 9 years old or more) and abortion (3.39 per cent); poisoning (1.07 per cent) and spastic paresis (1.02 per cent).

Cattle Tracing Scheme

A scheme operated by the BRITISH CATTLE MOVEMENT SERVICE by which cattle are identified and all their movements recorded on a 'passport'.

Cauda Equina

Cauda equina, meaning 'tail of a horse', is the termination of the spinal cord in the sacral and coccygeal regions where it splits up into a large number of nerve fibres giving the appearance of a 'horse's tail', whence the name.

Caudal

Relating to the tail. The caudal end of any part of the body means the posterior end.

Cavalier King Charles Spaniel

The smallest of the spaniels, the breed is said to have originated in the reign of Charles II. It is prone to heart conditions and shows 2 inherited conditions: cataract and 'fly catching phenomenon'. In the latter, a form of epilepsy, the dog behaves as if it were trying to catch flies when none is present.

Cell Count Service

A routine monitoring of the number of somatic cells in the milk (see under MASTITIS).

Cell-Mediated Immunity
(see under IMMUNE RESPONSE)

Cells

Cells are the microscopic units of which all the tissues of the animal and plant kingdoms are composed. Every cell consists essentially of a nucleus, a cell wall or membrane, and the jelly-like cytoplasm (protoplasm) contained within the cell membrane. The cytoplasm consists of water, protein, lipids, inorganic salts, etc.

(The circulating red blood corpuscles have in mammals no nucleus, and although commonly referred to as red cells are not typical cells, their nucleus having been lost.)

Classical descriptions of the cell (before the introduction of the electron microscope) referred to organelles (presumed living) and non-living inclusions.

Organelles include the nucleus which controls the activities of the cell and contains its genetic material (chromatin in the non-dividing cell; chromosomes in the dividing cell), Golgi apparatus; mitochondria (containing enzymes); ribosomes (granules containing RNA); and others.

The nucleus is bounded by the nuclear membrane and contains a nucleolus or 2 or more nucleoli. DNA and RNA are both present in the nucleus.

Cells vary very much in size, the smallest being about 0.002 mm in diameter, and the largest being the egg of a bird, which is still a simple cell although much distended with food.

It is estimated that mammalian cells contain about 10,000 genes, but only a small proportion of these will be active at any one time. Each cell of an animal contains a complete set of its genes. The function of the individual cell is determined by which genes are 'expressed' and which 'repressed'.

(See also CANCER; TISSUES OF THE BODY; BLASTOCYST; GIANT CELLS; BLOOD; LYMPHOCYTE; GENETIC ENGINEERING; B CELLS; T CELLS.)

Cellulitis

Usually refers to a diffuse swelling in the subcutaneous tissues. Sometimes implies a diffuse area of inflammation and suppuration, as compared with an abscess which is localised. Whereas an acute abscess tends to come to a head, or 'point', and then burst, this does not happen with cellulitis which, if untreated, is liable to spread beneath the skin.

Cause Bacterial infection of the tisue, usually by streptococcus or pasteurella.

Treatment Antibiotics are used. If, however, treatment has been delayed, it may be necessary to lance the lowest part of the area.

Cattle The term 'necrotic cellulitis' has been applied to cases of diffuse swelling beginning under the jaw and then, if untreated, extending down the neck to the brisket.

Horses Cellulitis occurs in a form referred to also as ULCERATIVE LYMPHANGITIS.

Cats Cellulitis is more common than an abscess, which is localised and comes to a head.

Animals in the tropics For a form of cellulitis occurring in many species, see under HAEMORRHAGIC SEPTICAEMIA.

CEM
(see CONTAGIOUS EQUINE METRITIS)

Central Nervous System (CNS)

This comprises the brain and spinal cord, each with its grey and white matter. The 12 pairs of cranial nerves from the brain and the 42 pairs of spinal nerves carry between them all the messages to and from the brain.

For descriptive purposes the CNS is divided into 2 further systems: (1) somatic, and (2) autonomic.

Somatic This system is concerned with the control of voluntary muscles, and with nerve impulses from the skin, eyes, ears, and other sense organs. Accordingly, this system includes both motor and sensory nerves.

Autonomic This system of the CNS maintains the correct internal environment of the body (e.g. see HOMEOSTASIS), and its functions lie outside voluntary control. This system regulates breathing and heart rates, for example, and likewise the activity of the liver, digestive tract, kidneys, bladder, etc. This autonomic system comprises sympathetic and parasympathetic nerves. Most organs receive nerve impulses from both these, and they have opposite effects. For example, sympathetic nerves increase heart rate, while parasympathetic nerves slow heart action.

The sympathetic nervous system prepares the body for 'flight or fright', i.e. for emergency action. Accordingly, under its influence breathing becomes more rapid, the heart's action faster, and blood is diverted from the digestive organs to heart, CNS and voluntary muscles; while the liver releases glucose for extra muscular activity.

The parasympathetic system restores the situation after the emergency, slows the heart, and relaxes the body generally, as it also does during sleep. (See also BRAIN; SPINAL CORD; NERVES.)

Central Veterinary Laboratory

The headquarters of the Veterinary Investigation Service, now the Veterinary Laboratories Agency, New Haw, Addlestone, Surrey KT15 3NB.

Cephaloids

These include clams, cuttlefish, mussels and octopuses. It is now accepted that some octopus species can experience pain and have a considerable memory. As a result, *Octopus vulgaris* is protected under the Animals (Scientific Procedures) Act 1976. It is quite likely that squid, nautilus, cuttlefish and other species of octopus can also feel pain but it has not been shown that they can remember the experience.

Cephalosporin Antibiotics

A range of bactericidal antibiotics related to penicillin. Earlier cephalosporins are active against both Gram-positive and Gram-negative organisms. Later ones are active against some Gram-negative organisms resistant to the earlier 'first generation' products.

Cercaria

Cercaria is an intermediate stage in the life-history of the liver-fluke, viz. the tadpole-like form, which is produced in the body of the freshwater snail *Limnoea truncatula*, bores its way out of the snail, and attaches itself to a suit-able blade of grass to wait for the arrival of a sheep which will eat it. In the sheep's stomach and intestines further development takes place. (See LIVER-FLUKES.)

Cereals

Cereals, such as wheat, barley, oats, rye, maize, millets, and rice, are all rich in starch and com-paratively poor in proteins and minerals, and mostly poor in calcium but richer in phospho-rus. Some dangers of cereal feeding for cattle are referred to under BARLEY POISONING. (See also MOIST GRAIN STORAGE; DIET; HORSES, FEEDING OF.)

Cerebellar Hypoplasia

A form of degeneration of the cerebellum char-acterised by ataxia, head tilting and nystagmus. In cats, it may be due to feline panleucopenia infection or (rarely) as a result of live vaccine. Use of such vaccines during feline pregnancy or in kittens less than 3 weeks old should be avoided. It is an inherited defect in some Airedale terriers.

Cerebellum and Cerebrum

(see BRAIN)

Cerebral Haemorrhage

Cerebral haemorrhage is, in human medicine, referred to as a stroke. An older name was apoplexy. It is characterised by loss of con-sciousness, and may arise from bleeding from an artery in the brain or following embolism or thrombosis.

Cerebrocortical Necrosis (CCN)

A condition found mainly in ewes and calves. It is also called POLIOENCEPHALOMALACIA. The cause is a thiamin deficiency due to endogenous thiaminase production in the rumen by, for example, *Clostridium sporogenes* and *Bacillus thiaminolyticus*. Symptoms include: circling movements, a staggering gait, excitement, opisthotonos and convulsions. Only a few ani-mals in a flock or group become affected, but nearly all of those die.

A differential diagnosis has to be made between CCN and bacterial meningitis, GID, BSE, listeriosis, and lead poisoning – each can give rise to similar symptoms.

At post-mortem examination, autofluores-cence is seen when the CCN-affected brain is examined under ultra-violet light.

The lesions consist of multiple foci of necro-sis of the cerebral neurones.

Cerebrospinal Fluid Sampling

A diagnostic technique.

Indications for cerebrospinal fluid sampling in the dog include the following:

Encephalitis	Intracerebral
Meningitis	haemorrhage
Myelitis	Subarachnoid
Toxoplasmosis	haemorrhage
Brain neoplasia	Spinal cord
Spinal cord neoplasia	compression caused by epidural abscess

Ceroidosis

A form of liver degeneration characterised by deposition of a pink/golden, fat-insoluble material within cells. It is associated with the use of rancid or vitamin-E deficient feeds. (See FISH, DISEASES OF; *also* LYOSOMES.)

Cervical

Cervical means anything pertaining to the neck or to the cervix (the neck of the uterus).

Cervical Spondylopathy

(see under SPINE AND SPINAL CORD, DISEASES AND INJURIES OF)

Cervicitis

Cervicitis is inflammation of the *cervix uteri*. (See UTERUS.)

Cervid

A member of the Cervidae, the deer family. The red deer is *Cervus elaphus*.

Cestode

A tapeworm.

Cetavlon

Another name for CETRIMIDE.

Cetrimide

An antiseptic of value in wound treatment and for cleaning cows' udders and teats; a 0.1 per cent solution being effective against *Streptococcus agalactiae*, a cause of mastitis. A 1 per cent solution acts as a detergent.

Chabertiasis

Infection of the colon with chabertia worms (*Chabertia ovina*); found in sheep and occasionally in goats and cattle.

Signs Usually mild: soft faeces, with mucus and sometimes blood-flecked. In severe cases, anaemia may occur.

Chagas Disease

An infection with *Trypanosoma cruzi*, mainly occurring in wild mammals (such as opossums, armadillos, and wood rats) of Central and South America, but also infecting man, dogs, cats, and pigs. (See TRYPANOSOMES – American trypanosomiasis.)

Chalazion

Chalazion is a small swelling of the eyelid caused by a distended Meibomian gland. It is commonly seen in dogs.

Chancre

In human medicine this term is reserved for the ulcer or hard 'sore' which is the primary lesion of syphilis. In a veterinary context it means the local skin reaction at the sites of bites by tsetse flies carrying trypanosomes. The chancre – the first sign of trypanosome infection – begins as a small nodule, developing into a hard, hot, painful swelling measuring up to 3 or 4 inches across.

Charlock Poisoning

The common charlock *Brassica sinapis* (wild mustard) is dangerous to livestock after its seeds have formed in the pods, although only when eaten in large amounts. The seeds contain the volatile oil of mustard and also a glycoside.

Signs are those of abdominal pain, loss of appetite, a yellowish frothy liquid at mouth and nostrils, diarrhoea. There is nephritis, and the urine may be blood-stained.

First-Aid Give milk and strong tea.

Charolais Cattle

This is numerically the second-largest breed of cattle in France, and they have been exported throughout Europe and the USA. The Charolais, white, is an excellent beef animal, a most efficient grazer, with a rapid growth-rate and a quiet disposition. The loin and thigh muscles are exceptionally well developed. The bulls are colour-marking and highly prized for crossing purposes. UK trials of this breed for crossing purposes were approved in 1961, and the British Charolais is now the third most important beef breed.

Charolais Sheep

This breed was developed in the 19th century by crossing Dishley Leicester with the local sheep of Central France, and has been recognised as a breed since 1974. Mature ewes weigh up to 79 kg and rams up to 109 kg. Both sexes are polled.

'Chastek Paralysis'

A condition of secondary vitamin B_1 deficiency, seen in foxes and mink on fur farms as a result of feeding raw fish. An enzyme in the latter has the property of destroying the vitamin, also known as THIAMIN. The condition is seen also in cats.

Check Ligament

This is joined to the Perforans tendon, and acts as a check on the movement of the pastern joint. The check ligaments are often strained in the racehorse.

Cheese

When cheese is made from raw milk, *Brucella*, *Listeria* and other organisms may infect the cheese. In the UK, pasteurised milk is used, although it is argued that the flavour may be less good. The unpasteurised form is widely produced in Europe; sheep and goat cheese is popular as well as cow's milk cheeses. (See BRUCELLOSIS.)

Cheilitis

Inflammation of the lips.

Cheilosis

Cracked and scaly lips, often also affecting the corners of the mouth. Characteristic of vitamin B deficiency.

Chelating Agents

Chelating agents are substances which have the property of binding divalent metal ions to form stable, soluble complexes which are non-ionised and so virtually lacking in the toxicity of the metal concerned. Derivatives of ethylene-diamine-tetra-acetic acid (EDTA) afford examples. EDTA itself is poisonous, as it removes calcium; but the calcium-EDTA complex has been recommended in the treatment of acute lead poisoning, being given repeatedly for several days. It would possibly be of service in mercury, copper, and iron poisoning.

Chemosis

Chemosis means swelling of the conjunctival membrane that covers the white of the eye, leaving the cornea depressed.

Chemotherapy

Chemotherapy means the treatment of disease by chemical substances. The use of antibiotics, sulfonamides, and the diamidines, useful in the trypanosome diseases, are examples. In the treatment of cancers, chemotherapy has come to mean the use of cytotoxic drugs, which are usually associated with severe side-effects.

Chelonians

Reptiles which have a CARAPACE, or shell; they include tortoises, turtles and terrapins. They may be subject to a variety of dietetic and parasitic problems. Clinical examination is restricted to those parts protruding from the shell, while laboratory examination of blood samples and faeces is necessary to confirm parastic infection. Infestation by nematode worms can cause failure to survive hibernation and worming beforehand is advisable. **Note. Ivermectin must not be used in chelonians.** Respiratory disease is not uncommon and animals suffering in this way must be prevented from hibernating.

Chest, or Thorax

Chest, or thorax, is the part of the body lying between the neck and the abdomen. It is a conical cavity, with the apex directed forwards. The base is formed by the diaphragm, while the sides are formed by the ribs, sternum, and vertebrae. Lying between adjacent ribs on the same side there are 2 layers of intercostal muscles, those on the outside running almost at right angles to those on the inside. The intercostal muscles fill up the spaces between the ribs and their cartilages, and are active agents in moving the ribs during respiration. The outsides of the chest walls are covered with the masses of the shoulder muscles, and the shoulder-blades or scapula lie one on either side, anteriorly over the rib-cage, but not attached to it by bony connections.

Within the thorax are the termination of the trachea, the bronchial tubes, and the lungs. Between the lungs, but projecting towards the left more than to the right, lie the heart and its associated vessels. The oesophagus, or gullet, runs through the chest, passing for the greater distance between the upper parts of the lungs,

and enters the abdomen through an opening in the diaphragm. The thoracic duct, which carries lymph from the abdomen, runs forwards immediately below the bodies of the vertebrae and ends by opening into one of the large veins in the apex of the cavity. Various important nerves, such as the two vagi which control the abdominal organs, the phrenics, which supply the muscles of the diaphragm, and sympathetics, pass through the chest in particular situations. The thymus gland lies in the anterior portion of the chest. Lining each of the 2 divisions of the chest cavity is the pleura, a fold of which also covers the surface of the lung, and the heart is enclosed in a special sac or pericardium. (See HEART; LUNGS; PLEURA; PERICARDIUM.)

Chest Injuries/Diseases

Injuries to the chest wall are often the result of dogs or cats being struck by a car; or of falls leading to fractured ribs and closed PNEUMOTHORAX. Puncture-type wounds from animal bites are less common and seldom lead to pneumothorax as they are self-sealing; but some subcutaneous emphysema may occur. Infection may lead to PLEURISY.

(See THORACOTOMY; DIAPHRAGMATOCELE; HYDROTHORAX; 'FLAIL CHEST'; PYOTHORAX; *also* BRONCHITIS; PNEUMONIA; HEART DISEASES; PARASITIC BRONCHITIS; 'BROKEN WIND'; LUNGS, DISEASES OF.)

Chestnuts

Flat oval areas of the horn on the inside of the fore- and hind-limb of the horse.

'Chewing Disease'

The colloquial name in the USA for a type of encephalomalacia in the horse caused by yellow star thistle (*Centaurea solstitialis*).

Cheyletlella Parasitovorax

A mite which infests dogs, cats, birds, rabbits, squirrels, etc. It gives rise to itching and scurfiness of the skin. In man *Cheyletiella* species (including *C. yusguri*) may cause urticarial weals of trunk and arms, together with intense itching.

C. blakei infests cats; *C. parasitovorax*, rabbits; *C. yasguri*, dogs.

Cheyne-Stokes' Respiration

Cheyne-Stokes' respiration is an abnormal form of breathing in which the respirations become gradually less and less until they almost die away; after remaining almost imperceptible for a short time they gradually increase in depth and volume until they are exaggerated; after attaining a maximum they again decrease until nearly imperceptible. This alternation proceeds with considerable regularity.

Cheyne-Stokes' breathing is always a very serious condition, which is generally associated with severe nervous disturbance, shock, and collapse, or with heart or kidney disease. It is most obvious in the dog and horse after they have sustained very severe injury but without internal haemorrhage (which induces what is generally known as 'sobbing respiration').

Chianina

These Italian cattle are named after their place of origin, the Chiana valley. Probably the largest cattle in the world, a mature bull can weigh over 1.75 tonnes and be 1.8 m tall at the withers. Formerly used as draught animals, they are an excellent beef breed, now present in the UK.

Chick Oedema

(see 'TOXIC FAT SYNDROME')

Chihuahua

One of the smallest breeds of toy dog, originating from Mexico. Frontal foramina are present, i.e., the frontal bones of the domed skull remain ununited. The breed is liable to suffer problems in parturition. Possible inherited conditions include pulmonary stenosis, dislocation of the patella, and hydrocephalus. Mange in this breed must never be treated with amitraz.

Chicken Anaemia Virus

Transmitted by breeder flocks to their progeny, chicken anaemia virus causes increased mortality with anaemia, lymphoid depletion, liver changes and haemorrhages throughout the body. Signs develop at 2 to 3 weeks old.

Chicks

The ambient temperature for rearing chicks must be kept above 18°C (60°F) during the first 5 weeks or so of life. Ambient temperature for rearing chicks should be 32°C (90°F). Chilling is one of the commonest causes of pullet chick mortality. Chicks require artificial heat for 3 to 8 weeks, depending upon the type of house, weather, etc. (See also POULTRY – Chick feeding).

Chilblain Syndrome in Dogs

This was first described as affecting Service dogs in Northern Ireland. These dogs had previously thrived in unheated, outdoor kennels, but were affected during a very cold winter. The first sign was biting of the tip of the tail – found to be red, swollen, warm and intensely

itchy. Ulceration, infection, and necrosis of the tail tip occurred in a few cases, necessitating amputation of the tip. It is not unknown for a dog to eat the affected part of its tail. Elizabethan collars, protective tail covering, and anti-inflammatory drugs were used in treatment.

Chilling

(see under CHICKS *and* HYPOTHERMIA)

Chimera

An animal having in its body, cell populations arising from different species; that is, cells with different KARYOTYPES which have originated from 2 or more zygotes with different karyotypes. A freemartin is, technically, an example of XX:XY chimerism. This is secondary chimerism. Primary chimerism occurs if 2 sperms fertilise the same ovum. (See CYTOGENETICS.)

Other examples which have been reported include a fertile female mule that had apparently inherited a mixture of both horse and donkey chromosomes, and was phenotypically a chimera rather than a hybrid. And a sheep-goat chimera found at the School of Veterinary Medicine, University of California, USA, was capable of oestrus cycles, producing fertile ova, and carrying pregnancy to full term.

Chimera is also a term used to describe an organism that has had foreign DNA inserted into its genome.

Chinchilla

Chinchilla laniger is a small rabbit-like rodent, prized for its fur. It originates from the South American Andes; those living at higher altitudes have better coats. Originally brought to the UK for fur farming, the project had to be abandoned because of the poor quality of the imported animals. Adults weigh about 400 to 500 g; the female is larger than the male. Pregnancy lasts 111 days; there are usually 2 in a litter but up to 5 may be born. Weaning is at 6 to 8 weeks. They are sexually mature at 8 months and can live for 10 years although the record is 18. Body temperature is 38 to 39°C. They can be active during the day but are mainly nocturnal in habit.

Chinchillas require ample room (about 4 m3) with a nest box about 30 x 25 x 20 cm within that. An ambient temperature of 10 to 20°C is adequate; as low as 0°C can be tolerated provided there are no draughts. Fine sand must be provided for sand-bathing to keep their coat in good condition.

If treated with sulfonamides, the coat colour may fade; it will eventually return to normal.

Chinchilla, Diseases of

Enteritis, pneumonia and impaction of the intestine are the most common diseases. Out of a series of 1000 post-mortem examinations made in the USA, 'epidemic gastroenteritis' was found in 23 per cent of the chinchillas, as against 25 per cent with pneumonia, and 12 per cent with impaction (blockage of the intestine). In a further series of 1000 examinations, the figures were: impaction, 20 per cent; pneumonia, 22 per cent; and enteritis, 24 per cent. *Yersinea paratuberculosis, Listeria monocytogenes,* proteus, pseudomonas, staphylococcus and salmonella infections have been recorded, as has *Clostridium perfringens* associated with diarrhoea, flatulence and prolapsed rectum. Acute and fatal gastroenteritis caused by *Yersinia enterocolitica* has caused severe losses among chinchillas on farms in California, and also in Europe. (See YERSINIOSIS.)

An important cause of pneumonia is *Klebsiella pneumoniae.* This may also produce loss of appetite, diarrhoea, and death within about 5 days.

Lying on one side and stretching the legs are said to be signs of impaction. A diet with too little roughage is believed to be a cause.

Intussusception is not uncommon and sometimes follows enteritis. Inability to retract the penis (paraphimosis) has also been noted.

Fur-chewing and associated skin problems – that bane of the North American chinchilla industry – has been attributed to 'environmental stress' associated with captivity. Of course, the wrong diet may enter into it too. High fibre pellets, timothy hay combined with some fresh greenstuff, with a little apple and a raisin or two now and then will also help prevent digestive disorders.

Chinchillas' teeth grow constantly; unless the animals are provided with materials to gnaw on, the teeth become excessively long, preventing a proper bite and causing injuries inside the mouth. Often the condition requires veterinary attention.

Chipmunks

A rodent (*Tamias striatus*), not dissimilar to the squirrel, with longitudinal stripes across its back. Adults weigh 72 to 120 g. When kept as pets they should be in pairs or a trio of 1 male and 2 females. A large, escape-proof enclosure should be provided. They become hyperactive if stressed and must never be kept near a television set. If outside, protection from adverse weather conditions must be given.

Body temperature is 38° C when awake, falling to a few degrees above ambient temperature when hibernating. Chipmunks are comparatively healthy animals provided they are well kept. Ectoparasites may be present, as may mange, fleas and harvest mites. Cataracts occur in older animals; emphysema has been recorded and is difficult to treat. If hypoglycaemia (milk fever) is seen after parturition, it can be treated with 0.5 ml calcium borogluconte given subcutaneously. Swellings due to collection of fluid (lymphoedema) may be seen. These usually regress during hibernation but can be treated with a daily dose of 0.5 mg frusemide.

Chiropractic

A technique which aims to relieve disease problems by manipulation of body structures, particularly the spinal vertebrae.

Chitin

The horn-like substance forming the main constituent of the body-covering of insects, ticks, mites, spiders, etc. A polysaccharide, it is also found in some fungi.

Chlamydia and Chlamydophila

Widespread Gram-negative bacteria containing species of veterinary and medical significance. They include *Chlamydophila psittaci*, responsible for psittacosis (see below) in birds (and man); *C. abortus,* a major cause of abortion in sheep and some other ruminants; and *C. felis,* which causes pneumonia, conjunctivitis and respiratory problems in cats. *Chlamydia suis* causes conjunctivitis, pneumonia and enteritis in pigs.

Psittacosis Sometimes called parrot disease, psittacosis affects virtually all avian species. There are several strains (serovars) of *C. psittaci,* some of which affect other species. Affected birds may show no signs initially but active infection is often triggered by stress. Parrots and other cage birds become listless, have diarrhoea, coryza, conjunctivitis and sinusitis. Pigeons develop respiratory signs and bronchitis. In poultry, egg production falls off; up to a third of a flock may die.

There is a considerable risk that people in contact with infected birds pick up the disease, sometimes with serious results.

In one Edinburgh outbreak, 100 out of about 300 budgerigars in an aviary died. Human cases followed and a dog was found to be excreting *Chlamydia* organisms and to have a lung infection.

Treatment Tetracycline or doxycycline, given to birds over a period of 7 weeks in the feed or on medicated seed.

Prevention Quarantine of imported birds; disinfection of infected premises.

Ornithosis is the name formerly given to the same infection in birds other than those of the parrot family.

Post-Mortem findings include enlargement of liver and spleen, together with pneumonia. Confirmation of diagnosis is by ELISA, immunofluorescent test or bacterial culture.

Measures to protect the UK's poultry against psittacosis infection from abroad are specified under the Importation of Birds, Poultry and Hatching Eggs Order 1979. All diagnoses of the disease in imported birds are notified by the State Veterinary Service to medical officers of environmental health.

Public health Human psittacosis in its milder forms resembles influenza. In children the symptoms are slight or absent altogether, but in older people the illness is more likely to be severe. Symptoms include shivering, headache, backache. Death from pneumonia may follow. Acute kidney failure has been recorded; also heart disease. Human infection comes through handling infected birds.

Abortion *C. abortus* (and some strains of *C. psittaci*) are responsible for abortion in ruminants.

Sheep usually show no signs of disease until they become depressed shortly before abortion occurs. Afterwards, most ewes recover uneventfully. When disease is established in a flock, 5 to 10 per cent of ewes will abort; immunity develops following infection. The infection is usually transmitted at lambing, through placenta, uterine discharges and faeces.

Vaccines are available against certain strains of chlamydial infection.

Cattle Animals show no sign of disease but sporadic abortions occur, usually in the 7th to 9th month of gestation. Sometimes, dead or short-lived weakly calves are born at full term.

Public health The infection is transmissible to humans. Cases in pregnant women who have assisted at lambing have been recorded. Difficulties during pregnancy, and in one case death, followed.

A farmer's wife who aborted in the 28th week of pregnancy, had helped with difficult lambings. Five of 200 ewes had aborted and a serum sample had shown high antibody titres to chlamydia.

Chlamydia spp. were detected in smears of liver, lung and placenta from the human fetus.

Chloral Hydrate

Chloral hydrate is a clear, crystalline substance with a sweetish taste; it dissolves rapidly in water. It was formerly used widely as a hypnotic, and occasionally for euthanasia.

Chloral Hydrate Poisoning

In the dog, poisoning has occurred after eating meat from horses humanely euthanased by means of chloral hydrate.

Chloramines

Chloramines are widely used as a disinfectant. Their activity depends upon the amount of available chlorine.

Chloramphenicol

An antibiotic which has a similar range of activity to the tetracyclines. It can be given orally (except to ruminants), by intravenous injection, and by local application, especially as an eye ointment. Because of its importance in the treatment of human typhoid and the avoidance of resistant strains, its use in veterinary medicine has been severely restricted, particularly in food-producing animals.

In human medicine, poisoning by chloramphenicol has led to aplastic anaemia, skin eruptions, and moniliasis. There are three main side-effects: allergy or hypersensitivity to the drug; damage to the blood or bone-marrow; and gastrointestinal upsets.

Intramuscular injections of chloramphenicol are painful.

Chlorate Poisoning

In acute cases cattle may die after showing symptoms suggestive of anthrax. In subacute cases, a staggering gait, purgation, signs of abdominal pain, and red-coloured urine may be seen. Cyanosis and respiratory distress are also symptoms.

Treatment Gastric lavage. If cyanosis is present, methylene blue should be given intravenously.

Chlordane

A highly toxic insecticide of the chlorinated hydrocarbon group. It is volatile and poisoning through inhalation may occur.

Chlorfenvinphos

An organophosphorus acaricide and insecticide. It has been used in sheep dips, etc. and against fly strike, keds, lice and ticks. Less toxic compounds are now preferred.

Chlorhexidene

Chlorhexidene gluconate is widely used as an antiseptic and surgical scrub; and in teat dips, sprays and udder washes.

Chlorinated Hydrocarbons

These insecticides include: chlordane, DDT, DDD, methoxychlor, benzene hexachloride, toxaphene, aldrin, dieldrin, isodrin, and endrin plus a range of others less well known. Ingested at toxic levels, or absorbed through the skin, they act primarily on the central nervous system causing excitement/frenzy at the outset followed by muscular tremors leading to convulsions in acute cases. Species capable of vomiting do so. Loss of appetite with marked loss of body weight is usual in subacute poisoning. Cats are especially susceptible. Wash off any residues from the skin and keep the animal warm, comfortable and sedated.

Most compounds – methoxychlor is an exception – can be stored in the body fat and excreted in the milk and so may constitute a public health problem. Their use in animals is now minimal because of the residue levels caused by this persistence.

Chloroform

Chloroform is a colourless, mobile, non-inflammable liquid, half as heavy again as water. It is much less used now than formerly as a general anaesthetic. (See ANAESTHETICS; EUTHANASIA.)

Four stages of chloroform anaesthesia are recognised:

(1) The stage of excitement begins immediately the drug is administered. Vigorous animals struggle violently, and when in the standing position may rear or strike out with their forefeet and shake their heads in an endeavour to dislodge the mask. Deep breaths are taken often in a gasping manner, and in from 3 to 6 or 7 minutes the second stage follows.

(2) The stage of depression follows the stimulation stage, and is marked by a quieting of the movements of the voluntary muscles, by a lessening of the force and volume of the pulse, and by slower and deeper breathing. Pain is still felt, and if inflicted induces reflex movement.

(3) The stage of anaesthesia produces complete muscular relaxation and unconsciousness. This is the safe or operating stage; all the centres of the brain are subdued except those that govern respiration and heart action.

(4) The stage of paralysis occurs when the anaesthetic is pushed beyond the safe stage. The centres of respiration and heart action, in common with all the other nervous centres, become paralysed. The heart stops beating about 2 minutes after respiration ceases, and any attempts at ARTIFICIAL RESPIRATION must be prompt.

Chocolate Poisoning

The feeding of waste chocolate bars to cattle has led to fatal poisoning in calves in the UK. The animals showed excitement, stared about in all directions, walked with exaggerated strides, and had convulsions.

It was suggested that the caffeine content would account for the excitement; the theobromine content may have caused heart failure.

In dogs, the signs include panting, vomiting, thirst, diarrhoea, excitement, fits, coma.

Treatment Use of an emetic or gastric lavage. (Activated charcoal is used in human medicine.) For control of the convulsions, diazepam is among the suitable drugs.

Autopsy findings include cyanotic mucous membranes, swollen and reddened gastric mucosa.

(See also COCOA POISONING.)

'Choking' (Obstruction of Pharynx or Oesophagus)

'Choking' is, by dictionary definition, an obstruction to respiration, but in a farming context the word has been misused to denote an obstruction to the passage of food through the pharynx and oesophagus, either partial or complete.

The domesticated animals, especially cattle and dogs, are very prone to attempt to swallow either foreign bodies or masses of food material too large to pass down the oesophagus (gullet), with the result that they often become jammed. Such substances hinder the free passage of solid or fluid food, give rise to pain and discomfort, and are very often attended by serious and even fatal consequences. Choking in cattle, dogs, and cats is usually due to a hard, large, sharp-pointed, or irregularly shaped object; while in the horse it is most often due to a mass of dry impacted food material, or to a portion of a mangold or turnip.

Cattle Choking is of comparatively common occurrence, particularly in districts where roots are fed whole to the animals, and where there is a quantity of rubbish scattered about the pastures.

Signs The animal immediately stops feeding, and becomes uneasy. A feature of nearly all cases of choking in cattle is the rapidity with which gas formation occurs in the rumen. (See BLOAT.)

In a number of cases of choking, relief occurs quite spontaneously after the lapse of from 30 minutes to 2 or 3 hours from the origin of the symptoms. This is because the muscles of the gullet, which have been tightly gripping the obstruction, gradually become fatigued and relax, thereby allowing the object to pass down into the stomach. Naturally, such a satisfactory termination cannot occur wherever there is a sharp projecting point on the object causing the obstruction, but it frequently happens with eggs, apples, potatoes, and other smooth bodies.

First-Aid In all cases of choking, no matter how simple they appear to be, the owner should seek veterinary assistance as soon as possible.

Professional treatment depends on the site of the obstruction. This may be palpable in the oesophagus and manipulation up to the mouth may be possible after giving hyoscine hydrobromide and metamizole dypirone (Buscopan; Boehringer) as a muscle relaxant. If in the intestine, passage of a probang or stomach-tube down the oesophagus may dislodge the obstruction; if not, it can be removed by rumenotomy or a trochar can be inserted into the rumen; in many cases, the blockage will reduce by maceration over 3 to 4 days.

Horses The horse is less often choked than the cow, but owing to the long and narrow equine oesophagus, the accident is more serious.

Treatment Avoid raising the head or giving drenches, lubricating or otherwise. It is imperative to secure professional assistance at once.

Dogs and cats

Signs At first there is usually a sudden pain, which causes the animal to cry out. If it has been feeding it immediately ceases, and becomes very restless. It may paw at its mouth. Salivation is often profuse.

When a threaded needle has become fixed in the throat or below it, the end of the thread may often be seen.

Treatment Swallowed objects which become jammed in a dog's oesophagus can be treated in one of two ways: surgically or conservatively. The latter includes the use of an endoscope, passed into the oesophagus and enabling the foreign body to be grasped with forceps and drawn out or, alternatively, pushed down into the stomach, whence it can, if necessary, be removed.

In a series of 90 cases treated by J. E. F. Houlton and others at the University of Cambridge, 85 of the foreign bodies were pieces of bone, and two were composed mainly of gristle. A potato, a fish-hook, and a ball were also found. The success rate of treatment by surgical and conservative means was 82 per cent.

A young African elephant died from obstruction of its oesophagus by an apple.

Cholagogues
Cholagogues are substances reputed to act on the liver, increasing the secretion of the bile.

Cholangiocarcinoma
Cancer of the bile ducts; it is associated with liver-fluke infestation of animals in Thailand.

Cholangiohepatitis
Inflammation of bile ducts and associated liver parenchyma.

Cholangioma
A benign tumour originating from the bile ducts, and occurring in cats, dogs, sheep, and poultry.

Cholangitis
Inflammation of the intra-hepatic bile ducts.

Cholecystitis
Inflammation of the gall-bladder.

Cholecystography
Cholecystography is the term used for X-ray examination of the gall-bladder after its contents have been rendered opaque by administration of lipiodol or pheniodol compounds.

Cholecystokinin
A hormone produced in the small intestine and causing emptying of the gall-bladder.

Cholecystomy
A surgical incision into the gall-bladder.

Cholera, Fowl
(see FOWL CHOLERA)

Cholesteatoma
An epidermoid cyst within the middle ear cavity of dogs, complicating simple otitis.

Cholesterol
A sterol present in blood, brain and other tissues, bile, and many foods. It is produced in the

liver and adrenal glands; it decreases in cows with fatty liver.

A high cholesterol level can be a precursor to high blood pressure, ATHEROMA, and THROMBOSIS.

Cholesthiasis
(see GALLSTONES)

Choline
Choline is an amine compound with important functions in the metabolic process. It is found in egg-yolk, liver, and muscle, and is associated with the vitamin B complex. Acetyl choline is essential for the transmission of an impulse from nerve to muscle.

Cholinesterase
Cholinesterase is an enzyme which inactivates acetylcholine. Some poisons, such as carbamates and organophosphates, cause cholinesterase inhibition, and it is inactivated by a substance isolated from occuring in white clover S.100.

Chondritis
Inflammation of cartilage.

Chondrocytes
Cartilage-forming cells.

Chondrogenesis
(see Growth-plate disorders under BONE, DISEASES OF)

Chondroma
A rare tumour, composed of cartilage-like cells, which has been seen in dogs, rats, and mink.

Chorea
Twitching or trembling caused by a succession of involuntary spasmodic contractions (clonic spasms) affecting one or more of the voluntary muscles. The spasm is of a rhythmic nature, occurring at fairly regular intervals, and between the individual contractions relaxation of the affected muscle takes place.

The condition affects dogs almost exclusively, although muscular spasms of a similar nature have been seen in horses, cattle, and pigs. In lambs, congenital chorea is described under 'BORDER DISEASE'. (See also SHIVERING.)

Causes In dogs, chorea generally follows a mild attack of distemper. It may appear within a few days after apparent recovery, or its appearance may be delayed. All dog owners would be well advised to regard cases of distemper as not cured until the lapse of at least 10 days after apparent recovery, and during this period to continue to treat the animal as though it were still sick, so far as exercise is concerned.

Signs Twitchings usually begin about the lips and face, or in the extremities of one or more limbs. Later, perhaps the whole head is seen continually nodding or jerking backwards and forwards, quite irrespective of the pose or position of the animal. As the condition progresses, there comes a time when it is unable to rest, loss of condition and weakness result, and the dog becomes exhausted. Ulceration of the affected limb, as the result of continual friction with surrounding objects, the ground, etc., is not uncommon. Chorea is always a serious condition.

Treatment is with ANTISPASMODICS.

Chorion
Chorion is the outermost of the three fetal membranes, the others being the amnion and the allantois. The chorion is a strong fibrous membrane, whose outer surface is closely moulded to the inner surface of the uterus. Chorionic villi are the vascular projections from the chorion which are inserted into the crypts of the uterine mucous membrane. (See also PARTURITION.)

Chorionic Gonadotrophin
(see HORMONE THERAPY)

Choroid, or Chorioid
Choroid, or chorioid, is the middle of the 3 coats of the EYE, and consists chiefly of the blood vessels which effect nourishment of the organ.

Choroiditis
Inflammation of the choroid.

Chow Chow
A stocky, medium-sized dog with a thick coat; the tongue is blue-black in colour. Originally bred in China for meat, the breed specification still reads as if that were its main purpose. They tend to be a 'one person' dog. Entropion and muscle spasm (myotonia) may be inherited.

Christmas Rose
(see HELLEBORES)

Chromobacter Violaceum
An organism, often regarded as non-pathogenic, which has caused a fatal pneumonia in pigs in the USA.

Chromosomes

Minute bodies, within the nucleus of cells, which carry the genes, and are composed largely of DNA. The number of chromo-somes is constant for any given species. (See under GENETICS.) The haploid number (n) represents the basic set found in the gametes, i.e. egg and sperm. The diploid number (2n) represents paired basic sets, one set from the sire, the others from the dam, and this number is found in all somatic cells.

(See also under CYTOGENETICS for chromosome abnormalities; *and* PLASMIDS.)

Chronic Obstructive Pulmonary Disease (COPD)

A name for a disease of horses affecting principally the small airways. It seems that *Micropolysporum faeni*, hay dust, and food mites are all potentially involved in causing COPD, which – in one survey – was found to have a higher incidence in stables with much ammonia and dust particles in the air. Dyspnoea is worse at night, as is the case with human asthma.

Chronic Respiratory Disease

Chronic respiratory disease is a complex problem in poultry. The signs include noisy breathing (rales), coughing and nasal discharge. It is usually set off by infectious bronchitis virus and if the birds also carry *Mycoplasma gallisepticum* the condition can be severe. Further infection by strains of *E. coli* usually follows and air sacculitis may develop.

Chyle

The milky fluid which is absorbed by the lymphatic vessels of the intestine. The fluid mixes with the lymph and is discharged into the thoracic duct. (See LYMPH; DIGESTION.)

Analysis of chyle can be helpful in the diagnosis of several diseases of the abdomen.

Chyloperitoneum

The presence of chyle in the peritoneal cavity.

Chylothorax

The presence of pleural fluid identifiable as chyle, following injury to, or a tumour of, the thoracic duct. Treatment consists of repeated drainage. The condition has been recorded in cats and dogs.

Chyme

Chyme is the partly digested food passed from the stomach into the first part of the small intestine. It is very acid in nature, contains salts and sugars in solution, and the food constituents in a homogenised semi-liquid state.

Cicatrix

Cicatrix is a scar.

Cilia

This term covers both the eyelashes, and the microscopic hair-like projections from the cells of the mucous membranes lining the larynx and trachea. Their rhythmic beating moves fluid over the cell surface.

Ciliata

Ciliated protozoa are found in the alimentary canal of animals. (See BALANTIDIUM.)

Circling Movements

Repetitive circling behaviour in an animal may be a symptom of meningitis or encephalitis. (See BRAIN DISEASES.)

Circulation of Blood

The veins of the whole body – head, trunk, limbs, and organs in the abdomen – with the exception of those in the thorax, pour their

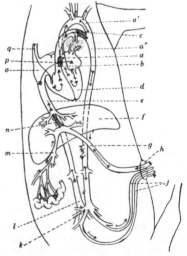

Diagram of fetal circulation. *a*, Origin of aorta; *a'*, arch of aorta; *a"*, posterior aorta; *b*, origin of pulmonary artery; *c*, the ductus arteriosus (shaded); *d*, left ventricle; *e*, caudal vena cava; *f*, liver; *g*, umbilical vein; *h*, the umbilicus; *j*, umbilical arteries; *k*, bifurcation of aorta; *l*, origin of caudal vena cava; *m*, portal vein; *n*, ductus venosus, which short-circuits blood from umbilical vein to vena cava without passing through liver; *o*, right atrium; *p*, foramen ovale (shaded); *q*, crania vena cava. (After Bradley, *Thorax and Abdomen of the Horse*.)

blood into one of the three great terminal radicles which open into the right atrium of the heart. This contracts and drives the blood into the right ventricle, which then forces the blood into the lungs by way of the pulmonary artery. In the lungs it is contained in very thin-walled capillaries, over which the inspired air plays freely, and through which the exchange of gases can easily take place. The blood is consequently oxygenated (see RESPIRATION), and passes on by the pulmonary veins to the left atrium of the heart. This left atrium expels it into the left ventricle, which forces it on into the aorta, by which it is distributed all over the body. Passing through the capillaries in the various organs and tissues it eventually again enters the lesser veins, and is collected into the cranial and caudal vena cava and the azygos vein (see VEINS), from where it passes to the right atrium once more.

In one part of the body there is, however, a further complication. The veins coming from the stomach, intestines, spleen, and pancreas, charged with food materials and other products, unite into the large 'portal vein' which enters the porta of the liver and splits up into a second capillary system in the liver tissue. Here it is relieved of some of its food content, and passes to the caudal vena cava by a second series of veins, joining with the rest of the blood coming from the hind parts of the body, and so goes on to the right atrium. This is known as the 'portal circulation'.

The circuit is maintained always in one direction by four valves, situated one at the outlet from each cavity of the HEART, and by the presence of valves situated along the course of the larger veins.

The blood in the arteries going to the body generally (i.e. to the systemic circulation) is a bright red in colour while that in the veins is a dull red; this is owing to the oxygen content of arterial blood being much greater than that of venous blood, which latter is charged with carbon dioxide. For the same reason the blood in the pulmonary artery going to the lungs is dark, while in the pulmonary veins it is bright red.

There is normally no connection between the blood in the right side of the heart and that in the left; the blood from the right ventricle must pass through the lungs before it can reach the left atrium. In the fetus, two large arteries pass out from the umbilicus (navel), and convey blood which is to circulate in close proximity to the maternal blood in the placenta, and to receive from it both the oxygen and the nourishment necessary for the needs of the fetus, while one large vein brings back this blood into the fetal body through the umbilicus again. There are also communications between the right and the left atria (the foramen ovale) and between the aorta and the pulmonary artery (the ductus arteriosus), which serve to 'short-circuit' the blood from passing through the lungs in any quantity. At birth these extra communications rapidly close and shrivel up, leaving mere vestiges of their presence in adult life. There are rare instances, however, in which one or more of the passages may persist throughout life.

Circulation of Lymph
(see LYMPH)

Cirrhosis, or Fibrosis
Cirrhosis, or fibrosis, is a condition of various internal organs, in which some of the non-parenchymatous cells of the organ are replaced by fibrous tissue. The name 'cirrhosis' was first used for the disease as it occurs in the liver, because of the yellow colour, but it has been applied to fibrosis in the lung, kidney, etc. Classic instances of cirrhosis are seen in the liver in chronic ragwort poisoning in cattle, in chronic alcoholism in man, and in old dogs.

Citrullinaemia
This disease occurs in some Australian Friesian cattle; also in dogs. It is hereditary in origin, and due to a deficiency of the amino acid Citrulline. In calves depression, recumbency, and convulsions result.

CJD
(see CREUTZFELDT-JAKOB DISEASE)

Claviceps
A fungus (see ERGOT, FUNGAL).

Clavicle
Clavicle is another name for the 'collar-bone' in man. This bone is not present in the domesticated mammals (except sometimes in a very rudimentary form in the cat), but is present in the fowl.

Claws
(see NAILS)

Clay Pigeons
Ruminants and outdoor pigs may eat these if found lying on pasture. The outcome can be fatal in pigs but in ruminants, chronic unthriftiness results as the material is digested only slowly. (See PITCH POISONING; LEAD POISONING.)

Clazuril

In racing pigeons, clazuril is given for the prevention and treatment of coccidiosis.

'Clean' Pasture
(see PASTURE)

'Cleansing'
(see PLACENTA)

Cleft Palate

Cleft palate is a hereditary defect of the roof of the mouth, generally seen in puppies of the toy breeds that have been in-bred. It consists of a gap in the structures forming the palate, often so extensive as to allow of communication between the mouth and the nasal passages. Puppies so affected are usually unable to suck, and die soon after birth unless given artificial feeding; others are able to obtain some small amount of nourishment, but never thrive as the rest of the litter. The condition of 'HARE-LIP', or 'split-lip', is often associated with cleft palate. The palate may also be cleft as the result of violence; for example, it is commonly seen in the cat which has fallen from a considerable height.

Cleft palate in cattle is referred to under GENETICS – Genetic defects.

Clenbuterol Hydrochloride

A specific β_2 agonist, used as a bronchodilator in coughing horses; and to suppress contractions of the uterus in cows to aid obstetrics.

Clenbuterol has also a metabolic effect, and is an effective growth-promoter in beef cattle, increasing the volume of skeletal muscle (as well as heart muscle) and decreasing fat. The size of other organs is not increased, as is the case with anabolic steroids such as trenbolone acetate. However, their use as growth promoters is prohibited in food animals in the UK and some other countries.

Climate in Relation to Disease
(see entries under ENVIRONMENT; *also* TROPICS)

Clindamycin

An antibiotic used in dogs and cats for the treatment of infected wounds, pyoderma, osteomyelitis and as supportive therapy during dental procedures. It is usually given by mouth; injections may also be used.

Clipping of Dogs

These animals are usually clipped for medical reasons, such as to allow better dressing of the skin during treatment of mange. Some owners however, particularly of long-haired breeds, have their dogs regularly clipped at the beginning of the summer to rid them of long matted, or thick winter, coats. In addition to this, certain breeds are clipped for show purposes, such as the French poodle and the Bedlington terrier.

Clipping of Horses

The covering of hair over the body of certain of the domesticated animals is liable at times to interfere with health if allowed to grow unchecked, and accordingly it is customary to remove it at certain periods of the year; in horses the long winter coat, if left to grow, hinders efficient grooming and drying, prevents the skin from excreting waste products, and causes the horse to perspire more. (See also SHEARING.)

Methods Clippers work best when used against the flow of the hair, and should be thoroughly and frequently lubricated. It is of course essential that the blades should be sharp. For racehorses, carriage-horses, ponies, etc., it is usual to clip 'down to the ground', as it is called, i.e. all the hair is clipped from the body, legs, and face, the mane is 'hogged' (clipped short), and the tail is thinned. For saddle-horses a 'hunter's clip' is preferred; in this the hair is taken from the body, except for a patch on the back which corresponds with the outline of the saddle ('saddle-patch'), and the legs, which are left covered with hair below the level of an oblique line running across the middles of the fore-arms and gaskins. The mane is hogged, and the tail is thinned and cut straight across about a hand's-breadth above the level of the points of the hocks.

Times for Clipping The time for clipping horses varies according to the weather, but should take place as soon as the winter coat has 'set', i.e. as soon as the summer coat has been fully cast off and the winter coat is well grown. It usually happens that in an ordinary autumn this condition is fulfilled about the end of October and the beginning of November, but in some years it is earlier and in some later. Sometimes horses are clipped twice during the winter, once before Christmas and once some time after; but this is only necessary in animals which have a luxuriant growth of hair.

Precautions Never clip a horse suffering from a cold or other respiratory trouble. Never clip during excessively severe weather. Always provide a rug when standing outside for the first week or 10 days to allow the heat-regulating mechanism to become accustomed to the more rapid radiation of heat from the body surface. Thoroughly dry a newly clipped horse after coming into the stable in wet or snowy weather, by means of straw or hay wisps. Do not allow newly clipped horses to stand in draughty places in a stable without protection. Give extra bedding for a few days after clipping. Give an extra ration of hay and oats to recently clipped horses to make good the loss of heat occasioned.

Clipping of Sheep
(see SHEARING; CLOTHING OF ANIMALS)

Clitoris
Clitoris is the small organ composed of erectile tissue, situated just within the lower commissure of the vulva. It is the homologue of the penis.

Clitoral sinusectomy The RCVS has ruled that veterinary surgeons who are asked to carry out clitoral sinusectomies on mares which are destined for export to the United States can be clear that they will not be held to be acting unethically, even if, at the time of the performance of the operation, there is no evidence that the mare is infected with the CEM organism (see CONTAGIOUS EQUINE ARTERITIS.)

It is contended by the United States Department of Agriculture that clitoral sinusectomy:

(a) could show up, on the subsequent culturing of the excised material, that CEM was present when swabbing proved negative;

(b) when accompanied by the prescribed follow-up treatments would eliminate the CEM organism if it was present; and

(c) was the method by which CEM outbreaks in Kentucky had been eliminated.

Enlargement of the clitoris may occur in bitches treated with androgens for the suppression of oestrus.

Cloaca
In birds and lower vertebrates the alimentary, urinary and genital systems have a common outlet; this is the cloaca. When an egg is laid, however, the alimentary outlet is closed, reducing the risk of shell contamination with enteric bacteria. (See VENT GLEET.)

Clones
A group of cells derived from a single cell by mitosis. (See CLONING.)

Clonic
Clonic is a word applied to spasmodic movements of muscles lasting for a short time only.

Cloning
A technique whereby genetically identical animals can be produced. The first sheep produced by transfer of the nucleus from cells from the mammary tissue of adult sheep was produced at Roslin Institute in 1997. The cell nucleus was transferred to an ovum from which the nucleus had been removed and which was then implanted into a surrogate mother. After a normal pregnancy the ewe produced a lamb genetically identical to the sheep from which the mammary cells were taken. The 'age' of a cloned sheep has been questioned. The original cloned sheep had aged centromeres in her cells from birth and developed arthritis at a younger age than normal.

A similar technique has been developed by the same workers to produce transgenic lambs containing therapeutic proteins which can be collected from the sheep's milk, a technique which it is believed will have important implications for the production of human medicines.

Rats, calves, cats and rabbits have all been successfully cloned.

Clopidal
A drug used to prevent or control coccidiosis in chickens, guinea fowl and rabbits.

Cloprostenol
A prostaglandin analogue, used for induction of oestrus or pregnancy termination in horses and in cattle. In the latter it is also used for endometritis, pyometra and removal of a mummified fetus. In pigs, it is used for induction of parturition. (See CONTROLLED BREEDING.)

Closantel
An antiparasitic drug. Among its applications are the treatment and control of fascioliasis, nasal bots (*Oestrus ovis*) and the barber pole worm (*Haemonchus contortus*) in sheep.

Clostridial Enteritis, or Enterotoxaemia
Clostridial enteritis, or enterotoxaemia, is a cause of sudden death in cattle. The deaths usually, though not invariably, occur shortly after calving. The animal, usually one, is found dead. Where death is not immediate, 'milk fever' may be suspected, but the elevated temperature at once rules this out. The cow may be in considerable pain before succumbing. On postmortem examination, acute inflammation of the intestine is found – such as might be expected with some types of poisoning. This enteritis is associated with the presence of a toxin, difficult to demonstrate in the laboratory, produced

by the organism *Clostridium welchii* type A. The same condition may account for the sudden death of pigs. *Cl. oedematiens* may likewise be a cause of sudden death in sheep, pigs, and cattle.

Clostridial Myositis
(see BLACK-QUARTER; GAS GANGRENE)

Clostridium
A genus of anaerobe spore-bearing bacteria of ovoid, spindle, or club shape. They include *Cl. tetani*, *Cl. perfringens* (*welchii*), *Cl. oedematiens*, *Cl. septicum*, *Cl. botulini* and *Cl. difficile* (a possible pathogen of piglets, especially if receiving antibiotics, and associated with enteritis). *Cl. chauvoei* may cause pericarditis and meningitis, as well as BLACK-QUARTER in cattle (and sheep). (See CLOSTRIDIAL ENTERITIS; TETANUS; LAMB DYSENTERY; BRAXY; BOTULISM.)

Cl. perfringens caused the sudden death from enterotoxaemia of 18 cats, aged 2 months to 3 years, in Saudi Arabia. They died within a few hours of scavenging on chicken remains, which caused vomiting and diarrhoea.

Clothing of Animals
As a general rule, only cow, horse, and dog, of the domesticated animals, are supplied with clothing. Sheep already possess protection in the form of wool sufficient except in severe weather on the uplands, although plastic and fabric coats may be used to prevent hypothermia in lambs; while pigs carry a deep layer of subcutaneous fat.

Horses Horses require clothing for the following reasons: (1) to provide protection against cold, chills, draughts, and sudden lowering of the temperature; (2) to protect parts of the body from bruises and abrasions, such as might occur while travelling by road, rail or on board ship; (3) to afford protection from sudden showers of rain or snow when at work in the open. For the latter purposes, waterproof sheets lined with woollen fabric on the inside are usually used.

Cattle Formerly, it was only for sick cattle, and for use at agricultural shows and upon similar occasions, that clothing was provided for cattle, but of recent years Jersey, etc., cows may wear coats. A large quarter-sheet, kept in position by a surcingle, and sometimes provided with fillet-strings, is most commonly employed. An ordinary horse-rug serves the purpose, but the buckle at the neck should never be fastened for cattle.

Sheep Jute coats for ewes were designed and introduced by William Wilson, a Carlisle farmer, who found them economic in his flock in severe weather on the Pennines. The idea is for the coats to be worn from mating to lambing. Five stitches secure the coat. Rugs or coats of man-made fibre have been used in Australia to protect the fleeces of sheep, and have proved economic, since buyers have paid more for the wool. Plastic coats have been used for lambs in the UK.

In Australia an estimated 800,000 sheep die each year during the first fortnight after shearing. Many of the deaths are associated with cold, wet, windy weather. The use of plastic coats during this period has saved many lives.

Head caps have been found to give good and sometimes complete protection against the headfly in the UK.

Dogs For the dog a coat made of woollen fabrics which wraps round the body and buttons or straps together is often used. Dog-coats or rugs are made according to various patterns, but whatever variety is selected should provide protection for the front and under part of the chest, as well as for the sides of the body. The elaborate garments which are used for coursing greyhounds and whippets are excellent articles of clothing, and may be copied with advantage for other breeds of dog.

Clotting of Blood
This is a very complex process, and an obviously important one since on it depends the natural arrest of haemorrhage.

The jelly-like clot consists of minute threads or filaments or fibrin, in which are enmeshed red blood corpuscles, white blood cells, and platelets.

When the injury giving rise to the bleeding occurs, thromboplastin is released from the damaged tissue and from the platelets, and reacts with circulating prothrombin and calcium to form thrombin. This reacts in turn with circulating fibrinogen to produce the fibrin.

The above, however, is only a part of the story, for several other factors are now known to be involved. For clotting to take place, adequate vitamin K is necessary; prothrombin supply being, it seems, dependent on this vitamin.

Clotting time varies in different species and under different degrees of health, but normally it takes between 2.5 and 11 minutes after the blood is shed. After some hours the fibrin contracts and blood serum is squeezed out from the clot.

Clotting may be inhibited by anticoagulants, such as heparin, dicoumarol, warfarin. In cases of haemophilia, a disease from which some dogs suffer, clotting is also inhibited. (See CANINE HAEMOPHILIA.)

'Cloudburst'

'Cloudburst' is a colloquial name for false pregnancy in the goat which, after an apparently normal gestation, suddenly voids from the vulva a large quantity of cloudy fluid – after which the size of the abdomen returns to normal. 'Cloudburst' is a fairly common condition.

Clover

A protein-rich pasture herb. (See INFERTILITY; BLOAT; LEYS; SILAGE; PASTURE MANAGEMENT.)

Cloxacillin

A semi-synthetic penicillin resistant to penicillinase (beta-lactamase). It is mainly used in the treatment and prevention of mastitis.

Clubbed Down

An abnormality of the down of newly hatched chicks and poults in which the ends of the down are shaped like clubs. It is caused by a deficiency of riboflavin in the breeder flock.

Coat Colour Change

(see CUSHING'S SYNDROME)

COB

COB is a short-legged horse, suitable for saddle work of a prolonged but not rapid nature; also used for light trade-carts. Cobs generally stand from 13.5 to 14.5 hands high.

The word 'cob' is also used for cubes made from unmilled dried grass.

Cobalt

Cobalt is one of the mineral elements known to be essential for health, but only required in minute amounts – a trace element. Its function is to act as a catalyst in the assimilation of iron into haemoglobin in the red blood corpuscles. Cobalt is essential to the synthesis of cyanocobalamin (vitamin B_{12}) and a lack of it leads to a deficiency of this vitamin. (See BUSH SICKNESS; 'PINING'; ANAEMIA; TRACE ELEMENTS; MOLYBDENUM.)

Cobalt deficiency occurs in parts of Scotland, Northumbria, Devon, and North Wales. Affected sheep may show symptoms such as progressive debility, anaemia, emaciation, stunted growth, a lustreless fleece, and sunken eyes from which there is often a discharge, with a mortality of up to 20 per cent.

However, symptoms are seldom as definite and clear-cut as the above description might suggest, and in many flocks a 'failure to thrive' is all that is observed or suspected. Sometimes poor performance comes to be accepted as normal, and yet could be remedied by preventive measures after soil analyses had indicated a cobalt deficiency.

Nowadays, 0.25 part per million of cobalt in the soil is regarded as an acceptable level; and 0.17 ppm as constituting a deficiency.

In a comparison of 2 methods of treatment – the administration of a single cobalt 'bullet', and 2 doses of cobalt chloride – both appeared to have been equally effective in alleviating the deficiency as judged from the liveweight response of the lambs. Treatment by cobalt bullet was, however, more effective in increasing and, more importantly, in maintaining serum vitamin B_{12} (closely related to cobalt) than was the cobalt-dosing regime.

Poisoning Overdosage must be avoided. Twelve beef stores on cobalt-deficient land died when they were not only offered a cobalt supplement in boxes, but drenched as well with cobalt sulphate 'measured' by the handful. (See also under TRACE ELEMENTS.)

Cocaine or Coca

Coca leaves are obtained from 2 South American plants, *Erythroxylon coca* and *Erythroxylon bolivianum*, and contain the alkaloid cocaine. This acts as a local anaesthetic by paralysing the nerves of sensation in the region to which it is applied. It has now been displaced by synthetic local anaesthetic agents which are less toxic.

Coccidian Parasites/Diseases

(see COCCIDIOSIS; HAMMONDIA; SARCOCYSTIS; TOXOPLASMOSIS)

Coccidian life-cycle The oocyst is passed in the faeces. It consists of the zygote, which results from the union of the male and female elements, enclosed within a protective membrane or cyst wall. On the ground and in the presence of moisture, oxygen, and a suitable temperature, development proceeds. The zygote splits into 2 or 4 sporoblasts (depending upon the genus), each of which becomes enclosed in a capsule to form oval sporocysts. The contents of each sporocyst divide into 4 (or 2) sporozoites. Once this process of sporulation is completed, the oocyst is 'ripe' and capable of infecting a host; unsporulated oocysts are not infective. When ripe oocysts are swallowed by a suitable host, the action of the digestive juices on the cyst walls allows the motile sporozoites to escape and each penetrates an epithelial cell. Here each parasite increases in size and finally becomes a large rounded schizont. This divides into a number of small elongated merozoites which, escaping from the epithelial cell into the gut, attack new cells, and the process is repeated. The massive feeding stage in the cell before it starts dividing is called a trophozoite, and is usually a young schizont. Under certain conditions, however, some trophozoites develop into large female forms or macrogametocytes which, when mature, become macrogametes. Meanwhile certain other trophozoites develop into male cells or microgametocytes, which divide into a number of small microgametes. One of these unites with each macrogamete, and the resulting cell is called the zygote. The fertilised macrogamete, or zygote, then secretes a thick capsule around itself, forming an oocyst which is discharged into the lumen of the organ intestine or bile-duct and thus escapes from the host in the faeces.

(a) *Levincia* (formerly *Isospora*) – the mature oocyst contains 2 sporocysts, each with 4 sporozoites.

(b) *Eimeria* – the mature oocyst contains 4 sporocysts, each with 2 sporozoites.

Coccidiomycosis

Coccidiomycosis is a fungal disease, involving chiefly the lymph nodes, and giving rise to tumour-like (granulomatous) lesions. It occurs in cattle, sheep, dogs, cats, and certain wild rodents, caused by infection with a fungus, called *Coccidioides immitis*. It has been recognised in many parts of the USA and Canada. It is seen in animals with immuno-suppression; especially young dogs.

Signs Loss of appetite, fever, weight loss, cough, enlarged lymph nodes.

Chiefly recognised in abattoirs during the inspection of meat for human consumption, or in other animals at post-mortem examination. The lesions are sometimes confused with those of actinomycosis or actinobacillosis. In the dog, the disease may involve several internal organs and also bone.

An imported baboon diagnosed with the condition had skin lesions on muzzle and tail consisting of raised, plaque-like ulcers. The lesions may resemble those of *Mycobacterium tuberculosis* and *Yersinia pseudotuberculosis*. Coccidiomycosis is communicable to man.

Coccidiosis

A disease of major economic importance affecting many species of farm and domestic mammals, poultry; also people and birds.

Cause Eimeria, a group of protozoan parasites. For the life-history of the parasites causing this disease, see under COCCIDIAN PARASITES/DISEASES.

Cattle (in which coccidiosis is called red dysentery).

Causal agent Eimeria zürnii. This is believed to be the most important species affecting cattle. Developmental forms occur wholly in the large intestine and caecum where considerable denudation of epithelium occurs, resulting in extensive haemorrhage. The oocysts are nearly spherical, and sporulation, under favourable conditions, takes place in from 48 to 72 hours. It is found in Europe, Africa, and N. America. It is prevalent during the warm season, and attacks especially animals of 2 months to 2 years.

Signs are first seen 1 to 8 weeks after infection. There is a persistent diarrhoea which becomes haemorrhagic. After about a week, emaciation is evident; the temperature rises, and there are digestive disturbances. Milk is diminished or stopped. Passage of faeces is attended by straining or even eversion of the rectum. Convalescence is slow. The lesions are mainly in the large intestine. Mortality varies between 2 and 10 per cent of affected animals, and, generally speaking, the younger the animal, the more likely it is to succumb.

Treatment consists of isolation of all sick animals and careful nursing, with the use of sulfadimidine or decoquinate.

Sheep and goats

Causal Agents At least 7 species of *Eimeria* occur in these animals, and mixed infections with 2 or more species are the rule rather than the exception. The various species are widely distributed and as a rule the clinical disease is seen in lambs and kids, but seldom in the old animals which, however, may harbour coccidia. However, new-born lambs are relatively resistant. Decoquinate, sulfadimidine or sulfamethoxypyridazine are used to treat or prevent coccidiosis.

Signs are those of a pernicious anaemia accompanied by diarrhoea and emaciation.

Pigs Coccidiosis is seldom reported as a serious disease in the UK, and its importance is debatable. However, reports of increasing losses from it in the USA led to a re-appraisal. Occasional outbreaks have been treated with amprolium, monensin or toltazuril.

Horses Diarrhoea, emaciation and death have occurred following infection. (See also GLOBIDIOSIS.)

Rabbits There are 2 forms of the disease: 1 attacking the intestines, and the other the liver. Young rabbits may have acute enteritis, leading to death. The hepatic form often takes a chronic course, with diarrhoea developing later. Affected livers show whitish spots at autopsy. Robenidine or clopidol may be used for treatment.

Dogs and cats The following species have been found in cases of coccidial infection: *Isospora felis; I. rivolta; I. bigemina; E. canis;* and *E. felina.*

Most of these parasites have been isolated from healthy animals. The majority of coccidial infections of dogs and cats are light, and there is little evidence of serious damage to the hosts. In a few cases, however, there is diarrhoea and occasionally fatal dysentery.

Coccidiosis in carnivores is commoner than was once believed, especially in young cats, where the parasite is *I. felis.* The disease causes no symptoms except diarrhoea when a heavy infestation has occurred. Death is rare. The rabbit parasite may be found in faeces when diseased rabbits have been eaten. *I. canis* was isolated from 4 per cent of 481 faecal samples from dogs in North Island, New Zealand; *I. ohioensis* from 9 per cent.

Fowls At least seven species of *Eimeria* have been implicated. The disease commonly affects chicks 5 to 7 weeks old, as well as older growing birds. In the former the mortality may be high. Diarrhoea, often with blood in the faeces, is seen.

Control A vaccine derived from the species of *Eimeria* that affect chickens (Paracox; Schering-Plough) is administered in the drinking water. A single dose gives effective control of coccidiosis and, unlike earlier live vaccines, does not carry the risk of causing the disease in non-vaccinated birds.

Before the introduction of this vaccine, control was dependent upon antibiotics such as monensin and SALINOMYCIN, or upon amprolium.

Turkeys Six species of *Eimeria* cause disease.

Ducks Coccidiosis occurs, but is of little economic importance.

Geese Three species of *Eimeria* occur in the intestine. Rather severe outbreaks have been ascribed to *E. anseris.* A 4th, important species is *E. truncata,* which causes a severe form of renal coccidiosis. The disease affects goslings from 3 weeks to 3 months of age, and in heavy infections goslings may die within 2 or 3 days after symptoms are first seen. The mortality is often very high.

Coccygeal
Coccygeal vertebrae are the tail bones. One or more may fracture if a dog, cat, etc., becomes caught by a closing door or gate. The coccygeal vein is often used to obtain venous blood in cattle.

Cockroaches
These insects may be responsible for the spread of salmonella, which they carry in their gut. A protein found in the faeces of European and North American cockroaches could induce an attack of ASTHMA.

Cocker Spaniel
The commonest and most popular of the spaniels. Originally used to retrieve game, the breed has blunt teeth which avoid damage when carrying birds, etc. They are liable to inherit distichiasis, entropion, glaucoma and retinal atrophy, among other conditions. A 'rage syndrome' is also associated with the breed (see 'JECKYLL AND HYDE' SYNDROME).

Cocoa Poisoning
Poisoning of pigs and poultry, as a result of feeding cocoa residues or waste, was recorded in the UK during the 1939–45 war. (See also CHOCOLATE POISONING.)

Cocoa Shells
Ground cocoa shells are sometimes used in animal feeds. The material contains traces of caffeine and theobromine and was blamed as the source of those drugs found in the blood of a winning racehorse, which was subsequently disqualified.

Cod-Liver Oil
A valuable source of vitamin A and D supplements for animal feeding. The best varieties contain about 1000 to 1200 International Units of vitamin A, and 80 to 100 Units of D, per gram. It should be stored in a dark-coloured container, preferably in a cool place, and if air

can be excluded until it is to be used, this will enable it to be kept longer. Both strong sunlight and oxygen cause a destruction of vitamin A. Overdosage can be harmful. (See also VITAMINS.)

Uses It has a particularly beneficial action in warding off rickets in young animals, and if this trouble has already started it may be checked, or cured, by the administration of cod-liver oil. Synthetic vitamins have largely replaced cod-liver oil.

Swabs of cod-liver oil are also useful in eye injuries and in simple burns.

Cod-Liver Oil Poisoning

This may occur through the use of oil which has been allowed to oxidise or become rancid. One result may be muscular dystrophy in cattle (see under MUSCLES, DISEASES OF).

Codeine

Codeine is one of the active principles of OPIUM, and is used as codeine phosphate, to check severe coughing in bronchitis, common cold, and in some cases of laryngitis. It is also used as an analgesic.

Coenuriasis

Infestation of the sheep's brain with cysts of the dog (and fox) tapeworm *Taenia multiceps*. (See under TAPEWORMS.)

Coffin Bone

The bone enclosed in the hoof of the horse. Also known as the pedal bone.

Coggins Test

The agar-gel immunodiffusion test. Useful in the diagnosis of, e.g., equine infectious anaemia.

Coit, Mal Du

Another name for DOURINE.

Coital Exanthema

(see VULVOVAGINITIS; *also* RHINOTRACHEITIS)

Coitus

(see REPRODUCTION)

Colbred

A cross between the East Friesland and 3 British breeds of sheep (Border Leicester, Clun Forest, and Dorset Horn). The aim of Mr Oscar Colburn, their breeder, was to produce ewes with a consistent 200 per cent lambing average and a sufficiency of milk for this.

Colchicine

The alkaloid obtained from meadow saffron (*Colchicum autumnale*). It is used in plant and experimental animal breeding as 'a multiplier of chromosomes'. It has been possible to produce TRIPLOID rabbits, pigs, etc., by exposing semen to a solution of colchicine prior to artificial insemination.

Colchicum Poisoning

(see MEADOW SAFFRON POISONING)

Cold

(see HYPOTHERMIA; EXPOSURE; FROSTBITE; SHEARING)

Colic

Colic is a vague term applied to symptoms of abdominal pain, especially in horses. In order to emphasise the large number of different conditions which may produce abdominal pain in the horse, the following list is included:

1. Acute indigestion, resulting from the feeding of unsuitable food, the presence of gas (flatulent colic).

2. Severe organic disorders, such as impaction of the colon, intussusception, volvulus, or strangulation of the bowel, rupture of the stomach, enteritis, and peritonitis, are among the serious causes.

3. The presence of large numbers of parasitic worms, horse bots, etc. (See under EQUINE VERMINOUS ARTERITIS.)

4. Calculi present in the kidney, urinary bladder, or urethra in the male, causing irritation of these organs.

5. Anthrax, where one of the common symptoms is abdominal pain.

6. Approaching parturition in the pregnant mare.

7. Grass disease.

8. See HYMEN, IMPERFORATE.

9. Uterine rupture.

10. Nephritis.

11. Various poisons (see POISONING).

12. In addition, in countries where RABIES is endemic, this disease should be borne in mind when presented with a horse which appears to have colic.

The horse has a peculiarity in the arrangement of its alimentary canal, in that while the stomach is comparatively small, the intestines, and especially the large intestines, are of great bulk and capacity. In addition to this, the stomach itself has the peculiarity that its entrance and exit are small; the former only allows escape of gas into the gullet under exceptional circumstances, and the latter, owing to the S-shaped bend of the pylorus and first part of the small intestine, is very liable to become occluded when there is any considerable pressure of gas within the stomach. These facts combine to make it difficult or impossible for gas collected in the stomach, as the result of fermentation, either to escape by the mouth or to pass on into the intestines. Fermenting or otherwise?unsuitable food may cause tympany of the stomach; while an excess of any food may lead to impaction of the stomach; and occasionally to its rupture.

Inflammation or volvulus may affect the small intestine, but most cases of colic involve the large intestine. Impaction of the caecum or colon may occur; likewise tympany.

The ileum, supplied only by a single artery, appears to be particularly vulnerable to ischaemia, following thrombosis often caused by *Strongylus vulgaris* worms.

Anaerobic bacteria and their toxins may exacerbate the situation after circulation defects have occurred.

(See also INTUSSUSCEPTION, another cause of colic.)

Signs

1. Spasmodic colic is typified by sudden and severe attacks of pain, usually of an intermittent character. Breathing is blowing and faster than usual; there is an anxious expression about the face; and the pulse is accelerated and hard. In a few minutes the attack may pass off and the horse becomes easier, or the pain may continue. In the latter case the horse lies down and rolls, after having first walked round about the box. In some cases rolling appears to afford some measures of relief, but in others the horse rises again almost at once. During an attack the horse may kick at its belly, or may turn and gaze at its flank.

In another form, ileus – often called flatulent colic – the pain begins suddenly, but there are not such distinct periods of ease. The horse walks round and round the box, kicks at the abdomen, gazes at its sides, breaks out into patchy sweating, and breathes heavily. The horse frequently crouches as if to lie down, but only actually lies in the less severe cases, and seldom or never remains lying for any length of time. Attempts at passing urine are noticed, but, as in the truly spasmodic colic, they are seldom successful. Faeces may be passed in small quantities, and are usually accompanied by flatus.

2. Obstructive colic may arise through impaction of the bowel with dry, fibrous, partly digested food material. Symptoms develop slowly, commencing with dullness and depression, irregularity in feeding, and abdominal discomfort. In 12 hours or so signs of abdominal pain appear. In some cases acute pain is shown, the horse rolling on the ground in agony. Small amounts of faeces are passed with considerable frequency at first, but when an attack is well established the passage of both urine and dung ceases. An attitude to which some importance may be attached, since it is very strongly suggestive of impaction of the colon, is one in which the horse backs against the manger or other projection, and appears to sit upon it, sometimes with the hind-feet off the ground. In other cases a horse with obstruction in the colon or caecum may sit with the hindquarters on the ground, but retains an upright position with the forelegs – somewhat similar to the position assumed by a dog. (See CALCULI for another cause of obstruction.)

3. Colic due to a twist (volvulus). There is great pain, during which the horse may become restless and violent. Sometimes the pain passes off, and sweating occurs, before a further period of pain. The temperature may be 41°C (105 or 106°F), becoming subnormal in the last stages. Pulse-rate may rise to 120. Death is usually preceded by convulsions.

Many colic cases end fatally, and it is certain that many horses might have been saved if a veterinary surgeon had been summoned at the outset.

A survey of 134 cases of colic, seen at the veterinary clinic, University of Zurich, included 34 which were symptomless on arrival, required no treatment, and were regarded as cases of spasmodic colic. Thirty-three horses had impaction of the pelvic flexure of the colon and were treated conservatively; as were 14 with impaction of the ampulla, coli (4), and caecum (1). There were 7 cases of tympany of the stomach and 2 of impaction. Of 53 cases of ileus, the prognosis was hopeless in 7 which were destroyed, and owners refused surgery in another 6 cases. Forty underwent laparotomy, and 24 were discharged. Surgical success rate was 60 per cent; overall success of treatment was 68 per cent. Suggestions included maintenance of a nasal stomach tube to eliminate possibly lethal consequences of secondary gastric distension by fluid and gas during the journey to the clinic; and 1 litre of 5 per cent sodium bicarbonate solution intravenously to help control the start of acidosis. (See also HORSES, COMMON CAUSES OF DEATH IN.)

Cattle Bovine colic occurs relatively infrequently. It is mainly caused by torsion of the caecum or abomasum, mesenteric torsion, intussusception, strangulation or phytobezoar.

Coliform

A convenient term used to describe several species of lactose fermenting bacilli which inhabit the gut. The most commonly encountered is *Escherichia coli* and approximately 80 per cent of coliform isolates tested at the National Institute for Research in Dairying are *E. coli*. Other coliform species implicated in bovine mastitis include *Klebsiella pneumoniae*, *K. oxytoca*, *Enterobacter cloacae*, *E. aerogenes* and *Citrobacter freundii*. All are 'gut associated' but some, notably *K. pneumoniae* and Enterobacters, may be free-living in forest environments or soil and be introduced into a dairy herd with sawdust or wood shavings used for cattle litter.

Coliform Infections

Coliform infections include mastitis, enteritis and septicaemia. Coliform organisms are frequently found in apparently healthy animals. An examination of cattle carcases at slaughterhouses showed that coliform organisms were isolated from surface swabbings from 208 out of 400 head of cattle (52 per cent); 81 of these being resistant to 1 or more antibiotics. Of 400 pig carcase swabs, 331 (83 per cent) were positive for coliforms; 246 being resistant to 1 or more antibiotics. Chloramphenicol resistance was present in 19 pig isolates and 1 cattle isolate. (See BEDDING – Sawdust; E. COLI; MASTITIS IN COWS.)

Colitis

Inflammation of the colon, or first part of the large intestine. (See INTESTINES.)

Collagen

(see FIBROUS TISSUE; *also* CUTANEOUS ASTHENIA)

Collateral Circulation

(see ANASTOMOSIS)

Colliculus Seminalis

This protrudes into the lumen of the urethra, and at its centre is a minute opening into a tiny tube (the uterus masculinus) which runs into the prostate gland.

Collie Eye Anomaly

A congenital disease occurring in some rough collies, smooth collies, and Shetland sheepdogs. In the worst cases, blindness may follow detachment of the retina or haemorrhage within the eye.

Collodion

Flexible collodion, a mixture of pyroxylin, alcohol and ether, is fairly elastic and does not crack with movement. It was used for application to lesions around joints. Medicated collodion contains substances such as salicylic acid and iodoform. A collodion preparation containing a caustic was used for destroying the horn-buds of calves. (See DE-HORNING.)

Colloid

Colloid is matter in which either the individual particles are single large molecules, such as proteins, or aggregates of smaller molecules are more or less uniformly distributed in a dispersion medium, e.g. water, oil. Examples: colloidal silver (used for eye infections), and colloidal manganese.

Coloboma

A congenital eye defect caused by an absence or fault in the tissue. (See under EYE, DISEASES OF.)

Colon

The part of the large intestine extending from the caecum to the rectum. (See COLITIS; INTESTINES.)

Colostrum

Colostrum is the milk secreted by the udder immediately after parturition and for the following 3 to 4 days. It contains 20 per cent or more protein, a little more fat than normal milk, and may be tinged pink due to blood corpuscles. It coagulates at about 80° to 85°C, and cannot therefore be boiled. This is sometimes used as a test. It is normally rich in vitamins A and D provided the dam has not been deprived of these in her food. It acts as a natural purgative for the young animal, clearing from its intestines the accumulated faecal matter known as 'meconium', which is often of a dry, putty-like nature. Of much greater importance, it is through the medium of the colostrum that the young animal obtains its first supply of antibodies which protect it against various bacteria and viruses.

Before the cow calves, her udder selectively withdraws these immunoglobulins from her blood into the colostrum. In the suckling calf, the immunoglobulins become active in the blood serum after absorption, and they also have a local protective action within the small intestine. If the calf is to survive, both the serum and intestinal immunoglobulins must be present in adequate quantities; for the serum immunoglobulin will protect against septicaemia, but not against the enteritis which leads to scouring and dehydration.

The importance of the calf receiving colostrum early has long been emphasised. This is recognised in the Welfare of Livestock Regulations 1994, which specify that colostrum must be fed within 6 hours of the calf's birth.

Research at Glasgow veterinary school found that beef suckler cows suckled their calf within 1.5 hours of birth whereas, on average, dairy cows suckled their calves after 4 hours.

Colour-Marking Bulls

Colour-marking bulls, e.g. Hereford, Aberdeen Angus, Charolais, and Galloway, for mating with cows in dairy herds which are of dual-purpose type and moderate to poor milkers, in order to increase the number of store cattle suitable for fattening for beef production. (See also BEEF-BREEDS AND CROSSES.)

Columnaris Disease

A disease in fish caused by *Chondrococcus columnaris*, an opportunist myxobacterium present in the water. Affected fish have greyish-white lesions on the skin. It is prevented by controlling water temperature to below 25°C and reducing stress on the fish.

Colt

A young male horse.

Coma

Coma is a state of profound unconsciousness in which the patient not only cannot be roused, but there are no reflex movements when the skin is pinched or pricked, or when the eyeballs are touched, etc. The cause is generally an excessively high temperature, brain injury, cerebral haemorrhage, some poisons, or too much or too little insulin in cases of diabetes, or the terminal stage of a fatal illness.

Comb

A projection of the skin, serrated at the top, running from front to back of the skull. In healthy poultry, it should be bright red and well developed. When birds go out of lay or are caponised, the comb becomes smaller and paler. Anaemia may also cause this. A pale comb of normal size suggests internal haemorrhage. Scurfiness is suggestive of favus; yellow scabs of fowl-pox.

Comeny's Infectious Paralysis of Horses

This condition, of unknown aetiology, was first described in French army horses by Comény. The reported signs are a sudden rise in temperature to 40°C (104° or 105°F), persisting for 5 days, and followed in some cases by paralysis after a period of hind-limb incoordination and difficulty in turning.

Commensalism

Commensalism is the association of 2 species in which 1 alone benefits, but the other does not suffer. The term is used to refer to a benign parasitism. Commensal micro-organisms are found on the skin surface, for example, and do not produce disease.

Commissure

Commissure means a joining, and is a term applied to strands of nerve fibres that join 1 side of the brain to the other, to the band joining 1 optic nerve to the other, to the junction of the lips at the corners of the mouth, etc.

Communicable Diseases

For diseases communicable to man, see under ZOONOSES. For diseases communicable from man to farm livestock, etc., see ANTHROPONOSES.

Companion Animal Welfare Council

An independent body established in 1999 to conduct and publish studies into the welfare, treatment and care of companion animals. It is funded by a charitable trust.

Comparative Test

(see TUBERCULIN TEST)

Compensation

Compensation is the term applied to the method by which the body makes good a defect of form or function in an organ which is abnormal in these respects.

Complement

A complex protein that is a constituent of serum and plays an essential part in the production of immunity. Bacteria are killed by the specific antibody developed in an animal's serum only in the presence of complement. Complement is also necessary for haemolysis.

An immune serum may contain antibodies which, together with the antigen, absorb or fix complement and are hence called complement-fixing antibodies. These form the basis for the Complement Fixation Test, which is used in the diagnosis of certain diseases, e.g. Johne's. As an indicator for the test, red blood corpuscles plus their specific antibody are used, i.e. the corpuscles plus the antiserum heated at 55°C to inactivate or destroy the complement. In the test, on adding the indicator, haemolysis will not occur if the complement has been fixed.

Compound Feeds

A number of different ingredients (including major minerals, trace elements, vitamins and other additives) mixed and blended in appropriate proportions, to provide properly balanced diets for all types of stock at every stage of growth and development. (See DIET; FLUOROSIS.)

Compulsive Polydipsia

The urge to drink excessive quantities of water, due to some psychological disturbance, is a recognised syndrome in human medicine, and it probably occurs in dogs as a result of stress; leading to urinary incontinence. (See also DIABETES INSIPIDUS.)

Conalbumin

An important constituent of egg-white. It makes iron unavailable to certain bacteria (*Salmonella* and *Arizona* spp) thus inhibiting their multiplication within the egg during incubation. (See also IRON-BINDING PROTEINS.)

Concentrates

The bulk of these in Britain today come from highly reputable compound feeding-stuffs manufacturers, and are expert formulations related not only to the current price of various ingredients but also to the proper balancing of these ingredients. Computers are often used in the formulations. The inclusion of trace elements, minerals, and vitamins makes these compound feeding-stuffs foods complete in themselves. Suitable mixes are obtainable for every class of farm livestock.

Farm-mixed concentrates are commonly used on large arable farms, using home-grown barley, oats, beans, etc. The expertise required for formulation may also be lacking, so that on the smaller farm, proprietary concentrates are often to be preferred.

(See DIET; CUBES; *also* ADDITIVES, COMPOUND FEEDS; SUPPLEMENTS.)

Conception Rates

Conception Rates following artificial insemination of cattle are stated to be in the region of 65 per cent in dairy breeds, and over 70 per cent in beef breeds. In the UK, the conception rate is usually based upon the number of animals which, in a 3-month period, do not return to the first insemination. In Denmark, the conception rate is based on the evidence of a physical pregnancy diagnosis carried out 3 months after insemination.

Conception rates are influenced by many factors. The best time for insemination is between 2 and 20 hours after 'heat' is observed; after that, delay will mean a lower conception rate. Health of male and female, and inseminator's skill also influence the rate. (See also FARROWING RATES.)

Conceptus

The embryo or fetus together with the tissues, such as the placenta, that nourish it.

Concrete

The precise composition of concrete may prove important where floor feeding is practised. Suspected iron poisoning from the licking of concrete made with sand rich in iron has been described in fattening pigs. Concrete floors of piggeries, etc., should be made with integral air spaces in order to have some insulating effect, and should not be abrasive. If they are, they can lead to injuries, followed by staphylococcal or other infection which may cause severe illness or death **even in a new pig pen**. Pigs should never be allowed to lie on freshly set concrete; skin burns may result from chemicals in the mix. (See under FOOT-ROT OF PIGS; HOUSING OF ANIMALS; BEDDING.)

Concussion

(see under BRAIN DISEASES)

Condensation in Buildings

(see NITRITE POISONING; CALF HOUSING; PNEUMONIA; YORKSHIRE BOARDING; VENTILATION)

Condition

(see under MUSCLE)

Condition Score

A method used to evaluate the thinness or fatness of cattle, sheep, goats, pigs and horses. It is used to monitor feeding and check that animals are fit to breed and maintain pregnancy.

Condyle

Condyle is the rounded prominence at the end of a bone; for instance, the condyles of the humerus are the two prominences on either side of the elbow-joint in animals, while the condyles of the femur enter into the formation of the stifle joint.

Conformation Assessment in the Cow

(see under PROGENY TESTING)

Congestive Heart Failure

(see under HEART, DISEASES OF)

Coniine
(see HEMLOCK POISONING)

Conjunctiva
Conjunctiva is the membrane which covers the front of the eye. It lines the insides of the eyelids of all animals, both upper and lower, and from each of these places it is reflected on to the front of the eyeball. The membrane is transparent in its central portion, where it is specialised to form the covering to the cornea, which admits light into the cavity of the eye.

Conjunctivitis
(see under EYE, DISEASES OF)

Connective Tissues
These include: (1) white fibrous (collagenous) tissue, having fibres of collagen produced by fibroblasts, e.g. in tendons, ligaments; (2) yellow elastic tissue, composed of kinked fibres; (3) reticular tissue, composed of fine fibres which form a framework for bone-marrow;.(4) adipose tissue or fat; (5) cartilage or gristle; (6) bone.

Consolidation
Consolidation is a term applied to solidification of an organ, especially of a lung. The consolidation may be of a permanent nature due to formation of fibrous tissue or tumour cells, or temporary, as in acute pneumonia.

Constipation
Difficulty or delay in passing faeces. The faeces are passed in a variety of ways among the domestic animals. In the horse, cow, and sheep, the excreta appears to be evacuated with very little or even no effort. The horse can defecate perfectly and naturally when galloping in harness, and seems only partly aware of the process. In the case of the dog and pig, on the other hand, the process involves a cessation of all other occupation, the assumption of a special position of the body, and an obviously conscious effort. This attitude towards the process is more nearly that of human beings, and it is easy to understand that the more involved and particular the process, the more likely is it to become upset when circumstances arise which alter the animal's mode of living. Consequently it is found that while dogs and pigs are liable to suffer from the true form of constipation, especially after exposure to some unusual factor, horses, cattle, and sheep, although they are liable to suffer from acute obstruction of the bowels, are seldom affected with true constipation.

Causes Anything which is likely to interfere with the normal peristaltic movements of the bowels, such as the use of too dry, bulky, or concentrated foods, overloading of the alimentary tract with unsuitable foods, tumours in the abdomen, pain originating from an enlarged prostate gland, or from obstructed anal glands, will at any rate predispose to constipation if not actually cause it. Inadequate exercise and too much food is a common cause. Changes from one owner to another, or from one district to another, or stress in the case of nervous individuals, are said to be a cause.

Treatment
(see LAXATIVES; ENEMA)

Cats It is important that owners do not mistake what may at first appear to be constipation for difficulty in passing, or inability to pass, urine owing to UROLITHIASIS.

Contagious Abortion of Cattle
(see BRUCELLOSIS IN CATTLE)

Contagious Bovine Pleuro-Pneumonia (CBPP)
This disease has decimated herds throughout Europe and in other parts of the world on several occasions, and probably has been directly responsible for the death of more cattle than any other single disease with the possible exception of cattle plague (rinderpest). It is a NOTIFIABLE DISEASE in the EU.

It is present in Asia, Africa, Spain and Portugal; while in recent years, outbreaks have occurred in Australia and South America.

Cattle, buffaloes, and related species, such as reindeer, yak, and bison, are susceptible.

Cause Mycoplasma mycoides. (See under MYCOPLASMOSIS.)

Infection may occur by direct contact. Buildings which have housed infected cattle may remain infective for long periods.

Incubation period 3 weeks to 6 months.

Signs The first sign of illness is a rise of temperature to 39.5° to 40.5°C (103° or 105°F). In the acute disease this rise of temperature is soon followed by signs of general illness, such as dull coat, debility, loss of appetite, cessation of rumination. Shortly afterwards a dry, short, painful cough makes its appearance.

Pregnant cows are liable to abort.

Death usually follows in 2 or 3 weeks after the symptoms have become pronounced and acute. Recovery is frequently more apparent than real, for a chronic cough remains, and the disease may again become acute and even end fatally.

Post-Mortem appearances Large or small areas of pneumonia in the lungs, which are often of a marbled appearance. The lesion is primarily one of interstitial pneumonia, with thickened septa dividing the lung up into lobules; some lobules show acute congestion, some are in a stage of red or grey hepatisation, while others consist of dead encapsulated tissue, known as 'sequestra'. Evidence of pleurisy with often much fibrinous deposit around the lungs is usual.

Diagnosis The slaughter of suspected animals may be essential for this. Corroboration may be obtained by laboratory methods.

Treatment is not allowed in most countries, but neoarsphenamine and tylosin have proved useful elsewhere.

Immunisation Live vaccines may be used in eradication and control programmes.

Contagious Caprine Pleuro-Pneumonia

A disease of goats, caused by a mycoplasma and occurring in Europe, Asia, and Africa. Acute, peracute, and chronic forms occur. Mortality may be 60 to 100 per cent. Antibiotics are useful for treatment where a slaughter policy is not in force.

Contagious Diseases

Certain of these are notifiable. (See under NOTI-FIABLE DISEASES.) The responsibilities of animal owners are discussed under DISEASES OF ANIMALS ACTS.

Contagious Ecthyma of Sheep

Contagious ecthyma of sheep is another name for ORF.

Contagious Epithelioma of Birds

(see FOWL POX)

Contagious Equine Metritis (CEM)

Contagious equine metritis (CEM) is a contagious venereal disease found in mares and transmitted by stallions. This is a NOTIFIABLE DISEASE in the UK, under the Infectious Diseases of Horses Order 1987.

Cause A Gram-negative coccobacillus, *Taylorella equigenitalis* (formerly *Haemophilus equigenitalium*). This has been isolated from the cervix, urethra and clitoris. The organism is apt to persist in the clitoral fossa after clearance from other parts of the mare's urogenital tract, and routine sampling at this site is therefore necessary or diagnosis may fail to be confirmed.

Control A code of practice for control of the infection was formulated by the Horserace Betting Levy Board in 1977, and supported by the Ministry of Agriculture and the Thoroughbred Breeders' Association. A list of laboratories authorised to test for the CEM organism is published annually in the *Veterinary Record.*

Cervical swab tests are a routine diagnostic and preventive measure on stud farms. Among

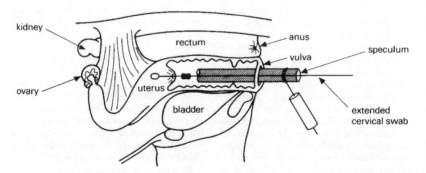

Diagram showing the technique of collecting a cervical swab via a tubular speculum. The swab is passed as far into the open oestrous cervix, and beyond, as possible.

techniques used for taking swabs is that shown in the diagram.

Measures to control the spread of CEM in non-thoroughbred mares have been in operation since 1978.

(See also CLITORIS – Clitoral sinusectomy.)

Contagious Ovine Digital Dermatitis (CODD)

A disease resembling, but distinct from, foot-rot which causes severe ulcerative lesions of the coronet that may lead to complete separation of the hoof case. It was first identified in the UK in 1997. The cause is a spirochaete similar to that responsible for bovine digital dermatitis. It is differentiated from foot-rot by the absence of interdigital sores (in most cases) and by failure to isolate *Dichelobacter nodosus*, the cause of foot-rot, from the lesions.

For treatment, see DIGITAL DERMATITIS.

Contagious Pustular Dermatitis in Sheep
(see ORF)

Contagious Stomatitis
(see FOOT-AND-MOUTH DISEASE; also VESICULAR STOMATITIS)

Contraceptives

Megestrol is one of the drugs used to stop dogs and cats coming on heat. An injection of oestradiol benzoate has been used in cases of misalliance in bitches; prostaglandins have also been used. Prostaglandins have been used to control the timing of pregnancy in cattle and to terminate an unwanted pregnancy. Attempts to develop a contraceptive for wild rabbits have been hampered by the problem of drug residues in wild rabbits caught for food. (See also STILBENES.)

Contracted Foot or Contracted Hoof

A condition of the horse in which some part of the foot, very often a quarter or heel, becomes contracted and shrunken to less than its usual size. It is brought about by anything which favours rapid evaporation of the moisture in the horn, such as rasping away the outer surface of the wall; or by conditions which prevent expansion of the hoof, such as paring away the frog so that it does not come into contact with the ground, cutting the bars, allowing the wall at the heels to fall inwards, shoeing with high calkins, etc.

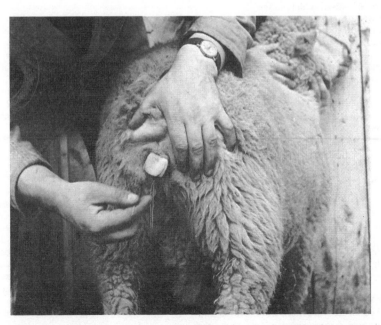

About to withdraw the progestogen-impregnated sponge at the end of the 2-week treatment period. At this time, the ewe receives a single intramuscular injection of PMSG – to complete the controlled breeding treatment.

Prevention consists in leaving the frogs as large and well developed as possible; reducing the overgrowth at the heels and bars to the same extent as at the toe and other parts of the foot; shoeing with shoes which allow the frog to come into contact with the ground.

Treatment In severe cases a run at grass with tips on the affected feet, and leaving the heels bare, is advisable. (See also HOOF REPAIR.)

'Contracted Tendons'

(1) A congenital condition, in which the foot is not fully extended, seen mainly in calves, lambs and foals. The causes are various and the condition may clear up without treatment in a few days. If it does not, splints may be applied to straighten the foot. Surgical correction by partially severing the tendon is sometimes carried out. (2) Chronic tendonitis in adult horses. The limb is not fully extended and the animal appears to be standing on its toes (sometimes called 'ballerina syndrome').

Control, Controlled Experiment

In any scientifically conducted experiment or field trial, the results of treatment of 1 group of animals are compared with results in another, untreated, group. Animals in the untreated group are known as 'the controls'.

Control of Dogs Order 1992

(see under LAW)

Controlled Breeding

The manipulation of ovarian activity to enable successful insemination at a predetermined time is widely practised in cattle, sheep and pigs. Synchronisation of oestrus enables groups of animals to be inseminated at a chosen time, and parturition planned to take place when convenient. A progestogen preparation is administered for 10 to 14 days according to a specific dosage schedule; the animal comes into heat when the progestogen is removed. Insemination, by natural mating or artificially, then takes place. The progestogen is administered orally, by injection, implant, or intravaginally, according to species and particular product.

An implant of MELATONIN will stimulate early onset of natural reproductive activity and improve fertility early in the season.

Cattle Two main systems are used. In one, used in beef animals or maiden heifers, an implant containing norgestomet is inserted under the skin of the ear and then an injection of norgestomet plus oestradiol given immediately.

The implant is removed after 9 or 10 days and the animal inseminated twice, 48 and 72 hours, or once, 56 hours later. In the other system, a spiral device incorporating progesterone, with a gelatine capsule containing oestradiol attached, is inserted into the cow's vagina and left for 12 days. The cow is inseminated twice, after 48 and 72 hours, or once at 56 hours.

Alternatively, a progestogen may be administered by injection.

Sheep A sponge impregnated with a progestogen (flugestone or medroxprogesterone) is introduced to the vagina and left for 12 to 14 days. The ewes are introduced to the ram 48 hours after removal. The sponge may be used in conjunction with an injection of pregnant mare serum gonadotrophin, given on removal of the sponge, to advance the breeding season by up to 6 weeks

Pigs A suspension of altrenogest is added to the feed once daily; for sows for 3 days, for gilts for 18 consecutive days.

Farrowing may be induced, within 3 days of the expected normal time, by an injection of a luteolitic agent such as cloprostenol or dinoprost. Farrowing then occurs between 24 and 30 hours later.

Mares Induction of ovulation in mares to synchronise ovulation more closely with mating can be achieved by an injection of buserelin, a synthetic releasing hormone analogue for both gonadotrophin and follicle stimulating hormone.

Warning: Progestogen products should be handled with great care, particularly by pregnant women. They must not come in contact with the skin.

Controlled Environment Housing

Temperature, ventilation, and humidity are controlled within narrow limits by means of electric fans, heaters, etc., and good insulation. Poultry, for example, are protected in this way from sudden changes in temperature; rearing can be carried out with the minimum loss throughout the year; and increased egg yields and decreased food intake can effect a considerable saving in costs of production. Some of these houses are windowless; artificial lighting being provided: respiratory disease may occur through overcrowding or ventilation defects.

Failure of automatic control Ventilation systems must have fail-safe alarms and back-up systems under UK law. If those are not effective, there may be fatal consequences, as the following examples show.

A thunderstorm blew the fuse in the fan circuit of a controlled environment house, and unfortunately 'fail-safe' ventilation flaps did not work. As a result 520 fattening pigs died of heat-stroke.

In another incident the heating system continued to function in a house containing 82 pigs. The fans failed, and minimal natural ventilation resulted in the temperature reaching 46°C (104°F), and the death of 65 pigs.

Convex Sole or Dropped Sole

The sole of the horse's foot, instead of being arched (concave) when viewed from the ground surface, is convex and projects to a lower level than does the outer rim of the wall in many cases. (See LAMINITIS.)

Convolvulus Poisoning

Another name for MORNING GLORY.

Convulsions

Convulsions are powerful involuntary contractions (alternating with relaxation) of muscles, producing aimless movement and contortion of the body, and accompanied by loss of consciousness. (See SPASM; FITS.)

Coombs (Antiglobulin) Test

Coombs (antiglobulin) test is a laboratory test used in the differential diagnosis of various blood disorders.

Coopworth

A breed of New Zealand sheep derived from the 'Border-Romney' cross.

COPD

(see CHRONIC OBSTRUCTIVE PULMONARY DISEASE)

Copper (Cu)

Copper (Cu) is one of the TRACE ELEMENTS which is essential in the nutrition of animals. It acts as a catalyst in the assimilation of iron, which is needed in the production of haemoglobin in the liver. Its absence from the foodstuffs eaten in some areas leads to a form of anaemia.

In several parts of the world a deficiency of copper in the herbage has been a major obstacle to livestock production, and appropriate dressings of the land have permitted dramatic increases in production.

In several parts of Britain, copper deficiency is a serious condition. (See HYPOCUPRAEMIA.)

Two types of copper deficiency are recognised: primary and secondary. The former arises from an inadequate intake of copper and, while herbage levels of copper below 5 ppm are uncommon in Britain, a survey showed that over 50 per cent of 1078 beef herds in mid-Wales had low blood copper levels, probably associated with low intake. Secondary copper deficiency is the more common form in the UK and occurs where absorption or storage within the animal body of copper is adversely affected by a high sulphate or molyb denum intake, even though there is adequate copper in the diet.

An excess of molybdenum in the 'teart' soils and pastures of central Somerset, and of areas in Gloucestershire, Warwickshire, Derbyshire and East Anglia, has long been recognised, giving rise to scouring (especially from May to October), a greyness of the hair around the eyes, staring coats and a marked loss of condition.

However, analysis of sediments from stream beds in many counties shows that herbage may contain excessively high concentrations of molybdenum.

Copper deficiency may be prevented by administering copper sulphate powder containing 254 g/kg mixed with feed at a dose of 2 g per head; or by a ruminal bolus containing small blunt rods ('needles') of copper oxide, once a season.

Treatment of copper deficiency is by parenteral injection of copper, usually in the form of copper edetate or heptonate.

Sheep Caution: Indiscriminate dressing of pasture with copper salts is likely to cause poisoning in sheep if the quantities used are too large, or if sheep are re-admitted to dressed pasture before there has been sufficient rain to wash the copper salts off the herbage.

Copper sulphate for pigs Copper sulphate, added to the fattening ration at the rate of 150–180 ppm, has produced an improvement in the growth rate in pigs. (See SWAYBACK; *also* MOLYBDENUM.)

Copper, Poisoning by

With the exception of sheep, which may be given an overdose to expel worms, animals are not likely to be poisoned through internal administration of copper sulphate as a medicine. Poisoning has occurred, however, in sheep given a copper-rich supplement, intended for pigs, over a 3.5-month period; in a heifer similarly, as well as in pigs given too strong a copper supplement. Poisoning also occurs when animals are grazed in the vicinity of copper-smelting works, where the herbage gradually becomes contaminated with copper, in orchards where fruit-trees have been sprayed with copper salts and also in sheep grazing land treated with copper sulphate (either crystals mixed with sand, or as a sprayed solution) as a snail-killer in the control of liver-fluke or as a preventative of swayback.

Signs are those of an irritant poison – pain, diarrhoea (or perhaps constipation), and weakness; staggering and muscular twitchings are seen in chronic cases. A fatal chronic copper poisoning may occur in pigs fed a copper supplement of 250 parts per million.

Failure to achieve accurate mixing of small quantities of copper sulphate into farm-mixed rations has led to fatal poisoning of pigs.

It has been pointed out that copper poisoning is almost specific to the housing of sheep. It occurs even in diets ostensibly containing no copper supplement. The capacity of the sheep for storing copper from the normal constituents of the diet is higher than that of other animals, and markedly higher in housed sheep. And lambs reared indoors have died because their hay was made from grass contaminated by slurry from pigs on a copper-supplemented diet.

It is dangerous to exceed 10 ppm of copper in dry feeds for sheep over a long period.

AFRC research has shown that the sheep's physiological response to copper is influenced by heredity, and that there are significant breed differences as regards swayback and copper poisoning.

Treatment Following some Australian research, it was shown at the Rowett Research Institute that 3 subcutaneous injections of tetrathiomolybdate (on alternate days) can remove copper from the livers of both sheep and goats without causing any apparent ill-effects.

'Copper Nose'

A form of LIGHT SENSITISATION occurring in cattle.

Copperbottle

Lucilia cuprina, the strike fly which attacks sheep in Australia and South Africa.

Coprophagy

The eating of faeces by an animal. In rabbits, this is a normal practice. The rabbit produces 2 types of faecal pellet: the normal black pellet, which is not eaten, and a soft brown pellet, produced in the caecum, which is eaten immediately on being expelled from the anus. The latter pellets are rich in B vitamins and amino acids, but can also serve to recycle parasites. Female parents of several species ingest the faeces of their offspring in order to keep the nursing area clean. Within 3 weeks of birth, foals will eat their dams' faeces and thereby acquire the various bacteria needed for digestive purposes in their own intestines. Overnight coprophagy has also been reported in adult horses in adjusting to 'complete-diet' cubes when no hay is on offer.

It has been suggested that foals may obtain nutrients, and that coprophagy may be a response to a maternal pheromone signalling the presence of deoxycholic acid which may be required for gut 'immuno-competence' and myelination of the nervous system.

Coprophagy also occurs in piglets, dogs, and non-human primates.

Copulation
(see REPRODUCTION)

Corgi

A long-backed, short-legged dog of medium size with erect ears. There are 2 forms: the Pembrokeshire, which is orange-brown in colour; and the Cardiganshire, which is black, white and tan. The long back can give rise to intervertebral disc problems and the breed may be susceptible to recurrent corneal ulceration.

Corium

The main layer of the skin, also known as the dermis. It lies below the epidermis and above the subcutaneous tissue (see SKIN).

'Corkscrew Penis'
(see under PENIS AND PREDUCE, ABNORMALITIES AND LESIONS)

Corn Cockle Poisoning

The plant *Lychnis* (or *Agrostemma*) *githago*, a weed of corn fields, is usually avoided by livestock; but they may be poisoned through eating wheat or barley meal contaminated with the seeds. The latter contain SAPONINS.

Dogs and young animals are most susceptible to poisoning; the signs of which are restlessness, frothing at the mouth, colic, paralysis and loss of consciousness.

First aid Large amounts of white of egg, starch paste, and milk may be given to calves and dog as a drench.

Cornea

Cornea is the clear part of the front of the eye through which the rays of light pass to the retina. (See EYE.)

Corns

A bruise of the sensitive part of the horse's foot occurring in the angle formed between the wall of the hoof at the heel and the bar of the foot.

Signs In the majority of cases the horse goes very lame either gradually or suddenly. When made to walk he does so by using the toe of the affected foot, keeping the heels raised. Sometimes the pain is so great that he refuses to place the affected foot on the ground at all, but hops on the sound foot of the other side.

Treatment The shoe should be removed as in all cases of lameness, and the hard dry outer horn pared away. Particular attention should always be paid to the region of the heels, for stones often become lodged there. If a corn is present the horse will show pain whenever the knife is applied to the affected part, and efficient paring will necessitate an analgesic.

Mild cases take about 5 days to a week to recover, while horses with severe suppurating corns may be as long as 6 or 7 weeks before they are fit to work. (See also FOOT OF THE HORSE.)

Coronary

Coronary is a term applied to several structures in the body encircling an organ in the manner of a crown. The coronary arteries are the arteries of supply to the heart which arise from the aorta, just beyond the aortic valve; through them blood is delivered to the heart muscle.

Coronary Band, or Coronary Cushion

Coronary band, or coronary cushion, is the part of the sensitive matrix of the hoof from which grows the wall. It runs round the foot at the coronet, lying in a groove in the upper edge of the wall. Its more correct name is the coronary matrix. (See FOOT OF THE HORSE.)

Coronary Thrombosis

Coronary thrombosis, associated with *Strongylus vulgaris*, is a cause of sudden death in yearling and 2-year-old horses. (See EQUINE VERMINOUS ARTERITIS.)

Coronaviruses

Coronaviruses cause diarrhoea in calves, foals, dogs, cats, turkeys, sheep, and pigs (see TRANSMISSIBLE GASTROENTERITIS OF PIGS); infectious bronchitis in chickens; hepatitis in mice, respiratory disease in mice; feline infectious peritonitis; and encephalomyelitis in pigs.

Coronet

(see FOOT OF THE HORSE)

Coronoid Processes

One of these is present on the mandible (lower jaw) where the temporal muscle is attached to it. On the ULNA they form protuberances which articulate with the radius and humerus.

Corpora Quadrigemina

Corpora quadrigemina form a division of the BRAIN.)

Corpus Luteum

Also known as the yellow body, this is formed by the cells lining the empty follicular cavity, under the influence of the luteinising hormone, as explained under OVARIES.

Corridor Disease

This affects the African buffalo and also cattle, and is caused by the protozoan parasite *Theileria lawrencei*, transmitted by ticks. It resembles East Coast fever, and has a 60 to 80 per cent mortality in cattle.

Corticosteroids

These comprise the natural glucocorticoids, cortisone, and hydrocortisone – hormones from the adrenal gland; and, in ascending order of potency, the more potent synthetic equivalents – prednisolone, methylprednisolone, triamcinolone, betamethasone and dexamethasone.

In veterinary medicine, corticosteroids are used in the treatment of a wide variety of inflammatory conditions. They have been used for the relief of lameness and navicular disease in the horse, and arthritic joints. They find application in a wide variety of conditions: shock, stress, ketosis, acetonaemia, respiratory diseases, colitis.

A corticosteroid given intravenously in late pregnancy is likely to induce abortion.

Corticosteroids are immunosuppressive and produce relief of symptoms without treating their cause. Their benefits in suppressing symptoms and allowing increased mobility must be weighed against the risks of increasing joint damage. Overdosage may bring out latent diabetes.

Corticotrophin

The hormone from the anterior lobe of the pituitary gland which controls the secretion by the adrenal gland of corticoid hormones. These corticosteroids, or steroid hormones, are of 3 kinds: (1) those concerned with carbohydrate metabolism and which also allay inflammation; (2) those concerned with maintaining the correct proportion of electrolytes; (3) the sex corticoids.

Cortisol
(see CORTISONE)

Cortisone
A hormone from the cortex of the adrenal gland. In medicine, one of its synthetic analogues is normally used.

Actions Cortisone raises the sugar content of the blood and the glycogen content of the liver, among many other actions.

Uses Cortisone has been used effectively in the treatment of rheumatoid arthritis, but when the drug is discontinued, symptoms return. However, because of potential side-effects its long-term use is not recommended (see CORTICOSTEROIDS).

Corynebacterium
A genus of slender, Gram-positive bacteria which includes the cause of diphtheria in man. In veterinary medicine *C. pyogenes* (now renamed *Actinomyces pyogenes*) is of importance, causing 'summer mastitis' and 'foul-in-the-foot' in cattle. A generalised infection has been reported, giving rise in cattle to lameness, slight fever, leg-swellings, lachrymation, and later emaciation and death.

C. suis (or *Eubacterium suis*) is responsible for infectious cystitis and pyelonephritis in pigs.

C. ovis (*C. pseudotuberculosis*) causes caseous lymphadenitis in sheep and some cases of ulcerative lymphangitis and acne in horses.

C. equi causes pneumonia in the horse and tuberculosis-like lesions in the pig.

C. renale is the cause of pyelonephritis in cattle.

Corynebacteria are also associated with disease in fish causing scattered white lesions throughout the spleen, liver and kidney. It can be severe in Atlantic salmon. Sometimes called Dee disease, after the river Dee at Aberdeen.

Costia
Costia necatrix is a serious parasite of freshwater fish. (See also FISH, DISEASES OF.)

Cotton-Seed Cake or Meal
Cotton-seed cake or meal may, if undecorticated, contain up to 25 per cent of indigestible fibre and lead to intestinal impaction if fed to calves or pigs. Gossypol poisoning may also result. (See GOSSYPOL.)

Cotyledons
(see PLACENTA *and* PREGNANCY)

Coughing

Horses Common causes of coughing in horses include equine influenza; other virus infections; laryngitis and bronchitis from other causes; an allergic or asthmatic cough often heard in the autumn; strangles; and 'broken wind'.

(For a list of viruses which cause coughing (and also other symptoms) in the horse, see EQUINE RESPIRATORY VIRUSES.) Where coughing occurs with a normal temperature, horses may prove to be infested with the lung-worm *Dictyocaulus arnfieldi*.

Clenbuterol is widely used for treatment.

Pigs Coughing may be due to dusty meal or to enzootic pneumonia. It also occurs during migration of the larvae in infection with *Ascaris* worms.

Dogs A cough is often a symptom of acute or chronic bronchitis. In the dog – often fat and middle-aged – chronic bronchitis may result in a cough persisting for weeks or months at a time and recurring in subsequent years, and is due to excessive secretion of mucus in the trachea and bronchi. It may follow an attack of pneumonia. A cough is also a symptom of valvular disease of the heart. (See also KENNEL COUGH.)

A sporadic yet persistent cough, noticed especially after exercise or excitement, may be a symptom of infestation with the common tracheal worm *Oslerus osleri*. Mortality among puppies of 4 to 8 months has been as high as 75 per cent in some litters, following emaciation. Less serious is infestation with *Capillaria aerophilia*, which may give rise to a mild cough.

Cats Coughing is (in addition to sneezing) one symptom of viral diseases such as feline viral rhinotracheitis and feline calicivirus infection; tonsillitis; as the result of grass seeds lodged in the pharynx; infestation by the cat lungworm; pleurisy; bronchitis; pneumonia; tuberculosis; and some cases of feline leukaemia. (See under separate headings.)

Cattle
(see CALF PNEUMONIA; IBR *under* RHINOTRACHEITIS; PARASITIC BRONCHITIS; 'SHIPPING FEVER'; TUBERCULOSIS)

Coumarin

A chemical compound present in sweet vernal grass, in sweet clovers, and in other plants. Although harmless in itself, coumarin may be converted to DICOUMAROL if hay containing such plants becomes mouldy or overheated.

Cowherds

Occupational hazards include ANTHRAX; BRU-CELLOSIS; LEPTOSPIROSIS; RINGWORM; Q FEVER; TUBERCULOSIS; cowpox (see under POX); MILK-ER'S NODULE; salmonella (see SALMONELLOSIS); SPOROTRICHOSIS; BUBONIC PLAGUE (not in the UK).

Cowbane Poisoning

(see WATER HEMLOCK)

Cow Kennels

These have become popular as a cheaper (first cost) alternative to cubicle houses, though some have been developed to the point where they are almost cubicle houses, with the wood or metal partitions forming an integral part of the structure. Slurry can be a problem, and sometimes exposure to draughts and rain requires protection with straw bales or hardboard at the ends. (See also CUBICLES FOR COWS.)

Cowpox

(see under POX)

Cowpox, Pseudo-

(see MILKER'S NODULE)

Cow's Milk, Absence of

In a newly calved cow giving virtually no milk, the cause may be a second calf in the uterus, and a rectal examination is accordingly advised. A normal milk yield can be expected, in such cases, to follow the birth of the second calf which may occur a few months later. (See SUPER-FETATION; also AGALACTIA.)

Cows

Gentle treatment Cows should at all times be quietly and gently treated. Hurried driving in and out of gates and doors, chasing by dogs, beating with sticks should not be tolerated. A cow in milk must have time to eat, chew, and digest her food in comfort, and rough treatment will not only interfere with digestion but will also disturb the nervous system which more or less controls the action of the milk-making glands, thus lessening the milk yield. (See STRESS.)

Gentle treatment should begin with the calf, and be continued with the yearling, 2-year-old, and in-calf heifer; where it is customary to approach and handle young stock at all ages there will be no difficulty in the management and milking of the newly calved heifer; her milk yield will be increased, and much time will be saved. (See MILKING; also VETERINARY FACILITIES ON THE FARM.)

Comfort and fresh air The housing provided should ensure comfort. In winter, sufficient bedding should be provided to keep the cows warm and clean. (See HOUSING OF ANIMALS; RATIONS.)

Cowper's Gland

The bulbourethral glands, which are situated one each side of the urethra (see SEMEN).

Coxalgia

Coxalgia means pain in the hip-joint.

Coxiella

Micro-organisms in the order Rickettsiae (see under Q FEVER).

Coxitis

Inflammation of the hip-joint.

Coxsackie B Virus

A group of enteroviruses which mainly infects horses. Infection in dogs may be a cause of diarrhoea; swine vesicular disease is antigenically related to coxsackie B7 virus. Infection in laboratory workers has caused influenza-like symptoms, and sometimes heart disease and meningitis.

Coyotes

Coyotes are rabies-vectors in the USA.

Crab Lice (Phthirus Pubis)

Crab lice (phthirus pubis) occasionally infest dogs, but this happens only in a household where people are infested.

Crabs

(see FOOD POISONING)

Cramp

Painful involuntary contraction of a muscle. Cramp is of importance in the racing greyhound, which is observed to slow down and drag both hind-legs, or – in severe cases – may collapse and struggle on the ground. The animal's gait and appearance are 'wooden'. The muscles of the hindquarters are hard to the

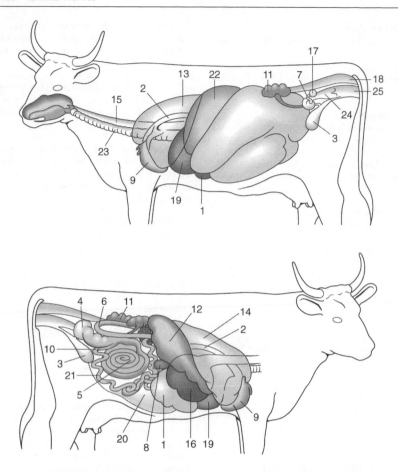

INTERNAL ORGANS OF THE COW

1 abomasum	10 ileum	19 reticulum
2 aorta	11 kidney, left	20 rumen
3 bladder	12 liver	21 small intestine
4 caecum	13 lung, left	22 spleen
5 colon	14 lung, right	23 trachea (wind-pipe)
6 duodenum	15 oesophagus (gullet)	24 uterus
7 Fallopian tube	16 omasum	25 vagina
8 gall bladder	17 ovary, left	
9 heart	18 rectum	

touch. Cyanosis may be present. Recovery usually takes place within a quarter of an hour, aided by rest and massage. Possible causes include: fatigue, defective heart action, bacterial or chemical toxins, sexual repression, a dietary deficiency, poor exercise, and cold. (See also 'SCOTTIE CRAMP'; MUSCLE – Action.)

Cranial Nerves

Cranial nerves are those large and important nerves that originate from the BRAIN.

Craniomandibular Osteopathy

An inherited proliferative condition of the skull and jaws in breeds of dog including Boston terriers and Cairn terriers. Symmetrical bony enlargements of the temporal bone, mandible, and occasionally the long bones, may be seen and pain experienced. There may be difficulty in breathing and swallowing. Steroid therapy may be effective although the condition can recur in dogs less than a year old. It is rarely seen in older animals.

Craniopagus

A double-headed monster. In a double-headed calf delivered by Caesarean section in Trinidad, major abnormalities involved skeletal structures and included: fusion of both crania at the parieto-occipital-temporal regions; presence of cleft palate involving both the palatine process of the maxilla and the horizontal plate of the palatine bone; and malalignment of the mandibles.

The cranial fusion resulted in the existence of a single complete occipital bone which articulated with both crania at their ventrolateral surfaces, and bounded a single foramen magnum articulated with the occipital bone interposed between them.

'Crazy Chick' Disease, or Nutritional Encephalomacia

'Crazy chick' disease, or nutritional encephalomacia, is caused by vitamin E deficiency associated with a diet too rich in fats, or containing food which has gone rancid, and vitamin E has been used in its prevention. It is seen at 2 to 4 weeks of age. Signs include falling over, incoordination, paralysis and death. Similar signs are seen in avian encephalomyelitis, a virus disease of chicks under 6 weeks of age.

Creatine

(see MUSCLE – Action of muscles)
Creatine kinase is an enzyme found mainly in muscle. The activity of this enzyme in serum or plasma is used as an aid to the diagnosis of skeletal or heart muscle lesions.

Creep-Feeding

The feeding of unweaned piglets in the creep – a portion of the farrowing house or ark inaccessible to the sow and usually provided with artificial warmth. Creep-feeding often begins with a little flaked maize being put under a turf, and is followed by a proprietary or home-mixed meal from 3 to 8 weeks. Creep-feeding of in-wintered lambs and calves is also good practice.

Housed calves usually creep-feed hay or silage plus concentrates from a few weeks of age. Excessive creep-feeding with concentrates before turnout of autumn-born calves depresses gains at grass.

Creep-feeding at grass from the late summer can improve calf performance. With autumn-born calves, creep-feeding a total of up to 100 kg barley will improve weaning weights by up to 23 kg. But as the calves grow larger it is difficult to allow them access to a creep while excluding smaller cows. Some producers wean early, graze the calves on high-quality aftermaths and use the cows to eat down rougher areas. Because milk contributes more to the growth of spring-born calves, creep-feeding can be delayed until later in the season. But in the last few weeks before weaning, a total of 40 kg barley can be expected to increase weaning weights by up to 15 kg.

Creep-feeding of calves prior to weaning also has the advantage of conditioning them for future diets and guarding against any check in growth rate that may occur as a result of weaning. (*See* table below.)

Creep-Grazing

Creep-grazing is a method of pasture management, enabling lambs to gain access to certain areas of pasture in advance of their dams.

Cremation and Burial of Pet Animals

This service is offered by a number of companies, or a veterinary surgeon can advise.

Crenosoma

A genus of lungworms. *Crenosoma vulpis* infects dogs and some wild carnivores.

Creosoted Timber

Creosoted timber may give rise to poisoning in animals, particularly young ones, where wooden housing has been freshly treated. For disease in cattle from this cause, see under HYPERKERATOSIS.

Cats are prone to creosote poisoning. Contaminated paws may be cleaned by coating them with cooking oil, and then washing this off with a mild detergent.

Crepitus

Crepitus means the grating sound of fractured bones when handled.

Cresol Solutions

(see DISINFECTANTS)

Cretinism

Dwarfism caused by an insufficiency of the hormone THYROXIN(E). (See also THYROID GLAND.)

Creutzfeldt-Jakob Disease (CJD)

Creutzfeldt-Jakob disease (CJD), which has a worldwide distribution, is characterised by

Effects of creep feeding on calf weaning weight		
	Supplementary feed (kg)	Extra calf weaning wt. (kg)
Autumn-born calves	76	19
Spring-born calves	30	10

spongiform degeneration of the brain. Once symptoms appear, it is invariably fatal. Transmission has occurred through a corneal transplant.

In 1996 a 'new variant' of CJD appeared in young people; it has been linked to the consumption of BSE-infected meat products.

Chronic Respiratory Disease (CRD)

Infection of poultry by *Mycoplasma gallisepticum*. Infected birds suffer a variety of respiratory diseases, coughing and nasal discharge. There is a reduction in egg yields; morbidity is low but carcases are rejected at slaughter.

Treatment is by administering an antibiotic by injection, in severe cases, or by addition to the drinking water.

Crib-Biting and Wind-Sucking

Crib-biting and wind-sucking are different varieties of the same vice, which are learned chiefly by young horses. In each case the horse swallows air. A 'crib-biter' effects this by grasping the edge of the manger or some other convenient fixture with the incisor teeth; it then raises the floor of the mouth; the soft palate is forced open; a swallowing movement occurs; and a gulp of air is passed down the gullet into the stomach. A 'wind-sucker' achieves the same end, but it does not require a resting-place for the teeth. Air is swallowed by firmly closing the mouth, arching the neck, and gulping down air in much the same way.

In crib-biters the incisor teeth of both jaws show signs of excessive wear.

Remedial measures are not always satisfactory. Crib-biters may cease the habit if housed in a bare loose-box, being fed from a trough which is removed as soon as the feed is finished.

Proprietary preparations, with an unpleasant taste, are available for treating woodwork.

Crocodiles, Farmed

Sudden loss of the righting reflex was the outstanding feature of a thiamine-responsive disease in softwater crocodiles (*Crocodylus porosus*). 'Affected hatchlings were found floating or lying on their sides, unable to right themselves.'

Treatment Two intramuscular injections of 30 mg thiamine hydrochloride 24 hours apart.

(Dr T. F. Jubb, Department of Agriculture, Kununurra, Western Australia.)

Crooked Toe Deformity

A condition seen in chicks brooded under infra-red lamps. The birds have difficulty in walking; the toes are turned out because of malformation of the lower metatarsal and foot bones. The cause is unknown.

Crop

Crop, of birds, is a dilatation of the gullet at the base of the neck, just at the entrance to the thorax. In it the food is stored for a time and softened with fluids. It acts as a reservoir from which the food can be passed downwards into the stomach, gizzard, etc., in small amounts.

Crop, Diseases of

By far the commonest trouble affecting the crop of the bird is that known as 'crop-bound', in which food material collects in the crop through the swallowing of bodies which cannot pass on to the stomach and gizzard. This may include feathers, wool, straw, small pieces of stick, etc. Other cases are due to a lack of vitality in the walls of the crop, which become too weak to force the contents onwards.

The dilated crop can often be noticed pendulous and distended. Death occurs from exhaustion unless relief is obtained. Massage of the impacted food material from the outside, along with the introduction of warm liquid in small amounts through a rubber tube, may be sufficient to dispel mild impactions, but usually surgical opening is required. (See under CAGE (AVIARY) BIRDS, DISEASES OF.)

Cross-Eye

(see STRABISMUS)

Cross-Immunity

Immunity resulting from infection with one disease-producing organism against another. For example, rinderpest virus infection in dogs gives rise to a degree of immunity against canine distemper virus.

Cross Pregnancy

Development of a fetus in the opposite horn of the uterus to that side on which ovulation occurred. Migration from one horn to the other may occur.

Croup

Croup of the horse is that part of the hindquarters lying immediately behind the loins. The 'point of the croup' is the highest part of the croup, and corresponds to the internal angles of the ilia. The crupper of the harness passes over the croup, and derives its name from it.

Crows

Carrion crows often cause injury to ewes and lambs, sometimes death, and in addition they may transmit CAMPYLOBACTER infection.

In India, house crows (*Corvus splendens*), which live in close contact with people and domestic animals, can be important in the transmission of Newcastle disease to domestic poultry. The crows themselves may show no symptoms, but can excrete highly virulent virus over a short period.

Cruciate Ligaments

Cruciate ligaments are two strong ligaments in the stifle-joint which prevent any possibility of over-extension of the joint. They are arranged in the form of the limbs of the letter X. Degenerative change leading to rupture of one or both ligaments in dogs engaged in strenuous exercise (e.g. police dogs, gun dogs, sheep-dogs) is common among all breeds and gives rise to lameness. If both ligaments are ruptured, instability of the joint follows, and surgery may be necessary if lameness is severe. However, strict rest for 8 weeks is often successful in itself, especially when only one ligament is involved.

A technique for repair of ruptured cruciate ligaments involves their replacement with multifilament polyester (Terylene) prostheses. The polyester is anchored distally through a hole in the tibial tuberosity and passed 'over the top' of the lateral femoral condyle.

Cruelty, Avoidance of

(see LAW; ANAESTHETICS, LEGAL REQUIREMENTS; CASTRATION; TRANSPORT STRESS; WATER; EUTHANASIA; DOCKING; NICKING; WELFARE CODES; NUTRITION, FAULTY; STRESS; TETHERING; OVERSTOCKING)

Crural

Relating to the leg.

Crush

A pen constructed of wood or tubular steel, and used for holding cattle, etc., in order to facilitate tuberculin testing, inoculations, the taking of blood samples, etc.

A wooden crush is less noisy than a metal one; clanging metalwork can be alarming to cattle. Nevertheless, metal is more often used, particularly for making mobile crushes. Collecting cattle in darkened pens or boxes an hour before testing is due to begin makes for better behaviour in the crushes.

An efficient type of crush is one constructed in a building through which the cows always come on leaving the parlour. The two ends are solid and fixed in concrete. The sides consist of iron gates hinged one on the front and the other on the back of the crush. Before an animal enters, the gate hinged on the front is opened back against the wall. This provides a wide space and she is not asked to enter a narrow confine. When she is in, the gate is shut and the neck secured with a rope. The other gate may now be opened and testing done without reaching through the side of the crush.

A funnel-shaped pen for filling the crush is useful, and if the crush is big enough to hold 2 animals, the second will enter more readily. Fast working can be achieved with a race to hold 7 or 8 cows; there being 2 men each with a rope on the side opposite to the veterinary surgeon. The whole batch is tested before release.

The traditional neck-yoking feature of cattle crushes is often abandoned for a design in which the animal is restrained by pressure from the sides of the crush moving together. Cattle are said to enter it more readily and to stand more quietly in it.

It is generally agreed that behaviour in crushes is partly dependent upon breed. For example, Dairy Shorthorns are generally docile, Ayrshires easily alarmed, and Friesians often more angry than frightened. Angus and Galloways seem to resent the crush rather than be alarmed by it.

Much also depends, of course, upon gentle treatment and avoiding the indiscriminate use of sticks. Some farm workers never learn to hold cattle properly by their noses, but push a thumb into one nostril and try and cram all their fingers into the other – naturally the animal struggles for breath! Even when it is done properly, Angus and Galloways seem to dislike this form of restraint intensely.

It may save a lot of time in the end if animals are accustomed to being put into a crush. An experiment at the Central Veterinary Laboratory involved weekly weighings of 60 adult heifers, which were obstreperous in the extreme. Each was led (with a head-collar, not a halter) from its standing in a cowshed to a crate mounted on the low platform of a large weighing machine in a yard. The first weighing occupied 2 strenuous periods totalling 135 minutes. The 37th weighing was accomplished in 38 minutes. The heifers not only learnt what was expected of them but seemed to relish this break in their routine; trotting into the crate, coming to a dead stop, and standing stock still while the weighing machine beam was adjusted. (See also VETERINARY FACILITIES ON FARMS.)

C

Crushed Tail Head Syndrome

A condition in dairy cows in which there is tail paralysis, hind-limb weakness and knuckling of the fetlock joint. It occurs suddenly, usually in healthy cows showing recent oestrus activity. The clinical signs follow damage to the sacral vertebrae which affects the sacral and coccygeal nerves, Vigorous mounting by a bull may be the cause of the trauma. Recovery is more likely in those cases less badly affected.

'Crutching'

'Crutching' means shearing of wool from a sheep's breech, tail, and back of hind-legs. It is done before May and in autumn as an aid to controlling 'STRIKE'.

Cryospray

The use of liquid nitrogen in cryosurgery.

Cryosurgery

Destruction of unwanted tissue (e.g. of a tumour) by the use of very low temperatures. For example, a metal rod, cooled in liquid nitrogen to −196°C, may be applied to the tumour.

Dogs Cryotherapy has been found useful in several conditions, including intractable interdigital cysts and 'lick granuloma'.

Cats It has been used for the relief of highly irritant eczema, and also eosinophilic granulomatous lesions; especially those involving the lips and hard palate, and in cats suffering from chronic gingivitis/stomatitis.

Horses Cryosurgery may be used in the treatment of sarcoids, squamous cell carcinoma and other neoplastic conditions of the skin, and for the removal of excessive granulation tissue. In ophthalmology it can be used for the treatment of retinal detachment, iris prolapse, glaucoma and the extraction of cataracts.

Cryptocaryon

A parasite inhabiting the skin of salmonid fish kept at high density in salt water.

Cryptococcosis

Infection with the yeast *Cryptococcus neoformans* occurs occasionally in all species. Lungs, udder, brain, etc. may be involved. It has been described as the least rare of fungal infections in the cat – in which it may give rise to sneezing, a discharge from the eyes, and sometimes to a nasal granuloma. Other signs include cough and dyspnoea.

Bone and eye lesions may be produced. (See also EPIZOOTIC LYMPHANGITIS.)

Cryptorchid

An animal in which 1 or both testicles have not descended into the scrotum from the abdominal cavity at the usual time. The condition may cause some irritability in the animal. The retained testicle(s) may be defective. (See also under GELDING.)

In several breeds of pigs it has been shown that some individual males start with 2 apparently normal testicles in the scrotum at birth, but that within a few weeks or months 1 testicle may decrease in size and then may disappear from the scrotum, ascending back into the inguinal canal inside the abdomen. Absorption of this testicle may occur, so that by the time the animal is 6 months old there may be no remains, or virtually none, of the missing testicle to be found.

The name 'late cryptorchids' has been given to such animals which have 2 testicles in the scrotum at birth, but subsequently only 1. A research worker at the Central Veterinary Laboratory, Weybridge, has referred to the finding of 44 such late cryptorchids out of 110 cryptorchid Lacombe boars. (See also under MONORCHID; CASTRATION.)

Cryptosporidiosis

Disease caused by protozoan parasites of the genus *Cryptosporidium* and of the order Coccidia. *Cryptosporidia* are not host-specific like other coccidia. The oocyst is the infective stage. It causes diarrhoea in mammals and may also cause respiratory disease in poultry. Both farm and companion animals may be affected. The disease is more severe in young animals; some older ones may become carriers. Infected animals grazing near rivers or on the banks of reservoirs may contaminate water supplies; the parasite is not usually removed in the normal filtering process. Diagnosis is by identifying the parasite in faecal smears; special staining techniques are required.

Public health In humans, cryptosporidiosis causes a severe and malodorous diarrhoea which may last up to 2 weeks. Cases usually arise from drinking contaminated water, although animal to human transmission has occurred. In Doncaster, an outbreak involving 220 persons was traced to a swimming pool, the parasite not being killed by the concentration of chlorine in the water.

Treatment Halofuginone is used for treatment and prophylaxis in calves.

Cubes and Pellets

Animal feed compressed into small cubes or pellets. A cow takes about 10 minutes to eat 3.5 kg (8 lb) of cubes: a fact of some importance if the animals are fed in the milking parlour where time may not permit of a high-yielder receiving her entire concentrate ration. (The figure for meal is about 2.75 kg (6 lb) in 10 minutes.) (Compare also with LIQUID FEEDING.)

It is sometimes suggested that cubes can replace hay for horses on pasture in winter, or for rabbits, chinchilla, etc. which are not out at grass. However, roughage is needed in addition for peristalsis and health of the digestive system. (See also HORSES, FEEDING OF; DRIED GRASS.)

The type of lubricant used in cubing and pelleting machines is important; hyperkeratosis can arise in cattle if an unsuitable one is used. (See LUBRICANTS.)

Cubicles for Cows

Cubicles were introduced over 35 years ago and have varied in size and design. One of the earliest was the Newton Rigg design, a type which allows the cattle to be loose housed but, once built, is difficult to alter to accommodate different sizes of cattle. Cubicles designed for Friesian cows have had to accommodate the larger Holstein animal, with resulting problems including lameness and mastitis.

The ideal cubicle will allow the cow to take up her normal resting positions and give room to get up and down easily. Cubicles are usually built from metal tubing or wood, although division rails are sometimes of wire or tensioned rope.

Dimensions are, typically, length 2.4 m (8 ft), width 1.2 m (4 ft), rear step not more than 150 mm (6 in), fall from front to rear 100–125 mm (4–5 in), division height 1.125 m (3 ft 9 in), lower division rail 400 mm (1 ft 4 in), brisket board 105 mm (4 in) deep, brisket board from rear 1.7 m (5 ft 8 in), brisket board from front 0.75 m (2 ft 6 in), head rail 150–250 mm (6–10 in) below average wither height. The passageway between the cubicles should be greater than 2.4 m (8 ft) wide to minimise build up of slurry. Comfortable, clean bedding should be provided. It is essential that both passageway and cubicle are kept clean to avoid transmission of faeces from the cows' feet to the udders when they lie down.

There are several types of cubicle. It appears that the type of heelstones, floor, and the width are important factors in determining whether cows take to cubicles or not. (See also COW KENNELS.) Bad design can lead to injury and lameness.

Cuboni Test

Cuboni test for pregnancy involves a single urine sample. It is an alternative to rectal palpation in the mare.

Cud and Cudding

(see RUMINATION)

Cuffing Pneumonia

A pneumonia of calves caused by a virus or mycoplasma. A chronic cough is the usual symptom. It is so called because a 'cuff' or sheath of lymphocytes forms around the bronchioles.

Culard

Muscular hyperplasia, or so-called 'DOUBLE MUSCLING'.

Culture Medium

That substance in or upon which bacteria and other pathogenic organisms are grown in the laboratory. Such media include nutrient agar, broths, nutrient gelatin, sugar media, and many special ones adapted to the requirements of particular organisms. Viruses cannot be grown in such media but require living cells, e.g. of chick embryos.

Curare

Curare is a dark-coloured extract from trees of the Strychnos family, which causes muscular paralysis. It is used by South American Indians as an arrow poison. Curare-treated arrow-heads were used by a veterinary surgeon in 1835 in treating tetanus in a horse and a donkey.

Curare, when injected, is one of the most powerful and deadly poisons known, but by the mouth it is harmless, since the kidneys are able to excrete it as rapidly as it is absorbed, and it does not collect in the system. Its action depends on the presence of an alkaloid, curarine, which paralyses the motor nerve-endings in muscle, and so throws the muscular system out of action yet leaving the sensory nervous system unaffected. A standardised preparation of tubocurarine is used to obtain muscular relaxation during anaesthesia. (See also under MUSCLE RELAXANTS.)

Curb

Curb is a swelling which occurs about a hand's breadth below the point of the hock, due to sprain, or local thickening of the calcaneocuboid ligament, or to similar conditions affecting the superficial flexor tendon. Lameness is usually present at first.

'Curled Tongue'

A deformity occurring in turkey poults, due to feeding an all-mash diet composed of very small particles in a dry state, during the first few weeks of life. If a change is made to wet feeding many of the poults will become normal.

Cushing's Syndrome (Hyperadrenocortism)

This has been recognised and treated in the dog, occurring usually after the age of 5 years, and the cat. It is also seen in old horses and ponies with hairy coats, lethargy, polydipsia or laminitis.

Cause Excessive production of corticosteroids by the adrenal cortex. In some cases there is a tumour affecting the adrenal gland or the pituitary; in others merely excessive growth of the adrenal cortex. It may result from over-administration of glucocortisoids.

Signs These include lethargy, premature ageing, baldness, skin eruptions, excessive thirst, 'pot belly', and a ravenous appetite. Wasting of the temporal muscles may be seen. Skin changes may not occur until up to a year after thirst becomes noticeable.

There may also be a change of coat colour and texture. A 6-year-old male poodle, clipped 8 months previously, developed a sparse and fluffy coat; instead of being an apricot colour it was now pure white. The dog was drinking over 800 ml of water per day, and scavenging for food. A diagnosis of Cushing's disease was confirmed by means of the adrenocorticotrophic hormone (ACTH) test.

Treatment Mitotane given orally is used in dogs. A daily dose calculated by weight is given until thirst becomes normal, followed by a weekly or fortnightly maintenance dose. (Mitotane is obtainable by a veterinary surgeon only on completion of a special Treatment Authorisation.) The drug trilostane has been used successfully in treating dogs with pituitary-dependent hyperadrenocortism.

This treatment is a preferable alternative to surgery, but success has followed surgical removal of both adrenal glands where intensive care has been provided both before and after the operation. Salt supplementation and implants of desoxycorticosterone acetate (DOCA) are necessary following the adrenalectomy.

Cutaneous
(see SKIN)

Cutaneous Asthenia

Cutaneous asthenia is associated with defects in the formation and maturing of collagen fibres. The skin becomes fragile and more elastic than normal, and a dog's skin may appear 'too big for its body'. (The human equivalent is the Ehlers-Danlos syndrome.)

Cutter

A pork pig weighing 64 to 86 kg (140 to 190 lb) liveweight or 45 to 64 kg (100 to 140 lb) deadweight.

Cutting
(see BRUSHING)

Cuttlefish

The internal bone of the cuttlefish is used as a dietary supplement and exercise toy for caged birds.

CVH
(see CANINE VIRAL HEPATITIS)

Cyanides

Cyanides are salts of hydrocyanic or prussic acid. They are all highly poisonous. (See HYDRO-CYANIC ACID.)

Cyanobacteria (Blue-Green Algae)

Cyanobacteria (blue-green algae) are microorganisms able to convert nitrogen from the air to ammonia, using the enzyme nitrogenase and sunlight as the energy source. The presence of cyanobacteria in plankton and scum accumulating along leeward shores of the UK, etc. is a cause of death among fish and birds. Dogs swimming in lakes affected by blue-green algae have died. In Spain, 579 out of 943 greater flamingo chicks died in a marsh lagoon in Donana National Park when a dense bloom of cyanobacteria occurred in 2001.

Cyanocobalamin

Cyanocobalamin is the water-soluble vitamin B_{12}. At the nucleus of molecules of cyanocobalamin is cobalt, a deficiency of which leads to a deficiency of the vitamin. Some intestinal parasites have a very large requirement for cyanocobalamin, to the extent that infected animals may show a vitamin deficiency. In such cases, cobalt should be given as well as anthelmintics.

Hydroxocobalamin is an antidote in cyanide poisoning.

Cyanosis

A blue or purple discoloration of the tongue, lips and gums when there is a shortage of oxygen in the blood. It sometimes results when excessive strain is put upon the heart, in animals that have been hunted or chased. It is a symptom of nitrite poisoning, and also occurs in a few cases of feline pyothorax, and in ASPHYXIA.

Cyathostomiasis
Infestation by one, or several, species concurrently of Cyathostome worms. They are a cause of chronic diarrhoea in horses.

Cyclonite Poisoning
A plastic explosive, known as PE4, has as its active ingredient cyclonite, and this has caused poisoning in a police dog trained to detect explosives. In both dogs and man the poison causes epileptiform convulsions, best controlled by diazepam given intravenously, plus barbiturates if necessary. In the above case, the dog bit into some of the PE4 which had been concealed for a training exercise.

Cyclophosphamide
A drug used in the treatment of lymphoma, and certain other cancers, in cats and dogs. It can cause severe side-effects and must be used only under strict veterinary supervision.

Cyclopropane-Oxygen Anaesthesia
A costly but otherwise useful form of anaesthesia for dogs and cats. It has also been used for horses and goats. Cyclopropane is an inflammable gas.

Cyclops
This genus of minute crustaceans acts as the intermediate host of the broad tapeworm of man, dog, and cat.

Cymric
The name, meaning Welsh, given to a breed of cat established from long-haired kittens born to Manx parents in Canada. The breed is known as Manx longhairs in the USA. It suffers from the same defects and problems as the MANX.

Cypermethrin
A pyrethroid ectoparasiticide. It is used in sheep dips and in insecticidal ear tags for cattle.

Cypress Poisoning
Leaves of the cypress are toxic, although poisoning is rare. Two yearling heifers died in a field where several cypress trees (*Cupressus sempervirens*) were felled one morning. One heifer was dead by the afternoon; the other 2 nights later.

Cystadenoma
(see CHOLANGIOMA)

Cystic Calculi
(see CALCULI)

Cystic Ovaries
(see OVARIES, DISEASES OF)

Cysticercosis
Infestation with TAPEWORM.

Cystine
An amino acid (and a constituent of some urinary calculi).

Cystitis
(see URINARY BLADDER, DISEASES OF)

Cystopexia
Surgical fixture of the urinary bladder to the wall of the abdomen.

Cysts
This term is applied to swellings containing fluid or soft material, other than pus, and to hollow tumours – usually non-malignant.

Varieties
(a) *Retention cyst* This may be no more than a swollen sebaceous gland, filled with its normal secretion which has been unable to reach the skin surface owing to blockage of its duct. Retention cysts of other glands arise similarly.

(b) *Ovarian cysts* (see OVARIES, DISEASES OF).

(c) *Developmental cysts* The most important of these is the DERMOID CYST.

(d) *Hydatid cysts* are produced in internal organs through the ingestion of the eggs of tapeworms from other animals. They occur in the peritoneal cavity, liver, spleen, brain, etc.

(e) *Hard tumour cysts* sometimes occur in tumours growing in connection with glands, such as the adenocarcinomata, which may occur in the mammary gland.

(f) '*Interdigital cysts*' in between the toes of dogs are in reality often granulomas or abscesses. (See INTERDIGITAL CYST.)

Cytoectes
(see EHRLICHIOSIS)

Cytogenetics
The study of chromosomes and the genetics of cellular constituents involved in heredity.

Chromosome analysis Usually, white blood cells are used, and these are inoculated into a liquid tissue culture medium, supplemented with serum and antibiotics. Phytohaemaglutinin, a plant extract which stimulates the white cells to

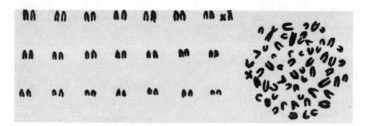

Cytogenetics. Left: the karyotype. Right: a bull's lymphocyte in metaphase of mitosis. (With acknowledgements to Dr C. R. E. Halnan and the *Veterinary Record*.)

divide, is added. The cultures are incubated for 2 days at 38°C. Then colchicine is added to arrest the dividing cells at the metaphase stage. Hypotonic solutions are used to swell the cells and spread out the chromosomes. The cells are then fixed, dropped on to slides, and stained.

Suitable cells containing well-spread chromosomes are selected on the slides after examining them under the microscope at 1000x magnifications. Some of the cells are then photographed, and the individual chromosomes cut out from the prints, paired and stuck on to a card. This is called the karyotype.

An example of chromosome abnormalities in cattle is the freemartin. Whereas the normal heifer calf has a karyotype 60, XX, the freemartin has a proportion of XY cells. The condition is technically known as XX:XY Chimerism.

Centric fusions (Robertsonian translocations) are the result of 2 chromosomes fusing to form 1, so that the total number of chromosomes in the cells is reduced. The 1/29 translocation was discovered by Gustavsson in about 1 in 7 of the Swedish Red and White breed of cattle, and has since been found in many other breeds. This autosomal abnormality, involving a member of each of pairs 1 and 29, has been found to be inherited through both the male and the female in Red Poll and Charolais cattle in Britain, and appears to be associated with lowered fertility in the female.

Another common centric fusion is the 13/21 translocation, first found in 1973 in a New Zealand bull of the Swiss Simmental breed, and in 1974 in that bull's sire in Scotland.

Many other chromosomal abnormalities have been found. (See MOSAIC; TRISOMY; TRANSLOCATION; POLYPLOIDY.)

Cytogenetics has also proved useful in confirming or detecting the origins of some breeds of cattle. For example, in Australia Dr C. R. E. Halnan and Professor J. Francis have stated: 'The Africander has anatomical and other characteristics of an animal of approximately 3/4 Bos indicus heredity. The fact that these cattle carry the Bos taurus Y chromosome supports this view and indicates that the local cattle in South Africa would have been crossed with 1 or more Bos taurus bulls. Droughtmaster and Braford cattle retain the *Bos indicus* Y chromosome because Bos indicus instead of Bos taurus bulls were used to establish these taurindicus breeds.'

Chromosome abnormalities have also been detected in infertile mares. One, which had never shown oestrus, was found to have the karyotype 63, X, i.e. lacking an X chromosome. Another mare, which had shown irregular oestrus, had the karyotype 63, X/64, X, i.e. containing both the abnormal cell line and normal cells.

Cytokines

Naturally occurring compounds which cause tumours either to grow more slowly, or to destroy the malignant cells. (See INTERFERON, the first to be discovered.) Genetic engineering has made possible large-scale production of cytokines.

Cytology

The study of cell function, origin, structure, formation and pathology.

Cytotoxic Drugs

Drugs which act on cell growth and division; they are used in the treatment of certain types of cancer. Their use in chemotherapy is limited by their toxicity, and dosage must be very carefully controlled.

Hazards Use of these drugs presents serious risks to health from residue disposal, spillage, etc. Miscarriage in nurses was twice as frequent in those who had been exposed to anticancer drugs, according to a study in Finland at 17 hospitals, as compared with unexposed nurses.

D

D-Value

This is the percentage of digestible organic matter in the dry matter of the feed.

D-value is used to assess or describe the digestibility of animal feeds, such as dried grass, hay, silage, etc.

'Daft Lambs'

Those affected with cerebellar atrophy – a condition associated with incoordination of head and leg movements. The lambs are normal at birth but have problems walking; there is incoordination of limbs, straddled leg stance, head arched backwards and muscle tremors. It is to due to a recessive gene. (See GENETICS – Genetic defects.)

Dachsunds

Small long-bodied breed of dog with very short legs; originating in Germany, where they were used for badger hunting. The long body makes them prone to intervertebral disc problems.

They are also liable to inherit cleft palate, deafness, diabetes mellitus and un-united anconeal process. Distichiasis is seen in the miniature long-haired dachsund. Over-shot jaw and progressive renal atrophy may be congenital.

'Dagging'

Removal of soiled wool by the shepherd from sheeps' hindquarters as an aid to preventing STRIKE.

Dairy Herd Management

In 1970, herd size averaged only 30 in the UK, and 80 per cent of cows were still tied up in cowsheds. There was, however, a growing movement towards larger herds, and many of those which formerly were 50 to 70 cows became 90 to 120 in size; today there are several 300-cow units, and a few larger still. The imposition of milk quotas by the EU led to herd sizes becoming static, but numbers are again increasing.

Increase in herd size has been accompanied by other changes: notably, milking in a parlour and housing in a cubicle house instead of in a cowshed. (See CUBICLES FOR COWS; COW KENNELS.) There has been a tendency to replace the tandem parlour by the herringbone. (See illustration.) Parlour feeding is now, in up-to-date units, related automatically to milk yield; this

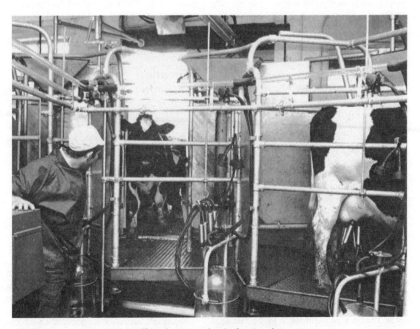

Milking in a rotary herringbone parlour.

both makes for economy and avoids the problem of cow identification in the big herd, so far as the milker is concerned. Identification is still necessary, however, for use in conjunction with herd records and in the parlour where the milker or relief milker (who will rarely know all the cows) must feed according to yield in the absence of automated equipment. Plastic numbered collars, anklets, discs on chain or nylon, freeze branding and even udder tattooing are among methods used.

In the UK, measures to deal with BSE have led to the introduction of a comprehensive system of herd and individual cow identification, with a national database; initially, this was to be based on a 'passport' that would follow the animal throughout its life.

Feeding outside the parlour has been mechanised in many large units. Feeding from silos is less popular than formerly. Many farms have mixer wagons to produce a complete diet made from forage, grass or maize silage, straw, concentrates or straights feeds. Fed ad lib, this system allows better utilisation of feed and increased dry-matter intakes. In others, side-delivery trucks are drawn by tractor down the feeding passages and deliver into the long mangers. Self-feed silage, with the clamp face in or near the cubicle house, is another labour-saver. Group feeding (e.g. of dry cows, high yielders, and low yielders) is convenient management practice but may give rise to stress (see BUNT ORDER). (See also under 'STEAMING UP' and the advice on feeding given under ACETONAEMIA – Prevention.)

ADAS advice stresses the need for adequate feeding in early lactation. 'Since appetite is often limited at this stage, only the highest quality food should be fed: whether it is good hay, early cut silage, or 1.5 kg ($3^1/_2$ lb) per gallon cake. This will allow optimum intake of nutrients at the responsive stage of the lactation – weeks 1–12 after calving.'

Zero-grazing, where cattle are kept in paddocks, and grass is cut and brought to them, is practised on some farms where poaching is a serious problem in wet weather, or where the movement of a large number of cows is involved. With a very large herd on a very small acreage (such as an American 550-cow herd on under 5 acres), zero-grazing obviously becomes essential. It is little used in the UK.

Paddock grazing now forms an important part of dairy herd management, and includes the two-sward system in which separate areas are used for grazing and for conservation.

Dung disposal presents difficulties with large herds. There are two options: it may be treated as a solid or as a liquid. Straw bedding lends itself to solid-muck handling, with the liquid (urine, washing-down water, rainwater) being taken separately to a lagoon or to an underground tank. Slatted floors can be used in a cubicle house, either over a dung cellar which is cleared out once a year, or over a channel leading to an underground tank. With the semi-solid method, dung may be spread on the land by tanker, or the slurry may pass to a lagoon or be pumped through an organic irrigation pipeline system. Where this is used, cows must not be expected to graze pasture until there has been time for rain to wash the slurry off the herbage. The use of organic irrigation is not entirely free from the risk of spreading infectious diseases.

Poaching must be avoided by the use of concrete aprons at gateways, by mobile drinking troughs, by wide corridors between paddocks with an electric fence dividing the 'corridor' so that one half can be kept in reserve, or by moveable ramps as are used in New Zealand.

In the large herd, one of the biggest problems is spotting the bulling heifer or the cow on heat. Properly kept herd records can be a help in alerting farm staff to the approximate dates. (See CALVING INTERVAL; OESTRUS, DETECTION OF; CONTROLLED BREEDING.)

On large units, regular weekly visits by veterinary surgeons help in the detection and treatment of infertility and the application of veterinary preventive medicine. (See HEALTH SCHEMES; VETERINARY FACILITIES ON FARMS, CALF HOUSING; also CONTROLLED BREEDING and CATTLE HUSBANDRY.)

Dalmation

A medium-sized dog, white with regular black or brown spots, that originated as a carriage dog in the Balkans. Unlike most dogs, it excretes uric acid in the urine and could be affected by gout. It may inherit deafness and atrophic dermatitis.

Damalina

A genus of biting lice.

Dangerous Dogs Act 1991

This requires that certain breed types (pit bull terrier, Japanese tosa, fila brasileiro, dogo argentino) must not be taken out unless on a lead, muzzled, and by someone at least 16 years old.

Owners of these dogs must register them with the police, and either comply with the exemption scheme or arrange for euthanasia to be carried out by a veterinary surgeon.

To comply with the exemption scheme, owners must take out 3rd-party insurance, arrange for the animal to be neutered, and to be identifiable by a tattoo and a microchip. The dog must also be kept under escape-proof conditions.

The Act has proved controversial; in a number of cases there has been confusion over identification of dogs as pit bull terriers. Several attempts have been made to have the Act amended.

Dangerous Wild Animals Act 1976
This requires people keeping lions, tigers, poisonous snakes, certain monkeys and other unusual pets, such as crocodiles and bears, to obtain a licence – authorised by a veterinary surgeon. Bison, wild boar, ostriches and emus are classed as dangerous wild animals under this Act. They are farmed in the UK and the farmer needs to register with the local authority. The premises must be inspected by a veterinary surgeon nominated by the local authority before a licence is granted.

Local authorities have power to refuse licences, on the advice of an authorised veterinary surgeon, on such grounds as safety, nuisance or inadequate or unsuitable accommodation.

Before a licence is granted, local authorities must be satisfied about arrangements for the animal's food, exercise and general comfort, fire precautions, and precautions against infectious diseases.

People with such animals must take out insurance.

Conviction for the keeping of an animal without a licence or contravening a condition of one could result in a fine of up to £400 and a ban from holding a licence.

Zoos, circuses, pet shops and research workers are exempted under the Licensing Act 1981.

Danish Red Cattle
More than half the cattle in Jutland, and 97 per cent of those in the Islands, belong to this breed, which is a very old one, though its official name (meaning Red Danish Milk breed) dates from 1878.

Danish Reds are strong, dual-purpose animals with a good 'barrel', teats and udders, and weigh between 500 and 770 kg (1100 and 1700 lb). (See also BRITISH DANE.)

Darnel Poisoning
The grass known as 'darnel' (*Lolium temulentum*) is a common weed in cereal crops and in pastures in some parts, but it does no harm when eaten before the seeds are ripe (or almost

so). Many instances are on record where harmful results to man and animals have followed the use of meal or flour which contained ground-up darnel seeds, and there are numerous references in classic literature to the harmful effect produced upon the eyes as the result of eating bread made from flour containing darnel.

Toxic Principle is a narcotic alkaloid, called temuline, which is said to be present to the extent of about 0.66 per cent; some authorities assert that a substance called loliine, and others that picrotoxin, should be considered responsible. A fungus called *Endoconidium temulentum* is very often found present in the seeds of darnel, living a life that is to a great extent one of symbiosis, and the poisonous alkaloid temuline is found in the fungus.

Signs Darnel produces giddiness and a staggering gait, drowsiness and stupefaction, dilatation of the pupils in the horse, and interference with vision in almost all animals. Vomiting, loss of sensation, convulsive seizures, and death follow when it is eaten by animals in large amounts. In some cases tremblings of the surface muscles are seen, and the extremities of the body become cold. Death usually occurs within 30 hours of eating the seeds.

First-Aid Strong black tea or coffee at once.

Darrow's Solution
Darrow's solution is used for fluid replacement therapy in cases of a potassium deficiency, and contains potassium chloride, sodium chloride and sodium lactate. It is rarely used in veterinary medicine; it is unsuitable for cases of neonatal diarrhoea. (See under DEHYDRATION.)

Dart Guns or Syringes
(see under PROJECTILE SYRINGE)

Daturine
An alkaloid. (See under STRAMOMIUM.)

Day-Old Chicks
(see CHICKS)

DDT
The common abbreviation for dichlorodiphenyl-trichlorethane, a potent parasiticide, lethal to fleas, lice, flies, etc. DDT was once used incorporated in dusting powders, for applying to animals; and dissolved in solvents for use as a fly-spray. DDT-resistant insects are now found in nearly all countries, unfortunately, and dangers

of DDT residues in human and animal tissues have led to its abandonment in the UK and elsewhere.

DDT preparations should not be applied to animals, owing to the risk of poisoning. The use of DDT with oils or fats enhances its toxic effects, and should be avoided. Symptoms of poisoning include coldness, diarrhoea, and hyperaesthesia. Minute doses over a period result in complete loss of appetite. DDT sprays may contaminate milk if used in the dairy; and may lead to poisonous residues in food animals when applied in livestock buildings, with consequent danger to human beings eating the contaminated meat. DDT can also contaminate streams and rivers, and prove harmful to fish.

However, in the control of human trypanosomiasis in Africa, both DDT and dieldrin have been extensively used for ground spraying, often by aircraft.

Dead Animals, Disposal of
(see DISPOSAL OF CARCASES)

Deadly Nightshade
Deadly nightshade is the popular name of *Atropa belladonna*, from which the alkaloid ATROPINE is obtained. It is a deadly poison, and parts of the plant are sometimes eaten by stock. (See also BELLADONNA.)

Deafness

Congenital deafness is common in white bull terriers and also in blue-eyed white cats. In the USA the Dalmatian breed is reported to have the highest prevalence of deafness of all breeds of dogs, with a risk factor of 40 to 50 per cent. One or both ears may be affected.

Conductive deafness is that caused by interference with the transmission of sound waves from the external ear to the organ of Corti in the inner ear. Such interference may be due to: (1) excess of wax in the ear canal; (2) perforation of, or infection involving, the eardrum. (In human medicine otosclerosis is another cause, being a loss of flexibility between the bones of the middle ear and the membrane connecting them with the inner ear, possibly due to hardening or ossification.)

Nerve deafness results from pressure upon, or damage to, the auditory nerve; it can also be a side-effect of antibiotics such as streptomycin and neomycin, and possibly chloramphenicol.

Deafness is or may be also a symptom of santonin poisoning, coal-gas poisoning, of a vitamin deficiency, and, in human medicine, a side-effect of streptomycin and aspirin. Other causes include damage to the internal ear, to the Eustachian tube, nervous system, etc.

Death, Causes of Sudden
In the majority of cases either failure of the heart or damage to a blood vessel (e.g. in cattle caused by a nail or a piece of wire from the reticulum) is the direct cause, but nervous shock following an accident or injury, cerebral haemorrhage, anthrax, black-quarter, lightning strike, braxy, hypocalcaemia in cattle, hypomagnesaemia (also in sheep), and over-eating of green succulent fodder in young cattle, are all capable of producing sudden death. In the case of pigs, sudden death has sometimes resulted from heat stroke. (See also BOWEL, OEDEMA OF THE.) In both cattle and pigs sudden death due to *Clostridium welchii* type A has been reported. In countries bordering the Red Sea, horses that have not been bred locally are sometimes attacked by a form of heat stroke with fatal results. (See also POISONING *and* (with reference to dogs) CANINE PARVOVIRUS; CANINE VIRAL HEPATITIS.) Sudden death, without obvious preliminary symptoms, may occasionally occur in cases of rabies, botulism, and foot-and-mouth disease. (See also ELECTRIC SHOCK).

Death, Signs of
The physical signs of death are well known, but there are occasions when it is difficult to state whether an animal is dead or not. In deep coma an animal may have all the superficial appearances of being dead, and yet recovery is possible if effective measures are taken. In the later stage of milk fever a cow has been mistaken for dead, has been dragged out of the byre preparatory to removal to the slaughterer's, has been examined by a practitioner, has been found to be living, has been suitably treated, and within 2 hours has been up on her feet again looking well. Foals have been discarded soon after being born and considered dead, have been removed to the outside of the loose-box while attention was paid to the dam, and later have been found living, the fresh cold air having revived respiration and stimulated the circulation, etc.

When an animal dies, the essential sign of the cessation of life is said to be the stopping of the heart. This, however, is not strictly correct, for it is possible by massage to resuscitate an already stopped heart, and to recover an apparently dead creature. Strictly speaking, it is almost impossible to say exactly when death takes place, but it is considered that when heart and respiration have ceased, when the eyelids do not flicker if a finger be applied to the eyeballs, when a cut artery no longer bleeds, and when the tissues lose their natural elasticity, life is extinct. A few of the common tests that are applied in uncertain cases are as follows. The animal is dead when (1) a piece of cold glass held to the nostrils for 3 minutes comes away without any condensed moisture upon it; (2) a superficial incision in the skin does not gape open; and (3) the natural elastic tension of the tissues disappears. Changes that follow death in a variable period depending upon the species of animal, and upon the weather at the time, are: (1) the clotting of the blood in the vessels; (2) the onset of rigor mortis (the stiffness of death); and (3) the commencement of decomposition of the carcase, usually first evident along the lower surface of the abdomen.

De-Beaking

De-beaking is done by poultry-keepers when birds are kept in groups and there is a potential problem of feather-picking or cannibalism. No more than one-third of the upper beak is removed; more than this can expose the sinuses and lead to infection. If performed when very young there are few after-effects. Older birds will develop neuromas at the cut tip, resulting in hypersensitivity of that region. Management practices should be improved to try to eliminate the need for de-beaking but the problem can be difficult to resolve.

There are moves to phase out the practice, on welfare grounds.

Debridement

The removal of dead tissue and infected material from a wound surface. This can be achieved by enzymes or combinations of organic acids. The use of maggots free from pathogenic organisms is an old method of wound treatment currently being revived in human medicine.

Decoquinate

A coccidiostat originally developed for use in poultry but mainly administered to control coccidiosis in lambs and calves.

Decubitus

Decubitus is the recumbent position assumed by animals suffering from certain diseases.

Decussation

Decussation is a term applied to any place in the nervous system at which nerve fibres cross from one side to the other; e.g. the decussation of the pyramids in the medulla, where the motor fibres from one side of the brain cross to the other side of the spinal cord.

Deep-Freeze

(see ARTIFICIAL INSEMINATION; LIFE AFTER FREEZING)

Deep Litter for Cattle

This is a very satisfactory system if well managed. It is mainly practised in straw yards. Straw, shavings and sawdust can be used, in adequate quantity. The bedding must be kept dry and no contact must occur between the udder and dung in the litter. Warmth given off as a result of the fermentation taking place in the litter makes for cow-comfort; and there is, of course, the added advantage of a thick layer of insulation between the cows and the concrete of a covered yard.

Deep Litter for Poultry

Chopped straw, shavings, and sawdust are commonly used. Musty straw could cause an outbreak of aspergillosis. Peat-moss is apt to be too dusty. Oak sawdust should not be used as it may discolour the egg-yolks. The depth should be at least 10 cm (4 in). The litter should be forked over, and added to from time to time. If it gets damp, the ventilation should be attended to. Many coccidia larvae get buried in the litter, and this is an advantage. After each crop of birds, the litter should be removed and heaped, so that enough heat will be generated to kill parasites. If deep litter is returned to a house, the succeeding batch of birds sometimes suffer from ammonia fumes, which may cause serious eye troubles. Compaction of the litter must be prevented by allowing the poultry to 'work' it; otherwise, the litter does not meet the definition specified by EC Directives.

Deep-Rooting Plants

Deep-rooting plants are valuable in a pasture for the sake of the minerals they provide. Examples of such plants are chicory, yarrow, and tall fescue.

Deer, Diseases of

Deer are susceptible to the following infections: BRUCELLOSIS; BOVINE VIRAL DIARRHOEA; ELAPHASTRONGYLUS; EPIZOOTIC HAEMORRHAGIC DISEASE; FOOT-AND-MOUTH DISEASE; JOHNE'S DISEASE; LISTERIOSIS; LOUPING-ILL; malignant catarrhal fever – see BOVINE MALIGNANT CATARRHAL FEVER; MENINGOENCEPHALITIS; PARASITIC BRONCHITIS; TICK-BORNE FEVER; TUBERCULOSIS; WARBLES; YERSINIOSIS; and also an enzootic ataxia resembling SWAYBACK in lambs.

Tuberculosis in deer Tuberculosis of deer is NOTIFIABLE in the UK. Tuberculin testing of deer and the establishment of tuberculosis-free herds was the basis of the Deer Health Scheme operated by MAFF. Tuberculin testing of deer and interpretation of the results are more difficult than in cattle; special training is required.

The Tuberculosis (Deer) Order 1989 provides for the individual marking of farmed or transported deer, and can be used for enforcing movement restrictions on affected or suspect animals.

Farmed deer Red deer (*Cervus elaphus*) and fallow deer (*Dama dama*) are the most commonly farmed.

Around 300 farms, mainly in Scotland, raise deer in the UK. Some 36,000 animals are farmed in total. Most (75 per cent) are red; the rest, fallow. All farmed deer must be identified by tagging; the British Deer Farming Association supervises a tagging scheme.

In Britain the harvesting of antler velvet from live stags is illegal.

In New Zealand, yersiniosis has become a serious disease of farmed red deer. It appears to be triggered off by stress, and most cases occur during the winter. The incidence of malignant catarrhal fever (MCF) in red deer herds in Canterbury, New Zealand, ranges from 0.2 to 10 per cent a year.

Meningoencephalitis, caused by *Streptococcus zooepidemicus*, has resulted in the death of farmed red deer exported from the UK and Denmark to New Zealand. Autopsy findings are typically congestion of lungs and liver, the presence of frothy fluid in trachea and bronchi, and acute meningoencephalitis.

Dictyocaulus viviparus is the most important parasite of red deer in New Zealand and frequent drenching with anthelmintics is used to control it. Development of resistant species is hindered by dosing strictly according to the manufacturers' directions and alternating the product used.

Another parasitic worm of importance in deer is *Elaphostrongylus cervi*. It is pale and thread-like, 4 to 6 cm long, and found in the intramuscular fascia and also in the meninges of the brain. This parasite occurs in Scotland, the mainland of Europe, and Australasia.

Eggs reach the lungs via the bloodstream and hatch in the alveolar capillaries, causing slight pneumonia. Nervous signs appear when the brain is involved.

In the UK, one of the most important infections of deer is Johne's disease, caused by *Mycobacterium paratuberculosis*. It may be seen in animals as young as a year old and results in wasting, with or without diarrhoea.

Defecation
Defecation is very differently performed in the various animals, and some diagnostic importance is attached to the manner of its performance. (See CONSTIPATION; DIARRHOEA.)

Deficiency Diseases
These form a group of diseases bearing no clinical resemblance to each other, but having the common feature that they result from omission from the diet of some substance or element essential for normal health and nutrition. The essential element may be one of the inorganic mineral substances, such as calcium, phosphorus, magnesium, manganese, iron, copper, cobalt, iodine, selenium or more than one of these; it may be a protein or an amino acid; or it may be a vitamin. In the last case the condition is often referred to as an 'avitaminosis', and the particular vitamin is specified, e.g. A, B, D or E. Starvation through inadequacy of general nutritive food intake is not classed as a deficiency disease. Some deficiency diseases are simple, such as iron deficiency in young pigs; while others are more complex, such as phosphate deficiency in South Africa, which is associated with botulism through the gnawing of bones of dead animals contaminated with *C. botulinus*. (See VITAMINS; TRACE ELEMENTS; NUTRITION, FAULTY.)

Definitive Host
This is the host in which an adult parasite with an indirect life-history lives and produces its eggs. A definitive host is the final host, as compared with the intermediate host or hosts. For example, an ant is one of the intermediate hosts of a species of liver fluke; the definitive host is a sheep or other grazing animal.

Deformities
Deformities of cattle and sheep, etc. are mentioned under GENETICS – Genetic defects. (See also HARE-LIP; MOUTH, DISEASES OF; MONSTER.)

DEFRA
Acronym for Department of the Environment, Food and Rural Affairs – the UK Government department that replaced the Ministry of Agriculture, Fisheries and Food (MAFF). Its responsibilities include notifiable diseases, food safety, and welfare of animals in transport, on farms and at slaughter. The Home Office is responsible for experimental animals.

Deglutition

Deglutition means the act of swallowing. During swallowing, breathing temporarily ceases (apnoea); otherwise food might enter the respiratory tract. (See CHOKING.)

Dehiscence

A breakdown in the union of a suture of adjoining bones of the skull. The condition can be treated successfully by surgery.

An example of this is a breakdown of the suture line in mandibular fractures. The term is also applied to the re-opening of wounds.

De-Horning of Cattle

Dairy cows are routinely dehorned to facilitate handling and to avoid injury to those handling them and to other cattle. The use of mechanised milking systems makes dehorning virtually essential. Fattening beef cattle in yards or pens are also often dehorned because there is usually 1 animal that obtains dominance; if it possesses horns it is liable to inflict wounds upon others or upon the attendants.

The most satisfactory method in calves is that known as 'disbudding'. This is best done when the horn bud is fully detectable, which takes a variable time to occur. The buds are then removed, under local anaesthetic, by cauterising with an electric or gas-heated dehorner.

An alternative method consists of painting the young buds of the horns, when they first appear in calves, with caustic compound. A little petroleum jelly or thick grease may be rubbed on the hair around the base of the bud and care is needed to ensure that no caustic gets into the eyes. The bud of the horn is first cleaned with spirit to remove grease – an essential preliminary – and a second coating of the caustic is given after the first has dried. A scab will form over the bud and drop off, carrying with it the cells which would have produced horn. Little or no pain is occasioned to the calf by caustic collodion (whereas caustic potash sticks, now largely superseded, do cause much pain) and the horn is effectively prevented from growing.

In Britain the operation of de-horning cattle requires the administration of an anaesthetic. (See ANAESTHETICS, LEGAL REQUIREMENTS.) A saw, an electric saw, cutting wire or special horn shears may be used when the horns are more developed.

Bleeding from the matrix and horn core can usually be controlled by using a figure-of-eight tourniquet around the roots of the horns.

Dehydration

Loss of water from the tissues, such as occurs during various illnesses, especially those producing vomiting or diarrhoea; in impaction of the rumen; and as a result of injury or serious burns.

Diarrhoea is one of the most common causes of dehydration. A scouring calf may lose 100 ml of water per kg bodyweight in 12 hours. As the metabolism attempts to conserve extracellular body fluid (ECF) volume, urine production decreases and blood urea levels rise while pH levels are lowered. Electrolytes are lost, particularly sodium, potassium and bicarbonate, and ketone bodies accumulate.

Treatment Restoration of fluid volume is the immediate priority, and replacement of lost electrolytes and blood nutrients.

Parenteral fluids In the severely dehydrated animal, the restoration of ECF by parenteral (usually intravenous) administration of plasma, if available, or infusion of a sterile istonic (0.9 per cent) solution of sodium chloride, compound sodium lactate infusion (lactated Ringer's solution) is indicated. In the case of blood or plasma loss through injury or burns, a plasma expander based on dextran or gelatin is added to the electrolyte solution; proprietary solutions are widely available.

The rate of administration of intravenous solutions should be carefully supervised. In severe cases of dehydration or profound shock, up to 50 ml per kg bodyweight per hour may be given initially, reducing to 5 to 10 ml/kg/hour. These high rates should not be continued for more than 20 to 30 minutes. A close watch must be kept for signs of too rapid administration: restlessness, lung sounds, tachycardia, tachypnoea.

A formula to convert ml/kg/hour to drops per minute is given in *The Veterinary Formulary*:

$$\text{Drops/minute} = \frac{\text{Drops/ml} \times \text{FR} \times \text{BW}}{60}$$

Drops/ml = number of drops delivered by the infusion set per ml
FR = Flow rate in ml/kg/hour
BW = bodyweight of patient in kg

The total amount given will depend on the amount of fluid lost and the condition of the animal.

Oral rehydration is usually satisfactory in most cases of diarrhoea. Solutions for this purpose usually contain sodium and glucose, which help the water uptake of the dehydrated animal. To help correct any acidosis, citrate should be included, and/or bicarbonate. Such solutions are suitable for calves and most mammals. Many proprietary formulations are available.

D

For first-aid purposes, glucose-saline may be given by mouth to all animals. UNICEF's 'Oral Rehydration Salts', intended for infants and children, may be used; the sachet contents being dissolved in 1 litre of (sterile or boiled) water (which must not be boiled thereafter). The formula is:

Sodium chloride	3.5 g
Potassium chloride	1.5 g
Sodium bicarbonate	2.5 g
Glucose	20.0 g

The effectiveness of the above glucose-saline solution can be enhanced by the addition of citrate and/or citric acid.

Glucose-saline can also be administered per rectum, or subcutaneously.

Delivery
(see PARTURITION)

Demephion
An organophosphorous preparation used as an insecticide and acaricide. Livestock should be kept out of treated areas for at least a fortnight.

Demodecosis
Another name for DEMODECTIC MANGE.

Demodectic Mange (Follicular Mange)
Demodectic mange (follicular mange) is caused by the demodectic mite *Demodex folliculorum*. This parasite, microscopic and cigar-shaped in appearance, with very short stumpy legs, lives deep down in the hair follicles, and is accordingly difficult to eradicate by dressings. It is a common cause of mange in dogs.

In cattle, *D. bovis* is in the UK responsible for mild and infrequently reported cases of demodectic mange, but in some parts of the world the disease may be severe. Fatal, generalised cases have been reported from Africa. *D. caprae* infestation of goats may also be severe in the tropics.

The parasites have been recovered from the eyelids of cattle, sheep, horses, dogs, and man (see MANGE).

Demulcents
Demulcents are substances which exert a soothing influence upon the skin or the mucous membranes of the alimentary canal, and in addition afford some protection when these are inflamed. Examples of demulcents for internal use are arrowroot, glycerin, bismuth subnitrate, and bismuth carbonate.

Demyelination
Destruction of the myelin, a lipid which surrounds the axis-cylinder of a medullated nerve fibre.

Dendrites
(see NERVES)

Dengue
(see EPHEMERAL FEVER)

Dental Plaque
(see TARTAR)

Dentine
Dentine is the dense yellow or yellowish-white material of which the greater part of the teeth is composed, and which in elephants, etc., constitutes ivory. The dentine is pierced by numerous fine tubules which communicate with the sensitive pulp in the hollow of the tooth-root, along each of which run tiny vessels and nerves which nourish its structure. In the young, newly erupted tooth the dentine is covered over with a layer of hard, dense, brittle enamel, which prevents too rapid wear of the softer dentine. (See TEETH.)

Dentition
Dentition refers to the configuration and conformation of the teeth, with special reference to their periods of eruption through the gums.

Horses The dentition of the horse consists of the following teeth:

	Incisors	Canines	Molars
Upper jaws	6	2	12, 13 or 14
Lower jaws	6	2	12, 13 or 14

Incisor teeth are 6 in number in the upper and lower jaws. The temporary incisors differ from the permanents in that while each of the former possesses a definite crown, neck, and root, the latter do not. Moreover, the temporaries are smoother, whiter, and smaller. When there are both temporaries and permanents present in the mouth it is not usually difficult to differentiate between them, but inexperienced persons sometimes confuse temporaries and permanents in yearlings and 5-year-olds, or in 2-year-olds and 6-year-olds. A typical unworn permanent incisor tooth from a horse possesses an infundibulum, or 'tucking-in' from its free edge or crown (see TEETH), and since this results in an infolding of the enamel, 2 rings of enamel, an outer and an inner, are seen in the partly worn tooth. However, as wear proceeds the inner ring of enamel eventually disappears, since the level of wear has passed the depth of the infundibulum. At the same time, the outline of the tooth is changing from an oval to a quadrilateral, and eventually to a triangle, since the tooth is tapered from crown to root. It is upon an examination of these factors that the estimation of the age of an adult horse is based.

The incisors are named centrals, laterals or intermediaries, and corners, according to their situation in the mouth.

Canines ('tushes', 'eye-teeth', or 'dog-teeth') number 2 in each of the jaws – 1 on the right and 1 on the left side. In horses, canine teeth are only typically present in the male, although rudimentary canines may occasionally be found in mares. They are situated between the last incisor and the 1st molar, 1 on either side, being nearer to the incisors than to the molars. The spaces between the canines and the molars are spoken of as the bars of the mouth. In the bridled horse, the bit runs across the bars.

	Incisors	Canines	Molars
Upper jaws	6	0	6
Lower jaws	6	0	6

Molars ('grinders', or 'cheek teeth') number 6 or 7 at each side of both upper and lower jaws, according to whether 'wolf teeth' are or are not present. The first 3 permanent molars are represented in the milk dentition and are therefore sometimes called premolars. Each tooth has a complicated folding of the enamel which bears some resemblance to the capital letter 'B'.

Eruption The 'eruption' means the time when the tooth cuts through the gums, and not when it comes into wear. It must be remembered that in the table, allowance has to be made for the time of foaling. All thoroughbreds are dated as having their birthdays on January 1 each year, and all other breeds of horses on May 1, so that with an early foal the teeth will appear sooner than the corresponding periods subsequent to May 1 or January 1 in any year, and with a late foal, later.

Time of eruption	Incisors	Canines	Molars
Birth to 1 week	2 temporary centrals	—	—
2 to 4 weeks	2 temporary laterals	—	Nos. 1, 2 and 3 temporary molars
7 to 9 months	2 temporary corners	—	No. 4 permanent molar
1 year 6 months to 1 year 8 months	—	—	No. 5 permanent molar
2 years 6 months	2 permanent centrals	—	Nos. 1 and 2 permanent molars
3 years 6 months	2 permanent laterals	—	No. 3 permanent molar
4 years	—	All 4 canines	No. 6 permanent molar
4 years 6 months	2 permanent corners	—	—

Usually, the teeth in the upper jaw erupt sooner than those in the lower jaw, although there are many exceptions to this.

An estimate of the horse's age from its teeth can only be approximate in later life. Galvayne's groove is practically the only definite guide, and even it may be indistinct or absent.

Cattle The permanent dentition of cattle consists of the following teeth:

	Incisors	Canines	Molars
Upper jaws	0	0	12
Lower jaws	8	0	12

In the upper jaw there are neither incisors nor canines, while in the lower jaw there are 8 teeth present in the incisor region. The most posterior of these (i.e. 1 on either side) are supposed to be in reality modified canines, which have moved forwards in the gums and have assumed the shape and the functions of incisors.

The temporary or milk dentition is as follows:

	Incisors	Canines	Molars
Upper jaws	0	0	6
Lower jaws	8	0	6

Incisors are absent from the upper jaw of cattle, their place being taken by the 'dental pad' – a hard, dense mass of fibrous tissue developed in the upper incisor region, against which the 8 lower incisor teeth bite. Each is a simple tooth possessing a spatulate (spade-shaped) crown, a constricted neck, and a tapered root or fang. The teeth are loosely embedded in the jaw so that a slight amount of movement is normally possible. They are named centrals, 1st intermediates or medials, 2nd intermediates or laterals, and corners; but it is perhaps more convenient to enumerate them from the central pair as 1st pair, 2nd pair, etc.

Canines are absent unless the corner incisors are considered as modified canines.

Molars are like those of the horse in number and arrangement, except that they are smaller and progressively increase in size from first to last, so that the 1st is quite small, and the length of gum which accommodates the first 3 is only about half that occupied by the last 3. One or more 'wolf teeth' may be present in rare cases.

Eruption In ruminants – whether domesticated or not – the eruption of the permanent teeth is subject to considerable variations.

Time of eruption	Incisors	Molars
Birth to 1 month	All 8 temporaries	All 12 temporaries
3 months	—	4th permanent
9 months	—	5th permanent
1 year to 1 year 3 months	1st pair permanent	
1 year 6 months	—	6th permanent
1 year 9 months	2nd pair permanent	1st and 2nd permanents
2 years	—	3rd permanent
2 years 3 months	3rd pair permanent	
2 years 9 months to 3 years	4th pair permanent	—

Sheep The terms which were used as applied to cattle, and the description of the various teeth, may be taken to hold good for sheep as well. The sheep has 8 lower incisor teeth but none in the upper jaw. There are 24 molar teeth, 12 in each jaw, of which half these numbers are represented in the temporary dentition.

Eruption The following is given as an average eruption table for improved breeds of sheep in Great Britain:

Time of eruption	Incisors	Canines	Molars
At birth	Corner temporaries	All 4 temporaries	—
1 month	Central temporaries	—	Nos. 2, 3 and 4 temporaries
2 months	Lateral	—	
5–6 months	—	—	No. 1, which remains through life, and No. 5 permanent
8 months	Corner permanents	—	—
9 months	—	All 4 permanents	—
10–12 months	—	—	No. 6 permanent
12–13 months	Central permanents	—	Nos. 2, 3 and 4 permanents
17–18 months	Lateral permanents	—	No. 7 permanent

Pigs There is probably no farm animal which shows such variation in the eruption of its teeth as the pig, but because of the demand for young pigs for killing by weight and size rather than by age, and because of the intractability of older breeding animals – sows and boars – the actual age of the pig is not of such very great importance, except perhaps for fat stock show purposes.

When the permanent teeth have all erupted they are distributed as follows:

	Incisors	Canines	Molars
Upper jaws	6	2	14 (i.e. 8 and 6)
Lower jaws	6	2	14 (i.e. 8 and 6)

In the molar region there is a little tooth in each of the four jaws, erupting at about 5 to 6 months, which is permanent from the very beginning. It is sometimes called the premolar, and in some cases is never developed. The next 3 teeth behind it are represented in the temporary dentition, the permanents replacing them in the usual way. The last 3 teeth are true molars, i.e. permanents only.

The temporary dentition is as follows:

	Incisors	Canines	Molars
Upper jaws	6	2	6
Lower jaws	6	2	6

Incisors: the upper incisors are small, and are separated from each other by spaces. The 1st pair (centrals) are the largest, and converge together. The 2nd pair are narrower and smaller; while the corner pair are very small and laterally flattened. The lower incisors are arranged in a convergent manner, and point forwards horizontally in the jaw. The 1st two pairs are large prismatic teeth deeply implanted in the jaw-bones and are used for 'rooting' purposes. The corner pair are smaller, and possess a distinct neck.

Canines, or tusks, are greatly developed in the entire male, and both upper and lower tusks project out of the mouth. The upper canines of a boar may be 3 to 4 inches long, while the lower ones may reach as much as 8 inches in an aged animal. Each has a large permanent pulp cavity from which the tooth continues to grow throughout the animal's life.

At 3 months the lateral temporary incisors are well up, and the temporary molars are well in wear.

At 5 months there are signs of the cutting of the premolars (i.e. the No. 1 molars), and the 5th molar (a permanent) is seen behind the temporaries. It is, however, not yet in wear.

At 6 months the premolars are cut and the 5th permanent molar is in wear.

At 7 to 8 months there are signs of the cutting of the corner permanent incisors, or they may already be through the gums. The permanent tusks are also often cutting through the gums at this age in forward animals.

At 9 months the corner permanent incisors are well up and the permanent tusks are through the gums, although in many cases there may be still one or two of the small temporary tusks in position. Where they are cut they are not far through the gums.

At 1 year it is generally held that the central permanent incisors cut through the gums, but there are a large number of animals which do not cut these teeth till about 13 months old. The 6th permanent molar cuts at this time, and is more reliable than the incisors for reference.

Shortly after 1 year the 3 temporary molars fall out and their places are taken by the permanents. They are into line with the other molar teeth 3 months later.

At 17 to 18 months, when the final changes occur, the 7th molar, the last permanent molar tooth, and the lateral permanent incisors are cut through the gums. By this time the pig has obtained its full permanent dentition, and the succeeding changes are not sufficiently reliable to warrant estimations of age being based upon them.

Dogs The average adult dog has 42 teeth. The upper jaw contains 6 incisors, 2 canines, 8 premolars, and 6 molars. The lower jaw has 6 incisors, 2 canines, 8 premolars, and 6 molars. (There is some breed and individual variation in the number of permanent teeth, short-skulled breeds, e.g. Pekingese, Boxer, and Bulldog, having fewer teeth.)

Cats The number of teeth in the adult cat averages 30. In the upper jaw there are 6 incisors, 2 canines, 6 premolars, and 2 molars; while the lower jaw has 6 incisors, 2 canines, 4 premolars, and 2 molars. Some cats have only 28 permanent teeth; lacking 2 premolars.

Rabbits are unique in that they are born with permanent teeth. Milk teeth are shed before birth and may be found in the placenta.

Deoxyribonucleic Acid
(see under DNA)

Depilation
Depilation is the process of the destruction of hair that takes place during certain skin or other diseases, or after the application of chemical or thermal substances to the surface of the body. (See MANGE; RINGWORM; 'BALDY CALF' SYNDROME; BURNS; CYCLOPHOSPHAMIDE, ALOPECIA.)

Depluming Scabies
Depluming scabies is a form of parasitic mange affecting the fowl, in which the feathers are eaten through close to the skin surface and fall or break off. It is caused by *Cnemidocoptes gallinae*. (See MITES.)

Depraved Appetite (PICA)
(see under APPETITE)

Dermatitis
Dermatitis means any inflammation of the skin. (See SKIN; ECZEMA; ALLERGY.)

Dermatophilus
Dermatophilus infection results in a chronic dermatitis, in which the hairs stand erect and matted in tufts, like a wet paintbrush. Many species of animals are susceptible, e.g. horses, cattle, sheep (also dog and cat).

Cause *D. congolensis*, which is a Gram-positive bacterium having some fungus-like characteristics, e.g. the production of branching filaments.

The disease, also known as cutaneous streptothricosis or mycotic dermatitis, follows the prolonged wetting of an animal and is widespread in the tropics, but occurs also in temperate climates such as Ireland, Britain, etc. (For examples in horses, see GREASY HEEL; 'RAIN SCALD'.)

In sheep, where it is also called 'lumpy wool', it can cause 'strawberry foot rot'.

Predisposing causes, other than wetting, include tick and insect bites, wounds from thorns, etc. Fly transmission is recognised. The bacterium can resist drying, but under wet conditions it invades the epidermis, with effects mentioned under 'greasy heel', where first-aid and precautionary measures are given. Antibiotics are helpful in treatment.

In the tropics, dipping to control ticks is regarded as important, and acaricide preparations used in sheep dips are effective against *Dermatophilus*. (See also SENKOBO; STREPTOTHRICOSIS.)

Dermatosis Vegetans
A hereditary disease of young pigs characterised by raised skin lesions, abnormalities of the hooves, and pneumonia. The semi-lethal recessive gene probably originated in the Danish Landrace. UK outbreaks occurred in 1958 and 1964.

Dermatosparaxis

A rare feline disease, resembling the human Ehlers-Danlos syndrome, and characterised by abnormal elasticity of the skin. The latter and its blood vessels also become fragile. Any wound healing takes longer than normal. The disease is inherited.

Dermis

The layer of the skin between the epidermis and the subcutaneous tissue (see SKIN).

Dermoid Cyst

Dermoid cyst is one of the commonest of the teratomatous tumours. It consists usually of a spherical mass with a surrounding envelope of skin. In this there are sebaceous glands and hair follicles from which grow long hairs. These, together with shed cells and sebaceous material, form the central part of the mass.

Dermoid cysts develop subcutaneously in various situations, and are also found in ovary or testicle. They arise through the inclusion in other tissues of a piece of embryonic skin, which continues to grow and produces hair, etc., just as does skin on the surface of the body. Owing to the cystic structure (i.e. the cavity being a closed one) there is no means of getting rid of shed hair, debris, etc., and these substances accumulating in the centre cause the cyst to continue slowly increasing in size.

A dermoid sinus is a common congenital abnormality of the Rhodesian Ridgeback dog.

Treatment No local treatment is of benefit. Surgical removal of the cyst wall and its contents, with the necessary means to obliterate the cavity, is desirable with subcutaneous dermoid cysts.

Derrengue

A paralysis of cattle occurring in El Salvador, and attributed to the ingestion of a weed, *Melochia pyramidata*, during periods of drought when scrub is the only available fodder. The symptoms resemble vampire-bat-transmitted rabies (*Derriengue*) and include a paralysis first of the hind legs, with knuckling of the fetlocks. Death usually follows.

Derriengue

The Mexican name for vampire-bat-transmitted rabies. (See VAMPIRE-BATS.)

Derris

The powder obtained by grinding the root of a South American plant. It contains rotenone, a parasiticide, useful against warbles, fleas, and lice. It will not kill the nits of the last, however, and hence the dressing must be repeated. Against fleas and lice it can be used as a constituent of a dusting powder, or with soap and warm water as a wet shampoo. It is safe for cats provided the normal precautions against licking are taken – i.e. the bulk of the powder is brushed out of the coat after 10 minutes or so, during which licking is prevented – but must be used with caution on young kittens.

Derris is highly poisonous to fish – a fact which must be borne in mind when disposing of the powder or solutions in circumstances which could lead to river pollution.

Derzsy's Disease

A form of viral hepatitis that can cause a high mortality among goslings. The cause is the goose parvovirus strain 1. Signs include dullness, loss of appetite, conjunctivitis and nasal discharge. A mutant virus is used to immunise layers and so protect their goslings.

Desmitis

Inflammation of a ligament.

De-Snooding

The removal of a turkey poult's snood, which may be pinched out or removed with a suitable instrument. De-snooding is done by turkey farmers because the snood is one of the first parts of the body to be attacked during a fight. It then provides an ideal site for invasion by *Erysipelothrix rhusiopathiae* or other pathogens.

Desquamation

Desquamation means the scaling off of the superficial layers of the skin, and is applied to the peeling process that accompanies some forms of mange and ringworm, as well as to the state of the skin in dry eczema.

Destruction (Humane) of Animals

(see EUTHANASIA)

Detergent Residue

Detergent residue in syringes used for spinal injections has caused serious demyelinating complications in humans. Similarly, an unrinsed 'spinal outfit' has led to paraplegia in a dog.

Detergents

Detergents are substances which cleanse, and many are among the best wetting agents (i.e. substances which lower the surface tension of water and cause it to spread over a surface rather than remain in droplet form). Detergents are inactivated by soaps, and the 2 must not be used together. Detergents are widely used in the cleansing of milking equipment, etc., and formulated in skin lotions and shampoos. They will remove gross contamination but are not themselves disinfectants, which, if necessary, must be applied after detergents. Examples of detergents are cetrimide and sodium lauryl sulphate.

Detomidine (Domosedan)

Given by intravenous injection, this drug has been found useful for the sedation of horses during radiography, endoscopy, etc. Sedation lasts for 20 to 30 minutes. An analgesic is needed in addition. It is also used as an equine anaesthetic, administered in conjunction with ketamine.

Dew Claws

Dew claws in cattle are sometimes torn off or injured by slatted floors. (For dew claws in dogs, see NAILS.)

De-Wattling

The removal of a fowl's wattles. (See also DUBBING.)

Dewlap

A loose fold of skin under the jaw or neck. It is found in some cattle and dogs, e.g, bloodhounds.

Dexamethasone

One of the synthetic CORTICOSTEROIDS. It is used as an anti-inflammatory agent in cases of shock, allergies, ketosis, etc.

Dextran

A water-soluble polysaccharide used as a plasma substitute. It may be infused intravenously instead of whole blood in cases of severe haemorrhage, etc.

Dextran Sulphate

An alternative anticoagulant to Heparin. Its effects last longer.

Dextrin

Dextrin is a soluble carbohydrate substance into which starch is converted by diastatic enzymes or by dilute acids. It is a white or yellowish powder which, dissolved in water, forms mucilage. Animal dextrin, or glycogen, is a carbohydrate stored in the liver.

Dextrose

Dextrose is another name for glucose.

Dhrek

An Asiatic tree of which the leaves and fruits are poisonous to farm animals. (See MELIA.)

Diabetes Insipidus (Polyuria)

Diabetes insipidus (polyuria) is a condition in which there is secreted an excessively large quantity of urine of low specific gravity. It results from a deficiency in the bloodstream of the antidiuretic hormone (ADH). It is treated with vasopressin or desmopressin. (See PITUITARY GLAND.) Diabetes has been reported to occur in dogs as a result of fright; symptoms include poor appetite, dull coat, and frequent urinating in the house. (See also POLYURIA.)

Diabetes Mellitus

Diabetes mellitus is a condition in which there is excessive glucose in the blood (hyperglycaemia). This produces various symptoms: thirst, polyuria, weight loss, recurrent infection; in more severe cases, diabetic coma (ketoacidosis), and progressive disease of the kidneys and retina, which may lead to blindness, may occur.

Cause Pancreatic disease in which the insulin-producing cells (islets of Langerhans) are deficient. A 2nd, less common, type of diabetes is caused not by a deficiency of insulin but by an excess of insulin antagonist in the boodstream. Insulin-dependent diabetes is seen in cats and dogs; the 2nd type is more usually seen in equines.

Treatment with certain medicines – for example, glucocorticoids and megestrol acetate – may predispose to diabetes.

A study in cats found that breed had no detectable effect on the risk of the animal developing diabetes, but bodyweight, age, sex and neutering had significant effects. Overweight cats were twice as liable to develop diabetes as those of normal weight. Male cats, those over 10 years old, and neutered cats are also more likely to become diabetic.

Signs These are vague at first. The diabetic animal develops an excessive thirst, and passes more urine than formerly. Appetite remains good, and sometimes becomes almost ravenous. Loss of weight occurs over a period of weeks or months. A previously active animal tends to become sluggish. The urine contains an abnormal amount of sugar. Sometimes the liver becomes enlarged.

These signs may progress to sudden depression and vomiting, which alert the cat- or dog-owner to the illness. Great weakness, a fall in blood pressure, prostration, and diabetic coma may ensue as the result of ketoacidosis.

(The temporary presence of sugar in the urine, due to a metabolic disorder, involving liver and other tissues, is encountered from time to time in the course of fever, some forms of poisoning or overdosage with chloroform, chloral or morphine, and when excessive amounts of sugars or starchy foods have been eaten. These cases return to normal with recovery from the cause.)

Treatment The only effective method of treatment is injection of insulin (which is ineffective if given by mouth), at regular intervals for the rest of the animal's life, together with attention to the diet. This is a matter which must be undertaken under expert supervision, and with dedication on the part of the owner.

There are 3 types of insulin injection: short acting (soluble insulin); intermediate (insulin zinc suspension and isophane insulin); and long acting (protamine zinc insulin). The duration of activity ranges from about 8 hours for soluble insulin to about 36 hours for protamine zinc insulin. Treatment is begun by establishing the correct dosage regime – individual animals differ in their response to a given dose. Small doses of 0.5 or 1.0 ml per kg bodyweight are given and the dose increased gradually until the optimum glucose level is reached. In many cases, a single daily injection of a longer-acting insulin will suffice. A regular, fixed routine of insulin, feeding and exercise must be observed, with meals being given when insulin activity is at a peak. It will take a few days to achieve stabilisation of dosage and routine. Animals vary considerably in their response to treatment but most dogs and cats tolerate the injection procedure quite well once they are accustomed to it.

Oral antidiabetic drugs such as chlorpropamide and tolbutamide, or biguanides may be effective in some cases where some insulin activity remains; control by diet alone is rarely effective.

Hypoglycaemia if mild, as after too strenuous exercise, is corrected by feeding the animal or giving glucose or sugar dissolved in water.

Severe hypoglycaemia must be treated as soon as possible in order to avoid irreversible brain damage.

In the emergency situation, when ketoacidosis is approaching the coma stage, dehydration must be countered by intravenous infusion of 50 per cent glucose solution at a rate of 1 ml per kg bodyweight, or by glucagon injection, 20 mcg/kg subcutaneously, intramuscularly or intravenously.

Diagnostic Imaging
(see X-RAYS; RADIOISOTOPES)

Diagnostic Tests
(see LABORATORY TESTS)

Diaphoresis
Diaphoresis is another name for perspiration (see SWEAT).

Diaphoretics
Diaphoretics are remedies which promote perspiration.

Diaphragm
Diaphragm is the muscular and tendinous structure which separates the chest from the abdominal cavity in mammals. It is an important organ in respiration. (See MUSCLES.)

Diaphragmatocele
A rupture in the diaphragm through which some of the abdominal organs, often the small intestine, stomach, and perhaps spleen and liver, have obtruded themselves, so that they become situated actually within the chest cavity. It occurs during falls, when jumping from a great height, and sometimes in cats and dogs hit by a car. The breathing becomes very much disturbed and the animal usually shows an inclination to assume an upright position, whereby the organs are encouraged to return to the abdominal cavity and pressure on the lungs is relieved. Treatment by surgical means has occasionally been effected in the dog and cat. (See THORACOTOMY.)

Diarrhoea
Diarrhoea is not, of course, a disease in itself, but merely a symptom, which may indicate nothing more than the result of an 'error of diet', or a 'chill'. A sudden change of diet, or the feeding of unsuitable, mouldy, rancid, or fermenting material will give rise to diarrhoea – a symptom of enteritis, and also of specific diseases in which enteritis is one symptom. Some drug treatments can also cause diarrhoea as a side-effect.

Continuing diarrhoea is always serious because not only are the digestive processes and the absorption of nutrients impaired, but the loss of fluid gives rise to DEHYDRATION – a frequent cause of death unless treatment is undertaken in time. If diarrhoea persists for 48 hours or more, veterinary advice should be sought by livestock-owners.

Other causes include poisons such as lead, arsenic and mercury; infection with tuberculosis in some part of the bowel wall; the presence of parasites such as worms, flukes, or coccidiae;

infection with specific diseases, such as Johne's disease, salmonellosis, lamb dysentery, white scour, etc.; or the excessive action of purgatives given in too large doses. In all of these instances there are other symptoms which help in the diagnosis of the condition, and examination of the diarrhoeic material will often show the presence of the agent responsible (see SALMONELLOSIS).

Treatment The treatment of diarrhoea from specific causes is dealt with under the appropriate headings. (See also WORMS, FARM TREATMENT AGAINST.)

If diarrhoea persists, the mere loss of large amounts of fluid from the body may itself become serious, and it becomes essential to replace this fluid. (See under DEHYDRATION.)

Irrigation of the bowel with warm saline is useful in some cases of severe diarrhoea in puppies.

Adult cattle The best first-aid measure is to feed hay only. If 'scouring' persists beyond 48 hours, obtain veterinary advice. Specific diseases in which diarrhoea is a symptom include AMYLOIDOSIS; FASCIOLIASIS; JOHNE'S DISEASE; SALMONELLOSIS; PARASITIC GASTROENTERITIS; TUBERCULOSIS; CRYPTOSPORIDIOSIS; BOVINE VIRAL DIARRHOEA.

Calves Neonatal diarrhoea is still regarded as the most important disease of young calves in both dairy and beef herds. Mortality varies widely from 0 to 80 per cent, and in non-fatal cases the resultant poor growth-rate and the cost of life-saving treatment can be a source of considerable loss to the farmer.

The causes are various. Although pathogenic strains of *E. coli* are important in the septicaemic and enterotoxaemic forms of the disease, there is doubt concerning the role of *E. coli* in all outbreaks of typical calf scours.

Of the many other bacteria which have been associated with the disease, few – with the exception of salmonella – can be shown to be the cause.

For viruses associated with diarrhoea in calves, see ROTAVIRUS; CORONAVIRUSES; REOVIRUS.

The coronavirus was originally isolated from scouring calves in Nebraska, USA, and shown to be present also in the UK. This virus resembles that causing transmissible gastroenteritis of pigs (TGE). (See also WHITE SCOUR; SALMONELLOSIS; COLOSTRUM.)

Sheep Lamb dysentery, *E. coli* infection, coccidiosis, parasitic gastroenteritis, salmonellosis, poisoning, and a sudden change to grain feeding are among the causes of diarrhoea. (See also JOHNE'S DISEASE; WORMS, FARM TREATMENT AGAINST; SOIL-CONTAMINATED HERBAGE; CAMPYLOBACTER; COCCIDIOSIS; COPPER, POISONING BY; ROTAVIRUS.)

Pigs The causes are numerous and include: iron deficiency; high fat content of sow's milk at about the 3rd week; stress, caused by e.g. long journeys; cold, damp surroundings; change of diet; vitamin deficiencies; poisons; transmissible gastroenteritis (TGE), swine dysentery, porcine intestinal adenomatosis and other disease. Viruses responsible include coronavirus and rotavirus. Bacteria include *E. coli* (some strains), *Campylobacter, Salmonella cholerae suis, S. dublin, Clostridium welchii, Erysipelothrix rhusiopathiae* (the cause of erysipelas); also protozoa, e.g. *Balantidium coli, coccidia*; fungi; yeasts; worms.

E. coli is regarded as being associated with a high proportion of outbreaks of scouring, though it can be obtained from the gut of virtually any healthy pig. Its precise importance and roles are explained under E. COLI. *E. coli* vaccines have been administered to sows before farrowing on farms where scouring is a problem. (See also K88 ANTIGEN.)

Scouring piglets need plenty of drinking water, for there is always danger of DEHYDRATION. (See also SWINE DYSENTERY; SOW'S MILK; SWINE FEVER; ILEUM; NECROTIC ENTERITIS.)

Dogs Diarrhoea may be associated with a number of infections, distemper, toxoplasmosis, tuberculosis, nocardiosis; occasionally with pyometra; with allergies; tumours; and poisoning.

Diarrhoea may also result from an infestation of dog biscuits or meal, stored in large bins, by flour/forage mites (see FLOUR MITE INFESTATION). (See also SALMONELLOSIS; E. COLI; STRESS; PANCREAS; WORMS; CANINE PARVOVIRUS; CAMPYLOBACTER; ROTAVIRUS; YERSINIOSIS; GIARDIASIS.)

Chronic diarrhoea is sometimes caused by *Clostridium difficile*. Metronidazole has proved useful in treatment, though relapses may occur.

Cats Similar causes (except distemper) apply. (See also FELINE INFECTIOUS ENTERITIS; FELINE INFECTIOUS PERITONITIS; COCCIDIOSIS; AEROMONAS; CORONAVIRUSES.)

Horses Clinical evidence has suggested a possible association between diarrhoea, stress, and antibiotic therapy. For example, a horse which is undergoing stress and happens to be a salmonella carrier may develop diarrhoea, and this may be exacerbated by tetracycline therapy which removes normal bacterial antagonists of the salmonella. Diarrhoea may, of course, be unassociated with stress, and among the many other causes is ulceration of the colon and caecum – probably caused by the thrombo-embolism associated with migrating larvae of the worm *Strongylus vulgaris.* (See also FOALS, DISEASES OF; SALMONELLOSIS; EQUINE INFECTIOUS ANAEMIA; EQUINE VIRAL ENTERITIS; HORSES, WORMS IN; GLOBIDIOSIS; CANCER; and POTOMAC HORSE FEVER.)

Whenever an apparently simple diarrhoea lasts for more than 1 or 2 days, it is wise to seek professional advice rather than attempt what must at best be only empirical treatment. The temperature is a useful guide to the severity of the condition, especially in young animals such as foals and puppies, and in all cases where it is high it is an indication that there is some serious condition complicating the diarrhoea which demands immediate attention.

Diastema

A gap between the front and cheek teeth in ruminants.

Diastasis

Diastasis is a term applied to separation of the end of a growing bone from the shaft.

Diastole

Diastole means the relaxation of a hollow organ. The term is applied in particular to the heart, to indicate the resting period that occurs between the beats (systoles) while the blood is flowing into the organ.

Diathermy

Diathermy is a process by which electric currents can be passed into the deeper parts of the body so as to produce internal warmth and relieve pain, or, by using powerful currents, to destroy tumours and diseased parts bloodlessly. Short-wave diathermy has been used in the treatment of muscle, tendon, and ligament strains. In horses with e.g. flexor-tendon trouble, 20-minute treatments over a period of a week may be effective.

Diazepam

A tranquilliser used in the treatment of epilepsy and some abnormal behaviours in the dog. Valium is a proprietary name.

Diazinon

An organophosphorus compound used in dips for sheep scab and other ectoparasites.

Diazinon granules are used for the control of wireworms on lawns and larger areas of grassland. If applied too liberally there is a risk of poisoning to birds, and also to young cattle.

In a case involving ornamental peafowl, adult birds fell forwards on to their chests, with legs stretched out behind when attempting to walk. Some could not walk at all. Diarrhoea and dyspnoea were evident. Sick birds remained alert but refused food. Two young birds were found dead; the ill adults recovered without treatment.

Dichlorophen

A drug of value against tapeworms in the dog. Dichlorophen ointment and a spray preparation have been used in the treatment of ringworm in cattle.

Dichlorvos

An organophosphorus insecticide and parasiticide used in a range of internal and external applications. For example, it has been used against fowl mites on laying hens and turkeys, and as an aerosol for treating flea infestations in cats and dogs. Strips of resin impregnated with dichlorvos have been used successfully for the control of dog and cat fleas, over a period of 3 months or so. (See FLEA COLLARS.) However, in common with other organophosphorus compounds dichlorvos must be used with care to avoid toxicity. In the UK the sale of products containing it is restricted.

Poultry have died after gaining access to the faeces of horses dosed with dichlorvos for anthelmintic purposes. Dichlorvos is effective against horse bots as well as round worms.

Diclazuril

A drug used for the treatment and prevention of coccidiosis in turkeys, meat-producing chickens and lambs.

Dicoumarol

Dicoumarol is chemically related to WARFARIN; it is an anti-coagulant and a cause of internal haemorrhage. The latter condition may develop after cattle have eaten mouldy hay containing sweet vernal or sweet clovers, the COUMARIN content of which has been converted to dicoumarol.

Dicrocoelium

(see under LIVER-FLUKES)

Dicrotic

Dicrotic pulse is one in which at each heartbeat, 2 impulses are felt by the finger that is taking the pulse. A dicrotic wave is normally present in a tracing of a pulse as recorded by special instruments for the purpose, but in health it is imperceptible to the finger.

Dictyocaulus Viviparus
(see PARASITIC BRONCHITIS)

Dicyclanil
Dicyclanil is used as a pour-on for the long-term prevention of blowfly strike in sheep and lambs. It stops the development of fly larvae by interfering with moulting and pupation.

Dieldrin
A persistent organochloride insecticide formerly used against the maggot-fly of sheep. Dieldrin is highly poisonous to birds and fish. The symptoms of dieldrin poisoning in foxes (which have eaten poisoned birds) are stated to resemble closely those of fox encephalitis. Dogs and cats have been poisoned similarly. (See also DOG, KENNELS.) Dieldrin has been suspected as a cause of infertility in sheep, and residues in the fat may be a danger to people eating the mutton or lamb. The use of dieldrin sheep-dips was banned in the UK in 1965, following similar bans in Australia and New Zealand. Dieldrin was also banned as a dressing for winter wheat early in 1975, but cases of dieldrin poisoning continued to occur among wild and domestic pigeons, and in kestrels, etc., fed on pigeons, during that year. Dieldrin is still used for ground spraying in Africa (see under DDT; and CHLORINATED HYDROCARBONS).

Diesel Oil Poisoning
Thirsty cattle have drunk diesel oil with fatal results. Cattle with access to canals may drink water contaminated with diesel oil from boats. The results are less severe and recovery is possible.

Symptoms include loss of appetite, depression, vomiting, tympany of the rumen, and emaciation. Death (sometimes from lung damage) may occur after several weeks.

Diesel poisoning occurred in a ewe after eating grass contaminated by oil from a fuel tank sited in a field. Breath, urine and faeces all smelt strongly of the oil.

Diet and Dietetics

The most important part of animal husbandry is sound feeding of the animals. This is not by any means, as might be supposed, a simple matter.

In order fully to understand rational feeding, owners of livestock (and of companion animals) must be conversant with the various food constituents and what part they play in the body; they must have an idea of the composition of the many foods that are available; and they must know how to make the best use of them. The importance of palatability should never be underrated.

Composition of foods By ordinary chemical analysis, foods can be split up and separated into water, proteins, fats or oils, soluble carbohydrates, crude fibre or insoluble carbohydrates, minerals, and trace elements. In addition to these there are vitamins.

Water Water, as an essential need for livestock, is discussed under the appropriate heading, and is found in greatest amount in roots, succulents such as cabbages and kale, wet brewer's grains, silage, and pasture grasses, which contain from 7 to 90 per cent. Cereal grains, such as wheat, oats, barley, etc. average 11 per cent. Meadow grass yields from 70 to 80 per cent of water, but when it is air-dried and made into hay under favourable circumstances this is reduced to 12 to 14 per cent.

Carbohydrates The carbohydrates in foods are divisible into 2 groups: the crude fibre, and the soluble carbohydrates.

Oats contain 10 per cent of fibre and hay and wheat-straw 25 per cent and 40 per cent respectively.

Crude fibre is a mixture of celluloses, lignin, cutin, and some pentosans (polysaccharides), etc. Cellulose forms the cell-wall of plants. In its simplest form it is easily digested, but with the growth of the plant, cellulose becomes associated with lignin, which gives stiffness to the parts of the plant requiring support, and also cutin, which is a waterproofing material.

The carbohydrates are made up of carbon, hydrogen, and oxygen. Foods containing much carbohydrate are called carbonaceous foods, e.g. the cereal grains, potatoes, molasses, etc.

The cereals contain from 60 to 70 per cent of carbohydrate. The simplest of the carbohydrates, such as the simple sugars, are absorbed directly from the gut, while the more complex sugars, and still more complex starches, have to be reduced by processes of digestion to more simple forms before they can be absorbed and be of use to the body.

Fats or Oils Fat is present in all foods, but the quantity varies greatly; thus in hay there is 3 per cent, in turnips there is 0.2 per cent, in cereals from 2 to 6 per cent, and in linseed as much as 40 per cent, while linseed cake, from which most of the fat has been expressed, contains on an average rather less than 10 per cent. In meals produced from fat-rich foods, such as cotton seed or linseed, by extraction with a solvent, all the oil except some 1 or 2 per cent is removed.

Cattle cakes and other foods in which the fat has gone rancid are dangerous for animals, and often cause diarrhoea. (See LIPIDS; COD-LIVER OIL POISONING.)

Proteins The proteins or albuminoids in a food differ from the other constituents, in that in addition to having carbon, hydrogen, and oxygen in their composition, they also contain nitrogen and usually sulphur and sometimes phosphorus. They are very complex substances, and are made up of AMINO ACIDS.

Mineral matter or ash Plants have their own mineral peculiarities; for example, the leguminous plants are rich in calcium which is so necessary for animals; other foods, such as maize, are deficient in calcium, but contain phosphorus; while others again, such as the wheat offals, have an unbalanced mineral content.

Vitamins (see under this heading)

Function of food constituents

Carbohydrates The carbohydrates are chiefly utilised for the production of energy and heat, and what is not required for immediate use is stored as fat which is to be regarded as a reserve story of energy.

Fibre A certain amount of crude fibre is necessary in the diet of all animals except those under $3^1/_2$ weeks of age, when all young domesticated animals are on a fluid diet and most are supported solely by suckling. If animals, especially herbivorous animals, are given insufficient fibre they fail to thrive, are restless and uncomfortable, and every cattle-feeder knows that without 'bulk' to the ration the animals do not do well. Breeding gilts and sows need extra fibre to stretch their stomachs so that they can accommodate enough concentrated feed during lactation to provide for their litters.

Adequate fibre is necessary to cattle and rabbits for proper muscular activity of the whole digestive system. Secondly, the proportion of fibre in the diet has an important bearing upon the actual digestion done by living organisms within the rumen. Thirdly, a high-protein and low-fibre intake may lead to bloat. Fourthly, adequate fibre is necessary in the cow's rations if she is to give a high yield of butterfat and solids-not-fat.

On the other hand, if too much fibre is given in the ration, the animals cannot digest enough food to get sufficient nutriment. Ruminants make the most use of fibre, then horses, pigs, and dogs, in that order. Fattening pigs, though requiring a certain amount of fibre, must have the allowance strictly limited, though sows and boars can do with more.

Fat The fat that is digested and absorbed may be oxidised to form energy direct, or it may be built up to form body fat. Speaking generally, fat has $2^1/_2$ times the value of carbohydrates or protein as an energy producer. While a certain amount of fat is necessary in the daily diet of animals, an excessive amount does harm.

Protein It is not only the amount of protein in the ration which is important, but also the quality of that protein.

Cereal protein is of poor quality, being deficient in lysine and methionine; and wheat is worse in this respect than barley. Accordingly, herring, (other) fish, and soya-bean meals are relatively good sources of the desirable AMINO ACIDS.

For substitution of some of the protein in a ration or diet, see under UREA.

For health in all animals, adequate protein of good quality is essential in the diet. Failure to provide it can result in economic loss to farmers; losses often being far higher than the cost of the 'extra' necessary protein. Excess protein, on the other hand, can bring its own problems. (See under ACETONAEMIA, for example.)

Minerals, trace elements These are essential for bone formation and maintenance, milk production, fertility, and the metabolism as a whole. The essential minerals and trace elements are phosphorus, calcium, sodium, potassium, magnesium, iron, manganese, copper, zinc, sulphur, iodine and cobalt. Not only are they essential, but the balance is important, too: the ratio of one to another. For example, as mentioned under CALCIUM SUPPLEMENTS, the ratio of this mineral to phosphorus can mean the difference between health and ill health.

Proprietary concentrates from reputable manufacturers ensure a feed for farm animals with well-balanced minerals and trace elements as a rule, and this is something which cannot always be achieved in a farm mix unless a proprietary minerals premix is used.

On some soils, deficiencies of certain trace elements may occur so that special supplements may be needed.

For further information, see under METABOLIC PROFILE TESTS; TRACE ELEMENTS; CONCENTRATES; FELINE JUVENILE OSTEODYSTROPHY; PIGLET ANAEMIA; IODINE DEFICIENCY; COBALT; SALT.

Vitamins (see under this heading)

Antibiotic supplements (see under ADDITIVES)

General principles of feeding There is no such thing as a well-balanced ration suitable for all animals and all needs.

Sudden changes, involving a major proportion of the ration, are to be avoided in all stock. Changes should be made gradually or involve only 1 or 2 out of several ingredients. In ruminants a sudden change to a predominantly cereal diet can prove fatal. (See BARLEY POISONING.)

Regularity in the times of feeding is essential for success. Only good-quality food should be used; there is no economy in feeding with inferior or damaged fodder. On the contrary, the use of such food has been the cause of much illness. There should not be long intervals between meals; with horses this is one of the common causes of colic. When compounding a ration it should be remembered that a mixture of foods gives a better result than the use of 1 or 2 foods. The ration should contain a sufficiency of energy-producing constituents, sufficient protein, fibre, and mineral matter. (See CONCENTRATES.)

Digestibility of foods Only that part of a food which is digested is of value to an animal. The digestibility of foods varies greatly, some being easily and completely digested, while others, especially those containing much fibre, are digested imperfectly and with difficulty; and, of course, some animals will digest a particular food better than others. (See D-VALUE.)

Preparation of foods Some foods are fed to animals in the natural state, while others are prepared in some such way as by grinding, bruising, cutting, chaffing, boiling, steaming, or soaking in water. Oats may be bruised for hard-working horses, for colts changing their teeth, and for calves; there is undoubtedly a slight increase in the digestibility of bruised over whole grain, but for an economic advantage the total cost of bruising should be less than 10 per cent of the whole grain. Beans should be split or 'kibbled' for horses, as the tough seed-coat makes them difficult to masticate. Maize also is more easily eaten if it is cracked.

Grinding grains to a meal is advisable for pigs, but it is important that the particle size be not too small. Absence of milk in the recently farrowed sow and bowel oedema may be associated with meal particles that are too fine.

Deterioration with storage Bruised or kibbled seeds do not keep well, especially if exposed to a damp atmosphere, and are liable to turn musty owing to fermentation. So long as the grain is whole and intact it is essentially still a living entity. When crushed, etc., it is killed, and the normal processes of deterioration and decomposition commence.

All feeds tend to deteriorate, and to become less palatable, on storage. With whole cereals this deterioration will be very slight, but with maize meal it can be rapid. It is recommended that the following storage periods should not be exceeded:

Maximum safe storage periods	
Vegetable proteins	3 months
Animal proteins	1 month
Molassine meal	2 weeks
Ground cereals	1 week
Mixed feed	1 week

Flour mite infestation This can very adversely affect the value of animal feed. At the National Institute for Research in Dairying it was suspected that infestation with flour mites of an experimental feed, during prolonged storage, was the cause of reduced performance of growing pigs in a diet trial. A comparison was made between deliberately infested feed and control samples. It was demonstrated that, as the mite-infestation increased, there was a considerable loss of dry matter, carbohydrate, and amino acids. Subsequent growth trials showed that the daily liveweight gain and feed:gain ratio were significantly reduced in the pigs on the mite-infested diet. Under the test conditions about one-fifth of the nutritive value of the diet was lost to the pig through progressive infestation with flour mites.

Palatability It is important that foods offered to animals should be palatable and appetising. Some foods are not very palatable, such as palm kernel cake or meal, but may be made more palatable by mixing with some molasses or locust bean meal. On the other hand, foods which are naturally palatable may become very unappetising if they have been allowed to get damp and musty. The inclusion of even a small quantity of musty food – such as foxy oats and mouldy hay – in a ration spoils the whole food. The greatest care should be taken to see that the food is fresh and wholesome and that food-troughs and water-troughs are kept clean.

For dangers of poisoning by mouldy food, see AFLATOXINS and MYCOTOXICOSIS.

Variety and mixtures Animals benefit from variety in their rations. It is often found that while a given ration may give excellent results for a time, there is a tendency for animals to eat the food without zest. This applies less to pigs and horses than to cattle, sheep, poultry, dogs and cats. A change, which may be quite simple, results in a return of the normal zest.

Also, as a rule, mixtures of several different foods are more palatable and are better digested than single food-stuffs. This is partly because during digestion, foods of different origins actually assist to digest each other, and partly because if there is any deficiency in a particular food substance in one food, it may be made good to the animal by being present in another one of the mixture.

Maintenance and production rations Rations given to animals can be divided into 2 parts, a maintenance and a production part. A maintenance ration may be described as that which will maintain an animal that is in a resting and non-producing condition and in good health, in the same condition and at the same weight for an indefinite period.

A production ration is that part of the daily diet which is given in excess of maintenance requirements, and which is available for being converted into energy, as in working horses, or into milk, or into fat or wool, or is used for growth.

It will be clear that a maintenance ration by itself is uneconomical, since it gives no return.

In devising a maintenance ration it should be clearly understood that any food will not do;

wheat straw does not contain sufficient protein for the maintenance of health in yearling bullocks, but wheat straw in combination with good quality hay will do so. (See RATIONS – Winter rationing.)

The most practical application of maintenance and production rations is in use where the cows are fed according to their milk yield.

Substitutional dieting A farmer who has fixed a daily ration for, e.g., his dairy cows, and desires to change some of the constituents in the diet by substituting other foods, should note that if foods are merely changed haphazardly weight for weight it is almost certain that the diet will be altered appreciably. For example, if 3.5 kg (5 lb) of maize is substituted for 3.5 kg of oats in a horse's ration, the animal will be getting more nutriment than formerly, as 36 kg (80 lb) of oats are equal to 27 kg (60lb) of maize. Again, oat straw, pound for pound, has rather less than half the nutriment found in meadow hay, and so on. (See STARCH EQUIVALENT; PROTEIN EQUIVALENT; RATIONS; DRIED GRASS; SILAGE; UREA.)

When substituting one food for another it is important that the change be made gradually. Disastrous results have followed the sudden change of a diet. (See also NUTRITION, FAULTY; VITAMINS; HORSES, FEEDING OF; DOGS' DIET; CAT FOODS.)

Diet During Illness or Convalescence
(see NURSING)

Digestibility
(see DIET)

Digestion, Absorption and Assimilation
Digestion, absorption and assimilation are the 3 processes by which food is incorporated into the body.

Salivary digestion begins as soon as the food enters the mouth and becomes mixed with saliva secreted by the salivary glands. It is not very thorough in animals, such as the dog, which bolt their food without careful chewing, but in the horse during feeding, and in the ox and sheep while rumination is proceeding, it is more effective, especially when starchy foods are eaten. Raw starches, which are very often enclosed in a matrix of cellulose or woody material, are not acted upon to any great extent until the cellulose covering has been dissolved, through the action of bacteria, in other parts of the system. Saliva has no digestive action upon proteins. In the domesticated dog, however, there seems little doubt that when given dry biscuits, which necessitate a certain amount of chewing, some salivary digestion does occur.

Saliva contains the enzyme ptyalin, an *a*-amylase, which actively changes the insoluble starch of carbohydrate foods into partly soluble sugars, but the process requires consummation by the enzymes of the small intestines. Ptyalin is only able to act in an alkaline medium, and its action therefore ceases as soon as the food has become permeated with acid gastric juice in the stomach.

Stomach digestion begins shortly after the food enters the true stomach and continues till it leaves this organ. There are great differences in the domesticated animals, due to the fact that some, e.g. ruminants, have a compound stomach.

In animals with a simple stomach, such as the horse, pig and dog, when food enters the stomach, 'gastric juice' is secreted from the digestive glands situated in its walls. This juice contains the enzyme pepsin, which, in the presence of dilute hydrochloric acid, also produced by these glands, acts upon the protein constituents.

Gastric lipase is another enzyme, present both in ruminants and in simple-stomached animals, which is concerned with preliminary digestion of fats.

In the horse, food stays in the stomach till it is about two-thirds full, and is then hurried through to the small intestine to make room for further amounts entering from the mouth. In spite of this the stomach is practically never found empty after death – unless the horse has been starved.

In the pig and dog, food is retained in the stomach for a variable time according to the state in which it was swallowed, and is thoroughly churned and mixed with gastric juice. During this time the softer portions along with fluids and semi-fluids are squeezed through the pylorus into the intestine.

In the ruminating farm animals – cattle and sheep – stomach digestion is complicated by the presence of 3 compartments before the true stomach, or abomasum, is reached. These are concerned with the preparation of the food before it enters the abomasum for true digestion. Although the rumen possesses no true digestive glands, a considerable part of the digestive process takes place in it through the activity of cellulose-splitting and other organisms. (See also RUMINAL DIGESTION.)

In the unweaned calf, the act of sucking apparently stimulates reflex closure of the oesophageal groove, so that the dam's milk by-passes the rumen (where it could not be effectively digested).

After the food has been subjected to the action of the organisms in the rumen, and has been chewed for a second time as 'cud', it is sent on into the 3rd stomach or omasum for further breaking up by trituration, and then into the true stomach or abomasum where digestive glands are present, and where a form of digestion similar to that which occurs in the stomach of other animals takes place.

Intestinal digestion The softened semi-fluid material which leaves the stomach is commonly known as 'chyme'; it has an acid reaction, since it has been well mixed with the hydrochloric or lactic acid in the stomach. Shortly after entering the small intestine it meets with alkaline fluids and its acidity is neutralised. This occurs through the action of the bile from the liver and of the pancreatic juice from the pancreas. These fluids are similar in that they are both alkaline, but differ greatly in their functions. The bile is partly composed of complex salts and pigments (see BILE). Its function is fourfold: it aids the emulsification of fats, dividing large droplets into tiny globules which are more easily split into their component parts by other enzymes prior to absorption; it assists in keeping the intestinal contents fluid and preventing undue fermentation and putrefaction through its slight antiseptic action against putrefactive organisms; it stimulates peristalsis to some extent; and it gives the faeces their characteristic colour. The pancreatic juice contains at least 3 enzymes which are probably sufficient in themselves to ensure complete digestion of a food. Trypsin is active in the further splitting up of protein substances which have been partly acted upon by the pepsin of the stomach. The next pancreatic enzyme is amylopsin. It acts on carbohydrate constituents, splitting them up into sugars and other substances, but not carrying the process far enough to allow of complete absorption. Amylopsin has an action similar to that of the ptyalin of saliva, but can act upon raw starch. Lipase, or steapsin, is the fat-splitting enzyme of the pancreatic fluid. It acts upon the tiny globules of fat which have been emulsified by the bile, etc., and splits them into their compounds – glycerol and a fatty acid, the latter depending upon the origin of the fat.

Secretions from the intestines contain a number of enzymes of which the most important are erepsin, enterokinase, maltase, lactase, and invertase. The 1st of these completes the

D

breaking up of any protein which may have escaped the action of the pepsin and trypsin. Enterokinase is concerned with the formation of trypsin from its fore-runner trypsinogen, and the last 3 complete the splitting up of carbohydrates into soluble sugars. Bacteria also have a most important digestive function in the intestines. In the large intestines of herbivorous animals they have a cellulose-splitting action, which is somewhat allied to fermentation, and is similar to the activity of the organisms present in the 1st stomachs of ruminants. They act upon fats in a similar manner to the pancreatic juice; they form certain volatile obnoxious substances (indole and skatole) from proteins, which give the faeces their characteristic odour; they produce lactic acid in certain cases; and they may even destroy alkaloidal poisons which have been formed during other stages of digestion.

Absorption Water passes through the stomach into the intestines almost immediately. But it is only after subjection to digestion in the intestines for some hours that the bulk of the food is taken up into the system. The chyme which leaves the stomach is converted by the action of the bile and pancreatic fluids into a yellowish-grey or a brownish-green fluid of creamy consistency called 'chyle', containing in the herbivorous animals particles of hay, oats, grass, etc. From this the fats are absorbed (after emulsification and breakdown) by the lymph vessels or 'lacteals' which occupy the centre of each of the 'villi' of the small intestines. (See VILLUS.) From the lacteals the fat globules are collected by the lymph vessels of the intestines and are ultimately passed into the bloodstream. Sugar, salts, and soluble proteins pass directly into the small blood vessels in the walls of the intestines, and are thence carried to the liver and so enter the general circulation.

The food is passed onwards through the various folds and coils of the intestines, each particular part of the bowel wall removing some portions of the food, and the residual, unabsorbable, useless constituents are eventually discharged from the rectum and anus during the process of defecation.

Assimilation takes place slowly. After the products of digestion have been absorbed into the blood- and lymph-streams they are carried round the body, ultimately reaching every organ and tissue, and the body cells extract from the blood in the capillaries whatever nutritive products they may require for growth or repair. For instance, cells in bony tissues

extract lime salts, muscles take proteins and sugars, etc. When the supply of food is much in excess of immediate requirements the surplus is stored up, e.g. as glycogen in liver or muscle fibres.

Digital Dermatitis

A condition in cattle usually affecting the skin above the bulb of the heel. The animal is very lame. The cause is probably a spirochete, *Borrelia burgorferi*.

Treatment Clean the affected area and use an oxytetracycline spray. For herd treatment, lyncomycin/spectomycin footbaths may be used. Antiseptic foot baths may help prevent the infection.

Digitalis

Digitalis is a preparation from the leaf of the wild foxglove, *Digitalis purpurea*, gathered when the flowers are at a certain stage.

The leaves contain glycosides, including digoxin, digitoxin, gitoxin, and gitalin; the seeds contain another glycoside, digitalin. The purified glycosides digoxin and digitoxin are used medicinally.

Digitalis is used in the treatment of chronic heart disease, in dogs mainly. The action of the heart is slowed down, the drug increasing the length of diastole, and at the same time it is strengthened.

Digitalis must be used with care, as the digitoxin is excreted only slowly and there is a cumulative effect which can readily lead to poisoning. Its use in cats is inadvisable, and liable to cause vomiting. This, together with loss of appetite, depression, and bradycardia, may occur in some dogs even with normal dosage.

The drug is usually used in the purified form as digoxin or digitoxin.

Digitalis poisoning may occur from a single, large dose or from prolonged administration. The heart's action may become irregular. Diarrhoea may occur.

In grazing animals poisoning may result from the eating of the plant rosettes. Foxgloves included in hay have also caused poisoning.

Dihydrotachysterol

An oil-soluble steroid used to raise the calcium level of the blood, and so treat or prevent hypocalcaemia.

Dihydroxyanthraquinone

A non-toxic laxative, acting chiefly on the large intestine, effective in all the domestic animals, including horses. It may be given in the food, when it acts in about 24 hours.

Dimethicone

An anti-frothing agent used in the treatment of 'frothy bloat' in cattle (see under BLOAT).

Dimetridazole

Dimetridazole is a drug used for the treatment and prevention of histomoniasis in turkeys, pheasants and chickens and trichomoniasis and histomoniosis in pheasants and partridges. It is the treatment of choice for trichomoniasis in pigeons as no staining of the tail feathers results. It is still used in the UK and elsewhere but is banned in many EU countries.

Dimidium Bromide

A trypanocide effective against *Trypanosoma congolense*.

Dinoprost

A synthetic preparation of prostaglandin $F_{2\alpha}$ (see PROSTAGLANDINS).

Dioctophymosis

Infestation with the kidney worm, *Dioctophyma renale*, a parasite of dogs encountered in Europe, America, and Asia. A survey of 500 dogs in Iran revealed an incidence of 1.3 per cent. Stray dogs and jackals have been found infested. Man may become infested through the eating of fish. (See also under ROUNDWORMS.)

Diodone

A contrast medium used in radiography of the kidneys.

Dioestrus

The resting, or inactive, phase of the sexual cycle in the female, during which progesterone is secreted by the corpus luteum. This causes the mare, for example, to reject the stallion and induces changes in the reproductive tract designed to provide a suitable environment for development of the embryo. In the mare, dioestrus normally lasts 15 to 16 days and is terminated by the release of 1 or more luteolytic factors from the endometrium which induces regression of the corpus luteum. (See OESTRUS.)

Dioxin

Dioxin is a toxic chemical formed as an impurity during the synthesis of trichlorophenol and its derivatives. Accidental exposure may lead to cancer; skin, eye, blood and liver damage; and also to abortion, fetal malformation and chromosomal aberrations.

Dioxin contaminated milk on a farm near a toxic waste disposal plant in the Netherlands. The dioxin was emitted during the destruction of polyvinyl plastic (PVC); it may be present in the exhaust from incinerators or other industrial processes. Dioxin contamination of animal feed in Belgium led to the condemning of meat and other food products during 1999.

Diphtheria, Calf

(see CALF DIPHTHERIA)

Diphtheria, Guttural Pouch, of Horses

(see GUTTURAL POUCH DISEASE)

Diplegia

Paralysis on both sides of the body.

Diplostomum

Diplostomum is a fluke which lives in the eye of salmonids. The intermediate hosts are snails and water birds, especially gulls.

Diprosopus

Duplication of the face. This is a type of conjoined twinning.

Dips and Dipping

In Britain mostly sheep are dipped, but beef cattle may also be dipped with advantage. Dipping is an important means of tick control in cattle, and is widely practised in the tropics.

Sheep are dipped in order: (1) to eradicate the commoner parasitic agents, such as keds, lice, ticks, etc.; (2) to act as a check upon the spread of mange in the sheep, commonly called 'sheep scab', and where that disease has broken out, to cure it; and (3) to prevent attack by the sheep-blowflies and consequent infestation with maggots. Dipping is no longer compulsory in Britain and a serious increase in outbreaks of sheep scab has resulted.

In Britain, dips contain the amidine, organophosphorus compounds, mainly diazinon or protemphos; or the pyrethroids, cypermethrin or flumethrin.

Precautions Purchasers and users of organophosphorus sheep dips must hold a certificate of competence in the safe use of sheep dips issued by the National Proficiency Tests Council. Protective clothing must be worn, care taken to avoid inhaling dust or spray, and splashes on the skin washed off immediately. All owners should ensure that any dips they purchase carry on their labels the statement that the dip has been approved by the Ministry of

Agriculture and Fisheries. The following precautions should be observed when sheep are dipped:

1. For 1 month or 5 weeks after service, ewes should not be dipped lest abortion result. Pregnant ewes require careful handling to avoid injury, but with care they may be dipped almost up to the time they lamb, provided that the weather is favourable.

2. Early spring washing or dipping must be carried out with a solution which does not harm the wool, making the fibres brittle or stained.

3. Summer dipping should take place when there is a sufficiency of fleece to carry and hold the dip, and when parasites may most easily be destroyed, i.e. from 3 to 5 weeks after clipping.

4. Autumn dipping should be finished before the 1st frosts of the season begin, and when the weather is so much settled that rain is not expected during the next 24 hours.

5. Sheep should be offered a drink of water before being dipped in hot weather, as there is some risk of thirsty animals drinking the dip, with fatal results if it is a poisonous variety.

6. Sheep should be rested before actual immersion, especially if recently brought in from a hill, or when they have walked a distance to the dipper. This is particularly important in hot weather.

7. Sheep with open wounds or sores, and those that have recently been attacked with maggots or have been ill, should not be dipped until the skin is whole and until they have otherwise recovered. This is another reason why dipping should not immediately follow shearing.

8. Sheep must not be turned out on to grazing land immediately after being dipped, for the drainage from the fleeces contaminates the herbage, and the sheep, being hungry, may eat sufficient dip-sodden grass to produce poisoning. They should be allowed about 15 minutes in the draining pens.

9. After dipping operations are finished the dip should be disposed of in such a way that there is no danger of it contaminating water-supplies, ponds, streams, etc. (See FISH, POISONING OF.)

Baths and Their Use The bath to be used depends on many circumstances, such as numbers to be dipped, land and materials available, and so on. The best material to use is concrete, and the most popular shape is that shown in the illustration. The dimensions for the various animals are as shown in the table (the figures are only given as a general guide).

In order to avoid waste of dip, the farmer needs to know how much liquid the bath will hold, and also needs a calibrated stick or sidemarking to indicate the volume of liquid still in the bath at all stages of dipping.

What is sometimes overlooked is the fact that a sheep with wool 2.5 to 4 cm (1 to 1½

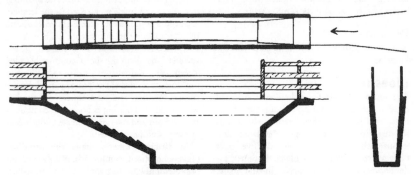

Plan of dipping bath. (*See* table for dimensions.)

	Horses			Cattle			Sheep			Pigs		
	metres	ft	in	metres	ft	in	metres	ft	in	metres	ft	in
Breadth at top	1.75	5	9	1.60	5	2	1.00	3	3	1.00	3	3
Breadth at bottom	1.00	3	3	1.00	3	3	0.75	2	6	0.75	2	6
Depth	2.60	8	5	2.30	7	6	1.75	5	9	1.75	5	9
Length at top	16.60	55	0	15.30	50	0	13.70	45	0	10.65	35	0
Length of well	9.15	30	0	9.15	30	0	9.15	30	0	6.10	20	0
Entrance slope	2.20	7	3	2.00	6	6	1.50	5	0	1.50	5	0
Exit slope	4.95	16	3	4.00	13	0	3.00	10	0	3.00	10	0
Depth of dip from bottom	2.00	6	6	1.70	5	6	1.20	4	0	1.20	4	0

inches) long will not merely remove permanently at least 2.25 litres ($^1/_2$ gallon) of liquid, but will strain off additional insecticide. This necessitates 'topping up' of the dip wash at double strength as compared with the liquid used for the first filling of the bath.

It is a false economy not to top up before the last 20 or 30 sheep are put through the dip, since any saving of money thereby could later be more than offset by those animals becoming victims of strike. Disappointing results of any dip can also follow if sheep are immersed for far short of 30 seconds; or if they are soaking wet when they enter the bath, for then their fleeces can carry much less than the normal quantity of wash.

Arsenic-dipped animals should never be allowed on to pasturage until there is no risk of contamination of grass.

In all cases the animal should be totally immersed at least once (hence the abrupt commencement of the bath), and special attention should be paid to the ears and tail. Dipping must be thorough.

One dipping will seldom (if ever) be effective in ridding an animal of parasites, as the dip may not affect the eggs. The dip must accordingly be repeated at suitable intervals. Against keds, dips should be repeated in 3 to 4 weeks, and against mange in about 7 to 10 days.

Lameness Especially in warm climates, where the dip has been allowed to remain in the tank and has become dirty, there is a danger of sheep becoming lame after dipping. This results from infection with *Erysipelothrix rhusiopathiae* (see under SWINE ERYSIPELAS) through any cuts or abrasions. Such lameness does not follow the use of a freshly prepared dip. It has been obviated by the addition to the dip of tetramethyl thiuram disulphide; this controls any bacteria which contaminate the dip liquid. Non-phenolic sheep dips have little or no action against bacteria.

Spraying Dipping of all animals involves considerable trouble, expensive equipment, and in most cases is static so that animals must come to the dipper. The use of modern sprays and jets, whereby the chemical agent is directed on to the animal's skin with considerable force, has some advantages over dipping and is partly replacing dipping in some countries (see SPRAY RACE; also JETTING). In Britain, those who practise spraying, as opposed to dipping, would be unwise to rely on more than 3 weeks' protection against strike. This is partly because less insecticide remains in the fleece after spraying; also, the organophosphorus insecticides move down

the wool but, apparently, not sideways, so that if a patch is left unsprayed it remains vulnerable to strike.

Protective clothing Operators engaged in dipping or spraying **must** use protective clothing. The latest guidance issued by the manufacturers or government agencies should be followed. Basically, protection such as coveralls, waterproof apron or leggings, wellington boots and elbow-length rubber gloves, a face shield and hat should be worn; details vary with the type of product used. There is a National Proficiency Test Council certificate in personal protection equipment for those regularly involved in the use of dips and sprays.

Farmers should familiarise themselves with the guidelines on the storage, use and disposal of dips issued by the manufacturers and the Veterinary Medicines Directorate.

Diquat
This herbicide has caused fatal poisoning in cattle, 4 years after the discarding of a container.

Dirofilariasis
(see HEARTWORMS)

Disbudding
Disbudding is the removal of, or the prevention of growth in, the horn buds in calves, kids, and sometimes in lambs. (See DE-HORNING OF CATTLE; GOATS, DISBUDDING OF KIDS.)

Disc, Intervertebral
(see under SPINE)

Discospondylosis
Inflammation of the intervertebral discs of the spinal column.

'Disease-Free' Animals (In Research)
The availability of animals born and reared free from infection is an important tool in the study of disease. The technique is used in laboratory animals and has had particular application in pigs, as described below.

Piglet mortality is one of the main sources of economic loss to the pig industry, and it is in the study of important piglet diseases that special laboratory pigs are necessary. Without such animals, research work may not only be hampered or even brought to a standstill by natural infections, but complications may also arise.

From the moment the piglet leaves the security of the uterus and enters the birth-canal it becomes exposed to an infected environment.

Under natural conditions it is protected, against this environment, to a greater or lesser degree, by the wide range of antibodies received from its dam in the first milk, the colostrum. When deprived of colostrum piglets almost always die. But the research worker wishes to avoid the feeding of colostrum, since it may well contain antibodies against the disease under investigation.

The problem is, then, to rear piglets which are both disease-free and devoid of antibodies. In principle, the solution to the problem is a simple one. All that needs to be done is to obtain the piglets before they reach the infected environment and to rear them away from possible infection, so that colostrum is unnecessary. In practice, these requirements are not easily met. However, by using a technique developed in the USA at the University of Nebraska, 'disease-free', antibody-devoid pigs have been produced.

The piglets are taken direct from the sow's uterus a day or 2 before the estimated farrowing date. The sow is anaesthetised, the whole uterus carefully but rapidly removed and passed through a bath of disinfectant, into a sterilised hood. The hood is supplied with warm, filtered air under slight pressure, and 2 operators, working through long-sleeved rubber gloves, take the piglets from the uterus. Their navel cords are tied off, and they are dried with sterile towels. The piglets are then transferred, by means of a sealed carrying case, to sterile incubator units kept in a heated isolation room. The incubators, each of which holds 1 pig, are equipped with filter pads so that both the air entering the unit and that passing out into the exhaust system is filtered.

During the first few days of their independent existence, great care is necessary to protect the young animals from bacteria in general. The attendant wears mask and cap in addition to rubber gloves and overalls. Subsequently, masks and caps are unnecessary. The diet, which consists of pasteurised milk, eggs and minerals, is sterilised by heat for the first 3 days of life, but not thereafter. The piglets are fed from flat-bottomed trays 3 times daily – morning, midday and late afternoon. There are no night feeds. After some 10 days in the incubator units the young pigs are transferred to individual open cages in another isolation pen. There they are rapidly weaned to solid food. Later, the pigs are mixed together and treated as ordinary ones except that, of course, precautions are taken to prevent accidental infection.

Pigs reared by this technique are in a state of minimal disease: they are not germ-free. In fact, non-pathogenic bacteria are deliberately introduced by feeding pasteurised, instead of sterilised, milk from the 4th day of life onwards. These pigs are not, therefore, in the same category as germ-free GNOTOBIOTIC animals. Production of 'disease-free' pigs was begun at Cambridge primarily to permit the critical investigation of pig diseases, particularly diseases of sucking pigs, but such pigs have obvious advantages for nutritional and genetic studies because the technique does eliminate that unpredictable variable, disease. (See also SPF.)

Diseases

(see NOSOCOMIAL; IATROGENIC; STOCKMEN/WOMEN)

Diseases of Animals Acts

Legislation relating to animal health, including the Diseases of Animals Act 1950, was consolidated under the Animal Health Act 1981, which also includes the relevant Orders made under the various Acts. It is administered by the Animal Health Division of the Ministry of Agriculture.

It covers the diseases listed under NOTIFIABLE DISEASES.

The Act and Orders provide for the compulsory notification of the existence or suspected existence of these diseases; for the immediate isolation or segregation of diseased or suspected animals; for the diagnosis of suspected disease by specially trained persons; for the slaughter, treatment or vaccination of diseased or suspected animals where appropriate and for the disposal of carcases and other waste where necessary; for the payment of compensation to owners in certain cases; for the apprehension and punishment of offenders; for the systematic inspection of markets, fairs, sales, exhibitions, etc., and for the seizure of diseased or suspected animals therein; for regulating the transit and transport of animals by land or water, both within the country and in the home waters; for controlling the importation of animals and things which may introduce one or other of these diseases from abroad; and for inspection at the ports and quarantine or slaughter where necessary.

The following regulations have a general application to all scheduled diseases, but in practically every case there is at least one Order applicable to the particular disease, in which there is set out more fully regulations dealing with that disease. These Orders can be obtained through the Stationery Office, and must be consulted individually if complete information is required.

Notification of diseases or suspected disease must always be made by the owner of an animal, or by the occupier or person in charge, and by the veterinary surgeon in attendance, to an inspector of the local authority or to a police constable, without undue delay.

Presumption of knowledge of disease. A person required to give notice if charged with failure to carry out his or her obligation shall be presumed to have known of the existence of the disease, unless and until s/he shows, to the satisfaction of the Court, that s/he had not knowledge thereof and could not with reasonable care have obtained that knowledge.

Separation of diseased animals. Every person having a diseased animal shall, as far as is practicable, keep it separate from animals not so diseased.

Facilities and assistance to be given for inspection, cleansing, and disinfection. Persons in charge of diseased animals are required to give every facility for the execution of the above, and must not obstruct or in any way hinder inspectors or other officers in doing their duty.

Prohibition of exposure of diseased animals. It is unlawful to expose a diseased or suspected animal in a market, sale-yard, fair, or other public or private place where such animals are commonly exposed for sale; to place an affected animal in a lair or other place adjacent to or connected with a market, sale-yard, etc., or where such animals are commonly exposed for sale; to send a diseased animal on a railway, or on any canal, inland navigation or coasting vessels; to allow one on a highway or thoroughfare, or on any common or unenclosed land or in any insufficiently fenced field; to graze one on the sides of a highway or to allow one to stray on a highway or thoroughfare or on the sides thereof, etc.

Digging up carcases. No person may dig up the carcase of an animal that has been buried, without official permission. (See also under each main heading of the scheduled diseases, e.g. ANTHRAX.)

Diseases of Animals (Waste Food) Order 1973

This Order, amended in 1987, makes it an offence for producers to feed, intentionally or inadvertently, untreated meat or meat products to livestock on their premises. Any litter spread on fields must be examined for the presence of carcases, which must be removed.

Diseases of Fish Act

This lists the notifiable diseases. (See FISH, DISEASES OF.)

Dishorning
(see DISBUDDING)

Dishorning of Cattle
(see DE-HORNING OF CATTLE)

Disinfectants

Disinfectants may be either physical or chemical. Among the former are heat, sunlight and electricity; while among the latter are solids, liquids, and gases. Steam may be used.

Chemical disinfectants At the present time these are numerous and diverse. The Deparment of the Environment, Food, and Rural Affairs tests them from time to time and issues its approval only to those that are maintained up to standard. Consequently, owners should examine the labels on containers and use only those that carry the official approval since this is a guarantee of potency.

The Diseases of Animals (Approved Disinfectants) Order 1970 governs the uses of disinfectants in the UK, and specifies those approved for use in connection with foot-and-mouth disease, tuberculosis, fowl pest, and general orders relating to disease control. Dilution rates are also specified.

A full list of disinfectants approved for use in outbreaks of foot-and-mouth disease is given under that entry.

Disinfectants act in 1 of 3 ways: (1) as oxidising agents or as reducing agents; (2) as corrosives or coagulants acting upon the protoplasm of bacterial life; or (3) as bacterial poisons.

Most chemical disinfectants are supplied in a concentrated form and must be diluted with water before use. The water should be clean, preferably soft, and if it can be used warm the efficiency of the disinfectant is increased. After the active agent has been added, the whole should be well stirred for a few moments to ensure thorough mixing. The solution must be applied so that it remains in contact with the offending material for a sufficiently long time to kill the bacterial life therein; generally 10 minutes to half an hour should elapse before disinfecting solutions are rinsed away.

When 2 or more disinfectants are mixed together, instead of an increased disinfecting power in the mixture they often enter into chemical combination with each other and a useless compound results. (See also ANTISEPTICS.)

For quaternary ammonium compounds, see under this heading.

Cresol solutions: there are many of these, e.g. the cresol and soap solution of the BP, the compound cresol solution of the USAP, lysol, isal, cyllin, creolin, cresylin, Jeyes' fluid, or one of the proprietary preparations. These are used as 3 to 5 per cent solutions for practically all purposes of disinfection about a farm premises, and very often as antiseptics also. Their action is enhanced by the use of hot water instead of cold. None is suitable for use in connection with food, for all are to a greater or lesser degree poisonous. Cresols are not very effective against many viruses or bacterial spores. The cresols are related to PHENOL.

Formalin is sometimes used as a solution for disinfecting floors, about 5 per cent strength being necessary. Formaldehyde gas may be used for fumigation of livestock buildings where viral or other diseases have occurred. (See under DISINFECTION.)

Sodium hypochlorite (bleach) is widely used and effective. Depending on the dilution and formulation it can be used as a general disinfectant and in, for example, sterilising milking machines. It has the advantage of leaving no taint, as it breaks down into salt and water.

Disinfection

Disinfection of buildings cannot be achieved by applying a disinfectant solution to walls and floors which are heavily contaminated with dirt. There are 2 reasons for this: (1) the disinfectant cannot reach most of the micro-organisms, which will be protected by layers of dirt; and (2) the latter may alter the nature of the disinfectant solution chemically, rendering it ineffective.

Preliminary cleaning is therefore essential. The building must first be thoroughly scraped, brushed, and cleansed. Concrete floors may be power-hosed, and scraped free from all dirt and debris. A hot detergent solution such as 2.5 to 4 per cent washing-soda is then thoroughly scrubbed into floors, walls, stall partitions, mangers, troughs, or other fittings.

Disinfectants After an outbreak of infectious disease, buildings and equipment must be treated to remove traces of infection before animals are rehoused. To be effective, the application of disinfectants is the 2nd stage of the process of disinfection – cleaning being the 1st stage.

In certain cases it may be desirable to fumigate the building. All air entrances and exits are securely closed, the inside of the walls and roof soaked with water, and formaldehyde gas generated (e.g. by pouring on to 250 g of potassium permanganate 500 ml of formalin per 1000 cu ft of air space.) All doors and windows are left shut for a day, and the building is then flushed out with clean water under pressure from a hose-pipe.

Steam cleaning may be carried out as part of a disinfection process.

Movable objects All pails, grooming tools, wheelbarrows, shovels, forks, etc. which have been used for the infected animals must also be disinfected before they can be considered safe for further use.

Dislocation

Dislocation is a displacement of a bone from its normal position in relation to a joint. Deformity is produced, and there may be intense pain if the part is interfered with. As well as displacement there is also bruising of the soft tissues around the joints, and tearing of the ligaments which bind the bones together.

Probably the most common dislocation is that of the patella, which becomes lodged on the uppermost part of the outer ridge of the patellar surface of the femur and is unable to extricate itself from this position. In the dog, dislocation of the shoulder joint is by no means rare.

The causes of dislocations are similar to those which produce fracture, e.g. violence applied in such a manner that the structures around the joint are unable to withstand the stress. (For inherited abnormality in dogs, see under PATELLA.)

Signs The injured limb is useless, and as a rule is held off the ground in an unnatural attitude. There is generally little or no pain so long as the parts are not forcibly moved; but if a nerve trunk is pressed upon, the animal may perspire with the pain. When the limb is compared with that of the opposite side there is seen a marked difference in its contours or outline – the joint affected shows hollows or prominences where none is seen in the normal limb. There is a loss of the power of movement, but there is no grating sound heard when the joint or the whole limb is passively moved, such as occurs when a fracture exists.

Treatment The reduction of dislocations necessitates the use of anaesthesia.

Displaced Abomasum

A condition encountered in cattle some weeks after calving and leading to a lack of appetite. Displacement can be left or right; left is more common. (See under STOMACH, DISEASES OF.)

Disposal of Carcases

Carcases must be disposed of under the Animal By-products Order 1999. It is an offence to leave the carcase of an agricultural mammal unburied for 48 hours. Carcases may be sent to a knacker's yard or a destructor. Burning on the farm is possible, but may only be done by permission of the Environmental Protection Agency. Moreover, where the cause of death has been a contagious disease there is always the risk of healthy animals becoming directly or indirectly affected, and of the disease spreading accordingly. In most progressive countries there are government regulations which provide for the safe disposal of the carcases of animals that have died from any of the notifiable contagious diseases, such as anthrax, foot-and-mouth disease, cattle plague, etc., but it is important that **all** carcases should be safely and efficiently disposed of, no matter what has been the cause of death.

The safest and most expeditious manner of disposal is for the carcase to be digested in a special destructor, either by heat (burning, or by live steam) or by chemical agents. In country districts, however, such plants as these are seldom available, and it is necessary to bury or burn the carcases.

Burial of carcases A suitable site should be selected where there will be no danger of pollution of streams, rivers, canals, or other water-supplies, and where there is a sufficiency of subsoil to allow a depth of 2 m (6 ft) of soil above the carcase. A pit is dug, about 2.5 to 3 m (8 or 9 ft) deep, in such a manner that the surface soil and the subsoil are not mixed, and a clear approach is left to its edge. Roughly, about 2.5 to 3 m² (2½ to 3 sq yd) of surface are required for a horse, 1.25 to 2.5 m² (1½ to 2½ sq yd) for an ox, and about 1 m² (1 sq yd) for each pig or sheep. The dead animal should be arranged upon its back with the feet upwards. The carcase is next covered with quicklime or a powerful disinfectant, and the pit filled in with the soil – subsoil first and surface soil last. If the weather is very wet, or if the soil is naturally loose and soft, the surface of the ground should be fenced off to prevent horses and cattle from passing over it and perhaps sinking into the loose soil. It is not safe to plough over a large burial pit for 6 months after it has been closed, nor should heavy implements or vehicles be allowed to pass over it.

Cremation of carcases Where a large coal boiler or furnace is used for heating supplies of water, there is no reason why, occasionally, the carcases of small animals that have died should not be burned in it. However, special incinerators are used where small animal carcases are routinely disposed of; they must be sited to conform with local environmental health rules.

Dead horses and cattle, and large sheep and pigs, should not be dismembered and destroyed in such a manner; they must be burned in a specially constructed cremation pit.

There are 3 methods of cremation: (1) the crossed trench; (2) the Bostock pit; and (3) the surface burning method.

In the crossed trench, 2 trenches 1.2 m (7 ft) long are dug so that they form a cross. Each is about 40 cm (15 in) wide and 45 cm (18 in) deep in the centre, becoming shallower towards the extremities of the limbs. The soil is thrown on to the surface in the angles of the cross, and upon the mounds so made, 2 or 3 stout pieces of iron, beams of wood, or branches from a tree are placed. Straw and faggots are piled in the trenches to the level of the surface of the ground, the carcase is placed across the centre of the trenches, and more wood or coal is piled around and above it. Two gallons of paraffin oil are poured over the whole, and the straw is lit.

In the Bostock pit, an oval pit 2.25 m (7 ft) long and 1.25 m (4 ft) wide is dug to a depth of 1 to 1.25 m (3 to 4 ft), and a crossed trench 20 × 20 cm (9 × 9 in) is dug in its floor. Upon the windward side of the pit a ventilation trench 1.25 m (4 ft) long and 50 cm (1 ft 6 in) wide, and a 30 cm (1 ft) deeper than the main pit, and at right angles to it, is dug. A field drain-pipe is placed in a tunnel connecting the trench with the pit, and this pipe is stuffed with straw. Straw is laid in the bottom of the main pit, wood or coal is piled above it so that about three-quarters of the pit is filled, and the carcase is next rolled into the pit. More wood or coal is piled around and above it, and paraffin oil poured over the whole. The straw is finally lit in the bottom of the ventilation trench. A carcase cremated by this method takes about 8 to 10 hours to burn away, and requires little or no attention. When burning is complete the soil is replaced and the ground levelled.

The surface burning method is mainly used where there are numbers of animals to be burned. One long trench is dug about 50 cm (1 ft 6 in) deep and 30 cm (1 ft) wide, and about 1 m (3 ft) length is allowed for each cattle carcase. At intervals along each side there are placed side flues to coincide with each carcase. Fuel (straw, wood, and coal) is placed around the central trench and the carcases are drawn across it. More fuel is heaped around and between them, and paraffin oil or petrol is sprayed over the whole. The straw is lit. More fuel needs to be added at intervals.

Instead of the trench and side flues, battens of stout wood are sometimes laid upon the ground, and the carcases pulled over them. Fuel is piled around them and lit, and more is added as required. This latter method is specially applicable where the ground is very wet, or where there is rock immediately below the soil and digging is impossible.

Precautions Where the carcase of an animal that has died from a contagious disease is being disposed of in one of the above ways, it is essential to ensure that blood or discharges are not spilled upon the ground in the process of removal. An efficient method of preventing this is to stuff tow saturated with some strong disinfectant into all the natural orifices – nostrils, mouth, anus, etc. – and to cover the surface of the improvised sleigh (door or gate) with pieces of old sacking which have been soaked with disinfectant, so that parts of the carcase do not become chafed through friction with the ground and so leave behind bloodstains. Everything that has come into contact with the carcase must be carefully disinfected before it is removed. Old ropes, sacking, and other objects used for handling the dead animal may be burned. The surface of the soil around the edge of the pit, upon which the carcase rests, should be scraped off and thrown into the fire or pit so that any blood or discharges may be rendered harmless. Finally, all attendants should be impressed with the risks they run in handling diseased carcases, and with the risks there are of contaminating other healthy cattle. Appropriate biosecurity measures, including the use of protective clothing, disinfected or discarded before leaving the premises, must be observed.

Disposal in the tropics (see TROPICS – Carcase disposal)

Disposal of Veterinary Clinical Waste (UK)

Such waste is defined by the Health and Safety Commission as including animal tissue and excretions, drugs or medicinal products, sharp instruments, or similar materials or substances.

Clinical waste must be separated from other waste in accordance with the system agreed by the local authority, e.g. yellow sacks and reinforced containers. (The Collection and Disposal of Waste Regulations 1989.)

Distemper

Distemper is a name applied to a specific viral disease. As a rule, all members of the Canidae and Mustelidae are susceptible to canine distemper. These classes include dog, fox, wolf, ferret, mink, weasel, ermine, marten, otter and badger.

Felidae (cats) are not susceptible except for lions. An outbreak in the Serengeti National Park in Tanzania appears to have been brought under control by vaccination of the dogs belonging to the local population. In the terminal stages of distemper in the fox, the animal becomes paralysed and froths at the mouth, giving rise to the suspicion of rabies.

Injection of dogs with measles or rinderpest virus confers immunity against distemper.

Canine distemper is an infectious disease mainly of young dogs, characterised usually by a rise in temperature, dullness, and loss of appetite, and in the later stages by a catarrhal discharge from the eyes and nostrils. The disease is often complicated by broncho-pneumonia, and in some cases nervous symptoms develop, either when the febrile conditions subside, or before this happens. The incubation period of the disease is from 4 to 21 days, though it may be longer.

Cause Canine distemper virus, a morbillivirus. There is only one antigenic type, though various syndromes (including 'hard pad') may be associated with various strains, some of which can suppress or impair the body's natural defence systems, and this has a bearing upon possible complications due to secondary bacterial infections.

Certain bacteria are responsible for secondary lesions; for example, *Bordetella* is often responsible for bronchitis.

Cases of distemper may be complicated by the coexistence of other infections such as CANINE VIRAL HEPATITIS, LEPTOSPIROSIS and TOXOPLASMOSIS.

Although it is chiefly in young dogs that the disease is encountered, older dogs are often affected; as a general rule, however, young animals between the ages of 3 and 12 months are the most susceptible.

KLEBSIELLA infection gives rise to symptoms similar to some of those of distemper.

Signs and complications In typical cases the dog becomes feverish, has a discharge from eyes and nose, and a cough. In some cases the eye inflammation become severe. (See KERATITIS.)

Complications include broncho-pneumonia with a hacking cough. (See BORDETELLA.)

Gastroenteritis, and mouth ulcers, complicate other cases.

Sometimes (apart from the fact that the dog has seemed unwell) the first sign of the disease to alarm the dog-owner is a fit. (See ENCEPHALITIS.) A change in temperament, with a tendency to viciousness, may occasionally be noticed.

Paralysis of face muscles, or of a limb, may occur, and sometimes hindquarter paralysis (see PARAPLEGIA) accompanied by incontinence indicate that the dog is unlikely to recover,

'Hard pad disease' may cause a dog to make a tapping sound as it walks on a hard surface, and this manifestation of distemper may be accompanied by pneumonia and/or diarrhoea.

Diagnosis and treatment An early diagnosis is important. A veterinary surgeon should be consulted as soon as any of the above symptoms appear, and will advise on the use of serum, sulphonamides, antibiotics, vitamin preparations, etc., as the situation demands. (See also NURSING.)

After recovery from distemper it is important to remember that, unless the dog is looked after with great care, relapses are liable to occur. For a week or 10 days after all symptoms have apparently subsided, the dog should be given only a limited amount of exercise. A vitamin preparation may be prescribed.

After-effects CHOREA may occur when the dog appears to be making a good recovery, and often after an otherwise mild illness. A syndrome has been described ('old dog encephalitis') in which, several months after being ill with distemper, even a young dog may become senile and forget its house training.

Prevention Various vaccines have long been available and have included:

1. *Live, egg-adapted distemper virus*
   (a) obtained from embryonated hens' eggs
   (b) obtained from cultures of avian fibroblastic tissues.
2. *Live distemper virus adapted to homologous tissue culture* obtained from cultures of dog kidney cells.

Combined vaccines against distemper, infectious canine hepatitis, canine parvovirus, leptospirosis and parainfluenza are on the market.

The timing of vaccination is crucial. Assuming an adequate intake of colostrum, puppies born to bitches immunised against distemper should have sufficient antibody to protect them during the initial weeks of life. The immunity provided by the antibody wanes: by the time the puppy is 12 weeks old, the level of maternal antibody is negligible. It will no longer protect against naturally occurring virus; equally it will not interfere with distemper vaccination.

Puppies inoculated when between 7 and 9 weeks old should therefore receive a 2nd dose of vaccine at 12 weeks of age.

A booster dose is often advisable when the dog is 2 years old.

These are general guidelines. Individual manufacturers' dosage instructions for specific vaccines may vary, and must be followed.

(See also COLOSTRUM; GAMMA GLOBULIN; ANTISERUM; MEASLES VACCINE; MATERNAL ANTIBODIES.)

Distichiasis

Distichiasis is the presence of a double row of eyelashes, of which one or both rows are turned in against the eyeball, causing inflammation. It may lead in dogs to EPIPHORA.

Distiller's Grains

A feed, relatively high in protein and energy, for dairy cattle. For hazards of storage, see BREWER'S GRAINS.

Distomiasis

Infestation with liver flukes.

Diuretics

Drugs which increase the amount of urine excreted. They are used mainly in the treatment of oedema (dropsy) in cases of heart failure. They act by inhibiting the reabsorption of sodium and chloride from the loop of Henle (loop diuretics) or the kidney tubule. (See KIDNEYS – Structure.) Furosemide is a powerful loop diuretic. Thiazides, which act in the distal part of the tubule, are less potent. The risk of excessive excretion of potassium presented by loop diuretics may be avoided by the use of potassium-sparing diuretics, which are often given in combination with loop diuretics to enhance their effect. Spironolactone is an example. A 2nd type of diuretic acts by osmotic action, which causes water retention in the nephron. Osmotic diuretics such as mannitol are used, for example, to promote urine flow in kidney failure.

While diuretics can help, they will not cure the condition which has given rise to the oedema.

Diverticulum

A small pouch formed in connection with a hollow organ. There are certain diverticula which are normally present in the body, e.g. the diverticulum of the duodenum, which is found at the point of entrance of the bile and pancreatic ducts, or the posturethral diverticulum, a little pouch behind the opening of the female urethra into the posterior genital tract in the sow and cow; while there are others which are found as the result of injury or disease, e.g. in the oesophagus, in the rectum, and sometimes in the intestines.

DNA

Deoxyribonucleic acid. This is found in the nucleus of every cell and carries coded information/instructions for reproducing other cells. 'DNA can be visualised as a long coded tape, divided into segments. These segments are individual genes, and each carries information for the assembly of a specific protein. The genes issue the instructions for the cell; the proteins execute the orders. Some genes code for structural proteins such as hair, horn, etc., but most code for enzymes which perform tasks in the cell, such as motility, metabolism, and secretion.' (Professor W. F. H. Jarrett FRS.)

A chromosome is composed of a giant molecule of DNA, plus supporting protein, and it is the DNA which is the very basis of heredity. (See CELLS; GENES; CHROMOSOMES; GENETIC ENGINEERING.) Bacteria, viruses, and plasmids contain DNA. (See also CANCER.)

DNA 'Finger-Printing'

DNA 'finger-printing' of human beings was first described by Dr Alec Jeffreys of Leicester University in 1985; and has since been used to prove the identification of sires of many different animal species.

The 1st case concerned a pack of Siberian huskies, and proving the true identity of puppies born to one of them, prior to registration with the Kennel Club.

Other applications of the technique are positive identification of thoroughbred horses, and of laboratory animals. The technique has been used in the prosecution of robbers of raptor nests by identifying the parents of young raptors found by the police.

Genetic fingerprinting can also provide an effective means of tracing the source of microbial contamination as it differentiates between closely related micro-organisms, making possible precise identification of individual strains.

DNOC

Dinitro-ortho-cresol, a yellow crystalline substance employed in agriculture as a weed-killer spray solution, acts as a powerful cumulative poison. In man the symptoms are excessive sweating, thirst, and loss of weight. Poisoning in domestic animals might well be encountered following contamination by the spray or residue.

DNP

Dinitrophenol, a product somewhat similar to DNOC.

Dobermann Pinscher

A medium-sized, muscular dog with smooth hair, most often black. The ears are naturally pendulous. The breed originates in Germany and is often used as a police or guard dog. It can be affected by Von Willebrand's disease, cervical spondolithesis ('wobbler syndrome') and polyostic fibrous dysplasia (bone cyst).

Docking

Docking is removal of the tail or a part of it. In Britain, docking of the horse (excluding amputation of the tail by a veterinary surgeon for therapeutic reasons) is illegal. (See also NICKING.)

Dogs Since 1 July 1993 it has been illegal for anyone other than a veterinary surgeon to dock puppies' tails in the UK. 47 of the 185 breeds registered with the Kennel Club have traditionally been docked. The RCVS has said it is unethical for a dog's tail to be docked except for therapeutic reasons. There is evidence that the docked end is more sensitive to pain than the rest of the tail. Tails are widely used in communication between dogs and between dogs and people. Dogs with docked tails cannot communicate adequately; their attitude and intentions might be misunderstood by other dogs and fighting may result. 'It is not mandatory for dogs to have their tails docked in order to be entered for Shows.' (BVA Animal Welfare Foundation.)

Sheep It is customary for sheep of lowland breeds to be docked, for if the tail is left long it accumulates dirt and faeces, and these predispose to the attacks of blow-flies. Enough tail must be left to cover the vulva, or anus in the case of the male. The use of rubber rings for docking without anaesthetic is allowed only within 48 hours of birth. (See ANAESTHETICS, LEGAL REQUIREMENTS.)

Many mountain breeds of sheep are left undocked; the long woolly tail helps to keep the hind part protected from frost and wind.

Docks, Poisoning by

Losses of sheep have been occasionally ascribed to eating either the common sorrel dock (*Rumex acetosa*) or sheep's sorrel (*R. acetosella*), both of which contain oxalates. A condition of staggering with dilated pupils, muscular tremors, and later, convulsions and prostration, has been noticed in horses which have eaten large quantities of sheep's sorrel. In sheep, there is a loss of appetite, rapid breathing, exhaustion, sometimes constipation and at other times diarrhoea, with an unsteady gait and occasionally death.

Milk of cows that have eaten docks is made into butter only with difficulty.

Dog Bites

Anti-tetanus injections should always be given in cases of dog bites. Various infections including *Pasteurella septica* infection in man can result from these. (See also RABIES, BITES.)

Dog, Feminisation of

(see SERTOLI CELL TUMOUR; also INTERSEX)

Dog, Kennels

Former kennels should not, unless they have been thoroughly cleaned and disinfected, be used for the temporary housing of lambs or goatlings; in both, deaths have followed from cysticercosis of the liver. (See TAPEWORMS; also BEDDING, HOOKWORMS)

Two sheep dogs died from dieldrin poisoning, their kennel having been washed weekly with old sheep dip.

Dog-Sitting Position

In pigs this may be a symptom of pantothenic acid (vitamin B) deficiency, or lameness due to *Mycoplasma hyosynoviae*. In the horse this position may be adopted during severe COLIC. With reference to the newborn Galloway calf, see GENETICS – Genetic defects. Re lambs, see SWAYBACK.

Dog Ticks

In Britain these include *Ixodes hexagonus* (common on suburban dogs and cats); *I. ricinus* (the sheep tick, commonly found on country dogs); *I. canisuga* ('the British dog tick'); and *Dermacentor reticulatus* (which may infest also cattle and horses). *I. canisuga* may establish itself in buildings, as may *Rhipicephalus sanguineus*, which has infested houses in Denmark as well as quarantine stations. Modern central heating may facilitate the survival of this tick in northern latitudes. In a house in England, a sitting-room sofa, and a bedroom chair used by a dog, were infested. This tick may arrive in travellers' luggage. Hedgehogs are a source of *I. hexagonus*.

Dogs, Breeds of

The reader is advised to consult textbooks on this subject. (See also WILD DOGS.)

Dogs' Diet

Most owners wisely feed their animals on a mixed diet, offering some variety and at the same time providing the essential nutrients. It is a misconception that dogs should be fed only on meat. However, some owners appear to believe that red (muscle) meat, cooked or raw, is a complete food for dogs and cats. It is not, since it does not provide, for example, enough calcium. Cooked meat should be mixed with biscuit meal or pasta, potatoes or vegetables, and fed at room temperature. Most dogs like one or other of the proprietary biscuits.

Dogs should be fed at regular times, once or twice a day; any food left uneaten should be removed. Fresh water should be available always. A bone, or one of the proprietary substitutes, is useful to exercise the jaws and help keep the teeth healthy.

Proprietary dog foods are very widely used nowadays; they may be moist (canned), semi-moist (packeted) or dry. Major manufacturers have carried out extensive research on the dog's nutritional needs and when fed according to their recommendations such prepared diets are perfectly adequate for the normal dog.

Any marked change in an animal's feeding or drinking habits may be an indication of disease; a veterinary surgeon should be consulted. Specially formulated diets are available for a wide range of disorders (for example, diabetes or kidney disease); they are prescribed by a veterinarian as necessary. (See also PET FOODS.)

Dogs, Diseases of

Several are listed under the prefix CANINE. Others include bacterial diseases such as brucellosis, 'kennel cough', salmonellosis, leptospirosis, tetanus, and tuberculosis. For skin diseases, see ECZEMA; MANGE; RINGWORM; HOOKWORMS; ATOPIC DISEASE. Other canine diseases are referred to under the following headings: RABIES; PARALYSIS; PYOMETRA; FUNGAL DISEASES; BLACK TONGUE; CANCER; LEUKAEMIA; CAMPYLOBACTER; ANAEMIA; ANTHRAX; AUJESZKY'S DISEASE; BOTULISM; ORF; CHLAMYDIA; CHOREA; CRAMP; CUSHING'S DISEASE; DIABETES; DIARRHOEA; HIP DYSPLASIA; HYDATID DISEASE; HYSTERIA; MYASTHENIA GRAVIS; PARASITES; TGE; TOXOPLASMOSIS; YERSINIOSIS; SPOROTRICHOSIS; COCCIDIOSIS; (See also under the various organs and tissues, e.g. HEART, EYE, PANCREAS, PROSTATE, KIDNEY.)

Dogs' pharyngeal injuries are often caused during retrieving, or playing with, sticks thrown by the dog's owner. These injuries can be avoided if a rubber 'bone' or ring is substituted for the sticks. (A rubber ball can also be used, provided that it is too big for the dog to swallow.)

Dogs, Mortality

Larger breeds of dog tend to have a higher mortality rate than smaller, according to insurance statistics. A Swedish survey based on more than

220,000 animals found that mortalities in Irish wolfhounds were 9 times greater than in the soft-coated wheaten terrier.

Dogs (Protection of Livestock) Act 1953

Dogs (Protection of Livestock) Act 1953 provides that the owner and also the person at the time in charge of a dog, which is worrying livestock on agricultural land, are guilty of an offence. The owner will not, however, be convicted if s/he proves that the dog was, at the time, in the charge of a fit and proper person other than him or herself.

Amendments to the 1953 Act made by the Wildlife and Countryside Act 1981 made it an offence for a dog to be at large in a field or enclosure where there are sheep unless it is on a lead or otherwise under close control. There are exceptions for a dog owned by, or in the charge of, the occupier of the field or the owner of the sheep or a person authorised by either of these; or a police dog, guide dog, trained sheep dog, working gun dog or a pack of hounds. This requirement applies only to fields or enclosures where there are sheep and not, therefore, to open hill areas.

Dogs, Transport by Air

This is governed by the Live Animal Board Regulations of the International Air Transport Association (IATA) 1989. In addition, any requirements of the various regulations governing the import and export of dogs must be observed.

Greyhounds are usually transported by air between Ireland and England in wooden kennels similar in size to greyhound racing starting traps.

A study of 12 greyhounds showed that stress varied greatly as between individuals. They were transported either in the wooden kennels or in wider Perspex kennels. These were stowed either in the belly hold or in the main cargo hold of jet freighter aircraft. Stress was greater in the belly hold.

Dogs, Working

(see also SHEEPDOGS). Working dogs include also guide dogs for the blind, hearing dogs for the deaf, avalanche rescue dogs, and dogs as predictors of human epilepsy. (The way in which some dogs can detect the imminence of fits in people is as yet unknown. Further investigation is being undertaken in Canada and the USA. The service is a valuable one, because it allows the epileptic time to get to a safe place, and to take appropriate medication; or for the dog to warn the person's family.)

Huskies are used in the Arctic for transport purposes (and bred back to wild wolf stock every few generations). Refuse collection is yet another service performed by dogs, and was introduced in Milan, Italy. In a demonstration, dogs were shown picking up plastic and soft drink cans; and 1 bitch learned to alert her handler by barking when she found a hypodermic syringe on the ground.

Dogs are widely used by customs authorities and police in the detection of cannabis and other substances. Trained 'sniffer dogs' can detect drugs concealed in packing cases, etc.

Dogs, Worms in
(see WORMS)

Dolichocephalic Skull

Dolichocephalic skull is one which is long and narrow, as distinct from one which is short and broad. Examples of the former are skulls of the greyhound and collie, and of the latter (brachycephalic), those of the pug and bulldog.

Dominant

That member of an allelic pair of genes which asserts its effects over the other dissimilar member (recessive) of a gene pair.

Donkeys

Descendants of the wild ass, donkeys are grey or sable in colour; they are widely used as beasts of burden in some countries. Their life-span in Turkey, Egypt, Tunisia, Ecuador and Peru is only 11 years. In the UK the figure is 37 years. (The Donkey Trust, Sidmouth, Devon.)

They are spared many of the leg and joint troubles common in the horse, but are very prone to lungworm infestation. This may not give rise to symptoms such as coughing, but the lungworms may lower the donkey's resistance to strangles and equine influenza, from which more young donkeys die than young horses. Donkeys often constitute a source from which horses become infested with lungworms. (See PARASITES.)

For gestation period, see under PREGNANCY. (See also JENNY; HINNY; MULE.)

Dopamine

Dopamine is involved in the transmission of 'messages' in the central nervous system. Early-weaned piglets which develop the 'vice' of nose-rubbing show evidence of decreased dopamine production in the brain.

Dopamine hydrochloride can be useful in overcoming the effects of anaesthesia with halothane, which depresses the cardiopulmonary system of horses.

Doppler
(see ULTRASOUND)

Dosing Injuries
(see DRENCHING; also X-RAYS – Ordinary radiography)

Double Muscling
Also called muscular hyperplasia or myofibre hypoplasia. An inherited conformation in which there is an increase in muscle fibres with a corresponding decrease in fat, as seen in Charolais and Belgian Blue cattle. It can give rise to dystokia; double-muscled cattle are more likely to develop respiratory problems or muscular dystrophy.

Double Pregnancy
A term applied to the existence of 2 sets of fetuses, of different ages and born with a corresponding interval between litters, in the sow, cow, etc. (See SUPERFETATION.)

'Double Scalp'
A condition seen in older lambs and young sheep, mainly on hill grazings, in autumn and winter. There is unthriftiness associated with a thinning of the bones of the skull. The cause is believed to be related to phosphorus-deficient pastures.

Dourine
Dourine is a venereal disease of horses, donkeys and mules caused by *Trypanosoma equiperdum* which is NOTIFIABLE throughout the European Union. Imported horses have to be declared free from the infection. It occurs in Africa, Asia, parts of Europe, and in areas in both North and South America. (See TRYPANOSOMES.)

Transmission appears to be by coitus only, and is spread by 'carriers' which themselves show no symptoms.

A discharge from vulva or penis may be the 1st symptom, followed by oedema of the genital organs, with the swellings extending forward along the abdomen. Fever, loss of condition, and painful micturition may be observed. A few weeks later chancres may be seen on the flanks and elsewhere, lasting for a few hours or sometimes days. Later the animal becomes weak, loses weight, may be lame or have paraplegia, and dies.

Identification of 'carrier' animals is of great importance in controlling and eradicating the disease, and depends on the complement fixation test (though this presents difficulties in areas where other trypanosomiasis occur). In most countries slaughter is obligatory.

Treatment Quinapyramine or suramin are medications used against trypanosomes.

Control (see TSETSE FLIES)

'Downer Cow' Syndrome
Sometimes in cases of 'milk fever' (parturient paresis, hypocalcaemia) a cow goes down and never gets up again, even though the 'milk fever' itself is treated successfully. The critical factor may be the length of time the cow is recumbent with one hind leg (usually the right) underneath her body. If that time extends to 6 hours or more, there may be permanent muscle or nerve damage to that leg. Nerve damage may be the factor determining whether a recumbent cow becomes a downer. It has been suggested that slight differences in body position can account for the fact that some animals suffer nerve damage but not others.

If a cow is found recumbent and showing signs of milk fever, the animal's position should be changed so that tissue damage can be minimised while veterinary aid is awaited. If the cow is in close, cramped quarters, with a floor not providing a good grip, she should be moved to a better place. This can be achieved by sliding her on to a large piece of plywood, which can be used as a sledge.

An inflatable bag, attached to a rigid base, and inflated by an air compressor, is marketed for lifting a cow on to its feet. The device is placed under the body of the cow (or the cow is dragged onto it); the animal is helped to rise as the bag inflates.

The syndrome may arise from a wide range of conditions; all the following have been implicated: metabolic disorders, such as hypocalcaemia, hypomagnesaemia, hypophosphataemia, hypokalaemia, and bloat; toxaemia, associated with mastitis, metritis, peritonitis, and aspiration pneumonia; rupture of uterus, reticulum, abomasum, and traumatic pericarditis; other injuries, such as a fractured pelvis, displacement of the sacrum, obturator or sciatic nerve paralysis, dislocation of the hip, and rupture of muscles (e.g. adductor, gastrocnemius).

About half of all downer cows get up within 4 days. After 10 days the prognosis is poor, but there have been cases of cows rising to their feet after 2 or 3 weeks, or even a month.

Doxapram
A respiratory stimulant used to aid recovery from general anaesthesia or in neonates after a caesarian section or a difficult birth.

Doxorubicin

An anthracycline anti-tumour antibiotic which is effective in treating certain types of cancer in cats and dogs. It can cause severe side-effects and must only be used under specialist supervision.

Dracunculiasis

(see GUINEA WORM)

Drenching

The giving of liquid medicine to animals by a bottle or a drenching gun. It must be done slowly, and with care, in all animals if the medicine is to be effective. The fluid must be directed over the back of the tongue to avoid some of the dose going straight into the abomasum. Pneumonia is a common sequel to liquid medicines 'going the wrong way'.

Another danger is associated with the use on pigs of a drenching gun intended for sheep. Unless these appliances are used with care, severe injury may result. In a series of cases reported in Australia, 24 pigs suffered rupture of the pharyngeal diverticulum – part of the throat – and 12 died. In sheep, rupture of the oesophagus has been caused.

Dressed Seed Corn

Any surplus should **not** be fed to farm livestock owing to the danger of poisoning. Pigs have been accidentally killed in this way after being given corn treated with mercury dressing. Dieldrin dressings kill birds.

Dried Grass

Dried grass has for long been incorporated by compounders into feeding-stuffs for poultry and pigs, but is also fed to dairy cows as part of a ration together with some roughage (straw, hay, silage) and some other concentrate feed, such as barley. Dried green crops are also fed on a small scale to sheep and beef cattle.

The dried grass can be either milled and made into pellets or cubes; or left unmilled and pressed into cobs or wafers, which saves the high cost of hammer-milling. Unmilled material may have other advantages, too, for it has been shown that hammer-milling and pelleting decrease the digestibility of the product and, while increasing the efficiency with which digested nutrients are used by non-lactating animals, depress butterfat production of those in milk.

The hardness of the pellets and cobs is an important factor; if too hard, they can give disappointing results. Particle size is also important.

Minimum protein content of dried grass for use without supplementary protein is considered to be 18 per cent; minimum digestibility figure about 60 per cent. Crude protein analysis is of little help in indicating digestibility. This (and hence energy equivalent) mainly determines milk production, not protein.

Work at the Grassland Research Institute and in Northern Ireland suggests that dried grass is as good as, or slightly better than, barley as a supplement for silage. Fed with cereals and minerals, dried grass has successfully provided a standard feed for MLC Bull Performance Tests, giving an average daily liveweight gain of 1.5 kg (3.3 lb) over the 200-day test, with individual gains well over 1.8 kg (4 lb).

Drinking Water

(see WATER)

Droncit

The trade name of a Bayer preparation used in dogs and cats against tapeworms, and for *Echinococcus* eradication schemes. The active ingredient is praziquantel. Preparations are available for oral dosing and also for subcutaneous and intramuscular injections.

Dropped Elbow

(see RADIAL PARALYSIS)

Dropped Sole

(see LAMINITIS)

Dropsy

(see OEDEMA)

Dropwort Poisoning

(see WATER DROPWORT)

Droughtmaster

A breed of cattle developed in Australia from Brahman and British (mainly Shorthorn) ancestors. It is claimed to be 10 times more tick-resistant than British breeds, and a more efficient beef producer under the relatively harsh grazing conditions of North Australia.

Drowning

Submersion in water for a period of about 4 minutes is sufficient to cause asphyxia and death, but shorter periods, while they may cause apparent death, usually only produce a collapse from which recovery is possible. Practically all animals, even the very young, are able to swim naturally, so that immersion in water for this period does not necessarily result in drowning. Animals falling into water are drowned from one of several causes: they may be exhausted by struggling in mud; they may be carried away by a swift current, e.g. during floods; they may be hindered by harness or other tackle from keeping their nostrils above the level of the water; or they may become panic-stricken and swim away from shore. Remarkable instances of the powers of swimming that are naturally possessed by animals are on record; one example being that of a heifer, which, becoming excited and frightened on the southern banks of the Solway Firth, entered the water and swam across to the Scottish side, a distance of over 7 miles, and was brought back the next day none the worse.

Recovery from drowning As soon as the animal has been rescued from the water, it should be placed in a position which will allow water that has been taken into the lungs to run out by the mouth and nostrils. Small animals may be held up by the hind-legs and swung from side to side. Larger ones should be laid on their sides with the hindquarters elevated at a higher level than their heads. If they can be placed with their heads downhill, so much the better. Pressure should be brought to bear on the chest, by one person placing all their weight on to the upper part of the chest wall, or kneeling on this part. When no more fluid runs from the mouth, the animal should be turned over on to the opposite side and the process repeated. No time should be lost in so doing, especially if the animal has been in the water for some time. (See ARTIFICIAL RESPIRATION.)

After-treatment As soon as possible the animal should be removed to warm surroundings and dried by wiping or by vigorous rubbing with a rough towel. Clothing should be applied, and the smaller animals may be provided with 1 or more hot-water bottles. The danger that has to be kept in mind is that of pneumonia, either from the water in the lungs or from the general chilling of the body, and the chest should be especially well covered. Sometimes the ingestion of salt water leads to salt poisoning in dogs, or to a disturbance of the digestive functions, and appropriate treatment is necessary.

Drug Interactions

For those in which one drug enhances the action of another, see SYNERGISM.

Adverse drug interactions or reactions are indicated by manufacturers in the product data sheet. Unexpected adverse reactions should be reported to the manufacturer or the Veterinary Medicines Directorate.

Drug Residues in Food

Drug residues in food are regarded as very important from the point of view of public health. The permitted maximum level of drugs remaining in meat, milk or eggs after medicines have been administered (maximum residue limit [MRL]) is specified by regulation for all EU countries. The manufacturer's recommended withdrawal period between the last dose of drug administered and the animal going for slaughter, or the milk or eggs being sold for human consumption, must be observed. Carcases in abattoirs are monitored to ensure that the residues are within allowable limits.

(See also HORMONES IN MEAT PRODUCTION; MILK – Antibiotics in; SLAUGHTER.)

Drug Resistance

(see under ANTIBIOTIC RESISTANCE; DIPPING; FLY CONTROL)

Drugs, Disease Caused by

(see IATROGENIC DISEASE)

Dry Eye

(see EYE, DISEASES OF)

Dry Feeding

Dry feeding of meal may give rise to PARAKERATOSIS in pigs; to 'CURLED TONGUE' in turkey poults; and to 'SHOVEL BEAK' in chicks.

Dry, Firm and Dark (DFD)

Dry, firm and dark (DFD) describes the meat of animals that have undergone stress in transport before slaughter. The condition is a result of glycogen depletion in the body. The meat's acidity is reduced but it is safe for consumption.

Dry Period

In cattle it is considered advisable on health grounds that after a period of lactation, cows should not be milked for about 8 weeks – the dry period. Cows are dry in the weeks before calving.

Drying-off Cows

After milking out completely, the teats should be washed and a dry-cow intramammary preparation inserted in each teat. The cows should be inspected daily.

If possible, keep the cows on dry food or very short pasture for 3 days after drying off.

Drysdale

A sheep with a very good fleece bred in New Zealand. A natural mutation of the Romney, it was identified and developed by Dr F. W. Dry of Massey University.

Dubbing

Trimming of the comb imay be performed, with scissors, by poultry keepers, and involves removal of a crescent of comb about 1.5 mm ($^1/_{16}$ inch) deep – in day-old chicks. It is credited with increasing egg production by 3 to 4 per cent per year. It is also advocated in intensive rearing, where a floppy comb may be a disadvantage if pecking and cannibalism are rife; and in order to reduce the risk of frost-bite. Dubbing can not be recommended from a welfare point of view; it is a cause of stress and an unnecessary mutilation.

Duck Virus Enteritis (Duck Plague)

The disease is caused by a herpesvirus. It appeared for the first time (so far as is known) in the UK in 1972 among birds on ornamental waters, not on commercial duck farms. One entire group of 72 Muscovy ducks died within 16 days.

Symptoms, which may not be observed before death occurs, include listlessness and very severe diarrhoea, drooping of wings, and a disinclination to take to water. Adult mortality may be high.

Prevention is by vaccination of healthy birds at 4 weeks of age.

Duck Virus Hepatitis

A virus infection which causes up to 90 per cent mortality among ducklings under 3 weeks of age, but in ducklings a month or more old losses are less. Duck strains resistant to the virus can be bred. A vaccine, administered at 1 day old to susceptible ducklings, has proved effective in most cases although mutant strains can arise in which the vaccine is ineffective (as in Norfolk in the 1960s). It is a NOTIFIABLE DISEASE. It should be suspected in cases of sudden death if the ducklings' heads are stretched upwards and backwards.

Research at the Animal Health Trust has shown that the fatty kidney syndrome can be reproduced in ducklings following infection with virulent duck hepatitis virus alone. Only birds which are dying or dead show the accumulation of lipid in the convoluted tubules of the kidneys.

Ducks, Septicaemia in

Two forms occur, one due to *E. coli* and one to *Pasteurella anatipestifer*.

The former may occur in ducklings 4 to 8 weeks of age. The latter infection causes losses in ducklings under 4 weeks old. Vaccines may prove the most effective method of control.

Ductless Glands

(see ENDOCRINE GLANDS)

Ductus Arteriosus

This connects the left pulmonary artery to the arch of the aorta. (See diagram of fetal circulation under CIRCULATION OF BLOOD.) If the duct remains open after birth, it is regarded as a congenital abnormality. (See HEART DISEASES; also LIGAMENTUM ARTERIOSUM for the remains of the duct in the normal animal.)

Dulaa

A reddish, balloon-like organ arising from the soft palate of male camels, it fills with air from the trachea when the nostrils are closed. The dulaa is blown out of the mouth during rutting.

Dung-Fouled Pasture

(see PASTURE MANAGEMENT)

Dung Heaps

To minimise the possibility of active infection persisting in dung, new dung should be buried under the older. Under natural fermentation conditions a temperature of 70° C can be reached, which will pasteurise the dung. Dung heaps should be fenced off as they are a source of parasites.

Duodenum

Duodenum is the 1st part of the small intestine immediately following the stomach. Into it open the bile and pancreatic ducts. (See INTESTINE.)

Dura Mater

Dura mater is the outermost and the strongest of the three membranes or meninges which envelop the brain and spinal cord. In it also are found the blood vessels that nourish the inner surface of the skull. (See BRAIN.)

Duraznillo Blanco

A poisonous plant of South America. (See ENTEQUE SECO.)

Duroc

A breed of pig, varying in colour from a light golden-yellow to a very dark red, originating in the eastern states of the USA.

Dusting Powders

Dusting powders form a convenient application for wounds in animals. They may be used for an antiseptic effect, to control infection, or for astringent and protective effects to dry up superficial lesions and encourage scab formation. Various active ingredients, in an inert base, are incorporated according to the intended use.

Dusting powders containing parasiticides are used to destroy fleas and lice on animals.

Dusty Atmosphere
In piggeries, this can be a cause of coughing, etc., simulating pneumonia. (See MEAL FEEDING.) Inoculations should not be carried out in a dusty shed. (See ANTHRAX.) Material in dust may give rise to an allergy (see BROKEN WIND) and to abortion if fungi are present (see UTERINE INFECTIONS).

Duvenhage
A rhabdovirus causing a disease similar to rabies. It is carried by fruit bats, which are widely distributed in Africa.

'Dwarf Tapeworm' (*Hymenolepis nana*)
This parasite sometimes completes its life-cycle in a single host (e.g. man or rodent), and sometimes the eggs are ingested by fleas or flour-beetles. Human infestation may follow the eating of contaminated food or, accidentally, a flea.

Dynamite
Poisoning from this has occurred in cattle and sheep in the USA, after they have found mislaid or discarded sticks of the explosive. They apparently relish its taste. Poisoning is due to its nitrate content. (Gelignite, a type of dynamite, could be expected to be similarly toxic.)

Dys-
Dys- is a prefix meaning painful or difficult.

Dysautonomia
A malfunction of the autonomic nervous system, such as occurs in 'grass sickness' in horses, and which is virtually always fatal. Signs include slowness of the heartbeat in dogs and cats. A similar condition has been described in wild hares in Great Britain and it has even been suggested that they could be the carriers of 'grass sickness'. (See also CANINE DYSAUTONOMIA; FELINE DYSAUTONOMIA.)

Dyscrasia
Any disease condition; it usually relates to an imbalance of component elements as in blood dyscrasia, which is a term for any pathological condition of the blood.

Dysentery
Dysentery is a condition in which blood is discharged from the bowels with or without diarrhoea. Dysentery is most commonly encountered in certain specific diseases such as anthrax, cattle plague, haemorrhagic septicaemia, purpura haemorrhagica, lamb dysentery, swine fever, and swine dysentery. It may occur when there are large numbers of strongyle worms or coccidiae present in the bowels. Dysentery in young pigs may be due to *Clostridium welchii* infection, which causes death within 36 hours of birth. (See also SWINE DYSENTERY; HAEMORRHAGIC GASTROENTERITIS OF PIGS.)

Dysphagia
A difficulty in swallowing. (See 'CHOKING'; BOTULISM; RABIES; MYASTHENIA GRAVIS; also, for one cause in horses, see under GUTTURAL POUCH DISEASE.) (See also 'GRASS SICKNESS'; DOGS' PHARYNGEAL INJURIES; ABSCESS; FOREIGN BODY; ACHALASIA.)

Dysplasia
Absence of some part of the body (but see HIP DYSPLASIA IN DOGS).

Dyspnoea
Abnormal, difficult or laboured breathing (see BREATHLESSNESS, RESPIRATORY DIFFICULTY).

Dystokia, or Dystocia
This means difficulty during parturition. (See PARTURITION; CALVING, DIFFICULT.)

Dystrophy
(see MUSCULAR DYSTROPHY)

Dysuria
An absence of or difficulty in excreting urine.

E. Coli

Escherichia coli, formerly known as *Bacillus coli*, is a normal inhabitant of the alimentary canal in most mammals. This bacterial family is a large one, comprising many differing serotypes which can be differentiated in the laboratory by means of the agglutination test. Only a few serotypes cause disease. However, *E. coli* infections can be severe and have become sufficiently prevalent for a range of vaccines to be developed for protection against the most common pathological strains in farm animals. (See also DIARRHOEA; JOINT-ILL; COLIFORM INFECTIONS.)

Sheep *E. coli* scours and septicaemia are common in newborn lambs and often fatal. Vaccines are available for protection and antisera may be used for treatment.

Pigs One serotype gives rise to oedema of the bowel; another to the death of piglets within a few days of birth.

Those strains of *E. coli* which cause diarrhoea in piglets only a few days old are able to do so because they are covered with an adhesive coat known as the K88 antigen. This enables them to adhere to the wall of the intestine where they induce disease by means of toxins, causing diarrhoea, dehydration, and death.

E. coli toxins are classified as (a) heat labile (LT), which may cause severe diarrhoea, dehydration and death of piglets; and (b) heat stable (ST) associated with only a mild enteritis.

Scouring in older pigs may often be caused by strains of *E. coli* having no K88 antigen.

The K88 antigen and related antigens can be prepared in the form of a vaccine, formulated with *E. coli* toxoids. This is injected into pregnant sows and gilts to provide protection (passive immunity) to the piglets when they are suckled, via the colostrum, by preventing the K88-coated *E. coli* from adhering to the intestinal wall. Oral and parenteral vaccines are available.

Cattle *E. coli* is an important cause of calf enteritis, enterotoxaemia and septicaemia, and of mastitis. Combined antiserum preparations, vaccines, and antisera-vaccine combinations are available.

Poultry Coliform septicaemia is a frequent cause of loss, and one difficult to control since infected birds are disinclined to eat or drink, which hinders drug administration.

Dogs *E. coli* is perhaps the most important pathogen of the bladder and urethra; it also causes enteritis.

Horse (see FOALS, DISEASES OF)

Public health A strain of *E. coli*, 0157, has been associated with outbreaks of disease in humans. Animals that carry this toxic strain do not usually show any signs of clinical disease and shedding of the organism by animals is erratic, making detection difficult. Young children and the elderly are most susceptible to the disease. In the mild form there is blood-tinged diarrhoea. Some of those cases will go on to develop haemorrhagic diarrhoea and a number develop neurological disease that is fatal. Following an outbreak involving more than 50 persons who had eaten contaminated meat, an investigation led by Professor Hugh Pennington of Aberdeen University resulted in a series of recommendations for good hygiene practices.

Ear

Sound is appreciated through the mechanism of the outer, middle, and internal ears. Sound waves are collected by the funnel-like external ear (pinna) and transmitted down into an external canal, across the bottom of which is stretched the ear-drum or tympanum against which these waves strike. Their impact causes a vibration of the tympanum, and the sound wave becomes transformed into a wave of movement. This movement is transmitted through a chain of tiny bones, called auditory ossicles, in the middle ear, and then to fluid contained in canals excavated in the bone of the internal ear. The vibration of this fluid stimulates the delicate hair-like nerve-endings which are found in the membranous walls of the canals, and impulses pass to the brain, whereby an animal is able to appreciate external sounds literally by feeling them.

Structure The middle and inner ears are essentially the same in all animals, but the external ears present certain differences in different species. (See also AURAL CARTILAGE.)

External ear

Horses The ears serve to some extent as an indication of the state of the horse's emotions –

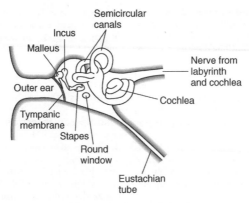

Outline of the structure of the ear.

anger or viciousness being shown by laying the ears flat back against the head, and surprise, anticipation, or pleasure being indicated by 'pricking' the ears. At the base of the ear a complete cartilaginous tube is formed, and this leads into the bony canal or external auditory meatus.

Middle ear The tympanic membrane, forming the 'drum', is stretched completely across the outer passage at its innermost extremity.

The cavity of the middle ear is a compartment excavated in the hard mass of the petrous part of the temporal bone which lodges the ossicles. These are the small auditory bones which carry impulses across its cavity and are called the malleus (hammer), incus (anvil), and stapes (stirrup). The Eustachian tube admits air from the throat, and so keeps the pressure on both sides of the tympanum equal.

Horses have a diverticulum (guttural pouch) of the Eustachian tube. (See GUTTURAL POUCH and GUTTURAL POUCH DISEASE.)

Internal ear This consists of a complex system of hollows in the substance of the temporal bone enclosing a membranous duplicate. Between the membrane and the bone is a fluid known as perilymph, while the membrane is distended by another collection of fluid known as endolymph. This membranous labyrinth, as it is called, consists of 2 parts: the posterior part, comprising a sac, called the utricle and 3 semicircular canals opening at each end into it, is the part concerned with the preservation of balance; the anterior part consists of another small pouch, the saccule, and of a still more important part, the cochlea, and is the part concerned in hearing. In the cochlea there are 3 tubes, known as the scala tympani, scala media,

and scala vestibuli, placed side by side (the middle one being part of the membranous labyrinth), which take 2½ spiral turns round a central stem, somewhat after the manner of a snail's shell. In the central one (scala media) is placed the apparatus known as the organ of Corti, by which the sound impulses are finally received, and by which they are communicated to the auditory nerve, which ends in filaments to the organ of Corti. The essential parts of the organ are a double row of rods and several rows of cells furnished with hairs of varying length.

The act of hearing The main function of the movement of the ears is that of efficiently collecting sound waves emanating from different directions, without the necessity of turning the whole head, although in some animals the ears may be flicked to dislodge flies.

When sound waves reach the ear-drum, the latter is alternately pressed in and pulled out; the movements being communicated to the auditory ossicles.

These movements are then transferred to the perilymph in the scala tympani, by which in turn the fluid in the scala media is set in motion. Finally these motions reach the delicate filaments placed in the organ of Corti, and so affect the nerve of hearing, which conveys the sensations to the auditory centre in the brain.

Ear, Diseases of

Diseases of the ears of animals should never be neglected, for although in the early stages most are amenable to treatment, in the later stages treatment is likely to be more difficult.

Inflammation of the outer ear (otitis externa) may be found in one or both ears. It is often due to the presence of a foreign body (a grasshopper in one case), parasites or bacterial infection.

The signs include shaking the head, often persistently for a few moments at a time, scratching, rubbing head rotation with the affected ear lowered, and a foul-smelling discharge.

Scratching the ears is also a symptom of ear-mange mite (*Otodectes*) infection of the external ear canal. (See MITES – Mange in dogs and cats, for first-aid and treatment of *Otodectes*.)

Other forms of mange may start at the ears and involve the pinna, e.g. psoroptic mange, notoedric mange.

Discharge from the ear, or the presence of pus within, is a sequel to a neglected case of parasitic otitis in the dog and cat and due to secondary infection by bacteria and/or moulds.

Excessive wax in the ear often leads to disease later. It is especially common in dogs which have large pendulous ear flaps, when ventilation is poor.

In some cases, dressing the inner parts of the ear is difficult or impossible because of the thickening and perhaps distortion. For these an operation, in which the cartilages at the lower parts are opened or resected, has been devised. Operation may also be needed where deep-seated ulceration of one or other of the aural cartilages has occurred, and even the mere initial cleaning of a very inflamed and painful ear must be done under an anaesthetic.

Foreign bodies, such as hay seeds, sand, pieces of glass, wood, peas, or parasites, may become lodged in the ears of animals and give rise to irritation occurring very suddenly.

Haematoma is common in dogs and in cats which are affected with ear mange, but it may occur in almost any animal. A large fluctuating swelling appears upon the flap of the ear and causes the animal to hang its head towards the same side. In many cases little or no pain is experienced once the swelling has appeared, and, in fact, a small swelling becomes larger in many cases through the continued shaking of the head even after its original formation. The swelling is caused by bruising of the skin and the blood vessels which lie between it and the cartilage, with a consequent extravasation of blood or serum under the skin. The condition is treated by opening the haematoma under conditions of surgical cleanliness, evacuating the fluid contents, and suturing the skin in such a way that the collection of more fluid is prevented.

Wounds of the flaps of the ears are usually caused by bites, or from barbed wire, etc., in the larger animals. The comparatively poor blood supply to the AURAL CARTILAGES means that, if torn or lacerated, necrosis may occur. In dogs it may be necessary to secure the ear-flaps by means of surgical adhesive tape, or a head-cap improvised to give several 'tails' which can be tied.

Deafness (see under this heading)

Middle-ear infection (otitis media) is always serious as it may lead to MENINGITIS. It is often found on one side but both ears may be affected. Signs are similar to those of external ear inflammation but the balance can be affected; there is swaying of the hind quarters and the head is carried abnormally. It may be caused by spread of external ear infection or by an infection carried in the blood.

Inner-ear infection (otitis interna): signs are – the head is often rotated; the animal may walk in circles and show a stumbling, swaying gait.

Tumours are occasionally found. Warts are not uncommon in horses and cattle. In cats a polyp is occasionally found, and in white cats a squamous-celled carcinoma may affect the tip of the pinna.

Mange Psoroptic and notoedric mange often begin on the pinna of the ear; auricular or otodectic mange involves the presence of mites (*Otodectes*) within the ear canal. (See MITES.)

Fly strike A dog brought to a veterinary surgeon in Cornwall was found to have a badly infected left ear, from which came a profuse purulent discharge. On auroscopic examination, Mr D. S. Penny BVetMed was surprised to see three faces staring back at him. Under anaesthesia 18 large maggots were removed.

Ear Tags

A permanent method of identifying animals. It is the main method of legal identification of cattle. Tags are also used in sheep, goats and pigs as well as other animals. They can incorporate an insecticide (see FLIES).

Ear Tipping

Ear tipping of feral cats has been advocated by animal welfare organisations and practised in America and Denmark, for example. The idea is to identify those cats which have been spayed, and prevent any 'rescued' cat from being subjected to unnecessary anaesthesia and laparotomy.

In Australia, ear tattooing is practised for the same purpose, but has the disadvantage that the spayed feral cat cannot be identified from a distance.

Early Weaning
(see under WEANING)

Ears as Food
Ears from beef cattle which had been receiving sex hormones as implants in the ear have been fed in breeding kennels with disastrous results.

Earthing
Earthing of electrical apparatus on farms, and especially in the dairy, is occasionally faultily carried out in such a way that in the event of a short-circuit, the water-pipes supplying the cows' drinking-bowls become 'live' – leading to the electrocution of the cows. (See ELECTRIC SHOCK.)

Earthworms
Earthworms are of veterinary interest in that they act as intermediate hosts to stages in the life-history of the gape-worm of poultry (see GAPES) and of lung-worm in pigs. They may also harbour viruses which cause disease in pigs. Earthworms can live for as long as 10 years. They can often be found at night in drains outside piggeries, and in crevices and cracks in the cement inside piggeries. (See also INFLUENZA.) An ARC research team at the Rothamsted Experimental Station found that earthworms, bred in animal manure, can provide a high-quality protein supplement for pigs, poultry, and especially fish. Several species of earthworm were used, of which *Lumbricus rubellus* was the one of choice. *Eisenia foetida* (the brandling worm) is easier to farm but contains a heat-labile toxin in its skin making it unsuitable as a raw food. Ideally, earthworms should be heat-processed into meal for use in animal diets.

East Coast Fever (Theileriosis)
An acute specific disease of cattle enzootic in certain parts of Africa, especially in the eastern provinces of South Africa, in Kenya and in Zimbabwe. In these areas the native cattle attain a certain amount of natural immunity, and only imported animals are affected. Animals which recover are commonly known as 'salted', but the mortality is very high (e.g. 90 per cent) in new outbreaks of the disease. Buffaloes are also susceptible.

Cause Theileria parva, which spends part of its life-history in cattle and part in ticks (*Rhipicephalus appendiculatus*).

Signs After an incubation period of a fortnight or so, the animal becomes dull, listless, loses appetite, and runs a high fever. Lymph nodes become enlarged. There may be a discharge from eyes and nose; laboured breathing and diarrhoea may be seen.

Prevention and treatment East Coast fever may be to a great extent prevented by systematic dipping of all newly purchased cattle, and quarantining them for at least 5 weeks before they are mixed with the rest of the stock.

Where the disease has broken out on a farm, the 'short-interval' dipping system first devised by Watkins-Pitchford has proved of immense benefit in eradicating it. (See under CONTROL OF TICKS.)

Since ticks responsible for the spread of East Coast fever can live for some time on other domesticated animals, it is advisable to dip sheep, goats, and horses at suitable intervals.

Clinically ill cattle may be treated by any antibiotics that can penetrate cell membranes, such as tetracyclines.

East Friesland Milk Sheep
This breed comes from NW Germany, and in England has been used to produce the COL-BRED. East Friesland ewes average 545 litres (120 gallons) at 6 per cent butterfat in a lactation, rearing their lambs, and a yield of 1000 litres (220 gallons) is not unknown. The lambs have a high growth rate and early maturity.

'Eastrip Special Blend'
A cross between Bluefaced Leicester and Poll Dorset sheep. A high lambing percentage is claimed.

Ebola Virus
This, together with the Marburg virus, is a member of the Filoviridae.

It is, in appearance, indistinguishable from the Marburg virus, but antigenically distinct. Infection of humans is very often fatal; cases have occurred in laboratory workers handling infected monkeys. It was found in 1976 in Zaire and Sudan; 500 people became ill and 350 died. (*See under* MONKEYS, DISEASES OF.)

An outbreak of disease caused by an Ebola-related filovirus, and by simian haemorrhagic fever, occurred in 1990 at an American quarantine station among cynomolgus monkeys imported from the Philippines. It was reported that this was the first case in which a filovirus had been isolated from non-human primates without deliberate infection.

EC
(see EUROPEAN UNION)

ECG
Electrocardiogram.

Ecbolics
Ecbolics are drugs which cause contraction of the muscle fibres of the uterus, such as ergot, pituitrin, etc. They are used to induce labour.

Ecdysis
Ecdysis is the shedding of an exoskeleton in arthropods, and of the old skin in crustacea and reptiles. Failure to shed completely can lead to problems.

Echinococcosis
(see HYDATID DISEASE; TAPEWORMS)

Echium Plantagineum
A poisonous plant, also known as Paterson's Curse, or Salvation Jane, which has caused the death of many sheep from copper poisoning in South Australia. In one outbreak, 1259 sheep died out of a total of 29,715 at risk. On one farm, 500 of 3000 ewes died. Merino × Border Leicester crosses appear to be especially susceptible. At autopsy, jaundice is evident; livers are friable and enlarged or, less frequently, shrunken and fibrotic. Kidneys are swollen, soft and blackish.

The plant contains up to 10 alkaloids, and is the first to show growth after a prolonged drought.

Eclampsia
Eclampsia is a disease occurring during the later stages of pregnancy or after parturition, and characterised by loss of consciousness or convulsions, or both. It occurs in the bitch and cat. A preferable name is lactation tetany. It is associated with HYPOCALCAEMIA. (See also MILK FEVER; FITS.)

Ecraseur
A surgical instrument used for castration of the larger domestic animals. Haemorrhage is largely prevented by crushing of the blood vessels of the spermatic cord.

Ecthyma
Ecthyma is a localised inflammation of the skin characterised by the formation of pustules. (See ACNE; IMPETIGO.)

Ecto-
Ecto- is a prefix meaning on the outside.

Ectoparasites
Ectoparasites live on the skin or the hair. (See FLEAS; FLIES; LICE; MANGE; MITES; TICKS.)

Ectopic
Ectopic means out of the usual place. An ectopic pregnancy is one in which a fetus is present outside the uterus. (See PREGNANCY, ECTOPIC.)

Ectopia cordis thoracoabdominalis A
very rare congenital abnormality characterised by protrusion of the heart to the outside of the body through a ventral body-wall fissure.

Ectromelia
Ectromelia means literally absence of a limb or limbs. The word is also used to describe a contagious disease caused by a pox virus, which affects laboratory mice, and in the sub-acute form causes necrosis of a whole limb, toe, tail or ear. Outbreaks are usually very severe at the outset, killing many of the affected mice, but later on the mortality becomes less, and the outbreak gradually fades and disappears; though a latent infection may persist.

Ectropion
Ectropion is a condition of the eyelids, in which the skin is so contracted as to turn the mucous membrane lining of the lid to the outside.

Eczema
An inflammation of the skin (dermatitis), occurring in both farm and domestic animals. Intense irritation or itchiness may accompany the acute form, and frantic licking of the affected area may exacerbate the condition. In chronic eczema there may be very little irritation.

Cats Eczema is often referred to as feline miliary dermatitis. Symptoms include reddening of the skin, with the appearance of papules (small blister-like spots) and, later, scabs. These may be easier to feel than to see. The area of skin involved may be small or large. Neck, shoulders, and back are common eczema sites. Occasionally a bacterial infection is a complication.

The most common cause is considered to be hypersensitivity to flea bites. Once a cat (seldom a young one) has become sensitised to flea saliva, the presence of only a single flea on the cat's body is sufficient to cause the allergic reaction.

Other allergies may produce eczema; for example, a 'hay-fever' type (see ATOPIC DISEASE), or a food allergy of some kind. Cat foods containing colouring agents or preservatives are sometimes involved. Skin contact with some chemicals should also be considered. It is likely that among some breeds or strains there is a family predisposition to eczema.

Treatment involves flea removal; the veterinarian may prescribe a change of diet, a vitamin supplement, megestrol acetate, an antihistamine, etc.

Dogs The causes, symptoms and treatment of eczema are similar to those described above. The disease is more common in dogs, however, and an acute form often involves the skin between the toes, resulting in constant licking. Other sites are around the eyes, and the scrotum.

First-Aid Calamine lotion may be applied if precautions can be taken to prevent its being immediately licked off.

In a few cases what a dog-owner assumes to be eczema may prove to be mange; a professional diagnosis should always be obtained.

Horses A common cause of eczema is sensitisation to midge-bites. (See 'SWEET ITCH' for preventive measures.)

Cattle and sheep Some cases of eczema affecting white-haired areas of skin are the result of LIGHT SENSITISATION. Overseas this condition is often referred to as 'facial eczema' and follows sensitisation to sunlight following the eating of certain plants.

Edema
Edema is another spelling of oedema.

Edta
Ethylenediamine tetra-acetic acid. Its salts (edetates) are chelating agents which are used to treat poisoning by heavy metals. For example, calcium edetate is used in cases of lead poisoning. Non-clinically, sodium edetate is used as an anticoagulant for blood samples.

Efferent
Efferent is the term applied to vessels which convey away blood or a secretion from a part, or of nerves which carry nerve impulses outwards from the nerve-centres.

Effluent
Liquid waste from an abattoir or slurry (see SLURRY; DAIRY HERD MANAGEMENT).

Egg-Bound
Egg-bound is the condition in laying poultry in which an egg (or eggs) may be formed in the oviduct, but the hen is unable to discharge it. The bird shows obvious discomfort, stands straining and pressing. A dose of liquid paraffin (2 ml) may be tried.

Egg Eating
Among intensively housed poultry, this may be a vice or sign either of boredom or of pain.

Egg Yield
In Britain, the average is approximately 130 eggs per bird per year. An annual yield of 200 is obtained in well-managed batteries; about 190 on deep litter; 170 in fold units. A Honegger has laid 305 in 350 days.

Ehlers-Danlos Syndrome
(see CUTANEOUS ASTHENIA)

Ehrlichia Canis
Ehrlichia canis, 'or a closely related species', has been identified in human patients who had recently been bitten by ticks. They were suffering from fever, rigors, myalgia, and gastroenteritis. Tests showed leukopenia and thrombocytopenia.

Ehrlichiosis
Infection with species of *Ehrlichia*, a rickettsia. *E. risticii* is one cause of abortion in mares. *E. chaffeensis* is a cause of human ehrlichiosis.

Canine ehrlichiosis has as its vector the brown dog tick. (See TICK-BORNE FEVER OF CATTLE.)

Eicosanoids
Arachidonic acid, a polyunsaturated fatty acid present in most body cells of domestic animals, can be oxidised to the prostaglandins, prostacyclin, thromboxanes and leukotrienes. These compounds, collectively known as the eicosanoids, are involved in inflammatory and allergic conditions; in reproductive and perinatal processes; with platelet aggregation and vascular homeostasis, kidney function, fever, and certain tumours; and with other normal and disease conditions.

Eimeria
(see COCCIDIOSIS)

Elaphastrongylus
A genus of nematode found in deer. *E. cervi* locates in the central nervous system; *E. panticole* in the brain; and *E. rangiferi* in the muscles and central nervous system.

Elastic Bands
(see RUBBER BANDS)

Elastrator

An instrument used to stretch a strong rubber ring so that it may be placed over the neck of the scrotum for the purpose of castration.

Elbow

Elbow is the joint formed between the lower end of the humerus and the upper ends of the radius and ulna.

Electric Fences

(see under PASTURE MANAGEMENT)

Electric Shock, 'Stray Voltage' and Electrocution

Faulty electrical wiring and earthing have led to drinking-bowls, water pipes, mangers, etc. becoming live. In some instances this has led to the death of cows from electrocution following a short circuit.

'Stray voltage' In one incident this led to cows refusing concentrates in the parlour – not because they were unpalatable, as at first thought, but because cows wanting to eat were deterred by a mild electric shock.

This 'stray voltage' has been associated with intermittent or unexplained periods of poor performance, increased milking time, and 'an increased prevalence of mastitis'. 'Stray voltage' was detected in 32 out of 59 dairy farms in Michigan, following investigations requested by dairymen or veterinarians.

Electrocution Deaths from electrocution may occur outside buildings. In one case 30 cows and heifers were found dead beneath an electric pylon. It seems that the cattle had used a metal stay as a rubbing 'post', which had become loose and then come in contact with the high-voltage lines that the pylon was carrying.

Pigs Metal troughs becoming electrically live led to 20 pigs becoming paralysed after a severe thunderstorm in England. Injuries apparently resulted from panic and crushing. In another case 22 out of 32 pigs in one pen were found piled up around the trough, close to which was a burnt-out live wire. The carcases were bloated and the skin bluish. Additional post-mortem findings may include external burns, numerous haemorrhages affecting many internal organs, black unclotted blood, congestion/oedema of the nervous system, and fracture of lumbar vertebrae or of the pelvis. In pigs, rupture of the urinary bladder may occur.

Horses A New York insurance agency has stated that 0.96 per cent of its claims in respect of the death of horses were for lightning strike, and 0.27 per cent for electrocution.

In Canada a veterinarian was asked to call to see a horse which appeared to be suffering from colic. On arrival at the farm he was told that the animal had died minutes after he had been telephoned. Earlier the same day, the owner explained, a mare in foal had died instantly in the same spot in front of a small barn; and another had died there too. Suspecting electrocution, she had switched off the barn's power supply.

Subsequently an inspector found that the builder of the barn had made a serious mistake when carrying out the electrical work, so that what was supposed to be the earth line was anything but safe. The situation had become more dangerous after recent excavation in front of the barn, where the earthing plate had been accidentally dug up and replaced horizontally across the path to the barn. The horses had died on the first wet day after the work was completed; but their owner recalled that previous to that they had shied or tended to bolt when passing the spot.

Dogs and cats Electrocution is not uncommon, and almost invariably results from puppies or kittens chewing through the insulation of electric wiring (e.g. of vacuum-cleaner, table-lamp, etc.). Burns to the mouth and lips are seen; a tan to grey discoloration is noticeable. Oedema of the lungs may be caused, with dyspnoea. In a survey of 26 dogs treated for electrocution, 16 survived and were discharged from hospital within 2 or 3 days. Mortality rate for all the dogs in the survey was 38 per cent. (See EUTHANASIA.)

Lightning strike Cattle, sheep, and horses are most often affected. Usually death occurs instantly, and the animal is often found with a bunch of grass between its teeth. Usually, but not invariably, there are external scorch marks, with subcutaneous lesions beneath. The other signs are as those given above under 'Electrocution'.

Static electricity can build up on equipment made from materials such as plastics. In one incident, turkeys refused to eat because of a build-up of static electricity on the chain feeders which gave the birds a shock when they attempted to feed. The situation was detected when it was noticed that wood shavings were attracted to the feeders where the chains were operated. Earthing the feeders removed the problem.

Electrocardiogram (ECG)

Electrocardiogram (ECG) is a record of the variations in electric potential which occur in the heart as it contracts and relaxes. This record is obtained by placing electrodes on either side of the chest wall or on the two forelegs, the skin being first wetted with salt solution. These are then connected to an electrocardiograph, which records the pattern of the heart's activity. The normal electrocardiogram of each heartbeat shows 1 wave corresponding to the activity of the auricle, and 4 waves corresponding to the phases of each ventricular beat. Various readily recognisable changes are seen in cases in which the heart is acting in an abnormal manner, or in which one or other side of the heart is hypertrophied. This record, therefore, forms a useful aid in many cases of cardiac disease.

Electrocardiography has been described as a useful aid to pregnancy diagnosis in the mare – 'where thoroughbred mares more than 5 months pregnant are presented for sale' (see under TWINS); and also for monitoring heart rate during anaesthesia.

Electrocautery

Electrocautery is useful for operations where space is restricted, such as removing small tumours, etc. in mouth, nose, or throat, and to check haemorrhage in the deeper parts of wounds. Also sometimes for disbudding. (See also CRYOSURGERY.)

Electrocution

(see under ELECTRIC SHOCK)

Electrolyte

Any compound which, in solution, conducts an electric current and is decomposed by it. (See under FLUID REPLACEMENT THERAPY; NORMAL SALINE; DEHYDRATION.)

Electrolyte Solutions

Electrolyte solutions contain sodium, potassium and other electrolytes in an ISOTONIC formulation. They are used, often with plasma substitutes or other additives, in restoring the body fluid volume in cases of shock, diarrhoea, injury and other conditions.

Electron Microscope

These instruments have made it possible to study and photograph viruses, bacter-iophages, and the structure of bacteria. Instead of light, the electron microscope uses a beam of electrons to scan the specimen. This is prepared as an extremely thin film and subjected to a high degree of vacuum. The electron image is focused on a video screen and may be recorded photographically or electronically. Magnification may be up to ×300,000, and by means of photographic enlargement and the use of projection slides a total magnification approaching ×1,000,000 can be achieved.

Electrophoresis

The movement of particles in a fluid under the influence of an eleric current. It is used, e.g., in the analysis of blood or serum constituents which form visibly identifiable patterns in a starch gel to which current is applied.

Electrotherapy

High-frequency currents are mainly used to produce muscular contractions as an aid to muscular re-education following injury or during transient paralysis. It can also be used for passive exercise when an animal is suffering from certain neurological conditions. The technique is painless and no control measures are necessary. Animals must not, however, be excited during periods of therapy, which vary between 5 and 20 minutes per day. Some chronic skin conditions may be controlled by this method. Where movement of painful joints or tendons is required, or where there is neuritis, administration of painkillers or use of nerve blocks by local anaesthetic may be considered.
Diathermy is a modified form of high-frequency current therapy in which warmth is induced deep in the tissues.
Repetitive stimulation is produced by cardiac pacemakers; these have been used in small animals and in horses.
Faradism is the use of electric currents to treat certain muscle, tendon and joint conditions, mainly in horses. It has also been used in working elephants.
(See also X-RAYS; IONIC MEDICATION; IONTOPHORESIS; CANCER.)

Electuary

Electuary is a soft paste made by compounding drugs with treacle, sugar, or honey. It is used as a convenient method of applying medication to the throat and pharynx of animals. To relieve sore throat in the horse, an electuary of extract of belladonna, potassium chlorate, and aniseed, made up into a paste with treacle, was formerly much used. The electuary is applied by means of a flat stick, and is smeared upon the back of the tongue and upon the teeth.

Elephants

(see MUSTH; SPEED OF ANIMALS). The height to the shoulder of the Asian elephant (*Elephas maximus*) is about 3 metres (10 feet); that of the African elephant (*Loxodonta africana*) 3.5 metres (13½ feet).

Elephants, Diseases of

These include anthrax (sometimes brought on by the breaking of a tusk where the disease has lain dormant in the dental pulp), multiple abscesses, blackleg, botulism, elephant pox, enzootic pneumonia, foot-and-mouth disease, influenza, myiasis, parasitic gastroenteritis, pasteurellosis, rabies, salmonellosis, steanofilarial dermatitis, schistosomiasis, surra, tetanus, trypanosomiasis, tuberculosis. Elephants imported into Great Britain may serve out their quarantine period for foot-and-mouth disease on board the ship transporting them.

ELISA

ELISA is the abbreviation for the system of enzyme-linked immunosorbent assay, developed by the Swedish scientists Engvall and Perlmann. ELISA tests are widely used in laboratories for the rapid detection of pathogens.

Elizabethan Collar

Often improvised from cardboard, the shape of a lampshade, and designed to fit over the dog's head and to be attached to its collar, with the object of preventing the animal from

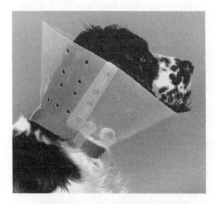

This Elizabethan collar is a transparent version, easy to adjust to the dog's neck diameter. An excellent way of preventing the canine patient from interfering with wounds, skin lesions, or dressings.

interfering with wounds, skin lesions or dressings. The illustration shows a proprietary version.

Elk

A species of large deer also called the wapiti (*Cervis elaphus*); the European elk is *Alces alces*; the American moose *A. americana*. This farmed animal was found to be a source of tuberculosis in people in Alberta, Canada, in 1990. *Mycobacterium bovis* was isolated.

Elkhound

A medium-sized dog with thick grey-black coat, pointed ears and a bushy tail curled over the back; it originated in Scandinavia. Inherited traits include progressive retinal atrophy, renal cortical hypoplasia and hip dysplasia.

Emasculator

An instrument to remove the testicles in horses, cattle and sheep. Most crush the spermatic cord to prevent haemorrhage as well as severing the testicle from it.

Embolism

The plugging of a small blood vessel by blood-clot fragments originating from elsewhere in the body, and carried along in the bloodstream. Bacteria, worm larvae, air-bubbles, and fat are other causes of embolism. The importance of the embolism depends upon the situation. In the brain it may cause apoplexy; in other organs, the area that was supplied by the little vessel before it became blocked by the embolism ceases to function, and if the blood supply is totally cut off it dies, or degenerates, becoming an 'infarct'. (See also GLASS EMBOLISM; THROMBOSIS; CATHETER EMBOLUS.)

Embrocations

(see LINIMENTS)

Embryo

(see EMBRYO TRANSFER; EMBRYOLOGY; FETUS)

Embryo Transfer

The technique of transferring an embryo from one animal and implanting it in the uterus of another has become a widely used method, particularly in cattle, of improving breed quality and herd reproductivity. Basically, the technique involves the collection of embryos from one cow (the donor), 7 to 8 days after insemination, by flushing out the uterus with a special medium such as phosphate-buffered saline. The donor cow is prepared by administering gonadotrophins to cause superovulation, the production of multiple eggs and therefore multiple embryos. The embryos are collected and transferred surgically, or non-surgically by a method similar to artificial insemination, to the recipient cow which must be at exactly the same stage of oestrus as the donor. Embryos may be preserved by deep-freezing and thawed for use when required.

A number of firms operate commercial embryo transfer services; success rates of up to 70 per cent are achieved.

Embryo transfer is also used in sheep and goats; it is possible, but little used in practice, in mares and pigs. (*See* illustration on page 162.)

The advantages of embryo transfer have been summarised as follows: (1) increased number of offspring from valuable females; (2) rapid progeny testing of females; (3) induction of twinning; (4) the investigation of causes of infertility; (5) transport of cattle ova from one state or country to another; and (6) an increased rate of genetic improvement.

Development The technique had already in the 1950s been successfully carried out in sheep – ewes having produced young of which they were not, in the full sense, the mothers; and it was extended to cattle later, by L. E. Rowson and colleagues at Cambridge, who were responsible for much of the research.

Development of a method of freezing the embryos greatly widened the scope of embryo transfer. Fertilised 10- to-13-day eggs (blastocysts) are treated with a protective agent (dimethylsulphoxide) to prevent damage by freezing and cooled to –196°C; they are then stored in liquid nitrogen until required for implantation.

The technique Five days before oestrus is due, the donor animal is treated with pregnant mare's serum gonadotrophin (PMSG) or a similar gonadotrophin to produce superovulation. When oestrus occurs, insemination is carried out 2 or 3 times, using fresh rather than frozen semen.

Surgical transfer On day 6, when the eggs are at the morula stage, consisting of 8 to 32 cells each, and looking under the microscope like blackberries, they are flushed out of the Fallopian tube. This may be done surgically or nonsurgically. In the former, a fine catheter is inserted through a blunt needle after surgical exposure of the uterus by means of a flank incision, the cow being under local anaesthesia. It may be possible to recover 8 to 12 ova, and an attempt is made to select the normal ones. (For example, by culturing them for 1 or 2 days after recovery. In that time further development will have occurred; eggs which do not show this are discarded.) The transfer is made by puncturing

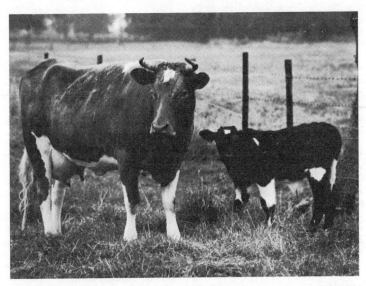

Transplantation. As a 7-day embryo, this calf was stored for a month at a temperature of –196°C before being transferred, non-surgically, to the recipient cow seen in the photograph. (ARC.)

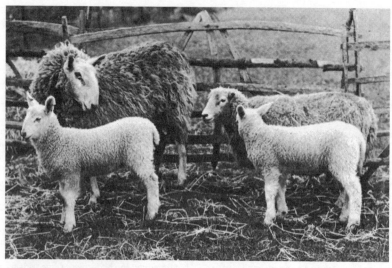

Twins from different mothers. One of 2 eggs was removed from the Border Leicester ewe and transplanted into the Welsh ewe.

one horn of the anaesthetised recipient's uterus with a small pipette containing one ovum in a synthetic medium. This liquid is forced out of the pipette, carrying the ovum with it.

Non-surgical transfer The eggs are collected by means of a 2- or 3-way catheter having an inflatable cuff. The catheter is passed through the cervix and into one of the horns of the uterus which is then sealed by inflating the cuff. Fluid is flushed into the horn and withdrawn through the catheter, with the eggs. The technique for transfer into the recipient cow is similar to artificial insemination. An egg is placed into a 'straw' and the embryo introduced into the uterine horn by means of an insemination 'gun'. With skilled operators, the results by this method are comparable with surgical collection and without the trauma of a surgical operation. This method is commonly used in the dairy industry.

The first inter-species transfer of embryos was carried out in 1979 at the Thoroughbred Breeders' Association's equine fertility unit at Cambridge. This resulted in a pony mare foaling a donkey (gestation period about 346 days or about 15 days longer than for a foal), and 2 donkeys giving birth to pony foals (born after 346 and 361 days' gestation period, respectively). (See PLACENTA.)

Embryology
Embryology is the study of the development of the embryo within the body of the female.

Embryotomy
The section and removal of a fetus in the uterus to facilitate parturition; most commonly undertaken in cattle and sheep.

Emesis
Emesis means VOMITING.

Emetine
Emetine is one of the alkaloids of ipecacuanha.

Emphysema
An abnormal presence of air in some part of the body. The term is applied to the presence of air in the subcutaneous tissues following a wound but, more commonly, to 2 abnormal conditions of the lungs: destructive (vesicular) emphysema and interstitial emphysema.

Destructive (vesicular) emphysema is a condition of the lung characterised by an abnormal enlargement of the air spaces, accompanied by destructive changes in the alveolar wall. This condition occurs in dogs with chronic bronchitis and in horses with chronic obstructive pulmonary disease (see 'BROKEN WIND'). Emphysema is irreversible and may progress to respiratory failure and death. The main symptom is respiratory distress on exertion, with a marked expiratory effort.

Interstitial emphysema Air is present in the connective tissue of the lung – a state of inflation of the interstitial (interlobular) tissue. The air is found in the lymphatics, under the pleura in the interlobular septa, and around blood vessels, sometimes in the form of large bullae 10 cm or more in diameter. Air may track as far as the hilum of the lung and gain access to the mediastinum from where, in exceptional circumstances, it may even spread to subcutaneous connective tissue – usually in the shoulder region or over the upper part of the chest.

Interstitial emphysema is a common condition in cattle, especially in association with parasitic bronchitis (HUSK) or with 'FOG FEVER'. Increased effort, in response to obstructed airways, over-exertion and violent struggling, causes a marked increase in pressure within the alveoli. Rupture then occurs, allowing air to escape into the interstitial tissue on inspiration, but impeding its leaving on expiration. When the lung lobules become surrounded by interstitial emphysema their ability to inflate during inspiration is restricted, and this may lead to respiratory distress.

Empyema
A collection of purulent fluid within a cavity. (See PYOTHORAX; PLEURISY.)

Emu
A large flightless bird, *Dromaius novae-hollandiae,* native to Australia. It is farmed in Britain but to a lesser extent than the ostrich. Severe enteritis resulting in death of up to 65 per cent of a flock has occurred in the USA from infection by eastern equine encephalitis virus. This is a NOTIFIABLE DISEASE throughout the EU.

Enamel
The very hard substance found on the external surface of the crowns of teeth (see TEETH).

Enarthrodial Joints
Enarthrodial joints are those of the ball-and-socket type which allow movement in nearly any direction. Examples include the shoulder joint between the scapula and the humerus; and the hip joint in which the nearly spherical head of the femur fits into the cup-shaped cavity called the acetabulum on the pelvis.

Encephalitis
Encephalitis is inflammation of the brain. It may be brought about through the activity of bacteria, such as those of strangles and listeriosis, but especially during infection with viruses, such as those of rabies, canine distemper, etc. (See BOVINE SPONGIFORM ENCEPHALITIS.)

Signs Symptoms of encephalitis include fever, excitement, delirium, convulsions, paralysis, and loss of consciousness. Several symptoms are common to MENINGITIS. (See also SLEEPER SYNDROME.)

First-Aid Keep the animal quiet – in a darkened room if showing excitement – and avoid noise or handling the patient.

Encephalitozoon Cuniculi
An intracellular protozoal parasite. It develops in macrophages, brain, kidney and other tissues of rabbits, dogs, rodents and primates.

In carnivores, severe nephritis, encephalitis and a high mortality are associated with transplacental infection.

In a Norwegian outbreak, 1500 blue fox cubs died (33 per cent of the litters), although the parents showed no signs of infection.

In the UK, foxhound puppies have died, and in Tanzania 2 spaniel puppies died which had shown rabies-like signs.

Diagnosis An ELISA test. In one study, 51 positive samples were identified out of 248 sera from stray dogs.

Encephalomalacia
A group name for the degenerative diseases of the brain. Causes include the copper deficiency of swayback, horse-tail and bracken poisoning, metallic poisoning, and mulberry heart disease of pigs. Another example of encephalomalacia is 'crazy chick' disease.

Encephalomyelitis
Inflammation of both the brain and the spinal cord.

Encephalomyelitis, Viral, of Pigs
This term covers the group of diseases known as Teschen disease, Talfan disease, and *Poliomyelitis suum.*

Believed to have originated in the former Czechoslovakia, viral encephalomyelitis of pigs is now encountered throughout most of Europe. In Britain and Denmark, only a small percentage of pigs become infected, and illness is far milder than in some other countries.

Symptoms include fever, stiffness, staggering gait, paralysis, and those of encephalitis.

Encephalomyocarditis Virus
Encephalomyocarditis virus is a picornavirus. Antibodies have been found in the serum of more than 28 per cent of normal pigs in the

UK. It is also a pathogen of rodents and human beings, and has caused outbreaks of illness in pigs in Australia, the USA, and Panama.

Enchondroma
A tumour formed of cartilage. (See TUMOURS.)

Encysted
Enclosed in a cyst.

Endangered Species Act 1982
Endangered Species Act 1982 lists measures for the protection of named animals.

Endarteritis
Inflammation of the inner coat of an artery. (See ARTERIES, DISEASES OF.)

Endemic
An endemic disease is one present in an animal population at all times.

Endo-
Endo- is a prefix meaning situated inside.

Endocarditis
Inflammation of the smooth membrane that lines the inside of the heart. It occurs especially over the heart valves. (See HEART DISEASES.)

Endocrine Glands
Endocrine glands are those which secrete hormones. (See HORMONES; also under the name of individual endocrine glands, e.g. ADRENAL, THYROID, PARATHYROID, PITUITARY, THYMUS, PANCREAS.)

Endometritis
Inflammation of the mucosal lining of the uterus (endometrium) (see UTERUS, DISEASES OF).

Endorphins
Morphine-like, natural analgesics produced in the body. Acupuncture is said to stimulate their release into the bloodstream. (See also TWITCH.)

Endoscope
An instrument used for viewing the interior of an organ, and for facilitating the extraction of a foreign body, e.g. from the oesophagus; and for assistance with other surgery, including embryo transfer. (See also LAPAROSCOPY.)

Endothelium
Endothelium is the membrane lining various vessels and cavities of the body, such as the pleura, pericardium, peritoneum, lymphatic vessels, blood vessels, and joints. It consists of a fibrous layer covered with thin flat cells, which render the surface perfectly smooth and secrete the fluid for its lubrication.

Endotoxins
Endotoxins are those toxins which are retained within the bodies of bacteria until the latter die and disintegrate.

Endotracheal Anaesthesia
(see ANAESTHESIA)

Endotracheal Tube
A tube introduced into the trachea to prevent its collapse; used in endotracheal anaesthesia.

Endrin
A highly toxic insecticide of the chlorinated hydrocarbon group. It has caused fatal poisoning in cattle, dogs, fish, and birds.

Enema
The introduction of fluid into the rectum to assist evacuation of faeces.

Energy
(see CALORIE; CARBOHYDRATES; METABOLISABLE ENERGY; JOULES)

English Springer Spaniel
Long-eared, medium-sized dog with silky coat, brown and white or black and white; originally bred as a gun dog. Retinal dysplasia, entropion, cutaneous asthenia and haemophilia may be inherited conditions.

Enrofloxacin
Enrofloxacin is a quinolone antibacterial active against a wide range of Gram-positive and Gram-negative organisms. As it may affect the development of load-bearing articular cartilage, it should not be administered to growing animals.

Ensilage
(see SILAGE)

Enteque Seco
A wasting disease of cattle, sheep and horses. It occurs mainly in Argentina, but also in Uruguay and possibly Brazil. It may be identical with Manchester wasting disease (Jamaica) and Naalehu disease (Hawaii).

Cause A plant, common on wet land, known as duraznillo blanco (*Solanum melacoxylon* or *glaucum*). Poisoning may arise from deliberate eating of the leaves or from the accidental consumption of dead, fallen leaves during grazing of the underlying pasture plants. It is particularly dangerous when growing in association with white clover.

It produces an arteriosclerosis, with calcification in heart, aorta, lungs, etc. Blood levels of calcium and phosphorus tend to be high as *S. malacoxylon* contains a potent metabolite of vitamin D.

Signs Emaciation occurring over weeks or months, and an abnormal gait.

Enteralgia
Enteralgia is another name for colic.

Enteritis
Inflammation of the intestines (see DIARRHOEA and INTESTINES, DISEASES OF).

Enterocele
(see HERNIA)

Enteroliths
Enteroliths are stones that develop in the intestines, being formed by deposition of salts round a hard metallic or other nucleus. (See CALCULI.)

Enterostomy
Enterostomy means an operation by which an artificial opening is formed into the intestine.

Enterotoxaemia
An acute disease of calves, lambs, goats, and occasionally of piglets and foals.

Cause Toxins emanating from the intestines and present in the bloodstream. The toxins involved are from 4 strains of *Clostridium welchii* and from some strains of *E. coli*.

Signs Severe enteritis, with dysentery in some cases, and sudden death in others.

Prevention A vaccine is available.

Calves seldom survive for more than a few hours.

Goats show a sudden drop in milk yield, dysentery, and death within 36 hours. There is also a subacute type of the disease lasting 7 to 10 days, and followed by recovery.

Sheep The disease affects both unweaned lambs and sheep 1 to 2 years old.

Enteroviruses
A group of smaller viruses pathogenic to animals and causing disease in cattle, pigs and ducks (duck hepatitis).

Entropion
The turning in, or inversion, of an eyelid. It can be congenital or acquired and is inherited in some breeds of lambs and dogs. It is very common in 'mini-pigs' (see EYE, DISEASES OF).

Enuresis
(see INCONTINENCE)

Environment
(see HOUSING OF ANIMALS; PASTURE MANAGEMENT; EXPOSURE; RAINFALL; ALTITUDE; HEATSTROKE; ANHIDROSIS; TROPICAL DISEASES; VENTILATION; CALF HOUSING)

Enzootic
Enzootic refers to a disease present (endemic) among animals in a particular region, country, or locality. For example, braxy and louping-ill are enzootic in the south and west of Scotland and the north of England. Compare EPIZOOTIC (epidemic), in which a disease spreads rapidly through large numbers of animals over a wide area.

For enzootic abortion of sheep, see under ABORTION, ENZOOTIC.

Enzootic Bovine Leukosis
(see BOVINE LEUKOSIS)

Enzootic Haematuria
A disease typically found in old suckler cows following the long-term ingestion of bracken. It results in various cancer problems of the bladder.

Enzootic Muscular Dystrophy
A disease in calves, lambs and foals caused by vitamin E and selenium deficiency. Acute cases may drop dead after exercise; mild cases are weak and breathe with difficulty.

Enzootic Ovine Abortion
Enzootic ovine abortion is caused by *Chlamydia psittaci*. (See under ABORTION, ENZOOTIC.)

Enzootic Nasal Granuloma
Obstruction of the nasal cavities of cattle by an eosinophilic granuloma. More common in Channel Island breeds.

Enzootic Pneumonia of Calves
Acute pneumonia usually seen in calves between 2 and 4 months old; it is caused

by environmental and management changes as well as viral, mycoplasmal and bacterial infections.

Enzootic Pneumonia of Pigs

This was formerly described as virus pneumonia of pigs (VPP), but the cause is now generally regarded as being *Mycoplasma hyopneumoniae*. However, other organisms may be involved to a varying degree. (See RESPIRATORY INFECTIONS OF THE PIG; SYNERGISM.)

Many pigs reaching the bacon factories are affected with some degree of pneumonia, so that the matter is of the very greatest economic importance.

Signs When the disease is first introduced into a herd, pigs of all ages (from 10 days upwards) go down with it, and many die. Where the disease is already present, deaths are few. Symptoms, which may easily be overlooked or ignored, then consist merely of a cough. There is, in addition, a certain degree of unthriftiness which in extreme cases may amount to stunted growth. In all cases one may expect the liveweight gain to be reduced. Sometimes pigs which contract the disease earlier in life quite suddenly develop acute pneumonia at 19 to 26 weeks of age, known as 'secondary breakdown'. Affected animals lose their appetite and often become prostrate, breathing rapidly with a temperature over 40.5°C (105°F). A number die if left untreated, but the majority have a fluctuating fever for a few days and then recover.

Prevention Vaccination at 1 to 10 weeks of age and management measures such as avoiding buying-in infected stock. Litters are best kept in arks on pasture, and any sows showing a cough eliminated. Weaned pigs should not be brought into a fattening house where pigs with pneumonia are present. (See DUSTY ATMOSPHERE; SWINE INFLUENZA.)

Diagnosis Confirmed by a complement fixation test.

Treatment Macrolide antibiotics, administered on a herd or individual basis, help to control the severity of outbreaks.

Enzootic Pneumonia of Sheep

(see PASTEURELLOSIS; PNEUMONIA OF SHEEP)

Enzymes

Enzymes are complex organic chemical compounds which facilitate or speed biochemical processes in the animal body, including those of digestion. Some enzymes are also produced by the normal bacterial inhabitants of the intestinal canal. Each has a specific use in splitting up proteins, carbohydrates, fats, or crude fibre. The best known are the ptyalin of saliva and diastase of the pancreatic juice, which break down starches into soluble sugars; pepsin from the gastric juice and trypsin from the pancreas, which break complex proteins into simple amino acids; and lipase in the intestines, which attacks fats. (See DIGESTION.) Enzymes are used in the cleaning of badly infected wounds. (See STREPTODORNASE.)

Some enzymes detoxify poisons, breaking them down into relatively harmless compounds. The differing susceptibility of cat and dog, for example, to phenol is due to the former animal lacking a particular enzyme which the dog has. (See TAURINE.)

Some enzymes are injurious (see under THIAMIN).

(See also BLOOD ENZYMES, and CREATINE KINASE for enzymes used in diagnosis.)

Eosinophil

Eosinophil is the name given to white cells in the bloodstream containing granules which readily stain with eosin, a histological dye. The nucleus of this leukocyte is lobular. Eosinophils, basophils, and neutrophils are collectively known as polymorphonuclear leukocytes. As well as these circulating cells, eosinophils are found in the pituitary and pineal glands.

In a normal horse, 2.5 ml^3 (1 cu in) of blood contains between 5 and 8 million eosinophil white cells – compared with about 160 million other white cells, and 128,000 million red cells.

Eosinophils increase in numbers during certain chronic infections and infestations with parasites. They contain hydrolytic enzymes. 'Unlike neutrophils, eosinophils have low phagocytic capacity and are not good at killing microorganisms.' (*Lancet.*) (See BLOOD.)

Eosinophilia

Eosinophilia means that an abnormally large number of eosinophils are present in the bloodstream. This may occur during severe parasitic infestation in horses and dogs, in certain wasting conditions, and in disease of the lymph system.

Eosinophilic Granuloma

A complex in cats. The name covers at least 3 different lesions, of a chronic nature.

Eosinophilic ulcers usually occur on the upper lip, or commissure of the lips, gums, palate, pharynx and tongue. Reddish-brown in colour, they have raised edges. They are not malignant (compare 'rodent ulcer' in man which is a basal cell carcinoma).

Eosinophilic plaques may occur anywhere on the body but are most common on the abdomen and inside of the thigh. The plaques are red, with raised edges, and ulcerate. They are extremely itchy.

Linear granulomas are seen mainly on the hind legs and in the mouth, and are yellowish-pink in colour. Itching is not usually present. As with the ulcers mentioned above, females seem more prone to this granuloma than are males. In the mouth, lesions are 'more nodular' and have to be differentiated from bacterial or mycotic infections and also carcinoma.

Eosinophilic Myositis
(see under MUSCLES, DISEASES OF)

Eperythrozoon Felis
A blood parasite found in cats in Britain, and first reported in 1959. (See FELINE INFECTIOUS ANAEMIA.)

Eperythrozoon Parvum
A blood parasite of the pig, which gives rise to fever, anaemia, and sometimes jaundice. It can be transmitted from pig to pig by lice. It occurs in Britain and the USA. Other species of this parasite affect sheep, and cattle in Africa. In the UK *E. wenyoni* has been isolated from anaemic cattle. (See also HAEMOBARTONELLA.)

Ephedrine
Ephedrine is an alkaloid derived from the Chinese plant *Ma Huang*, or prepared synthetically. It stimulates the heart and central nervous system, and relaxes the bronchioles. It has been used for asthma in dogs.

Ephemeral Fever (Three-Day Sickness)
An acute, infectious, and transient fever accompanied by muscular pains, and lameness which has a tendency to shift from limb to limb. The disease was first described in South Africa in 1867 and has been seen in Africa, Asia and Australia. Considerable economic loss has been caused among beef and dairy cattle in northern and eastern Australia.

Cause A rhabdovirus. The disease is sudden in onset and attacks a large percentage of the cattle in affected districts, taking the form of an acute epizootic; then, in a few weeks, it dies down again as quickly as it arose. The disease is transmitted by insects, including *Culicoides* midges. The incubation period is 2–10 days.

Signs The disease is ushered in by a suddenly occurring rise of temperature which may reach 41.6°C (107°F). This is accompanied by loss of appetite, cessation of rumination, rapid respirations, a quick and full pulse (which, however, may become very weak later), and a staring coat. The affected subject stands with head down. The attitude of the patient is rather characteristic, the 4 legs being placed far under the body and the back arched, suggestive of the position of a horse suffering from laminitis. There may be a discharge from eyes and nose.

In milking cows, the milk yield is much diminished. Many animals prefer to lie down rather than remain on their feet, and once down are most reluctant to get up again. The symptoms along with the elevated temperature continue like this for about 3 days – hence the name. There is usually a considerable loss of condition.

In Australia the mortality is seldom more than 0.5 per cent.

Prevention Vaccines may be available in some areas.

Epi-
Epi- is a prefix meaning situated on, or situated outside of.

Epidemic
A disease affecting a large number of individuals at the same time in the same area. The term is strictly applied to man, not animals.

'Epidemic Tremors'
'Epidemic tremors' is the colloquial name for a virus disease of poultry characterised by an unsteady gait. (See AVIAN ENCEPHALOMYELITIS.)

Epidemiology
The study of disease as it affects groups of animals. It can be used in predicting the pattern of an outbreak and in making plans to control the spread. International reporting services, as carried out by WHO and OIE, play their part; and the use of computers has greatly assisted the statistical analysis on which epidemiology relies.

Epidermis
The outer layer of the SKIN.

Epididymis

Epididymis is a structure situated within the scrotum and in which the sperms mature after leaving the testicle. It has 3 parts: the head (capus epidiolysis), the body (corpus) and the tail (cauda).The epididymis has as its outlet the vas deferens. (See TESTIS.)

Epididymitis

Inflammation of the epididymis. (See also under RAM.)

Epididymitis and 'Epivag' (Vaginitis, Contagious)

A venereal disease of cattle and sheep in Kenya and Southern Africa, and an important cause there of infertility and sterility.

Cause Possibly a double infection with a virus and a mycoplasma; possibly a campylobacter. In sheep, *Brucella ovis* is responsible (not in the UK).

Signs There may be a yellowish discharge from the vagina, or merely a redness of the mucous membrane. In the bull, enlargement of the epididymis occurs over a period of months.

Control Slaughter of infected bulls, and use of AI.

Epidural Anaesthesia

Epidural anaesthesia is a form of spinal anaesthesia induced by the injection of a local anaesthetic solution into the epidural space of the spinal canal. The technique is used, for example, in bovine obstetrics – the injection being made between the 1st and 2nd coccygeal vertebrae. (See also ANAESTHESIA; ANALGESICS.)

Epigastrium

Epigastrium is the region lying in the middle of the abdomen, immediately over the stomach. (See ABDOMEN.)

Epiglottis

Epiglottis is a leaf-like piece of elastic cartilage covered with mucous membrane, which stands upright between the back of the tongue and the entrance to the glottis, or larynx. It plays an important part in the act of swallowing, preventing solids and fluids from passing directly off the back of the tongue into the larynx.

Epiglottic entrapment in the horse is diagnosed more and more frequently due probably to the wider use of endoscopy and greater expertise in its use. Affected horses have a history of decreased exercise tolerance and they make abnormal inspiratory and expiratory noises.

Epilepsy

Epilepsy is a chronic nervous disorder characterised by a sudden and complete loss of consciousness, associated with muscular convulsions. This is particularly a disease of the dog, although other domesticated animals may be affected. Epileptic fits in the horse were formerly called megrims.

Cause The cause of primary or idiopathic epilepsy is a genetic one, whereas secondary epilepsy may be caused by trauma, neoplasia, infections, cardiovascular disease, or metabolic conditions.

The disease can be controlled completely in about one-third of affected dogs, and considerably improved in another third.

Secondary epilepsy may be the result of a head injury, and can occur whenever scar tissue is formed in the brain.

(See also FITS; HYSTERIA; ENCEPHALITIS; POISONING; HEART DISEASE.)

Signs Attacks usually commence without any warning. The limbs are sometimes held out rigidly, and sometimes moved as if the animal were running or galloping. The animal champs its jaws; the eyes are fixed and staring, or the eyeballs may roll, and the pupils are dilated. There is usually a good deal of salivation from the mouth. The rectum and the bladder are usually evacuated involuntarily. The dog regains consciousness in 1 to 2 minutes; in a few cases consciousness may not be completely lost. The 1st fit often occurs between the age of 1 and 3.

Treatment Barbiturates, phenytoin, diazepam and primidone are among drugs used for treatment. After consciousness returns, the dog should be placed in a quiet room away from other dogs or human beings. Treatment should be left to a veterinary surgeon.

Epinephrine

(see ADRENALIN)

Epiphora

Epiphora is a condition in which the tears, instead of passing down the tear-duct to the inside of the nose, run over on to the cheek. It may be due to a blocking of the tear-duct, generally from inflammation of its lining membrane following conjunctivitis, etc. or (in the smaller animals) by a grass seed. (See EYE.)

Epiphora is a symptom of naphthalene poisoning in cattle.

Epiphyseal Fracture

Epiphyseal fracture is one which occurs along the line of the epiphyseal cartilage, and results in the epiphysis of a bone becoming separated from the shaft or diaphysis. These fractures may occur in any young animals before complete ossification has occurred. (See FRACTURES; BONE, DISEASES OF.)

Epiphysis

The end of a long bone (see BONE, DISEASES OF).

Epiphysitis (Physitis)

Epiphysitis (physitis) may occur in young calves affected with joint-ill, and has been reported in adult cattle housed on slatted floors. The cattle were lame, and inflammation and necrosis were found involving the distal epiphysis of the large metatarsal bones. It also occurs in horses.

Episomes

(see PLASMIDS)

Epispastics

Epispastics are substances which produce blistering on the skin.

Epistaxis

Bleeding from the nose. (See GUTTURAL POUCH DISEASE; HAEMORRHAGE.)

Epitheliogenesis Imperfecta

An inherited condition in which there is a gap in the epithelium which readily bleeds and then heals by scar tissue. It has been seen in foals, calves, piglets, lambs, and kittens.

Epithelioma

Epithelioma is a type of malignant tumour. (See CANCER.)

Epithelium

Epithelium is the layer or layers of cells of which skin and mucous membranes are formed. The epithelial tissues take many forms. (See SKIN and MUCOUS MEMBRANE.)

Epivag

(see EPIDIDYMITIS; VAGINITIS)

Epizootic

Epizootic is a term applied to a disease which affects a large number of animals in a large area of land at the same time and spreads with great rapidity, e.g. foot-and-mouth disease and cattle

plague. It is the equivalent term to epidemic in humans.

Epizootic Cerebrospinal Nematodiasis

A disease of horses in Asia, caused by the migrating larvae of the roundworm *Setaria equina*. (See ROUNDWORMS.)

Epizootic Haemorrhagic Disease

A virus of deer; it may cause heavy mortality. The signs resemble those of BLUETONGUE in sheep.

Epizootic Lymphangitis

A chronic contagious NOTIFIABLE DISEASE disease of the horse family (Equidae). Rare cases have been recorded in cattle, and also in man.

Distribution It occurs widely in Asia, in Africa, and has also been described in America.

Cause A fungus, *Histoplasma* (*Cryptococcus*) *farciminosa*, which gains entry into the body through a wound, either on the skin or on a mucous surface. The disease is spread by flies, grooming tools, or by any materials which have come into contact with diseased animals or their infective discharges, such as cloths, sponges, and even pails of antiseptic solution.

Incubation period Under natural conditions at least 1 month, but more commonly 3 or more, may elapse from the time of contamination of a wound till the onset of the symptoms.

Signs Initial signs of the disease are often thickenings or 'cording' of a lymphatic vessel and the enlargement of the adjacent lymph nodes. A fore-limb is usually the site of the lesions, which include granulomas, nodules which discharge a creamy pus and ulcerate. Ulcers may form on the mucous membrane of the nose; occasionally on vulva or scrotum.

The disease, which runs a slow course lasting weeks or months, has to be differentiated from glanders. A few horses recover.

Treatment In the UK this is not allowed.

Epizootic Pulmonary Adenomatosis

(see under JAAGSIEKTE)

Epsom Salts

(see LAXATIVES). Epsom salts are also useful as a first-aid treatment of lead and carbolic acid poisoning.

Epulis

Epulis is a tumour of the gum (or involving the jaw bones).

Equid

(see under EQUINE)

Equine

Pertaining to the horse.

Equine Back Lesions

(see HORSES, BACK TROUBLE IN)

Equine Biliary Fever

This disease is caused by 2 distinct parasites: *Babesia caballi* and *B. equi*. The former species resembles *B. bigemina* in size and morphology, and causes a disease similar to Texas fever but which is milder and more amenable to treatment than that caused by *B. equi*. This is a smaller species than *B. caballi* and causes a disease which is highly virulent for adult horses and other species of the horse family, but is mild in young animals. Recovered animals are in a state of premunition, and inoculation of colts as a means of protection later in life is commonly practised.

Distribution The disease occurs in Russia and various parts of Europe, India, Africa, South America, and South Africa.

Signs At the beginning of the disease there is a sharp rise in temperature to about 41.5°C (107°F). During this period the parasites are multiplying in the blood. In a few days the temperature falls and anaemia sets in. In the horse this is usually masked by an intense icterus, though not in the donkey and mule. Haemoglobinuria, and constipation followed by diarrhoea, are frequent symptoms, and are succeeded by rapid emaciation. The animal may die during the initial fever (2 to 5 days) or from anaemia and emaciation about the 11th day or later. Complications are frequent.

Treatment Complete rest; an injection of a broad-spectrum antibiotic.

Transmission In Southern Europe, *B. caballi* is transmitted by *Dermacentor reticulatus* and *D. silvarum*; in South Africa *B. equi* is transmitted by *Rhipicephalus evertsi* and *R. bursa*.

Other species and genera of ticks probably act as vectors of *B. equi* in other countries.

Equine Blood Typing

Seven main blood groups are recognised in horses: A, C, D, K, P, Q and U. A further group, T, is listed by some authorities. There are numerous subgroups, or subtypes, some of which are important. For example, a mare which is Aa- must not be given blood that is Aa+ as this can lead to fetal haemocytolysis in subsequent pregnancies. For a first transfusion, blood need not be typed in an emergency as the horse rarely has natural isoantibodies. However, blood will have to be typed for any subsequent infusions; typing is also recommended if blood from a different breed is to be used.

Blood typing can be used to identify a horse's parentage but DNA 'fingerprinting' is more accurate.

Equine Coital Exanthema

A venereal disease of horses caused by a herpesvirus. (See table under HERPESVIRUS.)

Equine Contagious Metritis

(see CONTAGIOUS EQUINE METRITIS)

Equine Dysautonomia

(see GRASS SICKNESS)

Equine Ehrlichiosis

(see POTOMAC HORSE FEVER). The tentative name given to a transmissible disease of horses first recognised in California. The causal agent resembles that of tickborne fever of cattle. Oedema of the extremities is a symptom.

Equine Encephalitis

A virus disease occurring in North, Central and South America, Russia, the Far and Middle East. It affects horses, but chickens, pheasants, etc. act as a reservoir of infection. Man can be infected. Paralysis of the head and neck muscles is a feature. Mosquitoes transmit this disease, or group of diseases; the horse is an 'accidental' host. (see also BORNA DISEASE; NEAR EAST ENCEPHALITIS; VENEZUELAN EQUINE ENCEPHALOMYELITIS.) The viruses mainly responsible are the alphaviruses St Louis encephalitis (SLE), western equine encephalitis (WEE), and eastern equine encephalitis (EEE). In the Far East, the flavivirus Japanese encephalitis (JE) is the most important cause. Outbreaks usually follow a bird-mosquito cycle, with an occasional spill-over to mammalian hosts. SLE appears in humans, and WEE/EEE appear in both humans and horses. Rodents may be affected, too. The infections cannot be differentiated on clinical grounds; laboratory tests are essential. (For signs, see under ENCEPHALITIS.)

Control Mosquito control measures reduce transmission of the disease; stabling horses during outbreaks and applying insecticides can help prevent mosquito attacks. Vaccines are available for use in areas where the disease is prevalent.

Public health In man, the disease takes the form of an aseptic meningitis; outbreaks can be very serious, and mortality can be high. In one outbreak in Canada, 509 human cases were reported, with 78 deaths; 12 of them among children. Of 27 infants, many suffered brain damage, resulting in convulsions, spasticity, and hemiplegia.

Equine Filariasis
Infestation of horses with the filarid worm, *Seturia equina*, the larvae being carried by mosquitoes and biting flies. It occurs in South and Central Europe, and Asia.

Signs Malaise and anaemia, or fever, conjunctivitis, and dropsical swellings.

Equine Gait Analysis
A combination of photographic recording and computer analysis is used to study the motion of the horse's limbs as it trots or gallops on a treadmill. The system was originally devised by a Swiss, Bruno Kaegi. It helps to provide an objective measurement of the degree of lameness affecting a horse, and also a comparison between the limbs.

Equine Genital Infections in the Mare
A wide range of organisms may be found on taking cervical swabs. Some may be harmless, but others may cause abortion or disease in the mare or transmit infection to the stallion.

CONTAGIOUS EQUINE METRITIS (CEM), a NOTIFIABLE DISEASE, is an important uterine infection described in a separate entry. It is caused by *Taylorella equigenitalis*.

Other infections include beta haemolytic streptococci, *Klebsiella aerogenes, Pseudomonas* species (see also LISTERIOSIS; LEPTOSPIROSIS; BRUCELLOSIS). Fungal infections have rarely been reported, and include *Aspergillus fumigatus* and *Candida albicans*.

Abortion caused by the virus of equine rhinopneumonitis has also occurred in the UK

for several years, most outbreaks being associated with imported or visiting mares.

Equine Herpesviruses
These include EHV 1, the equine rhinopneumonitis or 'equine abortion' virus which has also caused ataxia and paresis. Primarily affecting the respiratory system, EHV1 is the cause of much illness in young horses. EHV 3 causes equine coital exanthema. (EHV 2 may be non-pathogenic.)

Equine Hydatid Disease
(see HYDATID DISEASE)

Equine Hyperlipaemia
A disease of ponies, with an average age of 9 years, affecting the liver, kidneys, and pancreas. Mortality may reach 67 per cent.

Equine Infectious Anaemia
A NOTIFIABLE DISEASE. Synonyms include: pernicious equine anaemia, swamp fever, horse malaria.

A contagious disease of horses and mules during the course of which changes occur in the blood, and rapid emaciation with debility and prostration are evident. It occurs chiefly in the Western States of America and the North-Western Provinces of Canada, as well as in most countries of Europe, and in Asia, and Africa. The first case in the UK was reported from Newmarket in 1975.

Cause A virus. The horse is commonly infected by biting insects, e.g. horse flies, stable flies, mosquitoes. Infected grooming tools if they cause an abrasion, syringes, hypodermic needles (or even contaminated vaccines) are other means of transmission. The virus may be present in urine, faeces, saliva, nasal secretions, semen, and milk.

The disease is prevalent in low-lying, swampy areas, especially during spring and summer months.

The virus may cause illness in man (who may infect a horse); also in pigs.

Signs After an incubation period of 2 to 4 weeks, equine infectious anaemia gives rise to intermittent fever (with a temperature of up to 41°C [106°F]), depression and weakness. Often there are tiny haemorrhages on the lining of the eyelids and under the tongue. Jaundice, swelling of the legs and lower part of the abdomen, and anaemia may follow. In acute cases, death is common. In chronic cases there may be a recurrence of fever, loss of appetite, and emaciation.

About 50 per cent of horses in a stud or stable may become ill with this disease, and the mortality rate can vary between 30 and 70 per cent.

Some horses do not show symptoms but become latent carriers of the infection, passing it on to others.

No treatment has so far been proved to be efficacious, and recovered animals become carriers. Vaccines are ineffective.

Diagnosis may be confirmed by the agar gel immunodiffusion precipitation (Coggins') test. Horses imported into the UK from the USA must have passed this test with a negative result. Equine infectious anaemia may be confused with other infections including trypanosomiasis, anthrax, equine rhinopneumonitis abortion, African horse sickness, the equine encephalitides, leptospirosis and piroplasmosis.

Control Where possible, test the animals and slaughter reactors in order to eradicate the disease.

Equine Influenza

A common and highly infectious disease of horses. Provided that the animals have not been worked while ill, mortality from influenza is usually nil, except in foals infected during the first few days of life. There is a danger in referring to equine influenza as 'The Cough' or 'Newmarket Cough' if those colloquialisms give rise to the idea that it is only a cough and not an illness. Owners should appreciate that influenza viruses need to be treated with respect; also that there are many other causes of coughing in horses. (See COUGH.)

Cause Viruses of the family Orthomyxoviridiae type A. A virus was first isolated in Prague in 1957; one of a similar type was isolated in the 1963 outbreak in Britain, and is now known as A/Equi/l. Also referred to as the 'Cambridge strain', it was found as well in the USA. In the 1963 outbreak in the USA another virus, believed to have come from South America, was isolated. This is called A/Equi/2 or the 'Miami strain'. This virus appeared in Britain for the first time in the 1965 outbreak.

A strain of equine influenza virus – influenza/ A/equine/Jilin (China) 1/89 – identified in the USA caused up to 20 per cent mortality in some herds. (See EQUINE RESPIRATORY VIRUSES.)

Signs The temperature rises to a degree or two above normal, or even as high as 41°C (106°F). Often the first symptom observed by the owner is the cough, initially of a dry type but later becoming moist. Coughing may last for 1 week, or persist for 3 weeks. In mild cases there may be virtually no other symptoms and – if rested – the horse makes an uneventful recovery.

In less mild cases the animal has a dejected appearance and very little appetite. Sometimes there is probably pain in the muscles, for the horse may show difficulty or clumsiness in lying down and getting up, or may appear stiff.

A foal born to a mare during an attack of influenza, or as the first symptoms are beginning to appear, will appear normal for 4 or 5 days; but then the temperature rises to 40.5°C (105°F) or more, the foal ceases to feed, and within a couple of days its breathing becomes very laboured. Death can be expected when the foal is about 9 or 10 days old.

Treatment First-aid measures call for rest, warmth and, if appetite fails, several small feeds a day. Professional advice should always be obtained. Antibiotics may be used in order to prevent any complications caused by bacteria.

When the disease has already appeared in a stable, it is wise to rely upon the thermometer rather than the cough as the first sign of infection in a horse. The temperature may occur up to 12 hours before coughing starts, and if the fever is detected early the animal can be rested with all the greater chances of the influenza remaining mild.

Prevention Vaccines prepared from a mixture of virus strains are available. It is recommended that foals born to vaccinated mares are vaccinated after 5 months of age. In-foal mares should be vaccinated at least 3 weeks before they foal. Horses should be vaccinated 3 weeks before they go to sales, etc., where they are likely to be exposed to infection. Horses entering a property or competing under the rules of the Jockey Club or Fédération Equine International must be vaccinated according to the manufacturer's instructions, certificated by a veterinarian and identified by a 'passport'. Newcomers to a stable, especially 2- or 3-year-olds, should also be vaccinated. Immunity is developed in 98 per cent of vaccinated animals within 2 to 3 weeks, and should last for about a year. Regular booster doses are essential.

Equine respiratory viruses

Some apparent 'breakdowns' in horses vaccinated against equine influenza may be due to the fact that some outbreaks of coughing are due to other infections, e.g. rhinopneumonitis.

	Equine respiratory viruses	
Virus classification	Virus	Disease produced
Myxovirus	Myxovirus influenzae A/equi 1 Myxovirus influenzae A/equi 2	Equine influenza
Picornavirus	Rhinovirus 1 Rhinovirus 2	Rhinitis; pharyngitis
Herpesvirus	Equine herpesvirus 1 and 4	Rhinopneumonitis; viral abortion
	Equine herpesviruses 2, 3, etc. ('Slow growing herpesviruses'; 'Cytomegaloviruses')	Pathogenicity uncertain; often present in the respiratory tract
Adenovirus	Adenovirus	Pneumonia and acute respiratory illness; enteritis
Paramyxovirus	Parainfluenza virus; Morbillivirus; Pneumovirus	Acute upper respiratory infection; canine distemper; rinderpest; respiratory diseases
Coronavirus	Infectious bronchitis-like agent	Acute upper respiratory infection, enteritis, etc.
Orbivirus	African horse sickness virus	African horse sickness; bluetongue
Pestivirus	Equine arteritis virus; BVD virus; Border disease virus	Equine viral arteritis; bovine viral diarrhoea /mucosal disease; border disease

Equine Lymphosarcoma

In cases involving the thoracic cavity, clinical signs may include dysphagia, inappetence, weight loss, pectoral oedema, dyspnoea, pleural effusion and distension of the jugular veins. Post-mortem examination may disclose lesions in the abdomen as well as in the chest.

Equine Motor Neuron Disease (EMND)

This was first recognised in 1990. A suspected case was seen in the UK in 1993 by researchers C. N. Hahn and I. G. Mayhew of the Animal Health Trust. Of 45 confirmed cases of the disease, none had previously been reported outside North America.

Signs Weight loss over a 6-week period, trembling, muscle atrophy, generalised weakness, head carried downwards, a short-strided gait.

Equine Myoglobinuria (Azoturia)

Equine myoglobinuria (azoturia) is seldom seen in horses under 4 years old.

Cause When horses that have been in continuous work are suddenly rested for a few days, fed very well meanwhile, and then returned to work or exercise, there is a risk of azoturia.

It has been suggested that the cause is an accumulation of glycogen in muscle, liberating excessive amounts of lactic acid during exercise.

Signs The hind-limbs suddenly become stiff and weak or staggering, and there is a tendency to 'knuckle-over' at the fetlocks. The muscles of the hindquarters become tense, hard, and often painful. They feel like wood to the hand.

Colicky symptoms are observed in some cases, but these pass off after a short time. The urine is a wine-red or coffee colour. In some cases the urine is retained, and it is necessary to relieve the bladder by the passage of a catheter. The temperature is generally elevated in severe cases, but seldom reaches more than 40°C (104°F).

The horse should be taken from work at once when the stiffness is noticed. It should be placed in a loose-box for preference with plenty of bedding, and if the weather is at all cold, 1 or 2 rugs should be applied.

If the horse has to be taken home, this should be done by horse box. **If the horse is walked for any distance, a fatal outcome is likely.**

Treatment An antihistamine or cortisone may be used in treatment; the application of hot packs, etc., to the loins and over the hard muscles, gives relief.

Prevention When horses are out of work they should be given some amount of exercise, and have their concentrated diet restricted.

Atypical equine myoglobinuria This syndrome affects mostly horses at grass. (Compare above.) There is a sudden onset of stiffness unrelated to exercise. Affected horses or ponies are reluctant to move, and many become recumbent; some die. Appetite is not lost and water is drunk. Pulse and respiration rates also remain normal as a rule. Dark chocolate-coloured or red urine is passed.

Equine Piroplasmosis

The virus is transmissible by both the respiratory and the venereal routes. (See EQUINE BILIARY FEVER.)

Equine Purpura Haemorrhagica (EPH)
(see PURPURA HAEMORRHAGICA)

Equine Respiratory Viruses
The table on page 229 shows the viruses known to cause disease of the horse's respiratory system.

E Equine Sarcoid
(see SARCOID)

Equine Verminous Arteritis
This is a swelling of the cranial mesenteric artery, commonly encountered in horses, and resulting from thickening and fibrosis of the arterial wall due to the effects of migrating strongyle worm larvae. Thrombosis and embolism may follow the stenosis, or reduced lumen, of the artery. Infarction and ischaemia of the bowel may result. Rupture of the artery at this site is very rare indeed. (The term 'verminous aneurysm', which persisted in the veterinary literature until the late 1970s, or beyond, is a misnomer.)

Signs often occur during or shortly after work and include the sudden onset of abdominal pain, fever, flaring of the nostrils, a pulse rate of 70–80, and turning the head towards the right flank. Following recovery from one attack, abdominal pain may return at frequent intervals over weeks or months. The horse may become bad-tempered, be unwilling to back or turn in a small circle, may remain recumbent for long periods, and may hesitate before jumping.

Prevention Dosing with a suitable anthelmintic, such as ivermectin paste, kills the larvae responsible for the condition.

Equine Viral Arteritis
This is a highly contagious NOTIFIABLE DISEASE in which damage is caused to the arteries, especially the smaller ones. The disease may be transmitted from acutely infected animals through the breath, or venereally in the semen of chronically infected stallions.

Signs include fever, conjunctivitis, oedema of the lungs and also affecting the legs and other parts of the body. Haemorrhagic enteritis, with abdominal pain and diarrhoea, may occur. Over 50 per cent of pregnant mares abort. Horses which recover are likely to become carriers. A vaccine is available. (See HORSES, IMPORT CONTROLS.)

Equine Viral Rhinopneumonitis
A disease caused by the equine herpesviruses 1 and 4. (See EQUINE RESPIRATORY VIRUSES.)

Signs include slight fever, cough, and nasal discharge. These are seen in weaned foals and yearlings, though some infections are subclinical. In the mare, abortion, often after the gestation period has passed the 8th month, may sometimes result – hence its alternative name of 'equine virus abortion'. Indeed the term 'abortion storms' has been used, since 40 to 60 per cent (or even more) of the mares in a stud may abort. Usually such an occurrence is a sequel to an outbreak of severe and extensive nasal catarrh when the in-foal mares were between 0.5 and 7 months pregnant. It must be emphasised, however, that these 'abortion storms' are exceptional, and have become more so, in recent years.

When abortion has occurred, subsequent foaling is nearly always normal.

The virus is present in the aborted fetus, fluids, and membranes. It cannot survive more than a fortnight in the absence of horse tissue. On straw, concrete floors, etc. it dies within a week, but when dried on to horse hairs it has been shown to be infective for up to 6 weeks. The stallion is not, it is believed, involved in the spread of the disease, which was first reported in the UK in 1961.

Cases of acute paresis and paralysis in horses have been attributed to this virus.

Equisetum Poisoning
(see HORSE-TAILS, POISONING BY)

Ergometrine
Ergometrine is the most powerful of the active constituents of ergot in producing muscular contractions of the uterus. It is used to stimulate a sluggish uterus during parturition and to control uterine haemorrhage following parturition.

Ergot
Ergot is the small mass of horn which is found amongst the tuft of hair which grows from the back of the fetlocks of horses. It is produced by cells which are similar to those which form the horn of the hoof.

Ergot, Fungal
There are several species of ergot, including *Claviceps fusiformis*, which infests the bulrush millet, and *C. purpurea*, which is a parasite of rye and other cereals such as maize.

Ergot of Munga

Ergot of munga, the bulrush millet, is in southern Zimbabwe an important cause of loss to the pig industry. The sow's udder fails to enlarge and does not become functional; piglet mortality is heavy as a result of the absence of milk (agalactia). Sows show no other signs of ill health. The alkaloidal composition of this ergot is believed to differ from that of *Claviceps purpurea*.

Ergot of Rye

Ergot of rye is a fungus which attacks the seed of rye or other cereal, subsists upon it, and finally replaces it. The fungus is called *Claviceps purpurea*, and is artificially cultivated on account of its medicinal properties. Its medicinal preparations are used to stimulate the wall of the uterus during parturition when there is inertia (in both humans and animals), and are also useful for checking haemorrhage by causing constriction of the arterioles. The crude ergot is unsafe to use.

Ergot Poisoning

Ergot poisoning occurs through eating cereals upon which the fungus is parasitic, such as rye and various kinds of maize, etc., and through taking foods made from affected plants (e.g. maize meals). Extensive outbreaks have occurred in various parts of the USA, in Germany, Austria, and other parts of Europe. Abortion and gangrene of the extremities in cattle have been seen in Britain.

Signs The characteristic feature of poisoning due to *Claviceps purpurea* is that there is irritation and pain in the extremities of the body. Later, areas of the skin of these parts become gangrenous, and may slough off.

Two forms are recognised: in the first, convulsive symptoms due to stimulation of the nervous system are seen; and in the second, gangrene occurs.

Horses that have eaten large amounts of ergotised hay develop symptoms during the first 24 hours after feeding. The animal becomes dull and listless, a cold sweat breaks out on the neck and flanks, the breathing is slow and deep, the temperature is below normal, the pulse is weak and finally imperceptible, and death occurs during deep coma. When lesser amounts have been taken over a longer period there may be diarrhoea, colic, vomiting, and signs of abdominal pain. Pregnant animals may abort, and lose condition.

Trembling, general muscular spasms, loss of sensation of the extremities, convulsions and delirium may be seen.

In the gangrenous form there is coldness of the feet, ears, lips, tail, combs and wattles of birds, and other extremities, a loss of sensation in these parts, and eventually dry gangrene sets in. After a day or two the hair falls out, teeth drop out, the tips of the ears and tail may slough off, and the skin of the limbs, or even the whole of the feet, may be cast off. Death occurs from exhaustion, or from septicaemia.

Ergot-contaminated feed may result in reduced fertility and agalactia in the sow. (See also under ERGOT OF MUNGA.)

Erysipelas, Swine
(see SWINE ERYSIPELAS)

Erysipeloid

Human infection with *Erysipelothrix rhusiopathiae*, the cause of swine erysipelas.

Erythema

Erythema is a redness of the skin, the surface blood vessels of which become gorged with blood.

Erythrocyte

Erythrocyte is another name for a red blood cell.

Erythrocyte Mosaicism

The mixture of 2 blood types in each of non-identical twins.

Erythroleucosis

This is a transmissible virus-associated type of cancer occurring in poultry. It is associated with the fowl paralysis group of diseases. It was described and named in 1908, 3 years before the Rous sarcoma made history. (See under LEUKOSIS.)

Erythromycin

An antibiotic which has a bacteriostatic action against Gram-positive organisms. It is used when penicillin-susceptible strains have developed resistance. It is administered by mouth, in drinking water or feed to poultry and farm animals, and by tablets to dogs, cats and foals.

Erythropoiesis

The formation of red blood cells in the bone marrow, stimulated by the hormone erythropoietin secreted by the kidneys.

Eschar

Eschar is an area of body tissue that has been killed by heat or by caustics.

Escherichia Coli

This is the modern name for *Bacillus coli*. (See E. COLI.)

Escutcheon

The anal region of an ox, with special reference to the direction of growth of hair.

Ester

A compound formed from an alcohol and an acid by elimination of water, e.g. ethyl acetate.

Estradiol and Estrone (oestradiol and oestrone)

Estradiol and estrone (oestradiol and oestrone) are hormones secreted by the ovary (interstitial cells and Graafian follicles) which bring about oestrus and, in late pregnancy, stimulate development of the mammary gland.

Estrumate

A proprietary name for the prostaglandin analogue cloprostenol. (See CLOPROSTENOL; CONTROLLED BREEDING.)

Estrus

(see OESTRUS)

Etamiphylline Camsylate

Etamiphylline camsylate is a smooth-muscle relaxant and cardiac and respiratory stimulant. It is used in the treatment of neonatal weakness in calves and lambs when this is associated with cardiac and respiratory distress after dystocia or caesarian section. In dogs, cats and horses it is also used as an aid in the management of coughing.

Ether

A volatile liquid formerly widely used as an anaesthetic. It forms an explosive mixture with oxygen, and precautions to avoid electrical or other sparks must be strictly adhered to.

Ethidium Bromide

A trypanocide given by intra-muscular injection. This drug is also used in the treatment of 'heather blindness' (contagious ophthalmia) in sheep, and of bovine keratitis.

Ethmoid

Ethmoid is a bone which separates the nasal cavity from that of the brain. It is spongy in nature and contains numerous cavities, some of which communicate with the nose and serve to carry the nerves of the sense of smell.

Ethology

The study of the behaviour of animals in their normal environment. Applied ethology is an important aspect of animal welfare, and includes experiments to determine animals' preferences and also their reactions to farming practices.

Ethyl Chloride

Ethyl chloride is a clear, colourless liquid, produced by the action of hydrochloric acid upon alcohol. Extremely volatile, it rapidly produces freezing of the surface of the skin when sprayed upon it. It is used to produce insensibility for short surface operations, such as the removal of warts or small tumours, the lancing of painful abscesses, the removal of thorns or foreign bodies, etc. It is packaged in a glass or metal tube provided with a fine nozzle.

Ethylene

Ethylene is a colourless inflammable gas which is sometimes used as an anaesthetic in small animals. Ethylene glycol, the antifreeze used for cars, is highly poisonous for dogs and cats. (See ANTIFREEZE.)

Etiology

Etiology is the study of the cause(s) of disease.

Etorphine

(see 'IMMOBILON')

Eubacterium Suis

Also known as *Corynebacterium suis*, it is a cause of cystitis and pyelonephritis in pigs.

European Brown Hare Syndrome

This has been reported from several EU countries. including the UK.

Cause Picorna-like virus particles have been isolated in the UK.

Signs Dullness, loss of fear of people, and nervous disorders such as ataxia. The death rate has been high.

European Union (EU)

Originally the European Economic Community (EEC), created by the Treaty of Rome in 1957, with 6 member states, it subsequently became known as the European Community (EC). The UK became a member in 1973. In 1992, in Maastricht, the member states signed the Treaty on European Union. By 2007 the number of member states was scheduled to be 27.

The EU has been defined as a group of nations which have abandoned a significant part of their national sovereignty in return for a share in a much larger trading block.

A large number of directives concerning all aspects of animal health, meat inspection, abattoirs and food hygiene have been issued.

EU legislation on animal medicines, intended primarily to minimise drug residues in food animals, has created some problems for prescribing medicines in small animal and equine practice because of the all-embracing nature of the regulations.

Eurytrema

A fluke. (See PANCREAS, DISEASES OF.)

Eustachian Tubes

Eustachian tubes are the passages, one on each side, which lead from the throat to the middle ear, and serve to maintain an even atmospheric pressure upon the inner surface of the 'eardrum' or tympanum. They open widely in the act of swallowing, and during a yawn. Each has a sac or diverticulum connected with it in the horse, and in certain conditions these become filled with pus from a strangles abscess or from some other suppurating source near, when an operation becomes necessary to evacuate the pus and prevent it doing damage by burrowing into the middle ear or surrounding parts. (See EAR.)

Euthanasia

As applied to animals, this is a means of producing death free from ante-mortem fear or suffering. The term mainly applies to dogs and cats and other pets which must be put down because of an incurable or painful condition, or because of severe persistent behavioural problems. The decision to euthanase an animal is not to be taken lightly and the informed consent of the owner should be obtained in writing wherever possible.

Strictly speaking, the humane slaughtering of animals for food purposes, and the humane destruction of horses or other animals kept for working purposes, should also fall within the meaning of the word.

Small animals An injection of an overdose of a barbiturate, usually pentobarbitone given by rapid intravenous injection, is the method preferred by most veterinarians. The method is painless; the animal quickly loses consciousness and death occurs by depression of the respiratory and vasomotor centres of the brain.

Minimising stress Veterinarian E. H. Shillabeer, writing in the *Veterinary Record*, offered the following advice: 'It has been my custom to show a surviving companion animal its euthanased former companion whenever possible.

'Acceptance of the situation by the surviving dog (or cat) certainly appears to shorten their period of "grief" or unsettled behaviour.

'I also press strongly for the owner's presence at euthanasia because I believe that the animal's stress is thus minimised. If a house call is feasible, that is preferable too as I am always helped by a veterinary nurse to make the procedure as stress-free as possible for all concerned.'

Horses and cattle are sometimes killed by barbiturate injection where other means are unavailable or inappropriate. A combination of quinalbarbitone and cinchocaine (Somulose; Arnolds) is said to produce rapid heart arrest thus avoiding the gasping which barbiturates alone may produce. The carcases should not be used for food. Hunting dogs fed on meat from a horse killed by barbiturate have been poisoned as a result.

Captive-bolt pistol Correctly used, this type of 'humane killer' can be a valuable means of euthanasia for the larger animals, and also for the dog – though the method has obvious disadvantages from the point of view of a dog-owner wishing to be present.

The following advice may be useful for animal-owners or others in remote places where no veterinarian is available and who have to shoot an animal.

For horses and cattle, the point aimed at is **not** in the middle of the forehead, between the eyes; a shot so placed passes into the nasal chambers or air sinuses, down into the mouth and throat, and misses the important vital centres. The correct spot is higher up than this. Two imaginary lines should be drawn, each running from one eye to the opposite ear across the front of the forehead, and the point of their intersection is the most vital spot. A shot aimed about parallel with the ground and directed at this spot enters the brain cavity, destroys the brain and the beginning of the spinal cord, and passes on into the neck, where its energy is expended. Otherwise, if for some reason this part is not accessible, the next best place to aim at is the base of one ear, the direction being again parallel with the ground. In the case of horned cattle, the presence of the horn may deflect the shot, and it is better to shoot into the base of the brain from behind, directing the charge downwards and forwards. When pigs have to be shot, the middle line of the head is not altogether the best place, because there is a strong crest of bone running downwards in this position; the shot should be placed a little above and a little nearer the centre of the skull than the eye. For dogs and cats the centre of the forehead should be aimed at, for in these animals the brain is of relatively larger size, and more easily accessible.

Shotgun May be used to kill animals humanely if the gun is held as close to the head as possible and pointed as for a captive-bolt pistol. The shot will emerge from the gun in a tight cluster, penetrate the skull and disperse within the cranial cavity, destroying the brain in the process.

Electrocution was formerly used to kill dogs and is still used to stun or kill pigs and sheep in abattoirs.

Cervical dislocation by a sharp blow to the back of the neck is, **in expert hands**, the quickest way of stopping brain function in small animals that are easily handled, such as rabbits and poultry.

A number of other methods, including gassing by carbon dioxide, are used on occasion. For further information about euthanasia, particularly of fish and of exotic species, the *Humane Killing of Animals*, published by the Universities Federation for Animal Welfare, 8 Hamilton Close, Potters Bar, Herts. EN6 3QD, is very useful.

Evening Primrose

The oil derived from this plant is a source of gamolenic acid, an essential fatty acid. Administered orally, it is used, alone or in combination with fish oils or sunflower oil, in treating allergic skin conditions in dogs and cats and can lead to improvements in coat condition. Tablets, capsules, powder or liquid preparations are available

Exanthemata

(see under VESICULAR EXANTHEMA; EQUINE COITAL EXANTHEMA)

Exchange Transfusion

(see BLOOD TRANSFUSION)

Excipient

Excipient means any more or less inert substance added to a prescription in order to make the remedy more suitable in bulk, consistency, or form for administration.

Exercise

Exercise is a matter of great importance in the preservation of health. It is obvious that the methods of domestication, which have made such enormous modifications in the characteristics of horses, cattle, sheep, pigs, and dogs, have also so altered their modes of life that exercise is a matter over which they themselves often have no control. Lack of sufficient exercise is most serious in young animals, especially calves, pigs, and puppies. They do not grow and develop as they should.

Females of all species must have regular exercise during pregnancy, for otherwise the tone of the uterine wall and other muscles of the body is lost, and there is a risk of trouble occurring at parturition.

Over-exercise, especially if an animal is not in a fit condition, is, on the other hand, equally bad. Efforts beyond the animal's strength are apt to bring about dilatation of the heart, or lead to exhaustion; even, rarely, to death if a horse is taken out hunting when unfit.

Heavy draught horses should get a short walk for 10 to 15 minutes twice daily when standing idle, or they may be turned out into a paddock or yard for the greater part of the day. Cattle tied up in stalls should receive a minimum of 10 to 20 minutes' exercise out of doors twice daily. Breeding sows and boars kept in pig-houses where space is limited always thrive better when allowed into a yard for some part of the day, or when allowed into a paddock to graze. House-dogs need different amounts of exercise according to their breeds and ages. Young dogs of the sporting breeds never do well unless they receive at least 1 hour's sharp walk morning and night when on the leash, or about half this period when allowed to range at liberty. Older dogs and those of pet breeds need less, but generally speaking, the more exercise the dog gets the better health it will enjoy. (See also SHEEP-DOGS; MUSCLE – Condition.)

Exercising Horses

Horses must be gradually introduced to exercise or work, because over-exertion of an unfit or of a partly fit horse may have serious and permanent consequences. To get a riding horse fit it is usual to begin with daily walking exercise, with only an occasional trot for the first month or so. As the horse becomes fitter the duration of the exercise is lengthened, and the animal is made to walk, then given a sharp trot or a short gallop, and finally another walk home each day for a further 2 to 4 weeks. From this stage it proceeds to one when the gallop is of longer duration on alternate days, and then, later, the horse gets a stiff gallop every day for perhaps half an hour or so. In some stables there is a system of morning and afternoon exercise for each horse, but much must be left to the individual requirement of each animal, and to the judgement of the trainer. After a time, varying up to 4 months or more in some cases, the horse arrives at its maximum pitch of perfection, and then begins to 'go stale'. The art of the race-horse trainer enables him to judge the length of time it takes for each individual horse to arrive at his best at such a time as will allow him to enter for the race for which he is being trained. Every horse-trainer has his own individual methods, and as these are by no means hard-and-fast rules, nothing more than the merest outline can be given here.

The 'condition' of a horse, by which is meant its capacity for doing work, cannot be retained indefinitely; there comes a time when it begins to perform less and less well, and is said to have 'gone stale'. This is an indication that a rest is required.

Overtraining in the racehorse This, and stress, are a common cause of poor performance, and could be regarded as a clinical entity. Affected horses appear to 'fade' at the end of a race. They also show signs of stress before racing. Once identified, such a horse should be exercised more slowly and gradually worked up to previous levels. (See also RACEHORSES.)

Exfoliation
The separation in layers or scales of dead bone or of skin.

Exocrine
(see GLANDS)

Exophthalmos
Bulging of the eyeballs. In America it has been observed as a hereditary defect in certain Jersey cattle; and in Britain in certain Shorthorn herds – the condition being preceded by a squint. It is also seen in certain breeds of toy dogs. (See EYE, DISEASES OF.)

Exostosis
An outgrowth from a bone. (See BONE, DISEASES OF.)

Exotoxins
Toxins which diffuse readily from the bodies of bacteria during their lifetime.

Explosive, Plastic (PE4) Poisoning
(see CYCLONITE POISONING; also DYNAMITE)

Exporting Animals
(see IMPORTING/EXPORTING)

Exposure
Exposure to intense cold can usually be well tolerated by the animal which is well fed. More food is required during very cold weather in order to maintain the body temperature. Windbreaks are important, but the tendency is for their number to decline in the interests of larger fields and units more suited to mechanisation. Animals denied shelter from very cold winds, and at the same time inadequately fed, are most liable to disease of one kind or another. (See also SHEARING; FROSTBITE; FEED BLOCKS; SHEEP.)

External Fixators
External fixators are a system of metal rods, clamps, screws, etc., used to create a frame to keep fractured bones rigid while they heal. It is claimed that there are several advantages over conventional splinting materials; namely, they are 'very adaptable to bone shape, fragment size, and owner-acceptance'. They also 'maintain limb length, and allow access to open wounds'. Practice is required to master their use, however.

Extravasation
An escape of blood or lymph from the vessels which ought to contain it.

Extrinsic Allergic Alveolitis
(see FARMER'S LUNG; 'BROKEN WIND'; ALLERGY)

Exudate
A fluid which seeps into a body cavity or the tissues, often as a result of disease.

Eye
The eyes are set in deep cavities known as 'bony orbits', whose edges are prominent and form a protection to the eyeball. In the pig, dog, and cat the edge of the bony orbit is not complete posteriorly, but in the other domesticated animals it forms a complete circle. The two orbits are separated from each other in the middle line of the skull by only a very small space, and posteriorly the nerves leaving each eye (optic nerves) converge and meet each other on the floor of the brain cavity. Around the eyeball there is 'periorbital fat' upon which the eye rests. It is protected by 2 main eyelids and in many cases by a small rudimentary '3rd eyelid', 'haw', or nictitating membrane, which is found at the inner corner. The eyelids meet at the outer and inner 'canthi'. Within the inner canthus and attached to the nictitating membrane

is a small rounded pigmented prominence known as the 'lacrimal caruncle', which is formed of modified skin, and which often bears 1 or 2 tiny hairs. (See also HARDERIAN GLAND.)

Eyelids Each of the 2 main eyelids consists of 4 layers: on the surface there is skin similar to that which covers the adjacent part of the face, but thin, loose, pliant, and bearing extremely fine hairs; below this is a layer of thin subcutaneous tissue, and then comes the 2nd or muscular layer which is instrumental in opening and shutting the eyelids; the 3rd layer is fibrous, and along the free edge of the lid this layer is denser and forms the 'tarsus' of the eyelid, in the substance of which is embedded a row of glands, called the 'tarsal glands', numbering 45 to 50 in the upper and 30 to 35 in the lower lid of the horse (small cysts are occasionally formed in connection with these glands, which appear as rounded swellings upon the surface of the lid); the 4th layer consists of the delicate mucous membrane called the 'conjunctiva', which rubs over the surface of the eyeball (also covered by conjunctiva) and tends to remove any dust, particles of debris, etc. that may collect on the moist surface. The 2 layers of conjunctiva are continuous with each other, being reflected off the eyelid on to the anterior surface of the eyeball, and forming little pockets (upper and lower) in which oat-chaffs sometimes lodge and are difficult to remove; normally these pockets should contain small amounts of fluid,

forming tears. Any excess secretion of tears reaches the nasal cavity by the 'lacrimal duct', the 2 openings of which can be seen towards the inner canthus along the free margins of each of the lids. The 3rd eyelid is situated at the inner angle of the eye, consisting of a semilunar fold of the conjunctiva, which is supported and strengthened by a small roughly crescentic plate of cartilage. Ordinarily this eyelid covers only a very small part of the surface of the eye, but in certain diseases, such as tetanus, the pressure by the muscles of the eyeball upon the orbital fat displaces the 3rd eyelid, and it may reach across the eye to the extent of almost 1 inch.

In the cat, the appearance of the 3rd eyelid (nictitating membrane), like a curtain partly drawn across a window, is a common sign of general ill health and is due to absorption of fat in the vicinity. It is not usually a disease of the eye. (See also EYE, DISEASES OF – 'Dry eye'.)

Front of the eye If the lids of a horse's eye be separated widely, the 'white' of the eye comes into view. The white appearance is due to the sclerotic coat, composed of dense white fibrous tissue, shining through the translucent conjunctival covering. In the centre of the white is set the transparent oval 'cornea', through which the rays of light pass on their way to the inner parts of the eye. (In the pig, dog, and cat the cornea is practically circular in outline.) Behind the cornea lies the beautifully coloured 'iris', with a hole in its centre, the 'pupil', which looks

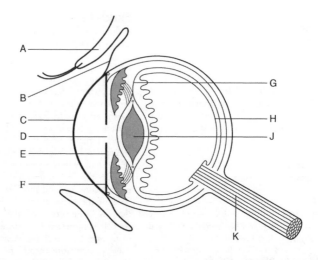

The eye: a sectional view. A, indicates the eyelid; B, conjunctiva; C, cornea; D, pupil; E, iris; F, ligament of the iris; G, ligament of the lens; H, retina; J, lens; K, optic nerve. Next to the retina (H) comes the hyaloid membrane, then the choroid coat and (the outermost) the sclerotic coat.

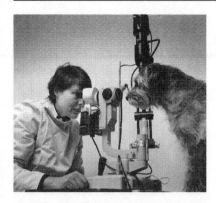

A senior ophthalmologist at the Animal Health Trust, Newmarket, examines a patient's eyes. She is using a slit lamp ophthalmoscope, a vital tool for identifying problems in the cornea and the front of the eye.

black against the dark interior of the eye. The edge of the pupil is often irregular in outline, owing to the presence of 'nigroid bodies'. The shape of the pupil and the colour of the iris vary in each of the domesticated animals and in individuals of the same or different breeds. In the horse and ox the pupil is roughly oval, or even egg-shaped, with the larger end inwards. In some horses, though rarely in cattle, there may be an absence of pigment matter in the iris, and the horse is then said to be 'wall-eyed' or 'ring-eyed'. In the pig, dog, and cat the pupil is rounded when fully dilated, but in the cat the contracted pupil (e.g. during the day or in a strong light) resolves itself into a vertical slit; the contracted pupil of the dog and pig is round. Lying between the anterior surface of the eye, the cornea, and the iris, in a space known as the 'anterior chamber' of the eye, which is filled with a clear lymph-like fluid – the 'aqueous humour'.

Coats of the eyeball

The eyeball, as already mentioned, rests upon a pad of fat within the cavity of the orbit, where it is held in position through the agency of seven ocular muscles and the optic nerve around which they are arranged. There are 3 layers forming the eyeball:

(a) *The Sclerotic Coat*, which is outermost, is composed of dense white fibrous tissue, which gives its appearance to the white of the eye in front. This coat completely encloses the ball, except for a small area through which emerges the optic nerve, while in front it is modified so as to form the transparent cornea. It maintains the shape of, and gives strength to,

the ball of the eye. The cornea, which has a greater curvature than the rest of the ball, bulges out in front. The whole cornea is somewhat like a window let into the front of the sclerotic coat.

(b) *The Choroid*, or vascular coat, lies within the sclerotic, and consists of 3 parts. The choroid membrane, which forms more than two-thirds of a lining to the sclerotic, consists mainly of a network of vessels which nourish the sclerotic coat and the interior of the eyeball. Its general colour is bluish-black, but an area a little above the level of the end of the optic nerve has a remarkable metallic lustre and is known as the 'tapetum'. The colour of the tapetum is variable, but generally it has a brilliant iridescent bluish-green colour shading imperceptibly into yellow. The choroid membrane is prolonged forwards into the 'ciliary body', a very complex structure which forms a thickened ring opposite the line where the sclera merges into the cornea. To this line of junction the ciliary body is firmly attached by the ciliary muscle, which by its contraction and relaxation moves the ciliary body to and fro over the sclerotic, so as to allow the lens of the eye which is suspended from, or rather 'set into', the ciliary body, to alter its shape in such a way that it is able accurately to focus rays of light, coming from an object before the eye, on to the retina. The farthest forward part of the choroid coat is the 'iris', lying in front of the lens and behind the cornea.

The iris consists partly of fibrous tissue and partly of muscle fibres, arranged radially and circularly, with pigment cells interspaced throughout. These fibres by their contraction serve to narrow or dilate the pupil, according to whether the light entering the eye is strong or weak, and according as the animal looks at a near or distant object.

(c) *The Retina*, or nervous coat, is the innermost of the 3 coats of eyeball. After the optic nerve has pierced the sclerotic and choroid coats, it ends by a sudden spreading out of its fibres in all directions to form the retina, which also contains some blood vessels and pigment cells. The retina, in microscopic sections, is seen to consist of no less than 10 layers.

The rods and cones convert light waves into nerve impulses. The rods are very sensitive under night vision and near darkness. The cones achieve (under good light) detailed vision and differentiate between colours.

The 'visual purple' is a pigment called rhodopsin, synthesised from retinene (a pigment related to carotene) and a protein. Under bright light, the fading of the visual purple involves a conversion of rhodopsin into vitamin A plus protein by means of an enzyme.

Contents of the eyeball, viz. aqueous humour, vitreous humour, and crystalline lens. Occupying the space between the iris and the cornea, i.e. the anterior chamber of the eye, there is a clear watery, lymph-like fluid. It is being constantly secreted and drained away, and eventually reaches the veins of the eye. Behind the iris lies the 'crystalline lens', which acts as does the lens of a camera, with the exception that it can alter the curves of its surfaces and therefore is able to change its refractive powers. It is composed of layers arranged like the leaves of an onion. The lens is held suspended by its capsule, which is attached to the ciliary body already mentioned. Behind the lens the cavity of the ball of the eye is filled with a viscid, jelly-like, tenacious fluid called the 'vitreous humour'. It maintains the intra-ocular pressure by which the eyeball retains its shape.

The lacrimal system provides a means whereby the eye surface is maintained free from dust and other foreign material. It consists of the lacrimal gland which secretes the clear fluid popularly known as 'tears'; excretory ducts, from 12 to 16 in number; and the 2 lacrimal ducts which open into a lacrimal sac from which begins the naso-lacrimal duct which carries the secretion down into the nose. The gland lies towards the upper outer aspect of the orbit; secretes the clear salty, watery fluid which flows out through the excretory ducts to reach the conjunctival sac and bathe the surface of the eye. The secretion is finally received by the 2 lacrimal ducts, the openings of which lie one in each eyelid about a third of an inch from the inner canthus. These open into the lacrimal sac, from which takes origin the long naso-lacrimal duct which conveys the secretion down into the lower part of the corresponding nasal passage, just within the nostril.

Accommodation All the rays of light proceeding from a distant object may be looked upon as being practically parallel, while those coming from a near object are divergent. The difference between distant and near in this connection can be taken as about 5 metres (20 feet) from the animal. A 'near' object can be seen anywhere between 5 metres (20 feet) and 10 to 12 cm (4 to 5 inches) from the eye, but nearer than this it loses its distinction. Parallel rays of light do not require any focusing on the retina other than is provided by the surface of the cornea; when an animal looks at a distant

object, the lens capsule (which is attached to the ciliary process) retains the lens in a temporarily flattened condition and the ciliary muscle is relaxed, so that no great strain is put upon the eye. Rays of light from an object near at hand, however, which are divergent, require to be brought to a point of focus upon the retina, and as they pass through the lens their direction is changed on account of the convexity of the lens. The amount of this convexity is determined by the divergency of the rays, and is automatically provided for through the pull of the ciliary muscle upon the ciliary body. As the function of the muscle is to pull the ciliary body forwards, the tension upon the ligament of the lens is lessened and the capsule of the lens slackens, so that the lens, by its inherent elasticity, is allowed to bulge with a greater convexity upon its anterior surface. The greater the convexity, the more are the rays of light refracted, and the more convergent do rays which pass through it become. (See also VISION.)

Lens (see illustration)

Eye, Diseases and Injuries of

All such diseases and injuries can be of economic importance to farmers, since the productive efficiency of affected animals is likely to be reduced, owing to stress, pain, or infection – or all of these. Milk yield may decline in the dairy cow. If the animal's sight is seriously impaired, feeding may become difficult, with consequent loss of bodily condition.

Blepharitis Inflammation of the edges of the eyelids; it usually accompanies conjunctivitis. Its causes, symptoms, and treatment are similar (see below).

Blindness There are many causes of this, including disease of the retina, of the optic nerve, and of the brain. Blindness may be congenital or acquired, temporary or permanent. Vitamin A deficiency may be responsible, and also poisoning by rape and other plants, and by substances such as lead. Blindness in the dog and cat may result from carbon monoxide poisoning, and persist for some time; it may also result from metaldehyde poisoning. (See also under QUININE; MALE FERN; BRIGHT BLINDNESS.)

'Day blindness' (Hemeralopia) is stated to be due to an autosomal recessive gene. This eye disease is common in the Alaskan malamute dog, and has been reported also in miniature poodles. The blindness occurs during bright light, although in dim light the animal can see.

Horses. The sudden onset of blindness in one or both eyes has been reported as a result of optic nerve atrophy, following trauma. Signs are dilated, fixed pupils, and a lack of the menace reflex. Within 3 to 4 weeks the optic disc becomes paler, and the retina's blood vessels markedly decreased. There is a rupture of the nerve axons.

'Night blindness' (nyctalopia) is a condition that sometimes affects horses and mules in countries where the glare of the sunlight is very intense during the day. At night such animals are quite unable to see, and will stumble into objects that are easily discernible to human beings.

Camels are seldom affected, owing to the effective protection afforded to the retina by the overhanging eyelids and deeply placed eyeballs.

Opacity of the cornea will, of course, prevent light rays from reaching the retina, as happens in keratitis, so that partial or complete blindness results. Similarly, partial or complete blindness may result from a cataract. Other causes are mentioned below, e.g. dislocation of the lens, glaucoma, etc.

Cattle and sheep Cerebrocortical necrosis (polioencephalomalacia), resulting from a thiamine deficiency, is a cause of blindness in ruminants. In sheep, other causes of blindness include: infectious keratitis or contagious ophthalmia ('heather blindness'); pregnancy toxaemia; and the effects of eating bracken, as described under BRIGHT BLINDNESS of sheep.

Poultry Blindness may be the result of excessive ammonia fumes from deep litter, or it may be associated with fowl paralysis, salmonellosis, aspergillosis, etc. Cataract, followed in some cases by liquefaction of the lens, occurs during outbreaks of avian infectious encephalomyelitis. (See also under LIGHTING OF ANIMAL BUILDINGS.)

'Blue eye' (see CANINE VIRAL HEPATITIS)

Cancer, either of sarcomatous or carcinomatous nature, is sometimes found in connection with the conjunctiva. Tumours appear as red hard swellings, painless when small, but not when large. These neoplasms often grow at a rapid rate, and may infiltrate the surrounding tissues, sometimes affecting the bones of the orbit. Cancer of the eye is a common condition in Hereford cattle. It has been suggested that several factors may contribute to the development of eye cancer in cattle. These include age, irritation of the eyes by dust, sand, insects or chemicals, sunlight, lack of eyelid pigmentation and viral infection. Some authorities believe that cattle may be genetically prone to the condition, while others feel that poor nutrition is another factor as the condition appears to occur more frequently following a drought. (See TUMOURS.)

The beginning of 'cancer eye', as it is sometimes colloquially known, may be a raised area of skin or a wart. Either may become malignant, developing into a typical carcinoma – the type of cancer occurring in this eye disease of Herefords. However, in the USA a survey was carried out; the eyes of 48 Hereford cows were examined at 6-monthly intervals for 2 years. Over half the cows showed preliminary signs of 'cancer eye', but – without any treatment – one-third of the growths had disappeared by the time of the last examination.

Cryosurgery has been used to treat cancer of the eye. The technique is a highly skilled one and requires special thermocouples to monitor the very low temperatures.

In a series of 718 cases of eye cancer treated by cryosurgery, 609 a single freeze caused total regression of 66 per cent of the growths. In 109, treated by a rapid freeze to –25°C, a natural thaw, and then a re-freeze, the cure rate was 97 per cent.

Cataract The condition is by far the most common in the horse and dog in old age, although it is also encountered in other animals, and it may occur at almost any time of life. It consists of a coagulation of the plasma of the cells in the lens with loss of transparency. A bluish, cloudy appearance of the eye results and vision becomes blurred.

Causes Cataract is primarily a change characteristic of old age. Other causes include diabetes. Cataracts have also resulted from naphthalene and other forms of poisoning, and from exposure to X-rays.

Treatment As in human patients, cataracts may be removed successfully in animals. In one study, cataracts were removed by phacofragmentation and aspiration from one or both eyes of 56 dogs. Vision improved immediately in 53 of the dogs: after 2 years, 25 of 29 dogs still had vision, and after 4 years, 5 of 7 dogs. The surgery was unsuccessful in dogs with severe anterior uveitis with secondary glaucoma, retinal detachments, and fibropupillary membrane formation.

'Collie eye anomaly' is an inherited condition in which there is underdevelopment of the choroid membrane of the eye.

Coloboma is a congenital and hereditary defect – a notch, gap, hole, or fissure in any of the structures of the eye. In other words, at birth a part of the eye is missing. Bilateral coloboma is common in Charolais cattle, often involving the optic disc. The condition can be recognised only with an ophthalmoscope, and does not deteriorate with the passage of time. Effect on vision varies from very slight to (rarely) blindness.

Conjunctivitis, or inflammation of the conjunctival membranes, is an extremely common condition among animals, and probably constitutes the commonest trouble to which the eyes are subject. In cattle, conjunctivitis is often the first symptom of cattle plague, ephemeral fever, and Ondiri disease (bovine infectious petechial fever).

Conjunctivitis is one symptom associated with many specific infections, such as distemper in the dog (*and see* EYEWORMS).

Causes The presence of dust, sand, pollen, seeds, lime, and pieces of chaff, in the atmosphere of a stable or field, is probably one of the commonest causes in the larger farm animals, but such agents as flies, worms, and ticks must also be noted in addition to the above. In the cat, 2 infections which cause conjunctivitis – *Haemophilus parainfluenzae* and *Moraxella lacunata* – are transmissible to man, in which illness may also be caused. (See FELINE EYE INFECTIONS.)

Chlamydia psittaci was isolated from 30 per cent of swabs from 753 cats suffering from conjunctivitis.

Signs The first signs of conjunctivitis are redness and swelling of the lining membranes of the eyelids, excessive discharge of tears, and a tendency for the animal to keep its eyelids shut.

First-Aid Clean away the discharges by bathing with a warmed eye lotion. (If only 1 eye is affected, the cause may be a foreign body that has lodged there.) The best way to apply lotions, whether to the horse, dog, or other animal, is to use a perfectly clean piece of cotton-wool soaked in the solution and squeezed above the eye so that the drops trickle into it. Cases of conjunctivitis should never be neglected, for the inflammation may spread to the cornea, resulting in keratitis (see below).

Dislocation of the lens is a condition in which the crystalline lens becomes displaced forwards into the anterior chamber. It occurs in dogs, especially Sealyhams and rough-haired terriers, and at first is very hard to recognise. The dog runs into stationary objects without any obvious reason. Casual examination of the eyes reveals no change and the condition may not be suspected for many months. Later, the owner becomes aware that sight is failing in the dog and careful examination reveals a 'wobbly lens' in the eye. Operation may do much to restore some degree of vision and save the eye, but neglect almost invariably results in the development of glaucoma (see below) and the affected eye may have to be surgically removed.

Technically, lens dislocation may be classified as congenital, primary, secondary, or traumatic. Secondary cases not uncommonly follow cataract or glaucoma, but most cases occur spontaneously in adult life.

'Dry eye' (keratoconjunctivitis sicca) is a condition in the dog arising from a partial failure of tear production and leading to roughening of the corneal surface with a consequent lack of lustre. 'Artificial tears' may have to be provided, or a surgical operation performed involving parotid duct transplantation. The condition has been linked to the use of sulphasalazine for the treatment of idiopathic colitis in dogs.

Ectropion means a turning-out of one or both eyelids, so that the conjunctiva is exposed. It is a common condition in bloodhounds and St Bernards, and is in them regarded as practically normal. It is also treated by operation, but a part of the conjunctiva from within the edge of the lid is removed instead of part of the skin from the outside, as in entropion.

Entropion Turning-in of the eyelid, often the lower one, so that it rubs upon the cornea, causing inflammation. The condition is common in dogs – often an inherited defect – occurring in many breeds. It is also seen in 'mini-pigs'.

In newborn lambs entropion is occasionally seen and, if bilateral, can lead to eventual blindness and starvation. It can be corrected by Michel clips (metal sutures). It is treated by a plastic operation such as is performed for trichiasis (see below).

Epiphora is another name for what is commonly called 'watery eye' or 'overflow of tears'. It is generally due to some obstruction to the drainage of tears through the lacrimal duct to the nose, but it is also an accompanying symptom of most forms of mild inflammation of the conjunctiva or cornea, of naphthalene poisoning in cattle, and of atopic disease in the dog.

Foreign bodies in the eye have already been referred to under 'Conjunctivitis' above. Severe irritation may be caused by a piece of grit or a grass seed or husk. Pain and irritation may be shown by the dog pawing its face.

Treatment If a hair, bristle or tip of an awn, for instance, can be seen on folding back the eyelid, or if a white spot (sometimes indicating the site of a thorn's penetration) or what

appears to be 'a white film' is visible on the surface of the eye, the best first-aid treatment is a drop of olive oil. (Cod-liver oil will do, but not any oil!) Boracic acid lotion is worse than useless (except for the mechanical washing-out of grit); what is needed is a lubricant to reduce the harmful friction, and this is where the oil helps. Removal of a foreign body is best accomplished with the aid of a local anaesthetic, and professional help should be obtained.

Occasionally the object may be removed by taking the corner of a clean handkerchief, winding it into a point, and lifting the offending body out with it. The use of a suitable eye lotion will be helpful afterwards.

Glaucoma is a condition in which the tension of the fluid contents of the eyeball is greatly in excess of the normal. It is associated with obstruction to the drainage system of the eye, in which fluid continues to be secreted but the excess is not removed. It may follow cases of progressive retinal atrophy. It eventually results in swelling and bulging of one or both of the eyes, and blindness results. Secondary glaucoma is more common and caused by an eye disease, of which the most frequent is lens dislocation. (See also under EXOPHTHALMOS.)

Harderian gland, displaced In the dog this gland sometimes becomes enlarged and displaced, owing to blockage of its ducts or to a nearby swelling, when it becomes visible at the corner of the eye as a reddish lump. It may then require surgical removal.

'Heather blindness' is a colloquial name for the equivalent of infectious bovine keratoconjunctivitis (IBK) in sheep. *Rickettsia conjunctivae* is a common cause.

Treatment Shade and fly-control aid recovery, but veterinary treatment of IBK is necessary.

Boracic and similar eye lotions are useless in treating IBK or 'heather blindness'. Chloramphenicol eye drops or cloxacillin may be effective in treatment.

Horner's syndrome The pupil of one eye appears smaller than normal, the upper eyelid may droop, the lower lid may be raised, and the nictitating membrane ('third eyelid') protruded across part of the eye.

The cause is some lesion affecting the sympathetic nerves of the eye, e.g. a tumour of the spinal cord, chronic otitis, bite wounds, bee stings. Some cases are transient, as with wounds and bee stings.

Infectious bovine keratoconjunctivitis (IBK)

Infectious bovine keratoconjunctivitis (IBK) is a convenient name for a group of eye diseases with a worldwide distribution, and includes New Forest disease (see below). What they have in common is conjunctivitis and keratitis.

Causes Bacteria, viruses, mycoplasmas, rickettsiae, fungi, and *Thelazia* worms – any of these alone or in combination may produce IBK. In addition, the sun's rays, dust particles, and chemical irritants may all predispose to, or exacerbate, the condition. IBK is commonly transmitted by flies and, in Africa, by two species of moth which feed on secretions and exudate from the eye. Some infective agents are present on the healthy eye, and become active only when the eye is damaged or irritated in some way.

Moraxella (Haemophilus) bovis is a common bacterial cause of IBK. Some American research has suggested that *Moraxella* may not cause keratitis unless the virus of bovine rhinotracheitis is present also. Cefalonium applied as an eye ointment is an antibiotic treatment.

Iritis means inflammation of the iris, a condition which is very often associated with inflammation of the ciliary body, when the term 'iridocyclitis' is used. The chief symptoms are dullness of the iris, congestion of the blood vessels around its margin, a lessened response to varying intensities of light, and usually a firmly contracted pupil. Occasionally, especially during inflammation of the cornea, the iris adheres to this structure – a condition known as 'anterior synechia'; while more frequently the iris adheres to the lens, which lies behind it, and the condition is spoken of as 'posterior synechia'. The aqueous humour is often cloudy and may appear purulent, little flocculi of lymph being seen floating in the anterior chamber or sticking to the posterior surface of the cornea. There is always great pain, fear of light (photophobia), and the animal hangs its head and is dull and listless.

Iritis is a common condition in cattle, usually caused by eating poor-quality big-bale silage.

Keratitis Inflammation of the cornea may follow conjunctivitis, or it may arise from an injury to, or infection of, the cornea itself. A thorn, for example, may pierce the surface layers of the cornea and remain invisible until a faint whitish ring appears around its protruding part. Should a larger area of the cornea be involved, opacity becomes obvious. (Animal-owners often refer to it as 'a film over the eye'; but in fact the opacity stems from inflammation below the surface.) Keratitis may be caused by trauma of various kinds, e.g. a whip lash, a kick or blow; or by irritant skin dressings which are not prevented from running into the eyes, or by lime, sparks, or by continuous irritation by a foreign body such as a grass awn, piece of glass or grit. It may arise during the course of certain diseases, such as distemper in dogs and influenza in horses; it can be produced by the presence of *Thelazea* worms, or by fly-borne infections; frost-bite is said to be the cause of it in ewes on hills during severe weather, when it is called 'snow blindness'; turning-in of the eyelids (entropion) may give rise to it in the dog.

Keratoconjunctivitis sicca is a condition seen mostly in small animals, and is caused by the inadequate production of tears. There is a tacky mucoid discharge round the eyes; the cornea appears dry and may be ulcerated. If untreated, corneal opacity vascularisation and pigmentation may result. Topical application of antibiotics is indicated; 'artificial tears', formulated for use in human medicine, are useful.

Keratomycosis is keratitis due to a fungus, and is uncommon. If, however, tissue resistance is reduced by treatment with corticosteroids (which are immunosuppressive), any fungi present on the cornea may become pathogenic. It may be only when corneal ulcers fail to respond to conventional treatment that keratomycosis is suspected. Natamycin may prove helpful. *Fusarium solani* is implicated in most equine cases, sometimes *Candida* species; but several other fungi may be involved. (See also HYPERKERATOSIS.)

In the early stages, inflammation of the cornea results in symptoms very similar to those seen in conjunctivitis; the production of tears, closing of the eyelids, pain and swelling being noticed. When the eye is examined, however, the surface of the cornea is found to have lost its lustre. There may be a bluish haze, and an opacity, varying from pin-head size to the whole of the cornea – when the animal becomes completely blind in that eye, for the time being, anyway. The appearance of blood vessels where none is normally seen is another feature of keratitis and occurs before opacity becomes complete. There may be ulceration of the cornea, and even penetration. If the latter should occur, a keratocoele (hernia) may form endangering the whole eye, since infection, or escape of the aqueous humour, may sometimes occur.

Microphthalmos is an abnormally small eye; it is seen in vitamin A deficiency.

Myiasis (see UITPEULOOG)

New Forest disease (infectious bovine keratitis). Success has been claimed for treatment involving the injection of 2 to 5 ml of an antibiotic preparation into the subconjunctival tissues of the upper eyelid. Antibiotics, parenterally, by subcutaneous injection or by long-acting antibiotic ophthalmic ointment are used in treatment; cortisone is contraindicated. Penicillin, oxytetracycline and chloramphenicol have been reported to give equally good results. A single treatment is usually sufficient.

Opacity of the cornea may result from oedema of the cornea following infection with CANINE VIRAL HEPATITIS; see 'Keratitis' above.

Ovine infectious keratoconjunctivitis
This occurs worldwide. In a field survey carried out by the University of Liverpool's veterinary staff, the microflora of 240 clinically unaffected eyes from sheep in 10 flocks were compared with those of 240 clinically affected eyes from 12 natural outbreaks. Totals of 16 and 17 genera of bacteria were recovered, including *Branhamella ovis*, *E. coli*, and *Staphylococcus aureus*. Mycoplasma and acholeplasma were isolated from both groups. *Chlamydia psittaci* can also be a cause.

Pannus is a complication of keratitis in which blood vessels bud out from the margins of the cornea and run in towards the centre of the eye, stopping at the edges of an ulcer if such exists. Pannus is a condition which always takes a long time to clear up, and even months after there may be seen a dullness of the cornea, due to the tiny vessels that still exist but are invisible to the naked eye.

Partial displacement Pekingese and other dogs with prominent eyes sometimes suffer a traumatic partial displacement of the eye from the orbit, as a result of being struck by a car or of some other accident. The globe may become trapped by the eyelids which become located behind it.

First-Aid The owner should bandage the eye with bandage moistened in saline solution (a teaspoonful of ordinary salt to a pint of water). Professional aid is urgently required.

Treatment This requires a general anaesthetic and re-positioning of the eye where possible. If the cornea, etc., has been badly damaged, the only course is enucleation of the eye. After suturing of the eyelids over the vacant socket, the result will not appear unsightly to the owner.

Periodic ophthalmia (*see under* this heading). (See also OPHTHALMIA.)

Progressive retinal atrophy, or so-called 'night blindness', is a hereditary condition common in some strains of Irish red setter. The blood vessels of the retina undergo progressive atrophy and the animal suffers from impaired vision in consequence. To endeavour to correct this the pupil dilates widely, even in daylight, and the dog's expression become staring. At night or at dusk, the dog is unable to avoid objects and blunders into them, but during full daylight it appears to see quite well.

No treatment can arrest the progressive degeneration and the dog gradually becomes blind. In severe cases puppies may show first symptoms soon after weaning.

Neither dogs nor bitches which show the condition should be used for breeding. Breeds affected include collies, griffons, poodles, retrievers, Sealyhams, cocker and English springer spaniels.

The disease also occurs in cats, e.g. Abyssinian and Siamese; 25 per cent of Abyssinian cats were found to be affected in a recent study. The earliest signs may not be seen until the cat is 18 months old or more; and the advanced form takes another 18 months to develop. (See also TAURINE.)

Ptosis is an inability to raise the upper eyelid, usually associated with some general disease, such as distemper in dogs or 'grass sickness' in horses. It may also arise after injuries when the nerve supplying the muscles of the upper lid (3rd cranial nerve) is paralysed.

Retention cysts are produced in the thickness of the eyelid owing to blockage of a tarsal gland.

Sclerotitis (scleritis), or 'blood-shot eye', is inflammation of the sclerotic coat of the eyeball. It often accompanies conjunctivitis when the latter is at all severe. It is treated as for conjunctivitis.

Stye, or hordeolum, is a condition in which a small amount of pus collects in the follicle around the root of one of the eyelashes. One after another may form in succession, owing to the spread of infective material from follicle to follicle.

E

Trachoma A term used in human medicine for a granular conjunctivitis, often followed by keratitis and pannus.

Trichiasis Turning-in of the eyelashes so that they irritate and inflame the conditions. The condition is common in dogs and is sometimes a hereditary defect. It is treated surgically, by means of an operation in which an elliptical piece of skin is removed from the outer surface of the eyelid, and the edges sutured together. This causes the lashes to turn outwards, where they will not irritate or inflame the cornea.

Warts occur in connection with the eyelids comparatively frequently in horses, cattle, and dogs, and sometimes become malignant, spreading at a rapid rate and causing interference with sight or the movement of the eyelids. Owing to the malformation which they may cause when numerous, warts should always be removed before they attain a large size or before they have time to spread.

Eye Diseases, Hereditary

The British Veterinary Association, the Kennel Club and the International Sheep Dog Society operate a joint scheme to identify the presence or absence of inherited eye disease in a number of breeds of dog to help ensure that only disease-free animals are used for breeding. The main conditions covered are central progressive retinal atrophy, collie eye anomaly, generalised progressive retinal atrophy, goniodysgenesis/primary glaucoma, hereditary cataract, persistent hypoplastic primary vitreous, and persistent pupillary membrane.

Eye Fluke
(see DIPLOSTOMUM)

Eyelids
(see under EYE)

Eyeworms

In cattle *Thelazia* worms are one cause of infectious bovine keratoconjunctivitis. Species include *T. skrjabini* and *T. gulosa*, found behind the 3rd eyelid and in the ducts of associated glands. From 1 to 67 worms were found in eyes examined at a UK abattoir in 36.9 per cent of 287 cattle heads examined. Other species of *Thelazia* infest dogs, cats, and man. *T. lacrymalis* was found in 28 per cent of horses whose eyes were examined at an abattoir.

Face Flies
(see under FLIES)

Facial Deformity
(see HOLOPROSENCEPHALY)

'Facial Eczema'
'Facial eczema' is a synonym used outside the UK for light sensitisation in cattle and sheep. (See LIGHT SENSITISATION.)

Facial Nerve
The facial nerve is the 7th of the cranial nerves, and supplies the muscles of expression of the face. It is totally a motor nerve.

Facial Paralysis
In the case of unilateral 'facial paralysis', which very often follows accidents in which the side of the face has been badly bruised. The muscles on one side become paralysed but those on the opposite side are unaffected. This absence of antagonism between the 2 sides results in the upper and lower lips, and the muscles around the nostrils, becoming drawn over towards the unaffected side, and the animal presents an altered facial expression. The ear on the injured side of the head very often hangs loosely and flaps back and forward with every movement of the head, and the eyelids on the same side are held half-shut. (See also under GUTTURAL POUCH DISEASE; LISTERIOSIS.)

Factory Chimneys
Smoke from these may contaminate pastures and cause disease in grazing animals. (See FLUOROSIS; MOLYBDENUM.)

'Fading'
'Fading' is the colloquial name for an illness of puppies, leading usually to their death within a few days of birth. Symptoms include: progressive weakness which soon makes suckling impossible; a falling body temperature; and 'paddling' movements. Affected puppies may be killed by their dams. One cause is canine viral hepatitis; another is a canine herpesvirus; a 3rd may be a blood incompatibility; a 4th Bordetella; a 5th is hypothermia or 'chilling' in which the puppy's body temperature falls. A possible 6th cause may be *Clostridium perfringens* infection.

Kittens A similar syndrome may be caused by the feline leukaemia virus.

Faeces, Eating of
(see COPROPHAGY)

Fainting Fits (Syncope)
Fainting fits (syncope) are generally due to cerebral anaemia occurring through weakened pulsation of the heart, sudden shock, or severe injury. It is most commonly seen in dogs and cats, especially when old, but cases have been seen in all animals. (See HEART STIMULANTS.)

Falcons, Diseases of
Avian pox has been found in imported peregrine falcons, giving rise to scab formation on feet and face and leading sometimes to blindness. Tuberculosis is not uncommon, and may be suspected when the bird loses weight. (A tuberculin test is practicable and worth carrying out, owing to the risk of infection being transmitted to other falcons and to people handling them.) 'Frounce' and 'inflammation of the crop' are old names for a condition, caused by infestation with *Capillaria* worms, which can be successfully treated. Frounce causes a bird to refuse food, or to pick up pieces of meat and flick them away again, swallowing apparently being too painful; there is also a sticky, white discharge at the corners of the beak and in the mouth.

Abnormal gait and spontaneous bone fractures may arise as a result of calcium deficiency through birds being fed an all-meat diet not containing bone. This deficiency may be prevented by sprinkling sterilised bone meal or oyster shell on the meat, or feeding the bird with small rodents.

In the Middle East, dosing falcons with ammonium chloride – a common if misguided practice believed to enhance their hunting qualities – has caused sickness and fatalities.

Fallopian Tubes
These, one on each side, run from the extremity of the horns of the uterus to the region of the ovary.

Falls from High Buildings

Cats 'They have an astonishing capacity for survival after falling from great heights,' according to a New York veterinary practice that recorded the injuries suffered by 132 cats which had fallen from a height of between 2 and 32 storeys on to pavements below. Ninety per cent of the cats survived after treatment.

Injuries increased, as would be expected, in proportion to the distance fallen – up to about 7 storeys. However, the number of fractures decreased with falls from a greater height than that. It is suggested that this was because the cats then extended their legs to an almost horizontal position, like flying squirrels, making the impact more evenly distributed. This resulted in more chest injuries than fractured ribs, however.

Emergency treatment was required in 37 per cent of the cats, non-emergency treatment in 30 per cent.

What causes them to fall? In a few instances, it seems, they lose their balance while turning on a narrow window-ledge. More often it happens while trying to catch a bird or insect. It has also been known for a cat to panic, and leap off the ledge, when threatened by a strange dog let into the room behind.

Dogs Of 81 dogs which had fallen from 1 to 6 storeys, all but 1 dog survived. 'The falls of 52 of the dogs were witnessed, and of them, 39 had jumped.' Injuries to face, chest, and extremities resulted in dogs falling 1 or 2 storeys. Spinal injuries were caused more often in falls from a greater height.

False Pregnancy
(see under PSEUDO-PREGNANCY)

Fan Failure
In buildings that are ventilated artificially, it is mandatory under the Welfare of Farmed Animals Regulations 2000 (2001 in Wales) to have an alarm and standby system in order to prevent heat-stroke or anoxia (see CONTROLLED ENVIRONMENT HOUSING).

Faradism
Local application of an electric current as a passive exercise which stimulates muscles and nerves.

Farcy
Chronic form of glanders (see GLANDERS).

Farm Animal Welfare Council (FAWC)
An independent body set up by the government in 1979 to keep under review the welfare of farmed animals. Farms, markets, abattoirs and vehicles are inspected and, where appropriate, recommendations made to government. Reports are issued from time to time on the welfare of particular species or aspects (transport, slaughter, etc.) of the use of farm animals. The address is: 1a Page Street, London SW1P 4PQ.

Farm Chemicals
(see SPRAYS USED ON CROPS; FERTILISERS; METALDEHYDE)

Farm, Operations on the
In the UK it is illegal for castration of horse, donkey, mule, dog or cat to be carried out without an anaesthetic. (See ANAESTHESIA, LEGAL REQUIREMENTS; CASTRATION.) Only a veterinary surgeon is permitted to castrate any farm animal more than 2 months old, with the exception of rams, for which the maximum age is 3 months.

Only veterinary surgeons are permitted to carry out a vasectomy or electro-ejaculation of any farm animal; likewise the de-snooding of turkeys over 21 days old, de-combing of domestic fowls over 72 hours old, and de-toeing of fowls and turkeys over 72 hours old. Nor can anyone but a veterinary surgeon remove supernumerary teats of calves over 3 months old, or disbud or dishorn sheep or goats.

Certain overseas procedures are prohibited in the UK, namely freeze-dagging of sheep, penis amputation and other operations on the penis, tongue amputation in calves, hot branding of cattle, and the de-voicing of cockerels. Very short docking of sheep is also prohibited (see DOCKING).

Farm Treatment Against Worms
(see WORMS)

'Farmer's Lung'
A disease caused by the inhalation of dust, from mouldy hay, etc., containing spores of e.g. *Thermopolyspora polyspora* or *Micropolyspora faeni*. Localised histamine release in the lung produces oedema, resulting in poor oxygen uptake. The condition has been recognised in humans, cattle, horses and turkeys. In chickens, a similar condition has been caused by inhalation of dust from dead mites in sugar cane bagasse. It is classed as an acute extrinsic allergic alveolitis. Repeated exposure causes respiratory distress, even when the interval between exposures is several years.

Farm, Veterinary Facilities on the
(see VETERINARY FACILITIES ON THE FARM)

Farrier
A person who shoes horses. Farriery is a craft of great antiquity and the farrier has been described as the ancestor of the veterinarian. In the UK, farriery training is strictly controlled.

Intending farriers must undergo a 5-year apprenticeship, including a period at an authorised college, then take an examination for the diploma of the Worshipful Company of Farriers before they can practise independently. The training is controlled by the Farriers Training Council and a register of farriers kept by the Farriers Registration Council, Sefton House, Adam Court, Newark Road, Peterborough PE1 5PP. Its website is at www.farrier-reg.gov.uk.

Farrowing

The act of parturition in the sow.

Farrowing Crates

A rectangular box in which the sow gives birth. Their use is helpful in preventing overlying of piglets by the sow, and so in obviating one cause of piglet mortality; however, they are far from ideal. Farrowing rails serve the same purpose but perhaps the best arrangement is the circular one which originated in New Zealand. (See ROUNDHOUSE.)

Work at the University of Nebraska suggests that a round stall is better, because the conventional rectangular one does not allow the sow to obey her natural nesting instincts, and may give rise to stress, more stillbirths and agalactia.

Farrowing Rates

In the sow, the farrowing rate after 1 natural service appears to be in the region of 86 per cent. Following a 1st artificial insemination, the farrowing rate appears to be appreciably lower, but at the Lyndhurst, Hants AI Centre, a farrowing rate of about 83 per cent was obtained when only females which stood firmly to be mounted at insemination time were used. The national (British) average farrowing rate has been estimated at 65 per cent for a 1st insemination.

Fascia

Sheets or bands of fibrous tissue which enclose and connect the muscles.

Fascioliasis

Infestation with liver flukes.

Fat

Normal body fat is, chemically, an ester of 3 molecules of 1, 2, or 3 fatty acids, with 1 molecule of glycerol. Such fats are known as glycerides, to distinguish them from other fats and waxes in which an alcohol other than glycerol has formed the ester. (See also LIPIDS [which include fat]; FATTY ACIDS. For fat as a tissue, see ADIPOSE TISSUE. A LIPOMA is a benign fatty tumour.

For other diseases associated with fat, see STEATITIS; FATTY LIVER SYNDROME; OBESITY, DIET.)

Fat Supplements

In poultry rations these can lead to TOXIC FAT DISEASE. (See LIPIDS for cattle supplement; also ECZEMA in cats.)

Fatigue

(see EXERCISE; MUSCLE; NERVES)

Fatty Acids

These, with an alcohol, form FAT. Saturated fatty acids have twice as many hydrogen atoms as carbon atoms, and each molecule of fatty acid contains 2 atoms of oxygen. Unsaturated fatty acids contain less than twice as many hydrogen atoms as carbon items, and 1 or more pairs of adjacent atoms are connected by double bonds. Polyunsaturated fatty acids are those in which several pairs of adjacent carbon atoms contain double bonds.

Fatty Degeneration

A condition in which there is an excess of fat in the parenchyma cells of organs such as the liver, heart, and kidneys.

Fatty Liver Haemorrhagic Syndrome (FLHS)

This is a condition in laying hens which has to be differentiated from FLKS (see next entry) of high-carbohydrate broiler-chicks. Factors involved include high carbohydrate diets, high environmental temperatures, high oestrogen levels, and the particular strain of bird. FLHS in hens is improved by diets based on wheat as compared with maize; whereas FLKS is aggravated by diets based on wheat. Death is due to haemorrhage from the enlarged liver.

Fatty Liver/Kidney Syndrome of Chickens (FLKS)

A condition in which excessive amounts of fat are present in the liver, kidneys, and myocardium. The liver is pale and swollen, with haemorrhages sometimes present, and the kidneys vary from being slightly swollen and pale pink to being excessively enlarged and white. Morbidity is usually between 5 and 30 per cent.

Cause FLKS has been shown to respond to biotin (see VITAMINS), and accordingly can be prevented by suitable modification of the diet.

Signs A number of the more forward birds (usually 2 to 3 weeks old) suddenly show symptoms of paralysis. They lie down on their breasts with their heads stretched forward; others lie on their sides with their heads bent over their backs. Death may occur within a few hours. Mortality seldom exceeds 1 per cent.

Fatty Liver Syndrome of Cattle

A 'production disease' which may occur in high-yielding dairy cows immediately after calving. It is then that they are subjected to 'energy deficit' and mobilise body reserves for milk production. This mobilisation results in the accumulation of fat in the liver, and also in muscle and kidney. In some cases the liver cells become so engorged with fat that they actually rupture.

An important consequence of this syndrome may be an adverse effect on fertility. Cows with a severe fatty liver syndrome were reported to have had a calving interval of 443 days, as compared with 376 days for those with a mild fatty liver syndrome.

Complications such as chronic ketosis, parturient paresis (recumbency after calving), and a greater susceptibility to infection have been also been reported.

Fatty Liver Syndrome of Turkeys

The only sign may be wattles paler than normal; the birds remain apparently in good condition. The cause may be varied – genetic, nutritional, management, environmental, and presence of toxic substances. Adding choline, vitamins E and B_{12}, and inositol to the diet can remedy the condition. Reducing the metabolisable energy level in the diet by about 14 per cent usually prevents it.

Fauces

Fauces is the narrow opening which connects the mouth with the throat. It is bounded above by the soft palate, below by the base of the tongue, and the openings of the tonsils lies at either side.

Faulty Nutrition

(see ACETONAEMIA; ACIDOSIS; KETOSIS; NUTRITION; FEED BLOCKS; DIET; LAMENESS in cattle; BLINDNESS)

Faulty Wiring of Farm Equipment

Faulty wiring of farm equipment has led to cows refusing concentrates in the parlour, not because they were unpalatable (as at first thought), but because the container was live so that cows wanting to feed were deterred by a mild electric shock. (See also EARTHING; ELECTRIC SHOCK.)

Favus

Favus is another name for 'honeycomb ringworm'. (See RINGWORM.)

FAWC

(see FARM ANIMAL WELFARE COUNCIL)

Feather Picking (Feather Pulling)

Feather picking (feather pulling) in poultry and in cage birds, particularly parrots, may be due to boredom or insecurity. It is in many cases due to the irritation caused by lice or to the ravages of the depluming mite. In such cases the necessary anti-parasitic measures must be taken. Insufficient animal protein in the diet of young growing chicks, especially when kept under intensive conditions, may cause the vice. Once the birds start pulling the feather they sooner or later draw blood, and an outbreak of cannibalism results. Treatment consists of isolating the culprit, if it can be found at the beginning, and of feeding the birds a balanced diet containing green food. The addition of blood meal in the mash is effective in many cases. The use of blue glass in intensive houses has stopped the habit in some cases.

Febantel

An anthelmintic used for the treatment of parasitic gastroenteritis and parasitic bronchitis in cattle, sheep, pigs and horses. Chemically, it is a probezimidazole which is converted in the body to benzimidazole.

Fedesa

The European Federation of Animal Health, an association of veterinary medicine manufacturers.

Feed Additives

(see ADDITIVES)

Feed Blocks

These 'self-help' lick blocks, placed out on pasture, are useful especially on hill farms for preventing loss of condition and even semi-starvation in the ewe.

Most feed blocks contain cereals as a source of carbohydrate, protein from natural sources supplemented by urea, minerals, trace elements, and vitamins. In some blocks glucose or molasses is substituted for the cereals as the chief source of carbohydrate. A 3rd type contains no protein or urea but provides glucose, minerals, trace elements, and vitamins; being especially useful in the context of hypomagnesaemia (and other metabolic ills) in ewes shortly before and after lambing.

Their effectiveness for providing specific ingredients is variable as animals differ in the extent to which they use feed blocks.

Feed Conversion Efficiency (FCE)

The gain in weight, in kg or lb, produced by 1 kg or 1 lb of feed; it is the reciprocal of the feed conversion ratio.

If FCRs are to be used as a basis of comparison as between one litter and another, or one farm's pigs and another's, it is essential that the same meal or other foods be used; otherwise the figures become meaningless.

Feed Conversion Ratio (FCR)

The amount of feed in kg or lb necessary to produce 1 kg or 1 lb of weight gain.

Feeding

(see DIET; FAULTY NUTRITION)

Feeding-Stuffs, Storage of

Feed must be stored separately from fertilisers, or contamination and subsequent poisoning may occur.

The safe storage period on the farm of certain feeds is given under DIET.

Poultry and rats and mice must not be allowed to contaminate feeding-stuffs, or SALMONELLOSIS may result. If warfarin has been used, this may be contained in rodents' urine and lead to poisoning of stock through contamination of feeding-stuffs. (See also TOXOPLASMOSIS.)

Unsterilised bone-meal is a potential source of salmonellosis and anthrax infections.

(See also ADDITIVES; CONCENTRATES; DIET; MOULDY FOOD; MYCOTOXICOSIS; CUBES; SACKS; LUBRICANTS.)

Feeding-Stuffs Regulations 2000

Feeding-Stuffs Regulations 2000 control the constituents of animal feed including pet food. They specify, among other items, permitted additives, colourants, emulsifiers, stabilisers, maximum amounts of vitamins and trace elements, and permitted preservatives.

Feedlots

Feedlots involve the zero-grazing of beef cattle on a very large scale. In the USA there are some feedlots of 100,000 head each, and many more containing tens of thousands of cattle. Veterinary problems arise when these cattle are brought to the feedlot from range or pasture, and fed on grain. Shipping fever is a common ailment; likewise liver abscesses.

Feline Anaemia

(see ANAEMIA; TOXOPLASMOSIS; HAEMO-BARTONELLA; FELINE LEUKAEMIA; FELINE BABESIOSIS)

Feline Babesiosis

Young cats may develop immunity to *Babesia felis*; older cats often have recurrent illness. Subclinical infections occur. When symptoms are present they include lethargy, loss of appetite, anaemia, and occasionally jaundice. The disease can prove fatal. (See also BABESIOSIS.)

Feline Bordetellosis

A disease of the upper respiratory tract of cats involving *Bordetella bronchiseptica*. Clinical signs can be mild, or fatal pneumonia can develop. Some animals may become symptomless carriers of the organism (which is also responsible for kennel cough in dogs). Treatment is by antibiotics.

Feline Calicivirus

One of the causes of FELINE INFLUENZA. Infection by calicivirus (of which there are several strains) may occur in combination with FELINE HERPESVIRUS. Signs include fever, discharge from the eyes and nose, and ulcers of the mouth and tongue. The virus is disseminated by sneezing cats, and on the hands and clothing of attendants, etc.

Feline Cancer

Cancer is an important disease of cats, and an American estimate suggests a rate of 264 per 100,000 cats per year. Cancer of the lymph nodes was most common (31 per cent), followed by 16 per cent involving the bone marrow. Skin cancer accounted for 7 per cent, mammary gland cancer for 5 per cent. (See also under CANCER for figures relating to mammary gland tumours, both benign and malignant.)

Feline Cardiomyopathy

Clinical signs of this heart condition include dyspnoea, weight loss and lethargy. Diagnosis is by radiography. Beta blockers, digitalis and diltiazem have been used in treatment. The cause is unknown.

Feline Chlamydial Infection

An acute upper respiratory disease caused by *Chlamydiophila felis*; also known as feline pneumonitis. Signs include conjunctivitis with severe swelling and redness, nasal discharge, sneezing and coughing. It commonly affects groups of animals, rarely single cats. Treatment includes topical and/or systemic antibiotics.

Chlamydiosis vaccine (available as a combination product) protects against clinical disease but not infection.

Feline Coronavirus

This is a common infection in cats. It may be linked to FELINE INFECTIOUS PERITONITIS (FIP).

Feline Diabetes

(see under DIABETES)

Feline Dysautonomia (Key-Gaskell Syndrome)

A condition in cats first recognised at Bristol University's department of veterinary medicine in 1981–2. It is also called feline autonomic polygangliopathy.

Signs include depression, loss of appetite, prominent nictitating membranes, dry and encrusted nostrils – suggesting a respiratory disease. Constipation and a transient diarrhoea have both been reported; also incontinence in some cases. The pupils are dilated and unresponsive to light. There may be difficulty in swallowing and food may be regurgitated; a key finding is enlargement of the oesophagus. The prognosis seems to depend on the degree of this 'megalo-oesophagus'; the greater the enlargement, the poorer the prognosis. Lesions include loss of nerve cells, and their replacement by fibrous tissue, in certain ganglia.

Cause The syndrome has some similarities with 'GRASS SICKNESS' in horses and, like the latter, appears to be prevalent only in the UK with a few cases reported from Scandinavia.

Treatment involves countering dehydration by means of glucose-saline, offering tempting food or feeding liquid foods by syringe, and use of eyedrops containing pilocarpine to obtain pupil constriction.

Prognosis The recovery rate is stated to be about 25 per cent, but recuperation may take weeks or months. Cats with a greatly enlarged oesophagus, persistent loss of appetite, or bladder paralysis are the least likely to survive.

(See also CANINE DYSAUTONOMIA.)

Feline Ehrlichiosis

A disease in which affected cats show anorexia, weakness, lameness (due to bleeding in the joints) and thrombocytopenia. The cause is infection by *Ehrlichia canis* in France and *E. phygocytophila* in the UK. Tick repellents help prevent infection; treatment is with doxycycline or tetracycline.

Feline Encephalomyelitis

This has been reported in Sydney, Australia, and is characterised by non-fatal cases of hind-leg ataxia, and sometimes by side-to-side movements of head and neck. On post-mortem examination, demyelinating lesions and perivascular cuffing involving the brain and spinal cord were found. The cause is thought to be a virus, but efforts to transmit the disease have failed.

Feline Eye Infections

Conjunctival swabs obtained from 39 cats with conjunctivitis and from 50 clinically normal cats were examined microbiologically. Non-haemolytic streptococci and *Staphylococcus epidermis* were isolated from both groups while beta-haemolytic streptococci, rhinotracheitis (feline herpes 1) virus, *Mycoplasma felis* and *Chlamydia psittaci* were isolated from cases with conjunctivitis. Organisms were isolated from 14 of the diseased cats and from 2 of the normal animals.

Feline Gingivitis

This can be mild and transient. Sometimes the term is applied not to an inflammation of the gums but merely to a hyperaemia – an increased blood flow – which 'may alarm the owner but does not hurt the (young) cat'.

Gingivitis can also be acute or chronic, easily treatable, or highly intractable.

One of the commonest causes of gingivitis in middle-aged or elderly cats is the accumulation of tartar on the surface of the teeth. If neglected, the tartar will gradually encroach on to the gums, causing these to become inflamed. Unless the tartar is removed, a shrinkage of the gums is likely to follow. As the gum recedes from the teeth it leaves pockets or spaces into which food particles and bacteria can lodge, exacerbating the inflammation, causing halitosis and leading to the roots of some teeth becoming infected.

The yellowish tartar deposits can become so thick and extensive that eventually they completely mask the teeth. A cat in this condition undoubtedly suffers much discomfort, finds eating a little difficult, and may have toothache. Health is further impaired by the persistent infection. The cat becomes dejected.

Even in such advanced cases, removal of the tartar (and of any loose teeth) can bring about almost a rejuvenation of the animal.

This form of chronic gingivitis can be successfully overcome by treatment and, indeed, prevented if an annual check of the teeth is carried out by a veterinary surgeon.

Intractable gingivitis Some cases of this are associated with a generalised illness rather than merely disease of the mouth. For example, chronic kidney disease, and possibly diabetes, may cause ulcers on the gums (as well as elsewhere in the mouth).

Some strains of the feline calicivirus may also cause gum and tongue ulceration. Bacterial secondary invaders are likely to worsen this, especially if the cat's bodily defence systems have been impaired by, say, the feline leukaemia virus, some other infection, or even stress.

Antibiotics or sulphonamides are used to control the bacteria; vitamins prescribed to assist the repair of damaged tissue and to help restore appetite, and other supportive measures taken. However, some cases of feline gingivitis do not respond.

It is likely that all the causes of feline gingivitis have not yet been established. Further research will no doubt bridge the gaps in existing knowledge, and bring new methods of treatment and a better prognosis. (See also FELINE STOMATITIS.)

Feline Herpesvirus

One of the causes of feline influenza. Infection may occur in combination with feline calicivirus. Clinical signs may be severe and include epiphora, coughing, dyspnoea and corneal ulcers. Secondary bacterial infection can lead to fatal pneumonia. Cats recovering from acute infection may develop chronic nasal disorders; they will also become carriers of the virus. Infection is spread by sneezing, and may be carried on equipment, clothing, hands of attendants, etc. (see FELINE VIRAL RHINOTRACHEITIS; FELINE INFLUENZA)

Feline Immunodeficiency Virus (FIV)

Formerly known as the feline T-lymphotropic lentivirus (FTLV). It was discovered in California by N. C. Pedersen and colleagues. Spread by the saliva of infected cats, or less often via the milk or placenta, it has a prolonged incubation period leading to permanent infection.

The virus is said to establish a permanent infection; the prognosis is poor. Clinical signs can be transient and mild – fever, depression, enlarged lymph glands. As the virus causes immunodeficiency, secondary infections account for many of the clinical signs.

Diagnosis is confirmed by laboratory demonstration of antibodies. Treatment is aimed at control of secondary infection by antibiotics; many cases, however, end fatally.

Feline Infectious Anaemia

This disease is caused by the bacterium *Mycoplasma haemofelis* (formerly classified as *Haemobartonella felis*). It is treated with antibiotics. Blood transfusions or fluid therapy may be required in severe, acute cases.

Adult cats may carry the parasite, the disease lying dormant until some debilitating condition (e.g. stress or immunosuppression) lowers the cat's resistance.

Signs are those associated with anaemia: loss of appetite, lethargy, weakness, and loss of weight. Anaemia may be severe enough to cause panting.

Diagnosis may be confirmed by identifying the causal agent in blood smears.

Feline Infectious Enteritis (Panleucopenia)

Formerly often known as feline distemper. Cats of all ages are susceptible; survivors appear to acquire lifelong immunity. The disease is less common than it was, as a result of successful vaccination programmes.

Cause A parvovirus, indistinguishable from mink enteritis virus. Resistant to heat and disinfectants, the virus can survive outside its host for a year.

Signs Loss of appetite, vomiting, intense depression, and prostration; the animal prefers to lie in cold places, cries out, and rapidly loses weight. The temperature, at first 40.5°C (105°F) or more, becomes subnormal in 12 to 18 hours, and death commonly occurs within 24 hours. Usually there is diarrhoea in the later stages. Dehydration is rapid. In newborn kittens, the brain may be affected giving rise to a staggering gait. In a few cases (which often recover) the tongue becomes ulcerated.

It seems that a mild form is common as many older cats have immunity without previous severe illness.

Diagnosis may be confirmed by laboratory tests – examination of bone marrow and blood smears. Poisoning, toxoplasmosis, intestinal foreign bodies, septicaemia and must be differentiated.

Prevention Live and inactivated vaccines are available; live vaccines, however, are not suitable for use in pregnant queens.

Treatment Whole blood given intravenously at 20 ml per kg or hyperimmune serum at 6 to 10 ml per kg, and lactated Ringer's solution, with anti-emetics every few hours, plus broad-spectrum antibiotics, vitamins, and an easily digested diet, such as baby food. In a cattery, isolation of in-contact animals and rigid disinfection must be practised. (See also NURSING.)

Feline Infectious Peritonitis (FIP)

A slowly progressive and fatal disease of young cats, and sometimes of older ones also, caused by a coronavirus. Although the coronavirus is commonly found in cats, most do not develop the disease. Where FIP develops, it usually does so in a 'wet' form in which fluid accumulates in the body cavities.

Clinical signs in the early stages are non-specific. Fever, depression, loss of appetite, gradual loss of weight, distension of the abdomen due to fluid. Occasionally, diarrhoea and vomiting occur. There may be distressed breathing.

There is also a much rarer 'dry' form, which may involve inflammation, and ultimately failure of the liver, kidneys, eyes, and brain. Both forms are fatal. Confirmation of a diagnosis of FIP depends on tissue biopsy or post-mortem examination.

Prevention is by avoiding overcrowding, culling of cats known to be infected (infected queens passing the disease to their kittens are a main source), and maintaining good hygiene in a clean environment. A vaccine is available in some countries.

Feline Influenza

The name is loosely applied to respiratory infections involving more than one virus, known as the feline viral respiratory disease complex. It commonly occurs in cat-breeding and boarding establishments, the infection(s) being highly contagious. Feline calicivirus and feline viral rhinotracheitis are commonly involved. Secondary bacterial invaders account for many of the more serious signs.

Signs Sneezing and coughing. The temperature is usually high at first; the appetite is depressed; the animal is dull; the eyes are kept half-shut, or the eyelids may be closed altogether; there is discharge from the nose; condition is rapidly lost. If pneumonia supervenes the breathing becomes very rapid and great distress is apparent; exhaustion and prostration follow. Diagnosis is confirmed by isolation of the virus from nasal swabs by a specialist laboratory.

Treatment Isolation of the sick cat under the best possible hygienic conditions is immediately necessary. There should be plenty of light and fresh air, and domesticated cats need to be kept fairly warm.

Antibiotics help to control secondary bacterial infection. Food should be light and easily digested. (See NURSING; PROTEIN, HYDROLYSED.)

Owing to the very highly contagious nature of the viruses causing feline influenza, disinfection after recovery must be very thorough before other cats are admitted to the premises.

Prevention Live and inactivated combined vaccines against feline viral rhinotracheitis and feline calicivirus are available; inactivated preparations are given parenterally and live preparations formulated for parenteral and intranasal use. Vaccines are generally effective, but as there are several strains of feline calicivirus, they may not protect against them all. Other controls include strict hygiene (of premises and attendants) and the segregation of carrier (infected) cats.

Feline Juvenile Osteodystrophy

Feline juvenile osteodystrophy is a disease, of nutritional origin, in the growing kitten.

Cause A diet deficient in calcium and rich in phosphorus; kittens fed exclusively on minced beef or sheep heart have developed the disease within 8 weeks.

Signs The kitten becomes less playful and reluctant to jump down even from modest heights; it may become stranded when climbing curtains owing to being unable to disengage its claws. There may be lameness, sometimes due to a green-stick fracture; pain in the back may make the kitten bad-tempered and sometimes unable to stand. In kittens which survive, deformity of the skeleton may be shown in later life, with bowing of long bones, fractures, prominence of the spine of the shoulder blade, and abnormalities which together suggest a shortening of the back.

Feline Leishmaniasis

This is a cause of ulcers, and small, palpable swellings under the skin. The disease is transmissible to human beings. (See LEISHMANIASIS.)

Feline Leukaemia

A disease of cats caused by a virus (FeLV) discovered by Professor W. F. H. Jarrett in 1964. The virus gives rise to cancer, especially lymphosarcoma involving the alimentary canal and thymus, and lymphatic leukaemia. Anaemia, glomerulonephritis, and an immunosuppressive syndrome may also result from this infection, which can be readily transmitted from cat to cat. Many cats are able to overcome the infection. The virus may infect not only the bone marrow, lymph nodes, etc., but also epithelial cells of mouth, nose, salivary glands, intestine, and urinary bladder.

Kittens of up to 4 months of age are more likely to become permanently infected with FeLV than older cats, but many cases do occur in cats over 5 years old.

Many cats which have apparently recovered from natural exposure to the virus remain latently infected, but keep free from FeLV-associated diseases. Such cats may infect their kittens via the milk.

Most deaths of FeLV-positive cats are not directly attributable to this virus, but to other viral or bacterial infections which, in the ordinary way, would not prove fatal to the cat; but which are rendered far more serious owing to the immunosuppression caused by the virus.

Significance of FeLV There is an association between FeLV infection and anaemia, tumours of the leukaemia/lymphoma complex, feline infectious peritonitis, bacterial infections, emaciation, FeLV-associated enteritis, lymphatic hyperplasia and haemorrhage. Links have also been established with icterus, several types of hepatitis, and liver degeneration.

Signs These vary with the age of the cat at infection; they include a gradual loss of condition, poor appetite, depression, anaemia. Breathing may become laboured due to the accumulation of fluid within the chest. A persistent cough, and vomiting, are other signs.

Diagnosis FeLV infection can be detected by a fluorescent antibody test, an ELISA test, electron microscopic examination of tissues, and by isolation of virus.

Control It is possible to prevent the spread of the disease to susceptible cats by a 'test-and-removal' system. Infected cats are removed from the household for euthanasia, and other cats in the same household are then tested. If FeLV-positive, they too are removed, even if clinically healthy. Retesting of the FeLV-negative cats is necessary after 3 and 6 months. If still FeLV-negative, they can be considered clear, and new cats introduced on to the premises, if desired.

The virus may persist in the bone marrow of cats which have ostensibly recovered. Such a latent infection can be reactivated by large doses of corticosteroid; the virus can be recovered by cultivation of bone marrow cells. FeLV is not transmitted from cats with a latent infection.

Vaccines will not protect cats that are already infected. Inactivated vaccines produced from the whole virus suitably processed, or by biotechnology from the 'envelope' of the virus which produces antigen but not infection, are available.

Feline Miliary Dermatitis
(see ECZEMA)

Feline Panleukopenia
(see FELINE INFECTIOUS ENTERITIS)

Feline Pneumonitis
(see FELINE CHLAMYDIAL INFECTION)

Feline Pyothorax
(see PYOTHORAX)

Feline Spongiform Encephalopathy (FSE)
This is similar clinically to BOVINE SPONGIFORM ENCEPHALOPATHY (BSE). The first signs are hypersensitivity to noise and visual stimuli. Ataxia follows and eventually the cat will not be able to get up. The cause is believed to be the eating of material from cattle affected by BSE. In a zoo, 2 pumas and a stray cat which shared their food were fed on split bovine heads. Both pumas and the cat died from FSE. At the height of the BSE outbreak in the 1990s, one case of FSE was being reported every 6 weeks.

Feline Stomatitis
Inflammation of the cat's mouth.

Causes Various. Viruses associated with stomatitis in the cat include the feline calicivirus in addition the rhinotracheitis virus; in addition, a chronic ulcerative stomatitis might be due to immunosuppression by the feline leukaemia virus, for example.

Signs These include difficulty in swallowing, halitosis, excessive salivation, loss of appetite, and sometimes bleeding.

Treatment The aim is to limit secondary bacterial infection by means of antibiotics. A supplement of vitamins A, B, and C may help. If the cat will not eat, subcutaneous fluid therapy will be required.

Chronic stomatitis in elderly cats may be due to EOSINOPHILIC GRANULOMA, or malignant growths such as squamous-cell CARCINOMA or FIBROSARCOMA. (See also FELINE GINGIVITIS.)

Feline T-Lymphotropic Lentivirus
(see FELINE IMMUNODEFICIENCY VIRUS)

Feline Urological Syndrome (FUS)

The name given to the several conditions causing painful and difficult urination as well as debility which, if untreated, can lead to death. Both cystitis and obstruction of the urethra may have a feature in common: the formation of sand-like material, composed of varying proportions of crystalline and organic matter. The crystals are usually struvite (ammonium magnesium phosphate hexahydrate). Calculi or 'stones' also sometimes occur in the cat, but less commonly than the sand-like deposits.

Cause Various theories have been advanced to account for FUS, which is much more common in male cats. It has been suggested that a virus or viruses may be involved, and that a high level of magnesium in the diet could cause FUS. The effects of heredity and castration have also been mentioned.

FUS is said to be more likely to occur when a cat is fed an ordinary commercial dry, rather than canned, food because these dry foods are lower in calories and digestibility than many canned foods. 'This increases the amount of dry food that the cat must eat to meet calorie requirements and, therefore, increases the amount of magnesium consumed and excreted in the urine.'

Excess magnesium can favour the formation of sand-like struvite crystals in the bladder. If the cat's urine is not sufficiently acidic (pH5 to 6), as it would be on a normal carnivorous diet, the formation of crystals is also encouraged.

Feline dry diets are now formulated to maintain urine at the correct degree of acidity to avoid the problem.

Signs The owners may notice the cat straining to pass urine, with only very little to be seen in the litter tray. The urine may be bloodstained. Cat-owners sometimes mistake FUS for constipation.

Other signs include loss of appetite, dejection, and restlessness. Signs of pain will be shown if the abdomen is touched, owing to distension of the bladder. Urethral blockage is an emergency requiring immediate veterinary attention, in default of which there is a great risk of collapse, leading to unconsciousness. The bladder may rupture, causing additional shock, and leading to peritonitis.

Treatment Skilled manipulation can sometimes free a plug (often a mixture of organic material and the struvite crystals) blocking the end of the penis. If this fails, or if the obstruction is further back, a catheter will have to be passed. If catheterisation fails, it will be necessary to empty the bladder by means of aspiration or incision.

Prognosis There are cases in which, after removal of the urethral obstruction, the latter does not recur. Unfortunately, in between 20 and 50 per cent of cases, recurrence does take place. After 2 or 3 such recurrences, the owner has to decide whether euthanasia would be best for the cat, rather than have it subjected to even more catherisations; or whether to opt for a URETHROSTOMY operation. (The potential benefits and risks are referred to under that heading.)

Post-operative treatment includes antibiotics and urine acid-alkali balance control in an attempt to dissolve the remaining crystals.

A low-magnesium, urine-acidifying diet, including taurine, is also recommended and proprietary preparations are on sale to meet this requirement. (See PRESCRIPTION DIETS.)

Feline Vestibular Syndrome, Idiopathic

The name given to a condition in which headtilt, ataxia, nystagmus, and occasionally vomiting were seen. Duration of signs was only up to 24 hours; 1 hour in 2 cats.

Feline Viral Rhinotracheitis

Feline viral rhinotracheitis is involved in the feline viral respiratory disease complex (FELINE INFLUENZA). The disease was discovered in the USA, and first recorded in Britain in 1966. Severe symptoms are usually confined to kittens of up to 6 months old. Sneezing, conjunctivitis with discharge, coughing and ulcerated tongue may be seen. Bronchopneumonia and chronic sinusitis are possible complications.

Cause A herpesvirus. Infection may occur in a latent form, and a possible link has been suggested between this virus and feline syncytia-forming virus.

Live and inactivated vaccines are available against feline calicivirus and feline herpesvirus which may be implicated in the infection.

Treatment May include the use of a steam vaporiser, lactated Ringer's solution to overcome dehydration, and antibiotics. Vitamins and baby foods may help.

Feminisation
In the male dog this may occur as the result of a SERTOLI-CELL TUMOUR of a testicle.

Femur
Femur is the bone of the thigh, reaching from the hip-joint above to the stifle-joint below. It is the largest, strongest, and longest individual bone of the body. The bone lies at a slope of about 45 degrees to the horizontal in most animals when they are at rest, articulating at its upper end with the acetabulum of the pelvis, and at its lower end with the tibia. Just above the joint surface for the tibia is the patellar surface, upon which slides the patella, or 'knee cap'.

Fractures of the head of the femur are common. Repair by means of divergent K wires, or lag screws, has been described.

Fenbendazole
A benzimidazole anthelmintic used in cattle, horses, pigs, dogs and cats. (See WORMS, FARM TREATMENT AGAINST.)

Fentanyl
An analgesic for use in small mammals (rabbits, ferrets, guinea pigs, rats and mice). It is usually combined with FLUANISONE for use as a neuroleptoanalgesic.

Ferns
Ferns other than bracken occasionally cause poisoning in cattle. For example, *Dryopteris filixmas* (male fern) and *D. borreri* (rusty male fern) give rise to blindness, drowsiness and a desire to stand or lie in water. Poisoning is occasionally fatal. (See also BRACKEN POISONING.)

Ferret
(*Mustela putorius furo*) These attractive creatures are increasingly popular as pets. They need careful and expert handling – a bite to the finger can penetrate to the bone. In the UK the breeding season begins in March and continues until the end of August. It is preferable that females ('jills' – males are 'hobs') not used for breeding are spayed. Unmated jills may be in oestrus for the whole of the breeding season, with the occurrence of persistently high levels of oestrogen. This can cause severe health problems, including a possibly fatal pancytopenia. The alternatives to spaying are injections of proligestone, given via the scruff of the neck, or

mating with a vasectomised male. The latter will result in a pseudo-pregnancy lasting about 42 days; the jill may need to be mated again if she returns to oestrus.

Other diseases of ferrets include hypocalcaemia, 3 to 4 weeks after giving birth; mastitis; ALEUTIAN DISEASE; CANINE DISTEMPER; BOTULISM (type C); abscesses; enteritis due to *E. coli* or campylobacter. Skin tumours are not uncommon. Periodontal disease is often caused by the accumulation of dental calculus. Urolithiasis can occur; the ferret can be fed food formulated for this condition in the cat. Ferrets are susceptible to zinc poisoning and any galvanised material can be a risk.

Ferritin
Ferritin is a form in which iron is stored in the body. Ferritin concentrations in serum are closely related to total body iron stores, and ferritin immunoassays can be used to assess the clinical iron status of human beings, horses, cattle, dogs, and pigs.

Fertilisation
(see REPRODUCTION)

Fertilisers
Fertilisers should not be stored near feedingstuffs, as contamination of the latter, leading to poisoning, may occur. In Australia, 17 out of 50 Herefords died after gaining access to the remains of a fertiliser dump. A crust of superphosphate and ammonium sulphate had remained on the ground.

For the risk associated with unsterilised bonemeal, see under ANTHRAX and SALMONELLOSIS.

Hypomagnesaemia is frequently encountered in animals grazing pasture which has received a recent dressing with potash. (See also BASIC SLAG; FOG FEVER.)

Fertility
(see CONCEPTION RATES; FARROWING RATES; INFERTILITY; CALVING INTERVAL)

Fescue
In New Zealand and the USA, a severe hindfoot lameness of cattle has been attributed to the grazing of *Festuca arundinacea*, a coarse grass which grows on poorly drained land or on the banks of ditches, and being tall stands out above the snow. In typical cases, the left hindfoot is affected first, and becomes cold, the skin being dry and necrotic. Symptoms appear 10 to 14 days after the cattle go on to the tall-fescue-dominated pasture. Ergot may be present, but is not invariably so.

It has been suggested that 'fescue foot' may be associated with a potent toxin, butenolide, produced by the fungus *Fusarium tricinctum*.

Fetal Infections

Examples of these are TOXOCARIASIS in bitches; and TOXOPLASMOSIS *in utero* of cows, ewes, sows, bitches and cats.

Fetal Membranes

(see CHORION; AMNION; ALLANTOIS; also UTERUS, DISEASES OF and EMBRYOLOGY)

Fetal Resorption

(see MUMMIFICATION)

Fetlock-Joint

The joint in the horse's limb between the metacarpus or metatarsus (cannon bones) and the 1st phalanx (long pastern bone). At the back of this joint are situated the sesamoids of the 1st phalanx. (See BONES.)

Fetus

For an outline description of the development of the fetus, see under EMBRYOLOGY. For fetal circulation, see the diagram under CIRCULATION OF BLOOD. (See also FREEMARTIN.)

Fever

Fever is one of the commonest symptoms of infectious disease, and serves to make the distinction between febrile and non-febrile ailments.

Examples of specific fevers are equine influenza, distemper, braxy, blackquarter, or swine fever.

When fever reaches an excessively high stage, e.g. 41.5°C (107°F), in the horse or dog, the term 'hyperpyrexia' (excessive fever) is applied, and it is regarded as indicating a condition of danger; while if it exceeds 42° or 42.5°C (108° or 109°F) for any length of time, death almost always results. Occasionally, in certain fevers or febrile conditions, such as severe heat-stroke, the temperature may reach 44.5°C (112°F). (See also under TEMPERATURE.)

There is usually a certain amount of shivering, to which the term 'rigor' is applied, but this is very often not noticed by the owner. The stage of rigor is followed by dullness, the animal standing about with a distressed expression or moving sluggishly. Later, perspiration, rapid breathing, a fast, full, bounding pulse, and a greater elevation of temperature are exhibited. Thirst is usually marked; the appetite disappears; the urine is scanty and of a high specific gravity; the bowels are generally constipated,

although diarrhoea may follow later; oedema of all the visible mucous membranes, i.e. those of the eyes, nostrils, mouth, occurs. (See also HYPERTHERMIA.)

Fever may perhaps have a beneficial effect. It was noticed in the 19th century that patients in a Russian mental hospital, suffering from neurosyphilis, improved as regards their paresis during a fever outbreak; and 'malaria therapy' was introduced at a later date. Experiments with newborn mice show that fatal infection with Coxsackie B1 virus can be modified to a subclinical infection if the animals are kept in an incubator at 34°C (93°F) and thus attain the same body temperature as mice of 8 to 9 days old. Similarly, puppies infected with canine herpesvirus survive longer and have diminished replication of virus in their organs if their body temperature is artificially raised to that of adult dogs.

Fibre, Importance of

(see under DIET)

Fibrillation

An involuntary contraction of individual bundles of muscle fibres.

Fibrin

Fibrin is a substance upon which depends the formation of blood clots. (See CLOTTING OF BLOOD; PLASMA.)

Fibrin is found not only in coagulated blood, but also in many inflammatory conditions. Later it is either dissolved again by, and taken up into, the blood, or is 'organised' into fibrous tissue.

Fibrinogen, Plasma

Concentration of this is increased in inflammatory conditions, especially lesions of serous surfaces and in endocarditis. (See also CLOTTING OF BLOOD.)

Fibroblast

A flat, irregularly shaped connective-tissue cell.

Fibroma

(see TUMOURS)

Fibrosarcoma

A tumour composed mainly of fibrous or connective tissue; often malignant.

Fibrosis

The formation of fibrous tissue, which may replace other tissue. (See also CIRRHOSIS.)

Fibrous Tissue

Fibrous tissue is one of the most abundant tissues of the body, being found in quantity below the skin, around muscles and to a lesser extent between them, and forming tendons to a great extent; quantities are associated with bone when it is being calcified and afterwards, and fibrous tissue is always laid down where healing or inflammatory processes are at work. There are 2 varieties: white fibrous tissue and yellow elastic fibrous tissue.

White fibrous tissue consists of a substance called 'collagen' which yields gelatin on boiling, and is arranged in bundles of fibres between which lie flattened, star-shaped cells. It is very unyielding and forms tendons and ligaments; it binds the bundles of muscle fibres together, is laid down during the repair of wounds, and forms the scars which result; it may form the basis of cartilage; and it has the property of contracting as time goes on so may cause puckering of the tissues around.

Yellow fibrous tissue is not so plentiful as the former. It consists of bundles of long yellow fibres, formed from a substance called 'elastin', and is very elastic. It is found in the walls of arteries, in certain ligaments which are elastic, and the bundles are present in some varieties of elastic cartilage. (See ADHESIONS; WOUNDS.)

Fibula

One of the bones of the hind-limb, running from the stifle to the hock. It appears to become less and less important in direct proportion as the number of the digits of the limb decreases. In the horse and ox it is a very small and slim bone which does not take any part in the bearing of weight; while in the dog it is quite large, and with the tibia, takes its share in supporting the weight of the body.

Filarial Worms

(see FILARIASIS)

Filariasis

Filariasis is a group of diseases caused by the presence in the body of certain small thread-like nematode worms, called filariae, which are often found in the bloodstream. Biting insects act as vectors. (See HEARTWORM and TRACHEAL WORMS for canine filariasis; also EQUINE FILARIASIS; BRAIN, DISEASES OF.)

Parafilaria bovicola causes bovine filariasis in Africa, the Far East, and parts of Europe. The female worm penetrates the skin, causing subcutaneous haemorrhagic lesions that resemble bruising. Eggs are laid in the blood there. Downgrading of carcases at meat inspection is a cause of significant loss. Ivermectin is useful for control.

Filovirus

(see MONKEYS, DISEASES OF)

Fimbriae

These are minute filaments with specific antigenic properties attached to the surface of bacteria. They can be used in vaccines against *E. coli*, for example. (See also under GENETIC ENGINEERING.)

Finnish Landrace Sheep

Finnish Landrace sheep are remarkable for high prolificacy, triplets being common, and 4 or 5 lambs not rare.

Fipronil

A drug applied topically for the treatment and prevention of flea and tick infestation in cats and dogs. In cats, one application is active for up to 5 weeks against fleas and for 1 month against ticks. In dogs, it is active for 2 months against fleas and for 1 month against ticks. It is not recommended for use on cats under 12 weeks or dogs under 10 weeks old, nor for animals suckling young. In view of the risk of animals becoming infected with tick-borne diseases abroad (see CANINE BABESIOSIS), it may be beneficial to treat them with such long-acting products before travelling.

Fire-Extinguishers

These are required in commercial kennels under the terms of the Animal Boarding Establishment Act 1963.

Fish, Diseases of

These are covered by the Diseases of Fish Act, and all are notifiable in Britain: furunculosis and columnaris (bacterial); infectious pancreatic necrosis, viral haemorrhagic septicaemia, infectious haematopoietic necrosis and spring viraemia (viral); whirling disease (protozoan); ulcerative dermal necrosis and erythrodermatitis (of unknown cause).

Yersinia ruckeri infection caused the death of yearling trout reared in an 'earth' pond in Scotland.

On a fish-farm in England, 4900 rainbow trout died from CEROIDOSIS over a 4-month period. Affected fish swam on their sides or upside down, and often rapidly in circles. A few were seen with their heads out of water, swimming like porpoises.

Aquarium fish may be affected with fish tuberculosis, caused by *Mycobacterium piscium,*

M. platpoecilus, or *M. fortuitum*. These cause a granulomatous condition which can prove fatal. Skin infection may develop in people handling diseased fish. (See also PETS; WHIRLING DISEASE; SPRING VIRAEMIA OF CARP.)

Fish-Farming

Fish-farming is a rapidly expanding industry, especially (in the UK) in Western Scotland. Rainbow trout and Atlantic salmon are the main species farmed. As the salmon cages are floated in sea lochs, the fishes come into close contact with wild fish attracted by the feed which may pass out of the cage. Thus disease may be spread from the wild fish to the farmed, with results that can be devastating. Fish lice are the greatest problem; they literally eat the fish alive.

In mainland Europe, carp and eels are farmed. Tilapia is an African fish which is farmed in various countries; it can be farmed in the warm water effluent from power stations. Sea bream and turbot are also farmed. In the USA, channel catfish are farmed in the southern states. The world's largest producer of farmed fish, however, is China, where more than 20 species are produced.

The Farm Animal Welfare Council has issued a report on the welfare of farmed fish.

Fish-Keeping

This very popular hobby mainly concentrates on tropical fish. Many of these are imported and may have travelled a considerable distance before arriving in the UK. The methods used for their capture in some countries may cause injury. The result of this and of subsequent mishandling may not be apparent until the fish are in the possession of the hobbyist. Deaths even then can still be due to the method of capture.

Fish Louse

(see ARGULUS)

Fish-Meal

Fish-meal is largely used for feeding to pigs and poultry, although it is also added to the rations for dairy cows, calves and other farm livestock. It is composed of the dried and ground residue from fish, the edible portions of which are used for human consumption. The best variety is that made from 'white' fish – known in the trade as white fish-meal. When prepared with a large admixture of herring or mackerel offal it is liable to have a strong odour, which may taint the flesh of pigs and the eggs of hens receiving it.

Fish-meal is rich in digestible, undegradable protein, calcium, and phosphorus; it has smaller amounts of iodine and other elements useful to animals. It contains a variable amount of oil.

It forms a useful means of maintaining the amount of protein in the ration for all breeding females and for young animals during their period of active growth. From 3 to 10 per cent of the weight of food may consist of white fish-meal. When pigs are being fattened for bacon and 'fattening-off' rations are fed, the amount of fish-meal is reduced; during the last 4 to 6 weeks it is customary to discontinue it entirely.

Many investigations have emphasised the very great economic value of fish-meal for animals fed largely upon cereal by-products. It serves to correct the protein and mineral deficiencies of these and thus enable a balanced ration to be fed. It serves a very useful purpose by enabling more home-grown cereals to be fed and largely replaces protein-rich imported vegetable products. (See also AMINO ACIDS; DIET.)

Fish Oils

Livestock owners should beware of feeding inferior fish oils, which often cause illness owing to their quickly becoming rancid, in place of good-quality cod-liver oil. (See RANCIDITY.)

Fish, Poisoning of

This may occur through liquor from silage clamps seeping into streams, etc. The following, in very small concentrations, are lethal to fish: DDT, Derris, BHC (Gammexane), Aldrin. Many agricultural sprays may kill fish, as will snail-killers used in fluke control. In one case, virtually all the 450,000 trout in a pond died. The owner of the trout farm reported that they had been leaping out of the water on to the banks. The Devon VI Centre's findings suggested that the inadvertent contamination by excessively chlorinated water, into the stream supplying the trout farm, was to blame. In Hampshire the flushing of drains with a chlorine preparation led to similar trouble in river trout. The autopsy findings were 'scalding of the flanks, fins, and gills'. (See also AFLATOXINS.)

Mortality among young salmon in cages was found to be caused by heavy colonisation of gills by *Trichophyra* species protozoa.

Alkaloids from a brightly coloured and luminescent plankton can cause a high fish mortality; though clams, oysters, scallops, and mussels can absorb the alkaloids without harm.

In people, paralytic shellfish poisoning can occur within 30 minutes; deaths from respiratory paralysis within 24 hours have been recorded.

Fish Solubles

Concentrated and purified stickwater; the liquid which is pressed out of fish during oil-extraction and meal-making processes.

Fistula

An unnatural narrow channel leading from some natural cavity, such as a duct of the mammary gland, or the interior of the rectum or anal gland, to the surface. A fistula may result from a congenital abnormality or, occasionally, may be created artificially by a surgeon. In cows, treads by neighbours, tears by barbed wire, bites or other injury to the teats sometimes result in a fistula through which milk escapes from the side of the teat. In a dental fistula, which occurs in cats and dogs most commonly but is also seen in the horse, an abscess develops at the root of a molar tooth, and the pus burrows upwards and bursts through the skin on to the surface of the face.

Occasionally a fistula heals, but often it is extremely hard to close, especially if it has persisted for some time. Surgery may be necessary.

Fistulous Withers

Fistulous withers is a condition in which a sinus develops in connection with the withers of the horse. It may follow an external injury and infection with bacteria, when, on account of the poor blood supply, local necrosis (death) of the ligaments above the vertebrae, or of the summits of the spinous processes, with suppuration, sets in. *Brucella* and *Actinomyces* organisms are often found. In other cases, filarial worms have been found embedded in the ligament, and are responsible for those cases which arise without any previous history of injury to this part of the body.

Signs There is pain and swelling over the withers, perhaps more obvious on one side than the other, and working horses resent the application of the collar, or may be reluctant to work. Later on the swelling usually bursts, but it may appear to subside in a few cases. The openings which are left when the purulent material is discharged may heal over in time, but other swellings form and burst as before. In many cases 1 or 2 openings remain permanently and a thin stream of pus is constantly discharged.

Treatment Fistulous withers is always a serious condition which should be treated before great and perhaps irreparable damage has been done to the tissues involved. Old-standing cases are notoriously difficult to treat, and many animals have to be destroyed.

The application of poultices and blisters to the outside is absolutely useless. Antibiotics may be effective; otherwise, extensive surgery may be necessary.

The treatment generally takes from 2 weeks (in very slight cases) to as long as 3 months or more, where the sinuses are deep and bone is involved.

Fits

Fits is another name for convulsive seizures accompanied usually by at least a few seconds of unconsciousness. Epilepsy is the commonest cause of fits in the adult dog. The animal may be relaxed or even asleep at the time when the fit occurs, and the 1st phase consists of a tonic spasm of voluntary muscle with arrest of respiration; this lasts 30 to 40 seconds and is succeeded by clonic contractions of limb muscles ('galloping'). After this the dog usually appears to be exhausted for a period varying from a few seconds to a few minutes, with a gasping form of respiration. Some dogs then get up and appear normal almost immediately, while others wander restlessly for half an hour or more, bump into furniture and eat greedily if they find any food. The pattern of the fit is reasonably consistent in any individual dog, but varies considerably from one dog to another. In between these fits, the dog appears to be entirely normal. (P. Croft)

Fits may also: occur during the course of a generalised illness such as canine distemper or rabies; follow a head injury; be associated with a brain tumour; or follow some types of poisoning. In puppies, hydrocephalus is a cause of fits, but more commonly cutting of the teeth or infestation with parasitic worms.

Deprivation of drinking-water may cause convulsions in dogs as in pigs. (See SALT POISONING.)

Treatment Anti-convulsant drugs, such as primidone or phenytoin, may be successful; the dose being the lowest found to control fits over a period. In dogs in which these drugs produce side-effects, phenobarbitone may be tried, though it may cause whining in some dogs. Diazepam is useful, given intra-muscularly alone, or with barbiturates. (See CONVULSIONS; EPILEPSY; HYSTERIA.)

Flagella

Whip-like processes possessed by certain bacteria and protozoan parasites and used for purposes of movement.

'Flail Chest'

A condition which may result when one or more ribs are fractured in 2 places; the damaged area moves slightly inwards on inspiration, and outwards on expiration.

Flashing

A term used to describe the behaviour of fish when suffering from skin irritation caused by parasites or other conditions. In trying to rub against stones or other objects in an attempt to relieve the condition, they often have to lie on their sides. When turning from the normal position to their side, and back again, 'flashing' is noticed by the observer.

'Flat Pup' Syndrome

'Flat pup' syndrome is a condition in which puppies can, at 2 to 3 weeks, use their front legs normally, but the hind-legs are splayed out sideways. The condition usually corrects itself. (See 'SWIMMERS'.)

Flavine Compounds

Among these are acriflavine, euflavine, and proflavine, derivatives of aniline. Acriflavine, the hydrochloride of diamino-methyl-acridinium, is an orange-red crystalline powder, soluble in water and forming a powerful antiseptic solution in strengths of 1 in 1000. It stains horn and skin tissues bright yellow. It has been used to control bacterial infection, and stimulate healing, in wounds.

Flavomycin

Proprietary name for the antibiotic flavophospholipol (bambermycin) marketed by Hoechst as an in-feed growth promoter. (See ADDITIVES.)

Flea-Collars

Flea-collars for dogs and cats are impregnated with a parasiticide, which varies with the manufacturer. Carbaril, propoxur and diazinon are among the insecticides used. All will kill fleas when used as directed; most are active for several months. They should be loosely fastened and the animal should not be allowed to chew them. Animal-owners should select a reliable make, for sometimes ineffective collars appear on the market; they should also watch for any signs of skin inflammation as a few animals are allergic to some of the chemicals used. Children should not be allowed to play with the collar.

Fleas

Fleas are members of the order Siphonaptera, and are degenerate forms of 2-winged insects.

The eggs are mostly laid on the floor or bedding; but a few may be laid on the body of the host, from which they fall. They appear as white specks, and pop when burst. Hatching takes from 2 days (in summer) to 12 days or so.

When fully grown, the legless larva spins a cocoon, in which the pupa develops. The adult flea emerges when conditions of temperature and moisture are favourable. It can remain alive in the cocoon for up to a year.

If infestation is suspected, but not a single flea can be seen, combing may gather some black or dark-brown flea faeces. These will form a reddish halo if placed on moistened cotton wool.

Pulex irritans is the human flea, but is frequently found on dogs and cats, and occasionally on pigs and horses.

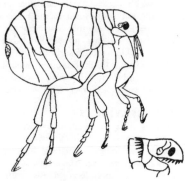

Pulex irritans. × 20.
Inset: head of dog flea.

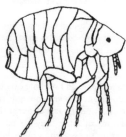

Echidnophaga gallinacea. × 30.

Ctenocephalides canis is the dog flea, but is often found on man and cat. It can transmit *Dipylidium caninum*, as also may the cat flea, *C. felis*, and the human flea, *P. irritans*. All these fleas cause severe irritation, and in young and debilitated animals may cause anaemia if numerous. Sensitisation to flea-bites is an important cause of ECZEMA.

In a survey, carried out at the Royal Veterinary College, London, fleas were recovered from 20 per cent of 193 dogs examined post-mortem. Three species were found: *C. felis*, *C. canis*, and *Orchopeas howardi*.

Spilopsyllus cuniculi, the European rabbit flea, infests also cats and occasionally dogs. It was introduced in 1966 into Australia, as a vector of myxomatosis, in order to reduce the rabbit population.

Reproduction of the flea is partly dependent on the reproductive hormones of the rabbit, and so the greatest numbers are present during the rabbit's pregnancy.

In cats *S. cuniculi* attach to the ear pinna causing an itchy dermatitis, but do not breed even on pregnant cats.

Archaeopsylla erinacei, the hedgehog flea, only occasionally and temporarily infests dogs, but may cause an allergic dermatitis in them. Cats might become infested too.

Echidnophaga gallinacea, the 'stick-tight' or chicken flea, is usually found attached in dense masses to the head of a fowl or the ear of a dog or cat. Man, horses, and cattle are occasionally infected. It is a common parasite throughout the tropics and is frequently the cause of death in poultry. The female flea, after fertilisation, inserts its mouth parts into the cuticle of the host, and remains there. Ulcers may form; and in any case the flea is difficult to move.

Tunga penetrans, the true jigger flea, differs only in slight details from the latter species. The female, however, penetrates the skin, and lying in an inflammatory pocket with an opening to the exterior, becomes as large as a pea. It is found in Africa and America in man and all the domestic mammals, especially the pig. The eggs are laid in the ulcers; and the larvae crawl out and pupate on the ground.

Destruction of fleas (see INSECTICIDES).

Bedding must be destroyed or disinfected and the surrounding floorboards and cracks cleaned thoroughly or the animal will shortly be reinfested. This is even more important than ridding the host of fleas.

Powders and aerosol sprays, applied externally; 'pour on' or 'spot on' formulations applied to the skin under the fur or coat; shampoos; and tablets to be taken internally are all available for the control of fleas. There are many preparations marketed: natural pyrethrins and their synthetic derivatives; organophosphorus compounds; carbamates and amidines are all used.

Cythioate, an organophosphorus compound, and lofenuron, a benzoyl urea derivative, are given as tablets or oral suspension.

Permethrin, a pyrethrin derivative, is formulated as a powder, 'pour on' and shampoo. Aerosol sprays often contain a mixture of piperonyl butoxide and pyrethrins. All are effective, properly used, but the manufacturers' directions must be followed carefully, with regard both to handling and to the suitability of the particular product for cats or dogs. Puppies and

kittens must only be treated with products recommended for use in young animals.

(See also 'FLEA-COLLARS'.)

Flies

Flies are mostly, but not exclusively, members of the order Diptera – the 2-winged flies.

Even the common housefly can transmit infection such as anthrax and tuberculosis, and also various species of parasitic worms. The stablefly's role in the production of summer mastitis is well known, and other flies, such as the sheep headfly, may be responsible for cases of this disease too. The autumnfly (and almost certainly others) can transmit an eye worm of cattle, and also the infective agent *Moraxella bovis* which causes the more commonly recognised contagious keratitis or New Forest disease.

The approach of a cloud of flies, such as the headfly, will cause cattle to cease grazing and huddle together. The movement or presence of a mass of even non-biting flies over the animal's body represents a further cause of 'worry' or restlessness; and both the headfly and the autumnfly feed on secretions from eyes, nose, etc., and on the serum exuding from small wounds.

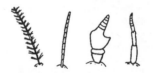

Culex Simulium Tabanus Chrysops

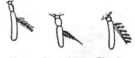

Musca Sarcophaga Glossina

Antennae of various flies. The small hair in the lower row is the 'arista'.

Cattle may become sensitised to the secretions poured into the bite wound, so that an allergy arises with sometimes the production of serious skin lesions which, in turn, may attract other flies.

Sawfly poisoning
Within 4 days of being moved to new pasture, a flock of 250 sheep on the Danish island of Sjaelland had sustained 50 deaths. The pasture had many birch trees, which were heavily infested with larvae of the blue-back sawfly (*Arge pullata*). Veterinary investigation confirmed that a toxin present in these was the cause of death, following internal haemorrhage and acute hepatitis.

The sawfly was first reported in Denmark in 1974, but sawfly poisoning of cattle and sheep has been recognised since 1955 in Australia, where heavy losses have occurred. Goats are susceptible also.

The sawfly larva is bright yellow with black dashed lines on the back. It defoliates birch trees, and then drops to the ground to pupate or search for more food.

Order Diptera Insects which have 1 pair of wings.

Simulium (buffalo gnats) The flies of this genus are small, thick-set hump-back flies – hence their name. They are often black or reddish-brown. The females at certain times appear in swarms and attack cattle, horses and other animals.

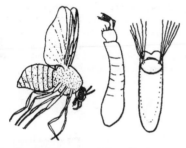

Simulium. Adult larva, and pupa. The adult fly is magnified × about 10.

The eggs are laid in water. The larvae, which are aquatic and creep about like leeches, can only live in well-aerated running water; in still water they are asphyxiated. The larva when mature spins a silky cocoon which is attached to water weeds. In this the pupa lies loosely, breathing by means of extruded gill-tufts. The fly is very active in Central Europe, where cattle may die in 2 hours after attack. They show laboured breathing, stumbling gait, rapid pulse, and swellings in pendulous places. In less severe cases loss of appetite, abortion, depression, and temporary or permanent blindness may result.

Sandflies Two-winged flies, of which the blood-sucking females transmit infections, including that of LEISHMANIASIS.

Mosquito The mosquito, the carrier of malaria and yellow fever to man, is also of importance in tropical veterinary medicine, transmitting diseases such as avian malaria (see PLASMODIUM GALLINALEUM), HEARTWORM of dogs, BLUETONGUE,

EQUINE ENCEPHALOMYELITIS, AFRICAN HORSE SICKNESS, AND RIFT VALLEY FEVER. In temperate climates, too, mosquitoes are important disease vectors.

Four genera of mosquitoes are of veterinary importance: *Aedes, Anopheles, Culex,* and *Mansonia.*

Eggs are laid on the surface of water or floating vegetation, either singly (*Aedes* and *Anopheles*) or as 'rafts' of eggs.

Larvae undergo 3 moults, and develop only in water, in which they are highly mobile.

Larvae-eating fish, such as *Alphanus dispar,* are being used in the Nile Delta and elsewhere for mosquito control. (See also DDT *and* DIELDRIN.)

Midges, biting (culicoid) (see under this heading)

Gadflies (tabanidae) The family of the gadflies is a large and important one, as the females are blood-suckers.

The eggs are laid in masses on leaves and plants near water. The larvae are more or less aquatic, but towards maturity they live in damp earth or decaying vegetation. The larva is cylindrical, pointed at both ends, and with most of the segments carrying pseudo-pods or false feet. The pupa resembles that of a moth. In temperate climates, development takes nearly a year. The males feed on plant juices, but the females are blood-suckers, and in addition carriers of various diseases – for example, trypanosomiasis, swamp fever in horses, and filariasis in man.

The bite is painful, and causes much irritation to horses and cattle, resulting in gadding, decrease in milk yield, and so on. No remedies are really satisfactory, although nets have been used with some success on horses.

If the pools most commonly frequented by these flies are covered with a thick layer of paraffin oil, the flies are killed. If this plan is adopted early in the season the numbers can be kept under control.

Tabanus can mechanically transmit surra and other blood diseases such as anthrax. Another species transmits swamp fever in horses.

Haematopota This is also a world-wide genus. The species has smoky wings, and include the British clegg or horse-fly which, in addition to being a veritable pest to horses, inflicts a very painful bite to man.

Chrysops is distinguished by its long slender antennae, and its green or golden eyes spotted with purple. It is found all over the world, including Britain. This genus is the carrier of the parasite of Calabar swelling in man. It also can inflict a very painful bite.

The non-biting 2-winged flies have an even greater significance to man and his animals than the biting flies.

Muscidae The flies belonging to this family are smallish to medium-sized flies. The type of this family is *Musca domestica*.

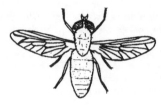

Tabanus. × 2.

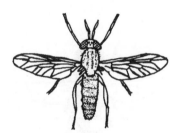

Haematopa. × 3.

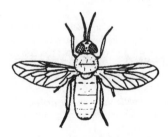

Chrysops. × 2.

Musca domestica The great majority of flies found in houses belong to this species. It is a medium-sized fly with 4 black stripes on its back, and a sharp elbow in the 4th wing vein. The eggs are laid; about 120 in a batch, preferably in horse manure, but occasionally in human or other excreta. They hatch in 24 hours, and the issuing larva (or maggot) feeds and moults and finally

becomes full grown in 4 to 5 days. It leaves the manure at this stage, and crawls to a dry spot where it pupates. The puparia are more or less barrel-shaped and dark brown in colour. In 4 or 5 days in summer the adult fly emerges. The shortest time on record between the laying of the egg and the appearance of the adult is 8 days; 10 to 12 days is more normal. In 3 to 4 days the female is ready to lay eggs. The fly lives over the winter in the pupal stage, although in kitchens and warm places adults may be seen at every season of the year.

The house-fly can transmit disease by swallowing bacterial spores, and either bringing them up in their vomit or passing them out in their faeces; or by carrying them about on its hairs and legs. Two species of stomach worm are carried by this fly, in which they pass part of their life-cycle. Among other organisms known to be carried by this fly are anthrax, tuberculosis, and many species of worm eggs. (See FLY CONTROL.)

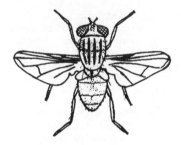

Musca. × 4.

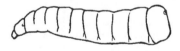

Larva

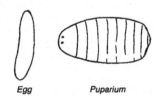

Egg   Puparium

Diagram to illustrate the life-history of *Musca domestica*.

Headfly This is a non-biting fly which, as its name *Hydrotaea irritans* suggests, is a cause of great irritation to cattle, sheep, etc., especially since so many headflies often settle on the same

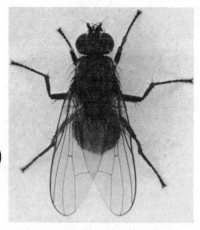

The headfly. (Crown Copyright photograph.)

animal. The fly will take advantage of any abrasion on the sheep's skin. Both fly-repellents and head-caps have been used and compared at the Redesdale Experimental Husbandry Farm. 'Head-caps gave good and sometimes complete protection,' but are inconvenient in use. Pine-tar oil is a useful repellent.

The headfly is responsible for carrying bacteria to cows' teats (especially when already damaged by biting flies or other causes), and appears to have an important role in producing 'SUMMER MASTITIS'. It is also involved in the spread of New Forest eye infection caused by *Morexalla bovis.*

Face flies These 'autumn flies' (*Musca autumnalis*) plague beef and dairy cattle, and horses, at pasture, feeding on watery secretions from nostrils and eyes.

Dipterous larvae or maggots—Myiasis

Of very great importance to the veterinary surgeon and the agriculturist are those non-biting muscid flies which have taken on a parasitic existence in their larval stages. Myiasis means the presence of dipterous larvae (or other stages) in organs and tissues of the living animal and the disorders and destruction of tissue caused thereby. (See 'STRIKE'.)

The myiasis-producing flies are now usually divided into 3 groups: specific, semi-specific, and accidental.

Specific: This group consists of flies which need to breed in living tissue. It includes *Chrysomyia bezziana, Cordylobia anthropophaga, Wohlfahrtia magnifica, Booponus intonsus,* and all the Oestridae.

Semi-specific: This group consists of flies which, normally breeding in carcases, may live in the living animal. It includes the blow-flies, the sheep-maggot flies, and some of the flesh-flies.

Accidental: This group includes all flies the larvae of which, accidentally swallowed with the food, may live in the intestine.

The more important of the above flies are considered below.

'Blow-flies' Calliphoridae are largish muscids of a metallic or yellow colour.

'Common blow-fly' or ***'Blue-Bottle'*** (*Calliphora* sp.) has reddish palps, black legs, and a bristly thorax. The general colour is dark blue with lighter patches on the abdomen. The colour, however, is not lustrous. The ova are usually deposited in decaying animal matter, but occasionally in living tissue.

'Green-bottle fly' (*Lucilia sericata*) is the British sheep-maggot fly. It is also found in Australia and America.

Lucilia. This fly is larger than the house-fly and smaller than the blow-fly.

L. caesar, a common species in Europe, does not 'blow' sheep in this country, but does so in countries such as Russia, where other species are absent. Other species of *Lucilia* in India and Australia occasionally are also implicated.

'Copper-bottle fly' (*Lucilia cuprina*) is the strike fly which attacks sheep in Australia and South Africa.

These are of a bright metallic or bluish-green colour, with many strong bristles on the thorax arranged in 2 parallel rows. There are no stripes on the thorax or abdomen. The cheeks are not hairy as in *Calliphora.*

This genus blows wool, but occasionally infects wounds.

Chrysomyia bezziana, found in India, Africa, and the Philippines, is a metallic greenish-blue blow-fly, closely related to *Lucilia,* but with dark transverse abdominal bands and with fewer and less-developed thoracic bristles. The metallic sheen is more brassy than in *Lucilia*. This fly breeds only in living tissue – it discharges from natural orifices, or in sores and cuts. Up to 500 eggs may be laid at one time. They hatch in about 30 hours, and the larvae rapidly reach maturity, crawl out and pupate on the ground. Several other species of this genus are semi-specific myiasis flies, normally breeding in decaying matter. These include *C. albiceps*, a notorious sheep-maggot fly in Australia.

'Screw-worm fly' (*Callitroga americana*) in America can be distinguished from the old-world species by the 3 well-marked blue dorsal stripes on the thorax and dark hairs on the abdomen. It is of a dark bluish-green colour, with a well-marked yellowish-red face. (See also FLY CONTROL.)

This species will lay eggs in decaying animal or vegetable matter, but will also oviposit in any diseased tissue, in wounds in the vulvae of freshly calved cows, the umbilical cord of calves, and so on. The ova hatch in 24 hours, and the maggot matures in 4 to 6 days. The pupal stage on the ground lasts 3 to 10 days. The maggot resembles a blue-bottle maggot, but the deeply cut constrictions between segments and the prominent rings of spines give it its popular name.

As soon as the egg hatches, the larva starts burrowing into the flesh. It can penetrate the sound tissue of living animals, and may even lay bare the bones.

'Tumbu fly' (*Cordylobia anthropophaga*) is a specific myiasis fly in Africa, attacking many hosts. It is a dirty brownish-yellow blow-fly with blackish markings. Eggs are laid in dust and rubbish on which the host, usually a dog, is accustomed to lie. The small larva may live apart from the host for 10 days, but it may eventually burrow into the epidermis or die. It moults in this position, and forms a 'tumbu' below the skin with an opening to the exterior through which it breathes. The 'tumbu' does not suppurate unless the larva dies. The larva emerges in about 7 or 8 days, and 2 or 3 days later it pupates. The adults emerge in about 20 days. This fly does not burrow into the deeper tissues. The scrotum is a common site of the maggot. Putting a drop of oil or Vaseline over the breathing hole will force the larva to protrude, when it can be removed.

Booponus intonsus is a light yellow specific myiasis fly found in the Philippines, which is somewhat allied to *Cordylobia*. It infects bovines and goats.

The eggs are laid on the hairs on the lower parts of the legs; and the larvae make their way

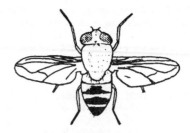

Cordylobia. × 2½.

to the coronet and bury themselves in the flesh. The larvae resemble the screw-worm. The larval period seems to last 2 or 3 weeks, when it leaves the host and pupates in the ground. The pupal life is 10 days.

The larvae cause a considerable lameness with numerous superficial wounds and distortion of the horn. The larva is called the 'foot maggot'.

'Flesh flies' (Sarcophagidae) are closely related to the Muscidae. The body is more elongated than that of the blow-flies, and they are usually grey in colour, with a mottled abdomen and a striped thorax. They generally bring forth living larvae instead of laying eggs. Two genera are important.

Sarcophaga spp. These are large grey flies with red eyes and square chequered markings on the abdomen. The 3rd segment of the antenna is long. All the species normally breed in decaying animal matter, but may be found in old festering wounds. They are found througout the world.

Wohlfahrtia magnifica resembles the preceding genus, but has well-defined round spots on the abdomen. The 3rd segment of the antenna is short and the arista is without bristles. It is widely distributed in Russia, Asia Minor, and Egypt. The larvae never attack carcases, but are always found in wounds and natural cavities of living animals. The fly deposits living larvae on sores and discharges.

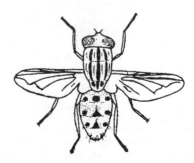

Wohlfahrtia. × 3.

In Australia the most important sheep-maggot flies are *Calliphora augur*, a large orange-coloured fly; *C. stygia*, the common sheep-maggot fly, often called the 'golden-haired blow-fly'; and *Chrysomyia albiceps* var. *putoni*, the larva of which is known as the 'hairy maggot'.

Injuries due to maggots The injuries due to maggots may be roughly divided into 2 classes – larvae attacking wounds and discharges, and larvae attacking the wool of sheep. The former type of injury is found on any animal, including man. The flies usually, but not always, select old sores. Some, such as *Chrysomyia americana* (the 'screw-worm') will penetrate into the sound tissue, and prefer fresh wounds or carcases. The infected wound usually has a watery discharge. Prevention is obviously most important. (See also under MYIASIS.)

Blood-sucking muscid flies These flies, which resemble the house-fly in general appearance, are responsible for an enormous amount of damage to farm animals. When one considers that they include such flies as the tsetse fly, the stable-fly, and the horn-fly, this is easily understood.

Stomoxys This genus is mainly confined to Africa and Asia, but one species, *S. calcitrans*, the stable-fly, is world-wide in its distribution.

Stomoxys breeds in stable manure and in other places where moisture and organic material found. The eggs hatch in 2 to 3 days, and the larva, which is similar to but smaller than *Musca*, becomes full-grown in 2 to 3 weeks. The pupal stage lasts 9 to 13 days. Development is more rapid in the tropics, where the time between egg and adult may be reduced to 12 days.

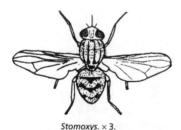

Stomoxys. × 3.

This fly is a serious pest to horses and other animals. It will also bite man. Apart from the extreme irritation of its bite, it can transmit anthrax, surra, and other diseases. It is also the intermediate host of *Habronema microstomum*, a worm parasite of horses.

Haematobia *H. stimulans* is a common blood-sucking parasite of cattle, and occasionally of horses and man, in Europe. It resembles *Stomoxys*, but has spatulate palps as long as the proboscis, and hairs on both sides of the arista. It breeds in fresh cattle dung. The larva becomes full-grown in 6 to 9 days, while the pupal stage lasts 5 to 8 days.

Lyperosia *L. irritans* is very closely related to *Haematobia*, but can be distinguished from it by the absence of bristles from the underside of the arista. It is found in Europe (including the UK) and America. It is a very serious pest to cattle, clustering round the base of the horns, a habit which gives the fly its popular name of horn-fly. The irritation caused by their bites is estimated to cause a drop in milk yield amounting in some cases to 50 per cent. The flies breed in fresh cow dung. Flies emerge in about 15 days after the egg is deposited. The maggots must have moisture, and can be destroyed by any means which will dry the manure quickly. The horn-fly seldom goes far from its host, and may be destroyed by attaching splash-boards to ordinary dippers. The fly leaves the cattle at the moment of entering the bath, but the dip, caught and flung back by the splash-board, drenches and destroys the flies. The hotter and more excited the cattle, the closer the flies stick and the greater the number killed. Any oily dip is suitable. (See also FLY CONTROL MEASURES.)

Tsetse flies (glossina) The flies of this genus are, with 1 exception found in Arabia, confined to Africa. They are the notorious carriers of trypanosomiasis in man and animals. *Glossina* resembles a large stable-fly but has a feathered arista, long slender palps, a slender shaft to the proboscis, and a peculiar wing venation. The life-history is unusual: the female produces 1 living larva at a time and deposits it when full-grown. It immediately pupates. One female produces only about a dozen larvae in her life.

More than a dozen species of *Glossina* are known. The most important are: *G. palpalis*; *G. morsitans*; *G. brevipalpis*; *G. longipalpis*; *G. pallidipes*; *G. tachinoides*.

Bot and warble flies The bot family Oestridae consists of hairy, heavy flies with rudimentary mouth parts. The female attaches the egg, or, in the case of the nostril flies, places the larva on a suitable host, and the remainder of the larval life is parasitic. When mature the larvae leave the host and pupate on the ground.

These flies may be placed in 3 groups according to the habitat of the larva:

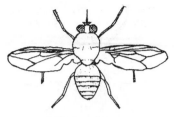

Glossina. × 2½.

(1) In the alimentary canal –
    Gastrophilus, the horse bot;
    Cobboldia, the elephant bot.
(2) In the head sinuses –
    Oestrus, the sheep nostril fly;
    Rhinaestrus, the horse nostril fly;
    Cephalomyia, the camel nostril fly;
    and others.
(3) In the subcutaneous tissue –
    Hypoderma, the warble-fly (see
    WARBLES);
    Dermatobia, the macaw worm fly;
    and others.

Bot flies The flies of the genus *Gastrophilus* are large and hairy, with large compound eyes and 3 ocelli. The females have an elongated ovipositor which is bent under the body when at rest. Four species are of importance.

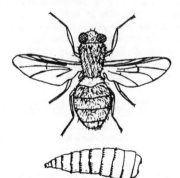

Gastrophilus. (Adult fly × 2½, and 'Bot' × 2.)

G. intestinalis (*G. equi*), the common horse bot, has cloudy wings; it deposits its eggs on any part of the horse, but especially on the distal ends of the hairs. The eggs require moisture and friction (supplied by licking) before they will hatch.

G. nasalis (*G. veterinus*) is smaller, more hairy, and has a rusty-coloured thorax. It oviposits usually at the proximal ends of hairs

under the jaw. It lays 1 egg and flies to a distance, returning later to lay another.

G. haemorrhoidalis has a bright orange-red tip to the abdomen. It deposits its eggs only at the base of the small hairs on the lips of the horse. The eggs may hatch without moisture or friction.

G. pecorum resembles *G. intestinalis*. In colour it is yellowish-brown to nearly black, with brownish-clouded wings. Its habits are similar to that species.

The distribution of the first 3 is universal, but the last seems to be restricted to Europe and South Africa.

The life-history of the species of this genus is not yet fully understood. Some of the newly hatched larvae may pierce the skin or buccal mucous membrane; in any case the larvae are found in various parts of the alimentary tract. Each species has its own special preference. *G. intestinalis* is usually found in the stomach, occasionally the duodenum; *G. nasalis* prefers the duodenum, but has been found in the pharynx and stomach; *G. haemorrhoidalis* is found in the stomach, duodenum, rectum, and even in the anus; while *G. pecorum* usually occurs in the pharynx or stomach, but may be recovered from any part.

Bots when present in large numbers in the stomach or intestine, or even in small numbers about the pharynx and anus, may cause a considerable suffering to their host by mere mechanical obstruction. The adult fly worries the horse considerably, especially the species *G. nasalis* and *G. haemorrhoidalis*, and may cause loss of condition.

Treatment Formerly, carbon disulphide, administered in autumn and early winter by stomach tube and followed by warm saline. This has been replaced by a haloxon formulation given in the feed and by ivermectin paste, which have both proved effective (also against roundworms). Withholding water 4 hours before and after dosing is recommended when treating against bots. (See AVERMECTINS; IVERMECTIN.)

Some control is possible by regular removal of the 'nits' from the lower limbs of grazing horses during summer.

Oestrus *O. ovis*, the sheep nostril fly, is somewhat larger than the house-fly and is greyish-yellow to brown in colour. It is found practically all over the world. It deposits eggs, or larvae. The hovering female 'strikes' at the nostrils, and the young larva crawls up the nose, and may lodge in one of the sinuses of the skull. It remains there until fully grown, when it is sneezed out and pupates in the ground.

Prevention is carried out by means of an application of tar to the nostrils. This may be applied by means of a salt lick, access to which may only be obtained by smallish holes (5 cm or 2 inches) smeared with tar. Ploughing a single furrow across a sheep pasture allows the sheep to protect their nostrils from the flies, 'strike', and gives some measure of protection. Some anthelmintics are effective.

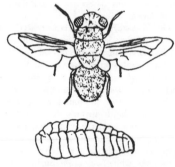

Oestrus. (Fly × 2; maggot × 1.)

Rhinoestrus *R. purpureus* (*R. nasalis*), the horse nostril fly, is common in Central Europe and North Africa. It is a smallish fly with the body covered with small tubercles, and is closely related to *Oestrus*. The female deposits a number of living larvae at one time in the eyes or the nose of the horse (and occasionally man). The larvae may be found about the cranial cavities or even in the pharynx or larynx. Russian gadfly is a synonym.

Hypoderma Two species of warble-fly, *H. bovis* and *H. lineatum*, are found in cattle (and occasionally in the horse). Both are very extensively found in Europe and America.

H. bovis is a largish fly with yellow hair just behind the head. The underpart of the abdomen is nearly black, while the tail end is orange-yellow. The legs have few hairs.

H. lineatum is rather smaller with a reddish-orange tail and rough hairy legs.

H. bovis lays its eggs one on the base of each hair at a time. The fly has a most terrifying effect on cattle, and causes them to gallop madly in all directions. *H. lineatum* irritates animals less than does *H. bovis*. The ova are generally deposited while the animal is lying in the shade. A number of eggs – up to 14 – are laid on the same hair, and are often in full view.

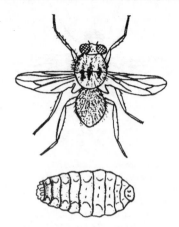

Hypoderma. (Fly × 2; and 'Warble' × 1½.)

In both cases larvae emerge in several days and pierce the skin. They travel up through the connective tissue and finally reach the back. Under the skin the larvae form a small swelling (about the middle of winter), which moves about at first, but gradually becomes still and enlarges. A small opening appears in the centre through which the larva breathes. In spring the larva falls to the ground and pupates. Several weeks later the adult fly emerges.

The presence of the larvae may decrease the milk yield by 10 to 20 per cent, cause a considerable depreciation in flesh near the points where the larvae are, and enormously reduce the value of the hide. The adult fly also causes loss through the mad chasing about of cattle. (See also under WARBLES.)

H. diana is a warble-fly affecting deer.

Dermatobia *D. hominis*, the macaw worm-fly, is a parasite of cattle and other domesticated animals (and occasionally man) in tropical America. It is a medium-sized fly, grey or steel-blue in colour, with pale brown wings. The female lays its eggs on the body of some blood-sucking arthropod, usually a mosquito. This carrier attacks an animal 5 or 6 days later, and the larvae, rapidly escaping from their shells, pierce the skin of the host, and form a local tumour near where they were deposited. In a month or so they emerge and pupate.

Pupipara This family, which includes the sheep ked and the horse ked (New Forest fly), was so called because live larvae are produced which pupate at once. The adults in this case are blood-sucking parasites with a hard integument with a broad neckless head and very stout

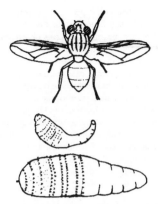

Dermatobia. (Fly and maggots × 1½.)

legs ending in grasping claws. Wings are present or absent.

Hippobosca equina, the New Forest fly or horse ked, has wings which, however, are seldom used, the fly preferring to run swiftly between the hairs of the host.

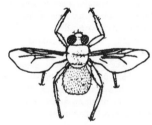

Hippobosca. × 2.

Paragle fly *Paragle redicum*, an anthomyiid fly, lays its eggs in canine faeces, and the white specks have been mistaken for tapeworm segments. Larvae may also be passed alive through the canine (and also the human) gut.

Hymenoptera Insects which have 2 pairs of wings.

Sawflies These have 4 wings and a saw-like ovipositor. The larvae are said to be poisonous if swallowed.

Fly control measures Perceptive farmers have for many years realised the harmful effects of fly infestation on livestock. Controlled field trials, comparing the productivity of treated and untreated cattle, have convincingly demonstrated the advantages that can be gained by modern fly-control methods.

Flies interfere with normal rest and feeding. The approach of a cloud of flies often causes cattle to cease grazing and huddle together. All countrymen are familiar with the sight of cattle 'gadding'; and swarms of black fly (*Simulium ornatum*) may not merely cause store cattle to break out of fields, or rush round them, but can actually kill the animals.

The horse fly (*Tabanus*), like the stable fly (*Stomoxys*), has a painful bite, and the wounds inflicted attract other flies; this exacerbates the 'worry' situation and often transmits even more infection. Some animals become sensitised to the secretions of biting flies, so that an allergy results. One example of this is the 'sweet itch' of horses caused by biting (*Culicoid*) midges.

Flies are notorious for spreading livestock diseases. Even the common housefly (*Musca domestica*) can transmit anthrax, tuberculosis, and the larvae of some parasitic worms. The headfly (*Hydrotaea irritans*) is among several species that may transmit the bacteria that cause 'summer mastitis'. This can lead to gangrene of part of the udder, usually with the permanent loss of use of one-quarter – and to great pain and occasionally death of the cow.

Besides interfering with grazing, the headfly causes infested sheep to scratch, rub and knock their heads, often breaking the skin. Open wounds then attract other flies, increasing the tendency to self-mutilation. Sometimes the whole poll region becomes raw. Pine-tar oil has been used as a repellent, and head caps for protection, but they are inconvenient to use.

Plastic tags impregnated with synthetic pyrethroids have been effective in the reduction of 'fly-worry' in cattle. For sheep too, tags containing cypermethrin and permethrin can be effective in controlling the severity of damage caused by headflies. Cyromazine, in a 'pour-on' formulation, is useful against blowfly larvae on sheep and lambs.

The activities of the autumn fly (*Musca autumnalis*) are very similar to those of the headfly. Both flies feed on secretions from nose, mouth, eyes and wounds and are among several species that transmit the various pathogens causing New Forest disease. This involves an acute and painful conjunctivitis, with inflammation also of the cornea, which becomes opaque, so that cattle are often rendered temporarily blind. Complications may result in permanent eye defects and impaired sight; but even without them the disease causes stress and, since it interferes with feeding, loss of condition can be appreciable.

Other bacterial diseases spread by flies include salmonellosis and brucellosis; while viral diseases such as swine fever and foot-and-mouth have in the past been similarly transmitted in the UK. The larvae of some flies also parasitise animals; for example, the 'green-bottle' fly causing 'strike' in sheep, the sheep nostril fly, and the horse bot flies. The mere approach of warble flies causes cattle to stampede, and the larvae undoubtedly cause pain during their migration through the cow's body, and probably irritation while present in the skin swellings, or warbles. In a few instances, cows have died following the accidental crushing of larvae in the warbles, and larvae occasionally seriously damage the spinal cord. In the UK, control measures have virtually eliminated warble infestation in cattle.

Deterring and killing flies The number of flies entering a milking parlour can be reduced by a spray-boom erected over the doorways, and a plain water mist, produced by ordinary sprinklers or misters, has been recommended for use in collecting yards where a spray-boom over the parlour entrance is impracticable. Such measures, however, do not reduce the total fly population of the farm – they do not kill. Electric fly traps do, and they can be useful when installed in piggeries and dairy cattle buildings. Which flies are electrocuted will obviously depend on the feeding and resting habits of the various species.

Of far wider application, and the most effective weapon against farm flies, is the insecticidal spray. This can be used to convert a livestock building into one big fly trap. A wide variety of effective insecticides is available.

For housed stock, spraying walls may suffice; but beef and dairy cattle at grass will be the target of flies coming from their resting places among trees. Fly control, if it is to benefit grazing animals, therefore requires application of an officially approved insecticide direct to their backs. For this purpose, the synthetic pyrethroids are effective.

These insecticides are chemically allied to the active ingredients of pyrethrum, but are more potent as fly-killers and are also light-stable so that they stay effective for longer in the sun.

Fly control for horses and livestock Numerous formulations based on cypermethrin and other synthetic pyrethroids are available, as both a spray and as pour-on applications, which are convenient to use.

A PVC fly band impregnated with cypermethrin, for threading on to either the browband or the crownpiece of a headcollar, and an ear tag impregnated with 8 per cent cypermethrin, are also available for cattle at pasture.

Whether measured in terms of reduced animal suffering, or farmers' incomes, or a lowered incidence of diseases – some of which are of public-health as well as economic importance – fly control is very worthwhile. If further evidence of its effectiveness were needed, any doubter should note the success of the UK government's 5-year plan to eradicate warble flies from the UK. Now, only sporadic outbreaks of warble infestation occur. Since horses, as well as cattle, suffer from warble-fly larvae (although to a much lesser extent), eradication has also benefited them and their owners.

Overseas Similar methods to those described above, suitably adapted for tropical climates, are in use. The spraying of ground with DDT and dieldrin has been very effective for the control of tsetse flies and human trypanosomiasis, but the practice was discontinued because of the development of resistance and the toxicity of those peparations to other species (see also under TROPICS).

The release of sterile male flies from aircraft has been used on a large scale in Puerto Rico to control the screw-worm fly.

Genetically engineered blowfly maggots have been used in attempts to eradicate sheep blowflies. The maggots were altered so that females which mate produce blind or sterile offspring – a hereditary characteristic which will 'confer genetic death on future generations'.

(See also DIPS AND DIPPING.)

Floods
(see PASTURE CONTAMINATION; SALMONELLOSIS; WATER-DROPWORT)

Floor
(see BEDDING AND BEDDING MATERIALS – Pigs; HOUSING OF ANIMALS)

Floor-Feeding of Pigs
This practice is attractive to the pig farmer since it eliminates the cost of troughs and also saves space – the normal feeding passage becoming a catwalk over the pigs' sleeping quarters.

From a health point of view, the precise composition of the concrete floor may prove important. In an outbreak of illness among pigs in Eire, with anaemia, gastric ulceration, and haemorrhage, the cause was thought to be the 'pit sand' (with a high iron content) with which the concrete was made, giving rise to iron poisoning once the surface layer had been licked off.

More important is the fact that loss of appetite in pigs – a common symptom of many diseases – may not be noticed. With trough-feeding, it is easy to see which pigs are uninterested in food.

Feeding pellets instead of meal may also cause trouble – digestive upsets. The method may involve more stress than conventional systems.

Floor Space
As a rough guide, the following minimum figures may be given: bacon pig, 2 m^2 (6 square feet); veal calf, 3.5 m^2 (12 square feet); laying hen on deep litter, 1 m^2 (2½ square feet).

Floor Sweepings
Floor sweepings in mill or barn have been added to feed and caused fatal poisoning. For example, pigs have died in this way from nitrate poisoning, and cattle from mustard seed poisoning.

'Floppy' Labradors
The colloquial name for an inherited muscle disease of both Black and Golden Labrador retrievers. The condition has been seen in both the UK and the USA. Inheritance is associated with an autosomal recessive gene, leading to a deficiency of type II muscle fibres.

Signs Poor exercise tolerance, especially in cold weather, a stiff hopping gait, with sometimes collapse. Signs have been shown as early as 8 weeks of age, but in other cases after several months.

Florfenicol
A chloramphenicol-like antibiotic which is used in cattle to treat infections caused by *Pasteurella*, *Mannheimia* and *Haemophilus* spp. It is also used in the treatment of fish, particularly in the treatment of furunculosis (*Aeromonas salmonicida* infection) in farmed Atlantic salmon. It is not recommended for use in breeding stock. The antibiotic is administered by injection in cattle and in the feed of fish.

Flour
(see AGENE PROCESS)

Flour-Mite Infestation
Infestation of animal feeds by flour mites (*Acarus farinae*; *A. siro*) can cause a significant loss of nutrient value, as explained under DIET. Like forage mites of various species, flour mites can also cause an irritating parasitic skin disease of animals. In one incident, 36 police horses were stabled in a building which was cleaned and whitewashed before their arrival. Unfortunately a feed barrow was overlooked and still contained

oats left over from the previous year. New oats of high quality were delivered in sacks, and the delivery man opened one sack and topped up the barrow. After he had gone, new oats continued to be put on top of what was left in the large feed barrow, which was never completely emptied. A fortnight after the horses' arrival, the last 4 in the line showed signs of head and neck irritation. One horse had rubbed the side of its neck bare; 2 others had dermatitis on the poll and alongside the mane.

Examination of the bottom layer of the barrow's contents revealed an enormous number of flour mites, and these were also isolated from the skin lesions.

An unsuspected cause of diarrhoea in dogs may be dog biscuits or meal, stored in large bins, and heavily infested with forage mites. As flies may carry nymphal forage mites, fly control is important in reducing such infestations.

Forage mites and/or their eggs may be found in dog faeces, where they may have been mistaken for the eggs of strongyle worms. However, the mite's egg is nearly twice the size of the worm's.

Flour mites (*A. siro* and *A. farinae*), the house/furniture mite (*Glycyphagus domesticus*), and the mould mites (*Tyrophagus putrescentiae* and *T. longior*) may also be involved.

Fluanisone
A neuroleptic drug used in small animals (ferrets. rabbits, guinea pigs, rats and mice). It is usually mixed with FENTANYL)

Flugestone
A hormone preparation supplied in impregnated sponges for the synchronisation of oestrus in ewes. It may also be used to induce oestrus and ovulation in the non-breeding season (see CONTROLLED BREEDING).

Fluid Replacement Therapy
(see under DEHYDRATION)

Flukes and Fluke Disease
(see LIVER FLUKES; LUNG FLUKES; SCHISTOSOMIASIS for blood flukes; PANCREAS, DISEASES OF; and RUMEN FLUKES)

Flumethrin
A synthetic pyrethroid compound used for the treatment of sheep scab and tick infestation. Impregnated in plastic strips, it is hung in beehives to treat varroasis in honey bees.

Flunixine Meglumine
A non-steroidal anti-inflammatory drug used for relief of pain and inflammation in horses, dogs

and cattle; formulated as granules, tablets or injection. Proprietary preparations are Finadyne (Schering-Plough), Cronyxin (Bimeda), and Binixin (Bayer).

Fluorescent

(see under TETRACYCLINES which make bone fluoresce, and under WOOD'S LAMP which shows ringworm-affected hairs fluorescing. For the fluorescent antibody test, see under RABIES and IMMUNOFLUORESCENT MICROSCOPY.)

Fluorescin (Fluorescein)

Fluorescin (Fluorescein) is a useful diagnostic agent in injuries and ulcers on the cornea of the eye. A weak solution is dropped into the eye and the injured area can be seen clearly demarcated from the surrounding healthy cornea.

Fluorine

This element occurs in body tissues and in some natural water supplies. Excess of fluorine causes mottling of the teeth. (For fluorine poisoning, see FLUOROSIS.)

Fluoroacetate Poisoning

Sodium mono-fluoroacetate is used to kill rats and mice, and it is in this connection that poisoning in domestic animals and man may arise. The drug causes distress, yelping, sometimes vomiting, and convulsions in the dog. Treatment consists in the administration of nembutal. A dose as small as 0.66 mg per kg body weight is fatal.

In 1963, 2 outbreaks of fatal poisoning involving numerous dogs, cats, cattle and a pony were attributed to the agricultural insecticide fluoroacetamide, a closely related compound.

Fluorosis

Fluorosis, or chronic fluorine poisoning, is of economic importance in cattle, sheep, etc., grazing pastures contaminated by fluorine compounds emanating from iron and steel works and other industrial plant. It has also been reported in dairy cattle receiving mineral supplements with a high fluorine content, the result of incorporation of rock phosphate. This is something which animal feed manufacturers should guard against, and they should offer guarantees concerning maximum fluorine content in their products.

Signs There is severe lameness, and a resulting loss of condition; milk yield is greatly reduced. The teeth may become mottled, and the bones particularly liable to fracture. Cows may stand with their legs crossed in cases of fracture of the pedal bones. Hip lameness is probably more common.

Antidote Calcium aluminate is of some limited value as an antidote to fluorine poisoning.

Fluothane

Fluothane is a trade name for HALOTHANE.

Flurbiprofen

Fluriprofen, Flurbiprofen and Ibuprofen are non-steroidal anti-inflammatory drugs used in human medicine, and sometimes given to dogs by their owners, or eaten by dogs with access to the tablets, with resultant poisoning (sometimes fatal). Stomach ulceration and kidney failure have been caused.

Eye drops containing flurbiprofen are used as pre-operative treatment for cataract extraction.

Flushing of Ewes

Flushing of ewes aims for rising metabolism in breeding ewes some 6 to 3 weeks before service, by putting them on to protein-rich feed. The purpose is to intensify subsequent oestrus and thereby ensure that each ewe is in fit condition to breed. Some trials, however, have failed to demonstrate the effectiveness of the practice.

Foaling

(see PARTURITION)

Foals

Foals are young horses of either sex until the time they are 1 year old. Male foals are known as 'colt foals', and female foals are called 'filly foals'. Most foals are born between March and June in Britain, although quite a number (especially thoroughbreds) are dropped earlier than this. Thoroughbreds are conventionally aged as from January 1 of the year in which they are born, and all other horses from May 1, irrespective of whether they were actually foaled before or after these dates.

Generally speaking, foals run with their dams at grass during the summer, and are weaned at 4 to 6 months of age. With weakly foals, however, and in the case of highly bred pedigree animals, it is not uncommon to allow them to run with their dams until nearly Christmastime, so that they may get an exceptionally good start in life.

As a rule, foals will begin to eat grass when they are between 3 weeks and a month old, although some start earlier and some later than this. At about 6 weeks to 2½ months they will begin to eat dry corn from mangers along with their mothers.

Foals, Diseases of

Diarrhoea may occur as a result of changes in the mare's milk, or as a result of the dam grazing avidly upon rich spring grass, etc.

Salmonella typhimurium may cause a subclinical infection; alternatively acute and severe diarrhoea or septicaemia may occur, the latter often following the former. (See SALMONELLOSIS.)

E. coli is another cause of acute diarrhoea in the foal. (See E. COLI.)

Corynebacterium equi is probably a more common cause of pneumonia than of diarrhoea; nevertheless the latter can be severe. Clostridial enterotoxaemia occurs; likewise campylobacter infections.

Viruses causing diarrhoea in foals include a CORONAVIRUS and a ROTAVIRUS. The latter may be associated with a profuse, watery diarrhoea and lymph-node enlargement, sometimes followed by death. (See also GLOBIDIOSIS.)

Navel-ill and joint-ill These are colloquial terms for dangerous infections which may attack the foal within the first fortnight of its life. Pain and swelling at the navel, with sometimes abscesses along the umbilical vein, may occur; but joint-ill (polyarthritis) symptoms may be noticed first. Often the hock and stifle joints are painful and swollen, there is fever, and the foal is obviously ill.

Treatment includes the use of appropriate antibiotics (but not corticosteroids, which have an immunosuppressive effect).

Septicaemia is always a danger likely to arise with or after the last 2 conditions. Septicaemia due to *Actinobacillus equuli* infection ('sleepy foal disease') may occur within the first 3 days of life. The foal becomes dull, disinclined to suck, has stupor and diarrhoea, and prostration and death quickly follow. Polyarthritis may occur in foals which survive a little longer.

Organisms causing septicaemia and joint-ill include *E. coli*, *Actinobacillus equi*, *Strep. zooepidemicus* and *Klebsiella pneumonia*.

Haemolytic disease This results from an incompatibility between the blood of sire and dam, and the consequent production of antibodies which reach the foal in the colostrum and break down the foal's red blood cells. These become so reduced in number that not only is there jaundice, but often also a fatal anaemia. If trouble from this cause were anticipated, the use of a foster-mother might save the situation but, obviously, this is seldom practicable. Moreover, unless the mare has previously had a

'jaundiced foal', there will be no indication of the problem. If she has previously had such a foal, however, it is possible to test her blood against the sire's during pregnancy and obtain a fairly good idea as to their incompatibility or otherwise. Treatment must be undertaken quickly and consists in exchange transfusion – the removal of up to 2.8 litres (5 pints) of the foal's blood and the simultaneous injection of up to 3.5 litres (6 pints) of a compatible donor's blood, previously collected. The transfusion requires special apparatus and takes about 3 hours to complete. Recoveries following this treatment have been spectacular.

Worms Both strongyles (red worms) and ascarids may cause trouble in foals. The former give rise to malaise, cough, unthriftiness, tiredness, and sometimes abdominal pain; the latter to diarrhoea and intermittent colic, among other symptoms. The Animal Health Trust recommends that foals be dosed every 4 weeks, alternately for ascarids and strongyles, until the age of 1 year.

Bone diseases in foals include valgus (see under BONE, DISEASES OF); and RICKETS which can render the growth-plate more vulnerable to injury.

Skin diseases Congenital or inherited conditions include *Epitheliogenesis imperfecta* and ICTHIOSIS. ALOPECIA is sometimes a complication of STRANGLES; to which URTICARIA is an occasional sequel.

Pneumonia, due to *Corynebacterium equi*, occurs sporadically in the UK. A suppurative broncho-pneumonia, with abscesses in the lungs and pulmonary lymph nodes, it may be associated with 'joint-ill' and osteomyelitis.

Rhinopneumonitis A congenital infection with EHV 1 virus is a case of early death in foals. (See EQUINE RHINOPNEUMONITIS.)

Muscular dystrophy (see under MUSCLES, DISEASES OF)

Pervious urachus, or 'leaking at the navel', is a condition in which the communication between the urinary bladder and the umbilicus or navel outside, which should close at the time of birth, remains patent and allows urine to dribble from it. The urine blisters the skin around, and ultimately results in considerable swelling and suppuration around the navel. The condition should be corrected by surgery.

Combined immunodeficiency (CID)

occurs in some Arab foals. (See IMMUNODEFI-CIENCY; also under HERNIA; VALGUS; TYZZER'S DISEASE.)

Fodder Beet

(see POISONING)

Fodder Mites

(see FLOUR MITES)

Foetal, Foetus

(see FETAL; FETUS)

Fog

(see under SMOG and 'FOG FEVER')

Fog Fever

The colloquial name derived from the word 'fog', meaning the second crop of grass taken from pasture already cut once that season for hay or silage, has caused much confusion, since it has been applied to several different syndromes in cattle.

True fog fever has been defined as acute pulmonary emphysema occurring in adult cattle (typically single suckler beef cows) which have been moved from poor to lush grazing in the autumn. It should be differentiated from parasitic bronchitis, and also from extrinsic allergic alveolitis caused by micro-organisms in mouldy hay.

It may be identical with the acute bovine pulmonary emphysema encountered in North American adult cattle moved from range to lush pasture.

Cause The probable cause is the conversion in the cow's lumen of the amino acid L-tryptophan in grass to 3-methylindole, a toxic substance.

Two clinical forms of fog fever may be seen. The mild form affects up to 50 or 60 per cent within affected groups of cattle, the animal remaining bright though breathing rather rapidly. In the severe form, the degree of respiratory distress varies greatly, is often severe, and results in a 30 per cent mortality, with death commonly occurring within the first 2 days of the illness.

Post-mortem Lesions include pulmonary congestion, oedema, and hyaline membranes, interstitial emphysema and diffuse alveolar epithelial hyperplasia.

A fog-fever-like condition in sheep, 6 months old, was seen in Sweden. All became ill within 3 days of being moved from poor to lush pasture.

Foggage

Aftermath, 'fog'. Grass grown for winter grazing.

Folic Acid

One of the vitamins of the B-complex. (See VITAMINS.)

Follicle

(see SKIN; OVARY)

Follicle Stimulating Hormone (FSH)

This stimulates the development of the Graafian follicles in the ovary, and controls the secretion of oestrogens from the ovary. It is secreted by the anterior lobe of the pituitary gland. In the male animal, FSH stimulates sperm production in the testicle.

Follicular Mange

Follicular mange is another name for demodectic mange due to the parasite *Demodex canis*, which lives in the hair follicles of the skin. (See MITES, PARASITIC.)

Fomentation

(see POULTICES)

Fomites

Fomites is a term used to include all articles that have been in actual contact with a sick animal, so as to retain some of the infective material and be capable of spreading the disease. Bedding material, fodder, mangers, stable or byre utensils, clothing, grooming tools, the clothes of an attendant, or even the attendant him or herself, may all be fomites.

Food Allergies

(see ALLERGIES; FATTY ACIDS)

Food Conversion Ratio

(see FEED CONVERSION RATIO)

Food Inspection

In countries such as Denmark and the USA, the inspection of meat and meat-derived products has long been carried out entirely by members of the veterinary profession. In the UK this has been only partly so, but to conform with EU regulations meat inspection, including pre-slaughter inspection of food animals, and the examination of organs and tissues as well as inspection of the dressed carcase are carried out by Official Veterinary Surgeons under the centralised control of the Meat Hygiene Service, a government agency. For conditions which render meat dangerous as food, see TUBERCULO-SIS; SALMONELLOSIS; ANTHRAX; TRICHINOSIS; HYDATID DISEASE, etc.

Food Poisoning in Man

(see E. COLI; SALMONELLOSIS; CAMPYLOBACTER; ROTAVIRUS; also BOTULISM). In the UK, salmonellosis is the most frequent cause of food poisoning but *E. coli* is becoming more common. *Clostridium prefringens, Staphylococcus aureus* and *Bacillus cereus* are also found. Yersiniosis and listeriosis, from infected milk or cheese, also occur.

Where meals are prepared for a number of people, as in homes for elderly people whose resistance is lowered, the risk of food poisoning is increased. The very young and immunologically comprised people are also more at risk. Following serious outbreaks of poisoning by *E. coli* 1057 in Scotland in 1997, a government report by Professor Hugh Pennington recommended a series of measures to raise hygiene standards in food shops, etc.

Food Safety Act 1990

This sets out regulations covering the whole of the food chain from retailers back to primary producers.

Food Standards Agency

An independent body established by the UK government with a brief to 'protect public health from risks which may arise with the consumption of food, and otherwise to protect the interests of consumers in relation to food'. The agency reports to government but can publish its advice independently. The Meat Hygiene Service, the agency responsible for meat inspection in all licensed abattoirs, reports to the FSA.

Foods and Feeding

(see DIET AND DIETETICS; NURSING OF SICK ANIMALS; RATIONS; also CAT FOODS)

Fool's Parsley,

Although a member of the natural order Umbellifera – very many of the members of which are poisonous (e.g. water hemlock, water dropwort, and hemlock) – the extremely common fool's parsley (*Aethusa cynapium*) is not a frequent cause of poisoning in animals. It is dangerous when fed to rabbits, if it is pulled in the early green succulent stage before the flowering tops are formed.

Under ordinary circumstances herbivorous animals do not readily eat fool's parsley, for at the time when its growth is most luxuriant (i.e. in spring) there is generally an abundance of grass, which they prefer.

Signs In cows, there have been seen a loss of appetite, salivation, fever, uncertain gait, and paralysis of the hindquarters. In horses, an instance has been recorded in which a number of animals ate the plant in quantity; those which had white muzzles and feet became attacked with diarrhoea and all white areas of the body became severely inflamed, but other horses of a whole-colour remained unaffected. (See LIGHT SENSITISATION.) In other cases stupor, paralysis, and convulsions have been noticed.

First-aid Drenches of strong black tea or coffee should be given so that the tannic acid in them may combine with the alkaloids of the plant and form inert substances.

Foot-and-Mouth Disease (FMD)

A very highly contagious NOTIFIABLE DISEASE that can affect all cloven-hooved species; other names are aphthous fever or epizootic aphtha. It is characterised by the formation of small vesicles (fluid-filled blisters) in the mouth and on the feet or, in the female, on the skin of the udder or teat. Economically, it can be devastating, particularly in cattle, pigs and sheep. The costs of eradication or control, involving diagnostic services, slaughter of infected or at-risk animals, compensation to farmers, disposal of carcases, or adoption of a vaccination policy, and loss of trade can be enormous. Where the disease is not dealt with and becomes endemic, failure to thrive and consequent loss of production and a total ban on export of live animals and, to a very large extent, animal products can be very serious. FMD has been considered the single most important constraint to trade in animals and animal products.

Foot-and-mouth disease has occurred in virtually every country in the world in which cattle, sheep or pigs are kept. It has been endemic in parts of South America, continental Europe, Asia and Africa. Except in young animals, where the death rate may be up to 50 per cent, the disease is not characterised by high mortality. Usually fewer than 5 per cent of infected adult animals die.

The disease is transmissible to humans but the infection is usually mild and transient. It is not the same as (human) HAND, FOOT AND MOUTH DISEASE.

Cause Foot-and-mouth disease is caused by an aphthovirus of which 7 types are recognised – including the 3 known as O (now named the PanAsia strain), A and C, which have caused outbreaks of the disease in Britain, and 4 more types which so far have been confined to Asia and Africa – Asia and Sat 1, Sat 2, and Sat 3. It is the PanAsia strain of type O, now dominant across much of Asia and the Middle East, that was responsible for the major outbreak in 2001. No cross-immunity is exhibited between types, and only partial cross-immunity between subtypes within a type. The virus has a high genetic variability.

The virus is present in the vesicles and in the fluid which comes from them when they burst; and since there is nearly always an excessive secretion of saliva from an animal affected with lesions in the mouth, it is through the medium of contamination with saliva that the disease is perhaps most readily spread. As well as this, however, the urine, faeces, and small amounts of serum from lesions in the feet, are factors in the spread to other animals; livestock markets and transport vehicles are particularly important in causing widening of an outbreak. But as the virus can survive for very considerable lengths of time, it may be picked up and spread by almost any object or animal that has been in contact with affected animals. Migratory birds in their flights from one country to another may act as carriers. Spread can occur by wind, watercourses, people and vehicles.

Bulk collection of milk has also been implicated. FMD virus may be excreted in milk before symptoms in the cow have appeared or become obvious.

The virus can survive in frozen liver or kidney for 4 months or more, and in bull semen stored at low temperatures.

The use of swill containing scraps of meat, bones, or other animal tissue for feeding to pigs is a very important factor in the spread of foot-and-mouth disease, and because of the number of outbreaks traced to swill, the (then) Ministry of Agriculture specified that swill shall have been boiled for at least 1 hour before being fed to pigs. It may have been neglect of this procedure that led to the 2001 UK outbreak. The feeding of swill is now completely banned.

The incubation period before signs of the disease appear after infection varies from 1 to 15 days, but the majority of cases show signs between the 2nd and the 6th day after having been exposed to infection. An important feature of the disease in relation to its infectivity is that virus may be excreted before symptoms become evident; thus the infection may spread before the farmer is aware that his stock are infected.

With pigs, 10 days may elapse between excretion of virus and the development of lesions. With cattle and sheep, the figure may be 5 days; or an average of 2½ days.

Signs

Cattle At first, animals become dull, refuse their food, lie about in a sluggish manner, and cows suddenly give a lessened flow of milk. Their temperatures rapidly rise to 40° or 40.5°C (104° or 105°F), and fever is maintained until the crop of vesicles form, after which it subsides. A few hours after the initial dullness has been noticed, affected animals usually commence to salivate profusely – long ropes of stringy saliva hanging from the mouth. Lameness may be the first sign of the disease. Foot lesions generally appear 4 or 5 days after the vesicles form in the mouth. In these, blisters form around the coronets, between the claws.

The animal frequently smacks its lips in a characteristic manner, yawns, and protrudes its tongue. Blisters are found in all stages of development: the most common locations are on the dental pad and in the upper incisor region; on the tongue, especially around its tip; and on the insides of the cheeks and gums. The blisters each run a similar course; for a few hours they gradually rise, then they burst, liberating a small amount of yellowish, straw-coloured serum (which should be regarded as highly infective and as containing the virus). There remains behind a shallow, eroded, red, raw, ulcer-like area, to the edges of which little pieces of mucous membrane adhere for a short time until they are removed by the movements of the mouth. Adjacent affected areas merge, and in bad cases large irregular, ragged, red patches form, from the surfaces of which the mucous membrane has disappeared. The lesions are always extremely painful, and in consequence the animal is prevented from feeding. Generally, it can still drink, and it will often take liquid or very soft food, but it refuses dry food entirely. In from 6 days to a fortnight or so, healing begins, the lesions disappear and the animal appears to have recovered. It is, however, still carrying the virus.

Sheep Foot-and-mouth disease may be difficult to detect. Onset of lameness is variable – between 2 days and a week – and may pass off quickly. Vesicles in the mouth rupture and heal quickly, leaving no sign of lesions. The sheep may not appear obviously sick and feet and mouth must be examined closely to detect signs of infection.

Pigs Foot lesions usually begin either at the coronet or at the heels instead of between the claws as in cattle. The muzzle and end of the snout may show lesions.

In all affected species, the illness may cause animals to lose much weight, or to cease to grow. Abortion, infertility and diabetes are occasional complications. Foot-and-mouth disease may be the cause of sudden death in pigs, cattle and sheep.

Animals in milk – cows, ewes and sows – may develop characteristic lesions upon their teats or upon the skin of the udder. The lesions are similar to those forming in the mouth, but they take longer to mature. In some cases the whole of the tip of the teat shows a single large blister, which is soon burst by milking or sucking. Subsequently an eroded appearance remains, until healing is established. Milk secretion rapidly diminishes. Permanent udder damage may result from the disease. The pain is usually acute, and the milk – contaminated with the exudate and with discharges from the lesions – is highly infective to young animals.

Differential diagnosis It is necessary to distinguish between foot-and-mouth disease, swine vesicular disease and vesicular stomatitis by laboratory tests. In the UK, tissue and blood samples from suspect animals are sent to the Institute of Animal Health (IAH) Pirbright laboratory for testing. If large quantities of virus are present, the test can give a positive result in 4 hours. In some cases, it may be necessary to multiply the virus by culture in cells and it may take up to 4 days to confirm that virus is not present. The cell culture technique is also used to provide material for identifying the precise type and strain of the virus.

Control A policy of slaughtering affected and in-contact animals is operated in the UK, Canada, the USA, Norway and countries throughout the European Union where the disease is not endemic. Such a policy, involving compensation to owners of compulsorily slaughtered animals, is normally far less costly than a long-term vaccination policy. Slaughtered animals are disposed of by burning or burial; affected premises are thoroughly disinfected and the holding and surrounding area subject to a period of quarantine. Vaccination is practised in countries where a slaughter policy is unworkable because the disease is endemic and its incidence high; not vice versa, as might be thought by those who condemn the slaughter policy without having studied the reasons for it. 'Overall' vaccination is seldom practicable in such areas for reasons of cost, so 'frontier', or 'ring', vaccination (of all susceptible animals within a given radius

of an outbreak) is usually practised. Israel is an exception; the high-yielding diary herds are vaccinated annually.

As a temporary measure, animals in areas surrounding outbreaks may be vaccinated to provide a 'ring fence' against infection. Contrary to its general policy, to protect Greece, the EU operates a vaccination policy in European Turkey and part of Turkey-in-Asia. The use of vaccination was seriously considered in the UK 2001 outbreak when the disease threatened to run out of control and the enormous numbers of animals slaughtered, and disposal of their carcases, created serious difficulties.

Vaccine bank The United Kingdom, Australia, New Zealand, Finland, Ireland, Norway and Sweden in 1985 formally established a foot-and-mouth disease vaccine bank. The participating countries are all free from the disease and do not normally vaccinate against it, but if an outbreak occurs, supplies of vaccine are held at the international vaccine bank, IAH Pirbright: 0.5 million doses of each of the 7 main strains of FMD are kept in store.

Foot-and-mouth disease in Britain A serious epidemic in 1967–8 involved 2397 outbreaks; the slaughter of more than 211,000 head of cattle, 108,000 sheep, 113,000 pigs, and 50 goats; and payments in compensation to owners of about £27 million. The policy and arrangements for dealing with the disease were subsequently reviewed by the Northumberland Committee, which recommended continuation of the slaughter policy with the option of ring vaccination.

Britain was free of FMD except for a minor, easily eradicated, outbreak on the Isle of Wight in 1981, until February 2001, when the worst outbreak ever broke out. Believed to have originated from a pig farm in Durham, where infected swill was fed, the disease spread to sheep which were mixed with others at markets in Hexham and Longtown. Transport of animals by dealers to Devon and other parts of the country caused rapid and widespread outbreaks; export to France and Holland caused further outbreaks which were rapidly contained. By the middle of the year, when the disease was subsiding, more than 3 million animals had been slaughtered. Cumbria, south west Scotland, Durham, Northumberland and Devon were the most seriously affected areas. Large parts of the countryside were out of bounds and the effects for the whole of the UK livestock farming industry, and for tourism, were devastating.

Foot-Baths for Cattle

A foot-bath with 3.75 cm (1½ inch) pipes laid horizontally 5 cm (2 inches) apart, even if filled with plain water, will help to detach mud; the pipes forcing the claws apart.

Caution A 5 per cent formalin foot-bath is often recommended for the control or prevention of foul-in-the-foot, but it is important not to exceed that strength or to put the cows through it too often. One veterinary investigation centre reported that on one farm, 90 out of 100 cows developed severe inflammation at their heels because they were walked through a 4.7 per cent formalin foot-bath twice daily for 2 weeks. Fifty of those cows developed further lesions, a few of which had not healed a month later.

Provision must be made in the planning stage for ease of filling, cleaning, and disposal of the formalin solution. It is convenient to have the foot-bath installed at the parlour exit, so that cows become completely familiar with it and readily walk through it, whether filled or empty. (It would not be desirable to have the foot-bath at the entry to the parlour, owing to fumes from the formalin.)

Suggested dimensions for the foot-bath are as follows: length, about 3 metres (10 ft); width 1 metre (3 ft 6 inches); depth 23 cm (9 inches). The ideal is to have 2 successive foot-baths, the first containing plain water, and the second a solution of 5 per cent formalin.

A more recent recommendation is a 1 per cent solution for routine use as an aid to reducing herd lameness.

Foot-Baths for Sheep

Foot-baths for sheep are used for the purpose of treating or preventing foot-rot and the foot lesions of orf.

The solutions most often used for foot-baths are 3 per cent formalin solution; or copper sulphate, 4 to 8 per cent. As a preventative of contagious foot-rot, a 3-weekly run through a foot-bath gives excellent results. (See FOOT-ROT.)

Caution A striking example of overdoing foot-bath use was the disastrous use of formalin in a foot-bath to treat lameness in a flock of 150 ewes. 'As the lameness increased,' MAFF stated, 'so did the frequency and strength of the formalin liquid until the entire flock was crippled and had to be slaughtered.'

Foot of the Horse

(see also CORNS; QUITTOR; LAMINITIS; SAND-CRACK; SEEDY TOE; BRUISED SOLE; INJURIES FROM SHOEING)

Skeleton of the foot consists of the lower part of the 2nd phalanx, the whole of the 3rd phalanx, and the sesamoid of the 3rd phalanx or navicular bone. (See under BONES.) From the posterior angles of the 3rd phalanx (coffin-bone) project 2 roughly quadrilateral plates of cartilage, one on either side, which are known as the 'lateral cartilages'. These are important structures in the absorption of shock and in preserving the elasticity of the foot as a whole. Under certain conditions they become ossified, when the name 'side-bones' is applied. The 3 bones mentioned above are bound together by a series of ligaments which, while they allow free mobility in normal directions, prevent unnatural movements which might rupture the capsules of the coffin-joint. Lying between the 2 lateral cartilages and behind the 3 phalanx there is a fibro-elastic structure known as the 'plantar cushion' or digital torus, which, although strictly speaking is not part of the skeleton of the foot, will be considered here for convenience. This plantar cushion is composed of extremely elastic, dense, fibrous tissue, poorly supplied with blood vessels and not greatly sensitive, and is one of the chief shock-absorbing structures of the foot. From above it is pressed upon by the descending deep flexor tendon, when the foot comes to the ground; from below it is pressed upwards by the horny frog. It cannot expand forwards to any great extent, because of the presence of the coffin-bone; and since it is practically a rubber-like buffer, it expands backwards and sideways. On either side of it, however, are the lateral cartilages, and these are pressed outwards in the process and carry with them the horny wall at the heels.

Sensitive structures Covering the parts described above and accurately moulded to them are the sensitive parts which nourish the horny hoof. These are: around the hoof-head above the coronary band, a perioplic matrix, the periople, which prevents undue evaporation from the wall; around the coronet, from one heel to the other, a structure about four-fifths of an inch wide, the coronary band, or coronary cushion, which nourishes and from which grows the horn of the wall; running down the inside of the wall all the way round and turning inwards and forwards at the heels, a laminar matrix, which is provided with laminae or 'leaves' which interdigitate with corresponding laminae on the inside of the wall; covering the lower surface of the coffin-bone, and nourishing the sole of the hoof, a solar matrix, or sensitive sole; and covering the lower surface of the plantar cushion and nourishing the frog, a furcal matrix, or sensitive frog. The term 'pododerm' is applied collectively to these sensitive structures. The pododermic tissues are in reality modified skin, and produce numerous minute tubular horn fibres which are firmly united to each other.

The hoof is composed of the wall, the sole, and the frog.

The wall is all that portion which can be seen when the foot rests upon the ground. It gives the foot its form. Its horn is hard, solid, only slightly elastic, and affords protection to the sensitive laminar matrix below it.

The inner surface of the wall has about 600 horny leaves or laminae, which dovetail with the sensitive laminae forming a firm union between wall and matrix. The upper edge of the wall is thin, flexible, and grooved for the lodgement of the coronary cushion. The lower edge is called the 'bearing surface', and is the part to which the shoe is fitted.

The sole is that part of the hoof which is nourished by the sensitive tissue covering the solar surface of the coffin-bone. It is divided into a body and 2 branches, and is roughly crescent-shaped. The sole is markedly vaulted in normal feet, especially in hind-feet, but in very many old horses it becomes flat or even convex; when excessively convex it is called a 'dropped sole'. The white line of soft horn acts as a kind of cementing substance between the wall and the sole. This line is of great importance in shoeing, as it indicates the thickness of the wall, and is used as a guiding line through which the nails can be driven with safety. In the posterior part of the sole there is a V-shaped notch, between the branches of which lie the bars and the frog.

The frog is an exact mould of the lower surface of the plantar cushion which it protects. It is a roughly triangular wedge-shaped mass filling up the space between the bars and the V-shaped notch of the sole. It projects downwards more than the sole, and receives the greatest amount of the concussion in the normal foot; it is only seldom injured, however, for its horn is of very elastic consistency. The ground surface presents a well-marked median cleft, which corresponds to an elevation in its upper (inner) surface.

Foot-Rot of Cattle

This name is used in the USA for what in Britain is called FOUL-IN-THE-FOOT. *Bacteroides nodosus* has been isolated from some foot lesions of cattle in Britain, but its role has not been established.

Foot-Rot of Pigs

Abscesses on the sensitive parts of the foot, often seen in pigs housed on rough concrete; this causes abrasions which become infected.

Thirty per cent of casualty pigs at one UK slaughter-house had abscesses (a common reason

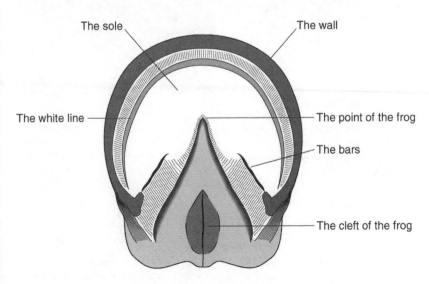

Diagram of the underside of a horse's foot. (With acknowledgements to *The UFAW Handbook on the Care and Management of Farm Animals*, Churchill Livingstone.)

for condemnation of meat) and 12 per cent of these abscesses were on the feet.

In a survey covering more than 6000 pigs, 30 per cent of the lesions were erosion of the heel, 24 per cent of the toe, and 21 per cent of the sole. Fine cracks to deep fissures constituted another 2.7 per cent of the lesions. (See diagram under BIOTIN.)

Causes These include excessively rough concrete, which can be abrasive. Softening of the horn under damp, dirty conditions is another factor; and nutrition may be involved in some instances.

Foot-Rot of Sheep

Foot-rot of sheep is a disease of the horny parts and of the adjacent soft structures of the feet. The organism primarily responsible is *Dichelobacter nodosus (Bacteroides nodosus, Fusiformis nodosus)*. The disease is commonly prevalent on wet, marshy, badly drained pastures, in old folds or sheep pens. Wet soil, however, does not cause foot-rot but merely facilitates infection. This is a mixed one, with *B. necrophorus* causing sufficient damage to permit the entry of *D. nodosus*.

In Australia 2 forms of foot-rot are recognised, in both of which *D. nodosus* is always present. The type of foot-rot which develops depends upon the proteolyptic capacity of the infecting strain of *D. nodosus*. In benign foot-rot the infecting strain is of low proteolytic activity; the resultant disease is limited and does not spread under the hard horn, although it might cause lifting of the sole of the foot. In virulent foot-rot the infecting strain is of high proteolytic activity and results in extensive separation of the hard horn, with uneven horn growth giving the clinical appearance of classical foot-rot.

It appears that transmission of foot-rot infection from cattle to sheep is possible.

D. nodosus cannot survive in the soil or on pasture for more than a fortnight.

Signs Lameness is the first noticeable feature. At first the sheep manages to put the foot to the ground, but after a time it goes on 3 legs only, the pain having greatly increased.

When the foot is examined either there will be found a swelling over the coronet, or an area of the horn of the hoof is found to be soft, painful on pressure, 'rotten-looking', with a variable amount of foul-smelling discharge present.

If neglected, the horn will begin to separate from the underlying sensitive tissues, and will eventually be shed. Sometimes the disease penetrates into the foot, affecting the ligaments or

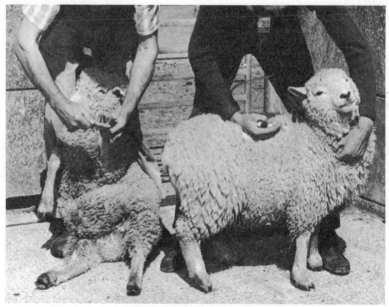

The old and the new in foot-rot treatment. Two injections with foot-rot vaccine at an interval of six weeks can help minimise the paring and cutting of feet necessary with traditional methods of control.

even the bone. One, 2, 3, or all 4 feet may be affected. If the 2 fore-feet are attacked, the sheep very often assumes the kneeling position for feeding. If the 2 hind-feet, any 3 feet, or all 4 feet are affected, standing becomes an impossibility, and the sheep, still retaining its appetite, will feed from the sitting position, crawling forward a few inches at a time to a new piece of grazing.

Prevention Foot-rot can be eradicated. Leave contaminated pasture free of sheep for 3 weeks. Isolate and treat all infected or suspected sheep. The feet of heavy sheep should not be allowed to get overgrown during wet weather; turning on to a bare fallow or stubble field, or walking along a hard road, is advocated by some to wear away the feet, but is not a very practicable proposition. The better way is to round up the sheep and pare each foot individually once every 6 weeks or 2 months.

Where the disease has not yet taken hold, the use of foot-rot vaccine may obviate much time-consuming work treating diseased feet; the manufacturer's directions must be followed if the vaccine is to be effective. Vaccines contain inactivated strains of *D. nodosus*.

Treatment It is advisable to separate the infected animals from the healthy, passing the latter through a foot-bath and changing the pasture to as high a ground as possible. If the lame sheep can be shut up in a dry, strawed yard, in pig-courts or in pens, and given hand-feeding and individual attention daily, they recover much better than if they are left out in the open and only attended to occasionally. The feet should be carefully trimmed, and all necrotic horny material removed. When all the 'rotten' substance has been removed, the sheep should be passed through a foot-bath. In severe cases, zinc sulphate solution is preferable to formalin, which can cause severe pain; proprietary formulations based on zinc sulphate heptahydrate are available.

The shepherd should take care not to spread the disease to other sheep through the medium of hands or knife; both should be washed after dealing with each case, and all parings, diseased tissue, and infected swabs collected in a pail and burned. Neglect of these precautions often results in a continuance of new cases in a flock.

Aerosol sprays containing the antibiotic oxytetracycline, and a purple dye as marker, are popular. Injection of a long-acting antibiotic can be highly effective.

The economic and welfare consequences of foot-rot can be severe. Losses of up to 15 per cent in weight can be shown in affected ewes with reduced growth rate in lambs.

(See also FOOT-BATHS; CONTAGIOUS OVINE DIGITAL DERMATITIS.)

Forage Mites
(see MITES)

Foramen
A hole or opening. The word is applied particularly to holes in bones through which pass nerves or blood vessels. The foramen magnum is the large opening in the posterior aspect of the skull through which passes the spinal cord to enter the foramina in each of the vertebrae of the spine. The nutrient foramina are the holes in the shafts, etc. of the bones which penetrate to the marrow cavity, by which blood and lymph vessels and nerves pass to and from the marrow cavity.

Foreign Body
Any object which becomes lodged in a body organ or tissue. The term includes a grass seed in the ear or nose, beneath the skin between the toes or beneath the eyelid, in the prepuce or penis of the cat; a needle embedded in the tongue or a chop bone wedged in a dog's mouth; a piece of bone lodged in the gullet; a piece of wire in the reticulum; pebbles in a dog's stomach; lead shot and airgun pellets. (See AWNS; under CHOKING; STOMACH, DISEASES OF, etc.)

Foreign bodies also include a broken-off portion of an intravenous needle within a vein, or of a catheter. Miniature 'button batteries', swallowed by small children, have caused an obstruction of the oesophagus, and also mercury poisoning; and a similar risk could be expected in dogs and cats.

Formalin
Formalin is a gas prepared by the oxidation of methyl alcohol. For commercial purposes it is prepared as a solution of 40 per cent strength in water. Formalin is a powerful antiseptic, and has the quality of hardening or fixing the tissues. The solution in water gives off gas slowly, and this has an irritant action on the eyes and nose.

Formalin is used for preserving pathological specimens, occasionally as a disinfectant, and for the production of formaldehyde gas for fumigation of buildings. A 3 per cent solution of formalin has been used in a foot-bath in the treatment of foot-rot in sheep. Its application, however, may cause considerable pain if it reaches sensitive tissues. Formalin gas has been used to fumigate eggs on farms and in the setters in the hatchery. The process carries some risk and must be done in special chambers; approved alternatives are available. Formalin gas must never be used to fumigate duck or goose eggs. (See also under FOOT-BATHS; DISINFECTION.)

Fossa

Fossa is an anatomical term applied to a depression in a bone which lodges some other structure, such as part of the brain in the skull. It is also used to describe grooves or pockets in soft tissues, such as the renal fossa of the liver in which is lodged the right kidney.

Foul-in-the-Foot

Called FOOT-ROT in the USA. A disease that affects cattle. Technically known as interdigital necrobacillosis, the lesion takes the form of a swelling which tends to force the claws apart. The whole length of the space between the claws may be involved, with 1 or 2 fissures in the skin evident, and a slough of dead tissue.

Cause Fusiformis necrophorus (*Fusabacterium necrophorum*) is the usual cause, entering tissues through a wound or through devitalisation of the skin from frost, mud, decomposing urine or faeces, or other irritants.

Signs There is nearly always well-marked lameness, with swelling of the interdigital tissues and a typical foul smell. Hind-feet are more often affected than fore-feet, probably owing to their greater liability to soiling from urine and faeces, in which the necrosis bacillus can generally be easily found. In many cases a cow will suddenly stop walking, and shake the affected foot as though she desires to dislodge a stone or other hard object which has become wedged between the claws.

A 'super foul' has been seen recently, which spreads very rapidly in the foot; it causes severe pain and deep erosion at the heel unless treated promptly. Tissue damage may be so extensive that the animal has to be culled.

Treatment This calls for prompt professional aid. The foot is dried and an oxytetracycline spray applied. In severe cases, parenteral antibiotics may be necessary and are essential in 'super foul'. Affected animals should be isolated. (See FOOT-BATHS.)

Fowl Cholera

Synonyms: cholera gallinarium, avian pasteurellosis, pasteurellosis of the fowl, haemorrhagic septicaemia of the fowl. This is a contagious disease of fowls, usually epizootic in type and characterised by sudden onset, high fever, extensive blood extravasations into the different organs, and severe diarrhoea. The disease occurs all over Europe, in North and South America, in most parts of Africa, and in Asia. All common fowls, including domestic poultry (chickens, ducks, geese, guinea-fowl, turkeys, pigeons, pheasants, and fancy birds), are susceptible. Most common wild birds are also liable to infection and serve to spread the disease. Rabbits and mice may also contract it under special circumstances.

Cause Pasteurella multocida.

Signs After a brief incubation period (usually 2 to 4 days) the birds may be seen to stagger and fall down, or more commonly are just found dead. In the less acute type, which perhaps is the more common, the birds are seen to look ill, to stand apart from the rest, droop their wings, and refuse both food and water. The combs, wattles, and ear lobes become discoloured, and there is great nervous prostration. A discharge comes away from the eyes and nose, a frothy saliva from the mouth, and there is usually severe diarrhoea. The respirations become rapid; the temperature may reach 43.3° or 43.9°C (110° or 111°F). The feathers are ruffled and draggled, and those of the hinder parts of the body are soiled with faecal discharges. Vomiting may take place, and in from 1 to 3 days the affected birds usually die. In other cases the symptoms are more subacute, and the disease may run on for from 7 to 9 or 10 days, but as a rule ends fatally. In the more chronic type, arthritis may be seen and it may take several weeks before death ensues. In acute outbreaks 90–95 per cent may die, although in others the death-rate may be only 20 per cent.

Treatment Tetracycline antibiotics are more useful than sulfonamides as these adversely affect egg production.

Prevention is by vaccination and avoiding contact with wild birds.

Fowl Paralysis

(*Neuro-lymphomatosis.*) (See MAREK'S DISEASE.)

Fowl Pest

This term usually refers to NEWCASTLE DISEASE, but also includes fowl plague (see AVIAN INFLUENZA)

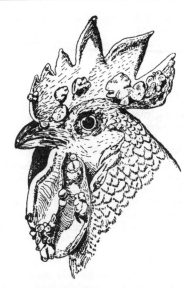

Head of cock affected with fowl pox (avian contagious epithelioma). Wattles and comb are mainly affected.

Fowl Plague

(see AVIAN INFLUENZA)

Fowl Pox

Also known as avian contagious epithelioma and avian diphtheria, this is a disease caused by the avian poxvirus in which wartlike nodules appear on the comb, wattles, eyelids, and openings of the nostrils.

The disease attacks the fowl most often, but other domesticated birds are all susceptible; likewise wild and domesticated pigeons. It occurs in almost all parts of the world. (See POX.)

The virus infects the skin through abrasions, and may be transmitted by insect vectors (especially mosquitoes). Various secondary organisms are usually responsible for deaths.

The period of incubation is usually between 3 and 12 days, and bad housing conditions, severe weather, and poor feeding serve to lower vitality and render an outbreak much more serious.

Signs There are 3 types of lesion: (i) nodular eruptive lesions on comb and wattles; (ii) a cheesy, yellowish membrane in the mouth and throat; (iii) oculo-nasal form (possibly due to a different virus).

The mouth lesions consist of patches of a greyish, fairly firm, cheesy-looking material,

which is of considerable thickness, and not easy to detach. This is the 'false membrane'. In many cases the entrance to the trachea is partially blocked with these deposits, and the breathing is consequently obstructed. The smell from the mouth is always foul.

Treatment is economically unsound. The best measures consist of the slaughter of all affected birds and the inoculation of the healthy ones with 'pigeon-pox vaccine'.

Prevention Newly purchased birds should be isolated for 3 weeks before being added to the flock, and after returning from shows, laying trials, etc., the same procedure should be adopted.

Vaccination (in regions where vaccine is available) can be done at 6 weeks of age; or, more usually, between 3 and 5 months of age.

Fowl Typhoid

This is an acute infectious disease of fowls (also of ducks, geese, turkeys, game and wild birds) caused by *Salmonella gallinarium*. The disease has a worldwide distribution, but has been virtually eradicated from the UK.

Most outbreaks occur in pullets near point of lay, but birds of all ages are susceptible – even chicks. The disease is usually introduced into a flock by the purchase of 'carrier' fowls, and thereafter spreads by contamination of food and water with the droppings of such birds. The incubation period is from 4 to 6 days.

Signs are not always characteristic. There is generally marked drowsiness, loss of appetite, and great weakness. The fowls prefer to sit about in dark corners. The comb and wattles are sometimes pale and anaemic; they may in other cases be markedly congested. Diarrhoea is usually present. Death, following progressive weakness, occurs in from 4 to 14 days after the onset of the symptoms. The percentage mortality varies from about 20 to 30 per cent, and many or most of the recovered birds become 'carriers', which serve to spread the disease to other birds.

Diagnosis If fowl typhoid is suspected, samples of blood from the surviving and apparently healthy birds should be submitted to the agglutination test, and all reactors should be isolated and destroyed – the carcases being burned or buried in quicklime. The remaining birds should be treated with antibiotics, moved to fresh premises, and retreated.

After removal of the reacting birds, the houses, utensils, etc. should be disinfected.

Fox, Diseases of

In Europe, North America and other parts of the world, wild foxes often become victims of rabies, and spread this disease to farm livestock which they may attack. A history of aggressiveness and atypical behaviour does not, however, point conclusively to rabies; distemper may be the reason. (See also FOX ENCEPHALITIS; 'CHASTEK PARALYSIS'.)

The fox acts as host of the roundworm *Toxocara canis* and of the *Toxascaris leonina*, and if silver fox cubs are reared by a cat, they may become infected with *Toxocara mystax* of the cat. The fox harbours the dog tapeworms *Taenia serialis* and *T. multiceps*, and *Echinococcus granulosus*. Leptospirosis occurs in foxes in the UK and may be spread to farm livestock (5 strains have been isolated). Flukes may infest foxes.

Fox Encephalitis

Fox encephalitis is of commercial importance on the fox ranches of North America, where these animals are bred for their fur. The disease is considered identical to Rubarth's disease of dogs.

Signs Young foxes in good condition are most frequently affected. A violent convulsion is followed by a lethargic or 'sleep-walking' state. This may be followed by excitability and more convulsions – during which the slamming of a door or any loud noise may prove fatal. The illness runs a very rapid course, from 1 hour to 3 days, 24 hours being the average duration.

Control By means of serum and preventive inoculation.

This disease, or one caused by a similar virus, may have accounted for the deaths of (wild) foxes in Britain, but the deaths may have occurred as the result of eating birds poisoned by dieldrin. Signs are similar.

Foxglove Poisoning
(see DIGITALIS POISONING)

Fox Terriers

Small, lively dogs classed as smooth-haired or wiry, according to the coat; tail usually short. In both breeds deafness and lens luxation may be inherited. Pulmonary stenosis and achalasia may be seen. Atopic dermatitis occurs only in the wire-haired terrier; cerebellar ataxia in the smooth.

Fractures

Simple fractures are the commonest variety, and consist of those in which the bone is broken clean across, with or without tearing and laceration of the soft parts surrounding it, but without any wound leading from the fracture through to the skin. They are spoken of as being transverse, longitudinal, or oblique, according to the direction of the break.

Compound fractures are those in which the skin is injured, so that a direct or indirect communication between the fracture and the outside air exists. The broken end of the bone

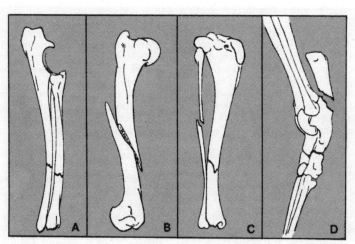

Classification of fractures. A. Transverse fracture with excellent stability after reduction. B. Oblique fracture with no stability after reduction. C. Slightly oblique fracture which, by virtue of the irregularity of the fracture lines, provides a useable degree of stability after reduction. D. A typical distracted fracture. (With acknowledgements to the British Veterinary Association.)

very often penetrates through the skin and is found exposed. Bleeding is apt to be severe; infection of the ends of the bones with pathogenic organisms may occur.

Incomplete fractures are those in which the bone is broken only partly across, or in which the tough periosteum (the tissue covering the bone) is not torn. This variety occurs in the shin-bones (tibiae) of horses which have been kicked, and in the bones of young animals. In these the bone cracks like a twig half-way across, and then splits for some distance along its length, just as does a branch which has been cut halfway through and then bent; these fractures are known as 'greenstick fractures'.

Fissured fractures are mere cracks in the bone which are found in the skull and face bones after blows or falls. They are usually not serious unless haemorrhage accompanies them and the blood clot presses upon a nerve or on the brain itself.

Deferred fractures occur when the bone has actually been fractured, but the fractions do not separate until or unless some extra severe strain is put upon the part.

Distracted fractures are those in which muscular contraction causes the detached fragment to be drawn away from the main body of the bone.

Depressed fractures also occur in the skull bones as a rule, and consist of fractures in which a fragment of bone is forced in below the level of the surrounding surface. They may give rise to very serious symptoms when the depressed portion presses upon the brain substance.

Complicated fractures are those in which there is some other serious injury produced in addition to the fracture, e.g. dislocation of the dog's hip along with fracture of the shaft of the femur; tearing of a large nerve; etc.

Comminuted fractures are those in which there is much splintering, the term 'sequestra' being applied to those splinters of bone which are separated and eventually die.

Impacted fractures are those in which, after the break has occurred, one fragment is jammed inside another, usually at an angle.

Ununited fractures are those in which, after the usual time has elapsed for the fracture to heal, it is found that union has not taken place. The failure to unite may be simply due to 'delayed union', on account of debility or illness or due to the fact that the limb or other member is not kept at rest sufficiently for the process of healing to occur. In other cases of ununited fracture, a piece of muscle or other tissue becomes placed between the broken ends of the bones and effectively prevents their union.

Causes Disease, such as osteomalacia, in which there is a reduction in the density of bone and of its tensile strength, is one cause. However, the common cause is external violence. (See also ELECTRIC SHOCK.)

Horses Fractures result from kicks, falls or blows; errors in judgement during jumping; the putting of feet into rabbit-holes when galloping; and accidents when the animal collides with some stationary object, or is struck by a vehicle.

Fractures incurred by 53 race horses at a New York track were found to be due to 3 lesions: osteochondrosis, chondro-osteo necrosis, and degeneration of tendons and ligaments.

Cattle Fractures result from injuries during fighting, slipping, and falling when struggling; from running, bulling and mounting or during service; from jumping fences, hedges, ditches; from crowding accidents at markets, etc.; and from crushes in cattle-trucks.

Fracture of the 3rd phalanx in a medial front claw is commonly associated with fluorine poisoning, and causes cattle to stand with their legs crossed. (See also SHOEING.)

Pigs and sheep The causes are usually similar, but legs are broken more easily. Careless use of the shepherd's crook is responsible for many. Falling over precipices and getting a limb fast in a gate, fence, or hurdle may also result in a broken bone.

Dogs and cats Of 298 cats brought, on account of fractures, to a small-animal hospital in London over a 2-year period, more than 90 per cent had been injured in road accidents. The bones most frequently broken were the femur (28 per cent of the cats), pelvis (25 per cent), and jaw (11 per cent).

In a survey of 26 feline fractures diagnosed at the Universiti Pertanian Malaysia, the femur, jaw, tibia, pelvis, and spine were the most common sites of fracture, in that order.

Of 61 dogs covered by the same survey, the femur, tibia, pelvis, radius and ulna were the bones most often involved. Nearly half the cases were the result of road-traffic accidents; with 6 being ascribed to nutritional causes, 4 to falls, and 1 to a bullet wound.

Signs The chief signs of a fracture are uselessness of the part, crepitus of the fragments, and sometimes unnatural mobility and deformity. If a limb is affected there is usually an unnatural mobility, inability to sustain weight, distortion or deformity, shortening of the length, a thickness or swelling at the seat of the fracture (due to overlapping of the fragments), and a variable amount of pain. (See also 'Fractures of special parts', below.)

Healing of fractures When the bone breaks, many blood vessels are torn, and accordingly a large clot of blood forms around the ends, between them, and for some distance up the inside of the bone. Later, great numbers of white blood cells find their way into this clot, which becomes 'organised' – blood vessels and, later, fibrous tissue being formed in it (soft callus). Next, lime salts are gradually deposited in this fibrous tissue, which thus develops into bone (hard callus). In this process a thick ring of new bone forms round the broken ends, filling up all crevices; and when union is complete, this thickening is again gradually absorbed, leaving the bone as it was before the injury.

In racing greyhounds, badly fractured scaphoids have been removed and replaced by plastic or metal prostheses. In one case, the use of a titanium-alloy prosthesis enabled a greyhound to race again 43 times before retirement from the track.

Treatment Reduction and apposition are brought about by manipulation of the fractured bones under anaesthesia. Immobilisation is then effected by means of plaster of Paris, and various proprietary mixtures impregnated into bandages. Splints of metal, leather, wood, or cardboard, padded with cotton-wool, are useful, especially with dogs and cats. (See SPLINTING MATERIALS.)

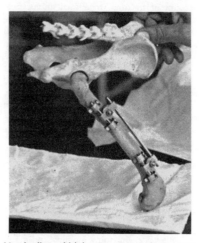

Metal splints which have transverse pins to penetrate and fix the bone are used in treating fractures in small animals, and have succeeded in cases where other methods would be ineffective.

Special types of extension splints, having transverse pins which transfix the bone, have been used with success in appropriate cases. Medullary pins, driven down the marrow cavity of long bones; wiring; and plating have all been used with success. (See BONE PINNING.)

Whenever splints, plaster, or other bandages are being applied to fractured limbs it is essential to ensure that the surface of the skin is well padded with cotton-wool, and that the pressure is evenly distributed. Failure in this respect may result in parts of the skin becoming gangrenous through obstruction to the blood-flow.

Bone Grafts These are used to a limited extent in veterinary surgery to repair fractures of the femur, humerus, tibia, radius and ulna; or to replace comminuted fragments, to lengthen bones, to correct delayed or faulty union.

The allografts are harvested aseptically from healthy dogs, autoclaved the same day, and may be stored at between –10° and –20°C (14° and –4°F) in a domestic freezer for use up to 1 year later. Ordinary bone-plating techniques are used to secure the implant.

Fractures of special parts

1. *The cranium* Cases of traumatic fracture of the skull result in concussion; if not severe they may recover with conservative treatment and nursing. Depressed fractures involving the cranial cavity or the cranial nerves are difficult to treat and usually carry a poor prognosis. (See also CONCUSSION.) Surgical treatment may be successful in cases in which fractures involve bones of the jaws and face.

2. *The face bones* Fractures may be simple or serious according to bones involved. Nasal bones, often fractured from accidents, may be accompanied by swelling, pain, haemorrhage, difficulty in breathing, and much watering of the eyes. Jaw-bones broken from falls, kicks, etc. usually interfere with feeding. Lower-jaw fractures usually result in an open hanging mouth, escape of saliva, and altered expression; frequently, loose teeth, torn lips, and haemorrhage are seen. Bones of orbit fractured by falls on to side of head, collisions, etc. interference with vision and with movements of the lower jaw, in most cases serious. Treatment usually necessitates operation – removal of broken pieces, elevation of depressed portions, removal of loose teeth, wiring or plating broken parts together. Feeding must be carefully undertaken when jaws are injured – sloppy food, mashes, etc., for horse; hand-feeding for dog.

3. *The vertebrae* Commonest in horse and dog through accidents (e.g. in horses getting cast in stall, casting for operation, road-traffic accidents in dogs, falls from heights, blows from sticks). If a vertebra is fractured, paralysis results. There is often a fatal termination, or a need for euthanasia. Tail-bones are often broken in dogs and cattle through getting caught in doors, gates, fences, etc.

4. *The ribs* Due to external violence usually, but the 1st rib is sometimes broken through muscular action in a side-slip and violent recovery, when it often results in RADIAL PARALYSIS. Otherwise broken ribs show little or nothing characteristic except local pain and deformity, unless many are involved, when breathing may be short and/or difficult. (See 'FLAIL-CHEST'; PNEUMOTHORAX.)

5. *The pelvis* In 123 cases of fracture of the pelvis in dogs in 1 practice, all were the result of road accidents. Twenty-eight of the dogs were treated surgically, and 66 conservatively. The conclusion drawn was that, although the majority of patients would recover without surgery, the latter could reduce the time taken for recovery, especially with multiple fractures on both sides of the pelvis. In bulls and stallions, pelvic fractures occur sometimes during service when their hind-feet slip from under them and they fall backwards on to buttocks. These are least serious when only the external angle of ilium ('point of hip') is involved.

6. *The scapula* Fractures are uncommon. Mostly, they occur through the neck of the bone, or on the projecting spine. The musculature covering the bone may impede diagnosis but assists recovery, acting as natural bandage.

7. *The humerus* Lameness, intense in all animals, follows fracture; the limb is usually quite useless. Horses and cattle do not make good recoveries except when young, but healing in small animals is more satisfactory. (See BONE-PINNING.) Absolute rest is essential; horses may be slung.

In a series of 130 cases in dogs and cats, most animals with proximal, shaft and supracondylar fractures had excellent results. The poor prognosis associated with distal articular fractures was most often because of failure of the fixation device in the supracondylar area. The best results were achieved with a plate on the caudal and medial surface of the distal humerus.

8. *The radius and ulna* One or both bones may be broken; fracture of the ulna is less serious unless the elbow-joint is involved. In dogs, if one is broken the other acts as a natural splint. Lameness is always marked, and there is pain on pressure. Local swelling is usually noticed, and deformity. Bandaging is advisable. Young horses should be placed in slings. Bone-pinning has been carried out successfully in the dog and the horse.

9. *Coronoid process* In 130 cases of fragmented coronoid process of the ulna in 109 dogs, 68 were treated surgically by medial elbow arthro-tomy and 62 with rest and anti-inflammatory drugs. Surgical treatment did not decrease the incidence of lameness after treatment, but the dogs treated surgically were more active and less lame than those treated without surgery. Young dogs with mild lameness due to fragmented medial coronoid processes probably do not benefit from surgery, but dogs with chronic, moderate or severe lameness do.

10. *Bones of knee* These are seldom fractured, but if they are it is usually impossible to bring about recovery without stiffening of the joint (ankylosis).

11. *The metacarpals* In the horse, good recoveries are made in cases of clean transverse fractures without complications or splinters. Prognosis is best in fractures occurring in the middle of the cannon. The limb is bandaged with a plaster or proprietary resin-impregnated bandage and the horse slung; the plaster is left in position for at least 6 weeks. In the dog, such fractures usually respond well after setting and supporting of the affected bone.

12. *The pastern bone* Fractures may be transverse, oblique, or longitudinal ('split pastern'), often comminuted. Severe lameness always results. Simple transverse fractures can be treated satisfactorily if the temperament of horse will allow rest and slinging; oblique, longitudinal, and all comminuted cases are unsatisfactory and if recovery occurs, usually some deformity or blemish is left.

13. *The second phalanx, coffin and navicular bones* Fractures in these bones are rare; they may be caused by direct violence, and sometimes follow an operation of neurectomy (un-nerving); may be seen in cattle as a result of weakening of bone through FLUOROSIS. Fracture of the coffin-bone, if simple and joint surfaces are not involved, makes good recovery as a rule, since hoof acts as splint and bandage. Fracture of the 2nd phalanx (short pastern bone) is usually difficult to resolve.

Most fractures of the navicular bone are

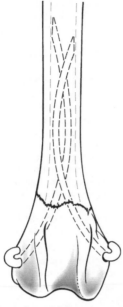

Two Rush-type intramedullary pins used to repair a supracondyloid fracture of the femur.

sagittal and minimally displaced, but the prognosis is usually poor because the fibrous callus causes permanent lameness. Such fractures have been repaired by inserting a 50 mm screw which exerts compression between the 2 fragments. The pilot hole is drilled and the screw is inserted precisely along the transverse axis of the navicular bone by means of a mechanical guide, the process being monitored by image-intensifying fluoroscopy. The fractures are said to heal without superfluous callus formation.

14. *The femur* Very commonly fractured in dogs after street accidents. Shaft, neck, or one of the trochanters may be involved. Frequently in dogs, dislocation of the hip-joint accompanies fracture. Extreme lameness, shortening of the limb, local swelling, and great pain on movement are usually seen. There may or may not be crepitus. In horses, fracture of pelvis very often accompanies fractured femur and makes diagnosis difficult. A fractured femur usually necessitates euthanasia in large animals, but in small animals recovery may be either partial or complete. (See BONE-PINNING.)

15. *The patella* Fracture is a very serious condition, resulting in a lowering of the affected stifle and inability to advance the limb. There is great pain. Treatment is union of the fragments by wire sutures; this may be difficult

to perform satisfactorily, and complete recovery may not occur.

16. *The tibia* Many fractures of tibia become compound from sharp points of broken bones penetrating through the skin. (See BONE-PINNING, which has been used successfully in dog, cat, and horse.)

17. *Bones of hocks* Fracture of os calcis (point of hock) – the epiphyseal summit becomes torn away from the rest of the bone by an undue pull of the Achilles' tendon (hamstring). Fractures of other bones of hock are less common (with the exception of the SCAPHOID in the racing greyhound).

Francisella
(see TULARAEMIA)

Free Radicals
Highly reactive molecules, formed in the presence of oxygen and capable of damaging living tissue. They have been implicated in human heart disease and arthritis. They may also be a cause of sudden death of pigs – those being transported for long distances or subject to other forms of stress. However, it has been suggested that protection may be given by feeding vitamin E, which 'scavenges' radicals.

Freemartin
Usually defined as a sterile heifer born twin to a normal bull calf; the most widely accepted explanation being that sex hormones from the earlier developing male twin pass across to the female twin, with the result that sexual differentiation of both male and female proceeds under control of male hormones.

However, as long ago as 1917 it had been suggested that hermaphrodites might occur in female single births, as a consequence of early fetal death and resorption of the male twin in the uterus. During the 1970s chromosome analysis had revealed the presence of both male and female cells in single-born bull calves. Dr W. V. S. Wijeratne and colleagues were the first to demonstrate this condition – technically known as secondary chimerism – in single-born freemartins. (Primary chimerism can occur where 2 sperms fertilise the same ovum.)

Not every female fetus having a male twin sharing the uterus will become a freemartin, because in some instances death of the male twin fetus occurs before about day 39 of pregnancy – when a common blood supply may become established. Moreover, in between 5 and 10 per cent of heterosexual twin pregnancies a common blood supply is not established.

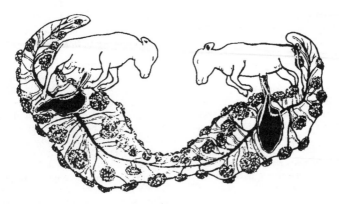

The bovine freemartin.

Blood samples were taken from 36 heifers not in calf after 3 or more inseminations or natural service; chromosome analysis of these animals' white cells showed that 12 of the heifers had both male and female chromosomes. Five of the heifers were single-born. In 3 which were slaughtered, abnormalities of the reproductive tract were formed.

Two of the slaughtered heifers had shown normal oestrous cycles, and had reproductive organs apparently normal on clinical examination; but 1 of them, with 5 per cent male cells, had her cervix closed by a fibrous band or hymen; the other, which had 12 per cent male cells, was sterile on account of fibrous bands blocking the horns of the uterus. Both heifers possessed functional ovaries. The 3rd heifer, with 45 per cent male cells, had a normal vagina, enlarged clitoris, seminal vesicles and sex organs having both ovaries and testes in primitive form.

'Presuming that 5 per cent of all heifers reared for breeding are infertile, the probable prevalence of single-born freemartins in this heifer population is about 0.9 per cent', (concluded Dr Wijeratne.)

About 90 per cent of heifer calves born twin to a bull calf are freemartins. Many freemartins can be detected on clinical examination, since the vagina is often only one-third of the normal length and, in addition, there is often an enlarged clitoris and a vulval tuft of hair.

The condition is associated with anastomosis of the placental blood vessels (see diagram).

Pig freemartins may also occur. (See also H-Y ANTIGEN.)

Freeze-Branding
(see BRANDING)

Fremitus
Fremitus is a sensation which is communicated to the hand of an observer when it is laid across the chest in certain diseases of the lungs and heart. Friction fremitus is a grating feeling communicated to the hand by the pleura or pericardium when it is roughened as in pleurisy or pericarditis.

French Bulldog
A small dog resembling the English bulldog of the 19th century. Haemophilia may be found as a sex-linked recessive trait. Ununited anconal process (elbow) is a dominant trait. Hemivertebrae, intervertebral disc disease, patellar luxation may occur.

Frog
(see FOOT OF HORSE)

Frontal Bone of the Skull
A roughly quadrilateral plate-like bone which forms part of the roof of the cranium and passes forward between the eyes to meet the nasal bones. In the horned breeds of cattle and sheep it is extended laterally to form the horn cores. (See BONES; also SINUSES OF SKULL.)

Frontal Sinus
(see SINUSES OF SKULL)

Frost-Bite
Frost-bite may affect any animal exposed for long periods to severe cold. As a result of this cold, the body reacts by a constriction of surface blood vessels, in order to minimise heat loss and maintain body temperature. This leaves exposed parts of the skin susceptible to freezing. The

part, such as the tips of ears, or the tail, becomes numb, and may be completely frozen. Pain is not felt at this stage (but occurs during the thawing process). In some instances natural recovery takes place, but in others gangrene follows and ear-tips, tails, and the wattles and combs of poultry may slough off.

An animal-owner may have no reason to suspect frost-bite until the appearance of gangrene and sloughing. (See GANGRENE.) Nowadays massage and rubbing the part with snow have been abandoned as likely to do more harm than good in human medicine; and immersing the part in warm or hot water is equally to be avoided. (See CHILBLAIN.)

Frounce
(see FALCONS)

Frozen Embryos
(see LIFE AFTER FREEZING)

Frusemide
A diuretic suitable for the treatment of some cases of OEDEMA.

'Frying Pan' Deaths
Overheated fat gives off acrolein, which can be highly poisonous and was, indeed, used in chemical warfare in 1914–18. A dog died after being shut up in a kitchen for half an hour with a smoking chip pan. Ante-mortem symptoms were distressed breathing and cyanosis.

Five cockatiels died within half an hour following exposure to fumes from a non-stick frying pan coated with plastic polytetrafluoroethylene. Within an hour the birds' owner became ill with 'polymer fume fever', but recovered. (See KITCHEN DEATHS.)

Fucosidosis
A lysosomal storage disease caused by the absence of an enzyme – alpha-L-fucosidase.

It is an inherited disease in the English springer spaniel, affecting mainly those between 18 months and 4 years old. The signs of this ultimately fatal disease include ataxia, change in temperament, depression, apparent deafness and impaired sight. Swallowing may be difficult. Loss of weight occurs.

Fumes
(see CARBON MONOXIDE; 'FRYING PAN' DEATHS; SLURRY; ANAESTHETICS; AEROSOLS)

Fumigation
(see DISINFECTION)

Fundus
Fundus is the base or innermost part of a hollow organ distant from its opening.

Fungal Diseases
Broadly speaking, these include both the invasion of tissues by fungi, and the effects on organs of fungal poisons (see MYCOTOXICOSIS).

Ringworm offers a good example of the invasion of tissues by pathogenic fungi; one should, perhaps, say potentially pathogenic fungi, for many are present in the alimentary canal of healthy animals, and cause lesions only when circumstances favour invasion or multiplication. (See MASTITIS IN COWS, Mycotic, for an example of the latter; also ASPERGILLOSIS; BLASTOMYCOSIS; HISTOPLASMOSIS; MUCORMYCOSIS; MONILIASIS; STREPTOTHRICOSIS; CRYPTOCOCCOSIS; FUSARIUM; MORTIERELLA; COCCIDIOMYCOSIS; RHINOSPORIDIOSIS; SPOROTRICHOSIS.)

Fungal Toxins
(see MYCOTOXICOSIS)

Fur Mites
(see MITES)

Fur, Swallowed
(see HAIR BALLS)

Furazolidone
A nitrofuran compound used against antibacterial and antiprotozoal infections. Its use in food animals is no longer permitted in the EU.

Furfuraceous
Furfuraceous is a term applied to skin diseases which produce a bran-like scaliness.

Furunculosis
The presence of boils (abscesses). In the dog, the term is applied sometimes to abscesses/ cysts between the toes. (See INTERDIGITAL CYSTS.) Perianal furunculosis also occurs in dogs.

Furunculosis in fish is caused by *Aeromonas salmonicida*. Raised furuncles can be seen all over the body and they may be complicated by secondary fungal infection. A sudden increase in water temperature can trigger the appearance of the disease.

Furunculosis in salmon is caused by *Aeromonas salmonicida* but may be triggered by a sudden rise in water temperature. Young fish stop feeding and may die soon afterwards. Older fish are more resistant; they develop large, boil-like swellings on the shoulder and back. If these burst, a reddish fluid rich in bacteria is released. The bacterium persists in some fish between outbreaks and is present in wild fish. Treatment is by medicating the feed with sulfonamides or tetracyclines but the fish may be reluctant to take medicated food. It is a NOTIFIABLE DISEASE under the Diseases of Fish Act 1937.

Furze (Gorse)

(*Ulex europaeus*.) A very common and plentiful shrub in waste lands in Britain, it was formerly often cut and used as fodder after chaffing or bruising. The plant contains a very small proportion of a poisonous alkaloid which is called *ulexine*, and is practically identical with cystine from broom. It is a nerve and muscle poison, but it is seldom present in dangerous amounts.

FUS

(see FELINE UROLOGICAL SYNDROME)

Fusarium

Mouldy shelled maize containing *F. monili-forme* has caused diarrhoea and ataxia in cattle; and in broilers the same species, contaminating maize and wheat, has with *F. culmorum*, *F. Tricinctum* and *F. nivale* been implicated in poor growth rate, poor feathering, and abnormal behaviour. *Fusarium* species may also cause keratoconjunctivitis. (See under EYE, DISEASES; also MYCOTOXICOSIS; ZEARALENONE.)

Fusiformis Necrophorus

Also known as *F. necrophorum*. An anaerobic bacterium causing foul-in-the-foot of cattle, calf diphtheria, abscesses in the liver and other organs. Also involved in foot-rot in sheep. (See table under BACTERIA, *and* FOOT-ROT.)

G

Gad-Fly

(see FLIES; WARBLES). In Britain, warble flies are on the wing from late May onwards.

Gadding

Excitement, restlessness, uncontrolled rushing around in horses or cattle due to the presence of biting flies; also, in the case of cattle, warble flies.

Gag

A device to facilitate oral examination or treatment by holding the mouth open.

Gait, Abnormal

(see ATAXIA; 'GOOSE-STEPPING'; LAMENESS)

Gall-Bladder

The little pouch-like sac in which bile produced by the liver is stored until it is required during the process of digestion. It is a hollow, pear-shaped organ lying in a depression on the posterior surface of the liver. The gall-bladder is not present in the horse and in animals of the horse tribe, but is found in the other domesticated animals.

Blockages of the bile-duct by liver flukes or by gallstones may result in jaundice as well as severe local inflammation. Acute inflammation of the gall-bladder is painful, and there is danger of rupture or gangrene.

'Gall Sickness'

(see ANAPLASMOSIS)

Gallstones

Gallstones, which are also known as biliary calculi (see under CALCULI), are concretions which are formed in the gall-bladder or in the bile-ducts of the liver. As a rule they are hard, brownish in colour, coated with mucus, and of a more or less rounded shape. They may be composed of cholesterol; of cholesterol and bile pigments; or of pigment and lime salts. One or several may be present, causing pain and jaundice.

Gallstones are more prevalent in sheep than in cows, dogs, cats, and horses.

In human medicine, ursodeoxycholic acid has been used to dissolve gallstones.

Galvanised Bins

Galvanised bins, used to store swill, have led to ZINC POISONING in pigs.

Galvayne's Groove

A vertical groove in the front surface of the horse's upper corner incisor teeth. It first appears at the gum margin at about 10 years old and gradually moves down the surface of the tooth as the horse ages until it grows out at about 30 years old. (see DENTITION – Horses)

Game Birds, Mortality

This may be considered under 2 headings:

From farm chemicals Many farm chemicals can cause poisoning in game and other birds. Deaths have resulted from the use, as seed dressings, of compounds such as dieldrin, aldrin and heptachlor, now banned in the UK. Some of the organophosphorus insecticides; dimethoate; and the 'nitro-type' of weedkillers such as DNC, which stains the carcase yellow; are among other chemicals hazardous to birds.

Pheasant poults have died as a result of being treated for lice with a 5 per cent gamma benzene hexachloride (BHC) dusting powder.

An organophosphorus insecticide does not necessarily act quickly. Death may occur 8 weeks after eating the poisoned food. The symptoms shown by poisoned birds include ruffled feathers, saliva around the beak, high-stepping gait or unsteadiness on the legs, distressed breathing, and paralysis. However, as their use is now reduced, problems caused by organophosphorus compounds are less frequent.

Spraying an orchard with either DDD or DDT (now banned) has caused heavy game-bird losses. A partridge was found dead in a field where blackcurrants had been sprayed with the insecticide endrin. It was reported from the farm that 8 or 9 partridges died within a few hours of eating earthworms which came to the surface of the soil soon after spraying. Rat poisons may perhaps be included in the term 'farm chemicals'. Owls die after eating poisoned rodents.

From natural causes Impacted gizzard, tuberculosis, aspergillosis, swine erysipelas, fowl-pox, fowl cholera, fowl typhoid, infectious sinusitis. Gapes is another cause of death; also in the USA, encephalomyelitis. Deaths from fowl pest (Newcastle disease) have been reported in the UK; blackhead in pheasants and partridges.

'Grouse disease' is the colloquial name for infestation with *Trichostrongylus tenuis*. Mortality

occurs when food is in short supply as a result of poor growth or overpopulation of birds on a moor. In some circumstances, it has been concluded that grouse have died because not enough were shot the previous year. Grouse tend to remain in a locality and not move to other moors.

Louping ill, transmitted by sheep ticks, is generally fatal to red grouse (*Lagopus lagopus scoticus*), the commonest game bird on British heather moorland, and can reduce stocks to very low densities.

Inclusion-body hepatitis A 9-day outbreak resulted in an 18 per cent mortality among 1000 intensively reared pheasant poults (19 days old when the outbreak began).

Salmonellosis An outbreak killed 50 per cent of 2800 pheasant poults, deaths beginning in 3-day-olds. The infection was one of S. typhimurium. An antibiotic achieved control later.

Coccidiosis is an important disease of pheasants and other game birds, in chicks 2 to 4 weeks old. Milky-white droppings are the most obvious sign (but these are also seen with excess urate excretion due to kidney disease).

Yersiniosis is another important disease of pheasants.

Moniliasis causes lethargy, stunted growth and a heavy mortality in partridges. Treatment with formic acid, sprayed on food, has proved successful. (See also BOTULISM.)

Gametes
These are the ova and spermatozoa, and contain half the number (haploid) of chromosomes present in all other body cells (diploid).

Gametocide
Gametocide for bird control. (See TEM.)

Gametocyte
An oocyte or spermatocyte, the cells which produce an ovum or spermatozoon.

Gamma Globulin
Gamma globulin is a protein fraction of the blood serum which contains the antibodies against certain bacteria or viruses. (See COLOSTRUM; IMMUNOGLOBULINS.) It can be prepared in a concentrated form and can be used to give protection against infection.

Gamma Glutamyl Transferase (GGT)
An enzyme that tends to increase in liver disease. Higher than normal concentrations are found in liver-fluke infection of sheep and cattle.

Gammexane
Gammexane products contain the gamma isomer of benzene hexachloride, a highly effective, persistent insecticide. Not now used in treating farm animals. (See BENZENE HEXACHLORIDE; also BHC POISONING.)

Ganglion
Ganglion is a group of nerve cell bodies.

Ganglioside
A glycolipid found in central nervous system (CNS) tissue.

Gangliosidosis
An inherited disease causing poor growth and progressive neuromuscular dysfunction. It results from an accumulation of gangliosides in CNS tissue and may be seen in cattle, pigs, dogs and cats.

Gangrene
The presence of dead tissue in a live animal. In primary gangrene, bacteria which cause the necrosis also bring about the putrefactive changes. In secondary gangrene the putrefaction is caused by organisms which have invaded dead tissue (e.g. following a burn). There are 2 varieties of gangrene, dry and moist; dry gangrene is a condition of mummification in which the circulation stops and the part withers up, while in moist gangrene there is inflammation accompanied by putrefactive changes.

Infection following necrosis may lead to gangrene after burns, scalds, frostbite, crush wounds, puncture wounds, etc.

Poisoning by ergot results in the same condition in the most distant parts of the body, e.g. the feet, tip of tail, ears, and the combs and wattles of poultry.

Signs There is at first a degree of pain when the affected part is handled, and in a short time it becomes reddened and swollen. Later it turns blue or black, the hair falls from it, and there is a distinct line of demarcation between the gangrenous and the healthy surface. Around the dividing line there is usually some degree of inflammation, and pus production.

Moist gangrene is considerably more serious, since it is accompanied by putrefaction and the absorption of toxins. The whole area turns black or greenish, the hair falls out, an offensive smell is evident, and much fluid exudes from the decomposing tissues. A high temperature, disturbed heart's action, and rapid breathing, are shown. (See also GAS GANGRENE.)

Treatment is mainly surgical, backed up by the use of appropriate antibiotics or sulfonamides. In advanced cases, euthanasia becomes necessary. (See also FROST-BITE.)

Gangrenous Dermatitis

A disease of poultry caused by *Clostridium septicum*; often associated with infectious bursal disease and inclusion-body hepatitis, it usually affects birds between 25 and 100 days of age. Mortality can be very high.

Ganjam Ulrus

The Indian name for a bunyavirus infection transmitted by ticks.

Gapes

Gapes is a disease of young chickens, turkeys, pheasants and other game birds particularly, although all the domesticated and many wild birds may also be affected. It is caused by infection with the gapeworm, *Syngamus trachea.*

The presence of worms in the bronchial tubes and trachea of the bird causes it to gasp for breath or 'gape', from which the name of the disease originated. Part of the life-history of the worm is passed in the body of the earthworm, and young chickens eating earthworms may become affected. Earthworms can live for 16 years. (See also under CAPILLARIASIS.)

Nitroxynil, given in the drinking water, is an effective treatment.

Garden Chemicals

Birds, dogs, and cats may be poisoned as a result of the use of pesticides. For the poisoning of birds, see preparations listed under GAME BIRDS, MORTALITY. Dieldrin is highly toxic for cats, and like DDT, should not be used on them or in their vicinity. In fact, all the CHLORINATED HYDROCARBONS are best avoided in places where small domestic animals or their food may become contaminated.

For the dangers of slug-baits, see METALDEHYDE POISONING. (See ORCHARDS for the dangers of fruit-tree sprays. For seed dressings, see under SEED CORN. See also PARAQUAT; HERBICIDES.)

Garden Nightshade Poisoning

Garden nightshade poisoning results from animals eating *Solanum nigrum*, which is found

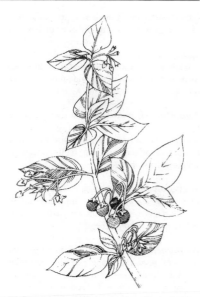

Garden nightshade (*Solanum nigrum*), also known as black nightshade, has small purple flowers, and large black shiny berries, several of which are attached to a single stalk. Height: 1.3 to 2 m (4 to 6 ft).

in many parts of the world. Its toxicity appears to vary in different localities. The berries contain an active alkaloidal glycoside called solanine, which is readily converted into sugar and the poisonous solanidine by the action of the gastric juices in the stomach.

Signs Staggering, loss of sensation and consciousness, and sometimes convulsions. First-aid: strong black tea or coffee.

Garron

A useful type of horse for hill-farm work and carrying deer. Garrons do not constitute a separate breed, but were a cross between Western Island ponies and the Percheron. Nowadays, the Garron is regarded as a larger version of the Highland pony.

Gas

(see AIR; BLOAT; CARBON MONOXIDE; OZONE; ANAESTHETICS; SLURRY; NITROGEN DIOXIDE.)

Gas Bubble Disease

A condition in which fish swim 'belly up' vertically; the cause is supersaturation of gases in the water in very intensive farming. It can be prevented by proper maintenance of pumps and normal (not pressurised) aeration of the water.

Gas Gangrene

Gas gangrene is an acute bacterial disease due to the inoculation of wounds with organisms belonging to the 'gas gangrene' group.

Gas gangrene may attack any of the domestic animals and man. The horse is least resistant and the cow least susceptible.

Causes Gas gangrene is produced by *Clostridium oedematiens, Cl. welchii, Cl. septicum* and *Cl. chauvei* gaining access to the tissues of an animal through a small wound; after castration or docking, or parturition, etc.

Signs A few hours after the organisms gain entrance, the area of invasion is found swollen, hot, painful on pressure, and may crackle when handled. This latter effect is due to gas formation below the skin. The skin and underlying tissues rapidly become discoloured.

In a series of 9 cases in horses, the signs were fever, depression, painful muscular swellings, and toxaemia. All were dehydrated. Colic had been evident in 6 of the horses; laminitis in 2. Infection had followed intra-muscular injections in 8 of the horses, and a puncture wound in 1. The *Clostridia* isolated were: *chauvei* (1); *septicum* (6); and *perfringens* (6).

Prevention Vaccination is effective (See also BRAXY; BLACKQUARTER; GANGRENE.)

Gastralgia

Pain in the stomach.

Gastrectasis

Dilatation of the stomach.

Gastrectomy

Gastrectomy is an operation for the removal of the whole or part of the stomach.

Gastric

Gastric means anything connected with the stomach, e.g. gastric ulcer, gastric juice.

Gastric Ulcers

These are seen in pigs in some cases (but not all) of SWINE FEVER. They have also been found in piglets under a fortnight old, due to *Rhizopus microsporus*, isolated from both stomachs and bedding. (See MUCORMYCOSIS.) Associated with this infection may be another fungal one – MONILIASIS – caused by the yeast-like organism *Candida albicans*.

Gastric ulcers may also be produced by the toxin of *Aspergillus flavus* (see AFLATOXIN), and by COPPER POISONING.

In mini-pigs, gastric ulcers are quite common when the diet lacks roughage.

For gastric ulcers in cattle, see under STOMACH, DISEASES OF.

In the USA, gastric ulcers have been an important cause of foal mortality.

Gastritis

Inflammation of the stomach.

Gastrocnemius

Gastrocnemius is the large muscle which lies behind the stifle-joint and the tibia and fibula, and ends in the Achilles tendon or 'hamstring' which is attached to the 'point of the hock'.

Gastrodiscus

Amphistome flukes, e.g. *G. aegyptiacus*, are common parasites of horses and pigs in the tropics and subtropics. A heavy infestation has caused collapse in the horse.

Gastroenteritis

Inflammation of the stomach and intestines, causing vomiting and diarrhoea. It is an acute condition commonest in young animals. It may be specific or due to irritant organic or inorganic poisons. (See also HAEMORRHAGIC, PARASITIC, and TRANSMISSIBLE GASTROENTERITIS; also DIARRHOEA.)

Gastropexy

A surgical operation in which the stomach is fixed, usually, to the abdominal wall to prevent a recurrence of torsion. In dogs it has been carried out after spot coagulation of the surface of the fundus by diathermy. The stomach is fixed in its normal position against the diaphragm by 7 to 10 rows of silk sutures (7 or 10 to a row).

The incision into the abdominal wall is closed by absorbable synthetic sutures.

This operation is also known as fundupexy.

Gastrotomy

An operation to open the stomach, usually to remove a foreign body.

Gavage

Feeding an animal by means of a stomach tube.

Gel

Gel is a colloid substance which is firm in consistency, although containing much water, e.g. ordinary gelatin.

Gelatin Sponge

Gelatin sponge is prepared as a haemostatic, and can be left in a wound; complete absorption taking place in 4 to 6 weeks. The sponge may be sterilised in dry heat, and applied either dry or moistened with normal saline, an antibiotic solution, or a solution of thrombin. Absorbable gelatin sponge complies with the requirements of the *British Pharmacopoeia.*

Gelatin, Succinylated

A modified, fluid, gelatin used as a plasma substitute to restore body fluid volume in cases of hypovolemic shock.

Gelbviehs

This German yellow breed of cattle, as it is also known, was evolved by crossing Swiss breeds with German breeds, and is dual-purpose, averaging nearly 3640 litres (800 gallons) of milk at 4 per cent butterfat. Fattening stock give a daily liveweight gain of 1.1 kg (2.5 lb) and are ready for the butcher at 405 days in Germany.

Gelding

A castrated horse. Occasionally a horse which has had both testicles completely removed shows stallion-like behaviour, when it is known as a 'false rig'. Such an animal may mount mares and achieve both erection and intromission. The chasing, or rounding up, of mares, and nipping them, may also occur. This behaviour is not hormonally induced or hormone dependent; it has been suggested that it is part of the normal social interaction between horses. 'False rigs' and cryptorchids may show similar behaviour.

Blood samples from 104 horses with either sexual and/or aggressive male behaviour, but which had no palpable or visible testes, were assayed for testosterone levels 30 to 100 minutes after an intravenous injection of human chorionic gonadotrophin. All but 8 horses were classified as either geldings (<40 pg/ml) or cryptorchids (τ100 pg/ml). Surgical investigation confirmed the diagnosis in 23 geldings and 47 cryptorchids; the remaining horses were not operated on. (See also CASTRATION – Immuno-castration, for treatment of an aggressive cryptorchid stallion.)

Generic Products

Those sold under their *Pharmacopoeia* names rather than brand names.

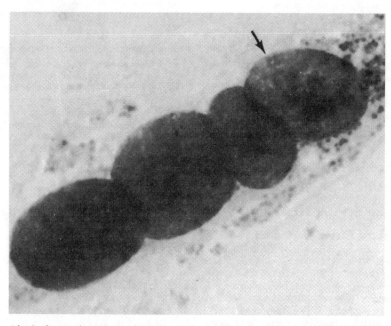

A bovine/hamster heterokaryon formed by the fusion of *Theileria parva*-infected bovine lymphoid cells and baby hamster kidney cells. The cell contains 3 hamster nuclei and 1 bovine nucleus (arrowed) with a prominent nucleolus. The intracytoplasmic masses are macroschizonts of *T. parva.* (× 1600). (With acknowledgements to the Institute for Research on Animal Diseases.) Monoclonal antibodies from mouse hybridomas have been produced for use in blood typing in cattle.

Genes

The biological units of heredity, arranged along the length of the CHROMOSOMES. (See also CELLS.)

Genetic Engineering

This may be defined as the recombination of genes from different organisms into 1 organism in a way that would never occur naturally; e.g. from a plant into an animal. However, in practice, the terminology also includes genetic manipulation, although some changes brought about by manipulation may also occur quite naturally.

Advances in knowledge of nucleic acids led to the creation in the laboratory of new combinations of genetic material. This was achieved by splicing together DNA from entirely different sources to form hybrid molecules that are less likely to occur during evolutionary processes.

Micro-organisms virulent for cattle (for example) will, if they can be adapted to grow in laboratory animals, become less virulent for

HYBRIDOMA TECHNIQUE FOR PRODUCING ANTIBODIES TO PARASITE ANTIGENS (DIAGRAMMATIC)

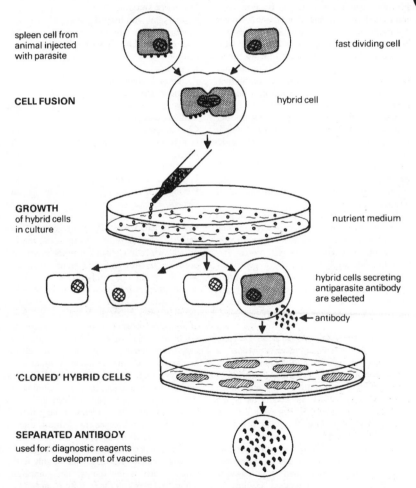

spleen cell from animal injected with parasite

fast dividing cell

CELL FUSION

hybrid cell

GROWTH of hybrid cells in culture

nutrient medium

hybrid cells secreting antiparasite antibody are selected

← antibody

'CLONED' HYBRID CELLS

SEPARATED ANTIBODY
used for: diagnostic reagents
           development of vaccines

Spleen cells from mice previously injected with parasite, and secreting antibody to the parasite, can be fused with other cells to form hybrid cells that live and multiply. From these a cell line is selected by 'cloning' (i.e. a colony that represents the progeny of a single cell is isolated) which secretes appropriate antiparasite antibody. (With acknowledgements to *WHO Chronicle*, **36.**)

the original host, and may have usefulness for later vaccine purposes. One method of adapting the micro-organisms to grow in laboratory animals is to fuse, artificially, cells to form a HETEROKARYON. (*See* illustration.)

Uses Genetic engineering has provided information on the molecular basis of gene action, on bacterial virulence and bacterial resistance. In agriculture it offers the hope of being able to transfer from bacteria to plants the genes which confer the ability to fix nitrogen – and so reduce farmers' dependence on scarce and costly nitrogen fertilisers.

In the UK, at the AFRC's Unit of Nitrogen Fixation, genes for nitrogen fixation were transferred with the aid of a PLASMID from a naturally occurring nitrogen-fixer *Klebsiella pneumoniae* to *E. coli*, which had never fixed nitrogen before. The plasmid, of the exchangeable class, was able, when transferring, to take along fragments of its host's chromosomes, including pieces bearing the nitrogen-fixation genes.

Some of the new nitrogen-fixing *E. coli* strains converted these fragments of *Klebsiella* chromosome into new, separate plasmids. Geneticists in the unit therefore constructed, by ordinary genetic manipulations, plasmids carrying nitrogen-fixation genes which would transfer themselves alone, without the aid of another plasmid.

In veterinary medicine the greatest potential lies in the preparation of completely safe viral vaccines. One of the first successes was with foot-and-mouth virus. The specific viral protein, free of infectivity, was produced by a genetically manipulated *E. coli*. This protein from a bacterial culture is capable of stimulating antibody production in animals. The technique is used also in the production of a number of other vaccines.

Recombinant DNA techniques Development of such techniques involved 3 lines of research: (1) recognition and isolation of extra-chromosomal DNA, or plasmids; (2) the manipulation of DNA with 'restriction' enzymes which selectively split DNA into fragments which could then be rejoined; (3) reinserting the fragmented DNA into living cells so that it became part of the genetic material of the cells.

In this way, genetic instructions for producing mammalian enzymes could be transferred into *E. coli*, the cell most used for propagating such plasmid vectors to produce insulin, for example.

The next step was to develop synthetic nucleotides, actually to construct genes. This

has been done successfully and nucleotides of up to 500 characters have been constructed.

Another technique in genetic engineering involves monoclonal antibodies. These are produced by fusing antibody-producing cells from an immunised donor with another type of white blood cell, thereby producing hybrid cells which in tissue culture could provide the desired antibodies. Among potential uses are, again, vaccines, but also diagnostic reagents; for blood-typing, in race-horses, for example.

Genetics, Heredity and Breeding

Introduction The science of genetics deals with the physiology of heredity – the mechanism by which resemblance between parent and offspring is conserved and transmitted; and with the origin and significance of variation – the mechanism by which such resemblance is modified and transformed. It seeks to define the manner in which the hereditary characters of the individual are represented in the fertilised egg in which the individual has its beginning.

Stock-breeding is a craft concerned with the maintenance of the desirable qualities of a stock, the improvement of these qualities generation by generation, and the elimination through breeding of qualities which are held to be undesirable. The problems of the geneticist and of the stock-breeder are identical, though their interests are dissimilar.

The geneticist has made much progress by studying, quickly maturing, very highly fertile animals such as the mouse, rat, guinea-pig, rabbit, and above all the fruit fly *Drosophila*.

A better understanding of heredity was rendered possible by the concept that the individual as a whole was not the unit in inheritance, but could be regarded as a definite orderly combination of independently heritable units.

Breed was now interpreted as signifying different combinations of independently heritable characters, all drawn from the common source of the stock in which modern domesticated cattle had their origin – just as different arrangements and combinations of letters make different words, though all words are made up of letters derived from a common source: the alphabet.

The breeder has employed the methods of hybridisation and inbreeding associated with selection in the creation of the modern breeds. He has practised inbreeding with selection in order that the desired type of his stock may be fixed, and he has sought hybrid vigour in outcrossing. The geneticist has employed these very same methods in his studies. The method of genetics is character-analysis. The object of the breeder is character-synthesis.

Instead of the hereditary mechanism being a simple affair as was first thought, it is one of the most complex.

Phenotype and genotype

Allan Fraser MD, DSc, when senior lecturer in animal husbandry at Aberdeen University, once drew a helpful analogy between heredity and a game of cards, with each card representing a gene, and Honours cards representing genes most desirable to a breeder.

A game of cards is preceded by the shuffling of packs, and so also is the conception of an animal preceded by a shuffling of genes. Each pack is then halved – just as before sperm and ovum meet, and the number of genes in both is halved by what is called the reduction division. Fertilisation then reunites the 2 half-packs to form 1 new pack. The cards in this represent the genes in the new individual animal.

'The cards in any one hand or the gene sample in any individual animal are the result of pure chance – no one can predict how the run of the cards or of the genes will go.'

Of 2 animals, sharing the same sire and dam, 1 may have a much better genotype, be a more valuable breeding animal than its full brother or sister.

If the cards dealt at conception be called the unalterable genotype of the animal, the playing of that hand may be called the environment, which includes climate, nutrition, exposure to infections, stocking rates, and every aspect of husbandry and animal management.

Some stockmen can make a surprisingly good job with poor genetic material; others a sorry job with the best stock; but of course the

most skilful stockman cannot improve upon the hand of genes once dealt.

Genotype can be defined as the entire array of genes carried by an individual (or, in another sense, the genetic constitution of an individual with respect to any limited number of genes under examination).

Phenotype is the appearance and/or the performance of an individual animal. Phenotypic variation of a population results from the combined effects of inheritance and environment. Genetic variation is that part of the phenotypic variation which is due to genes.

Homozygous and heterozygous

In order to illustrate one of the simpler aspects of heredity in relation to stock-breeding, the appearance of red calf in a herd in which the fashionable coat colour is black, and in which all red animals are eliminated, will serve as an example.

Black-and-red coat colours in cattle constitute a typical pair of Mendelian characters, black being the dominant and red being the recessive member of the pair. A red calf can only be produced by black parents when both of these are heterozygous in respect of their coat-colour character. For the character black-coat colour, there is a determiner or factor: this factor may be present in the zygote in the duplex state, having been conveyed thereinto by both egg and sperm. When the factor for black is present in the duplex state, the individual that arises for that fertilised egg or zygote is spoken of as being 'homozygous' for the character black-coat colour. On the other hand, into the zygote there may have been brought a factor for black from 1 parent and a factor for red, the alternative character, from the other parent. Under these circumstances, of these 2 factors (that for black and that for red) it is the former alone that determines what the coat colour shall be. Black is said to be dominant in its relation to red. Homozygous and heterozygous blacks will be indistinguishable on inspection. If 2 heterozygous blacks are mated there will occur on the average in every 4, 3 black calves to 1 red. To explain this 3:1 ratio it is assumed that half of both male and female gametes of such heterozygous individuals (i.e. sperm and ovum) carry the factor for the dominant character black, and the other half the factor for the alternative recessive red, and the 2 sorts of egg and of sperm occur in equal numbers. If it is assumed that for every pair of factors that correspond to a pair of characters, only 1 can pass into the ripe gamete, it follows that a 3:1 ratio in the next generation will be obtained, and of the individuals exhibiting the dominant character, 1 will be homozygous for that character and 2 heterozygous, whilst the individual exhibiting the recessive character must of necessity carry the factor for that character in the duplex state, since if in its hereditary constitution it carries a factor for the dominant, it will exhibit the dominant character. It is possible by examining the records of the coat colours of the offspring to define the hereditary constitution of the parent in respect of the coat colours black and red. The following matings are possible:

Homozygous black to homozygous black will give none but blacks, all homozygous.

Homozygous black to heterozygous black will give all blacks, of which 50 per cent will be homozygous and 50 per cent heterozygous.

Homozygous black to homozygous red will give all heterozygous blacks.

Heterozygous black to heterozygous black will give 25 per cent homozygous blacks, 50 per cent heterozygous blacks, and 25 per cent reds.

Heterozygous black to red will give 50 per cent heterozygous blacks and 50 per cent red.

Red to red will give all reds, of necessity homozygous. The only mating of blacks that can yield a red calf is that of two individuals heterozygous in respect of this coat-colour character.

The coat-colour character has to be considered quite apart from all the rest of the characters that in their association make the animal what it is. An individual is a pure black when it is in respect of this character homozygous, when in its hereditary constitution the determiner or factor for this character has been received from both its parents.

Inheritance through multiple genes

The above example shows how a character – coat colour – may be inherited through single genes. This is the mechanism of heredity at its simplest. Most characters, however, including

many of economic importance to the farmer, are inherited in a far more complex manner through multiple genes.

Multiple genes may have an additive effect as regards the expression of some character; or they may interact, one with another, in the production of a character, inheritance of which is even more complex.

Inheritance and high milk yields

It seems that it is easier to increase the butter-fat content and solids-not-fat content than it is to increase the milk yield through breeding. The heritability of milk yield is not as high as that of some other characters.

There is a correlation between high yields and body size, but conformation is by no means always associated with high yields. A few of the highest-yielding cows have had, to put it mildly, an unfashionable conformation.

The diagram below shows how 2 bulls, full brothers, may influence milk production in their daughters in opposite ways. It also shows how the 'gene lottery' can make nonsense out of the expectations of a breeder.

For this reason, progeny testing has proved of the greatest importance in the selection of bulls, each of which – through AI – may have not 100 offspring but tens of thousands.

It is possible for a farmer to use (by means of AI) a bull with the proved ability to produce daughters with a high milk yield, as compared with the yield resulting from use of an improved or average bull. Proven bulls are listed in terms of 'a bonus of 50 or of anything up to 100 gallons' and also in terms of a butterfat bonus. (See also PROGENY TESTING.)

Researchers have reported an association between blood groups and production characters in cattle and other animals. The work on transferrin and milk yield is an example; that of blood groups and milk yield another. However, the results were not sufficiently significant to be of practical value in selecting for productivity.

Selection

is the systematic choice of animals in a population (defined in the genetic sense as a group of interbreeding animals sharing a common gene pool, e.g. a closed herd, an AI district, a breed) as parents for the next generation.

Family selection means the selection of individuals on the performance of their relatives (sibs, half-sibs, or progeny), i.e. selection between families instead of between individuals.

Genotypic selection is that based on progeny testing with a very large number of progeny, so that the breeding value of the parent is exactly known.

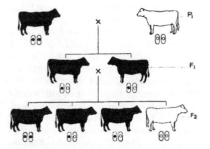

Black × Red. (Red is necessarily white in the diagram.)

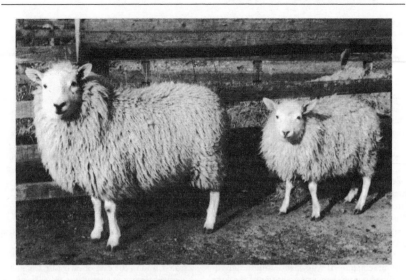

The effect of inbreeding and crossing. These 2 sheep were sired by the same ram, but the smaller one was highly inbred (59 per cent) and when 10 months old had attained little more than 40 per cent of the weight of its half-sib (left), which was a 3-way cross of inbred lines, its dam being a 2-way line cross. These hoggs are of Chevoit × Welsh extraction. (Animal Breeding Research Organisation photograph.)

Inbreeding may be defined as the mating of individuals more closely related than the average relationship of the population.

Both crossbreeding and inbreeding are methods of bringing about genetic change.

Inbreeding was practised by the early developers and improvers of livestock breeds in order to fix the type of their animals. Inbreeding can be expected to increase the proportion of animals homozygous for a given desired character. As the process proceeds, however, individuals with undesirable characters are likely to appear – animals which are abnormal in some respect, sterile, or weak. Inbreeding could prove disastrously expensive if the proportion of such animals were high. (Test mating of a bull to related or carrier females may be carried out in order to detect specific genes such as lethal factors; the carriers then being culled from the herd.)

Prolonged inbreeding will lead to disappointing regression, diminution of vigour, decreased fertility, and a reduction in body size.

The fusion of 2 inbred lines By inbreeding for a specific character, and by practising rigid selection for 2, 3, or more generations, a strain of relatively homozygous individuals for the selected character can be created. If 2 such strains are developed separately but simultaneously for 2 different but highly desirable characters, and if these 2 strains are then crossed, the resulting progeny can be expected to possess both desirable characters to a useful degree. The mechanism has been notably successful in producing strains of poultry with large egg size and high annual yields, and has been exploited commercially.

When the generation in which the 2 desirable characters are expressed is bred from again, an immediate reassortment of characters occurs, and only in a small percentage of the individuals will the desirable characters be expressed. The others are most likely to be useless.

Hybrid vigour (Heterosis), usually demonstrated by increase in size, better liveweight gains and greater resistance to disease and in the earlier attainment of sexual maturity, occurs in the first cross-bred generation out of the mating of 2 widely dissimilar pure-bred parental stocks. Hybrid vigour is an indication of heterozygosis. The 2 parental breeds must be within reason as dissimilar in their characterisation as possible; then in the pooling of those hereditary constitutions there will be a very considerable degree of heterozygosis in the 1st cross-bred offspring; the desirable characters are pooled, and in respect of those characters exhibited by the 2 parents the offspring will be heterozygous. Generally, a characteristic with poor heritability is enhanced more than one of high heritability.

If the 1st crosses which exhibit this hybrid vigour so markedly are interbred, their offspring will not exhibit this vigour to the same extent.

'Nicking' Two individuals not remarkable in themselves may produce superior offspring. This fact can be explained on the assumption that the mating brings together the chance association of factors which are complementary or supplementary, and that these in conjunction determine characters that are greatly esteemed.

'Pedigree and purity' Pedigrees and registration in the appropriate herd book have been an essential part of breeders' work in all but 'commercial' herds. The system has been of service, though not free from abuse. Pedigrees have from time to time been falsified or genuine mistakes made (including use of the wrong semen in AI work), and until the advent of blood typing there was no means of checking such errors.

It is easy to exaggerate the importance of 'family name' or of remote ancestors; and in terms of production traits or characters it has been stated that 'the concept of "purity" of pure breeds is not only something of a myth, but might actually be detrimental to the possibilities for improvement'.

Chromosomes A male can be distinguished from a female not only by external appearances and by differences in the architecture of the reproductive system, but also by differences in the organisation of the cells of which their bodies are composed.

The nucleus of the resting cell appears in stained microscopic preparations as a vesicle containing a network of delicate threads upon which are borne, like beads upon a tangled skein, minute masses of a deeply staining material known as chromatin. As the cell proceeds to divide into 2, this tangled mass of fine threads resolves itself into a constant number of filaments of definite shape and these become progressively shorter to assume the form of stout rods known as chromosomes. The number of chromosomes is usually some multiple of 2, and is constant and characteristic of the species to which the individual belongs, e.g. dog 78; horse 64; cow 60; sheep 54; pig 38; cat 38.

(The study of chromosomes is known as CYTOGENETICS.)

The gametes, egg and sperm respectively, differ remarkably in size and form, but they are alike in that each contains half the number of

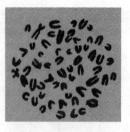

A bull's lymphocyte showing chromosomes in the 2nd stage (metaphase) of cell division (mitosis). (With acknowledgements to Dr C. R. E. Halnan and the *Veterinary Record*.)

chromosomes that is characteristic of the somatic cells of that species.

At fertilisation, the characteristic number is restored, and in the case of each pair 1 member is derived from one parent, the other from the other. In this distribution of the chromosomes one finds a mechanism by which offspring may inherit from both parents by means of the constituent genes.

It is possible to distinguish male from female by differences in the chromosome content. While all other pairs of chromosomes consist of 2 chromosomes exactly alike in size and shape, 1 pair differs in the 2 sexes. As they influence sex determination, these chromosomes are referred to as the sex chromosomes.

The ovum (or egg) contains the X chromosome.

The sperm may contain either the Y chromosome, which will produce male offspring (XY), or the X chromosome, which will produce female offspring (XX).

In most female mammals the paired sex-chromosomes are identical, and called the X chromosomes on account of their shape.

In the male, the sex-chromosomes are dissimilar, one being the X chromosome and the other the Y.

The autosomes are all the other chromosomes except the sex-chromosomes.

Genetic aspects of infertility These are briefly discussed in the following paragraphs. Chromosome screening (see CYTOGENETICS) and, to a lesser extent, blood-typing are likely to be of increasing value in eliminating a proportion of bovine infertility due to hereditary causes. (See also INFERTILITY.)

Inheritance of twinning It is mainly cows over 3 years old which have twins, and although twinning may be a desirable character for the farmer it is not one which is easy to obtain through breeding. It seems that there is a rather low level of genetic variation in frequency of twinning, and that prospects for rapidly increasing litter size in dairy cattle do not at present seem good. In some breeds of sheep, and perhaps also in cattle, it may not be the ovulation rate which is the limiting factor but, as indicated above, the survival rate of fertilised eggs.

Heritability of certain traits The following table, compiled at the Animal Breeding Research Organisation, shows the degree of heritability of certain traits sought by the pig breeder.

Trait	Heritability %
Litter size at weaning	7
Average weaning weight	8
Daily gain, after weaning	0
Food conversion	5
Average back fat	50
Percentage of lean meat	45

It will be seen that litter performance has a low heritability, and must be achieved by suitable crossbreeding. The crossbred sow has a marked superiority in this respect.

Lethal and semi-lethal factors Lethal factors have been defined as genes which, when present in the homozygous condition, cause the death of the embryo and when present in the heterozygous conditions cause a serious impairment in the individual often leading to non-survival.

Lethals may be dominant or incompletely dominant, but many are certainly recessive. They are not always recognised since they may cause death of the embryo early in development, and the mating may be regarded as having been infertile – another illustration of the difficulty of defining the genetics of infertility.

Several lethals are met with in cattle, such as parrot-mouthed, in which calves die at a few hours of age, or amputated, in which calves are born dead with legs and lower jaws absent.

Semi-lethals include over-shot jaws in calves.

Heredity and disease Diseases exhibit a spectrum according to the genetic influence. Canine haemophilia is entirely genetic. Swedish gonad hypoplasia is mainly genetic, mastitis is mainly environmental and injuries are entirely environmental. Simply dividing diseases into genetic and non-genetic is, therefore, inaccurate.

Recessive inheritance: many diseases are inherited as autosomal recessives. Neither parent is usually affected, but the disease comes from both; the sexes are affected equally, inbreeding is often being practised, the incidence is generally low and exact genetic ratios are obtainable. Few diseases, however, fulfil all the criteria of simple recessives.

Diseases due to sex-linked recessives, e.g. canine haemophilia, are uncommon in domestic mammals and, not being transmitted by unaffected males – the carrier female transmits the disease to half her male offspring – are unlikely to be a major problem. In poultry, however, sex-linked abnormalities such as familiar cerebellar degeneration are transmitted by the male to half his female progeny and are relatively common.

Diseases such as cryptorchidism and inter-sexes are sex-limited and sometimes regarded as due to recessives, the homozygote only expressing itself in 1 sex. While both parents are probably involved, their exact inheritance is unknown and cryptorchidism is certainly subject to environmental modification.

Irregular inheritance: many defects have a complex inheritance. Sporadic abnormalities, which increase on inbreeding, such as chicken 'crooked toes' or pig 'kinky tails', are called pheno-deviants, and are probably caused by recessives exhibiting a threshold of manifestation.

Dominant inheritance: the disease usually comes from 1 affected parent, and half its offspring are affected. Few dominant diseases are known in livestock, except in poultry. Irregular dominants, exemplified by 'curved limbs', where an unaffected male transmits a gene producing defective offspring out of unrelated females, and less than half are affected, do, however, occur. Environment or modifying genes may cause the defect inherent in the gene to develop.

Semi-dominant inheritance: several diseases are due to semi-dominants, the heterozygote being distinguishable from both homozygotes. A single dose of a semi-dominant gene produces a Dexter, a double dose a bulldog calf, and the homozygous normal allele produces a long-legged Dexter. Some American dwarf cattle result from semi-dominants (with acknowledgements to Dr G. B. Young, Animal Breeding Research Organisation).

Genetic defects All breeds of livestock may harbour some genetic defects, but their incidence is usually low. However, specific defects sometimes become more frequent in certain breeds, and give cause for concern.

Cattle Examples of genetic defects include the following:

Arthrogryposis in Charolais cattle. This defect is characterised by twisted limbs, cleft palate, and twisted spine. In France about 1 per cent of Charolais cattle are affected. AI records show that while many bulls transmit an occasional defect of this nature, a few sire about 5 per cent of offspring having this abnormality. Another defect encountered in some Charolais cattle involves the eyes. (See EYE, DISEASES OF – Coloboma.)

Decapitated sperms. This defect causes the rejection for AI in Britain of many Hereford bulls 'with superior test performance' because their semen contains a high percentage of sperms with the head separated from the tail.

Tibial hemimelia. A dog-sitting position in the newborn Galloway calf is suggestive of this defect, which involves bones missing from the hind legs (but has to be differentiated from another defect involving the pelvis, which also prevents the calf from standing on its hind legs). It is estimated that about 16 per cent of Galloways now carry the gene which transmits this defect. (The Galloway Breed Society has an excellent scheme, requiring compulsory insurance and compulsory slaughter of any bulls leaving offspring with this defect.) (See also MANNOSIDOSIS.)

Sheep Genetic defects include achondroplasia in some South Country Cheviot flocks. A 'squashed-in' face, shortened forelimbs and defective hooves are characteristic of these 'dwarf lambs'.

Cerebellar ataxia is seen in some Border Leicester flocks, and these 'daft lambs' have a staggering gait and incoordination of the head. This is due to a recessive gene.

Genital Organs
(see diagrams for PENIS and UTERUS)

Genome
A complete set of chromosomes derived from 1 parent; or the total gene complement of a set of chromosomes.

Genotype
This can mean the entire array of genes carried by an individual; or the genetic constitution of an individual with respect to any limited number of genes under examination; or (more loosely) the individual within a given genotype. (See also under GENUS.)

Genotypic Selection
Genotypic selection is that based on progeny-testing with a very large number of progeny so that the breeding value of the parent is exactly known. The expression is also loosely used as a synonym for progeny testing without this proviso.

Gentian
The dried and powdered root of the yellow gentian plant (*Gentiana lutea*). It is a bitter tonic used as an appetiser.

Gentian Violet
A stain used in microscopical work and a valuable antiseptic, of use against fungal and bacterial skin infections. (See also ANTISEPTICS – Crystal violet.)

Genus
Genus is a group of species. One of the species is chosen as being typical, and referred to as the genotype.

Gerbil
A small burrowing rodent, originating in deserts, popular as pets.They live for 3 to 5 years; adults weigh 50 to 90 g, the females being larger than males. Sexual maturity occurs at 10 weeks. The gestation period is 24 to 26 days and the young are weaned at 21 to 24 days. Rectal temperatue is 37.4 to 39°C. They are naturally healthy animals, remarkably free from infectious diseases: Tyzzer's disease is usually the only finding. In the wild they 'play dead' when attacked; this is a self-induced epileptic seizure and may occur when they are handled. (See also PETS.)

Geriatrics
The study of the problems and diseases of the older animal.

German Shepherd Dog
Previously known as the Alsatian, this is a medium to large-sized dog with a tan and black coat. The breed is extremely popular and, to fulfil demand, many unsuitable animals were used for breeding. In consequence a number of inherited defects are associated with the breed. These include achalasia, calcinosis circumscripta, cleft palate and epilepsy. A campaign to eliminate hip dysplasia, which is very common, requires all potential breeding dogs to be X-rayed for evidence of the defect. Dogs in which it is found are not used for breeding.

Germ Cells
The gametes, i.e. ovum or sperm.

Gestation
(see PREGNANCY)

Getah Virus

A mild infectious disease of racehorses, characterised by fever, dermatitis, and oedema of the limbs, appeared in Japan in 1978, and was found to be due to Getah virus. Antibodies to it had previously been detected in man, horses, pigs, and birds; none showed symptoms.

Giant Cells

Seen in various infections, e.g. the poxes, tuberculosis and Johne's disease, these multinucleate cells are formed by cell fusion, stimulated by viruses. Giant cells can be obtained *in vitro* in cell cultures, as well as being found in the body.

Giant Hogweed (Heracleum Mantegazzianum)

This plant grows to a height of up to 3.65 metres (12 feet), and has white flowers. The stem is hollow, and has reddish/purple blotches. Human contact with the plant, and subsequent exposure to sunlight, leads to dermatitis; the poisoning is a result of LIGHT SENSITISATION. A suspected case of this was seen in a goat, which was subdued, refusing food or water, and salivating profusely. Severe ulceration was found in its mouth. Two sheep were sensitive to the cut stems of the plant and developed mouth ulcers.

In another case, circumstantial evidence suggested involvement of this plant in week-old ducklings which had foot and beak lesions. Two ducklings with white beaks could manage only 'open-beak' breathing; whereas the beaks which were pigmented, in the other five ducklings, were not affected. The foot lesions consisted of large blisters.

Giardia

A genus of flagellate protozoa.

Giardiasis

In dogs a low-grade infection with *Giardia canis* may interfere with the absorption of fat and vitamin A; while if large numbers of *G. canis* are present there is likely to be chronic diarrhoea (sometimes dysentery), with resulting dehydration.

The flagellate parasite occurs in 2 forms: the trophozoite, which divides by binary fission, and is seldom seen in the faeces; and the cyst form which is found in the faeces but is not easy to identify.

Metronizadole is used in treatment.

In the USA *G. lamblia* is a common cause of human gastroenteritis. The infection is usually via drinking-water.

Gid (Sturdy)

Gid (sturdy) is a condition in sheep, and occasionally in cattle, caused by tapeworm cysts lodged in the brain. The sheep become infected through swallowing unhatched eggs of the dog tapeworm *Taenia multiceps*. The eggs are passed out in the dog's faeces. As the cysts (coenuri) develop, they press upon brain cells and give rise to nervous signs, such as staggering, circling, blindness. The name 'sturdy' derives from the 'sturdy' manner in which an affected sheep may struggle when caught. (See COENURIASIS.)

Gilchrist's Disease

Infection in man with *Blastomyces dermatitidis*. (See BLASTOMYCOSIS.)

Gills

The external breeding apparatus of fish and some other water dwelling creatures. They are delicate structures, prone to damage, infection and parasites. Chemical pollutants in the water cause fusion of the lamellae of the gills, reducing the absorptive surface.

Gill Maggot

(see SALMINCOLA)

Gilt

A female pig intended for breeding purposes before she has her 1st litter.

Gimmer

A ewe lamb up to its 1st shearing, or ewe which has not yet produced offspring (see under SHEEP).

Gingivitis

Inflammation of the gums. (See MOUTH, DISEASES OF; also FELINE GINGIVITIS.)

Gizzard (Ventriculus)

The thick-walled, muscular stomach in a bird; it has a tough keratin lining. The gizzard's main function is to grind food, and in this it is assisted by swallowed grit and small stones. (See under GRIT.)

Glanders

Glanders is a NOTIFIABLE DISEASE throughout the European Union. It is a specific, contagious disease of the horse family (Equidae), but also liable to be contracted by other mammals, including man. It is characterised by the formation of nodules in the lungs, liver, spleen, or other organs; ulcerations occur of the mucous membranes, especially those of the upper air passages, accompanied by changes in the lymphatics and also by skin lesions. The condition is due to the entrance and growth in the body of the glanders bacillus *Pseudomonas mallei* (formerly known as *Pfeifferella mallei*).

History Glanders has been known as a serious disease since about 450 BC, when it was mentioned by Hippocrates, and its contagious nature was pointed out by Vegetius (a veterinary writer) in the 4th century.

Distribution Glanders has been distributed to practically every country in the world at some time or other, and was once a usual concomitant of wars. It became prevalent, both in the United Kingdom and in South Africa, after the South African war (1899–1902). In the year 1892 there were more than 3000 cases of glanders recorded in Britain; in 1904 between 2000 and 3000; while only 9 outbreaks were recorded in the year 1923, and none since 1926.

Glanders is still endemic in Mongolia, other parts of Asia, East Africa and South America and, recently, it has been spreading from enzootic zones.

The donkey is the most susceptible to the disease and nearly always suffers from the acute form, from which it dies in from 2 to 3 weeks.

In the horse, glanders occurs in an acute or a chronic form, the latter existing for months or even years before it finally kills its victim; however, under modern conditions it is rare to allow the disease to run its natural course. The mule is intermediate in susceptibility between the donkey and the horse, but usually shows the acute type. Dogs and cats may become infected if fed upon meat from a horse which had glanders. The camel is susceptible, though natural cases are very rare.

Horses can be infected naturally by 3 different channels:

1. By the digestive tract, through the medium of infected food and water. This is by far the commonest method of spread.

2. By inhalation (rarely) when some abrasion of the respiratory passage is present.

3. By skin infection.

Incubation period This may last several months in the horse.

Signs The signs of glanders in the horse are very varied. The disease may run an acute course of only 2 to 3 weeks, but by far the greatest number of cases met with are of a subacute or chronic nature. A horse may be affected and show no outward sign of disease, and yet it may have nodules in 1 or both lungs.

Glanders may be of the nasal, pulmonary, or glandular form, of the type producing skin lesions (farcy), or an admixture of these, and it may also become generalised. One of the dangers of the disease is that a horse may work for weeks or even months with 'open' lesions – not losing a great deal of flesh nor appearing very ill – and so spread the disease to healthy horses with which it comes into contact.

When farcy is present the glands inside the axilla or inside the groin may be somewhat enlarged and even painful to the touch. In entire horses the testicles often become enlarged and painful, or even the seat of glanderous abscesses.

There may be a nasal discharge, thin and watery in the early stages, but later becoming thick, greyish, or yellow and oily. Examination of the nose in these cases is dangerous; strict hygenic precautions should be taken, as man may easily contract the disease by this means.

Farcy: in this form of the disease, the skin is involved. It is usually chronic in nature, but farcy buds and subcutaneous swellings may complicate the most acute form of the disease shortly before death. This complication is especially common in the mule, which often succumbs to the disease before the farcy buds have time to burst. In chronic farcy there is usually swelling of one or more limbs, more frequently a hind one. The lymphatic glands of the affected limb become enlarged, the lymph vessels corded, and usually a chain of farcy buds develops along their course.

In acute glanders there may be all the signs of an acute broncho-pneumonia, a high temperature, a rapid loss of flesh, rapid and sometimes noisy breathing, followed by death in a few weeks; in fact, this is the common form seen in the donkey and often in the mule, with or without the complication of farcy.

Diagnosis This is confirmed by means of the mallein test.

Treatment Sulfathiazole has been used, but in most western countries treatment is not permitted; the policy being one of slaughter and eradication.

Glanders in man is a distressing and nearly always fatal disease, and may be contracted by grooms and others working with infected horses. Laboratory workers handling infected material or pure cultures of the organism are especially liable to infection, so that every precaution against this contingency has to be taken; in fact, the glanders bacillus is amongst the most dangerous of all disease-producing bacteria cultivated.

The causal organism is present in all the lesions, though it does not – except the rare cases – circulate in the blood-stream.

Glands

A term loosely applied to a number of different organs. In each there are epithelial cells which have a secretory function (e.g. tear production). Glands are often classified as either *endocrine*, which are ductless, or *exocrine*, which usually have ducts to carry their secretion to an epithelial surface. (See ENDOCRINE GLANDS, HORMONES.)

A description of the various glands will be found under headings such as THYROID, LIVER, MAMMARY GLANDS, OVARIES, PANCREAS, SALIVARY GLANDS, TESTIS. Sweat and sebaceous glands are referred to under SKIN.

Lymphatic glands are nowadays more often referred to as *lymph nodes*.

Glass Embolism

Fluids for injection may contain glass particles. Glass gets in not during manufacture of the vial, but when the neck of the viual is snapped off to insert the hypoermic needle . In human medicine the risk of glass embolism has been stressed, and it has been suggested that, as a wise precaution, time should be allowed for glass particles to settle before filling the syringe.

Glass, Soluble

Soluble glasses containing cobalt, copper and selenium have been used in BOLUSES.

Glasser's Disease

An infection which causes swelling of the hock or knee joints, or both, in the pig. There is fever, lameness and a disinclination to move; it can also cause pericarditis, pleurisy and peritonitis. Death is usually a sequel, unless early treatment with, e.g., penicillin is undertaken. Glasser's disease is differentiated from joint-ill. Pigs of 5 to 14 weeks old are chiefly affected. The cause is *Haemophilus parasuis*, or a mycoplasma, or both.

Glauber's Salts

Glauber's salts is the popular name for sodium sulphate, a saline purgative.

Glaucoma

An increase in the pressure within the eye (intraocular pressure). (See under EYE, DISEASES OF.)

Glenoid Cavity

Glenoid cavity is the shallow socket on the shoulder-blade into which the humerus fits, forming the shoulder joint.

Glioma

Glioma is a tumour which forms in the brain or spinal cord. It is composed of neuroglia, which is the special connective tissue found supporting the nerve cells and the nerve fibres. (See TUMOURS.)

Gliosis

A proliferation of ASTROCYTES. It may follow a brain injury.

Globidiosis

A disease characterised by enteritis and closely resembling coccidiosis. It occurs in Africa, SW Europe, the USA, and Australia. The cause is a species of *Globidium*. Cysts may be formed in the skin or underlying tissue. Horses, cattle, and sheep are affected; in horses, severe diarrhoea may be caused. Fatal cases of *Globidium (Eimeria) leuckarti* have occasionally been recorded in horses in the UK and Ireland.

Globulin

Globulin is a protein fraction of the blood plasma, associated with immunity. (See also GAMMA GLOBULIN.)

Glomerulonephritis

Also called glomerula disease. (See KIDNEYS, DISEASES OF.)

Glomerulus

Glomerulus is a small knot of blood vessels, and from which the excretion of fluid out of the blood into the tubules of the kidney takes place. (See KIDNEY.) Glomerulonephritis is referred to under KIDNEYS, DISEASES OF.

Glossectomy, Partial

A surgical operation to remove part of the tongue. It has been found necessary in a horse following severe laceration by a sharp bit.

Glossitis

Inflammation of the tongue.

Glossopharyngeal Nerve

This is the 9th cranial nerve, which in the main is sensory. It is the nerve of taste for the back of the tongue, of sensation in a general way for the upper part of the throat, as well as for the middle ear, and it supplies the parotid gland.

Glottis

Glottis is the narrow opening at the upper end of the larynx. (See AIR PASSAGES; CHOKING; LARYNX.)

Gloves, Surgical

Sterile gloves of fine rubber or polyethylene worn during surgical procedures. A sleeve-length glove is worn by veterinary surgeons for carrying out e.g. rectal examinations in cattle.

Surgical glove powder (sterilised maize starch) can cause an iatrogenic starch peritonitis. In a comparative study of various methods of washing, brushing and rinsing, a routine involving a 1-minute povidine-iodine surgical scrub followed by a rinse under sterile running water (500 ml) for 30 seconds removed 99.8 to 100 per cent of the original starch grain count; this routine also provided the surgeon with a reassuring autotactile stick signal (separation of opposing forefinger and thumb as total removal of starch is about to be achieved). Glove stickiness disappears when tissue fluid of patient coats gloves. Rinsing gloves in water alone leaves about 10 per cent of the original starch on the gloves. Hypersensitivity to latex has been recorded in people who have used such gloves frequently.

Glucagon

This is a polypeptide hormone secreted by alpha-cells in the islets of Langerhans of the pancreas, and increases the amount of glucose in the blood.

Glucocorticoids

Hormones, from the cortex of the adrenal gland, concerned with the formation of glucose. Cortisol (hydrocortisone) is one of the most important of these. Excessive secretion of glucocorticoids is a feature of Cushing's disease.

Glucose

Glucose is the form of sugar found in honey, grapes, fruits, etc., and in diabetes mellitus it is passed in the urine. It is the form in which sugar circulates in the bloodstream, and is very useful as an injection or drench when there is a deficiency of circulating sugar in the blood or an excess of ketones. (See ACETONAEMIA.) Glucose is a most valuable food to give during the course of acute illnesses, since it puts no strain upon the digestive system yet provides fuel for the muscles, etc. Glucose saline is given as a drink or administered *per rectum* or by subcutaneous injection during the course of jaundice, gastroenteritis, etc. (See SUGARS.)

Glucosinolates

...es found in *Brassica* spp that are bro-
...in the rumen to form thiocyanates,
...nterfere with iodine absorption. If
...ten to excess during pregnancy,
... in the offspring.

Glucosurea

The presence of glucose in the urine. It is seen in diabetes mellitus (see DIABETES), and in some other conditions, and in all animals after severe shock. (See also under URINE – Abnormal constituents of.)

Glutamine

An amino acid important in brain and muscle metabolism. High levels of exercise, as in racing or endurance riding, can seriously deplete levels of glutamine in the muscle. If extreme, anabolism (growth and repair of muscle) is prevented and muscular exhaustion occurs.

Glutaraldehyde

A disinfectant. Used in dilute solution in preparations for cleaning udders.

Gluteal

Gluteal is the scientific name applied to the region of the buttocks, and to associated structures, such as gluteal arteries, muscles, nerves.

Glycerides

Organic esters of glycerin. (See FAT.)

Glycerin (Glycerol)

Glycerin (glycerol) is a clear, colourless, odourless, thick liquid of a sweet taste, obtained by decomposition and distillation of fats. It dissolves many substances and has a great power of absorbing water.

Uses Given by the mouth, diluted, it has been used with success in the treatment of pregnancy toxaemia in ewes and of acetonaemia in cattle. Internally, glycerin acts as a laxative to the dog in moderate doses. It is soothing and antiseptic to inflamed mucous membranes in the mouth and throat. In amounts of 15 to 30 ml (½ to 1 ounce) it is useful as a rectal injection to induce passage of impacted faeces in obstinate constipation in the dog, and it may be used for the same purpose in foals and calves. For these purposes it may be given diluted with a little water, or it may be used in the pure state. It is also used as a basis for the compounding of various electuaries for the horse and dog, and it is sometimes incorporated into cough mixtures for the smaller animals. It is used in certain skin dressings when it is desired to soften the skin surface and encourage the absorption of other drugs. It is also used as a diluent for semen. (See under ARTIFICIAL INSEMINATION.)

Glycogen

Glycogen is an animal starch found particularly in the liver as well as in other tissues. It is the form in which carbohydrates taken in the food are stored in the liver and muscles before they are converted into glucose when needed. Glycogen can become depleted when animals are stressed, as by travelling over long periods. If not replaced, animals slaughtered after a long journey may have dry, firm, dark (DFD) meat.

Glycol, Ethylene
(see under ANTIFREEZE for poisoning in dogs and cats)

Glycol, Propylene
(see PROPYLENE GLYCOL)

Glycosides
Glycosides are potent naturally occurring substances, combining a sugar with a hydroxy compound. Many are found in plants and are of great value in medicine. The cardiac glycoside digitalis, found in the foxglove (*Digitalis purpurea*), is a prime example. Cyanogenetic glycosides are found in linseed and *saponins* in 'lords and ladies' (*Aurum maculatum*).

Aminoglycosides are powerful antibacterials; streptomycin was the first widely used aminoglycoside antibiotic.

Glycosuria
(see GLUCOSUREA)

Gnathostoma Spinigerum
A roundworm infecting dogs, cats, wild carnivores, and man. It forms a nodule about 1.5 cm (½ inch) in diameter in the gastric mucosa. In a cat suspected of having rabies it caused anorexia, nausea, and convulsions, coma and death.

Gnotobiotics
Gnotobiotics is the name given to germ-free laboratory animals reared according to techniques developed by Professor J. A. Reyniers of Notre Dame University, Indiana. Such animals have been used in the investigation of certain diseases. (See also SPF; 'DISEASE-FREE' ANIMALS.)

Goads, Electric
Batons with electrodes at one end which give a mild electric shock when they touch an animal. They are preferable to the use of carelessly or sadistically wielded sticks. The points should be blunt and spring-loaded, as otherwise they can be jabbed into the animal – when the purpose and object of an electric goad are defeated.

It is illegal to use electric goads on calves and piglets. They may only be applied to the hindquarters of cattle over 6 months of age, and

to adult pigs. There must be a way clear for the animals to move forward. The Welfare of Animals (Slaughter or Killing) Regulations 1995 state that electric goads should be applied for no more than 2 seconds at a time and that there should be adequate time between applications.

Goat Warble Fly (Przhevalskiana Silenus)
Goat warble fly (Przhevalskiana Silenus) parasitises goats and horses in many European and eastern countries. *Hypoderma aeratum* and *H. crossi* are other species.

Goatling
A female goat between 1 and 2 years old.

Goats as Grazers with Sheep
(see PASTURE MANAGEMENT)

Goats, Disbudding of Kids
This is carried out under general anaesthesia (see ANAESTHESIA, GENERAL; GOATS); and the iron used for disbudding is heated by gas (or electricity) to a 'cherry-red' heat. Great care is needed in this operation as the skull is very thin in the area concerned.

Goats, Diseases of
(see under ACETONAEMIA; AGALACTIA; BRUCELLOSIS; CAPRINE ARTHRITIS-ENCEPHALITIS; CONTAGIOUS CAPRINE PLEURO-PNEUMONIA; CASEOUS LYMPHADENITIS; CHLAMYDIA (for abortion); 'CLOUDBURST'; COCCIDIOSIS; CRYPTOSPORIDIOSIS; CYSTICERCOSIS; ENTEROTOXAEMIA; JOHNE'S DISEASE; MASTITIS; ORF; PARASITIC BRONCHITIS; PARASITIC GASTROENTERITIS; PREGNANCY TOXAEMIA; Q FEVER; RICKETS; RINDERPEST; SALMONELLOSIS; SWAYBACK; TUBERCULOSIS; YERSINIOSIS; LOUPING ILL; SCRAPIE; OSTEODYSTROPHIA FIBROSA; MANNOSIDOSIS; LISTERIOSIS; MYCOPLASMOSIS; RINDERPEST; LIVER FLUKES; GOITRE; PULPY KIDNEY DISEASE)

Goats' Milk, Cheese
Goat's milk is often substituted for cow's milk for children suffering from a suspected allergy to cow's milk. However, unless the milk is pasteurised, there is a risk of human illness arising; especially from infection with *Brucella melitensis*, but also from *Yersinia pseudotuberculosis* – one cause of mastitis in goats. Goat's milk may contain louping-ill virus, *staphylococci*, *E. coli*; and, since goats are not immune to tuberculosis, even tubercle bacilli. Goat's milk cheese is also a source of *B. melitensis* infection.

Goitre

Goitre is an enlargement of the thyroid gland, associated with an iodine deficiency; rarely, it can be the result of a persistently high intake of iodine by the dam affecting the fetal thyroid. It is seen in puppies, foals, and lambs, and also in calves, and it appears to be commoner in some districts than in others. Swellings may appear below the larynx, usually one on either side, and beyond the local enlargements there may be no definite symptoms shown. Some cases respond to the administration of thyroid extracts, and iodine internally, while some clear up spontaneously without treatment. (See IODINE; CALCIUM SUPPLEMENTS; THYROID GLAND.)

Lethargy is a notable symptom of goitre in the dog, in which the disease often occurs in the 3 to 5 year age group, especially in the bigger breeds.

Some pastures and foodstuffs may give rise to goitre. (See GOITROGEN.) Goitre seems particularly common in Dorset horn sheep.

A number of cases of supposed 'goitre' prove upon careful examination to be tumour growth in some part of the throat, not necessarily in connection with the thyroid gland – though cancer of the thyroid is not uncommon in the dog.

Goitre also occurs when, instead of a deficiency of thyroxin, there is a state of hyperthyroidism, or too much thyroxin. (See THYROID GLAND, DISEASES OF.)

In goat kids, some supposed cases of goitre prove to be hyperplasia of the THYMUS gland.

In other animals 'goitre' may be a misdiagnosis for neoplasms in the throat region.

Goitrogen (Goitrogenic Factor)

Goitrogen (goitrogenic factor) is one which gives rise to goitre. Both kale and cabbage contain goitrogens (glucosinolates) and must therefore not constitute too large a proportion of an animal's ration over a period. The same applies to turnips. Iodine licks may be advisable. (See IODINE DEFICIENCY.)

Golden Retriever

Popular dog of medium or larger size with a flat, wavy coat, blonde or gold in colour. Cataract, progressive retinal atrophy and entropion are inheritable. Retrievers may also be susceptible to hip dysplasia and myopathy.

Goldfish (Carassus Auratus)

Ornamental fish of the carp family, originally domesticated by the Chinese in the Sung dynasty (960–1279). More than 120 breeds are recognised, as well as the common goldfish. They vary in colour and markings, and in conformation of the fin, tail and head. Their lifespan can range from 2 years to 25 years. Size may vary from 5 cm (2 inches) to 30 cm (12 inches) or more. If the diet is too rich in oil, deficiency of vitamin E may result. This can cause anaemia, poor growth, muscular dystrophy, exophthalmia and other conditons.

Gonad

Gonad is a sex gland which produces a gamete (the ovary or testis).

Gonadotrophic

Gonadotrophic indicates something which stimulates the gonads – testes and ovaries. (See GONADOTROPHINS; HORMONES.)

Gonadotrophins

Gonadotrophins are hormones which have a gonadotrophic effect in the body. (See HORMONES.)

Chorionic gonadotrophin effects luteinisation and is used in the treatment of functional uterine haemorrhage, cases of habitual abortion, and to induce descent of the testes in cases of cryptorchidism.

Serum gonadotrophin contains a follicle-stimulating hormone which affects the gonads of both sexes. It is used in the treatment of sterility, anoestrus, and hypoplasia of the gonads.

Goose Influenza

A disease of goslings (and ducklings) caused by *Pasteurella anatipestifer*. Signs include discharge from the nose and eye, and air sacculitis. The liver, heart and central nrevous system may also be affected.

'Goose-Stepping'

In the pig this can be a symptom of a deficiency of pantothenic acid, one of the B group of vitamins. In cattle it may be a symptom of familial ataxia. (See GENETICS – Defects.)

Gossypol

Gossypol is a toxic substance present in cottonseed. Cake or meal made from cottonseed is poisonous unless gossypol is removed efficiently before manufacture.

Gossypol poisoning gives rise to loss of appetite, gastroenteritis, ascites, pulmonary oedema, convulsions and death. These problems are probably due to lack of vitamin A in animals fed gossypol.

Contraceptive effect Already in the 1950s it was known that gossypol could impair spermatogenesis, but not ovulation, in rats.

In the 1980s research workers in China, in a search for possible male human contraceptives, included gossypol in their list, and sought to enhance the depressive effect on spermatogenesis while at the same time reducing gossypol's toxicity. The World Health Organisation was encouraging this research, which led to a highly purified acetic acid preparation of gossypol being offered to scientists in other countries.

Previously, gossypol had been considered as a contraceptive for possible use in dogs and cats.

Gout

Gout, the metabolic disorder hyperuricaemia, of man, is associated with an excess of urates in blood and tissue fluids which in some, but by no means all, cases leads to the deposition of crystals of sodium urate in joints. Subsequently an acute gouty arthritis may follow. A genetic factor, associated with an enzyme deficiency, may be involved. Gout has to be distinguished from lead poisoning.

In most animals (except primates), uricase converts urates into allantoin, which is highly soluble and is excreted in the urine. It is therefore extremely rare to find articular gout in domestic mammals, though some breeds of dog can be affected. In Dalmations the cause is different, being a defect in liver metabolism. Visceral gout in birds and reptiles is usually due to renal failure. (See also 'VISCERAL GOUT' in poultry.)

Calcium gout (*Calcinosis circumscripta.*) This has been recorded in dogs and monkeys as well as in man, and involves the deposition of calcium salts and the appearance of fibrous tissue around the deposits. Firm, painless nodules occur under the skin of the limbs and feet and at the elbow, and may ulcerate. Diagnosis may be assisted by radiography. Calcium gout occurs mainly in large breeds of dog, e.g. Alsatians.

An outbreak occurred in 32 piglets of 17 herds in Switzerland at the age of several days to 4 weeks. Signs were cough and dyspnoea in all cases; some showed weight loss and hunched backs. The respiratory and circulatory system evinced severe changes, with calcinosis in elastic fibres of lungs, atrial walls, and arterioles. Older piglets also showed inflammatory changes. Milder changes were seen in stomach, kidneys, and muscles.

Graafian Follicle

The mature ovarian follicle. (See OVARIES.)

Grafts

(see SKIN GRAFTING; IMMUNITY; H-Y ANTIGEN; MAJOR HISTOCOMPATIBILITY SYSTEM)

Grains, Brewers'

Brewers' grains are a by-product of brewing, consisting of the exhausted malt, and are used wet in some cases, where they can be easily obtained from a nearby brewery, or as dried grains. They are useful as a feeding-stuff for cattle, pigs, and sheep, providing protein as well as carbohydrate, but must be introduced gradually into the ration. Wet grains must be used fresh as they deteriorate on keeping. Dried grains keep well, and are suitable for horses, about 2.25 to 4.5 kg (5 to 10 lb) daily, and sheep, up to 225 g (5 lb).

Grains, Distillers'

Distillers' grains are produced as a by-product during the manufacture of whisky in a manner somewhat similar to brewers' grains in the manufacture of beer. They are sold either wet or dry, but are much to be preferred dry, since the wet grains are liable to contain considerable amounts of raw alcohol, which may lead to intoxication of animals eating them. The amounts and uses are similar to those of brewers' grains.

Gram-Negative

Gram-negative bacteria are those which do not retain the violet of Gram's stain (haematoxylin, eosin, and aniline methylene violet). Bacteria which do retain the violet are called Gram-positive. This staining differentiation provides an important means of classifying bacteria into 2 groups. (Nuclei are stained blue, cytoplasm red, and Gram-positive bacteria purple by this staining method, devised by a Danish physician.)

Gram-Positive

Gram-positive bacteria are stained purple by Gram's method.

Gramoxone

The proprietary name of a herbicide containing PARAQUAT.

Granular Vulvovaginitis

(see under VULVOVAGINITIS)

Granulations

Granulations are small masses of cells of a constructive nature containing loops of newly formed blood vessels which spring up over the surfaces of healing wounds (what is commonly called 'proud flesh'). Granulation tissue also occurs internally, forming GRANULOMAS at the site of lesions. (See also WOUND TREATMENT.)

Granuloma

A tumour composed of granulation tissue. (See EOSINOPHILIC GRANULOMA, and 'LICK GRANULOMA' for important conditions in cats and dogs; also 'SWAMP CANCER').

Occasionally a granuloma is seen as the result of a *Staphylococcus aureus* infection involving the skin of cats and dogs, or the mammary glands of cattle and goats, or the equine spermatic cord. One case involved a gastric ulcer in a cat.

Grass

(see under PASTURE MANAGEMENT; LEYS; DRIED GRASS; HAY; 'HAYFLAKES'; HAYLAGE; SILAGE)

Grass seeds as foreign bodies (see AWNS).

Grassland Management

(see under PASTURE MANAGEMENT)

Grass Sickness

A DYSAUTONOMIA which occurs in horses after they are put on to the grass between the months of April and September. Practically all breeds of horses and ponies may be affected. A very similar condition occurs in hares, but whether it is the identical disease is not known.

Cause Various theories advanced include: (1) degeneration of certain ganglia of the sympathetic nervous system due to a virus; (2) a fungal toxin; (3) a drastic reduction in peptide-containing autonomic nerves, though what produces this is not known.

Pathognomic lesions in the autonomic nervous system can be experimentally produced by intra-peritoneal injection of 500 ml serum from acute cases of grass sickness into normal horses. The serum injections do not, however, cause the stasis of the gastrointestinal tract which is typical of the disease. Examination of sera from acute cases of grass sickness revealed a compound of small molecular weight which does not occur in the serum of normal horses or in cases of colic. This substance may be a neurotoxin but this was not confirmed.

A 4th cause has been suggested, namely over-activity of the sympatho-adrenal system and stress, e.g. sweating, muscle fasciculation, tachycardia and increased plasma catecholamines. It is known that many types of stimuli caused by environmental, emotional or physical (trauma, disease) factors act as stressors and that general arousal will cause a common response in both parts of the sympatho-adrenal system.

Two sets of circumstances are thought to be involved in its aetiology: stress caused by travel to new surroundings, particularly in excitable young thoroughbred mares about to foal; and changes in the external environment such as cold and wet weather following warm and sunny weather. Similar changes are known to cause stress and increases in both plasma catecholamines and corticosteroids in laboratory animals.

Signs The disease may be:

1. Peracute. Death occurs in 8 to 16 hours, and periods of great violence are shown, at which times the animal may be a danger to people looking after it.

2. Subacute. The horse becomes dull and listless and off its food. It may have an anxious expression, and roll from pain. Later there may be a discharge from the nostrils, and an excessive amount of salivation. Swallowing is difficult. There may be localised twitching and sweating. No faeces are passed. Attempts at vomiting are made. Food material becomes impacted in the large intestine. The illness lasts from 2 to 5 days, when death or the chronic stage supervenes. The mortality is high.

3. Chronic. The signs are similar, except that constipation is not complete, and also some food may be eaten. The horse becomes progressively thinner, until in the later stages it has a tucked-up 'greyhound' appearance. The horse may live for a variable period in this state; some last only a few weeks, but others linger on for 6 months or more.

Diagnosis Administration of a barium preparation, followed by radiography, demonstrated serious malfunction of the oesophagus. 'Taken in conjunction with other clinical findings, this evidence was specific enough to confirm the diagnosis, without the need for an exploratory laparotomy, enabling euthanasia to be effected without delay.' (Animal Health Trust.)

Treatment Recovery is uncommon, and seldom complete. Euthanasia is usually indicated.

Grass, Turning Out to

(see under YARDED CATTLE)

Grave's Disease

Grave's disease is another name for exophthalmic goitre.

Grazing Behaviour

A study, made at Cornell University, of Aberdeen Angus and Hereford cows at pasture (receiving no supplementary feed) showed that

1. The average grazing time was 7 hours and 32 minutes, of which 4 hours and 52 minutes

were spent in actual eating, and the balance in walking and selecting herbage during the process of grazing. During the hours of darkness the cattle grazed for 2 hours and 28 minutes.

2. In a pasture of 6 acres the cow travelled 2.45 miles, of which 1.96 were during daylight hours and 0.49 during darkness.

3. The cows lay down for 11 hours and 39 minutes, but this was divided into 9 periods ranging from less than 1 hour to more than 6 hours. The time spent in chewing the cud averaged 6 hours and 51 minutes.

4. The calves, which were about 3 months old, were suckled 3 times a day at intervals of 8 hours, and for 15 minutes at a time.

5. Droppings were deposited on an average 12 times a day and urine, 9 times.

6. Under the conditions prevailing, the cows drank water once a day only. This may be accounted for by the luxuriant pasture herbage consisting of Kentucky bluegrass and wild white clover with an average water content of 72 per cent.

7. The cows showed no inclination to extend the grazing period beyond 8 hours even when the amount of herbage consumed fell to 20 kg (45 lb) a day. 'It is evident that a mechanical factor is involved in grazing management, and that one of the basic principles of good pasture management is to provide the livestock with pastures in a condition which will permit them to gather the optimum amount of food within a normal period of 8 hours' grazing.

'We may speculate upon the potential productivity of British pastures if we ever achieve a degree of efficiency in grazing management which will permit mature cattle to consume daily the normal maximum of about 68 kg (150 lb) of green herbage. This should be sufficient for maintenance and the production of about 22 kg (50 lb) of milk or possibly for the production of 2.25 kg (5 lb) liveweight increase daily.' (Professor D. R. Johnstone-Wallace.)

More recently, however, it has been shown that the time dairy cattle graze and ruminate is very flexible, and that the feed intake varies much less from day to day than the time spent in grazing. The cow has, in fact, a capacity to change her grazing habits to suit both her environment and her own bodily needs.

The quartering of a field by horses into parts for grazing and parts for defecation has been described by E. L. Taylor, who adds that cattle avoid the grass in the proximity of faecal pats. 'The fineness of this perception of contamination is shown by a helminthologist's observation that cattle were able to detect minute traces of faeces such as he was not able to see.'

Grazing Management
(see PASTURE MANAGEMENT)

Greasy Heel
This is a chronic fungal skin infection seen in horses mainly during the winter; with lesions occurring below the fetlock.

Cause *Dermatophilus congolensis*, which 'invades the epidermis but does not destroy the germinating layer', so that regeneration occurs, to be followed by renewed invasion and desquamation. Lesions extend and there is pus formation; the hair becoming matted and tufted.

Greasy heel occurs in horses with marked feather, such as Shires, stabled in unhygienic, damp stables, or grazing pasture liable to flooding. In ungroomed horses at grass, the tufting may be mistaken for normal coat condition.

First-aid Pending veterinary advice: Clip all the hair away from the affected areas, and thoroughly wash the leg with soap and water containing washing soda. Burn the hair. Wash the hands, as the infection is transmissible to man. Isolate horse under dry conditions. (See also POX; DERMATOPHILUS.)

'Greasy Pig Disease'
'Greasy pig disease' is now regarded as a staphylococcal infection. Bites, abrasions, tattooing, and lice infestation may facilitate entry of the organism through the skin.

Often only some piglets in a single litter on the farm are affected. Symptoms include dullness, loss of bloom, and soft, greasy spots on the reddened skin of the snout, ears, around the eyes, and sometimes on the abdomen. The spots join up and spread, and after a few days the piglet may have a largely greasy and brown body, with thickened and cracking skin. Severely affected cases die within a few days; survivors are seldom an economic proposition as recovery takes several weeks and may be incomplete.

Prevention Clipping the teeth of piglets, boiling tattooing instruments, and providing covered, non-abrasive flooring. To be successful, veterinary treatment with a suitable antibiotic has to be undertaken very promptly. Long-standing cases are best slaughtered.

Great Dane
A large dog of German orgin with broad head, short, folded-over ears, a long neck and tail. The lifespan is comparatively short. Ununited anconeal process (defective elbow development), hip dysplasia and 'wobbler syndrome'

(cervical spondolithesis) may be inherited. Deafness, distortion of the nictitating membrane and osteochondritis dissecans and calcinosis circumscripta may also develop.

'Green-Bottle' Fly
(see FLIES)

Greenstick Fracture
A greenstick fracture is one in which the bone fractures incompletely somewhat similar to the break of a green stick. They mostly occur in young animals. (See FRACTURES.)

Greyface
The term often applied to a Border Leicester × Scottish Blackface cross.

Greyhound
Medium to large dog, bred for racing, with smooth coat, small head and abdomen, long legs and deep chest. It has acute vision but a less good sense of smell than some other breeds. The racing life is short and dogs not selected for breeding may be abandoned or destoyed when comparatively young. Rescued greyhounds make good pets as they do not require more exercise than the average dog; they tire easily after a short burst of speed. Haemophilia and calcinosis circumscripta may be inherited.

Griffon Bruxellois
A breed of toy dog with wiry coat, prominent chin, short nose and erect folded-over ears. Patellar luxation may be inherited.

Griseofulvin
An antibiotic, which can be given by mouth, effective against ringworm and other fungal diseases. Dosing over a 3-week period may be necessary in the treatment of ringworm in calves. It is advisable not to use griseofulvin in pregnant animals, as there is some risk of malformed offspring resulting.

Grit for Poultry
Insoluble grit – sand, flint grit, tiny pebbles – is necessary for the grinding of the food in the gizzard (poultry possessing no teeth). Flint grit should be provided at the rate of 500 g (1 lb) per 100 birds, and is best broadcast with the grain every 2 or 3 months; except for battery birds, which require a monthly ration.

Soluble limestone grit is given in order to supply calcium for bone formation and eggshell production, and it dissolves in the gizzard within 48 hours. It is not necessary for chicks, growers or birds in early lay if they are receiving commercial mash or pellets without corn. Too much limestone grit can be harmful.

Grooming
The purpose of grooming horses, cattle, and dogs, especially when kept shut up in buildings, is fourfold: it is undertaken for the purpose of cleanliness, for the prevention of disease of the skin; to stimulate the skin circulation; and to remove waste products of metabolism.

Horses

Quartering This consists of going over the horse's body with a dandy-brush and removing the coarse adherent particles of bedding, dried dung, etc., as a preliminary before the horse leaves the stable for morning exercise. At the same time a cloth and a pail of water are used to wipe away discharges from the eyes, nose, and dock, in this order, and to remove any urine stains from other parts of the body. Quartering is usually only carried out in high-class stables, where the horses go out for a short walk before the stablehands have had their breakfasts, or when a horse is not going to work but is to be turned out to grass for the day. (See SPONGES.)

Dandy-brushing The dandy-brush is made of stiff, coarse, whisk fibre, generally of the yellow variety, with the bristles not close together. It removes the coarser particles of matter from the coat, and stirs up the finer debris, as well as disentangling matted hairs. Owing to its stiffness it is not used over the head, but each side of the neck, the whole of the body, and the 4 quarters are well brushed. It should be used in the left hand for the near side of the animal and in the right hand for the off-side. It is advisable to make short, vigorous sweeps, turning the wrist at the end of each sweep, so that the material collected in the bristles is thrown out of the coat. Care is necessary when the undersides of the body and the insides of the legs of thin-skinned or ticklish horses are being groomed with the dandy, for they may kick if this rough brush is used carelessly.

Body-brushing and curry-combing The body-brush is made from finer whisk fibre than the dandy, the bristles are set much closer together, and they are softer and more flexible. There is usually a strap across the back of the brush into which the hand is thrust, so that a better grip can be obtained. The curry-comb is made of metal, either in the form of a square plate with a series of alternately toothed and smooth ridges set across it, or it may be oval with crenated ridges running round it. The former variety is provided with a handle, and the latter has a strap across its back like the body-brush. The body-brush is used all over the horse's body, head, and neck. It picks up the finer particles of matter left behind by the dandy-brush and holds them between the fine bristles. To clean the brush it is necessary every 3 or 4 sweeps to draw it across the face of the curry-comb and transfer the dirt to the latter. The body-brush should be used in long firm sweeps, without any turn of the wrist. While grooming the near side, the body-brush is held in the left hand and the curry-comb in the right, and for the off-side the positions are reversed.

Wisping A wisp is a small mat of plaited straw or hay, which is used to remove fine dust from the coat, scour and polish the surface hair, and to promote a better skin and superficial circulation. When properly applied it acts as massage to the surface of the body, and gives the coat a fine shine.

Combing the mane and tail For this purpose a bone or metal comb is used, fashioned after the familiar manner of a toilet comb, with stouter teeth. The mane is combed a few strands at a time, both from the outside and also from the inside (with the teeth through the whole thickness of the mane), so that the hair may be laid straight and all tangles removed. Afterwards the tail is treated similarly. When a few unruly strands will not lie in position it is usual to damp the fibres of the water-brush (which is not unlike a small, fine dandy-brush pointed at each end) and lay the strands with the damp brush. Neither the mane nor the tail, however, should be soaked.

Rubbing or shining is carried out either with a stable-rubber, which is a piece of towelling about 45 cm (18 inches) square, or with a chamois leather. During this process the hairs of the coat are laid straight all over the body, any loose pieces of hay or straw from the wisp are removed, and the final gloss is put on to the coat.

Cleaning-out of the feet The last operation of grooming consists of picking up each of the feet and removing any adherent dung, etc., by means of a hoof-pick, and brushing out the sole of each foot with the water-brush. If desired, the walls of the hoofs may also be blackened or oiled at this time. This operation should be left till last, just before the horse

leaves the stable, for otherwise he may collect fresh dung in his feet. It is an important matter not to neglect this cleaning-out of the feet, for if there is a cake of dung in the soles of each foot, not only is it extremely untidy, but small stones are liable to be picked up and may cause injury to the soles.

Parts often neglected When examining a horse to discover the thoroughness or otherwise of the grooming, it is usual to take a white handkerchief and to rub it along the coat; the size of the particles of grey debris which adhere to its surface are in inverse ratio to the efficiency of the grooming – i.e. the larger the particles, the less efficiently has the horse been groomed. The following parts should be carefully examined: under the forelock, the poll, jowl, under the mane, between the fore-legs, behind the elbows, along the belly, inside the thighs, in the hollows of the heels, and around the dock and between the buttocks.

To dry a wet horse When a horse returns to a stable soaked with rain, snow, or sweat, it is advisable that it be dried to avoid the risk of chill through too-rapid evaporation of the moisture in the coat.

First of all it should be given a warm drink. The harness is next removed and the surface of the body scraped down with a sweat-scraper. This is a flexible ribbon of copper provided with a handle at either end. The scraper removes the excess water from the coat, and may be used to scrape away adherent mud from the legs and belly, but it should not be used over bony prominences owing to the danger of abrading the skin. Two or 3 hay wisps are made ready, and the horse is vigorously wisped down all over. As 1 wisp becomes wet it is discarded and another taken. Sometimes a coarse, rough towel is used instead of a wisp. In about 10 minutes all the moisture that can be removed by this means will have been eliminated, and the rest must be allowed to evaporate. An armful of straw is arranged across the horse's back; a rug is thrown over all, and girthed up. The straw allows a certain amount of ventilation under the rug, and prevents too-rapid cooling and chilling. In about 2 hours' time the rug should be removed, a second wisping should be given, and a new dry rug should be applied. If the feet and legs are very wet, especially if there is much feather, they should be bandaged with woollen stable bandages, and a little bran or sawdust may be sprinkled on to the wet hair below the bandage. Sometimes a horse's feet are washed immediately after coming in from work, especially if they are coated with mud; when this is carried out, care should be taken to see that they are well dried again afterwards, for frequent washing predisposes to grease, eczema, and other skin conditions, through maceration of the surface epithelium.

Dogs When grooming it is always advisable to begin by combing and brushing the coat in the wrong direction (against the lie of the hair), so as to remove pieces of dirt, debris, etc. which have become lodged under a lock of the coat. Finish by brushing and combing in the direction in which it is desired that the hair shall eventually lie.

In the spring, and again in the autumn, when the coat is changing, both dogs and cats require more careful grooming than they do at other times of the year.

Cats benefit from regular grooming. With long-haired breeds, this is essential.

Grootlamsiekte

A disease of sheep in SW Africa, associated with a prolonged gestation period, and caused by a poisonous shrub (*Salsola ruberculata*).

Groundnut Meal

Groundnut meal may be infected by a mould, *Aspergillus flavus*, which produces a toxin (aflatoxin). In an outbreak of fatalities among turkeys fed in Britain on proprietary feeding-stuffs, the cause was traced to Brazilian groundnut meal (not all samples of which, however, proved harmful). Calves and pigs also died. In calves, groundnut poisoning resembles that of ragwort.

The mould can grow on decorticated groundnuts when their moisture content exceeds about 9 per cent, or on meal at about 16 per cent. It usually develops on the nuts after they are harvested, particularly if drying is delayed and the shells damaged. However, if harvesting is delayed the nuts may become toxic in the ground, and if the nuts are stored at a moisture content in excess of 9 per cent they can also become toxic.

Pigs of from 3 to 12 weeks are particularly susceptible, and pregnant sows to a lesser extent.

It was found that cows fed on hay and a concentrate ration containing 20 per cent toxic groundnut meal excreted a toxin in the milk which produced the same biological effect in ducklings as aflatoxin. There is evidence strongly suggesting that aflatoxin may be a carcinogen, giving rise to cancer of the liver or bile ducts. A 100 per cent incidence of carcinoma of the liver was found in pigs which survived illness following the feeding of a mixture of oil-cakes. The same effect has been observed in rats. Toxicity trials in ducklings produced carcinoma of the bile ducts.

Groundnut meal contains an alkaloid, arachine, which can cause a fatal hepatitis in dogs, and temporary paralysis in frogs and rabbits. (See also AFLATOXINS.)

Grouse Disease

A wasting disease caused by heavy infestation with *Trichostrongylus tenuis*, a nematode parasite. Grouse tend to remain on the moor where they were hatched and a build-up of the parasite results. If the grouse population increases too much, food may become short. Coupled with the infestation, survival of chicks may become very difficult. Further, an ageing population of birds becomes less fertile. Paradoxically, in the proper management of a moor efficiently regulated shooting maintains the numbers of grouse. (See TRICHOSTRONGYLOSIS.)

Growth Hormone
(see SOMATOTROPHIN)

Growth Plates

Growth plates (for growth-plate defects, see BONE, DISEASES OF)

Growth Promoters

Substances which, given in animal feeds, increase feed conversion efficiency or result in better daily liveweight gains, or both. Although very useful when given properly, there have been problems in the past caused by the misuse of some hormonal growth promoters, particularly in Italy, which led to the banning in Europe of some potentially useful products. (For types and examples, see under ADDITIVES; see also SOMATOSTATIN; STILBENES; SURFACTANTS; HORMONES IN MEAT PRODUCTION; WORMS, FARM TREATMENT AGAINST.)

Growths
(see TUMOURS; CANCER; GRANULOMA)

Guarnieri Bodies
(see INCLUSION BODIES)

Guernsey

Cattle originating from the Channel Islands yielding milk of a high butterfat content. The coat is pale brown and white in colour.

Guide Dogs
(see DOGS: WORKING)

Guinea Fowl

Large bird (50 cm; 20 inches long) of the Numidiae family with featherless head and neck. Widely distributed in savannahs of Africa; introduced elsewhere. Used for food, and as an 'intruder alarm' because of the loud gobblng noise it makes if disturbed.

Guinea-Pig

Also known as a cavy, the guinea-pig is technically a rodent, *Cavia porcella*, originating from South America; it is better known as a children's pet, a laboratory animal, and as an animal bred for show purposes.

Breeds include English, Abyssinian and Peruvian.

Diseases include tuberculosis, pseudotuberculosis (yersiniosis), salmonellosis, leptospirosis, streptococcal pneumonia, toxoplasmosis, a viral infection of the salivary glands, and fascioliasis. Mange due to *Trixacarus* and lice infestations also occur. (See PETS.)

Guinea-pigs cannot synthesise vitamin C and so, like people, are liable to have scurvy if the diet is deficient in this vitamin. They practise coprophagy, swallowing the soft brown pellets produced in the caecum. these are rich in B vitamins and amino acids.

Guinea Worm

A nematode parasite (Dracunculus medinensis) which infects man, subhuman primates, dogs, cattle and horses. This parasite is found in Africa, the Middle East, India, Pakistan and Iran. The intermediate hosts are several species of the crustacea *Cyclops*, which live in ponds and wells, etc.

D. insignis infects carnivores in the USA and southern Canada.

The pads of a dog's feet may be severely affected by female guinea worms and may ulcerate.

Gullet

(see OESOPHAGUS)

Gumboro Disease

Properly called avian infectious necrosis or infectious bursal disease, Gumboro disease takes its name from a town in Delaware, USA. It affects broiler chickens of 1 to 5 weeks of age. The disease has been recorded in Britain since 1962. Because it destroys the cells of the bursa of Fabricius, the immune system of the birds is severely impaired, leaving the birds susceptible to other diseases after recovery from Gumboro disease. For this reson it has been called 'chicken aids' but this is incorrect as the mechanisms of the 2 are quite different. Vaccines are available for its control; administration must be planned strictly in accordance with the manufacturers' schedules. (See INFECTIOUS BURSAL DISEASE.)

Gums

The colour of these is dependent on the blood circulating within them, and provides useful clues to the veterinarian engaged on the detective work which goes into each diagnosis. Very pale gums suggest anaemia or internal haemorrhage. Gum pallor may be seen too in cases of leukaemia, shock after an accident, in warfarin poisoning, or failure of the left side of the heart. A yellowish tinge suggests jaundice. A blue or purple discoloration (CYANOSIS) indicates a shortage of oxygen in the circulating blood. (For inflammation of the gums, see MOUTH, DISEASES OF – Gingivitis. For a common tumour of the gum, see EPULIS.)

Gunshot Injuries

In the small-animal practice teaching unit of the University of Edinburgh, records showed that over a 5-year-period there were 23 cases in which the animal had been shot, as detected by surgical and radiological means. Of 11 canine cases, 7 involved shotgun pellets and 4 airgun pellets. One poodle died following lacerations to abdominal organs, and a lurcher developed a fatal fungal disease of the chest after shotgun injuries.

Of 10 feline cases, 7 were injured by airguns. One cat had a femur fractured by a single pellet. Of 3 cats wounded by shotguns, 1 was put down because of spinal injury; another had a urethral obstruction.

Many animals are wounded without their owners knowing, and the pellets are often detected only when X-rayed for some entirely different reason.

A cat found lying in the street was thought to have been hit by a car; however, a veterinary examination revealed only a slight puncture wound on the right side of the chest. The cat was in pain, and there was no femoral pulse. A metallic object was suggested on radiography, and found to be a BB shot inside the aorta, which was incised and sutured. The cat was able to walk with difficulty after 2 weeks, and appeared completely recovered after 5 months.

In Canada the owner of a Labrador took it to a veterinary clinic on account of a swollen leg with skin wounds explaining that the dog had been struck by a car 2 or 3 days previously. However, radiographs showed that, while there were multiple fractures, their cause was not a car but a shotgun.

Accidental or malicious shooting of dogs and cats often leads to serious eye injury, usually with some permanent impairment of vision. To give some examples, an 11-month-old dog, shot with a 12-bore, suffered injury to the iris of 1 eye; the iris became partly adherent to the lens (*posterior synechia*). Six weeks after the accident the rest of the iris was mobile, and the pupil able to respond to light. An opaque pigmented spot remained on the cornea where it had been penetrated.

Another dog received a lead shot in the lens and another in the vitreous body of 1 eye. Seven months later a cataract had developed.

A 3rd dog needed amputation of a part of the iris protruding through the shot wound in the cornea, which needed sutures.

'Gut-Tie'

'Gut-tie' is the colloquial name for a type of hernia in which a piece of bowel becomes entangled in the spermatic cord following castration of cattle.

Guttural Pouch

A diverticulum of the Eustachian tube developed from the pharynx.

Diseases of the guttural pouch include fungal infections, which may be followed by paralysis of the cranial nerves; and also a haemangioma, which may have a similar result. With both, the signs include difficulty in swallowing and the return of food and water through the nostrils. (See also GUTTURAL POUCH MYCOSIS; EAR – Middle.)

Guttural Pouch Disease (GPD)

Sometimes known as guttural pouch diphtheria, GPD is a general term for a number of diseases in horses locating in the guttural pouch. Empyema, mycosis or tympany have all been involved. GPD of one kind or another has been encountered in horses from 2 months to 18 years old – in ponies, cobs, hunters, and thoroughbreds. It may prove fatal within a week, or may be chronic, with symptoms shown over a period of 7 months or more.

Signs Clinical signs vary. Epistaxis (nosebleeding) is often seen. Haemorrhage occurs spontaneously while the horse was at rest in the stable. It is generally recurrent and may be mild, severe, or fatal. Other signs may include:

Dysphagia (difficulty in swallowing). Attempts to eat solid food result in coughing and the discharge of food material from mouth and nostrils. Drinking may be difficult. Water is conveyed back into the bucket via the nostrils.

Laryngeal hemiplegia. Paralysis of one side of the larynx, resulting in abnormal inspiratory noise when exercised.

Soft palate paresis. In racehorses this is shown by the sudden onset of respiratory obstruction during a race.

Diagnosis This involves an examination of the guttural pouches by endoscope.

Guttural Pouch Empyema

Caused by bacterial infection of the guttural pouch, empyema produces a painful swelling near the ear. Raised temperature, nasal discharge and anorexia may also be seen. Treatment with antibiotics and lavage of the guttural pouches is often effective; surgical drainage and removal of purulent material may be required in some cases.

Guttural Pouch Mycosis

Guttural pouch mycosis is usually caused by infection with *Aspergillosis* spp. Nosebleeding, which may be very severe, is common but dysphasia and other signs may be seen. Mycosis can usually be successfully treated with benzimidazole drugs given by mouth. A specially designed catheter has been used for local treatment with antifungal agents.

Guttural Pouch Tympany

Found mainly in young foals. Usually only 1 guttural pouch is affected, which becomes distended with air, causing a painless swelling near the ear. Breathing may be noisy and in severe cases empyema may develop. Surgical treatment involves an incision in the membrane between the two pouches to release trapped air. Prognosis is usually good.

Gyrodactylus

A fluke living on the skin of freshwater fish. It is viviparous and a developing embryo may be seen within an adult. It can invade the gills and the eyes, causing behavioural changes such as 'flashing' followed by skin erosin and secondary fungal infections. Although apparently harmless to fish stocks in its native habitat, the rivers of the Baltic, *G. salaris* has had severe effects on salmon in Norway. Gyrodactylosis is a NOTIFIABLE DISEASE.

Gyrus

A convolution of the brain.

H-Y Antigen

This histocompatability antigen is present in the gonads of the bovine freemartin. It causes XX cells in the female gonad to assume testicular organisation. It is responsible for the rejection of male grafts by females of the same species.

Habronemiasis

Infection of horses with worms of the genus *Habronema*, the cause of 'summer sores' and a usually mild chronic gastritis. (See ROUNDWORMS – Horses.)

Haemangioma

Haemangioma is a tumour composed of blood vessels. In the liver of adult cattle small haemangiomata are not uncommonly found, but they are seldom of any practical importance. (See also under GUTTURAL POUCH for haemangioma in horses.)

Haemangiosarcoma, Cardiac

A malignant tumour which may give rise to fatal internal haemorrhage, and has been found in the lung, spleen, liver, kidney, brain, etc. of dogs. Thirty-eight cases of this were seen at 1 veterinary hospital. In 16 dogs it was found on exploratory thoracotomy; in 22 the diagnosis was made only at autopsy. In 9 dogs in which the tumour could be resected, survival time averaged 4 months. Metastases were found in 16 of the dogs.

Haematemesis

Vomiting blood. When the blood is from a lesion of the stomach or oesophagus it is bright red; but when it has lain in the stomach for some time, and been partly digested, it resembles coffee-grounds.

Haematidrosis

The presence of blood in the sweat.

Haematocele

A haematocele results when blood collects in a body cavity. It often refers to the testicle following an injury which has ruptured the smaller blood vessels. Blood from them then collects in the cavity of the scrotum, in the loose fascia, or in the outer coat of the testicle itself.

Haematocrit Value

The percentage by volume of whole blood that is composed of erythrocytes. It is determined by filling a graduated haematocrit tube with blood – treated so that it will not clot – and then centrifuging the tube until the red cells are packed in the lower end. As a rough guide, values range as follows: sheep, 32; cow, 40; horse and pig, 42; dog, 45.

Haematoma

A swelling containing clotted blood under the skin, or deeper in the musculature, following serious bruising; for example, after an animal has been struck by a car. Haematomas also occur in cases of warfarin poisoning and canine haemophilia, and may result from shaking the head or scratching the ear. They are also seen in pigs and sheep. (See also under EAR, DISEASES OF for haematomas in the ear in cats and dogs.)

Haematopedesis

(see HAEMATIDROSIS)

Haematopinus

A genus of sucking lice. (See LICE.)

Haematophagous

This adjective applies to parasites which feed on blood, such as ticks, fleas, and vampire bats.

Haematopoesis

The formation and development of blood cells; usually takes place in the bone marrow.

Haematothorax

An effusion of blood into the pleural cavity.

Haematozoa

Haematozoa is a general name applied to the various parasites of the blood.

Haematozoon Canis

A coccidia-like parasite found in countries where the tick *Rhipicephalus sanguineus* is present.

Signs Anaemia, fever, hindleg weakness, dyspnoea; sometimes epistaxis.

Haematuria

Haematuria is any condition in which blood is found in the urine. When urine is allowed to stand, the red cells gravitate to the bottom of the container. (See URINE, ABNORMAL CONDITIONS OF.)

Haemobartonella

Also known as eperythrozoon, it is a single-celled parasite of the blood. *H. felis* (also known as Mycoplasma felis)is the cause of FELINE INFECTIOUS ANAEMIA; *H canis* of the corresponding disease of dogs, in which the parasite complicates many cases of canine parvovirus infections. (See also EPERYTHROZOON for the infections in farm animals.) Diagnosis is not easy as the parasites may not be present in the first blood samples examined. Antibiotic treatment is usually successful; a vitamin B_{12} preparation is often given simultaneously.

Haemocyte

A blood cell. Red blood cells are called erythrocytes; white blood cells, leukocytes.

Haemoglobin

Haemoglobin is a complex organic compound containing iron, and gives the red colour to the red blood cells. (See METHAEMOGLOBIN.) Haemoglobin has the function of absorbing oxygen from the air in the lungs and of transporting oxygen to the tissues.

It exists in 2 forms: carboxyhaemoglobin, found in venous blood, and oxyhaemoglobin, found in arterial blood that has been in contact with oxygen. This oxyhaemoglobin, a weak compound of haemoglobin and oxygen, is broken down in the tissues, yielding to the cells its oxygen, and becoming once more haemoglobin. In some forms of anaemia there is a great deficiency in haemoglobin. (See BLOOD; ANAEMIA; RESPIRATION.)

Haemoglobinuria

The presence of haemoglobin in the urine, such as occurs in azoturia, red-water fever, leptospirosis of calves and poisoning by an excess of kale or cabbage. When the urine is allowed to stand, the red pigment remains in solution (differentiates from haematuria).

Haemolymph

In invertebrates, haemolymph is the blood-like fluid that functions as does blood and lymph in vertebrates.

Haemolysis

The breakdown of red blood cells and the consequent release from them of haemoglobin. It occurs gradually in some forms of anaemia and rapidly in poisoning by snake venom. Some chemical and bacterial toxins cause haemolysis.

Haemolytic

Relating to haemolysis. For haemolytic disease of foals, see FOALS, DISEASES OF. Haemolytic disease in pigs and dogs is similar in its effects. In cattle, it may account for some cases of abortion.

Haemonchosis

Infection of the abomasal wall with *Haemonchus contortus* or *H. placei*. It causes acute anaemia, anasarca and sometimes death in sheep and goats but is often less severe in cattle. Usually seen in the summer.

Haemophilia

A condition in which clotting of the blood is impaired (see CANINE HAEMOPHILIA; FELINE HAEMOPHILIA).

Haemophilus Infections

Haemophilus infections include *H. somnus* causing the ' SLEEPER' SYNDROME in feedlot cattle in the USA. The organism has also been isolated from cases of pneumonia, metritis, and abortion in cattle; in Canada it is commonly found in the genital tract of bulls. *H. somnus* has been found in semen samples from Danish bulls. In pigs in the UK, *H. parasuis*, *H. parainfluenzae* and *H. parahaemolyticus* are often associated with chronic respiratory disease, including a painful pleurisy. *H. parahaemolyticus* may also cause an acute illness and sudden death.

Infection with *H. pleuropneumoniae* has been increasingly detected in Britain, as have the reported number of outbreaks of acute pleuropneumonia due to this organism.

Haemopoiesis, Haemopoietic

Relating to the formation of red blood cells.

Haemoptysis

The expulsion of blood from the lower air passages, generally by coughing. The blood so expelled is bright red in colour and is frothy, thus differing from that which has been expelled from the stomach. It is seen in tuberculosis.

Haemorrhage

(see BLEEDING; PROTHROMBIN; INTERNAL HAEMORRHAGE; and HAEMORRHAGIC DISEASE)

Haemorrhagic Diathesis

An inherited tendency, transmissible to either sex, to bleeding from the nasal and other mucosa. It has been reported in the dog (as well as in man).

'Haemorrhagic Disease' of Dogs

(see DIARRHOEA; HAEMANGIOSARCOMA; CANINE HAEMOPHILIA; HAEMORRHAGE)

Haemorrhagic Enteritis of Turkeys

This acute, often fatal, disease is seen in birds over 4 weeks old. The droppings are bloody and the disease spreads rapidly through a flock. It has appeared in the UK, the USA, Australia and Southern Africa. There is an increased incidence during hot weather. An adenovirus is usually the cause.

Haemorrhagic Fever with Renal Syndrome (HFRS)

An important human disease caused by Hantaan or related viruses, and occurring in Europe, the USA, and the Far East. Human mortality varies from 0.5 to 185 per cent. In Belgium, staff at a research institute were infected by laboratory rats; but voles are the main source. In the USA, urban rats have been implicated. (WHO.)

Signs These can be like the effects of a mild influenza attack; but in many cases they are those of a serious illness characterised by dizziness, vomiting, back pain, haematuria, acute kidney failure, and shock.

Haemorrhagic Gastroenteritis of Pigs

Haemorrhagic gastroenteritis of pigs can be caused by bacterial infections or parasitic infestations. One syndrome with a non-infectious artiology involves the sudden death of growing pigs, with autopsy findings of haemorrhage into the small intestine, and sometimes volvulus.

Whey-feeding is especially associated with this syndrome, but it can occur also in meal-fed pigs. It has been suggested that rapid gas production by fermenting whey in the colon leads to distension, displacement and sometimes volvulus. Haemorrhage may result from the twisting and occlusion of the mesenteric veins.

Haemorrhage from the intestine is an important feature of another syndrome seen in Australia. An outbreak involved 372 adult pigs in the breeding units of a minimal-disease piggery; 186 pigs died. Some had been seen to be passing blood; others died without any symptoms being observed.

This syndrome has the somewhat cumbersome name of proliferative haemorrhagic enteropathy (PHE), and has been described also by several research workers in the UK. PHE is associated with adenoma-like changes in the small intestine similar to those seen in necrotic enteritis and inflammation of the ileum, the last part of the small intestine. (See also PORCINE INTESTINAL ADENOMATOSIS.)

Haemorrhagic Septicaemia (Pasteurellosis)

This is present in most tropical countries, and is especially important in Asia. Outbreaks tend to occur at the beginning of the monsoon rains. Buffaloes and cattle are the animals mainly affected, but the disease occurs also in camels, goats, sheep, pigs and horses.

Cause *Pasteurella multocida* type 1, and possibly other serotypes. Stress due to exhaustion, underfeeding, and transport may predispose animals to infection.

Signs After a very short incubation period (2 days or less), buffaloes and cattle become dull, lose their appetite, salivate profusely, and have a high fever. Visible mucous membranes become dark red. The tongue may swell and protrude from the mouth. Oedema results in hot, painful swellings in the regions of the throat, brisket, and dewlap. Death, in this most acute form, usually follows dyspnoea, and occurs in from a few hours to 3 or 4 days. Mortality is very high. In less acute cases there may be dysentery or broncho-pneumonia.

Treatment can seldom be carried out in time to save life, but sulfonamide drugs and antibiotics may help if given early.

Control Specific and combined vaccines are available. (See also PASTEURELLOSIS; 'SHIPPING FEVER'.)

Haemosiderin

An iron-protein compound. It appears to be the form in which iron is stored until needed for haemoglobin.

Haemostatics

Haemostatics are means taken to check bleeding, and may be drugs applied to the area, mechanical devices, etc.

Hair-Balls

Hair-balls (also called trichobesoar) are masses of impacted hair or fur caused by animals licking their own or other animals' coats. They sometimes cause indigestion in calves, especially those aged about 6 weeks to 4 months. The hair may be in the form of a ball or in loose masses, sometimes mixed with milk curds, sand, binder twine, etc. Bad management encourages calves to lick their own or other animals' hair. The condition rarely proves fatal either in calves or in pigs. (However, the owner of an animal, on finding a hair-ball, may erroneously decide that this is the cause of death, which may in fact have been caused by some infection.)

Signs are usually vague, but may include grinding of the teeth, an unnatural gait, and in chronic cases a general loss of condition, although the appetite remains fairly good. Convulsions may also occur.

Prevention Ensure a well-balanced diet, adequate minerals and roughage, and attend to any skin disease. (See SALT – Salt licks.)

Treatment is surgical and often successful if carried out early.

Cats Particularly in long-haired varieties, hair/fur-balls sometimes result in impaction of the intestine. Less commonly this occurs also in the dog.

Hair, Clipping of The
(see CLIPPING OF ANIMALS)

Hair, Diseases of
(see ALOPECIA; RINGWORM; DERMATOPHILUS; SKIN DISEASES)

Hair Dryers
Hot air from these has been used for removal of maggots from wounds following the desired debridement.

'Hairy Shaker' Disease
'Hairy shaker' disease, or border disease, is a transmissible disease of lambs (see ' BORDER DISEASE' OF SHEEP).

Half-Bred
In sheep, this term usually means the cross of a Cheviot ewe × Border Leicester.

Half-Life
The time taken for the concentration of a drug in the animal's body to be reduced by 50 per cent.

Halitosis
Bad breath may be indicative of a number of disease conditions. Checking for offensive odour in the breath is routine in the clinical examination of many animals, particularly dogs and cats.

Halofuginone
A coccidiostat for the prevention of coccidiosis in turkeys and chickens reared for meat. It is also used for the treatment of *Cryptosporidium parvum* infection in calves.

Halothane (Fluothane)
A widely used, potent, non-irritant inhalation anaesthetic used for horses, dogs, cats, laboratory animals and, to a lesser extent, in cattle. It offers smooth induction, and gives moderate to good analgesia and muscle relaxation. Side-effects are usually dose-dependent and can include vasodilation, hypotension, cardiac arrythmia and hypothermia. High inspired concentrations can lead to cardio-respiratory depression. Halothane is usually administered in a mixture of oxygen and nitrous oxide.

Halothane Test
The ability of halothane to detect a single gene affecting stress susceptibility and production traits can be used to identify animals susceptible to PORCINE STRESS SYNDROME.

Pigs of around 8 weeks of age are made to breathe the anaesthetic through a face mask for a total of 3 minutes. If they remain relaxed throughout this period, they are scored as negative, or stress-resistant. If the muscles of the hind leg become rigid during the 3 minutes, the pigs are scored as positive, or stress susceptible. In this case the halothane must be turned off immediately, or the reaction may reach an irreversible stage which can kill the pig. Positive and negative reactors normally recover fully within 5 minutes of the test.

Ham
(see GLUTEAL, MUSCLES *and*, for abscesses, INJECTIONS)

Hamartoma
A tumour-like malformation composed of an abnormal mixture of the normal tissue components of the organ from which the hamartoma arises. Pulmonary hamartomas have been found in animals, with either vascular or cartilaginous tissue predominating. It is a rare congenital defect.

Hammondia Hammondi
A coccidian parasite, antigenically related to *Toxoplasma gondii*, of cats. The parasite has a 2-host life-cycle. Hosts also include rodents and dogs.

Hampshire
A black pig with a white belt, from Kentucky, USA. The origins of the breed were probably 19th-century Old English.

Hampshire Down
A short-wooled breed of sheep with brown/black face and legs used for meat production.

Hamsters

Small brown rodents popular as domestic pets: the dwarf Russian (*Phodopus sungorus*) and the golden (*Mesocricetus auratus)* hamsters. The former, also known as the striped, hairy-footed hamster, comes from Siberia, central Asia, and northern China.

Diseases include tumour formation affecting mouth, skin, and mammary glands, and leading to rapid loss of weight; indeed, to emaciation in many cases.

Weight loss as a result of broncho-pneumonia or of tooth-trimming also occurs.

Cystic ovaries, in hamsters prevented from breeding, result in an enlarged abdomen and a haemorrhagic discharge from the vulva.

Synthetic-fibre bedding material sold for hamsters has caused severe injury, sometimes necessitating euthanasia.

In the *M. auratus* species, the main health problem is 'wet tail', a fairly common and often fatal disease so-named because of diarrhoea and consequent staining of the tail.

Anaesthesia Halothane and isoflurane appear to be well tolerated, with rapid recovery.

Hamsters and human health They occasionally carry the virus of cymphocytic choriomeningitis (LCM).

Sixty people, aged from 3 to 70, became ill following the despatch by an Alabama breeder of LCM-infected hamsters (via wholesalers) to shops in 7 states of the USA. Of 60 patients, 55 kept hamsters as pets, and 4 worked for wholesalers or retail shops. An outbreak, involving 48 people, was also reported from Germany, the cause being medical laboratory hamsters. (See also under LYMPHOCYTIC CHORIOMENINGITIS, and PETS.)

Hand

A unit of measurement for the height of a horse, as measured at the withers. A hand is 4 inches. Under 1981 UK legislation, metrication was introduced, resulting in rounded equivalents, e.g. 12 hands = 122 cm, 10½ hands = 107 cm. (See HORSES, MEASUREMENT OF.)

Hand, Foot and Mouth Disease

A disease of man, first described in 1957, which has to be differentiated from rare human infection with foot-and-mouth disease. The cause is Coxsackie A9 virus (or A5, A10 or A16).

Hantavirus

A genus containing the Hantaan and related viruses. (See HAEMORRHAGIC FEVER WITH RENAL SYNDROME.)

Hantavirus infection in animals A single feline case in the UK was recorded in 1983, but since then the veterinary faculty of Liverpool University has carried out a survey of serum samples taken from 41 pet cats brought for treatment, and from 12 young cats for neutering. Six were shown to have antibody to the virus in their bloodstream.

One of 7 stray cats from Leeds, and 7 of 85 feral cats in various parts of England and Wales, were likewise *Hantavirus* antibody-positive.

The virus can cause chronic illness in cats, especially in those infected also with the feline leukaemia virus or the feline immunodeficiency virus.

Sources of infection Voles and rats.

Human hantavirus infection In many parts of Europe a mild form, *Nephropathia epidemica*, has been recorded; but a severe form appeared in Greece and Bulgaria. There may be internal haemorrhage and kidney disease in some cases.

Sources 'probably include' aerosols of the virus from saliva, urine, faeces, and lung secretions; also bites by rodents.

Laboratory infections from rats kept there, and from Hantaan tissue culture, are a recognised hazard.

Farm workers, water sports enthusiasts, sewage farm workers, and laboratory personnel have seropositivity rates of up to 21 per cent.

Signs, appearing 2 or 3 weeks after exposure, comprise conjunctivitis, with erythema of face, neck and upper chest. In the severe form, fever, headache, nausea and vomiting are typical; with moderate or severe kidney disease.

It has been suggested that people with suspected leptospirosis should have their blood tested also for *Hantavirus*.

Haploid

Haploid refers to the reduced number of chromosomes in the ovum and sperm − half the (diploid) number in the somatic cells. (See MEIOSIS.)

Hapten

A small molecule that cannot by itself initiate an immune response, but which can do so when linked to a 'carrier', e.g. a protein such as albumin. (See IMMUNE RESPONSE; B-CELLS.)

Hard Palate

(see PALATE)

Harderian Gland

A sebaceous gland associated with the 3rd eyelid which, in some animals, acts as an accessory to the lacrimal gland. Normally the Harderian gland is completely covered by the 3rd eyelid, but in dogs, obstruction to the flow of material from the gland not uncommonly causes its enlargement and projection beyond the 3rd eyelid, when it appears as a red, roundish mass. In some cases it may be necessary for the gland to be removed under local or general anaesthesia. (See also EYE, DISEASES OF.)

'Hardware Disease'

The colloquial American name for traumatic pericarditis of cattle caused by metal objects, such as nails or pieces of baling wire. (See under HEART DISEASES.)

Hare-Lip

This deformity is seen in puppies of the toy breeds, and in sheep. When the cleft in the lip is wide, sucking is impossible and the young puppies often die from starvation. In less severe cases they obtain some nourishment, but never thrive as well as the others in a litter. The malformation is generally associated with CLEFT PALATE.

Hares

(*Lepus* spp.) may harbour the liver fluke of sheep, *Fasciola hepatica*, and the cystic stage of the tapeworm *Taenia multiceps packi* of the dog, and of *T. pisiformis*. In some countries (e.g. Denmark), hares are a source of *Brucella abortus suis* infection to pigs. Some European hares also harbour *B. melitensis*.

In the UK, orf-like lesions have been seen (and confused with myxomatosis). Other diseases include aspergillosis, streptococcal endocarditis, toxoplasmosis, and coccidiosis. Louping-ill virus and/or antibody has been found in English hares, and also Q fever antibody. Avian tuberculosis is another occasional finding. European brown hare syndrome (leporine dysautonomia), a disease similar to grass sickness, has been diagnosed in East Anglia. Its cause is not yet known.

In order to prevent the introduction of *B. suis* and also of *Pasteurella tularensis* infections, the Hares (Control of Importation) Order 1965 was enacted in the UK. (See TULARAEMIA.)

Harvest Mites

(see under MITES)

Hassall's Corpuscles

(see THYMUS GLAND)

Haverhill Fever

The name given in human medicine to sporadic cases of rat-bite fever resulting from contamination of food. The causal bacteria are *Streptobacillus moniliformis* and *Spirillum minus*. Rats are usually subclinical carriers.

Haw

A number of eye conditions in dogs and cats may be called by this name. They include drooping of the lower eyelid, and protrusion of the 3rd eyelid (nictitating membrane).

Hawks

(see FALCONS)

Hay

There are 2 general classes of hay: that from grasses only; and that containing leguminous plants such as clover and lucerne. (See LEYS; PASTURE MANAGEMENT.) Hay is a very important, but nowadays perhaps a somewhat underrated, article of diet for cattle. (See under DIET – Fibre.) Hay is sometimes put down on very lush pasture where bloat is anticipated. As well as assisting in bloat prevention, it will help to obviate hypomagnesaemia and acetonaemia. The feeding of hay together with green fodder crops is said to reduce the risk of scouring, especially when large quantities, of the fodder are being eaten and during wet weather. When kale or rape are being fed in quantity, hay is most necessary in the diet. Hay made from leys is evidently not very palatable, for it is refused by the sick cow which will often relish even not very good hay made from old pasture.

'Tripoded hay has 4 or 5 times as much carotene as good hay made in the swathe, and barn-dried hay is even better. On the other hand, swathe hay has more vitamin D than other types if made in good weather. Badly damaged swathe hay is deficient in both carotene and vitamin D, and there may well be a case for adding vitamins A and D as well as minerals to any cereals used to make good the losses in poor hay.' (T. H. Davies.)

There would certainly seem to be more scope now for barn hay-drying, though the relatively high costs of this and also of hay-towers are likely to limit wide application of these 2 methods. The first essential, in any event, is of course high-quality grass to make into hay.

The nutritional quality of hay can vary widely. An ADAS study found that three-quarters of the 2,800,000 acres of hay made in England was of sub-maintenance quality. 'Average quality is inadequate for the bare maintenance of an average Friesian cow, which will require 0.9 kg (2 lb) of cereal supplement.' At the other extreme is hay with a crude protein content of 19.98 per cent which obtained for the Hillsborough Research Station, Northern Ireland, a daily liveweight gain of 1 kg (2.14 1b) daily in bullocks fed hay only.

Mouldy hay can be dangerous. (See ASPERGILLOSIS and FARMER'S LUNG.) Hay which contains sweet clovers, or vernal, and has become overheated or mouldy, may have a dangerously high DICOUMAROL content. Fatal poisoning has also occurred in stock fed hay containing RAGWORT or FOXGLOVES.

Hay, soaking Contrary to popular belief, dampening hay does not control mould and fungal spores. However, it reduces the amount of dust produced and thus may help respiratory conditions in horses fed hay. The hay is netted, then soaked for about 15 minutes; longer soaking is of no benefit and may be detrimental to the quality of the hay.

Hay Fever
(see ATOPIC DISEASE)

Hayflakes
In appearance, hayflakes resemble chopped hay but retain the quality of dried grass. They are not chopped so short that the fibrous quality of grass is destroyed, nor so long that storage space becomes difficult. They can be stored loose in the barn for self- or easy feeding; alteratively they can be baled.

Haylage
Haylage is a registered trade name for material which has been wilted down to 40 to 50 per cent dry matter, precision-chopped to 12 cm (½ inch) nominal length, and processed through a Harvestore tower silo.

Hch
Hexachlorocyclohexane. (See BHC, which consists of 5 isomers of HCH.) In Britain HCH-containing sheep dips have been withdrawn from the approved list.

Headfly
(see under FLIES)

Head Injuries
These may result in concussion (see under BRAIN, DISEASES OF) or secondary EPILEPSY in the dog. Lesions may include an intracranial haematoma, a depressed fracture of the skull, scar tissue, etc.

Head-Tilting
In cats this sign occurs in cases of a foreign body present in an ear. (See EAR, DISEASES OF – Shaking the head; also FELINE VESTIBULAR SYNDROME.)

Healing of Wounds
(see WOUNDS)

Health Schemes for Farm Animals
Private or officially run programmes by which the veterinary surgeon is closely involved in the health and productivity of livestock. In consultation with the farmer, all aspects of health and nutrition are monitored and medication prescribed on the basis of preventing disease, rather than curing it after an outbreak. Such schemes can lead to increased profitability, especially in the large units which are commonplace today.

Currently on farms in the UK a variety of health schemes are in operation, either private, government, or operated in conjunction with large retailing groups. For example, many large dairy units receive routine weekly or fortnightly visits, when cows are presented to the veterinary surgeon for pregnancy diagnosis and treatment of disease or advice on preventive measures, and testing and certification of freedom from infectious bovine rhinotracheitis (IBR), bovine viral diarrhoea (BVD), *Leptospirosis hardjo* and *Mycobacterium paratuberculosis* (as well as officially notifiable diseases).

In sheep, testing is possible for enzootic (chlamydial) abortion, maedi/visna, ovine pulmonary adenomatosis. Advice on management and nutrition, worming programmes and disease prevention can be routinely part of any health programme.

Pigs had the first official health scheme. The pig health scheme evolved into Farm Assured British (FAB) pigs, in which private and ministry veterinarians visit farms quarterly to assess the health status and welfare of pigs.

The importance of maintaining good health in their flocks has long been recognised by poultry farmers. Routine visits are the norm and some large producers employ their own veterinarians to produce protocols for maintaining the health of their flocks.

In the USA, Canada and other parts of the world where large-scale farming is practised, many dairy, poultry and pig farmers have produced, with their veterinarians, management and health protocols for their stock. These set out in detail how the animals are to be looked after and treated, and when veterinary assistance has to be sought.

Hearing
(see EAR – The act of hearing; also ULTRASOUND and TELEVISION SETS)

Heartbeat
(see PULSE RATE)

Heart Diseases
As in man, heart troubles are very much more common in old age. However, even young animals may suffer from faulty heart action due to congenital defects.

Signs Irregularity in the heartbeat, some difficulty in breathing without obvious changes in the lungs or pleura, breathlessness when the animals are compelled to exert themselves, a tendency to swelling of the dependent parts of the body (e.g. along the lower line of the chest and abdomen and 'filling' of the limbs), are among the signs. A cough is sometimes a symptom of valvular disease.

Congestive heart failure Disease of the right side of the heart often gives rise to ascites, sometimes to swelling of one or more limbs due to oedema. Engorgement of the veins often occurs, with enlargement of the liver. The animal becomes easily tired and may lose weight. Ultimately congestive heart failure is likely to occur. This may also result from left-sided failure due to myocarditis or mitral valve incompetence. In small animals, treatment consists in reducing exercise and giving diuretics.

A common cause of heart failure in dogs is degeneration of a MITRAL VALVE.

Pericarditis is an inflammation of the membrane covering the exterior of the heart. It may be 'idiopathic', when its cause is not known; it may be 'traumatic', when it is due to a wound; or it may follow a general infection (e.g. 'heartwater') or a local infection (e.g. pleurisy) or an abscess in a remote part of the body. Pericarditis may be 'dry', in which case the 2 opposing surfaces of the membrane are covered by a layer of fibrin; or oedema may accompany this condition, in which case fluid fills up the pericardial sac and, when no more distension of the sac can occur, presses upon the outside of the heart itself.

Pericarditis has been reported in very young pigs at grass. The piglet, often in good condition and not anaemic, dies suddenly at about 2 to 3 weeks of age. (See also 'MULBERRY HEART'.)

Tamponade A rapid accumulation of blood in the pericardium, suddenly arresting heart function.

Acute or chronic tamponade was the presenting sign in 42 cases of pericardial effusion in a series of large dogs with an average age of 9 years. Twenty-four of the cases were associated with neoplasia, 8 with benign idiopathic effusions, 6 with primary heart disease, and 2 with trauma.

Echocardiography was found to be the best way of detecting pericardial effusion; and the idiopathic effusions responded well to pericardiectomy.

Congenital heart disease in dogs and cats is usually indicated by a cardiac murmur, the site and nature of which shows whether a valve or a shunt is involved.

Shunts include 'holes' in the heart, and patent *ductus arteriosus*.

Radiography and Doppler ultrasound are helpful in diagnosis.

Surveys of a total of 580 dogs with congenital heart disease showed that 28 per cent had patent *ductus arteriosus*; 16 per cent had pulmonary stenosis; 9 per cent had persistent right aortic arch; over 7 per cent had a ventricular septal defect; and over 7 per cent had stenosis of the aorta. (See also HEARTWORMS.)

Deficiency of vitamin E is one cause of sudden cardiac arrest in cattle.

Signs These are not always characteristic, but they include breathlessness, pain on pressure of the left side of the chest, a jugular pulse (seen along the jugular furrow with each heartbeat), and oedema. On listening to the heart a variation in the normal sounds may be heard, or they may be altogether masked by the presence of the fluid. A tinkle is sometimes audible over the region of the heart; friction sounds indicate the presence of dry pericarditis; and irregularity or even palpitation may be noticed.

Traumatic pericarditis of cattle Sometimes when the animal is thought to be suffering from simple digestive disturbance, it is found that a nail or piece of wire has been swallowed and arrives in the reticulum.

A distance of about only 5 cm separates the heart from the reticulum, so that the foreign body is liable to penetrate the pericardium.

Attacks of pain may occur, the appetite is irregular, but after a time the animal regains its normal health, since an adhesion has occurred around the hole in the reticulum wall, and the inflammation subsides. A cow may die suddenly before symptoms of pericarditis appear, or soon afterwards.

Treatment is sometimes feasible by surgically opening the rumen and removing the piece of metal.

Prevention In Switzerland the percentage of cows slaughtered on account of traumatic pericarditis was reduced following the use of magnets for the treatment of traumatic reticulitis. Magnets weighing 114 g, 90 mm long and 15 mm in diameter were used orally 10 minutes after a subcutaneous injection of atropine sulphate. Without this it was found that only 53 per cent of the magnets dropped at once into the reticulum. The correct siting of the magnets was checked with a compass.

Myocarditis is inflammation of the heart muscle. In the pig it is seen in HERZTOD disease, for example; in cattle, in MUSCULAR DYSTROPHY. (See also CANINE PARVOVIRUS; MYOCARDIUM.)

Endocarditis is an inflammation of the membrane lining the heart. It frequently leads to the development of nodules on the valves.

The nodules result in an incomplete closing of the valves, and since the fibrin deposited upon them tends to become converted into fibrous tissue ('organised'), the growths slowly increase in size. They are seen in chronic erysipelas of pigs. (See SWINE ERYSIPELAS.)

The valvular insufficiency can be diagnosed by auscultation. Congestive heart failure may be the outcome (sometimes embolism); but compensation takes place, and the animal may live a long time with faulty valves.

Bacterial endocarditis is a cause of death in cattle, especially in South Wales. (See HEARTWORMS for another cause of endocarditis in the dog.)

Valvular diseases form a most important and common group of heart disorders, and although the power of compensation already referred to may so neutralise the ill-effects of a narrowed valve, or one which leaks, severe strains or exertion – or even trying conditions such as parturition – may precipitate ill-effects. Very often when an animal 'drops dead', perhaps after running a race or while undergoing some departure from its normal mode of life, the actual cause is afterwards found to be a diseased heart valve. Fainting fits are not by any means rare in incompetence of the tricuspid valves. Congestion of the lungs may be brought about by incompetence of the auriculo-ventricular valve on the left side of the heart (mitral insufficiency); this same condition may lead to a chronic asthmatical cough in old dogs, which is occasionally mistaken for bronchitis.

Canine heart repair Skeletal muscle transplants were used to replace or repair defects in the left ventricle of dogs, some of which were kept alive for over a year. At autopsy the transplants were found to be in good condition, according to a report in *Circulation*.

Hypertrophy, or enlargement of the heart, takes place as the result of some constant simple strain, such as occurs in racehorses, hunters, and sporting dogs; or as the result of backward pressure from a diseased valve, and which entails the heart muscle 'compensating' for the effects of valvular disease. Alternatively it may be due to resistance to the flow of blood in some diseased organ or tissue which results in high blood pressure. (See COMPENSATION.)

Hypertrophy of the left ventricle, leading to heart failure, may in the dog follow *Leptospira canicola* infection.

Dilatation of the heart may precede hypertrophy, i.e. when it occurs before the heart muscle has had an opportunity to increase to meet the extra demands upon it; and it very frequently follows hypertrophy, especially when there is some disease process at work which hinders the proper nutrition of the heart muscle.

Hypertrophy may be a beneficial condition in any animal, and, except when it is due to valvular trouble, need not cause any worry to the owner. It is sometimes excessive in horses; in some instances the heart may weigh as much as 11 kg (25 lb) instead of the 3 or 3.5 kg (7 or 8 lb) of the normal. Degenerative changes may follow hypertrophy when the animal becomes less active during later life.

Congenital defects These include a patent *ductus arteriosus*. (*See diagram of fetal circulation under* CIRCULATION OF BLOOD; also LIGAMENTUM ARTERIOSUM; ECTOPIA CORDIS.) Tetralogy of Fallot consists of: (1) stenosis of the pulmonary valve; (2) a defect in the septum which separates the 2 ventricles; (3) the aorta over-riding both ventricles; (4) marked hypertrophy of the right ventricle.

The signs are often vague: in kittens, for example, these may be a failure to thrive, and inability to cope with exercise. More serious defects result in the death of newborn kittens.

Functional disorders Palpitation is a condition in which the heart beats fast and strongly, due to fright, for example(*see* tachycardia, below).

Bradycardia is a condition of unusually slow action of the heart. Intermittency or irregularity is an exceedingly common condition among animals, and as a rule appears to cause them no

H

inconvenience whatever. In some horses at rest in the stable the heart constantly misses every 3rd, 4th, or 5th beat, a long pause taking the place of the pulsation, but when at exercise or work the normal rhythm is restored.

Heart-block is a condition in which the conducting mechanism between atrium and ventricle (atrio-ventricular bundle of His) is damaged in whole or part, so that the two beat independently of each other.

Rapid heart action (tachycardia) may have a number of causes including exertion or excitement. It is normally harmless in such cases. It is also seen in diseases which affect the transmission of the heartbeat stimulus.

Cardiac flutter and fibrillation are conditions of great irregularity in the pulse, due to the atria emptying themselves, not by a series of regular waves, but by an irregular series of flutters or twitches instead, which fail to stimulate the ventricles properly.

Five cases of atrial fibrillation were described in horses after racing. In 4 of them, which had performed poorly during their races, the arrhythmias disappeared spontaneously within 24 hours; these cases were regarded as paroxysmal. In the 5th horse, which won its race, the arrhythmia persisted for at least 45 hours after the race and it was regarded as an example of persistent atrial fibrillation. Treatment with quinidine sulphate restored the sinus rhythm. Paroxysmal atrial fibrillation may cause a sudden decrease in racing performance.

Diagnosis of heart disease is based largely on the character of the pulse and heart sounds. Murmurs, for example, indicate valvular incompetence, cardiac dilatation, or congenital lesions. Muffled sounds may indicate fluid in the pericardium (or pleurisy).

Additionally radiography and cardiography are used in diagnosis. (See PACEMAKERS as a possible treatment of some canine patients.)

Heart Stimulants

Drugs used as cardiac stimulants include theophylline, adrenaline, isoprenaline and dobutamine.

Heartwater

Heartwater, also known as BUSH SICKNESS (Boschziekte), VELD SICKNESS, and INAPUNGA, is a specific disease of cattle, sheep, and goats transmitted by the bont-tick (*Amblyomma hebraeum*) in South Africa, and *A. variegatum* in Kenya. The disease is characterised by the accumulation of a large amount of fluid in the pericardial sac and nervous symptoms.

In 1980 the existence of heartwater in many islands of the Caribbean was discovered; previously the disease had been known only in Africa. The tick involved is *A. variegatum*, introduced into Guadeloupe with cattle from Senegal.

Cause Infection of the nymphal or larval stages of the bont-tick with *Rickettsia ruminantium* (*Cowdria ruminantium*) which is transmitted to other animals upon which the tick feeds at a later state of its life-history.

Incubation After sheep and goats have been bitten by infected ticks, a period of between 11 and 18 days elapses before any symptoms are shown; in cattle the disease appears between 20 and 25 days after infestation with ticks. These periods are influenced by the stage of the disease in the animal supplying the infected blood to the ticks, and also by individual susceptibility, which is less in native-bred cattle than in those imported from other countries, and especially those brought from Britain.

Signs

Sheep and goats Sheep and goats at first show nothing more than a rise in temperature (which gradually increases to 41.7°C (107°F), falling each evening a few degrees lower), a general dullness, prostration, and lack of appetite. As these conditions are common to many other diseases, the difficulty of diagnosis is great. The affected animals isolate themselves from the rest of the flock, lie about in secluded spots, cease to ruminate, and when handled or driven are very easily tired and lie down.

Many animals show peculiar nervous symptoms, which vary in different individuals; some may bleat almost continuously; others champ the jaws as if feeding, moving the tongue backward and forward between the lips; others lick the ground; some turn in circles until they finally fall to the ground and lie prostrate or perform galloping movements with their limbs; while others show profuse salivation. Convulsions are not uncommon, especially when the animals are handled. Death usually follows soon after convulsions make their appearance. magesty

Cattle The symptoms in cattle are very similar to those seen in sheep. The nervous form in which peculiar masticatory movements are made by the mouth is common. Animals show a tendency to bite at their feet or legs, especially when lying on the ground, and biting the ground is also seen. A number of animals in the early stages may show a dangerous tendency to charge any human being approaching them. In cattle the disease is usually at its height about the 4th day after the first rise in temperature, and death usually occurs about the 6th day. Hyperacute cases occur in cattle, and the animal is found dead on the veld.

Autopsy Fluid in the pericardial sac surrounding the heart (hence the name 'heartwater'); but while this is usually found in sheep and goats, it may be absent in the case of cattle. In typical instances there is also a collection of similar fluid in the thoracic and abdominal cavities. Both the pericardium and the endocardium which lines the heart may show several small or a few large 'petechiae', i.e. areas where a slight amount of haemorrhage has taken place.

Prevention Entirely successful results have followed measures taken against the ticks which transmit the disease. These consist in '5-day dippings'.

Antibiotics and sulfonamides are used in treatment.

Heartworms

Dirofilaria immitis is a common parasite of dogs in Central Europe, Russia, Australia, America, and Asia. The disease has been introduced into the UK by dogs returning from travel in mainland Europe via the Pet Travel Scheme. The worm larvae are transmitted by various mosquitoes and gnats. They are present in the bloodstream of infected animals as microfilariae. The adult worms reach a length of up to 30.5 cm (12 inches) (females) and inhabit the right side of the heart, causing some degree of endocarditis and a variety of symptoms, e.g. cough, hind-leg weakness, collapse on exercise, laboured breathing, anaemia, emaciation.

This infestation is known as canine filariasis or dirofilariasis. The kidneys and urinary tract may be affected. (See also EYE, DISEASES OF.)

In a survey in Canada, 560 dogs (1.79 per cent of those tested) were found to have heartworms.

About 20 per cent of dogs may be infected with adult worms without having microfilariae.

Heartworms can cause devastating cardiopulmonary effects in cats. The disease may be present without microfilariae, not only during the prepatent period, for adult worms may be males, 'geriatric females', or of 1 sex only.

There have been reports of *dirofilaria* worms being recovered from the brains of cats. One such report referred to a cat with ataxia which died 48 hours later. At autopsy, 3 heartworms were found in the heart, 3 in the brain, and 4 in a kidney.

Diagnosis An ELISA test, based on the detection of antibodies to heartworms, is useful when no microfilariae are present. Radiography has also been recommended as a diagnostic aid.

Treatment and control of 5 dogs dosed with ivermectin 1 day after artificial infection with 50 infective larvae of *D. immitis*, none harboured any heartworms when killed 201 days later. The 5 control dogs had an average of 11 worms each at post-mortem examination. It is suggested that treatment with ivermectin at monthly intervals would prevent heartworm disease.

In the UK selamectin, a derivative of ivermectin, is licensed for use in dogs and thiacetamide has been used on imported dogs.

Another canine heartworm is *Angiostrongylus vasorum* which inhabits the pulmonary artery and the right ventricle of the heart. Symptoms include malaise and large subcutaneous swellings. Slugs and snails may act as intermediate hosts.

In a case seen at the Liverpool School of Tropical Medicine, a 3-year-old dog, which died suddenly after an acute attack of dyspnoea, was found to have an *A. vasorum*.

Heat

A female animal is said to be on heat when it will accept the service of a male (see OESTRUS; for the suppression of 'heat' in the bitch, see OESTRUS, SUPPRESSION OF).

Heat Detection in Cows
(see under OESTRUS, DETECTION OF)

Heat Exhaustion

A syndrome in which there is a depletion of electrolytes and water in the body. (See HEAT-STROKE.)

Heat Loss

Heat loss from the body occurs by radiation, by conduction and convection from the skin, and by evaporation from the skin and lungs. The normal body temperature is controlled partly by alteration of the rate of metabolism, and partly by constriction of the surface blood vessels when the animal is exposed to cold, as well as by shivering which generates heat. There comes a point, however, as body temperature falls still further, at which shivering ceases. Then the danger of hypothermia may not be recognised. (See BEDDING for pigs; also HYPOTHERMIA.)

Sensible loss of heat This is the heat which animals lose by convection, conduction, and radiation. It does not include heat lost by vaporising water from the skin and respiratory passages.

Heat-Stroke

Heat-stroke is a condition associated with excessively hot weather, and especially under conditions of stress. It occurs in domestic animals when taken to tropical countries from temperate countries, especially when recently unloaded from transport ships and subjected to great excitement in unfamiliar surroundings; it is seen in cattle, sheep, and swine travelling by road or rail, and it frequently occurs at agricultural shows; dogs may be affected when they have been left in a car parked in the sun, and with windows closed or almost closed. There is a failure to lower body temperature. (See CAR, PARKED; also HYPERTHERMIA; TROPICS.)

Signs The animal is usually suddenly overcome by a great lethargy and inability to work or move. The gait is staggering, and if the animal is made to move it falls to the ground. Convulsions may occur, and if the temperature is taken it is found to be very high, perhaps as much as 42.2°C (108°F) in the horse. Death often takes place in a few hours, but some cases last as long as 3 days. If recovery occurs, great dullness for a number of weeks is liable to follow.

Treatment Removal to a cool place; douching the head and neck with cold water from a hosepipe. Ice cubes may be used for the smaller animals.

An animal may die as a result of combined heat-stroke and heat exhaustion, or either separately. (See also HEAT EXHAUSTION.)

Hebdomadis Serogroup
(see LEPTOSPIROSIS)

Hedgehogs

Hedgehogs are of veterinary interest in that they are susceptible to natural infection with foot-and-mouth disease, which they transmit to other animals.

Hedgehogs, like horses, are the natural hosts for *Leptospira bratislava*. A possible case of this infection occurred in a dog, previously vaccinated against leptospirosis, but known to have access to hedgehogs.

A UK survey of mortality in hedgehogs (*Erinaceus europaeus*) showed that 47 per cent were road casualties; 39 per cent had salmonellosis. Other zoonoses were ringworm (*Trichophyton erinacei*) and *Yersinia pseudotuberculosis* in a very small proportion of the hedgehogs. Lungworms, flukes (*Brachylaemus erinacei*), tapeworms (*Rodentolepsis erinacei*), ticks, fleas, and mange mites (*Caparinia tripilis*) were other parasites found. Deaths have

been recorded after hedgehogs ate slug bait (metaldehyde).

A safe, simple method of dealing with 'rolled-up' hedgehogs, for the purpose of examination or treatment against external parasites, was described by Dr Nancy Kock, International Wildlife Veterinary Services, California. Her method is to place the animal in an aquarium tank (containing a parasiticide dip solution if needed), when it will immediately unroll and begin swimming. Using protective gloves, the hedgehog can then be grasped by the scruff of its neck like a kitten. Once held firmly like that, it is unable to roll up again, making examination easy.

Anaesthesia Fentanyl citrate + fluanisone (Hypnorm; Janssen) by subcutaneous injection is suitable for anaesthetising hedgehogs.

Heifer
A year-old female up to her 1st calving.

Heinz Bodies

Heinz bodies in red cells are seen in cases of haemolytic anaemia caused by, e.g., an excess of kale in dairy cattle. Heinz-body anaemia has also been seen in cats as a result of poisoning by methylene blue, formerly used in America as a urinary antiseptic. This form of anaemia has been linked with onions, and a case was reported in a puppy which preferred raw onions and other vegetables to conventional dog foods. After a change of diet the puppy became well, and no longer tended to collapse after exercise. Heinz bodies are present in cats poisoned by paracetamol.

Hellebores

There are 4 hellebores of importance to the owners of animals because of their toxicity. *Black hellebore* is the dried rhizome and rootlets of the Christmas rose, or bear's-foot, *Helleborus niger*. It may be eaten by livestock when garden trimmings are thrown out on to fields to which livestock have access. It contains 2 very irritant glycosides – *helleborin* and *helleborein*. *Stinking hellebore* (*H. fetidus*) and *green hellebore* (*H. viridis* or *Veratrum viride*) are sometimes the cause of livestock poisoning. The latter, along with *white hellebore* (*V. album*), contain several alkaloids. They are depressants of the motor nervous centres.

Poisoning by hellebores Symptoms are stupor, convulsions, and death when large amounts have been taken, and purgation, salivation, excessive urination, attempts to vomit, great straining and the evacuation of a frothy mucus, when smaller amounts have been eaten. Cows give milk which has a bitter taste and which is liable to induce diarrhoea or purgation in animals and man drinking it. Rumenotomy in cattle and sheep may be indicated, in order to remove parts of the swallowed plant.

'Western false hellebore' (*Veratrum californicum*) is teratogenic, due to the presence of cyclopamine in its roots and leaves. It causes the deformity known as 'monkey face lamb disease', which can be avoided by preventing pregnant ewes from foraging on the plant. The fetus is also at risk on days 19 to 21 from early embryonic death, and between days 28 and 33 when stenosis of the trachea may result, together with shortening of metacarpal and metatarsal bones. Sheep should be prevented from feeding on the plant until 33 days after the rams have been removed from the flock.

In Idaho, USA, ewes eating 'Western false hellebore' gave birth to lambs with harelip and hydrocephalus.

Helminths
(see ROUNDWORMS; TAPEWORMS; FLUKES)

Hemeralopia
Defective vision in bright light caused by degeneration of the retina (see EYE, DISEASES OF).

Hemimelia
Congenital absence of some or all of the distal part of a limb.

Hemiplegia
Hemiplegia means paralysis limited to 1 side of the body only. (See under GUTTURAL POUCH DISEASE for facial and laryngeal hemiplegia in horses.)

In the cat (and dog), paralysis limited to 1 side of the body may be the result of cerebral thrombosis, haemorrhage, or embolism – plugging of an artery in the brain. The affected cat may fall over (always to the same side), or move in a circle. A tilting of the head and nystagmus (a jerky involuntary movement of the eyeball) have also been recorded. Fortunately, extremely few cat owners will ever encounter these conditions.

Hemivertebrae
Hemivertebrae ('wedge-shaped' vertebrae) are inherited in some breeds of dog. The mechanism of inheritance is not yet known. (See SPINE, DISEASES OF.)

Hemlock Poisoning
As a rule animals will not eat hemlock on account of the mousy odour and disagreeable

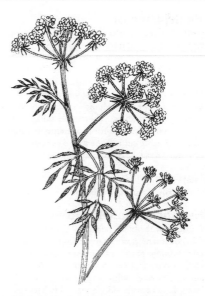

Hemlock (*Conium maculatum*). The flowers are creamy white, and the stem is distinguished by purplish spots. Height: 1.3 to 2 m (4 to 6 ft).

taste, but in the spring, when green herbage is scarce and when the fresh shoots of the plant are plentiful, young cattle are sometimes affected.

The toxic principles of hemlock are a group of volatile alkaloids, the most important being coniine. Others include N-methyloconiine, coniceine, and conhydrine. They are present in the flowers, fruits, and leaves.

Hay containing hemlock is not likely to cause poisoning, owing to the volatility of the alkaloids.

Signs Initial stimulation and then depression of the central nervous system. Dilation of the pupils, weakness and a staggering gait are seen first; later breathing becomes slow and laboured. Before death the animal may be paralysed and unable to rise from the ground, though consciousness usually remains.

The mousy odour, detectable in the breath and urine of poisoned animals, assists diagnosis.

Hemlock poisoning in the pregnant cow can result in deformity in the calf, and the same cause was suspected in piglet deformities where the sow had access to rough grazing.

First-aid (see ALKALOIDS)

Hen Yards
(see under POULTRY)

Henle, Loop of
The U-shaped loop connecting the ascending and descending tubules in the kidneys.

Henneguya
A group of parasites found in the skin and muscles of fish, notably sea trout and salmon. The parasites are seen as tadpole-shaped cysts containing two 'eye-spots'. They cause 'milky flesh disease'. This is seen in fish, apparently healthy, which on being cut into are found to have areas of muscle replaced by a milky fluid.

Heparin
A naturally occurring anticoagulant.

Hepatic Encephalopathy
A disease of the brain caused by cirrhosis of the liver; or it may possibly result from a congenital condition, portosystemic shunt. It is usually seen in dogs and cats but can occur in other animals. Affected animals are lethargic, become blind, have convulsions, ataxia and behavioural changes. The disease is clinically indistinguishable from FELINE SPONGIFORM ENCEPHALOPATHY but blood samples show high ammonia levels. Neomycin may improve the liver condition and a low-protein diet is recommended.

Hepatisation
Hepatisation means the solidified state of the lung that is seen in pneumonia, which gives it the appearance and consistence of the liver.

Hepatitis
Inflammation of the LIVER.

Hepatitis in the horse occurs after infectious equine encephalomyelitis, especially where vaccines or sera have been used. In cattle and sheep, it can occur after liver fluke, ragwort poisoning and aflatoxicosis.

For hepatitis in dogs, see CANINE VIRAL HEPATITIS *and* also under DUCK HEPATITIS.

Hepatozoon
A single-celled parasite transmitted by the tick *Rhipicephalus sanguineus*. *Heptazoon canis* infects both dogs and cats, often causing anaemia, fever, and occasionally paraplegia. Other species infect rodents.

Heptachlor
A constituent of chlordane, a chlorinated hydrocarbon, and used also as an insecticide on its own. It is not used on animals. It is stored in the body fat, and in the tissues is converted into heptachlorepoxide, 4 times as toxic to birds as heptachlor itself.

Herbicides
(see PARAQUAT; DIQUAT; MONOCHLOROACETATE; WEEDKILLERS; POISONING)

Herdsmen
Occupational hazards of those looking after cattle include BRUCELLOSIS; Q FEVER; TUBERCULOSIS; COWPOX; MILKER'S NODULE; SALMONELLOSIS; SPOROTRICHOSIS; BUBONIC PLAGUE (not in the UK).

Heredity
The transfer of genetic traits from parent to offspring (see GENETICS).

Hermaphrodite
An animal in which reproductive tissue of both sexes is present. A lateral hermaphrodite has an ovary on one side, and a testicle on the other; whereas a bilateral hermaphrodite has an ovary and testicle (or a combined ovary-testis) on each side. (See also INTER-SEX.)

In one case, a hermaphrodite rabbit served several females and sired more than 250 young of both sexes. In the next breeding season the rabbit (housed in isolation) became pregnant and produced 7 healthy young of both sexes.

Hernia
The protrusion of part of an organ through the membrane which contains it. In a typical abdominal hernia there are always the following parts: a 'ring', or opening in the muscular wall of the abdomen, which may have been brought about as the result of an accident or may have been present at birth; and a swelling appearing below the skin, composed of the 'hernial sac' and its contents.

The contents vary according to the situation, size, and nature of the hernia, but the following organs or parts of them are most commonly herniated: a loop of bowel with its attached mesentery omentum, either the whole or a part (very common in dogs); the stomach; the urinary bladder; the spleen or liver (through the diaphragm); the uterus, either when non-pregnant or with its contained fetus or fetuses; and sometimes a kidney in the cat.

(For strangulated hernia, *see under* 'Signs', below.)

Umbilical hernia The opening in the abdominal wall is a natural one which should, however, have closed at birth. If given time, it may still do so. In the puppy, for example, only a persistent or irreducible umbilical hernia will need surgical intervention owing to the risk of a piece of omentum having its blood circulation interfered with, or bowel becoming obstructed or strangulated – both serious conditions requiring immediate surgery.

Inguinal hernia, which is practically the same as scrotal hernia, but at a less advanced stage, is almost wholly confined to the male sex in all animals, except the bitch, where a horn of the uterus may, upon occasion, come down through the inguinal canal. Inguinal and scrotal forms of hernia may be either congenital or acquired; congenital forms (most common in young animals) result through some failure of the inguinal canal, through which the testicle descends, to close properly; while acquired forms (commoner in adults) result from such accidents as slipping sideways with the hindfeet, injuries to the abdomen from falls, blows, and kicks.

Femoral hernia is very rare, but sometimes occurs in performing dogs which have been trained to walk upon their hind legs for considerable periods of time. The vertical position of the body imposes an unusual strain upon the muscles at the fold of the thigh, and they give way. It is always acquired.

Perineal hernia is almost exclusively confined to the dog. It may occur in either sex, usually as the result of much straining occasioned by constipation or diarrhoea, chronic coughing or asthma, bronchitis, etc., and in old male dogs suffering from enlarged prostate glands.

Ventral hernia is almost invariably the result of a serious injury to the muscular portion of the abdominal wall. It is commonest in mares, especially those used for breeding purposes. Very often there is little or nothing to be noticed if the mare is injured when nonpregnant, but when pregnancy follows and the tension upon the abdominal wall increases, the muscular part gives way and a large mass appears along the lower line of the abdomen. In cows it very often results from horn-gores from neighbours; in such, the skin remains intact but the muscle is torn and a swelling appears at the seat of the injury. Hernia due to a gore is probably commonest in the region of the flank, where the muscle is naturally thin.

Mesenteric hernia is rare in cattle ('probably because of the thickness of the mesentery') but not in horses. In a case involving a cow, intestine was herniated through a tear or defect in the mesentery, resulting in incarceration. A laparotomy was performed, and the defect

enlarged to permit extrication of the intestine. The cow recovered.

Diaphragmatic hernia may occur in any animal, but is commonest in the dog and the cat. It usually results from jumping downwards from a great height – an act which throws the full weight of the abdominal contents forward against the diaphragm when the animal lands on its feet; it may also occur in road accidents.

The rent may be in the muscular or tendinous portion of the diaphragm, but it very frequently involves one or other of the natural openings (*hiati*), giving passage to the oesophagus, the vena cava, or the aorta, (although a hernia through an enlarged aortic hiatus is very rare on account of the powerful nature of the diaphragm in its upper parts).

Signs The symptoms vary greatly, depending upon the particular organ which is protruded, upon the size of the opening, which may or may not compress the hernia, and upon the condition of the latter. In very many cases among animals, herniae contain either omentum or a loop of bowel, or both. The swelling may be present at birth, or it may appear suddenly or gradually at almost any time during life. To the touch it may present one of several sensations: (1) in the simple form it feels soft, fluctuating (as if it contained fluid), painless, neither hot nor cold, and causes no discomfort to the animal when being handled. If it be pressed upon it can usually be returned to the abdominal cavity, though it will reappear as soon as the pressure is released. In small animals it will disappear when they are laid upon their backs, and remain out of sight until they regain their feet; (2) when the structures are adherent to the skin which covers them, return to the abdomen is impossible, no reduction can be achieved by manipulation, no definite ring can be determined as a rule, and there is no increase in size with exertion, but otherwise an adherent hernia presents the same appearances as a simple one; (3) in the strangulated form, which may supervene upon a hitherto simple hernia, there are very definite and serious symptoms of general disturbance: breathing is fast and distressed, an anxious expression is visible on the face, and the swelling shows a marked tenseness and pain when being handled. It may be red and inflamed-looking at first, but later it frequently becomes bluish. After about 12 to 24 hours gangrene sets in; the swelling becomes cold and painless to the touch; the temperature falls subnormal, and the animal becomes alarmingly weak. Death usually follows shortly after, unless the strangulation is relieved by operation and perhaps amputation of the strangulated portion of bowel. An obstructed hernia is usually merely the preliminary of strangulation.

Treatment Palliative treatment, such as is common in human beings consisting in the application of trusses, bandages, etc., is of no use whatever where animals are concerned. With young animals of any species it is usual to leave herniae alone provided that they are not acute, for it often happens that during the growth and development of the young creature the hernia disappears of its own accord, and the hole in the abdominal wall heals over. There is, however, always a danger that, as the result of some extra exertion, heavy feeding, boisterous playfulness, fighting, etc., strangulation may occur.

The most rational method is one in which the animal is anaesthetised, skin incised, the contents returned to the abdomen, the peritoneal sac obliterated if it is present, the edges of the ring carefully sutured so that they will form a strong union, and finally the skin wound closed.

The operation for a strangulated hernia differs from that for a simple one in that it is necessary to enlarge the tight ring, to allow restoration of the circulation.

Fifty-two perineal hernias in dogs have been successfully repaired by transposing both the internal obturator muscle and the superficial gluteal muscle together. The technique results in a strong pelvic diaphragm and good long-term results. Fewer post-operative complications are claimed to occur than with other techniques.

Herpesviruses

Herpesviruses cause, for example, Aujeszky's disease, jaagsiekte, feline rhinotracheitis. (*See the table above; also under* MONKEYS and FADING.)

Some of the herpesviruses of man, domestic animals and poultry*

Recommended label	Traditional name	Associated disease
Human herpesvirus 1	Herpes simplex type 1	Herpetic sores, etc.
Human herpesvirus 2	Herpes simplex type 2	Genital herpes and cervical cancer
Human herpesvirus 3	Varicella-zoster	Chicken pox and shingles
Human herpesvirus 4	Epstein-Barr virus	Burkitt's lymphoma and infectious mononucleosis (glandular fever)
Canine herpesvirus 1	Canine herpesvirus	Herpes of dogs (neonatal deaths, respiratory infection, genital lesions)
Feline herpesvirus 1	Feline rhinotracheitis virus	Respiratory disease
Equid herpesvirus 1	Equine abortion virus	Abortion
Equid herpesvirus 2	Cytomegalovirus	Nothing or respiratory disease
Equid herpesvirus 3	Coital exanthema virus	Coital exanthema
Equid herpesvirus 4		Respiratory disease
Bovid herpesvirus 1	Infectious bovine rhino-tracheitis/infectious pustular vulvo-vaginitis	Upper respiratory tract infection; vaginitis, abortion, etc.
Bovid herpesvirus 2	Bovine mamillitis virus	Mamillitis and pseudo-lumpy skin disease
Bovid herpesvirus 3	Malignant catarrhal fever virus (wildebeeste herpes virus)	Malignant catarrhal fever in cattle (Africa)
Bovid herpesvirus 4	Jaagsiekte virus pulmonary adenomatosis	Metritis, abortion, respiratory disease
Pig herpesvirus 1	Pseudorabies virus	Aujeszky's disease
Pig herpesvirus 2	Inclusion body rhinitis (cytomegalo) virus	Rhinitis
Phasianid herpesvirus 1	Infectious laryngo-tracheitis virus	Laryngotracheitis in poultry
Phasianid herpesvirus 2	Marek's disease virus	Marek's disease (fowl paralysis)

*Based on the recommendations of the Herpesvirus Study Group, International Committee for the Nomenclature of Viruses, and updated.

Herztod Disease

A heart condition in pigs, it has similarities to MULBERRY HEART. (See PORCINE STRESS SYNDROME.)

Heterokaryon

A cell containing nuclei of 2 different species (an example of genetic engineering). (See GENETICS.)

Heteroplastic Tissue

Heteroplastic tissue is that which is abnormal, different in structure, or different from another individual in the case of a graft (heteroplastid). Heteroplastic bones are those which are not parts of the skeleton, e.g. the *Os penis* in the dog, and the *Os cordis* (one of 2 small bones in the cow's heart). Heteroplasm is normal tissue found in an abnormal situation.

Heterosis

Hybrid vigour.

Heterotopic

Wrongly positioned.

Heterozygous

Relating to a heterozygote, which is produced from unlike GAMETES and has 1 gene (see ALLELES) dominant and the other recessive for a particular characteristic.

Hetp

An organophosphorus insecticide used in agriculture and horticulture. Similar to TEPP.

Hexachlorobenzene

A fungistat used as a seed-dressing, it has given rise to a form of PORPHYRIA in children in Turkey, and might similarly affect livestock.

Hexachlorocyclohexane

The group name for several isomers each having the formula $C_6H_6Cl_6$. The most important of them is BENZENE HEXACHLORIDE. (See HCH; BHC.)

Hexachlorophane

An antiseptic used as an ingredient of medicated soap to kill bacteria on the skin.

Hexamine

Also called methenamine. It is excreted by the kidneys, and as it sets free formalin in an acid medium it has antiseptic qualities when the urine is acid. It may be combined in a tablet with sodium acid phosphate for this purpose in treatment of cystitis in dogs.

Hexamitiasis

An infectious enteritis of turkeys occurring in the USA and Britain.

Cause *Hexamita meleagridis.*

Signs Day-old poults may be affected, but more commonly the disease attacks turkeys a few weeks old. The feathers become ruffled, the birds are listless with drooping wings. The droppings become liquid and frothy. Birds stand silent and motionless with eyes closed. Loss of condition is rapid, with marked dehydration. In young birds mortality may reach 100 per cent. Recovered birds may act as carriers.

Treatment Antibiotics, furazolidone.

Hexoestrol

A synthetic oestrogen said to be more active than stilboestrol. It is banned from use in animals in the EU. (See STILBOESTROL; HORMONES IN MEAT PRODUCTION; STILBENES; CAPONIEATION.)

Hexoses

Hexoses are monosaccharide carbohydrates and include GLUCOSE, fructose, galactose, and mannose. Monosaccharides also include the pentoses, e.g. arabinose, ribose. (See SUGAR.)

Hexylresorcinol

Formerly used as an anthelmintic for roundworms and for fluke.

Hiatus Hernia

Protrusion of (usually) part of the stomach through the diaphragm at the oesophageal hiatus (see under HERNIA).

Hibitane

Chlorhexidine, a valuable disinfectant effective against some bacteria which cause mastitis in cattle.

Hidrosis

Sweat secretion, either normal or abnormally profuse.

High-Rise Syndrome

(see FALLS FROM HIGH BUILDINGS)

Hilum (Incorrectly, Hilus)

Hilum (incorrectly, hilus) is a term applied to the depression on organs such as the lung, kidney, and spleen, at which the vessels and nerves enter or leave, and round which the lymph nodes cluster.

Hinny
The offspring of a stallion and a female ass.

Hip Dysplasia in Dogs
This term covers a number of abnormal conditions of the acetabulum and head of the femur.

Some of these conditions are hereditary. They include:

(1) Subluxation, in which the head of the femur is no longer firmly seated within the acetabulum. Deformity of the head of the femur gradually develops. The symptoms include a reluctance to rise from the sitting position, and a sawing gait, observed when the puppy (most often an Alsatian, sometimes a golden retriever or boxer) is 4 or 5 months old.

(2) Osteochondritis dissecans is seen in terriers with short legs, poodles, and Pekingese. It is possibly identical with Perthe's disease. Muscular wasting and lameness are observed, usually in 1 limb.

(3) Slipped epiphysis. This also causes pain and lameness at 4 to 6 months, but is difficult to distinguish from (2).

(4) Congenital dislocation, in which the acetabula are too shallow to retain the heads of the femurs in position. Reported in the Black Labrador. A false joint forms in time. (See also PERTHE'S DISEASE.)

The BVA and the Kennel Club jointly run a scheme whereby X-rays of a dog's hip-joint are examined by a panel of experts and given a score according to the condition of the joint. The intention is that dogs showing a tendency to dysplasia will not be used for breeding.

Hip-Joint
The joint formed between the head of the femur, or thigh-bone, and the depression on the side of the pelvis called the acetabulum.

Histaminase
An enzyme obtained from extracts of kidney and intestinal mucosa, capable of inactivating histamine and other diamines. It has been used in treating anaphylactic shock and other allergic conditions due to, or accompanied by, the liberation of histamine in the body.

Histamine
An amine occurring as a decomposition product of histidine (see AMINO ACIDS) and prepared synthetically from it. Histamine is widely distributed in an inactive compound form in the body, particularly in the lungs, liver, and to a lesser extent in blood and muscle. As a result of trauma, burns, or infection, it may be liberated from the skin, lungs, and other tissues.

Histamine dilates capillaries, reduces blood pressure, increases any tendency to oedema, stimulates visceral muscles and gastric and pancreatic secretions. Histamine toxicity is shown by engorgement of the liver, shock, and a tendency to urticaria-like skin lesions. (See also ANTIHISTAMINES; ALLERGY; MAST CELLS.)

Histidine
An amino acid from which histamine is derived by bacterial decomposition.

Histiocytes
Another name for macrophages. (See under BLOOD – Leukocytes.)

Histiocytosis A condition resulting from an excess of histiocytes in the bloodstream. It affects some breeds of dog, e.g. Bernese mountain dogs. Clinical signs vary from anaemia and respiratory disease in the malignant form to itchy skin patches.

Histocompatibility
The ability of a cell or tissue transplant to be accepted by a different animal. Histocompatible antigens are present in most tissue cells. They are the cause of the rejection of transplants. (See MAJOR HISTOCOMPATIBILITY SYSTEM.)

Histomoniosis
(see BLACKHEAD)

Histoplasmosis
A fungal disease, caused by *Histoplasma capsulata*, which gives rise to loss of appetite, diarrhoea, emaciation, and liver enlargement. It occurs chiefly in dogs and man. In man, often infected by venturing into bat-infested caves in Central and South America, and in Africa, lesions first occur in the lungs, but – in serious cases – other organs may be affected.

The mycelial phase, found in soil, produces 2 kinds of spore: *microconidia* and *macronidia*. The latter enter the body by inhalation.

Hock
Hock is the tarsus, a joint composed of 6 or 7 bones, between the tibia and the cannon bone of the hindlimb. (See under BONE.)

Hodgkin's Disease
Hodgkin's disease is a form of cancer involving the lymph nodes, bone marrow and sometimes other tissues.

Hog
A male pig after being castrated.

Hog Cholera
(see SWINE FEVER)

Hogg
Sheep up to the 1st shearing. (See also under SHEEP.)

Hogget
(see under SHEEP)

Hogweed
(see under GIANT)

Holly (Ilex)
Holly leaves eaten by lambs have caused deaths by obstructing the pharynx and larynx. One farmer lost 5 good lambs in 3 weeks while they had been grazing under holly trees.

Holoprosencephaly
A rare congenital brain malformation, accompanied by various facial deformities. The condition appears to be inherited in an autosomal recessive manner.

Holstein-Friesian
This breed of cattle in the USA and Canada has its origin in animals imported from the Netherlands mostly between 1857 and 1887. They are also known as American or Canadian Holsteins or Friesians.

Homatropine
Homatropine is an artificial alkaloid prepared from atropine. It is used to dilate the pupil of the eye for careful examination of the deeper parts of that structure. It does not interfere with vision for such a length of time as does atropine.

Homeostasis
Maintenance of the body fluids (as opposed to fluid within cells) at the correct pH and chemical composition.

Homograft Reaction
The process by which an animal rejects grafts of another's tissue. (See IMMUNE RESPONSE and KIDNEYS – Function.) The term 'allograft' is now regarded as preferable to 'homograft'.

Homozygous
(see GENETICS)

Honey
This appears to have an antibiotic effect and to be a successful dressing for bed sores in human patients. Some honeys contain PYRROLIZIDINE ALKALOIDS.

Hoof
(see FOOT OF THE HORSE)

Hoof-Prints
Hoof-prints, and other places where the soil is exposed below the turf, are on wet pastures a common habitat of the snails which act as intermediate hosts of the liver-fluke. Dressing with 12.5 kg (28 1b) of finely powdered bluestone (copper sulphate), mixed with 50 kg (1 cwt) of dry sand, to the acre (0.4 hectare), will reduce the snail population if done each year in June and repeated in August.

Hoof Repair with Plastics
Plastic material, consisting of acrylic resin with a filler, can be bonded with the horn, so that this can be built up. Cracks, deformities, and cavities can be repaired, using one or other of the proprietary preparations marketed. With one type, the acrylic assumes in about 5 minutes the hardness of wall horn; with the other, that of the frog tissue. The former can be rasped and nailed; the latter rasped or trimmed with a knife. Large defects should be repaired with a series of layers in order to avoid damage from heat generated by the process.

Hookworms
These include *Uncinaria stenocephala*, present in temperate regions (including the UK), and the more pathogenic *Ancylostoma caninum* in warmer climates. Infestation occurs either through skin penetration or by ingestion of larvae in bitch's milk, etc. (See also ROUNDWORMS.)

Hoose
(see PARASITIC BRONCHITIS)

Hordeolum
A stye. (See EYE, DISEASES OF.)

Hormone Therapy
Hormone therapy is of value in cases where a true endocrine failure or imbalance is at fault, but it is obviously not a panacea. Moreover, the indiscriminate use of hormones is fraught with danger, and if persisted with may give rise to the production of ANTIHORMONES. Therapy should be carried out by a veterinary surgeon only.

The uses of insulin, thyroxine, adrenaline, and pituitrin are described under these headings, and extracts of thyroid and parathyroid gland are similarly dealt with. Apart from these, considerable use is made in veterinary practice of the sex hormones. (See HORMONES.)

Chorionic gonadotrophin is used in the treatment of nymphomania due to cystic ovaries, of cryptorchidism, and also of pyometra and of some cases of infertility due to a deficiency of luteinising hormone. In the mare and cow a single dose given intramuscularly will usually correct nymphomania.

Serum gonadotrophin (PMS) is used in cases of anoestrus and infertility, and to obtain an extra crop of lambs. (PMS = pregnant mare's serum.)

Progesterone is used to prevent abortion or resorption of the fetus occurring as a result of luteal deficiency. It is also used to treat cases of cystic ovaries, and may be tried to relieve uterine haemorrhage. Luteal hormone preparations are given either intramuscularly (if in oil) or by implantation (if in tablet or pellet form).

Synthetic oestrogens were formerly used in cases of retention of the afterbirth, in some cases of pyometra, uterine inertia and dystokia, and in order to cut short lactation. Some synthetic oestrogens can be given by the mouth. In the dog, stilboestrol was used in treating enlarged prostate; in the bitch stilboestrol diproprionate may be used by intramuscular injection after mating to prevent conception.

Testosterone propionate is of use in sexually underdeveloped young males, and in adult males it may be given to improve fertility or to overcome impotence. In castrated or androgendeficient males it may be of service in obesity, alopecia, and possibly eczema. In the female it may be used to cut short oestrus in racing bitches and mares, to suppress lactation, and in the treatment of pyometra. It has been used with success in the treatment of alopecia (baldness) in spayed cats and also in the bitch (non-spayed). (See CORTICOSTEROIDS; SYNCHRONISATION OF OESTRUS.)

Hormones

Hormones are substances which upon absorption into the bloodstream influence the action of tissues or organs other than those in which they were produced. The internal secretions of the ovary, testicles, thyroid, parathyroid, adrenal, pituitary body, and the pancreas are examples of hormones. (See ENDOCRINE GLANDS.) The placenta is also a source of one or more hormones.

Most animal hormones are either polypeptides (small proteins) or steroids, and the 2 groups have different modes of action.

The interaction of the hormones is far-reaching and complex. In health, a delicate balance – the 'endocrine balance' – is maintained. In ill-health this balance may be disturbed by an insufficiency of a particular hormone or by excess of another. Some hormones are antagonistic to

each other, so that an excess of one amounts to much the same thing as too little of another. In some conditions, such as 'milk fever' in the cow, a number of endocrine glands are believed to be involved – the imbalance being far from a simple one. The thyroid might be regarded as the 'master gland'; its secretion profoundly influences growth, sexual development, immunity, and the rate of metabolism. Yet the thyroid is itself stimulated by a hormone secreted by the anterior pituitary gland – an example which illustrates the interdependence of the whole endocrine system.

An animal's disposition and its hormone secretions are closely linked. Fear or anger, for example, will cause an outpouring of adrenaline – the 'fight or flee' hormone. And, probably, the animal's 'endocrine make-up' determines to some extent its capacity for, or tendency to, anger, fear, etc., as it does for sexual appetite.

Insulin (see PANCREAS; DIABETES; HORMONE THERAPY).

Glucagon (see PANCREAS).

Thyroxine (see under this heading and THYROID GLAND).

Adrenaline (see under this heading and ADRENAL GLANDS).

Aldosterone (see under this heading and ADRENAL GLANDS). (See also GLUCOCORTICOIDS.)

Hormones of the anterior pituitary lobe stimulate the gonads (gonadotrophin), thyroid, adrenals, the skeleton, milk secretion, etc.

Pituitary gonadotrophin influences both the ovary and the testis. In the latter it stimulates development of the sperm-secreting tissue and of actual sperm production, and of the interstitial tissue and the secretion of male sex hormones. In the ovary it stimulates growth of the ovarian follicles and development of corpora lutea. Pituitary gonadotrophin is thus considered as having 2 parts or principles: FSH (follicle stimulating hormone) and LH (luteinising hormone).

Chorionic gonadotrophin. This is a hormone resembling that of the anterior pituitary, but formed in the placenta and excreted in the urine of pregnant women. The action of this hormone is predominantly luteinising.

Serum gonadotrophin (PMS) is a hormone similar to the above but predominantly folliclestimulating, obtained from the serum of pregnant mares.

Pituitrin is the hormone from the posterior lobe of the pituitary, and comprises a pressor principle (vasopressin), which acts upon the heart and circulation, causing a rise in blood pressure, and an oxytocic principle (oxytocin) which stimulates involuntary muscles such as those of the intestines and of the uterus (when pregnant). (See also under ANTI-DIURETIC HORMONE.)

Natural oestrogens are hormones obtained from the follicles of the ovary and include oestrin and its chemical variants oestrone, oestriol, oestradiol, etc. At puberty oestrin brings about development of the teats, udder, vagina, etc. Oestrin is, to some extent, antagonistic to luteal hormone and the parathyroid secretion.

Synthetic oestrogens have a similar effect to the above. They include stilboestrol, hexoestrol, and dienoestrol.

Progestin, progesterone, or the luteal hormone is produced by the corpus luteum. This hormone, stimulates preparation of the lining of the uterus for pregnancy, and by counteracting other hormones ensures the undisturbed maintenance of the gravid uterus; meanwhile suppressing oestrus, and – with the oestrogens – stimulates development of the udder and onset of lactation.

Androgens are sex hormones, e.g. testosterone secreted by the testes, and hormone(s) secreted by the adrenal supplementing, it seems, the action of testosterone. The latter is responsible for the development of secondary sexual characters, is capable of counteracting the female sex hormones, and apparently inhibits the deposition of fat.

Hormones in Meat Production

Hormonal preparations, such as stilboestrol, were formerly used to improve meat production. Often administered in unauthorised doses, serious health problems resulted in the animals and in the humans consuming the meat produced. The use of stilboestrol and similar hormones was banned.

ANABOLIC STEROIDS such as trenbolone became popular in the 1970s. They were claimed to have only slight side-effects, and improved food-conversion efficiency. However, their use as growth promoters is banned in livestock in the EU. They are used clinically in debilitating diseases, anaemia, renal failure and to promote tissue repair.

(See GROWTH PROMOTERS.)

Horn Fly

Lyperosia irritans is a parasite of cattle in America, Hawaii, and Europe. Heavy infestations of cattle have been reported in the UK. (See FLIES.)

Horner's Syndrome

(see EYE, DISEASES OF)

Horns, Injuries to

In the horned breeds of cattle, sheep, and goats, injuries to the horns are not uncommon. In spite of the great strength of the horns of cattle, fracture of the horn cores, from fighting, collision, etc., may arise with comparative ease when the force has been applied in a lateral or transverse manner. Frequently the horn itself remains apparently intact, but the bony core is fractured, and the injury is not suspected until it is noticed that the animal is bleeding profusely from 1 nostril, i.e. that on the same side as the injured horn. Sometimes the tip of a horn may be broken clean off, and the external haemorrhage is liable to be alarming.

Horse Bots

Maggots of the common horse bot fly. Horse bots have been known to infect the liver, causing hepatitis and jaundice.

As bot flies have only 1 generation per year, it has been suggested that a single annual treatment of horses, preferably during early winter, would remove most, if not all, the bots. (See under FLIES.)

Haloxon in the feed or paste preparations of IVERMECTIN are used for the control of bots.

A survey carried out in Ireland showed that during the months of October to May (inclusive), 90 per cent of horses slaughtered at an abattoir near Dublin, and just under 67 per cent of those at an abattoir near Belfast, were infected with *Gastrophilus intestinalis*. Over 28 per cent of horses at the former abattoir harboured *G. nasalis*; but none of those in the Ulster abattoir.

Horse-Meat

Uncooked liver, lungs, etc. may be a source of the hydatid cysts of the tapeworm *Echinococcus granulosus* of the dog. The diaphragm may harbour *Trichinella spiralis* and, though this parasite is unknown in the UK, horse-meat may have to be examined for it.

Dogs and cats have occasionally been poisoned, some fatally, after being fed horse-meat containing barbiturates or chloral hydrate (administered to the horse for purposes of euthanasia). Signs include drowsiness and muscular incoordination.

Human cases of TRICHINOSIS have followed the eating of horse-meat served rare.

Horse-Pox

(see POX)

Horse-Sickness, African

This is a NOTIFIABLE DISEASE throughout the EU. It is a viral disease transmitted by midges.

In Africa, the species is *Culiodes imicola*; with climate changes, this midge has expanded northwards and the disease is present along the north African coast. *Culicoides nebeculosus* can also transmit the disease, but not so successfully; however, it is able to spread into more temperate areas. Europe is at risk via the Straits of Gibraltar, the Middle East or the Balkans.

Signs The acute form of the disease is a severe respiratory condition with the horses literally 'drowning in their own juices'. A chronic form is seen as a cardiovascular problem. Subacute forms show both cardiac and respiratory symptoms.

Treatment All that can be done is to treat the symptoms.

Prevention Horses must be protected against night-flying insects. Vaccines can be used but they must be prepared from local strains of virus. **NB The statutory surveillance zone around an infected horse is 150 km: it follows that disease does not have to reach the UK before a surveillance zone has to be established there.**

Horse-Tails, Poisoning by
In different localities and under different conditions there may be considerable variation in the chemical composition of species of *Equisetum*, with results accordingly. It would appear that on the continent of Europe and in Britain, *E. palustre* and *E. sylvaticum* are the most dangerous, and that in America *E. arvense* is most to be feared, particularly when they are fed among hay. (See also BRACKEN POISONING; THIAMIN.)

Horses, Back Troubles in
A deterioration in a horse's performance or ability to jump may be the result of chronic back pain or discomfort. This may alter the animal's behaviour or temperament. Some may become fractious when handled or worked; some may resent any weight on their backs at all. When investigating back problems, it is essential for a complete history of the animal to be taken, since problems in schooling and equitation may be the real trouble, and to rule these out details of management, tack, performance, and previous temperament need to be studied.

The thoracic and lumbar regions of the spine are commonly involved. Lesions may be grouped as shown in the table.

In one study, 3 types of ACUPUNCTURE were found to be equally useful in the treatment of horses with chronic back pain. Three groups of 15 horses suffering from this condition for between 2 and 108 months were treated by: (1) needle acupuncture (once a week for 8 weeks); or (2) laser acupuncture (once a week for 11 weeks); or (3) injection acupuncture (once a week for 9 weeks). Pain was reduced in 13 horses in group l; in 11 in group 2; and in 13 in group 3; they were able to resume training and competition work.

Horses, Common Causes of Death in
Records of consecutive post-mortem examinations, carried out at the University of Liverpool Veterinary Field Station between 1958 and 1980, showed that in 480 horses the following conditions accounted for 10 or more deaths:

Alimentary system. Perforations, 21; specific and non-specific enteritis, 21; volvuli, 18; strangulated hernias, 15; malabsorption due to atrophic enteropathy, 14; intestinal obstructions, 13; parasitic enteritis, 12; (e.g. cyathostome larvae).

Nervous system. Grass sickness, 51.

Cardiovascular system. Verminous arteritis, 14; haemorrhage, 13.

Haemopoetic system. Lymphosarcoma, 12.

Miscellaneous. Pyaemia or septicaemia, 14.

The following conditions were not considered to have caused death in the 480 horses, but were found 30 times or more:

Alimentary system. Parasitic peritonitis, 93; gastrophilus larval infestation, 82; parasitic enteritis, 54; hepatic hydatidosis, 44; gastric ulceration with no gastrophilus present, 37.

Major causes of back troubles in horses. (With acknowledgements to Professor L. Jeffcott.)

DEFORMITY OF VERTEBRAL COLUMN	Scoliosis, lordosis, kyphosis, synostosis (congential vertebral fusion).
SOFT-TISSUE INJURIES	Strain/damage to supraspinous ligament of the back; myositis; or cramp; sacroiliac strain.
FRACTURES	Dorsal spinous processes – single or multiple; bodies of vertebrae and neural arch.
OTHER BONE DAMAGE	Ossifying spondylosis; crowding or overriding of the dorsal spinous processes; osteoarthritis and fusing of the dorsal spines, transverse and articular processes.
MISCELLANEOUS	Skin lesions – sitfasts; warbles beneath saddle area.

H

Cardiovascular system. Verminous arteritis, 146.

Respiratory system. Pneumonia, 31.

Horses, Diseases of

These include: acne, contagious; aneurysm; anhidrosis; anthrax; asthma; azoturia; blouwildebeesoog; blue nose disease; borna disease; 'broken wind'; brucellosis; chronic catarrhal enteritis; colic; Comeny's infectious paralysis; coronary thrombosis; cyathostomiasis; dourine; entéqué seco; epizootic lymphangitis; equine biliary fever; equine contagious metritis; equine contagious pleuropneumonia; equine ehrlichiosis; equine encephalomyelitis; equine filariasis; equine genital infections; equine infectious anaemia; equine piroplasmosis; equine rhinopneumonitis; equine verminous arteritis; equine viral arteritis; fistulous withers; foals, diseases of; glanders; grass sickness; grease; guttural pouch diphtheria; horses, back diseases in; horses, loss of condition in; horses, spinal cord disease in; horses, worms in; horse sickness, African; hyperlipaemia;

Japanese B encephalitis; Kimberley horse disease; laminitis; louping-ill; mal de caderas; mal du coit; periodic ophthalmia; 'poll evil'; potomac horse fever; pox; purpura; rabies; rhinosporidiosis; senkobo; strangles; stringhalt; summer sores; tetanus; tuberculosis; Tyzzer's disease; ulcerative lymphangitis; urticaria. (See under these headings and also under RACEHORSES; 'ROARING'; EPIGLOTTIS; TRANSIT TETANY.)

There have been cases of Q FEVER in Iran.

Diseases of the equine liver (see RAG-
WORT POISONING; LIVER-FLUKES; AFLATOXINS; HYDATID DISEASE)

Horses, Feeding of

Horses at grass are likely to be contented horses, for they can feed at intervals during both day and night (as they do in the wild state), with exercise as an appetizer. A stabled horse is denied these opportunities. (However, horses do need shelter in winter – or at least to be rugged.)

Horses are fussy feeders, and can be affected by the age, composition and type of pasture – all of which influence dry matter intake. (For grasses most suitable for horses, see PASTURE MANAGEMENT – Grass varieties.)

With concentrate feed, the aroma, freshness, and physical characteristics influence both initial acceptance and continued consumption.

(See DIET for preparation of feeds, palatability, and deterioration in storage, etc.; also LUCERNE; LINSEED; HAY; HYDROPONIC 'GRASS'.)

The horse can only eat relatively small quantities of feed at a time. The number of feeding times per day should therefore be increased with increasing workload because otherwise the horse cannot get enough feed to cover requirements. In addition, the horse chews its feed thoroughly and therefore requires relatively long feeding times (about 1 hour). A horse under an average workload requires per day about 2 kg feed (air-dry weight) per 100 kg (4 lb 6 oz per 220 lb) bodyweight.

Horses in all phases of life can largely cover their nutrient requirements by sufficiently long daily grazing on a good pasture. If the pasture is of poor quality then the nutrition of horses will be deficient unless supplemented.

Oats are the most widely used cereal for feeding horses; they do not need processing for adults, but should be crimped or rolled for foals. Barley, wheat and maize are used to a lesser extent. Barley should be crimped or rolled, wheat should be rolled, and maize cracked. If included in horse feeds, beans should be split or kibbled.

Cereals are rich in starch, comparatively poor in protein, and mostly provide too little calcium but too much phosphorus. This mineral imbalance is also found in bran, which should not form a significant proportion of the ration.

Hay and oats feed rations are sufficient to cover the requirements of adult horses both for maintenance and for work, gestation and lactation, only if the feed rations are of good quality. If of poor quality, mares in the late phase of gestation may suffer from a deficiency in minerals, whereas lactating mares and young horses may suffer from a deficiency not only in minerals but also in energy and in high-grade digestible crude protein.

For safety reasons (as a safeguard against undetected poor quality of feed rations) it is therefore advisable to supplement both grazing and hay and oats feeding of horses in all phases of life with minerals and trace elements (mineral supplement feed).

Mares at the peak of lactation and young horses up to 6 months after weaning, if they are fed on hay and oats, require feed supplementation with high-energy low-fibre concentrate feed containing high-grade protein, e.g. dried skimmed milk.

Regardless of the stage of life and of performance requirements, all horses should be given all necessary vitamins as a supplement to the feed. This is the only way to avoid uncertainties or actual deficiencies in vitamin supply which may arise owing to the variability of vitamin contents of feedstuffs. In addition, over and above a sufficient supply of minerals, all horses should have free access to common salt in the form of mineral licks.

A way 'to avoid deficiency situations when feeding horses on hay and oats rations is to replace the oats partly or entirely by a compound feed for horses. With such hay/oats/compound feed rations or hay/compound feed rations, no further supplementation is required provided the compound feed contains the necessary ingredients'. (Roche Information Service.)

Maintenance rations Crude protein requirements are relatively low, and can be met by cereal grains. More than half the diet can be hay. Horse hays in the UK average between 4 and 7 per cent crude protein. Energy requirements can be met by good-quality hay.

Growth, lactation and work each have different nutrient requirements. For a horse in work, or lactation, gut capacity is insufficient for energy requirements to be met from bulky, but good-quality, hay.

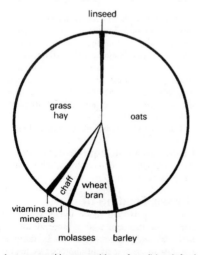

Average weekly composition of traditional feed given to thoroughbreds in training – percentage by weight. (With acknowledgements to David Frape in *In Practice*.)

For growth The protein requirements of a young, growing horse are much greater than those referred to under 'Maintenance rations' above. Both digestibility and amino-acid content are important. Diets containing only poor-quality protein should be supplemented with LYSINE, or some soya could be substituted for linseed.

Pregnant/lactating mares In America under poor range conditions, where grazing provides inadequate protein, feed blocks supplying 50 g urea daily improve a pregnant mare's condition.

During the last 3rd of pregnancy, energy requirements increase above those of maintenance. The mare should still be able to consume daily 1 kg of hay and 0.25 to 0.5 kg cubes per 100 kg of bodyweight. (Levels of feed for thoroughbreds need to be 30 per cent higher than those for pleasure horses.)

During peak lactation a 500 kg mare may produce over 13.5 litres (3 gallons) of milk daily and, if she is also undertaking some work, her energy demands are considerable. Requirements for concentrate cubes during the 3rd month of lactation may reach 250 g to 500 g per 100 kg bodyweight.

Proprietary concentrates are widely used. For novices, these concentrates are a boon, since they are likely to be well balanced. Some concentrates contain soya-bean meal, which is a good source of lysine in which home-mixed rations are often deficient.

Horses do need some long hay in addition to concentrates to provide bulk, assist peristalsis, and mitigate the boredom which can lead to habits such as crib-biting.

In recent years silage has, to a very limited extent, become an item of horses' diet. Care must be taken to avoid any mouldy samples, and it may take a week for a horse to accept silage.

Hydroponics have been used by a few horse-owners, who lay down 8 trays to grow mats of barley seedlings. These are harvested at the 8-day stage, when the flag is 8 or 9 inches high, and growing from a 2-inch accumulation of roots and barley husks. This food is relished, and parasite-free.

Food preferences of ponies Studies of the feed preferences of ponies should help to predict the acceptability and intake of rations containing sucrose, grains or by-product feedstuffs. Given a choice between oats, maize, barley, rye and wheat, 6 mature pony mares preferred oats, with maize ranking 2nd and barley 3rd. Wheat

and barley were liked least, but when the choice was restricted to these 2 grains the ponies' feed intake was not greatly depressed. Given oats or oats plus 2 per cent or 10 per cent sucrose, 4 of 6 pony geldings selected the sweetened oats but 1 disliked sucrose and the other selected from 1 feed bucket regardless of its content. The 6 pony mares preferred a basal diet containing 54 per cent maize, 20 per cent whole oats, 10 per cent wheat bran, 8 per cent soyabean meal, 7 per cent molasses and 1 per cent limestone when it was supplemented with 20 per cent of distillers' grain, but not when it was supplemented with 20 per cent beet pulp, 20 per cent blood meal or 20 per cent meat and bone meal. They did not prefer the same basal diet containing 20 per cent alfalfa meal, although horses are reported to prefer alfalfa pasture to other legumes.

The following rules should be adhered to as far as the feeding of horses in Britain is concerned:

(1) Water before feeding (see WATERING).

(2) Feed in small amounts and as often as the nature of the work or other circumstances will allow.

(3) Do not work immediately after the horse finishes feeding. An hour should be given for a full feed.

(4) Give the 1st feed of the day early, and give the majority of the bulky food at the last feed of the day, so that the horse can eat it at its leisure.

(5) Always buy the best quality of food obtainable; it is false economy to use inferior food-stuffs.

(6) Inspect the teeth periodically, and have any errors corrected at once.

Horses, Identification of

Under the Horse Passports Order 1997, the keeper of any horse born in the UK after January 1, 1998 must have the horse registered with an authorised organisation and receive a passport for it. This has to accompany the animal when it is moved in or out of Great Britain, when it goes to competitions, when it is moved for veterinary treatment, when it is moved to new premises, or for any other purpose. The passport contains an outline silhouette of the animal properly filled in and details of all vaccinations it has been given.

From 1999 it became a requirement of entry into the *General Stud Book* and *Weatherbys Non-Thoroughbred Register* that foals had to be identifiable by means of a microchip implanted in the neck at the same time that the blood sample (for typing) was taken and marking recorded for the animal's passport.

Freeze branding or hoof branding are also used for identification. Semi-feral equines, such as Dartmoor ponies, must be registered on capture.

Horses, Import Controls

There is free movement of horses throughout the EU. Importation of horses into Great Britain is allowed only through 1 of 4 Border Inspection Posts: Heathrow Airport, Immingham Port, Luton Airport and Tilbury Port. Unregistered equidae can be imported through Bristol. Importing a horse elsewhere is an offence, but factors such as the designated airport being fog-bound and the aircraft diverted will be taken into account. Each animal is examined, and if found clinically free from evidence of infectious disease, is free to travel anywhere in the EU. Each horse has to be accompanied by a health certificate. The health certificate accompanying competition horses is valid for 90 days' stay in the EU and does not require proof of freedom from venereal disease, whereas the certificate for permanent residency does.

Horses from the USA must have been tested for evidence of NOTIFIABLE DISEASE. Restrictions may be applied in the case of a new equine disease being identified. For example, in 1996 a respiratory disease was linked to certain race meetings in New England. No horse which had been in contact with any horse involved in those meetings was allowed into the UK until the matter had been cleared up.

The Animals and Animal Products (Import and Export) Regulations 1998 specify the terms of importation.

Horses, Infectious Diseases of
(see HORSES, IMPORT CONTROLS)

Horses, Infertility in
(see CONTAGIOUS EQUINE METRITIS; UTERINE INFECTIONS)

Horses, Loss of Condition in

When ponies and other riding horses lose condition, a veterinary surgeon should be consulted, for the possible causes are many and a professional diagnosis is important. Some pony-owners, inexperienced or otherwise, may be underfeeding their animals, not supplying enough drinking water, or overworking them. Appetite may be depressed because of pain – perhaps in the joints or feet, perhaps associated with brucellosis. The teeth may need attention. Chronic grass disease will result in loss of condition. Migrating red worm larvae may be causing circulatory disturbance, or the animal may have a severe infestation of worms in the intestine. Bots may be present in the stomach. Chronic disease of liver or kidneys may be present; or cancer or tuberculosis. These and many other conditions may be causing the pony to be unthrifty.

A scheme of regular visits by a veterinary surgeon (often on a contract basis) can help to keep horses and ponies in good condition. (See HORSES, DISEASES OF.)

Horses, Lung Haemorrhage

A study carried out at the Animal Health Trust's equine research station confirmed the high incidence of blood pigment present in tracheal washes from 'normal' racehorses, and indicated that exercise-induced subclinical bleeding from the lungs occurs in British as in other racehorses. (See RACEHORSES, EXERCISE.)

Horses, Measurement of

As equine veterinarian D. F. Oliver has pointed out, the precise height of a horse may determine whether it is worth thousands of pounds or only hundreds. 'The value of a horse which "measures in" may well be in the order of £35,000; if "measured out" only £500,' he said. Consequently, there is great pressure on the measurer. The use of a spirit level, to check the level of the ground, is now required in the UK. The horse must be measured from both sides, and the mean taken. Some horses resent the slightest pressure on their withers; others are taught to crouch at such pressure – both making accurate measurement extremely difficult. Horses should be familiarised with the measuring standard. (See HAND.)

Horses should be examined for 'over-preparation of the foot' and measuring postponed if they are found in this condition.

In one study, the heights of 89 horses were measured at the withers before and after half a furlong of trotting exercise. The average height-increase after the exercise was 1.75cm; the horses returning to their 'resting height' within 7 minutes.

Horses, Motor Neuron Disease

This is characterised by a considerable loss of weight, trembling, sweating, and a stiff gait.

Horses, Shoeing

In the UK, horses may only be shod by a farrier registered with the Farriers Registration Council after completing an approved apprenticeship and passing the examination for the Diploma of the Worshipful Company of Farriers.

Horses, Spinal Cord Diseases in

A survey based on 81 horses examined at the New York State College of Veterinary Medicine,

Cornell University, revealed 20 (25 per cent) cases of injury including cervical vertebral stenotic myelopathy (CSM – 11 cases), compressive myelopathy (4), occipitoatlantoaxial malformation (2), cervical vertebral osteomyelitis (2) and cervical injury (1). Of the 37 (45 per cent) inflammatory lesions, equine protozoal myeloencephalitis (EPM) as the most common. Organisms were seen in 16 of the 32 cases. There were also 23 (28 per cent) cases of equine degenerative myeloencephalopathy (EDM).

CSM occurred particularly in young male thoroughbreds and horses that were large for their age and breed. They were identified accurately by measuring (on radiographs) the minimum saggittal diameter at the level of each vertebra (it should exceed 16 mm) and also between adjacent vertebrae in the flexed position (it should exceed 13 mm).

EDM was characterised by the onset of progressive symmetric ataxia, spasticity and paresis in animals, particularly Arabs, under 2 years of age. EDM was distinguished from CSM and other conditions with focal lesions because of differences in the patterns of pelvic and thoracic limb gait deficits.

EPM was most frequent in young mature standardbred and thoroughbred horses in the spring and summer. In addition to ataxia and paresis there is frequently acute to chronic progressive asymmetrical defects in the gait and evidence of sensory deficits, loss of reflexes and muscle atrophy. Tetraplegia was associated with severe lesions in the spinal cord or brain stem. The protozoon parasite involved is probably a coccidian; morphological and serological evidence mitigates against the suggestion that EPM is a form of toxoplasmosis.

Horses, Worms in

The following list shows those adult worms regarded as of most importance.

Adult worms in the intestines:
Strongylus edentatus
S. equinus
S. vulgaris
Triodontophorus spp.
Oesophagodontus robustus

Adult worms mainly in other tissues:
Echinococcus granulosus (larval stage)
Dracunculus medinensis
*Draschia megastoma** (larval stages in the skin)
Dictyocaulus arnfieldi
Fasciola spp.
Habronema spp. (larval stages in the skin)

(See ROUNDWORMS; IVERMECTIN; FLUKES; TAPEWORMS.)

* Frequently, but incorrectly, called *Habronema megastoma*.

Hospital-Acquired Disease
(see NOSOCOMIAL; IATROGENIC; ANTS (Pharaoh's); SALMONELLOSIS)

Hounds
(see MEAT, KNACKER'S; HOOKWORMS; ORF; BOTULISM; HORSE-MEAT; SALMONELLOSIS; AUJESZKY'S DISEASE)

House Decorating, Poisoning
In one case, old lead primer was stripped by means of an electric sander, which dispersed particles of the primer so that the air soon contained a toxic amount of lead. An infant and a cat suffered lead poisoning as a result.

In another case, the purchaser of a house had the downstairs floors professionally treated against woodworm. Six pedigree cats were accordingly kept upstairs for 6 weeks. Even so, 4 weeks after being admitted to the downstairs rooms, 5 of the cats died from dieldrin poisoning.

House Plants
Poisoning in cats and dogs may be caused by the needles from Christmas trees, holly, mistletoe, laurel, oleander, azalea, lily-of-the-valley, rhododendron, honeysuckle and hydrangea. Ingestion of dumb cane (*Dieffenbachia* spp.) causes swelling of the mouth and throat and difficulty in breathing.

Housing of Animals
This is, obviously, a vast subject, and for detailed information reference should be made to specialist texts. (See also TROPICS.)

Two things must be said at the outset. The first is that, generally speaking – given windbreaks, the possibility of shelter in inclement weather and of shade in summer, the avoidance of muddy conditions and of overstocking – animals kept out-of-doors are likely to be healthier than those which are housed for long periods. In the past, housing of animals so often meant overcrowding in dark, damp, draughty or ill-ventilated buildings. Under such conditions disease is almost inevitable – pneumonia or scours in calves; infertility in the bull; agalactia in the sow; mastitis in the dairy cow; respiratory disease in poultry. Parasitic conditions such as lice and mange tend to spread in housed animals, as does ringworm in cattle and horses. Some modern and costly buildings still have ventilation defects, leading to condensation inside and resulting in ill-health of the housed stock. The use of Yorkshire boarding can obviate both the condensation problem and much of the pneumonia.

The second thing is that, from a health point of view, not every 'development' is an advance. Commercial competition may dictate the over-crowding of chickens to the point where feather-picking has to be counteracted by red lighting or de-beaking; this may lead to short-term economic gains, but it is the antithesis of good animal husbandry, and the solving of the veterinary problems raised must be viewed accordingly. Intensivism can surely be pushed to a stage where only a return to good husbandry will succeed in reducing the incidence of disease – and also, incidentally, the size of the drug bill.

On the other hand, the dairy cow has undoubtedly benefited from another dictate of economy – the change from cowshed to the yard-and-parlour system – for instead of being yoked or closely chained for long periods, she is free to move around; and such exercise is in itself important. (See CUBICLES FOR COWS.)

Cattle were housed on slatted floors in England in 1860 – with straw. Their use without straw may lead to welfare problems such as hygromata, damaged teats or injured legs, and housing on wholly slatted floors is not recommended.

Intensivism has led to development in forced-draught ventilation, and to the efficient insulation of walls and roof of animal houses by means of polystyrene, fibreglass, and other substances. Insulated roofs are not usually used for cattle or calves. Housing for poultry and pigs, however, should have roof insulation as well as wall insulation as these animals have a higher critical temperature than ruminants. (See under CONTROLLED ENVIRONMENT.)

It costs over 4 times as much to keep an animal warm by feeding concentrates – 'an internal fuel' – as by warming the livestock house. Minimum economic temperatures are given below.

Housing has an important bearing upon the feeding of animals. Pigs, for instance, confined on concrete have no opportunity for the normal scavenging which can obviate mineral or vitamin deficiencies, and special rations accordingly become necessary for such housed animals. Vitamin A and E deficiencies are particularly likely to occur.

Residual infection is obviously important, and advice is given on this under SALMONELLOSIS and DISINFECTION. In a building used, successively, for calves and pigs, or pigs and turkeys, for example, a cross-infection between the species may arise with a particular strain of *E. coli*. Buildings in which pigs and sheep are

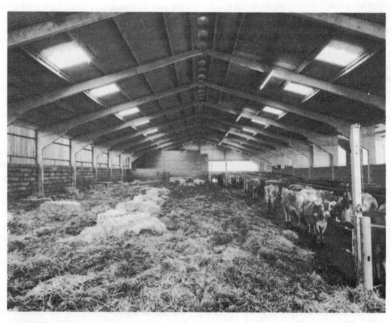

A dairy unit, with lying area, parlour and dairy under one roof. Note the Yorkshire boarding to the left of the picture – a means of ensuring good ventilation and an absence of condensation.

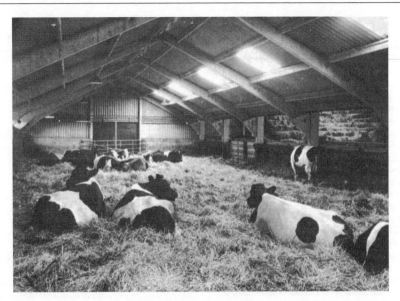

Cattle on deep litter in a covered yard.

housed may carry-over erysipelas; ringworm can pass from cattle to sheep, pigs or horses via an infected building. On land surrounding buildings it is worth remembering that the worm *Trichostrongylus axei* is common to cattle, sheep, horses, and goats.

Cattle An open-ridge method of ventilation is still recommended as the best for cowsheds. In winter, the optimum temperature inside appears to be within 6 and 13°C (44–55°F). Milk yields are said to be depressed when the temperature falls below freezing point. In summer, there is an upper limit of about 25°C (77°F), at which point cattle begin showing distress. High humidity at a temperature above 15.5°C (60°F) appears to diminish milk yield.

For covered yards, ventilators should be provided at the highest point, with a gap of 60 cm (2 ft) between the top of the walls and the eaves. Open-fronted covered yards should not have a gap. About 2 tonnes of straw per cow is required for straw yards in winter.

Pigs Given adequate straw, the most primitive arks on range will yield better results than a cold, damp house. A warm environment will reduce the risk of overlying by the sow. While different optimum temperatures have been given by different research workers, it seems that 21°C (70°F) is about the figure to aim at in the farrowing house. For artificial rearing, a temperature of 30°C (86°F) has been recom-

mended for the first 4 days. Cold, damp floors result in liver disorders which do not appear in buildings where the pigs have a warm, dry bed. Pregnant sows are better not housed. (See CONCRETE; HYPOTHERMIA.)

For fattening pigs, an optimum temperature would appear to be about 18°C (65°F); 15.5°C (60°F) should be the minimum. Humidity does not appear to have an adverse effect, though few authorities recommend it. Good ventilation is advocated.

Sheep In general, the disease problems associated with the housing of sheep have been less serious than might have been expected, and there is a credit side as well as a debit side. For example, if lambs are born and reared to market weight indoors, there is far less risk of worm infestation causing trouble. It is recommended that pens should not contain more than 15 to 25 ewes, grouped according to lambing dates.

Ewes and hoggs housed for the winter after grazing should be wormed during the 1st week. If it is a liver-fluke area, dosing against flukes is advisable 6 weeks after housing.

Lambs must be protected against lamb dysentery, and any from unvaccinated ewes should be given antiserum.

Infestation with lice may be aggravated by housing and spread more rapidly. Since it can cause serious loss of condition, dipping or spraying before housing is recommended.

E. coli infections are as much a threat to the housed lamb as to the housed calf. Overcrowding and dirty conditions at lambing predispose to *coli* septicaemia, which is usually a sequel to navel infection. In early weaned lambs, the quality of the milk substitute is important if scouring is to be avoided; measures should be taken to minimise contact between housed sheep and their dung. Slatted floors, regular cleaning, copious use of bedding material and periodical disinfection all help in this direction.

Good ventilation can go a long way towards reducing the risk of acute pneumonia. In lambs and older sheep this is often associated with *Pasteurella* infection, sometimes aggravated by lungworm infestation. *Pasteurella* pneumonia vaccine may be effective in prevention, but is useless against other forms of pneumonia – which can be caused by other bacteria, moulds, and viruses.

Infections which give rise to abortion may prove more troublesome indoors than out, and vaccination against enzootic (*chlamydial*) abortion seems worthwhile. (See also COPPER POISONING and under SHEEP BREEDING and INTENSIVE.)

Poultry Chickens probably do best at temperatures between 13 and 18°C (55° and 65°F). Egg-production declines at temperatures below 5°C (40°F) or above 23°C (75°F). A relative humidity of 50 per cent is considered the optimum for grown birds. A cold, dry house is better than a warm, wet one. Ventilation requirements vary; for example, a bird may need as much as 300 cm³ (1 cubic foot) per minute per 450 g (1 lb) bodyweight in the hottest weather, but only one-sixth of this in the coldest weather. (See also under CHICKS; NIGHT LIGHTING.)

For other aspects of housing, see under CONCRETE; LEAD POISONING; WOOD PRESERVATIVES; CUBICLES; BULL HOUSING; LOOSE-BOXES; DEEP LITTER; INTENSIVE LIVESTOCK PRODUCTION; YORKSHIRE BOARDING; WATER.

Huckleberry Poisoning
(see GARDEN NIGHTSHADE POISONING)

Humane Destruction of Animals
(see EUTHANASIA)

Humerus
Humerus is the bone of the foreleg between the shoulder-joint and the elbow-joint. It has a rounded head which, with the corresponding depression of the scapula, forms the 'ball-and-socket' shoulder-joint. At the opposite extremity it forms with the radius and ulna the hinged elbow-joint.

Humoral Immunity
Humoral immunity is that conferred by the immunoglobulins derived from the B-cells of the reticulo-endothelial system and is differentiated from cell-mediated immunity associated with T-CELLS. (See also IMMUNE RESPONSE; COLOSTRUM; IMMUNOGLOBULINS.)

Humour
Humour is a term applied to any fluid or semi-fluid tissue of the body, e.g. the aqueous and vitreous humours in the eye.

Husk
Husk is a disease of cattle, sheep, and goats characterised by bronchitis, which is caused by lungworms. (See PARASITIC BRONCHITIS.)

Husky
A muscular, medium-sized dog with a thick double coat. The breed is used to pull sleds in Polar regions and carts in warmer climes. Cart-racing is quite popular; it must not take place on public roads as this would contravene the Protection of Animals Act 1911. Huskies are prone to corneal dystrophy, glaucoma and ventricular heart defects. Haemophilia has been recorded.

Hyaline Membranes
A fibrinous exudate from the epithelium which lines the alveoli of the bronchioles, found in stillborn animals and those dying soon after birth. It is also referred to as hyaline membrane disease.

Hungarian Visla
A medium-sized dog with short, reddish-brown coat and pendulous ears. Few genetic defects are known other than haemophilia A.

Hyaluronidase
An enzyme which breaks down the hyaluronic acid forming part of the material in the interstices of tissue, and so facilitates the absorption of injected fluids. It assists the rapid distribution of drugs injected either subcutaneously or intramuscularly. It has been used in the treatment of urinary calculi.

Hyaluronate
A mucopolysaccharide used as an injection into the joint to treat arthritis.

Hybrid
At one time this word meant a cross between two inbred lines; now it is used to describe a simple cross between 2 different strains or breeds.

For a comparison between a hybrid and a chimera (with reference to fertile mules), see CHIMERA.

Hybrid Vigour

The improved performance produced in the offspring by mating 2 breeds (see GENETICS; BLOOD-TYPING; T-CELLS).

Hybridoma

(see GENETIC ENGINEERING; also under RABIES – Diagnosis)

Hydatid Disease

Hydatid disease is caused by the cystic larval stage of the tapeworm *Echinococcus granulosus*, of which the dog and fox are the usual hosts. Eggs released from tapeworm segments passed in the faeces by these animals are later swallowed by grazing cattle, sheep and horses, which may become infested also through drinking water contaminated by wind-blown eggs.

In Australia an anti-hydatid disease campaign has proved successful; though in New South Wales there is a sylvatic strain which circulates predominantly between wild dogs and wallabies.

Swallowed eggs hatch in the intestines and are carried via the portal vein to the liver. Some remain there, developing into hydatid cysts; others may form cysts in the lungs or occasionally elsewhere, e.g. spleen, kidney, bone marrow cavity, or brain. Inside the cysts, brood capsules, containing the infective stage of the tapeworm, develop, and after 5 or 6 months these can infest dog or fox.

People become infested through swallowing eggs attached to inadequately washed vegetables; eggs may possibly be inhaled in dust or carried by flies to uncovered food. The handling of infested dogs is an important source. In Beirut the risk is put at 21 times greater for dog-owners than others, by the World Health Organisation, which states also that in California, nomadic sheep-rearers are 1000 times more likely to have hydatid disease than other inhabitants of the state.

There have been successful campaigns to control human hydatid disease in both Cyprus and Iceland, by compulsory treatment and/or banning of dogs.

In Wales, where the incidence of hydatid disease is relatively high, farm dogs and foxhounds are important in its spread.

Only some 7 people are known to die from this disease in England and Wales each year – a figure which would probably be higher were diagnosis less difficult. Condemnation of sheep

and cattle offal from this cause runs into hundreds of thousands of pounds annually. Routine worming of dogs is essential for control. *E. granulosus* is far from being a typical tapeworm, as it has only 3 or 4 segments and a total length of a mere 3 to 9 mm, so that the dog-owner will not notice the voided segments.

A problem of diagnosis also arises, in that this worm's eggs are indistinguishable from those of *Taenia* tapeworms. Previously, one could dose dogs with arecoline hydrochloride and examine the faeces for the presence of the intact tapeworm, but in Britain this anthelmintic is no longer obtainable, having been replaced by more modern drugs which destroy the tapeworm but leave it unrecognisable.

Equine hydatidosis in Britain is caused by a strain of *E. granulosus* which has become specifically adapted to the horse as its intermediate host, and is often referred to now as *E. granulosus equinus*. This apparently is of low pathenogenicity for man.

In a survey covering 1388 horses and ponies examined at 2 abattoirs in the north of England, 8.7 per cent were infected. Prevalence of infection was closely related to age – rising from zero in animals up to 2 years old to over 20 per cent of those over 8 years old.

Sixty-six per cent of the infected animals had viable cysts. Prevalence appeared to be greatest in central and north-west England.

Treatment of human patients Hydatid disease has been said to be one of the rare parasitic conditions that can be treated only by surgery. However, the result is often incomplete, with frequent local recurrences or accidents of secondary dissemination. Repeated interventions are often mutilating and do not guarantee a definite cure. Mebendazole has been used successfully in some patients, but is not always effective.

Hydralazine

An arterial dilator, useful in treating dogs with failing heart due to mitral regurgitation (usually caused by fibrosis of the valve) and left-sided congestive heart failure.

Hydrargyrum

(see MERCURY)

Hydraulic Fluid

Intense generalised pruritis was suffered by animals grazing in a field beneath the flight path to an airfield after they ate grass contaminated by hydraulic fluid leaked from an aircraft.

Hydrocele

Hydrocele means a collection of fluid present within the outer proper coat of the testicle (tunica vaginalis) or within the spermatic cord.

Hydrocephalus

Hydrocephalus is a condition in which a large amount of fluid collects within the brain cavity of the skull. It may be present before birth (congenital hydrocephalus), in which case the large size of the head may present an obstruction to parturition. In the congenital form which is met with in foals, calves, and puppies, there is a large prominent swelling over the forehead, and a rounded dome-like cranium. Animals born in this condition are usually dead, or if they are living they die soon after birth. It may become necessary to puncture the swollen skull and evacuate the fluid before delivery can be effected.

In the acquired form, which is chiefly met with in the horse and dog, the fluid collects in the ventricles of the brain, or under the meninges, as the result of meningitis, or the presence of a tumour which has interfered with the free circulation of the cerebrospinal fluid, or has produced an exudate from the engorged blood vessels.

When due to meningitis, hydrocephalus is usually an acute condition, and its symptoms are masked by those of the meningitis; when due to other causes in which there is obstruction to the flow of cerebrospinal fluid it is usually chronic, and the symptoms are those of pressure on the brain. The animal becomes gradually dull, sleepy, insensitive to its surroundings. Convulsions may occur, and during one of these death is liable to take place. (See under HELLEBORES.)

Hydrochloric Acid (HCl)

Hydrochloric acid (HCl) is normally present in the gastric juice, to the extent of about 2 parts per 1000. (See DIGESTION.) In the concentrated form it is a corrosive poison.

Hydrocyanic Acid (HCN)

Hydrocyanic acid (HCN) and its salts – sodium and potassium cyanide – are among the most deadly poisons, and very rapid in their effects.

Signs If taken by mouth, or given by injection, there is a rapid acceleration of the breathing (and occasionally coughing). A poisoned dog or cat will utter a cry and collapse, the limbs extended fully. There is an odour of bitter almonds. There may be convulsions. Respiratory failure ensues, and death may occur within seconds.

Hydrocyanic poisoning may occur from the ingestion by grazing animals of plants containing a cyanogenetic glycoside. (See GLYCOSIDES.) Poisoning is then less acute, and signs are not always indicative of the cause.

Treatment In acute cases, death occurs in dogs and cats before treatment can begin. If a smaller quantity of the poison has entered the body, or if poisoning is the result of the cyanogenetic glycosides (and this is known in time), an intravenous injection of a 1 per cent solution of sodium nitrite, followed by 25 per cent sodium thiosulphate, has been recommended for the dog and large animals. Repeat doses at half that rate.

Hydrogen Peroxide

An antiseptic, with some effect against viruses, due to the release of oxygen. Available as a 3 per cent (10 volume) or 6 per cent (20 volume) solution, it is used, usually diluted, for cleansing the skin and disinfecting wounds. It is unsuitable for the irrigation of cavities or deep wounds. (See OXYGEN EMBOLISM.)

Hydrometra

Another name for pseudopregnancy, it is the accumulation of a watery fluid within the uterus, sometimes sufficient to push other organs aside and to cause swelling of the abdomen of rabbits. This idiopathic condition has also been seen in cats.

Hydronephrosis

Hydronephrosis is a condition in which the capsule of the kidney, or even the kidney itself, becomes greatly distended with urine which is unable to pass along the ureter into the urinary bladder owing to some obstruction in that channel, such as calculus, a twist, or owing to the pressure of some organ nearby. The kidney swells in size, and causes pressure upon the surrounding organs with pain over the lumbar region, and in severe cases a bulging of the muscles just behind the last rib. It is treated by either the removal of the whole kidney (provided the other one is healthy), or else by the removal of the obstruction.

Hydropericardium

The accumulation of clear, straw-coloured fluid in the pericardial sac, a swollen and discoloured liver and enlarged kidneys with distended tubules. This syndrome (Angaria disease) has had a devastating effect on the broiler poultry industry of Pakistan. The disease has typically been seen in 3- to 6-week-old growing broiler chicks and results in up to 60 per cent mortality.

Cause An unidentified infectious agent which appears to require the presence of an adenovirus to produce the lesions.

Hydrophobia
Rabies.

Hydroponic Grass
Hydroponic grass, consisting of a mat of barley seedlings harvested at the 8-day stage, has been used for horse feeding, and is usually eaten with relish. It is highly nutritious, very digestible and parasite-free. (See under HORSES, FEEDING OF.)

Hydrops Amnii and Hydrops Uteri
(see UTERUS, DISEASES OF)

Hydrosalpinx
An accumulation of serous fluid in the Fallopian tube. It has been stated to be a common cause of sterility in gilts in America.

Hydrothorax
Hydrothorax means a collection of exudate in the chest, i.e. in the pleural cavity. This is one of the results of certain forms of pleurisy.

'Hyena Disease'
A condition in cattle in which the hind part of the animal grows more slowly than the fore part, producing a silhouette said to resemble that of the hyena. The cause is unknown but bovine virus diarrhoea has been suggested. It has not been reported in the UK.

Hygiene
(see INFECTION; VENTILATION; HOUSING; WATER-SUPPLY; DIET AND DIETETICS; DISINFECTION; SLURRY)

Hygroma
Hygroma is a swelling occurring in connection with a joint, usually the knee or hock, and the result of repeated bruising against a hard surface. (See CAPPED HOCK.)

Hygroma in cattle may arise through an insufficiency of bedding, or through faulty building design. (See also CALLOSITY.)

Hygroma of the elbow in large dogs has been successfully treated by means of the following technique. A 6 mm diameter Penrose drain was passed through incisions made dorsally and ventrally into the hygroma, and secured firmly to the skin. Dressings were changed every 4 to 5 days, and the drain taken out after 2 or

3 weeks. The wounds healed satisfactorily, and the hygroma was obliterated in all 18 cases.

Hygromycin B
An antibiotic used in the USA as an anthelmintic, and claimed to be effective against large roundworms and whipworms.

Hymen, Imperforate
Imperforate hymen in thoroughbred fillies, with consequent accumulation of fluid in the uterus, has led to symptoms varying from acute abdominal pain, sweating, and attempts to lie down and roll, to discomfort when urinating. Immediate relief followed necessary surgery in the more serious cases. Pulse and respiration rates returned to normal within 10 minutes, with feeding resumed. (See also 'WHITE HEIFER DISEASE'.)

Hyoid
Hyoid is the name of the bone which gives support to the root of the tongue and to the larynx. It has some similarity to the letter 'U'.

Hyostrongylus Rubidus
A parasitic worm of pigs.

Hyper-
Hyper- is a prefix indicating excess.

Hyperadrenocorticism
(see CUSHING'S SYNDROME)

Hyperaemia
Congestion. An excessive amount of blood in a part of the body.

Hyperaesthesia
Oversensitivity to bright light, sudden noise or touch. It occurs in diseases such as rabies, tetanus and hypomagnesaemia. It is the main consistent clinical sign in bovine spongiform encephalopathy (BSE).

Feline hyperaesthesia may result also from poisoning by, for example, benzoic acid.

Signs Aggressiveness, excitement.

Hyperbaric
(see OXYGEN)

Hypercalcaemia
An excess of calcium in the blood.

Causes In dogs these include cancer, an excess of vitamin D, osteolytic lesions, kidney failure, excess parathyroid hormone, Addison's disease, severe hypothermia, and, rarely, blastomycosis.

In man, additional causes of hypercalcaemia include acromegaly, increased thyroid gland activity, long-term immobilisation, too much vitamin A, treatment with thiazide diuretics, tuberculosis, sarcoidosis, histoplasmosis, coccidiomycosis, and silicone-induced granuloma.

Hypercapnia
The presence in the blood of a raised level of carbon dioxide.

Hyperchlorhydria
Hyperchlorhydria is a form of indigestion associated with excessive secretion of hydrochloric acid.

Hyperglycaemia
An excess of sugar in the blood. (See DIABETES MELLITUS.)

Hyper-Immune Serum
The serum of an animal which has been hyperimmunised by repeated injections of a toxin or vaccine. It is rich in antibodies, and is used for curative treatment of, e.g., tetanus.

Hyperkalaemia
High concentration of potassium in the blood.

Hyperkeratosis
Hyperkeratosis means an excess of horn or KERATIN. The specific disease is also characterised by hardening of the skin.

Cause In cattle, the disease has been caused by poisoning by minute quantities of chlorinated naphthalene compounds (and possibly other chemical substances also). These are found in many wood-preserving compounds in insecticides, lubricants, and electrical insulation material. These substances bring about a secondary vitamin A deficiency. In America the disease has followed the feeding of pellets prepared by machinery lubricated with grease or oil containing naphthalene compounds – an indication of the minute quantities sufficient to cause trouble. Usually, however, the disease is a sequel to housing stock in recently creosoted buildings. (For the disease in pigs, see also ZINC and CALCIUM SUPPLEMENTS.)

Signs A thickening of the skin, sometimes with loss of hair, on neck and shoulders. In calves, stunted growth, a discharge from the eye (often with a corneal opacity), frothing at the mouth, weakness and emaciation occur,

and death may precede any obvious skin changes.

Treatment Vitamin A will assist recovery.

Hyperkinesis
Overactivity that may be caused by dietary or environmental factors. It can be accompanied by aggression, especially in the reaction to attempted restraint (e.g. putting on a lead). The heart and respiratory rates may increase; sedation may be a temporary measure. Expert evaluation of the diet may be necessary and the animal may have to be referred to an animal behaviour specialist.

Hyperlipaemia
An excess of lipids in the blood, which can be fatal in ponies and donkeys. It was first reported in Europe, then in Australia. Mares are affected in late pregnancy or early lactation.

Signs Depression, weakness, loss of appetite, diarrhoea, and terminal convulsions.

Autopsy findings: liver much enlarged, yellow and friable.

Hypermetria
A high-stepping gait. (See COENURIASIS.)

Hyperoxaluria
An excess of oxalates in the urine. This accompanies L-glyceric aciduria in kidney disease of kittens 5 to 9 months old.

Acute kidney failure develops together with atrophy of nerves supplying muscles.

Signs Extreme weakness, affecting standing and walking.

Cause A recessive gene.

Hyperparathyroidism
Of 21 dogs suffering from this, 20 had an adenoma, and 1 a carcinoma. (See PARATHYROID GLANDS.)

Signs Thirst, listlessness, weakness, loss of appetite.

Hyperplasia
Hyperplasia is the term applied to abnormally great development of some organ or tissue.

Hyperpotassaemia
Too high a level of potassium in the bloodstream. This may be brought about artificially, with fatal results, by the mistaken use of potas-

sium iodide intravenously instead of sodium iodide.

Hyperpyrexia

Hyperpyrexia means a high degree of fever. (See FEVER; TEMPERATURE.)

Hypersensitivity

Once an animal has been 'primed' or sensitised by an antigen, further contact with this will boost the immune response – but may also provoke tissue-damaging reactions. (See IMMUNE RESPONSE; ALLERGY; PENICILLIN, SENSITIVITY TO; ANAPHYLAXIS; SERUM SICKNESS.)

Hypersexuality

Hypersexuality is usually found in males with excessive testosterone production; it may also be the result of a malfunction of the cerebral cortex. Administration of short-acting progesterones may help diagnosis but, long term, castration is often the answer.

Hypertension

High arterial blood pressure. In dogs, kidney disease is the most common cause of hypertension.

Signs Detachment of the retina, or bleeding from it, may be the first indication. The dog may suddenly go blind. Long-term effects may include enlargement of the left ventricle of the heart, and kidney failure.

Hyperthermia

A body temperature greatly in excess of the normal, as occurs in fevers.

Hyperthermia, Malignant

When some dogs of the Great Dane breed, some pigs of the Piétrain breed, and some human beings (about 1 in every 10,000 people) are anaesthetised with halothane, their body temperature rises to a point at which, unless the anaesthesia is discontinued, the hyperthermia is likely to prove fatal.

Hyperthermia may occur in animals poisoned by chlorinated hydrocarbon insecticides. (See also HEAT-STROKE; TROPICS; FEVER.)

Malignant hyperthermia may also develop as a result of stress.

Hyperthyroidism

Excessive activity of the THYROID GLAND.

Hypertonic

(see under ISOTONIC)

Hypertrophic Osteopathy (Marie's Disease)

This was first described in man in 1890. It has been reported in the dog (see also ACROPACHIA) and in the horse. In Africa, the roundworm *Spirocera lupi* has been reported as associated with the condition in the dog.

In the dog the disease takes the form of a non-oedematous swelling of all 4 legs. It is associated with tumours of the lung. Severing of the vagus nerve has been recommended in cases (the majority) where surgical removal of the lung lesions is not possible, and has led to a reduction of the bone enlargement in the limbs, and of the swelling, pain, and lameness. Euthanasia may, of course, be preferable.

Hypertrophy

Hypertrophy means extra size or development of an organ or tissue.

In certain valvular diseases of the heart when obstruction to the free flow of blood occurs, the muscle wall of the heart becomes increased in thickness and strength, and a compensation results. In the training of horses the trainer aims at getting the maximum efficiency from the skeletal muscles, which under the influence of judicious training and feeding become hypertrophied.

After 1 organ of a pair has been removed – as, for instance, the kidney or the ovary – the remaining organ becomes increased in size so as to be able to perform practically the same amount of work as was previously done by the pair.

Hypervitaminosis

Disease associated with an excess of a particular vitamin. For example, chronic hypervitaminosis A occurs in cats fed exclusively, or virtually so, on an all-liver diet. (See under CAT FOODS.)

Hyphaemia

An infusion of blood into the anterior chamber of the eye.

Hypo-

Hypo- is a prefix indicating a deficiency.

Hypoadrenocorticism

(see ADDISON'S DISEASE)

Hypoalbuminaemia

A low level of albumin in the blood. It may be indicative of kidney or liver disease, or malnutrition.

Hypocalcaemia

(see MILK FEVER; TRANSIT TETANY; LAMBING SICKNESS IN EWES; ECLAMPSIA; METABOLIC PROFILES). An insufficiency of blood calcium. This occurs also in mares. The signs are a stiff gait, with the hind legs placed forward when standing still, trismus, and dyspnoea.

Hypochlorites

Effective disinfectants widely used in milking machines, dairy equipment and food premises; preparations are marketed under a number of trade names. They leave no persistent odour or taint. Their efficacy depends upon the amount of available chlorine, which is more active against viruses than most disinfectants. Hypochlorites are unable to penetrate grease and are often combined with detergents. Sodium hypochlorite is useful for disinfecting premises after an outbreak of a virus disease. (See also TEAT-DIPPING.)

Hypocupraemia

A condition in which there is too little copper in the bloodstream. This occurs in SWAYBACK in lambs, and is also associated with serious ill-health in cattle. On the Shropshire–Cheshire border, for example, hypocupraemia is accompanied by scouring and stunted growth. Two-year-old heifers have been mistaken for 8-month-old calves. In Caithness, hypocupraemia is liable to occur on 75 per cent of the farms unless precautions are taken. Scouring is not a common symptom there but calves of the beef breeds show a stilted gait and progressive unthriftiness. (See also COPPER.)

Hypocuprosis

A disease caused by a copper deficiency. (See HYPOCUPRAEMIA and COPPER.)

Hypodermic

(see INJECTIONS)

Hypoglossal Nerve

The hypoglossal nerve is the 12th cranial nerve and supplies the muscles of the tongue, together with others nearby.

Hypoglycaemia

Hypoglycaemia is a deficiency of sugar in the blood. It causes acetonaemia in ruminants and pregnancy toxaemia in sheep. It may occur in states of starvation, but is of special importance in connection with the administration of insulin, which is injected to lower the blood sugar from an abnormal amount, and which, if given in too large doses, may produce too great reduction with symptoms of nervousness,

breathlessness, and excitement. In human medicine hypoglycaemia may be a sequel to the use of sulfonamides, e.g. sulphadiazine. These symptoms are relieved by taking some food containing sugar and by an injection of adrenaline, which checks the action of insulin.

Hypokalaemia

A deficiency of potassium in the blood. (See 'DOWNER COW' SYNDROME.)

In cats, hypokalaemia results in weakness, the neck bending downwards.

Hypomagnesaemia

Also known as 'grass staggers' or Hereford disease, it is caused by too little magnesium in the bloodstream.

Hypomagnesaemia is of particular importance in cattle. It occurs when a herd is turned on to lush spring grass after being stall-fed during the winter, and often follows a frosty or wet spell; an interval of a few days may elapse before symptoms appear. The problem is particularly common where potash (potassium) and nitrogen fertilisers have been used, but the causes are complex. The low blood magnesium often results from a reduced intake of magnesium, while the absorption of that mineral is inhibited by the presence of potash and the rapid movement of feed through the gut. Hypomagnesaemia can also occur in the autumn in dry cows or suckler cows at grass and not receiving supplementary feed.

Hypomagnesaemia has apparently been more common in the Ayrshire than in other British breeds of cattle. Cows which have had several calves are more prone to it than heifers.

It is more common in ewes in the first 4 weeks after lambing than before lambing.

In calves, hypomagnesaemia can occur where the diet consists mainly of milk, which is not by itself an adequate source of magnesium for a rapidly growing young animal. The condition is thus seen mainly in suckler calves and those being reared for veal. (See OMASUM.)

Signs Animals are often recumbent; if on their sides, they paddle with their legs when stimulated, the head extends backwards and they froth at the mouth and defecate. The heart rate, which is rapid, may be heard several paces from the animal. Unless treated early they often die. If not recumbent, shivering, a staggering gait, excitement, convulsions, and paralysis may precede death. In less acute cases, the animals appear 'nervy' – responding violently to sensations of touch or sound – and there may be muscular tremors.

Treatment This must be prompt. A 25 per cent solution of magnesium sulphate is given subcutaneously. Intravenous injection may kill the animal; if it is used intravenously, magnesium should be given combined with calcium borogluconate. Great care is necessary, however, in giving the injection and even approaching the animal – which may otherwise die at the prick of the needle.

An enema of up to 5 tablespoonfuls of magnesium chloride in 250 ml of warm water is recommended by the Tennessee State University.

Magnesium can also be given in the drinking water, using a proprietary product.

Prevention The feeding of magnesium-rich supplements 3 weeks before early spring grazing and for up to 6 weeks after turnout or, in sheep, the use of a magnesium lick, from a month after service till a month after lambing. (For adult cattle a daily dose of 60 g (2 oz) per head of calcined magnesite, mixed with damp sugar-beet pulp, is recommended.) A mixture of magnesium acetate solution and molasses may be offered ad lib from ball feeders on pasture, as an alternative. Magnesium 'bullets' are also used. Top-dressing pasture with calcined magnesite is helpful. (See MAGNESIUM; MILK FEVER.) Magnesium can also be given in the drinking water; proprietary preparations are available.

Hypomyelinogenesis Congenita in Sheep

A congenital disease of lambs, characterised by trembling or twitching, staggering, and sometimes shaking of the head.

Hyponatraemia

A deficiency of sodium in the blood.

Hypoparathyroidism, Nutritional Secondary

(see CANINE and FELINE JUVENILE OSTEODYSTROPHY)

Hypophosphataemia

A condition in which the level of blood phosphorus is too low. (See MILK FEVER; 'DOWNER COW' SYNDROME.)

Hypophysis

The pituitary gland. Hypophysectomy is removal of the pituitary.

Hypoplasia

Under-development. Hypoplasia of the genital organs is a cause of sterility.

Hypotension

Low arterial blood pressure. It is not common in animals except following shock, for example after an accident.

Hypotensive Drugs

Hypotensive drugs are those which reduce high blood pressure.

Hypothalamus

A part of the brain below the thalamus which acts as a thermostat, maintaining body temperature. It also influences blood circulation, urinary secretion, and appetite. (See BRAIN.)

Hypothermia

An abnormally low body temperature; it is a common cause of lamb mortality. It can be caused by exposure in the first few hours after birth or, after about 12 hours, because of starvation. Affected lambs should be warmed; starved lambs must receive food or 20 per cent solution of glucose, injected intraperitoneally, before warming.

Piglets are also susceptible to hypothermia and will often die if creep areas are not adequately heated.

In human surgery, hypothermia is deliberately induced, by various means, for operations on heart or brain. A technique is used in human surgery for operations within the dry heart. The venous blood is cooled in a circuit outside the body (a method now preferred to the use of ice packs or refrigerated blankets) until a body temperature of 20° to 25°C (68° to 77°F) is obtained, when the flow of blood to the heart can be stopped for several minutes to allow the operation to proceed.

Hypothermia, Accidental

The chilling of newborn animals, or of those under a general anaesthetic, is a life-threatening condition. Warmth is essential. (See also under SHEEP BREEDING – Lamb survival; HOUSING OF ANIMALS.)

Hypothyroidism

A condition caused by underactivity of the thyroid gland. It is not uncommon in dogs and causes lethargy, weight gain and also alopecia. It is treated with thyroid preparations such as thyroxine. It is associated in cattle with a high incidence of aborted, still-born or weakly calves. (See also GOITRE.)

Hypovolaemia

A diminished volume of blood. (See SHOCK.)

Hypoxia

A reduced level of oxygen-supply to the body tissues. It can occur in newborn animals deprived of oxygen during birth. The animal is dull and weak, often unable to suck.

Hysterectomy

A surgical operation for removal of the uterus. Usually the ovaries are removed at the same time. (See OVARIO-HYSTERECTOMY.)

Hysteria (Canine)

A decline of this condition in the UK has been attributed to the abandonment of the use of agenised flour in the manufacture of dog biscuits. (The agene process involved the bleaching of flour with nitrogen chloride.)

It has been suggested that some cases may have been due to the use of flour, containing the spores of *Tilletia tritici*, in dog-biscuit manufacture.

Signs The dog would suddenly 'appear to go mad', racing round with a fixed stare, barking or howling.

(For distemper-like signs, see MENINGITIS.)

Iatrogenic Disease

Any illness resulting from treatment, such as the side-effects of some drugs. Adverse drug reactions were suspected in 130 of 39,541 cases treated at the Veterinary Hospital, University of California, Davis. In 66 cases there was reasonable evidence to link the reaction observed to the drug. Antibiotics and antiparasiticides were incriminated 21 times, with anaphylaxis being the most commonly observed reaction. There were 3 deaths following the administration of procaine penicillin (inadvertently intravenously) to a lamb; potassium penicillin (10,000 units/kg) to a cat; and oxytetracycline (25 mg/kg) to a cow. Anaesthetic and related agents were involved 20 times. Severe clonic convulsions developed in 5 cats receiving more than 80 mg ketamine hydrochloride; cardiac arrest, hypotension, dyspnoea and muscular rigidity in 2 horses given xylazine (1 mg/kg intravenously); and severe bradycardia and respiratory arrest in 2 dogs given fentanyl-droperidol. Anti-cancer drugs were implicated in 10 cases with the most dramatic reactions being observed in 5 dogs treated with 5-fluorouracil. One of these died as a result of neural toxicosis. (See also SIDE-EFFECTS; DRUG INTERACTIONS.)

IBK

Infectious bovine keratitis (infectious ophthalmia of cattle). (See EYE, DISEASES OF.)

IBR

Infectious bovine rhinotracheitis. (See RHINO-TRACHEITIS.)

Ibuprofen

A non-steroidal anti-inflammatory drug, much used in human medicine. It has a narrow margin of safety in dogs, in which it can cause a sometimes fatal gastric ulceration. The same is true of flurbiprofen.

Ice, Ice Cubes

Of use in cases of haemorrhage from the stomach, as an aid to control bleeding from wounds, and as an application in cases of meningitis and paraphimosis; also in cases of hyperthermia and sunstroke.

Icelandic Pneumonia

(see PULMONARY ADENOMATOSIS; also MAEDI/VISNA)

Ichthyophonus

A fungus that usually infects marine fish but is pathogenic to salmon in both sea and fresh water. It is caused by feeding salmon infected dead fish which have not been processed properly.

Ichthyosis

Ichthyosis is a condition of the skin in the dog, especially over the elbow and hocks in which large and irregular cracks appear. These become filled with dirt, and infection results.

Icterus

(see JAUNDICE)

Identichip

An electronically coded microchip, the size of a grain of rice, encased in implant-grade glass. It is inserted in the loose skin of the neck of the animal (under local anaesthesia).

The microchip is encoded with the animal-owner's address, etc., kept on a central computer register. Electronic scanners ('readers') are used to read the data in the chips.

A database of animals so identified is kept, under the name Anibase, by Animalcare Ltd., of Common Road, Dunnington, York YO1 5RU (see also MICROCHIP).

Identification of Cattle

This is controlled by law in the UK. The Bovine Animals (Records, Identification and Movement) Order 1995, as amended by the Cattle Identification (Amendment) Regulations 1999 and the Cattle (Identification of Older Animals) Regulations 2000, requires that all cattle be identified by an ear tag in each ear. Each animal must have a 'passport' that must accompany it wherever it goes and in which the following details must be entered: date of movement on to a particular holding, or date of birth on the holding; eartag number; breed; sex; dam's identification number (replacement ear tag where applicable). When the animal is moved off a holding, its age or date of birth, the holding from which it is moved, and that to which it is moved are recorded. Ear tags must be applied to dairy cattle within 36 hours of birth and, in other cattle, within 30 days of birth.

Identification of Goats

Identification of Goats is controlled by the Sheep and Goats (Records, Identification and Movement) Order 1996, as amended. Requirements are essentially the same as for sheep (*see* below) except that plastic ear tags are not recommended as goats will chew them.

Identification of Horses

Under the Horse Passports Order 1997, as amended, each horse must have a passport prepared as specified. The document must be in French and English. Details of the individual horse are given and a silhouette of the animal is filled in with the markings. Information of vaccinations and dates of administration must also be stated in the passport. There is also provision for the results of veterinary examinations to be included and signed by the veterinary surgeon in charge of an event in which the horse is entered, or when the animal is about to undertake a journey.

Identification of Pigs

All pigs must be identifiable to the pemises of origin, under regulations set out in the Pigs (Records, Identification and Movement) Order 1995. Breeding stock are usually ear-tagged before leaving the breeding farm. Pigs for slaughter are usually identified by a slap mark; those travelling across an EU frontier must be ear-tagged. Records must be kept of pigs born on a holding. Very strict measures have been taken to control disease transmission, because many viruses multiply rapidly in an infected pig and the quantity of virus shed can be much more than is the case with cattle, sheep or goats with the same infection. All movements of pigs must be recorded in a specified manner. Regulations set out the format for the declaration of pigs moved off a holding, moved from a farm for breeding, exhibition, artificial insemination or veterinary treatment, and returned to the farm after having left it for breeding purposes. The form of declaration is also specified for the movement off a farm of pigs that have been fed waste food (NB feeding of catering waste, including swill, is banned), and for those moved from a collection centre to a farm. Pigs must not be moved to an abattoir within 72 hours of their arrival on a holding; normally, pigs can only be moved after at least 20 days.

Identification of Sheep

Identification of Sheep is controlled by the Sheep and Goats (Records, Identification and Movement) Order 1996 (as amended). Sheep moving into the EU and sheep leaving Britain must be identifiable by ear tag. Animals must be marked before they are moved off the holding where they were born.

Idiopathic

Idiopathic is a term applied to diseases to indicate that their cause is unknown.

Idiopathic feline vestibular syndrome (IFVS) (see under FELINE VESTIBULAR SYNDROME)

Idiosyncrasy

An atypical reaction to a drug or to a food; in a behavioural sense, a quirk.

IgA, IgE, IgG and IgM

IgA, IgE, IgG and IgM are antibody/immunoglobulins found in the blood serum and also in secretions from mucous membranes. (See IMMUNOGLOBULINS; SECRETORY IgA.)

Ile De France

A French breed of sheep.

Ileitis

Inflammation of the ileum.

Ileocaecal

Ileocaecal refers to the junction between ileum and caecum, between the end of the small intestine and the commencement of the large. The so-called ileocaecal valve is formed by the caecum in such a manner that while food material may readily travel from ileum into caecum, it is difficult for it to pass in the opposite direction.

Ileum

Ileum is the last arbitrary division of the small intestine. (See INTESTINES.)

Inflammation of the ileum – which becomes thickened and stiff, almost like a piece of rubber hose – is a cause of death in piglets 2 to 4 months old. It has been suggested that there is a hereditary predisposition to this condition, which often affects the whole litter. In many instances, the trouble is recognised only at the bacon factory, having caused no apparent illness in the pigs. Those that die, on the other hand, do so from perforating ulcers and peritonitis, after showing evidence of thirst, a bluish colour of the skin, and collapse. (See PORCINE INTESTINAL ADENOMATOSIS.)

Ileus

The intestinal obstruction which can follow failure of PERISTALSIS.

Iliac

Relating to the flank. (See ARTERIES.)

I/M or Im

Short for intramuscular; usually refers to route of injection.

Ilium

Ilium is another name for the haunch-bone, the outer angle of which forms the 'point of the hip'. The ilium is the largest and most anteriorly situated bone of the pelvis. (See BONE.)

Imbalance

A term used to describe, for example, a faulty calcium to phosphorus ratio in the food of an animal, or an excess of one hormone in the bloodstream, or a deficiency of another – with resulting disease. (See RICKETS; INFERTILITY; METABOLIC PROFILES; CALCIUM SUPPLEMENTS; DOGS' DIET.)

Imidocarb Dipropionate

A drug used for the treatment and prevention of bovine babesiosis (Redwater fever, *Babesia divergens* infection). It is given, by subcutaneous injection in the neck, at the first clinical appearance of the disease; all animals in the same group should be treated as a precaution. Some animals may have an anaphylactic reaction that could be fatal. Imidocarb has also been used for treatment of canine babesiosis, although it is not registered in the UK for this purpose. In the dog it is given by slow intravenous injection or intramuscularly at a dose of 5 to 6 mg per kg bodyweight, repeated after 2 to 3 weeks.

Immobilon/Revivon (Large Animal)

(Novartis) is a neuroleptanalgesic, i.e. combines sedation with analgesia. It combines etorphine hydrochloride with acepromazine. Given by intravenous injection in the horse, it provides immobilisation and analgesia useful for restraint and minor surgical procedures. Immobilon does not, like morphine, cause excitement, vomiting or defecation. It does, however, act as a respiratory depressant, and slows heart action.

Immobilon is reversible in its effects by means of Revivon (diprenorphine hydrochloride). It is absolutely essential that the manufacturer's directions are followed.

Precautions Immobilon is rapidly fatal for man and must be used with great care. A veterinary surgeon died within 15 minutes after accidental self-inoculation when a colt made a sudden violent movement. Unfortunately the antidote, Narcan (naloxone), was not available. Donkeys are more sensitive to Immobilon than are horses and it is not licensed for that species. If used, about half the dose recommended in the horse is adequate.

Recommended precautions include the wearing of gloves to avoid skin contamination (which has required hospital treatment), and protection of the eyes. Once the dose has been withdrawn from the container into the syringe, the needle should be discarded and a fresh one inserted into the injection site; the syringe containing Immobilon is then attached to the needle and the dose injected. An assistant capable of administering the antidote must always be on hand.

Immune-Mediated Disease

Immune-Mediated Disease include PEMPHIGUS; FELINE INFECTIOUS PERITONITIS; MYASTHENIA GRAVIS. THROMBOCYTOPENIA and POLYARTHRITIS may also, in some instances, be immune-mediated diseases. (See AUTO-IMMUNE DISEASE.)

Immune Response

This is a term used in immunology, which is the study of the body's reaction to the presence of foreign substances.

Such substances (usually polysaccharide or protein) are present in bacteria, viruses and other parasites, but are dissimilar to any substances occurring naturally in the host's body. The foreign substances act as antigens and give rise to antibodies. This is the immune response.

When antigen enters the body, the immune response may take 2 forms: (1) humoral immunity, which involves the synthesis and release of antibody into the blood and other body fluids; and (2) cell-mediated immunity, involving the production of 'sensitised' lymphocytes which have the antibody on their cell surfaces. (See IMMUNOGLOBUUNS; INTERFERON; INFECTION.)

Antibodies combine with (and for all practical purposes neutralise) the antigens. In this way an animal may overcome infection.

Lymphocytes play an important part in the immune response, attacking cells containing the antigens. This happens in graft rejection and organ transplants, in reaction to malignant tumours, and in infections where bacteria, viruses or other parasites are present inside host cells.

B lymphocytes are the precursors of the plasma cells which secrete antibodies. B cells have antibody-like receptors on their surfaces which aid in the recognition of specific antigens. (See under BLOOD; B CELLS; T CELLS; RETICULO-ENDOTHELIAL; ANTIBODIES; IMMUNOGLOBULINS; SECRETORY IgA.)

Immunisation

Immunisation is the process of artificially producing resistance to a given infection – generally by means of a vaccine, sometimes by means of

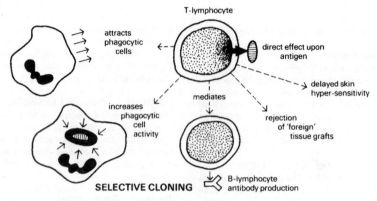

Specific immunity: humoral antibody production.

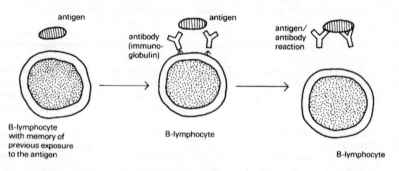

Specific immunity: cell-mediated immune response.

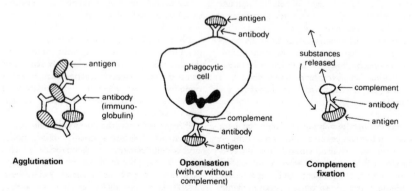

Specific immunity: immunoglobulin activity.

an antiserum or antitoxin. (See IMMUNITY; VACCINES; ANTISERUM.)

Side-effects

Immunisation is not always attained without side-effects. (See SERUM SICK-NESS; ANAPHYLACTIC SHOCK.) In human medicine both serum shock and serum neuritis may occasionally follow the use of equine antitetanus serum or of antitoxin made from this.

Immunity

Immunity is the power to resist infection or the action of certain poisons. This immunity is (1) inherited; (2) acquired naturally; or (3) acquired artificially.

Natural immunity

There are some species of animals that are not affected by diseases or by poisons that are dangerous to others. The snake-killing mongoose of India possesses an immunity against cobra venom; the pigeon can withstand large doses of morphine without harm; fowls are resistant to tetanus; the horse does not become affected with foot-and-mouth disease; rats are not attacked by tuberculosis; the ox is immune from glanders; man is not affected by swine fever and many other diseases that are fatal to the lower animals, while, with the exception of the monkey, animals are not susceptible to syphilis. It is probable that species immunity cannot be broken down even by massive inoculation of the causal agent.

A degree of immunity to locally occurring infections is transmitted to it by the medium of the colostrum in its mother's milk. (See COLOSTRUM; IMMUNOGLOBULINS.)

Acquired immunity

results from an attack of some disease from which the animal has recovered. It is probable that most diseases confer a certain amount of immunity, but this varies greatly. It may be life-long, or virtually so, as in sheep pox, swine fever or erysipelas; in most instances, however, its duration is less, and in some only temporary. For example, cattle may be attacked by foot-and-mouth disease several times during their lives, and horses after recovery from one attack of tetanus may have a second natural attack. The immunity conferred by recovery is liable in many of the viral diseases (e.g. blue-tongue), and in some protozoal diseases to break down in the presence of massive infection subsequently. Recovery from a disease involves a process of natural immunisation against that disease, the toxins or other antigens present in the body being destroyed by antibodies elaborated by the body tissues.

Artificially acquired immunity

is of 2 varieties, either active or passive.

(a) Active immunity may be artificially produced by inoculating an animal with a vaccine (i.e. dead or attenuated bacteria or virus) or with a toxoid.

(b) Passive immunity is that form of artificial immunity obtained by injecting into the body of 1 animal, blood serum drawn from the body of another animal which has previously been rendered actively immune by injecting particular antigens. The serum contains antibodies or 'antitoxins', which enable an in-contact animal to resist an infection, or enable an already infected animal to overcome the infection, so that an attack of illness – if it occurs at all – is milder than it would otherwise have been. (See ANTISERUM.) A young animal may acquire passive immunity through the colostrum of its dam which had been immunised with this purpose in mind. (For an example, see LAMB DYSENTERY.)

The immune system normally 'learns' to discriminate between self and non-self antigens early in development, leading to the normal state known as self-tolerance. A newborn mouse or rat injected with large numbers of cells from a genetically foreign individual will grow up tolerant of the foreign allo-antigens of the donor, so that, for example, it will accept a skin graft from the donor which would normally be rejected. It has been shown that this induced state of 'neonatal tolerance' is maintained by suppressor T-cells.

There are many complexities involved in immunity, which is far from being the simple subject it may here appear. (See IMMUNE RESPONSE; ORIFICES.)

Immunodeficiency

This may involve a specific factor, such as antibody or lymphocytes; or a non-specific factor such as a complement component. In either case the deficiency results in some failure of the IMMUNE RESPONSE, so that viral, bacterial or fungal disease may ensue.

Deficiencies of immunity can be either primary, due to congenital dysfunction of the immune mechanism, or secondary.

Primary immunodeficiency

has been studied more fully in humans than in animals, although a condition of foals called 'inherited combined immunodeficiency in foals of Arabian breeding' has been documented in America.

Theoretically, if the deficiency is mainly of B-lymphocytes, the animal is likely to have measurably low levels of immunoglobulins and a deficiency of lymphoid follicles in lymph nodes. Such an animal would be susceptible to pyogenic bacterial infection, but would be able to cope with most viral infections.

Conversely, if the deficiency is mainly of T-lymphocytes, the animal will have reduced 'delayed skin hypersensitivity' and will be more susceptible to viruses.

Foals affected by the inherited combined immunodeficiency frequently suffer from adenoviral pneumonia due to their inability to resist infection.

Secondary partial immunodeficiency is much more common, and is being increasingly recognised as an important cause of failure to recover completely from certain diseases.

Severe malnutrition, certain viral infections, exposure to X-rays, and corticosteroid therapy can all lead to a reduction in the immune response. (See also IMMUNOSUPPRESSION.)

Immunofluorescent Microscopy

This is a useful laboratory method of diagnosis, described as specific and very sensitive. It enables a virus to be identified during the course of an unknown infection. It can demonstrate the presence of swine fever virus, for example, even before the appearance of symptoms. Results can be obtained within a matter of hours.

The principle involved is that antigens in tissues are identified by using their ability to respond to, and fix, the homologous antibody previously labelled with a fluorescent tracer which does not affect its properties.

The method has demonstrated swine fever virus using impressions from lymph nodes taken from pigs killed during the first 60 hours after experimental infection. The virus is revealed first in the cytoplasm as a diffuse granular fluorescence; later bright, fluorescent particles become visible within the nucleus.

The term 'fluorescent antibody test' is applied to this technique. (See also under RABIES.)

Immunoglobulins

Immunoglobulins – found in blood, colostrum, and most secretions – are proteins produced by PLASMA CELLS in response to stimulation by antigens, and play an important part in the IMMUNE RESPONSE. Immunoglobulins inactivate or destroy antigens. In cattle, 4 main classes of immunoglobulin are recognised: IgA, IgE, IgG, and IgM.

IgA is mainly secreted locally in mammals. Its function is aimed at combating micro-organisms entering the body at a specific site, e.g. upper respiratory tract, lungs, intestines.

IgE is present in increased amounts in animals with allergies. It is attached to the mast cells and, on exposure to the antigen, anaphylactic and allergic mediators are released.

IgG is the main circulating immunoglobulin and the one responsible for transferring passive immunity from parent to offspring.

IgM is found in the serum and is the 1st antibody produced in an immune response. It is the only antibody produced by fish.

All domestic animals have IgA, IgG and IgM; a 5th immunoglobulin, IgD of uncertain function, is found in some other species, including man.

Immunoperoxidase Test

A method of staining tissue to show the presence of specific antigens.

Immunostimulation
(see LEVAMISOLE; BCG)

Immunosuppression

Suppression of the immune response, leading to greater susceptibility of an animal to pathogens, such as may occur in trypanosomiasis, influenza, distemper, and brucellosis. (See under CORTISONE; ANERGY; LEVAMISOLE; SPLEEN.)

The occurrence of anergy following certain viral infections is worth emphasising; affected animals show a reduced cell-mediated response, especially following infections by viruses having a cytotoxic effect on lymphoid cells, e.g. Newcastle disease virus.

Immunosuppressants include CORTICOSTEROIDS *and* cytotoxic drugs such as CYCLOPHOSPHAMIDE.

Impaction

Impaction is a condition in which 2 things are firmly lodged together. For example, when after a fracture 1 piece of bone is driven within the other, this is known as an impacted fracture; when a temporary tooth is so firmly lodged in its socket that the eruption of the permanent tooth below is prevented, this is known as dental impaction. Impaction of rumen or of colon means that food materials have become tightly packed into these organs, causing a blockage. (See STOMACH, DISEASES OF; INTESTINES, DISEASES OF; and COLIC in horses.)

Impetigo

A staphylococcal infection of the skin seen on the teats and udders of cows, facial skin in pugs and abdomen in puppies. It is characterised by the formation of painless pustules, shallow, thin-walled, and usually projecting upwards above the level of the surface of the skin. It is seen in puppies affected with worms, distemper, and teething troubles, in bitches and cows after parturition, and in other animals. (See also ACNE.)

Implantation

This term is used in connection with the application beneath the skin of pellets containing medication released gradually to provide a long-lasting effect. Microchips coded with identity data are also implanted. (See HORMONES IN MEAT PRODUCTION; CAPONISATION; also IDENTICHIP.)

Implant

Any material, tissue, or object inserted into the body on a more or less permanent basis. Implants may be prosthetic, such as replacement hip-joints; biodegradable, such as long-acting medicinal preparations; or for the purposes of identification, such as electronic microchips.

Importing/Exporting Animals

Many animal-owners – including sophisticated travellers completely familiar with passports, visas, and vaccination certificates – overlook the fact that they cannot legally take their pet animals with them across any and every national frontier. Some governments exercise a total ban on the import of certain species of animal; others require prior vaccination and production of a certificate; others insist upon an animal going straight into quarantine on arrival. Australia and New Zealand, for example, will admit dogs only from each other's territories or from the UK.

Pet animals Dogs and cats may travel to and from certain countries and the UK, without the need for quarantine, provided that strict conditions for vaccination against rabies and health checks are observed. For details, see under PET TRAVEL SCHEME.

The Export of Animals (Protection) Order 1981 laid down certain welfare requirements for the export of cattle, sheep, goats, and pigs from Britain.

There are restrictions on the import of cattle and semen on account of BLUE-TONGUE and other diseases.

Sheep Animals imported to Britain from outside the EU require a period of month-long on-farm isolation following release from the reception/quarantine station. During the isolation period, testing for maedi/visna, *Brucella ovis*, and *Mycoplasma agalactiae* is carried out; with slaughter or re-export required for positive reactors.

(See also HORSES, IMPORT CONTROL; BIRDS, IMPORT CONTROL; RABIES; QUARANTINE.)

Impotence

Inability of the male to mate successfully. Causes include malformation of the genital organs, weakness, starvation, and constrictions resulting from injuries or operations. Impotence may be only a temporary phase in the life of the animal from which it recovers with rest and good food. (See also PENIS; INFERTILITY.)

Imprinting

This is a mental process in which an inborn tendency in the animal causes it to attach itself to a set group of objects or a single object within a few hours after birth. It is a very important process if the young lamb or calf is to be properly suckled and cared for.

In Vitro

In the test-tube.

In Vivo

In the living body.

Inactivated

Made inactive. The term may be used to describe bacteria or viruses whose virulence has been removed, without destroying the antigenic properties. This may be achieved by heat, ultra-violet light or chemicals. Many vaccines are manufactured using inactivated micro-organisms.

Inbreeding

Mating of closely related animals. It may be practised deliberately to preserve desirable characteristics, but tends to encourage undesirable and enfeebling ones.

Incidence

In relation to disease outbreaks, incidence describes the number of new cases in a particular area in a specific time period (see also PREVALENCE).

Incision

A surgical incision is a cut made by a surgeon with a sharp instrument such as a scalpel.

Incisor

There are no upper incisor teeth in domesticated ruminants. (See TEETH.)

Inclusion Bodies

Round, oval, or irregular-shaped structures of a homogeneous or granular nature, found in cells during the course of viral infections, e.g. Negri bodies in nerve cells in rabies; Bollinger bodies in epithelial cells in fowl pox.

Inclusion Body Hepatitis

A viral disease of chickens, and also of intensively reared pheasant poults. In broilers the disease may appear at about 5 to 7 weeks of age, giving rise to an increased mortality but with some birds remaining healthy.

Incompetence

Inability to function effectively. The term is, applied e.g. to the valves of the heart when, as a result of disease in the valves or alterations in the size of the chambers of the heart, the valves are unable to close the orifices which they should protect. (See HEART DISEASES.)

Incontinence

Inability to control faecal and urinary function. Incontinence may follow injury to the spinal cord. (See PARALYSIS.) Faecal incontinence alone in the dog and cat may result from DIARRHOEA, STRESS, or possibly weakness of the sphincter ani in old animals.

Urinary incontinence may be associated with a dog with an enlarged prostate gland relieving bladder pressure indoors. (See also under DIABETES INSIPIDUS.) Old dogs may be unable to avoid incontinence at night, owing to kidney lesions. A rare cause is an ectopic URETER.

Occasionally urinary incontinence is a sequel to spaying of the bitch, and is attributed either to a hormonal effect or to adhesion between the vaginal stump and the bladder or urethra.

In the cat, as in the dog, chronic nephritis in the elderly animal is a common cause. The animal is obliged to drink more, and to pass urine during the night-time. Stress may be a factor too; for example, the appearance of an aggressive entire tom cat in the neighbourhood, being left alone for long periods, or the addition of a baby or another cat to the household. (See also POLYDIPSIA.)

Incoordination

Incoordination is a term meaning irregularity in movement. Various muscles or, in some instances, portions of 1 muscle contract or fail to contract without relation to each other or to the whole. Deliberate purposive movements are no longer possible or are carried out imperfectly.

Incubation Period

The time that elapses between infection and appearance of symptoms of a disease.

The average incubation periods for the commoner infectious diseases are:

Anthrax	12 to 24 hours or more
Black-quarter	1 to 5 days
Braxy	12 to 48 hours
Distemper	3 days to 3 weeks
Dourine	15 to 40 days
East Coast fever	10 to 20 days
Erysipelas (swine)	2 to 3 days
Foot-and-mouth disease	2 to 12 days
Heart-water	11 to 18 days
Influenza	3 to 10 days
Lymphangitis, epizootic	8 days to 9 months
Piroplasmosis, British bovine	14 days at earliest
Piroplasmosis, other forms	Up to 3 weeks
Pleuro-pneumonia, contagious bovine	3 weeks to 3 months
Pleuro-pneumonia, contagious equine	3 to 10 days
Rabies	10 days to 5* months
Rinderpest	4 to 5 days
African horse-sickness	6 to 8 days
Strangles	3 to 8 days
Surra	5 to 30 days
Swine fever	5 to 15 days
Tetanus, horse	4 days to 3 weeks
Tetanus, ox	5 to 8 days
Texas fever	6 weeks
Tuberculosis	2 weeks to 6 months

(*but see under RABIES)

Caution It is always wise to allow at least a week more than the longest incubation period given before allowing an animal that has been in contact with an infection and has not developed the disease to resume its place with other healthy animals. (See also INFECTION; ISOLATION; QUARANTINE.)

Indicator

A substance used in chemistry, etc., to show by a colour change that a reaction has taken place. Litmus is an example. (See also COMPLEMENT.)

Inductotherm

An electrical apparatus used in the treatment of sprained tendons, etc. (See DIATHERMY.)

Infarct

A localised area of necrosis resulting from the blockage of a blood vessel. (See EMBOLISM.)

Infection

The presence in the body of micro-organisms capable of causing disease; the passing on of disease from one animal to another. Exposure to infection may or may not be followed by disease, depending upon whether the potential host animal has or has not a useful degree of immunity against that particular infective agent, whether the animal is well nourished, not under stress, and has not any other major infection, disease, or defect which might lower its power to resist the new infection. (See IMMUNOSUPPRESSION; IMMUNODEFICIENCY.)

The virulence or otherwise of the infective agent, and the quantity of it, will also have a bearing upon whether disease will follow. For example, a heifer vaccinated against *Brucella abortus* will normally be able to resist exposure to these organisms; but her immunity might break down if challenged by a massive dose of *B. abortus*.

With rabies, for example, there is a 'threshold' dose of virus, and below this the infected animal will not become rabid (at any rate in the absence of stress).

Susceptibility to infection is also influenced by genetics. For example, see K88 and MAREK'S DISEASE.

Concurrent infections The average farm animal is host to several different parasites at one and the same time – including viruses, mycoplasmas, bacteria, fungi, and worms. Accordingly, when one speaks of a calf having pneumonia, it is unrealistic to imagine that, say, the parainfluenza 3 virus (causing the inflammation of the lungs) is the calf's sole resident parasite.

Some parasites may be present in relatively small numbers and not be causing active disease. Some, owing to the host's powers of resistance (the immune response), may be on the decline. Others may have a sudden opportunity for multiplication and increased activity as the host's resistance becomes lowered by some additional infection or by stress arising from cold, insufficiency of good food, poor ventilation, or the rigours of transport, etc.

Again, infections should be thought of as not merely mixed but changing all the time, developing, and with complex interactions between a number of factors, including management ones. (See under RESPIRATORY DISEASE IN PIGS.)

In respiratory diseases there is often a synergism between viruses and certain bacteria. In canine distemper, for instance, *Bordetella bronchiseptica* is quick to invade in the wake of the canine distemper virus and produce bronchitis. Foot-rot in sheep is often a mixed bacterial infection, with *Fusiformis necrophorus* causing

sufficient damage to permit the entry of *Bacteroides nodosus*. Liver-flukes and bacteria may both be involved in production of BLACK DISEASE.

Experimental work at the Institute for Research on Animal Diseases, Compton, has shown that fluke-free cattle can withstand an intravenous dose of 10^8 *Salmonella dublin*, whereas those infested with live-fluke are killed by this same dose.

Clinical and subclinical infections

Exposure to infection may lead to overt or clinical disease in which symptoms are in evidence; or there may be a subclinical infection in which few if any symptoms – detectable without laboratory aids – are shown. A good example is subclinical mastitis. (See MASTITIS IN THE COW.)

Infection may persist in an animal which has recovered from a disease and is no longer showing symptoms but is excreting the infective agent. Such an animal is known as a carrier. For example, a bull may be a carrier of brucellosis; a dog of leptospirosis; a horse of equine infectious anaemia; a cat of feline leukaemia.

Routes/modes of infection An animal may breathe in air containing droplets in which the infective agent is present, e.g. influenza virus or tubercle bacillus. This is sometimes called an aerosol infection.

The oral route provides a common mode of infection. Infective material may be licked, an infected carcase eaten, or a cow may eat feed contaminated with salmonella organisms or anthrax spores. (In some instances, an infective agent, such as salmonella, is already in the intestine but becomes pathogenic when its bacterial competitors are mostly destroyed by an antibiotic. See DIARRHOEA – Horses.)

Spirochaetes and hookworm larvae are examples of parasites which can enter the host through unbroken skin. Small, even insignificant, wounds can be followed by tetanus. Biting flies can transmit diseases (see under FLIES), and ticks are notorious vectors. Dog bites and cat scratches can lead to rabies, the virus of which can penetrate intact mucous membrane.

Infection may be transmitted at mating, e.g. brucellosis by the carrier bull. Dourine in the horse, and venereal tumours in the dog, are 2 other examples of infections transmitted at coitus. Congenital infections also occur.

Inter-species infections Many microorganisms have a wide range of possible hosts, e.g. the rabies virus, the influenza viruses, the anthrax bacillus. Infections from man to farm animals are ANTHROPONOSES. Farmers may also be interested in diseases which arise in one species following their use of buildings which previously housed another species. For example, turkeys have become infected in this way with swine erysipelas, which also affects game birds. (See also under HOUSING OF ANIMALS.) With cattle kept in association with pigs (as in North America), acute interstitial pneumonia may occur in cattle due to the pig worm *Ascaris suum*. (See also DOG KENNELS.)

Infections transmissible from animals to man are listed under ZOONOSES. In Britain, those of importance to farmers and stockmen include brucellosis, Q-fever, canicola fever, Weil's disease (leptospiral jaundice), louping-ill, anthrax, erysipelas, tuberculosis and salmonellosis.

Blood cells which counter infection
When bacteria gain entrance through a wound in the skin, for example, they are attacked by white blood cells (leucocytes). The first to attack are neutrophils, which have their origin in the bone marrow. They pass through the walls of the capillaries and engulf the bacteria. Monocytes perform a similar task when they have turned into macrophages, but in addition to engulfing bacteria they dispose of disintegrating neutrophils. Lymphocytes (T-cells or B-cells) also reach the site of infection. (See LYMPHOCYTES; also INTERFERON, IRON-BINDING.)

Other aspects of infection are dealt with under separate headings such as ANTIBODY; COLOSTRUM; FOMITES; IMMUNE RESPONSE; IMMUNITY; ISOLATION; NOTIFIABLE DISEASES; NURSING; DISINFECTION.

Infectious Bovine Keratoconjunctivitis
(see EYE, DISEASES OF)

Infectious Bovine Rhinotracheitis
(see under RHINOTRACHEITIS)

Infectious Bronchitis of Chickens

Cause A coronavirus.

Signs Breathing difficulties which may be evident only when the birds are at rest. A reduced egg yield. Misshapen eggs may be laid; this may persist following recovery. Mortality is usually

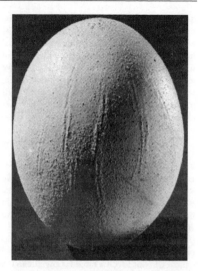

Infectious bronchitis can result in a marked deterioration in egg quality with consequent heavy economic loss. The illustration shows some of the effects, which include roughening and scoring of the shell. Shells may also be distorted and thin, or soft-shelled eggs may be laid by infected birds.

low and due to secondary infections such as mycoplasma or *E. coli*.

Prevention Live vaccines are available to control the disease; compound vaccines offer protection against other avian viral diseases as well as infectious bronchitis.

Infectious Bursal Disease (IBD)
Infectious bursal disease (IBD) of chickens affects the Bursa of Fabricius, an important part of the avian immune system, leaving the birds with lowered resistance to infection. It is also known as Gumboro disease from the town in Maryland, USA, where it was first identified. Young birds between 1 and 5 weeks are affected, with a peak at 3½ weeks. Mortality from IBD may be high; because of subsequent infections, high rates of mortality will continue. The main signs of disease are listlessness and diarrhoea. Post-mortem examination shows haemorrhage or a caseous plug in the bursa. Prevention is by vaccination of breeding stock.

Infectious Canine Hepatitis
(see CANINE VIRAL HEPATITIS)

Infectious Coryza of Chickens
Infectious coryza of chickens is caused by *Haemophilus paragallinarum*. The disease is sudden in onset and spreads so rapidly that it

seems as if all the birds have been infected simultaneously. Clinical signs include swelling of the head, wattles and sinuses, discharges from the eyes and nose, coughing, noisy breathing, lack of appetite and depression. Mortality is low but recovery takes time.

Infectious Haematopoietic Necrosis

A viral disease of salmonid fish, at present confined to North America and Japan.

Infectious Laryngotracheitis

(see under AVIAN)

Infectious Nasal Granulomata in Cattle

In certain parts of India, cattle in restricted areas (sometimes in single herds only) may become affected with this condition. Large tumour-like masses develop in connection with the frontal sinus and the turbinated bones in the nasal passages.

The cause is a schistosome, *Schistosoma nasalis*, which is present in the veins of the nasal mucous membrane.

Treatment Injections of various antimonial preparations have been used, but they have toxic side-effects. Praziquantel is among other drugs that may be effective, but regular administration is required. Prevention by control of the intermediate snail hosts is preferable.

Infectious Necrotic Hepatitis

(see BLACK DISEASE)

Infectious Pancreatic Necrosis

A viral condition of salmonids that is a NOTIFIABLE DISEASE throughout the EU. The clinical disease lasts only about 4 days. Affected fish often swim on their sides or with slow spiral movements and sink to the bottom of the pond. They may be darker than normal in colour and have swollen abdomens. It is mainly, but not exclusively, a disease of young fish. Losses are around 20 per cent but the survivors do not thrive. There is no treatment.

Infectious Salmon Anaemia

A NOTIFIABLE DISEASE of viral origin. Infected salmon are pale and lack energy. They may try to gulp air to make up for a lack of oxygen in the blood. There is no treatment; affected pools or cages of fish are slaughtered and any eggs, etc. destroyed under the provision of the Animal By-products Order 1999 for high-risk material.

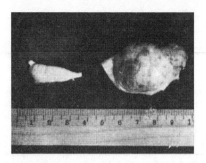

Hypoplasia of the left ovary of a cow of the Swedish Highland breed. Compare its size with that of the normal right ovary from the same animal. (The ruler is graduated in centimetres.)

Infectious Pustular Vulvovaginitis

A reproductive disorder caused by infectious bovine rhinotracheitis (see under RHINOTRACHEITIS, INFECTIOUS).

Infectious Tracheobronchitis

(see KENNEL COUGH)

Infective Drug Resistance

Resistant strains of bacteria may arise as a result of chromosomal mutation. More commonly, drug resistance is carried by PLASMIDS. (See ANTIBIOTIC RESISTANCE.)

Infertility

Inability of the female or male to reproduce. Insidious but great losses are directly due to failure to breed on the part of otherwise promising animals. The immediate loss to the individual owner of livestock is not so apparent as with certain specific diseases, but it is infinitely greater than the loss accruing from any other single specific or non-specific disease. This loss is made up by the keep of the barren animals, the absence of offspring, reduction of the milk supply, and interference with breeding programmes. (See also CALVING INTERVAL.)

Causes The most common and important causes of infertility can be grouped for convenience under the following headings.

1. *Feeding and Condition* Under-feeding is a common cause of infertility in heifers. The diet must include adequate protein of good quality and sufficient vitamins, especially vitamin A, plus essential trace elements including copper and iodine.

Excessive fat in cows, heifers or bulls may lead to infertility problems or to inability on the part of the male to accomplish coitus. (See also FATTY LIVER SYNDROME.)

In cows, temporary infertility may apparently be closely associated with the feeding at about the time of service. Cows losing weight are likely to be affected, especially if fed on poor-quality hay or silage. With ad lib feeding systems, heifers and more timid cows may not be receiving enough roughage. Kale is sometimes responsible.

In ewes, infertility and fetal death are always serious in many hill areas, the result – to quote Dr John Stamp – 'of keeping pregnant sheep under conditions of near-starvation during the winter months when weather conditions are atrocious'. (See DIET; FLUSHING OF EWES; STILLBORN PIGS; REPRODUCTION; VITAMINS; KALE; SELENIUM.)

2. *Environment and Management* A sudden change of environment, close confinement in dark quarters (formerly the lot of many a bull), and lack of exercise may all predispose to, or produce, infertility. Abnormal segregation of the sexes and the use of vasectomised males (for purposes of detecting oestrus) are other factors. A low level of nutrition may cause a quiescent or dormant state on the part of the ovaries. At the same time there are seasonal cycles of sexual activity, and a 'failure to breed' during the winter months may be natural enough, even if the farmer regards it as infertility. This 'winter infertility', as it is often called, may be influenced by temperature, length of daylight, lack of pasture oestrogens, underfeeding, etc. At this season, heifers often have inactive ovaries, while in cows irregular and 'silent' heats give low conception rates.

Infertility may result from the oestrogenic effects of red clover in the UK, as well as from subterranean clovers in Australia.

In outdoor pig herds, 'summer infertility' is common, partly due to seasonal loss of fertility in the boars.

The most frequent reason for poor fertility is poor management. In cows, poor oestrus detection or timing, or bad technique if artificial insemination is used, are common. Similar problems occur in pigs. In cattle and, particularly, pigs, when natural service is used, all matings must be seen and at least 2 undertaken within the heat period. In sheep, fertility problems often follow when too few rams are used, or those which are too young or unproven.

3. *Diseases of the Genital Organs in the Female* While there is a very long list of such diseases, their overall importance in causing infertility is much less than that of management problems such as poor oestrus detection.

Inflammation or other disease of the ovaries: ovaritis; the non-maturation of Graafian follicles, from any cause, and the presence in the ovary of cysts (which often form from a corpus luteum), are causes of infertility; another is blocked Fallopian tubes.

Persistent corpora lutea: as a true clinical condition, these are not very common. Where they do exist, the animals may have a uterine infection. The persistence of the corpus luteum prevents the ripening of the Graafian follicle, so the animal does not display oestrus and is not mated. (See under OVARIES, DISEASES OF; HORMONES; HORMONE THERAPY.)

Inflammation of the uterine mucous membrane: a large number of cases of infertility can be ascribed to infection of the uterus (metritis) or the oviduct by organisms. (For a list of the infections which cause infertility, see under ABORTION. For infections causing infertility in the mare, see under EQUINE GENITAL INFECTIONS.)

When the condition is mild, following a previous calving, it may disappear spontaneously, but in many instances it persists and becomes chronic. Associated with inflammation of the mucous membrane of the uterus or oviduct is often a persistent corpus luteum in the ovary. Carelessness during parturition, the use of unclean instruments or appliances, decomposition of retained membranes, and other similar factors, also bring about infection of the uterus. Brucellosis though not necessarily itself a cause of sterility, by lowering the vital resistance of the uterus, favours infection by a multitude of other organisms which normally may be non-pathogenic. The details of uterine infection, including salpingitis (inflammation of the oviduct), in the causation of sterility, are highly technical, but, generally speaking, it may be said that the presence of organisms in the uterus, or the presence of the products of their activity, either kills the spermatozoa, or renders the locality unsuitable for anchorage of the fertilised ovum (or ova), with the result that it perishes.

Abnormalities of the cervix may prevent conception – mechanically when the lumen is occluded or plugged by mucus of a thick tenacious nature; and pathologically when there is acute inflammation of the mucous membrane of the cervix, or even of the whole uterus. Scirrhous cervix – where much fibrous tissue is laid down in the cervix – when very advanced may cause sterility, but by itself is not usually of great importance. It is much more serious as a hindrance to parturition (*see, for example,* 'RINGWOMB' of the ewe).

Cysts and fibrous bands in the os are seldom sufficiently extensive to occlude the passage through the cervical canal. Occlusion may, however, occur as the result of swelling and congestion of the mucous membrane, due to infection and inflammation. In such cases the sperms are unable to penetrate into the uterus, and fertilisation does not occur. This may also be the result of acidity (and thickened mucus) following a mild infection, and sometimes syringing the vagina a short time before service with a weak alkaline solution (e.g. 5 per cent potassium bicarbonate) proves successful. (See 'WHITES'; 'EPIVAG'.)

Tumours – either malignant or benign.

Specific disease, such as tuberculosis in cattle, or in mares. Contagious equine ureritis. (See VULVOVAGINITIS.)

4. *Hereditary Abnormalities in the Female* (see FREEMARTIN).

Hypoplasia of the ovaries of cows may occur as an inherited condition in the female. It may involve 1 or both ovaries, causing either infertility or complete sterility. The uterus, also, may be hypoplastic. (See also under GENETICS.)

Endocrine failure: heredity may be involved.

Hermaphroditism.

'White heifer disease' (*see under this heading*).

It has been estimated that up to 10 per cent of female pigs are sterile. Group studies have shown that 25 to 50 per cent of infertile gilts had abnormalities of the genital tract sufficient to cause sterility, and two-thirds of these were regarded as hereditary.

5. *Disease of the Genital Organs in the Male* Orchitis, or inflammation of the testicle, and epididymitis, inflammation of the epididymis, due to injury from kicks, or to infection from external wounds, or from specific infection, such as *brucellosis* or *trichomoniasis* in the bull. (See TESTICLE, DISEASES OF; VENEREAL DISEASES.)

Tumours of the testicles may destroy the tubules or prevent spermatogenesis, and on the penis, or in connection with the prepuce, may act as purely mechanical agents, which prevent coitus by the male.

Adhesions between penis and prepuce, the result of acute or chronic balanitis, though rare, may cause mechanical inability to protrude the penis and fertilise the female. (See also under PENIS.)

Inflammation in the secondary sexual glands – i.e. in prostate, seminal vesicles, or other glands – may occlude the *vasa deferentia* or ejaculatory ducts, and cause inability to

pass semen, while in other cases the semen may be so altered as to cause death of the sperms in the female passages.

Affection of the prepuce, such as balanitis, and injuries accompanied by laceration or severe bruising, may cause temporary sterility, but when recovery occurs fertility returns. (See also under PENIS.)

6. *Hereditary Abnormalities in the Male* Cryptorchidism, in which 1 or both testes do not descend into the scrotum, is a well-known cause of infertility in the male. When 1 testis properly descends, and is fully developed, conception may follow service, and a sire suffering from this disability has upon some occasions been regularly used in a flock or herd; but when the rig animal has both organs retained, although sexual desire may be emphatic, service is usually unsuccessful. The condition unfits a male animal for use as a breeding sire, since there is evidence that it is a hereditary unsoundness. (See HORMONE THERAPY.)

Hypoplasia or under-development of the male sex organs, particularly of the testis, is an important cause of sterility. It may involve both testicles or only 1.

Endocrine failure may arise as a result of an inherited predisposition. In bulls this may occur in later life, rendering them sterile after they have produced a number of progeny which, in their turn, may perpetuate this form of infertility.

Hermaphrodism, or hermaphroditism, in which an animal possesses both male and female organs, but is without a full complement of either, is usually, but not always, associated with sterility. (See also GENETICS; INTERSEX.)

7. *Physical or Psychical Inability or Disturbance* Under this heading are grouped a number of conditions which are difficult to classify elsewhere. Some occur in the male, some in the female, and some are common to both sexes.

Incompatibility between the blood of sire and dam may be responsible for some cases of abortion in cattle, etc. (See HAEMOLYTIC DISEASE.)

Old age: when an animal reaches a certain age, reproduction becomes impossible. The periods of oestrus cease. Breeding ceases earlier in the female than in the male.

Discrepancies in size between male and female may result in failure to breed. The penis may be too short or too large; the vagina may be too long or too small; the female may not have the strength to carry a heavy male; or the male may not be tall enough to reach the female.

Injuries to the back, hips, hind legs, or feet of the male, and sometimes to the same regions of the female, may be severe enough to prevent successful coitus. Progressive spinal arthritis is a common condition in bulls. (See also BREEDING OF ANIMALS; REPRODUCTION; EMBRYOLOGY; UTERUS, DISEASES OF; HORMONE THERAPY; GENETICS; VENEREAL DISEASES; ANOESTRUS; ABORTION; MUMMIFICATION.)

Inflammation

Inflammation may be briefly defined as the reaction of the tissues to any injury short of one sufficiently severe to cause death. There are 4 cardinal symptoms of inflammation – heat, pain, redness, and swelling – to which may be added interference with function. (See ABSCESS; WOUNDS; ALLERGY.)

For the inflammations of special organs, see under PNEUMONIA; PLEURISY; PERITONITIS; MAMMARY GLAND.

For anti-inflammatory drugs, see CORTICOSTEROIDS; CORTICOTROPHIN; CORTISONE; NSAIDs; IBUPROFEN; FLURBIPROFEN; ANTIHISTAMINES; CALAMINE.

Influenza

Scientifically, this term is now applied only to diseases caused by a myxovirus.

The World Health Organisation (WHO) was much exercised as to what happens to the virus of human influenza between epidemics. It has long been known that there is a relationship between this disease and swine influenza. The human influenza virus (type A) was isolated from the parasitic pig lung-worm. Larvae of these lung-worms are harboured by earthworms – the only known intermediate hosts – which live for as long as 10 years.

Between epidemics, the virus is not found in the tissues of the pigs. However, earthworms taken from infected pig farms seem to carry inapparent viruses, and these can develop, in pigs eating the worms, into normal viruses capable of being isolated from the respiratory system. The question, therefore, arises whether the pigs are, in fact, the virus reservoirs, rather than being secondarily infected by the human virus. (See also SWINE INFLUENZA.)

There is evidence that influenza viruses of mammals and birds play an important part in the emergence of new viruses which cause outbreaks of illness in man in several continents.

The recovery from pigs in Taiwan in 1970 of influenza virus indistinguishable from that causing type A Hong Kong influenza epidemics in man in 1968 provided the first direct evidence of the inter-species transfer of influenza viruses. Pigs experimentally inoculated with that virus transmitted it to pen-mates. Moreover, the Taiwan virus taken from pigs readily infected human volunteers, who developed antibodies effective against virus from both pigs and people.

It is now suggested that the Hong Kong human influenza virus did not arise by mutation from a pre-existing human strain, but that it probably arose from the mixed infection in a mammal or bird with an animal influenza virus and a human type A Asian strain. The animal virus may have provided certain subunits or components; the other subunits having come from a human strain.

For influenza in the horse, see under EQUINE INFLUENZA.

Pneumonia in calves may be caused by a virus of influenza-type.

In the dog, parainfluenza virus SV5 has been isolated in the USA and the UK from dogs with upper respiratory disease. (See 'KENNEL COUGH'.)

Avian strains of type A influenza virus cause a number of diseases in hens, ducks, turkeys, etc. During 1980 and 1981, 9 subtypes of influenza A virus were isolated from birds in Britain, usually as a result of investigations of disease or death. However, these viruses were shown to be of low virulence for chickens. Highly pathogenic avian influenza virus has caused serious outbreaks among turkeys.

Avian influenza is a NOTIFIABLE DISEASE throughout the EU. Waterfowl are the main reservoir host for both avian and mammalian strains but they are not themselves much affected by the disease. The slaughter of all chickens in Hong Kong in 1997 was justified as the strain of virus present transmitted fairly easily to the human population. (See AVIAN INFLUENZA.)

'Influenza', Cat

(see FELINE INFLUENZA)

Infra-Red Lamps

Infra-red lamps are used as a source of heat in the creeps of piggeries and in poultry brooders; also for sickly lambs and calves. Either 'bright' or 'dull' emitters are available, the latter being preferred for chick-rearing. They have many advantages, but a power-cut can cause severe losses. (See also under TOES, TWISTED.)

Inguinal Canal

Inguinal canal is the passage from the abdominal cavity to the outside, down which pass the spermatic cords and their associated structures in the male, and in the female, the round ligament of the uterus. It is a slit-like opening, about 12.5 cm (5 inches) long in the horse, and is directed downwards, inwards, and forwards. It is bounded behind by a strong band called the inguinal or *Poupart's* ligament. The canal is important, because if it is dilated from any cause, some part of the small intestines may pass through it, resulting in inguinal hernia. (See HERNIAS.) It serves as the opening through which retained testicles are removed in the 'rig' or cryptorchid animal.

Inguinal Region

Inguinal region is the region of the inguinal canal, i.e. that part of the posterior and upper-most division of the abdominal wall which lies below the brim of the pelvis. The scrotum, penis, and their vessels, etc., are situated in the inguinal region in the male horse, and in the female the mammary glands with the vessels that supply them. In some animals such as the dog and boar, the scrotum is farther back, i.e. in the perineal region, while in the bull and ram the penis is farther forwards.

Inherited Defects/Diseases

Inherited defects/diseases are referred to under GENETICS. (See also DEFORMITIES and HORSES.)

Injections

Parenteral administration of medicines may be hypodermic or subcutaneous (sc), intra-articular (into a joint), intradermal, intramus-cular (im), intravenous (iv – into a vein) intraperitoneal (into the abdominal cavity), epidural, or subconjunctival (beneath the eyelid). Precautions must be taken against the introduction of bacteria, dirt, etc. The hair should be clipped away at the site of injec-tion, and the skin cleaned with spirit or an anti-septic. Needles and syringes should be sterilised before use, unless of the disposal type intended for once-only use and already sterilised and in a sealed wrapper.

Where the material to be injected is already fluid, this is generally guaranteed sterile by the manufacturers, and is put up in sealed vials. In cases where the drug has to be dissolved in water first, sterile water must be used. Manufacturers usually supply ampoules of sterile water with drugs that have to be dissolved; their instructions for use must be followed carefully. Neglect of these precautions is likely to be followed by the formation of an abscess at the point of injection or even by septicaemia.

For subcutaneous injections, a fold of the skin is picked up between the thumb and forefinger of the left hand, and the needle is inserted into the middle of this fold. The nozzle of the syringe, preloaded with the injec-tion fluid, is slipped into the head of the needle and the piston is slowly but firmly pressed home so as to expel the contents into the loose tissues under the skin. Care should be taken that all air-bubbles are excluded from the barrel of the syringe, as it is unwise to introduce them.

A number of proprietary multi-injection devices are manufactured for herd inoculations.

Precautions Restless animals should always be secured so that they will not make a sudden plunge when the needle is introduced, and break the stem of the needle. Abscesses in hams are common in pigs, and doubtless result from anti-anaemia intramuscular injections made without due precautions as to cleanliness and to broken-off needles.

The sciatic nerve may be damaged as the result of an intramuscular injection into a pig's ham, with paralysis of the limb possibly follow-ing. This site should be avoided, and it has been recommended that the injection be given into the muscles of the neck, just behind the ear, and not into fatty tissue.

Care must be taken not to make what should be a subcutaneous injection into the chest. This danger was illustrated when a farmer injected 500 lambs, using a multidose syringe intended for cattle, and with a 6 mm needle. Within a week 17 of the lambs had died; autopsy showed pyothorax and a pure growth of *Actinomyces pyogenes*. It has been demonstrated that it is pos-sible to reach the pleural cavity with a cattle syringe, especially in thin lambs; many other 'vaccine failures' may have been due to inadver-tent injections into the chest. Alternative sites, such as the side of the neck, would appear to offer a much reduced chance of complications.

With intravenous injections of certain prepa-rations, severe tissue damage may follow if some of the drug enters the vein wall or surrounding tissue; the manufacturers' instructions must be followed.

Inoculations should not be carried out in a dusty shed.

(See ANTHRAX; also AMPOULE; DETERGENT RESIDUE; ENEMA.)

Large-bore needles Use of these is not without risk, especially when liver biopsies are carried out by means of suction through a needle, inserted intraperitoneally and attached to a syringe.

Accidental self-inoculation may occur owing to the sudden violent movement of a large animal. People have been infected with BRUCELLOSIS in this way; and veterinary surgeons have died from IMMOBILON. **Accidental self-injection with oil-based vaccines requires prompt hospital attention.**

Injuries
(see ACCIDENTS; WOUNDS; FRACTURES; BLEEDING; SHOCK)

Injuries from Shoeing
These are not always the fault of the farrier. There are some horses with such bad feet that it may be quite impossible to shoe them without running the risk of injuring the sensitive structures in the process. The nails, toe-clips, or even the shoe, may inflict damage.

1. *The Nails* either may produce lameness by actually penetrating the sensitive laminae – a condition called 'pricking'; or, by being driven too close to the laminae, by pressing upon the sensitive structures – a condition known as 'binding'.

Pricking may be only slight when the farrier knows that the nail has stabbed the quick and immediately withdraws it. All nail injuries should receive prompt attention, for they are usually amenable to treatment in the early stages; but if neglected they rapidly suppurate, causing the horse great pain and often permanent damage.

Binding is not so serious. Generally it suffices to remove the shoe, to allow the horse to remain barefooted for a day or so, and then to replace the shoe, taking special care that the nails are not driven too coarsely upon the 2nd occasion. The lameness in this case very often only appears 2 or 3 days after the horse has been shod, and is attributed to some other cause.

2. *The Clip* may produce lameness by being driven too coarsely, and either burning the sensitive structures when being fitted, or pressing upon them unduly when hammered into position afterwards. When side-clips are used, i.e. 1 on each side of the foot, if they are forced home too far the foot is jammed in between 2 rigid structures which will not allow it to expand and contract with each movement of the foot, and lameness results. The shoe should be removed, the horse given a day or two's rest, the clips altered, and the shoe reapplied, when he will usually go sound. If burning is suspected, the same procedure may be adopted. If the shoe loosens until it is only holding by one nail, or if the shoe is partially torn off, the horse may tread on the clip which penetrates the sole of the foot and inflict a very severe wound. This is treated as for pricking, the area being pared out.

3. *The Shoe* may cause injury if it has an uneven surface and presses upon a part too much. This is particularly liable to happen when the horn of the foot is weak and thin. Horses with flat feet, or those with dropped sole, may develop bruises of the sole if the web of the shoe presses upon the outer circumference of the sole, where it joins the white line. In such cases the shoe should be removed and the unevenness corrected, or the bearing surface of the foot should be eased. Some horses may require to be shod with a bar shoe, so that the frog may take some of the weight off the affected part, and others need a run at grass.

Burning of the sensitive parts of the foot may occur through the carelessness of the farrier, not by making the shoe too hot, but by holding it in position on the foot for too long a time, so that it may 'bed itself in'. This is a most reprehensible practice and should not be tolerated. The injury usually results in a separation of the horn from the sensitive tissues below, and some weeks pass before the horse can resume his work again. (See CORNS; BRUISED SOLE.)

Innominate
Innominate is the bone of the pelvis and the structures associated with it. The pelvis is composed of 6 separate bones, 3 on either side: ilium, pubis, and ischium.

Inoculation
(1) Introduction into an animal or culture medium of micro-organisms. (2) To induce immunity by introducing a vaccine or serum. (See INJECTIONS; VACCINATION; INFECTION; IMMUNITY.)

Insecticides
A wide range of effective insecticides is available for both external application and systemic use. Some, such as the organophosphorus compounds, may be toxic if not used properly. They have been implicated in causing illness in humans. General notes are given below; more detail will be found in the cross-references listed.

Large animals Insecticides for the protection of large animals are discussed under FLIES and FLY CONTROL. They may be administered as sprays, by immersion (dipping), as 'pour-ons' or, in some cases, by mouth. IVERMECTIN is an example.

Small animals Insecticides are available in numerous formulations for application as wet shampoos, aerosol sprays, dry dusting powders, 'spot-on' formulations and 'flea collars'. Active ingredients include permethrin, dichlorvos, fenthion and carbaril. There are many others. Dichlorvos and diazinon (both organophosphorus compounds) are used in 'flea collars'.

Manufacturers' instructions should be strictly followed, and **only preparations stated to be safe for cats** should be used on those animals.

Over-exposure of animals to insecticides, either through too frequent use or use of excessive quantities, can lead to poisoning. (See CHLORINATED HYDROCARBONS; ORGANOPHOSPHORUS POISONING; PERMETHRIN.)

Accidental poisoning DDT fell into disrepute in the UK, the USA, Australia and New Zealand, but is still used for ground spraying in parts of Africa (see DDT). The use of unsuitable insecticides can lead to fatal poisoning in cattle, etc. (See TEPP.) Poisoning may occur following absorption of an unsuitable insecticide spray through the skin. This, or inhalation of spray droplets, may lead to dangerously contaminated milk. The following insecticides are not recommended for dairy and cowshed use on account of this risk: DDT, aldrin, dieldrin, chlordane, lindane, methoxychlor, toxaphene, and heptachlor. (See CHLORINATED HYDROCARBONS.)

Some insecticides may be safe for one species of animal but fatal to another. For example, on a farm in New York State, an insecticide spray containing thiophosphate had no effect on 50 chickens, but killed more than 7000 ducklings.

Dieldrin, used as a seed dressing, has caused fatal poisoning in wood-pigeons and other wild birds. Lambs have been killed by ALDRIN. (See BHC; DDT; DIELDRIN; DERRIS; TEPP; PARATHION; PYRETHROIDS; FLY CONTROL; CARBAMATES; CHLORINATED HYDROCARBONS; GAME-BIRDS.)

Insecticide resistance Extensive use of an insecticide can encourage resistance among the target species. Only a few years after its introduction in the 1940s, house flies showed resistance to DDT, and by 1970 some 250 species of fly affecting man, his animals or crops, had developed resistance to one or more of the organochlorines, e.g. dieldrin; organophosphates; or carbamates.

Most cases of resistance apparently depend on a single gene, and are developed mostly following large-scale use of insecticides in control programmes. (See also under FLY CONTROL.)

Insects
For a general description of these, see FLIES.

Insemination
The introduction of semen into the vagina or cervix. (See ARTIFICIAL INSEMINATION.)

Insulation of Buildings, Floors
(see under HOUSING OF ANIMALS)

Insulin
Insulin is a hormone secreted by part of the pancreas, where it is produced by the islets of Langerhans. It is used in the treatment of diabetes in dogs and cats. (See DIABETES.)

Insulinoma
A tumour affecting cells of the islets of Langerhans in the pancreas, which may lead to collapse, convulsions, coma and death in the dog as a result of hypoglycaemia.

Insurance
In the UK there is now a wide choice of comprehensive insurance policies available to animal-owners. Farmers can insure against the risks of foot-and-mouth disease or brucellosis, for example. There is insurance for horses, and dog- and cat-owners can avail themselves of policies covering veterinary fees, third-party liability, theft or death of an animal from illness or accident. Policies can be issued through veterinary surgeons. With the possibility of having to pay for a major operation or prolonged treatment, such policies can minimise the owner's financial outlay, and are a safeguard against unexpected and sometimes large expenses.

Intensive Livestock Production
This means, generally speaking, having farm animals indoors to a greater extent, and also having them within a smaller space inside a building. All intensive systems require skilled management and veterinary input to prevent the problems intrinsic among large concentrations of livestock.

The economic advantages claimed for intensive livestock production are the economies of scale through reducing costs of labour and equipment per animal housed; lower feed costs through bulk buying and home mixing; the ability to afford skilled management and labour; also a saving in acres of valuable land.

The disadvantages are the effect on stock of large concentration, disease, cannibalism and all the problems of stress, and intensive feeding methods.

The following describes potential hazards and health problems, and should not be regarded as condemnation of all current farming methods.

Poultry De-beaking, to prevent feather picking and cannibalism, if badly done can cause injury and reduce resistance to infection. Birds de-beaked and unable to take a dust bath are prone to severe infestation with lice and mites, which may be resistant to the commonly used parasiticides; and infestation can be a problem in battery houses. Lack of exercise is conducive to fatty degeneration of the liver in battery birds. Among birds crowded together on deep litter, coccidiosis and worm infestations are apt to be serious. Faulty ventilation often gives rise to a harmful concentration of ammonia in houses where there is litter, and also predisposes to infectious bronchitis and other respiratory infections. The greater the concentration of birds, the greater the stress, it seems; and the more chance of an increasing proportion both of susceptible birds and of 'carriers' of various infections.

Beef cattle In calf-rearing units, salmonella infections cause a high proportion of the deaths of bought-in calves. Bronchitis is also an important cause of losses, which often amount to 7 per cent.

In units taking in 12-week-old calves, respiratory disease, principally viral infections, is important. Other conditions encountered include foul-in-the-foot, infectious bovine keratitis, and bloat.

If trough space is too limited, inflammation of the eyes may be caused by cattle flicking their ears into their neighbours' eyes – simulating the effects of infectious bovine kerato-conjunctivitis.

Among veal calves, pneumonia, bronchitis and a peracute coliform septicaemia are major causes of losses. Anaemia, parasites, and a form of anaphylactic shock are also among the hazards of rearing.

Pigs These animals are particularly prone to the effects of STRESS, and of confinement in poorly ventilated buildings which favours respiratory infections such as enzootic pneumonia.

The use of farrow-to-finish pens which accommodate pigs from birth to slaughter day has been advocated. These obviate 4 or 5 moves to strange surroundings with its accompanying stress.

Sheep Respiratory troubles, including various forms of pneumonia, are a danger in buildings where ventilation is poor. There are some very successful flock houses, with one end virtually open, where disease problems have been minimal – foot-rot being controlled by regular use of a foot-bath. In such buildings, the ewes lamb indoors, to the great advantage of the shepherd. Straw is used for bedding. Yorkshire boarding assists ventilation.

Lameness Intensive systems of farming tend to ignore the social behaviour of animals to the detriment of their health. Two examples involving lameness in cattle may be given. In the first case 12 heifers accustomed to being in a small social group outside in a straw yard were abruptly transferred at calving and put in with cows in modern concrete-based cow cubicles. Five became acutely lame with septic and aseptic laminitis and solar ulceration. In 2, the condition was so severe that they had to be slaughtered, but the other heifers improved when they were transferred to straw yards.

The outbreak was attributed to the sudden introduction to concrete surfaces and uncomfortable cubicles which reduced the time that the animals lay down. Increased activity caused by behavioural interactions with the established cows was probably also a factor.

The 2nd case involved an outbreak of solar ulcerations in 90 per cent of a small herd of dairy cows. It coincided with the occupation of a new cubicle house with concrete-based lipless cubicles. When given an opportunity the cows 'voted with their feet' and returned to their old earth-floored cubicles.

(See also HOUSING OF ANIMALS.)

Intercostal
Between the ribs.

Intercurrent
Intercurrent is a term applied to a disease which occurs during the course of another disease already present, and modifies its course or increases its severity.

Interdigital
Between 2 toes or digits.

Interdigital Cyst (Interdigital Abscess)
Interdigital cyst (interdigital abscess) is a condition commonly affecting the feet of dogs, in which abscesses about the size of a pea or larger appear in the spaces between the digits of the paws. It most often affects spaniels,

Airedales, Scots terriers, Sealyhams, and Dandie Dinmonts.

Causes are generally held to be an infection of the hair follicles between the toes, or to grit penetrating the skin there. In some instances the lesion may be a true cyst.

Signs The dog licks its foot, and upon examination a swelling (which is painful) is noticed in the interdigital space. Within a couple of days or so, the swelling may discharge a little blood-stained pus. If the lesions have been repeatedly forming, they may suddenly cease, and the dog remains free from them for perhaps months at a time. Unfortunately, recurrences are likely at varying intervals.

Treatment The foot is bandaged to keep the wound clean, and dressed daily until there is no more discharge and the wound has healed. Some encouraging results have been obtained by the professional use of CRYOSURGERY.

Interdigital Necrobacillosis
(see FOUL-IN-THE-FOOT)

Interferon
A glycoprotein which inhibits the multiplication of viruses within living cells.

Many types of cells can produce interferon as a means of defence against further viral infection.

Recombinant DNA techniques have made possible the production of interferons for therapeutic use.

Interferon is being used in several countries as an adjunct to post-exposure prophylaxis of human rabies.

Internal Haemorrhage
Internal haemorrhage may result from rupture of some large blood vessel; or it may be the result of an injury to some organ that is richly supplied with blood, such as the liver or spleen. In either case the bleeding occurs into one of the body cavities and the blood is lost to the tissues of the animal. (See also HAEMANGIOSARCOMA; diseases with names beginning with the word HAEMORRHAGIC; WARFARIN.)

Signs of severe internal haemorrhage include extreme pallor of mouth and mucous membrane lining the eyelids, coldness of the skin, rapid breathing, or a series of gasps, collapse, and a pulse becoming weak, slow, and then imperceptible. (See SHOCK.)

Treatment of severe internal haemorrhage can seldom be undertaken in time to save life. When the internal bleeding is less profuse, success may be achieved with ADRENALINE, BLOOD TRANSFUSION or DEXTRAN, VITAMIN K.

Intersex
An individual with characteristics intermediate between those of a male and a female. In cattle, examples include the FREEMARTIN; XY gonadal dysgenesis (in which there are no gonads); and testicular feminisation. A case of the latter, described by Dr S. E. Long, was a single-born cow showing signs of virilism and found to have abdominal testes, some undeveloped Mullerian duct derivatives, a normal vagina, and a 60XY genotype in all tissues examined.

In a canine example of intersex, the *os penis* was absent, the penis could not be extruded from the prepuce, and no testicles were present in the scrotum. A laparotomy revealed a uterus and ovaries.

(See under TRISOMY for the case of an intersex Spanish-bred horse, 'considered to be a mare', which had the characteristics of a pseudo-hermaphrodite male.)

Interstitial
Interstitial is a term applied to cells of different tissue set amongst the active tissue cells of an organ. It is generally of a supporting character and formed of fibrous tissue. The term is also applied to diseases which specially affect this tissue, as interstitial nephritis. (See under KIDNEYS, DISEASES OF – Chronic nephritis.)

Intervertebral Disc Protrusion
(see under SPINE)

Intestinal Adenomatosis
(see under PORCINE)

Intestine, Obstruction
This may result from an impacted mass of food material. (See IMPACTION.) In the dog, for example, a hard mass containing spicules of bone may render defecation impossible, and an enema will be necessary if a dose of medicinal liquid paraffin does not achieve the desired result. In the cat a mass of fur (fur ball) may similarly cause obstruction. FOREIGN BODY of many kinds, including string, are another cause.

Wood chewing A bad habit of some horses, whether stabled or at grass, which can lead to obstruction of the small intestine.

Signs Colic, passage of stomach contents down both nostrils.

Treatment Enterotomy under a general anaesthetic; and removal of the obstruction.

Duodenal obstruction in cattle is not common but can occur. In most cases the obstruction is due to decreased motility of the duodenum, caused by inflammation of the duodenal wall and preperforative peritonitis, resulting from duodenal ulcers or penetrating foreign bodies respectively.

Other causes A strangulated HERNIA is a serious cause of obstruction, compression of blood vessels and nerves making matters worse. INTUSSUSCEPTION, in which a part of the intestine becomes turned in on itself (like the finger of a rubber glove may do), is fraught with similar dangers. VOLVULUS, or the twisting of a loop of intestine, is another cause. All these conditions may be followed by GANGRENE and PERITONITIS. Prompt surgical treatment is necessary to save life.

A growth affecting either the lumen of the intestine so blocking it, or the exterior and so constricting it, is another possibility. (See TUMOURS; CANCER.)

Signs Intestinal obstruction can be expected to cause depression, loss of appetite, dehydration, fever, some degree of toxaemia, vomiting, and pain.

TYMPANY (distension of the intestine with gas) may occur in some cases of intestinal obstruction. In brood mares, tympany of the large intestine may predispose to rupture of the caecum (or other part) from pressure exerted by the fetal hind feet at the onset of parturition. (See also COLIC for diseases in horses.)

Intestines

Horse (1) Small intestine. This measures about 20 metres, (70 feet), and is divided into a fixed portion – duodenum and a more or less free portion – jejunum and ileum. Its diameter varies from 4 to 8 cm (1½ to 3 inches) when moderately distended, and its capacity is about 55 litres (12 gallons). (2) Large intestine. This extends from the end of the ileum to the anus, and measures about 8 metres (25 feet) in length. Its diameter varies in different parts from about 8 cm (3 inches) in the small colon to nearly 50 cm (20 inches) across the widest part of the caecum. It is divided into caecum, large colon, small colon, and rectum.

The caecum is a large blind sac lying on the right side of the abdomen and extending downwards and forwards to within a hand's-breadth from the sternum. It is shaped somewhat like a reversed comma, having both its entrance and its exit near the base, and has a capacity of about 36 litres (8 gallons). Foodstuff enters it by the ileo-caecal valve, and leaves by the caeco-colic valve, which opens into the large colon.

Cows The intestines lie entirely to the right of the middle line of the abdomen. (1) Small intestine, measuring 40 metres (130 feet) in length, lies in the lower part of the right side of the abdomen, filling in the spaces left between more fixed organs. (2) Large intestine is much smaller than in the horse, and not so complicated. The caecum lies in the upper posterior part of the abdomen, with its blind sac posteriorly in or near the pelvic inlet. The caecum is about 75 cm (2½ feet) long and is followed by the colon (there is no small colon in the ox), which has a length of about 11 metres (35 feet). The colon is arranged like the coils of a watch-spring, with each coil double, consisting of one part running towards the centre (centripetal), and a corresponding part running from the centre (centrifugal).

Sheep The intestines of the sheep are similar to those of the cow.

Pigs (1) Small intestine. This varies from 15 to 20 metres (50 to 65 feet) in length, and mainly lies on the left side and floor of the abdomen, with some coils pushed across on to the right side of the body. (2) Large intestine is about 4.5 metres (15 feet) long and considerably wider than the small bowel.

Dogs The intestines are short in this animal, only reaching a length of about 4.5 or 5 metres (15 or 16 feet), of which the small intestine measures 3.75 to 4.25 metres (12 to 14 feet). The small intestine occupies the right side of the abdomen and part of the floor. From here the colon has a short course upwards towards the head, turns across to the left side of the body, and then runs backwards to end in the rectum.

Structure In all animals the intestines, both small and large, are constructed of 4 main coats. They all consist of an inner mucous membrane lining, a submucous coat, a middle muscular coat, and an outer peritoneal one.

Mucous membrane coat: this is the soft, moist, velvety lining which is found in all parts of the intestine. (See BRUSH BORDER; PEYER'S PATCHES; VILLUS.)

Muscular coat: there are 2 definite layers of muscle fibres in the wall of the bowel. The innermost of these has its fibres all running in a circular manner round the submucous coat, and the outer layer has fibres running lengthwise. In the large intestine some of these longitudinal fibres are collected into distinct bands called 'taenia', which, being somewhat shorter than the other fibres, cause a certain amount of puckering of the bowels. The muscular arrangement of the intestines is very important, as it is responsible for all the movement of the bowels. In health it is continually contracting and expanding, shortening and lengthening, and moving the food either onwards or backwards. During the process the food is squeezed and churned and most thoroughly mixed with the digestive juices. The movement is called 'peristalsis' when it tends to move the food towards the anus, and 'antiperistalsis' when it is in the opposite direction.

Peritoneal coat: this forms the outermost covering of the bowel. It is continuous for the whole length of the canal from the pylorus to the anus, except for certain comparatively small regions where, for example, the duodenum and the caecum are bound directly to the roof of the abdomen or to other organs by fibrous tissue. It is a tough membrane with a layer of smooth glistening cells on its outer surface which rub against similar cells on the surfaces of adjacent organs and reduce friction to a minimum. (See PERITONEUM.)

Attachments The intestines are hung or held in position by folds of peritoneum which bind them, directly or indirectly, to some part of the abdominal wall. The fold in which the free part of the small intestine hangs is called the 'mesentery of the small intestine', and it is through this that the blood and lymph vessels and the nerves enter and leave the bowel. It is composed of 2 layers, in the middle of which pass the vessels.

Functions (see DIGESTION)

Intestines, Diseases of

Intestinal inflammation, or ENTERITIS, is a common disease in all animals, and may take an acute or chronic form. In either case the chief symptom is diarrhoea. In acute enteritis, diarrhoea leads to DEHYDRATION; while in the chronic form, the animal ceases to thrive and the abdomen becomes permanently 'tucked up'. The causes and treatment of enteritis are given under DIARRHOEA.

PERFORATION of part of the intestine may follow ulceration, itself a complication of some cases of enteritis. Perforation injuries received in battle used to be common in cavalry horses; they may follow stabbing injuries such as goring by bulls, farm and road accidents, or the swallowing of sharp-pointed objects. (See FOREIGN BODY.) Perforation of the wall of the intestine is obviously a very serious condition and an immediate threat to the animal's life, since bacteria which accompany partly digested food escaping from the intestine will cause PERITONITIS.

Necrosis and infarction may be detected by assessing the serum levels of CREATINE kinase. (See also VOLVULUS; INTUSSUSCEPTION; COLIC.)

Intracranial

Intracranial is the term applied to structures, diseases, or operations associated with the contents of the cranium.

Intradermal

Into the thickness of the skin as in intradermal injections.

Intramedullary

Within the marrow cavity of long bones. Thus, intramedullary pins – used in the treatment of fractures.

Intramammary

Within, or into, the mammary gland (udder).

Intramuscular

Within a muscle, e.g. intramuscular injection.

Intraperitoneal Injections

Intraperitoneal injections are those made direct into the abdominal cavity.

Intrathecal

Into a sheath; intraspinal.

Intratracheal

Into the 'windpipe'. (See also ENDOTRACHEAL ANAESTHESIA.)

Intravenous Injection

An injection direct into a vein, a technique employed in anaesthesia and where much fluid has to be injected. (See also INJECTIONS.)

Intussusception

Intussusception is a form of obstruction of the bowels in which a part of the intestine turns in on itself like the finger of a rubber glove. It usually follows increased gut motility and often results from diarrhoea. It occurs mostly in horses, puppies and kittens, causes obstruction of the intestine and great pain.

If the condition is not relieved it leads to stopping of the blood supply in that part of the bowel which is enclosed, and death. Signs include loss of appetite, uneasiness due to abdominal pain, straining, and blood in the faeces. In the dog a sausage-like swelling may be palpated in the abdomen, or there may be protrusion from the anus of a turgid, cylindrical mass having four thicknesses of bowel wall. Treatment involves manipulation under anaesthesia (after laparatomy in most cases), and sometimes the surgical removal of the innermost portion of the bowel and an end-to-end anastomosis.

Caecal intussusception In 2 ponies, intussusception led, respectively, to pain followed by sudden death; and to pain lasting 3 weeks from the time of a veterinary examination. The 1st case was found at autopsy to have intussusception of the base of the caecum; the 2nd had the entire caecum invaginated into the colon. In both animals the lesions had been present for a long time.

Invertebrates

Animals without backbones. Some of these are kept as 'pets' (tarantula spiders, scorpions, millipedes, praying mantis, etc.). It should be noted that where they are kept as captive animals they fall under the Protection of Animals Act 1911 and action has been taken in cases of neglect. In New Zealand, 2 classes of invertebrate (molluscs and crustaceans) are covered by the Animal Welfare Act 1999. In the UK, the common octopus (*Octopus vulgaris*) is protected under the Animals (Scientific Procedures) Act 1986.

Involution

A change back to its normal condition which an organ undergoes after fulfilling its normal function, e.g. involution of the uterus following pregnancy.

Iodides

Iodides are salts of iodine. Sodium iodide is used in the treatment of actinobacillosis, and formerly it was used with other drugs in the treatment of oedema, and of ringworm. Taken in excess, iodides cause a condition known as 'iodism' or iodine poisoning. The symptoms of this are diarrhoea, loss of appetite, emaciation, total refusal of water, a dry, scurfy condition of the skin with a loss of hair, and in some cases catarrh of the nasal mucous membranes.

Iodine

Iodine is a non-metallic element which occurs naturally in seaweed, brine, etc. It is prepared in the form of dark violet-brown scales, which are soluble in alcohol and ether.

Uses Pure iodine in the form of scales is never used. The ordinary tincture of iodine that is a common household remedy contains 2.5 per cent of iodine. Solubilised formulations of iodine known as IODOPHORS, e.g. Iosan CCT, are used for teat-dipping in dairy hygiene for the prevention of mastitis. (See also MASTITIS IN COWS – Teat-dipping.) Iodophors are also used in treating minor skin wounds and abrasions.

Internally, iodine is a violent irritant poison. (See also under RADIOACTIVE IODINE.)

Iodine Deficiency on the Farm

Iodine is required by the body for the formation of thyroxine, the hormone produced by the thyroid gland, and the common sign of iodine deficiency is goitre. Acute iodine deficiency occurs in 14 states of the USA. In Britain, typical iodine deficiency is not common in farm stock, although in some areas the question of iodine intake below the optimum for health and fertility is of economic importance. The remedy is to provide salt licks or mineral mixtures containing traces of iodine. This is particularly important when large quantities of kale, cabbage, or turnips are fed. (See TRACE ELEMENTS.)

Iodophor

(see under IODINE)

Ionic Medication, Iontophoresis

A form of treatment involving the use of an electric current to cause ions of soluble substances to pass through the skin and subcutaneous tissues. Electrolytes which have been used include sodium chloride, magnesium sulphate, copper sulphate, methylene blue, quinine sulphate, and adrenaline. These are made into solutions in which pads of felt or lint are soaked, and the pads are applied to the area to be treated. One electrode is laid over the pad, and another applied to some suitable part of the body and the current is applied. This causes a disintegration of the electrolyte into its constituent ions which are driven through the skin.

Uses Ionisation has been used to stimulate the healing of ulcers, in the treatment of demodectic mange, to soften scars, to exert local antiseptic or germicidal actions, to allay

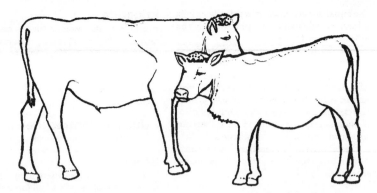

Iodine deficiency – comparison of body size between the normal and deficient animal.

pain, and to induce local construction of vessels in treating inflammatory changes.

Ionised Calcium

In horses treated surgically for colic, the concentration of calcium ions (Ca^+) was lower in 71 horses with strangulating and non-strangulating infarctions of the caecum, ascending colon, or small intestine than in 76 horses with non-strangulating obstructions of the ascending or descending colon. Treatment with 23 per cent calcium gluconate restored the ionised calcium concentration to within the normal range. Calcium has an important role in mediating the contractile activity of intestinal smooth muscle. It is recommended that ionised calcium should be monitored after surgery for colic in horses, and that calcium gluconate be administered intravenously as required.

Ionising Radiation Regulations 1985

These were introduced in the UK and cover the inspection of X-ray equipment in veterinary practices, from a safety point of view.

Ionophores

These include the antibiotics monensin, narasin, salinomycin, and lasalocid. They are so-called because they have the capability to combine with particular ions and to transport these ions through biological membranes. They are used as growth promoters and to control protozoal infections such as coccidiosis.

Ionophore poisoning (see MONENSIN SODIUM)

Iris

Iris is the muscular and fibrous curtain which hangs behind the cornea of the eye and serves to regulate the amount of light that is allowed to reach the inner parts of the eye. It possesses radiating and circular fibres which, when they contract under the influence of light, enlarge and decrease the size of the pupil respectively. (See EYE.)

Iridectomy An operation by which a part or the whole of the iris is removed.

Irish Setter

This largish dog with pendulous ears and a silky chestnut coat was originally a gun dog. Inherited defects include quadriplegia, amblyopia and progressive retinal atrophy. Other conditions that may possibly be inherited are haemophilia, spondylolithesis ('Wobbler syndrome'), and mega-oesophagus.

Irish Wolfhound

A very large, tall dog with long head, deep chest and rough wiry coat; usually grey or beige in colour. Ununited anconeal process (incompletely developed elbow-joint) and calcinosis circumspecta may be inherited. The breed is prone to rhinitis.

Iritis

Inflammation of the iris. (See EYE.)

Iron

Iron is a nutritional TRACE ELEMENT – essential for life. Over half the body's iron is contained in the haemoglobin of the red blood cells and myoglobin of muscles. Iron is additionally present as beta-globulin transferrin in the blood plasma, in the myoglobin of muscles, and in enzymes.

Iron deficiency results in anaemia, often seen in fast- growing piglets reared indoors; there is paleness, dyspnoea and diarrhoea. It is also found in calves and lambs fed milk or milk substitute without iron supplementation and little or no roughage.

Iron also has a role in bodily resistance to infection. IRON-BINDING PROTEINS can be shown to inhibit the growth of bacteria *in vitro*. The ability of some micro-organisms to bind iron to themselves, depriving the host animal, is a feature of pathogenicity, and ability of the host to limit availability to the pathogen is associated with resistance to infection.

Bacteria (e.g. salmonellas and tubercle bacilli) and some fungi produce iron-binding substances.

Iron-Binding Proteins

Iron-binding proteins include conalbumin, a constituent of egg-white; transferrin, in blood plasma; lactoferrin, in milk, tears, saliva, bile, seminal secretions, cervical mucus, and in the granules of neutrophils. All these proteins inhibit the growth of bacteria, including salmonella.

Iron-Dextran

A compound of iron used in injectable form to prevent iron-deficiency anaemia in piglets.

Iron Poisoning

This may occur from overdosage, or from the eating by a pet animal of an iron preparation left within reach. (See also under FLOOR FEEDING OF PIGS, for the danger of concrete made with sand rich in iron.)

Horses have died very soon after receiving an intramuscular injection of an organic iron preparation.

Piglets have been poisoned by iron-dextran preparations given to prevent anaemia and ASYMMETRIC HINDQUARTER SYNDROME may develop following organic iron injections.

In the dog, ferrous sulphate or ferrous gluconate in doses as low as 0.3 or 0.75 g respectively of ferrous iron per kg body-weight, have caused severe illness with diarrhoea, vomiting and ulceration of stomach and intestine.

Irradiation

Exposure to X-rays, radio-active material, ultra-violet, or infra-red rays. Irradiation with measured doses of X-rays is used therapeutically in treating tumours; and to attenuate lungworm larvae for use as an oral vaccine against husk. Irradiation with ultra-violet light is used to sterilise, e.g. milk to extend its usable life. (See PARASITIC BRONCHITIS; also 'RADIATION SICKNESS'; IONISING RADIATION.)

Irrigation

Irrigation is the washing-out of wounds or cavities of the body by means of large amounts of warm water containing some antiseptic in solution.

Ischaemia

Local anaemia.

Ischaemic Contracture
(see under MUSCLES, DISEASES OF)

Ischium

Ischium is the bone which forms the most posterior part of the pelvis, and forms the point of the buttock.

Ischuria

Ischuria means insufficiency in the amount of urine passed, due either to suppression of excretion in the kidneys or to retention in the bladder.

Islets of Langerhans
(see PANCREAS)

Isoflurane

A colourless liquid with an ether-like smell, non-explosive and non-inflammable in clinical concentrations, used as an inhalation anaesthetic for most species. Induction of anaesthesia and recovery are more rapid than with halothane. It is useful in high-risk cardiac cases.

Isolation

Isolation is an important procedure in the control of the spread of infectious disease. On a farm it is advisable, where practicable, to keep newly bought stock separate from previously existing stock for 2 or 3 weeks, so that if infectious/contagious disease occurs it may be possible to prevent its spread to the old stock. (See INCUBATION; INFECTION; QUARANTINE; NOTIFIABLE DISEASES.)

Isoquinolinium

Isoquinolinium chloride lotion has been used in the treatment of ringworm in cattle.

Isospora

A genus of protozoal parasites which cause coccidiosis. *I. suis* is a cause of coccidiosis in pigs.

Isotonic

Isotonic is a term applied to solutions which have the same power of diffusion as one another.

An isotonic solution used in medicine is one which can be mixed with body fluids without causing any disturbance. An isotonic saline solution for injection into the blood, so that it may possess the same osmotic pressure as the blood serum, contains 0.9 per cent sodium chloride. This is also known as normal or physiological salt solution. An isotonic solution of glucose for injection into the blood is one of 5 per cent strength in water. Solutions, which are weaker or stronger than the fluids of the body with which they are intended to be mixed, are known as hypotonic and hypertonic respectively.

Itchiness
(see PRURITUS)

'Itchy Leg'
A common term for choriotic mange.

-Itis
A suffix added to the name of an organ to signify inflammation of that organ.

IV
Short for intravenous; usually refers to that route of injection.

Ivermectin
Ivermectin, an AVERMECTIN, is a potent anthelmintic, effective at very low dosage, which can be given orally, by subcutaneous injection or as a pour-on (transdermally). Ivermectin also gives control of lungworms in addition to external parasites such as warbles, lice, and sarcoptic mange mites on pigs; it is an effective treatment for sheep scab, given as 2 injections, 1 week apart. It is effective against mature and immature roundworms of cattle, including *Ostertagia* larvae; against ticks, mange mites, warbles, etc. Horses can be dosed orally with a paste formulation of ivermectin for the control of roundworms and horse bots. (See WORMS, FARM TREATMENT AGAINST; HORSE BOTS.)

Formulations of ivermectin (Ivomec from MSD Agvet) are available in the UK for sheep, pigs, cattle and horses; but not for dogs or cats.

A pour-on formulation of Ivomec is available for the control of internal and external parasites of cattle. The product contains isopropyl alcohol which is highly inflammable. Protective clothing (including gloves) must be worn when liquid Ivermectin products are applied.

Ivermectin poisoning in dogs has occurred as a result of ignoring manufacturers' recommendations.

A dog which had been injected with ivermectin by a friend of the owner was in a coma for 7 weeks. On veterinary examination the day after the injection, the signs were dilated pupils, ataxia, and depression, with no response to sound and apparent blindness. Four days later, complete coma had developed. Only the swallowing reflex was present. The animal was maintained, after preliminary treatment, on oral glucose and hydrolised protein solution given by the owner

Twitching of an ear when spoken to was the first response on day 26. By 5 weeks the dog was eating, able to stand if lifted, but still blind. At 7 weeks, sight had returned and the dog appeared normal again.

Ixodes
Ixodes is the generic name of one of the varieties of ticks that infest animals. (See TICKS.)

J

Jaagsiekte
A disease of adult sheep, first recognised in South Africa. (See PULMONARY ADENOMATOSIS.)

Jack
A male donkey.

Jack Beans
Jack Beans may cause poisoning if fed raw. (See LEGUME POISONING.)

Jack Russell Terrier
A small, lively dog, having a white coat with brown or black patches. Originally a cross-breed, it now breeds true. Prone to patellar luxation, it may inherit ataxia, lens luxation and Perthe's disease.

Jacobson's Organ
Also known as the vomeronasal organ, this is associated with the detection of flavours such as those of food, but is thought also to be able to detect pheromones. The organ has 2 small tubes which extend from the floor of the nasal cavity to the level of the 2nd/4th cheek tooth. It is active in most mammals, but even more highly developed in certain reptiles, especially snakes.

Janet
A female mule.

Japanese B Encephalitis
This disease is present in Nepal and other regions of Asia.

Cause A flavivirus. The disease is transmitted by mosquitoes from avian species which act as reservoirs of infection but are themselves asymptomatic.

Signs In horses, the sight is affected first. Later they become drowsy. Many die, and the recovery of others is seldom complete. Pigs are also susceptible; abortion and stillbirths result from infection.

The disease is a zoonosis, and for its prevention in people a vaccine has been used.

Japanese Bobtail
A breed of cat of 'foreign' conformation with a rudimentary tail. The hind-legs are longer than the fore-legs but are kept angled so that the back is level. There are similarities with the Manx, but there does not appear to be the same frequency of defects as occurs in that breed.

Japanese Tosa
A breed of dog raised in Japan for fighting. Importation into the UK is banned under the Dangerous Dogs Act.

Jaundice
Jaundice is a yellowish discoloration of the visible mucous membranes of the body (eye, nose, mouth, and genital organs). The discoloration is caused by bilirubin, an orange-yellow pigment produced following the breakdown of erythrocytes due to liver disease or obstruction of the bile flow from the liver and gall-bladder.

The symptom of jaundice (icterus) may also follow the destruction of red blood cells by parasites, such as may occur in cases of biliary fever and surra in the horse; red-water in cattle; malignant jaundice (canine babesiosis); it is seen also in leptospiral jaundice (see LEPTOSPIROSIS), and canine viral hepatitis.

In cats, jaundice is seen in the dry form of feline infectious peritonitis, toxoplasmosis.

Jaundice may indicate an incompatibility between the blood of sire and dam causing haemolytic jaundice of the newborn foal or piglet.

When bile cannot enter into the small intestine by the bile-duct from the liver in the usual way, it becomes dammed back, is absorbed by the lymphatics and the blood vessels, carried into the general circulation, and some of its constituents are deposited in the tissues. (See GALL-STONES, also under GALL-BLADDER; CIRRHOSIS; LIVER, DISEASES OF; EQUINE BILIARY FEVER.)

It may be seen during poisoning with copper, mercury, phosphorus, chloroform, or lead, and after some snakebites. Aflatoxins may cause jaundice.

(See also LEPTOSPIROSIS; JAUNDICE; FOALS, DISEASES OF; and BILIARY FEVER.)

Jaundice, Leptospiral
(see under LEPTOSPIROSIS for the appropriate animal)

Java Bean Poisoning
The Java beans, *Phaseolus lunatus*, were once imported in large amounts. The beans are of varying origin, and differ in colour, thus: Java beans are as a rule reddish-brown, but they may be almost black; Rangoon or Burmah beans are

smaller, plumper, and lighter in colour (so-called 'red-Rangoons' are pinkish with small purple splashes).

The active poisonous agent in the beans is a substance called phaseolunatin, which is a member of a group of cyanogenetic glucosides.

Signs These are exactly the same as those given under HYDROCYANIC ACID.

Jaw

The upper jawbones are 2 in number and are firmly united to the other bones of the face. The lower jaw – mandible or coronoid process – is composed of a single bone in horse, pig, dog, and cat, but in the ruminants the fusion between right and left sides does not occur until old age. Each of the jaws presents a number of deep sockets or 'alveoli' which contain the teeth. (See DISLOCATIONS; FRACTURES; MOUTH; TEETH; also MUSCLES, DISEASES OF; ACTINOMYCOSIS (LUMPY JAW).

Jaw, Diseases of

For overshot and undershot jaws, see under TEETH, DISEASES OF.

'Lion jaw' (craniomandibular osteopathy): a disease seen mostly in West Highland terriers. Eating becomes difficult; mouth-opening, painful.

(See 'BOTTLE-JAW'.)

Jejunum

Jejunum is the central portion of the small INTESTINE.

'Jeckyll and Hyde' Syndrome

Also known as 'rage syndrome', this is a condition seen in cocker spaniels, especially those of a golden or dun colour. For no apparent reason a quiet dog will suddenly become very aggressive. The dog then returns to its normal behaviour.

Jenny

A female ass.

Jequirity Poisoning

This is caused by the red and black seeds of the climbing plant *Abrus precatorius*, which grows in Australia, Asia, and South America. It gives rise to cyanosis and pinpoint-sized haemorrhages from the skin, as well as diarrhoea.

Jersian

Also known as a F–J hybrid, this is a beef cross obtained from a Jersey bull on a Friesian cow. (In New Zealand, the reverse cross is used.)

Jetting

Jetting is a technique developed in Australia, involving the application of insecticide under pressure by means of a jetting gun – a handpiece with 4 needle jets for combing through the wool. The pressure used is 10 to 14 kg/cm^2 (60 to 80 lb per sq in), which can be achieved by an ordinary medium/high-volume agricultural sprayer.

Jetting is not displaced dipping to any extent in the UK, where spraying has been found inefficient in the control of sheep scab.

Jigger Flea

(see under FLEAS – *Tunga penetrans*)

Jill

A female donkey or ferret.

Johne's Disease (Paratuberculosis)

Johne's Disease (Paratuberculosis) is a chronic infection, involving the small and large intestines. It affects cattle particularly, but sometimes sheep, goats, and deer, and is characterised by the appearance of a persistent diarrhoea, gradual emaciation, and great weakness. The infection has been set up experimentally in the rabbit. It may occur naturally in the pig, and post-mortem findings may at first suggest tuberculosis.

Cause *Mycobacterium johnei* (*M. paratuberculosis*).

Experimentally, sheep can be infected with as few as 1000 *M. johnei* bacilli. These then multiply in the intestinal mucosa for the first 2 or 3 months after infection. Some animals are able to overcome the infection completely; others become carriers, with the bacilli remaining in the intestinal mucosa and lymph nodes. Some of the carriers eventually become clinically ill with Johne's disease.

Signs The disease is very slow in onset. Cattle that have become infected may not show symptoms for as long as 2 years after the last case occurred on that farm.

Pointers to the disease are an unexplained drop in milk yield (often months before other symptoms appear); and diarrhoea in an individual adult animal.

Loss of condition, general unthriftiness, a harsh, staring coat are then seen, with diarrhoea. The temperature fluctuates a degree or two above normal. Appetite is variable. In the last stages emaciation becomes very marked, and the animal becomes progressively weaker.

In sheep, diarrhoea is not a major symptom.

Treatment When well established, Johne's disease is invariably fatal, and no treatment is effective or worthwhile.

Prevention Attention should be paid to the prevention of infection in other animals, especially calves. Pastures that are suspected of being heavily infected should be left without stock for 4 or 5 months. All infected litter should be stored in a dung-pit which is not accessible to other animals, and should be used for cultivated land. Loose-boxes, sheds, etc., that have housed a case should be carefully disinfected and diseased animals should be fed after healthy ones. Ponds and water-courses should be fenced to prevent fouling by faeces, water for drinking being pumped out.

Calfhood vaccination may prevent clinical disease but interferes with subsequent tuberculin tests.

Vaccination is being practised in Iceland, the Netherlands, Belgium, and France.

In Norway a vaccination campaign to control the disease in goats reduced the infection rate from 53 to 1 per cent. Kids are vaccinated at the age of 2 to 4 weeks.

Diagnosis The disease can usually be diagnosed on clinical evidence, with some confirmation afforded by microscopic examination of the faeces. Typical clumps of acid-fast bacilli may be found, and the complement fixation test is positive in about 90 per cent of cattle with advanced disease. The fluorescent antibody test is equally useful.

Unfortunately, diagnosis of the carrier state is not possible with any certainty. There is no single test which can conclusively detect the presence or absence of *M. johnei,* although laboratory tests can identify the presence of *Mycobacteria* spp. The complement fixation test is positive in only a small proportion of carriers and can give false positive results.

The difficulty in identifying 'carriers' makes Johne's disease a difficult one to control.

Johnin

A diagnostic agent derived from *M. paratuberculosis* used for JOHNE'S DISEASE. Cutaneous injection results in thickening of the skin in positive cases. While insufficiently sensitive for individual diagnosis, the test is useful for identifying infected herds.

Joint-Ill

Also called NAVEL-ILL or POLYARTHRITIS, this is a disease of foals, lambs, and calves, in which abscesses form at the umbilicus and in some of the joints of the limbs, due, in the majority of cases, to the entrance of organisms into the body by way of the unclosed navel. There are numerous organisms associated with the disease, the commonest of which are streptococci, staphylococci, *Pasteurella, E. coli,* the necrosis bacillus, and see under FOALS, DISEASES OF.

Signs Usually the young animal becomes dull, takes no interest in its dam, refuses to suckle; the breathing is hurried; the temperature rises from 0.6° to 1.2°C (2° to 4°F) above normal; the foal prefers to lie stretched out on its side, and may have attacks of either diarrhoea or constipation. If the navel is examined it is found to be wet and oozing with bloodstained serous material, or it may be dry, swollen, painful to the touch, and hard, owing to abscess formation within. In cases that appear later in life there may be no umbilical symptoms. In the course of a day or so, one or more of the joints swells up. The joints most commonly attacked are the stifle, hip, knee, hock, shoulder and elbow, but it may be seen in any of the others. The swelling is tense, painful, hot, and oedematous. There is the danger of a fatal septicaemia.

A chronic form of infection resulting in internal umbilical abscesses is sometimes seen. The primary infection occurs at, or soon after, birth; but once the umbilicus has sealed over, external signs are not evident, and the umbilical remnant appears normal.

The calves are usually presented as unthrifty, depressed and slow in their movements. Their temperature invariably normal.

Prevention Attention must always be paid to the cleanliness of the foaling-box, the calving-box and the lambing-pen. Where climatic and other conditions are favourable, the pregnant females should be allowed to give birth to their young out of doors. Lambing-pens should without fail be changed to a fresh site every year.

Investigations undertaken by the Animal Health Trust suggest that thoroughbred foals in the UK suffer severe illness as a result of being deprived of a not inconsiderable volume of blood when the navel cord is severed prematurely by attendants. Severance of the cord, it seems, is always best left to the mare. The use of strong disinfectants applied to the stump of the navel cord is likewise deprecated.

An application of a sulphanilamide or other antibiotic dry dressing may be safer than iodine solution.

When cutting the cord, it is necessary to maintain the strictest cleanliness. Scissors should be sterilised, and tape scrupulously clean.

Treatment Antibiotics and, if available, anti-serum for the causative micro-organisms. Surgically, the umbilicus is opened up, evacuated, and disinfected. Isolation and other hygiene measures are needed.

All pails, and other feeding utensils that are liable to get infected, should be thoroughly cleaned using boiling water or steamed before future use, and the pen or box that houses a case should be occasionally washed out with disinfectant. (See also FOALS, DISEASES OF.)

Joints

Joints fall into 2 great divisions, namely movable joints and fixed joints. In a movable joint there are 4 main structures. Firstly, there are the 2 bones whose junction forms the joint; secondly, there is a layer of smooth cartilage covering the ends of these bones where they meet, which is called 'articular' cartilage; thirdly, there is a sheath of fibrous tissue known as the 'joint capsule', which is thickened into bands of 'ligaments' which hold the bones together at various points; and finally, there is a closed bladder of membrane, known as the 'synovial membrane', which lines the capsule and produces a synovial fluid to lubricate the movements of the joint. Further, the bones are kept in position at the joints by the various muscles passing over them. This type is known as a diarthrodial joint.

Some joints possess subsidiary structures such as discs of fibro-cartilage, which adapt the bones more perfectly to one another where they do not quite correspond, and allow of slightly freer movement, e.g. the stifle-joint. In others, movable pads of fat under the synovial membrane fill up larger cavities and afford additional protection to the joint, e.g. the hock-joint. In some the edge of one bone is amplified by a margin of cartilage which makes dislocation less of a risk than otherwise, e.g. the hip and the shoulder-joints.

In the fixed joints a layer of cartilage or of fibrous tissue intervenes between the bones and binds them firmly together (synarthrodial joint). This type of joint is exemplified by the 'sutures' between the bones that make up the skull. Classified among these fixed joints are the amphi-arthrodial joints, in which there is a thick disc of fibro-cartilage between the bones, so that, although the individual joint is capable of only limited movement, a series of these, like the joints between the bodies of the vertebrae, gives the column, as a whole, a very flexible character. In this connection it is noticeable that the movement in the region of the neck may be much more free than in some of the true movable joints, such as between the small bones of the hock or carpus.

Varieties Apart from the division into fixed and movable joints, those that are movable are further classified. Gliding joints are those in which the bones have flat surfaces capable only of a limited amount of movement, such as the bones of the carpus and tarsus. In hinge-joints like the elbow, fetlock, and pastern, movement can take place around one axis only, and is called flexion and extension. In the ball-and-socket joints, such as the shoulder and hip-joints, free movement can occur in any direction. There are other subsidiary varieties, named according to the shape of the bones which enter into the joint.

Joints, Diseases of

Arthritis means inflammation which involves all the structures of the joint – viz. synovial membrane, capsular ligaments, cartilages, and the ends of the bones that take part in the formation of the joint. Arthritis is a general term which includes osteoarthritis and rheumatoid arthritis. Arthritis often begins as a synovitis (see below), but the degree of inflammation is severe enough to extend to the structures around the synovial membrane. Its causes, symptoms, and treatment are similar to those given for synovitis, but it sometimes leads to ankylosis and fixation of the joint. (See CORTISONE.) The joints that are most often affected are the stifle, hock, knee, and fetlocks, but the shoulder, hip, elbow, and the lower joints of the digit are not infrequently the seat of disease as well. Among diseases that are associated with joints, and which are treated separately, are NAVICULAR DISEASE; SLIPPED SHOULDER; SLIPPED STIFLE; HYGROMA; CAPPED ELBOW; CAPPED HOCK; KNUCKLING OF THE FETLOCK; JOINT-ILL; see also below and BURSITIS; ANKYLOSIS; FRACTURES; DISLOCATIONS; GLASSER'S DISEASE; HIP DYSPLASIA IN DOGS; SWINE ERYSIPELAS.

Rheumatoid arthritis This can be important in the dog, and may occur at any age from 2 years. Symptoms may be vague at first; the animal appears depressed, with a poor appetite and often some degree of fever, but with no lameness. Eventually the latter symptom appears, sometimes involving several joints, sometimes affecting only one limb and then shifting to another. There may be crepitus – a grating sound – when the limb is moved.

Diagnosis depends upon radiography and – as in human medicine – there are certain laboratory tests, the results of which provide additional criteria for deciding whether the condition really is rheumatoid arthritis or not.

Intractable arthritis of the hip-joint in dogs, as in human beings, may be overcome by major surgery involving removal of the top of the femur and replacement of the ball part of the ball-and-socket joint with a plastic prosthesis.

Synovitis is the name given to any inflammation of the membrane lining a joint cavity. It may be acute, sub-acute, or chronic.

Generally this is not a separate condition but occurs during the course of rheumatism, rickets, gout (in poultry), severe sprains and bruises, and in a variety of specific infections such as brucellosis, swine erysipelas, tuberculosis. Tubercular joint disease often produces a chronic synovitis in the neck bones of the horse, which leads to an arthritis later.

Conditions such as wind-galls, curb, bog spavin, etc., are really only synovitis that have become chronic or are complicated with other pathological conditions.

The synovial membrane becomes inflamed, thickened, and secretes an excessive amount of fluid into the joint. As a result the joint becomes hot, swollen, and painful. The animal goes lame in greater or lesser degree according to the extent of the inflammation. When at rest, the joint is usually kept flexed with the toe of the affected leg just resting on the ground. If it is a simple condition, such as a mild sprain, these symptoms last for a few days and gradually pass off. In more severe cases, such as in joint-ill, there may be pus formation, septicaemia, and death. In the chronic type the swelling persists. The animal is able to use its limb as usual, but the accumulated fluid in the cavity does not disappear (e.g. bog spavin, wind-galls, etc.).

Open joint is a condition in which, by accident or other trauma, the inside of the joint is exposed to infection.

The seriousness of an open joint is not so much due to the initial injury as to the danger of infection. This may cause tissue destruction within the joint, and even lead to a fatal SEPTICAEMIA.

The most striking signs of open joint are, first, the excessive degree of pain that seems out of all proportion to the visible amount of damage that has been inflicted; secondly, the great amount of swelling that is usually seen; and thirdly, the discharge of a thin, straw-coloured or blood-stained sticky synovia which has a tendency to coagulate around the skin opening.

Veterinary advice should be sought at once. Prompt treatment with antibiotics, and surgery if required, is necessary to prevent or limit infection.

Dislocations (see main dictionary entry)

Bursitis, an inflammation of a bursa, commonly occurs in the region of a joint. The prominences of the hock, elbow, knee, stifle, etc., are protected by bursae – lined on their insides by synovial membrane. These sometimes become inflamed and lead to the formation of fluctuating swellings which have a tendency to become chronic. Capped elbow, capped hock, and hygroma of the knee, are of this nature. (See also OSTEOARTHRITIS; MAST CELLS; OSTEOCHONDROSIS; RHEUMATISM.)

Joule

A derived SI unit of metabolisable energy. (See CALORIES and STARCH EQUIVALENT, which it replaced; also SI UNITS.)

Jugular Veins

Jugular veins carry the blood back to the chest from the head and anterior parts of the neck. The jugular vein is often used for taking blood samples and for intravenous injection. The jugular furrow is the groove between the trachea and the muscles of the neck, in the depths of which lies the jugular vein.

Jungle Fowl

(*Gallus gallus*) A native of the rain forests of South-East Asia, it is the species from which the domestic fowl originated. In its normal environment it prefers hot, humid, shady conditions with frequent rain showers. A broiler-producing company has replicated the climate found in the rain forest in its broiler houses. Mortality was very low and lameness almost non-existent, although the birds took a little longer to reach market weight.

Juvenile Cellulitis

Also known as 'puppy strangles', this condition affects pups between 3 weeks and 4 months of age. The cause is unknown but a hypersensitivity reaction may be involved. Clinical signs are cellulitis on the face and head, prepuce and anus, accompanied by lethargy, anorexia and, possibly, raised temperature. There may be lymphadenopathy. Steroid and antibiotic therapy is indicated; affected parts may be bathed in aluminium acetate solution. Permanent scarring may result.

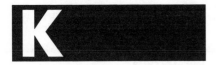

K88 Antigen

This is possessed by certain strains of *E. coli* which cause diarrhoea in piglets during their first few days of life. (See E. COLI; BACTERIAL ADHESIVENESS.)

K99 Antigen

K99 Antigen is found in strains of *E. coli* which cause diarrhoea in calves.

K Value

This is used as a measure of the insulating value of building materials such as glass fibre, wood.

Kala-Azar (Dumdum Fever)

A human disease caused by LEISHMANIA.

Kale

Kale contains a factor which gives rise to goitre if fed in large amounts, without other foods, over a long period. Haemoglobinuria sometimes follows the grazing of frosted kale by cattle, which may suffer anaemia without showing this symptom. The illness can be serious, resembling POST-PARTURIENT HAEMOGLOBIN-URIA, and may result in sudden death. The frothy type of bloat may also occur in cattle eating excessive quantities of kale – especially, it seems, during wet weather and when no hay is fed. There is some evidence to suggest that the feeding of large quantities of kale may lead to low conception rates, and to mastitis. (See also BLOAT.)

It should be added that kale anaemia and haemoglobinuria are by no means always associated with frosted kale, but merely with an excessive (probably over 18 kg (40 lb) per cow per day) intake of kale. The symptoms of kale anaemia include lassitude and rapid breathing and pulse-rate.

'Kangaroo Gait'

'Kangaroo gait' in ewes, both in New Zealand and in the UK, appears to be associated with disease of the radial nerves, which causes difficulty in advancing the front feet. When made to move rapidly, they do so with a bounding gait. The condition is seen in ewes during lactation; it normally resolves after weaning.

Kaolin (China Clay)

Kaolin (China Clay) is a native aluminium silicate, which is used as a protective and astringent dry dusting powder. Kaolin is sometimes given internally as an adsorbent in intestinal disorders. Mixed into a paste with glycerine and some antiseptic, it is applied as a poultice to acute sprains of tendons, etc.

Karyotype

This is, roughly speaking, a plan showing an animal's chromosomes. In technical terms, a karyotype is a presentation of the metaphase chromosomes characteristic of an individual animal or species. (See CYTOGENETICS.)

'Kebbing'

(see ABORTION, ENZOOTIC, OF EWES)

Ked

Melophagus ovinus, the sheep ked, is wingless, and lives on the wool and skin of the sheep. It is much larger than any of the lice, being 0.6 cm (¼ inch) long. It can easily be distinguished from the ticks by its tripartite body. It is a dark brown colour with a sharp biting proboscis. The nearly mature larvae are laid on the wool and they at once pupate. The pupa may remain in the wool or fall to the ground. The young hatch in 19 to 24 days, and the females start to deposit larvae in 12 to 23 days after emergence, and lay a larva every 9 days. The fly can live for about 12 days away from the sheep, while the pupa can live for 6 weeks on the ground. The whole life-cycle may be completed on the sheep within 1 month.

The sheep ked can cause severe anaemia if present in large numbers, and also leads to a damaged fleece. Shearing aids control, which is achieved by means of a sheep dip.

The ked may attack men while shearing and inflict a very painful bite.

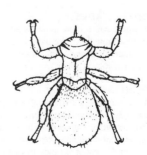

Melophagus × 4.

Keeshond

A medium-sized breed of dog, originally from Flanders, with a very thick coat, fox-like face and a tail that curls over the back. It is prone to hip dysplasia. The incidence of tetralogy of Fallot (a potentially fatal heart defect) in the breed is 1 in 10,000 births, the highest known in any animal.

Kemps

Coarse hairs, the presence of which reduces the value of a fleece.

Kennel Cough

Kennel cough is a convenient term for those outbreaks of respiratory disease, distinct from canine distemper, which are troublesome in boarding kennels and dog pounds. Other names are canine infectious tracheobronchitis and bordetellosis.

Usually only the upper air passages are involved in kennel cough, the chief symptom being a fit of coughing which is aggravated by exercise or excitement. The cough is a harsh, dry one. It has to be differentiated from infestation with TRACHEAL WORMS.

Causes *Bordetella bronchiseptica* is the principal cause (hence the name bordetellosis). Other organisms involved are the canine parainfluenza virus (CPI), a canine herpesvirus, two adenoviruses, a reovirus, and a mycoplasma. Bacterial secondary invaders may complicate the syndrome.

Prevention Vaccination is advisable a fortnight before a dog is taken to a show or left in boarding kennels. An intranasal live *B. bronchiseptica* vaccine is available.

Kennel Lameness

A colloquial term for lameness arising from a nutritional deficiency, such as may occur in a dog fed entirely on dog-biscuits. (See RICKETS.)

Kennel Sickness

A colloquial name used in the USA for outbreaks of salmonellosis, the symptoms of which may include pneumonia and convulsions. (See also under SALMONELLOSIS.)

Keratin

Keratin is the substance of which horn and the surface layers of the skin are composed. It is a modified form of skin which has undergone compression and toughening. It is present in the hoof of the feet of animals, in claws, horns, and nails.

Keratitis

Inflammation of the cornea. (See EYE, DISEASES OF.)

Keratocoele

Keratocoele is a hernia through the cornea. (See EYE, DISEASES OF.)

Keratoma

Keratoma is a horn tumour affecting the inner aspect of the wall of the hoof.

Kerosene Poisoning

(see PARAFFIN)

Kerry Blue Terrier

A medium-sized dog, born with a black coat that gradually lightens to grey, and an upright tail. It is predisposed to cerebellar abiotrophy, a degeneration in the cerebellum, that manifests as ataxia.

Ketamine

Ketamine is a non-barbiturate, non-narcotic anaesthetic. It can be administered by intravenous, intramusuclar or subcutaneous injection and is used in various species including cat, dog and horse. Ketamine is often used in conjunction with other agents, such as xylazine, medetomidine and detomidine, to improve muscle relaxation during surgical procedures.

Ketoconazole

An antifungal compound used to treat systemic candidiasis and ringworm in dogs and cats. It is administered orally.

Ketone Bodies

Ketone bodies arise from acetyl coenzyme A. The 3 main ketone bodies are acetone, acetoacetate and beta hydroxybutyrate. While acetone is not part of the metabolic process in the healthy animal, the others are involved in the energy metabolism of ruminants. If the diet provides insufficient energy sources in the diabetic, excess ketone bodies arise, producing ketosis (acetonaemia). Professor Sir Hans Krebs describes the process thus: 'The severe forms of ketosis of the diabetic coma or of the lactating cow are connected with the high rates of gluconeogenesis which occur under these conditions. Oxaloacetate, which is an intermediate in gluconeogenesis, is diverted from the tricarboxylic acid cycle to gluconeogenesis, owing to the high activity of the enzyme converting it to phosphopyruvate. The liver compensates the loss of energy from a reduced rate of the tricarboxylic acid cycle by an increased rate of oxidations outside the cycle. The main reaction of this type is the oxidation of fatty acids to ketone bodies. These arise grossly in excess of needs, as a by-product of reactions which satisfy the requirements for energy.'

Ketonuria is the term applied to the presence of ketone bodies in the urine. (See also ACETON-AEMIA.)

Ketoacidosis. A condition leading to diabetic coma. (See DIABETES.)

Ketosis
(see ACETONAEMIA)

Key-Gaskell Syndrome
(see FELINE DYSAUTONOMIA)

Khat
This plant (*Catha edulis*) contains 2 compounds – cathine and cathinone – which are both structurally related to amphetamine.

Chewing of khat leaves, popular in Arabia and East Africa, appears to be on the increase in the UK. Addicts esteem khat for the euphoria and extra energy which it provides, but over-use can lead to mental illness.

Veterinary surgeons in small-animal practice will need to be on the lookout for cases of khat poisoning in dogs and cats – as they already are for the effects of CANNABIS.

Kicking
(see 'VICES')

Kidney Worm (Stephanurus Dentatus)
Kidney worm (stephanurus dentatus) is a parasite of pigs. Affected animals fail to thrive. Occasionally migration of the larvae in the spinal canal causes some degree of paralysis. The intermediate host is the earthworm. In the USA the advice is to breed from gilts only, as a means of eradicating the parasite – anthelmintics so far not having proved effective. (For the kidney worm of dogs, see DIOCTOPHYMOSIS.)

Kidneys
Kidneys are paired organs situated high up against the roof of the abdomen, and in most animals lying one on either side of the spinal column.

Horse The kidneys of the horse differ from each other in both shape and position. The right has the outline of a playing-card heart, and lies under the last 2 or 3 ribs and the

transverse process of the first lumbar vertebra, while the left is roughly bean-shaped and lies under the last rib and the first 2 or 3 lumbar transverse processes. They are held in place by the surrounding organs and by fibrous tissue, called the renal fascia. Each of them moves slightly backwards and forwards during the respiratory movements of the animal.

Cattle The kidneys are lobulated, each possessing from 20 to 25 lobes separated by fissures filled with fat in the living animal. The right kidney lies below the last rib and the first 2 or 3 lumbar transverse processes, and is somewhat elliptical in outline. The left occupies a variable position. When the rumen is full, it pushes the left kidney over to the right side of the body into a position slightly below and behind the right organ, but when it is empty the left kidney lies underneath the vertebral column about the level of the third to the fifth lumbar vertebra. It may lie partly on the left side of the body in this position in some cases.

Sheep In the sheep the kidneys are bean-shaped and smooth. In position they resemble those of the ox, except that the right is usually a little farther back.

Pig In this animal the kidneys are shaped like elongated beans, and they are placed almost symmetrically on either side of the bodies of the first 4 lumbar vertebrae. They sometimes vary in position.

Dogs and cats In these animals the kidneys are again bean-shaped, but they are thicker than in other animals, and relatively larger. As in most animals, the right kidney is placed farther forward than the left, the latter varying in position according to the degree of fullness of the digestive organs. In the cat the left kidney is very loosely attached and can usually be felt as a rounded mass which is quite movable in the anterior part of the abdominal cavity.

Birds have paired kidneys, seen as elongated brown organs closely attached on each side of the vertebrae.

Fish have a single kidney which is seen in salmonids as a long black strucure in the dorsal part of the abdomen extending from the back of the head to the vent. The vena cava runs through the centre of the organ. The kidney also has a role in the development of blood cells and in combating infection.

Structure The organ is enveloped in a fibrous coat continuous with the rest of the peritoneal membrane, and attached to the kidney capsule. This capsule does not permit of much swelling or enlargement of the organ, and consequently any inflammation of the kidney is attended with much pain. On the inner border there is an indentation called the hilus, which acts as a place of entrance and exit for vessels, nerves, etc. Entering each kidney at its hilus are a renal artery and renal nerves; leaving the kidney are renal vein or veins, lymphatics, and the ureter. If the kidney is cut across, there are 2 distinct areas seen in its substance. Lying outermost is the reddish-brown granular cortex, which contains small dark spots known as Malpighian corpuscles.

Within the cortex is the medulla, an area presenting a radiated appearance, whose periphery is of a deep red colour.

The kidney tissue contains many thousands of filtration units called nephrons. Each of these comprises the glomerulus (almost a spherical arrangement of capillaries on an arteriole); Bowman's capsule, the blind end of a proximal tubule which expands so as almost to surround the glomerulus; the convoluted tubule itself (with its loop of Henle); and the distal convoluted tubule which leads on to an arched collecting tubule. The latter continues with a straight tubule in the cortex of the kidney, and on into the medulla, where papillary ducts are formed to take the urine to the pelvis of the kidney.

The Malpighian corpuscle, comprising the glomerulus and inner and outer layers of Bowman's capsule, is where most of the filtration of fluid from the blood occurs; but only a small percentage of this fluid is finally excreted as urine.

In birds, the glomeruli are of 2 different kinds; 1 type is similar to mammalian glomeruli; the other is more akin to the type found in reptiles.

Function The kidney's 2 main functions are:first, the excretion of waste (and excess) materials from the bloodstream; and, second, the maintenance of the correct proportions of water in the blood, the correct levels of its chemical constituents, and the correct pH. (See HOMEOSTASIS.)

Blood pressure in the arteries determines pressure in each glomerulus and has an important bearing on the quantity of fluid filtered from the blood.

For its controlling effect on the kidney, see ANTIDIURETIC HORMONE.

The proximal tubules reabsorb a high percentage of the water, sodium chloride and bicarbonate. The distal tubules reabsorb sodium, or exchange sodium ions for hydrogen, potassium or ammonium ions; determining thereby the pH of the urine.

The kidney also secretes the hormone erythropoietin (see under ERYTHROPOIESIS) and produces RENIN. Additionally, the kidney converts vitamin D1 into its active form.

Kidneys, Diseases of

These are particularly common in the dog, and must account for a high proportion of deaths in dogs and cats.

Exact diagnosis is based almost entirely upon macroscopic, microscopic, and chemical examination of the urine in the laboratory. Blood urea nitrogen (BUN) and serum creatinine concentrations are used to evaluate renal function in several species.

Nephrosis/nephrotic syndrome This may be a stage in nephritis and involves damage to the tubules of the kidneys, resulting in defective filtering, so that albumin is excreted in the urine to the detriment of albumin levels in the blood. Oedema occurs.

Nephrosis may be caused by poisoning with the salts of heavy metals, and with various toxins; or it may follow certain other diseases. In lambs, clostridial infections have been suggested as a cause of the disease, while nematodirus infestation may be responsible in older animals. (See also MEMBRANOUS NEPHROPATHY.)

Acute nephritis is a rapid inflammation of the kidney tissues as a whole, or of the glomeruli and the secreting tubules only. The latter is much the more common among all animals. Since the diagnosis and symptoms of each are clinically the same, and as their differentiation is only possible by microscopic examination after death it will suffice to describe the commoner type only.

Dogs Acute and subacute nephritis is often associated with LEPTOSPIROSIS, especially with *Leptospira canicola* infection; it may follow the nephrotic syndrome, and may co-exist with distemper or canine viral hepatitis. A predisposing cause is often, it seems, exposure to cold, wet conditions, which lower the animal's resistance and so exacerbates any existing infection.

Signs may include depression, loss of appetite, thirst, vomiting. The back may be arched, and there may be stiffness. There is fever, and sometimes ulcers are present in the mouth.

Lambs Acute kidney failure was diagnosed by clinical examination and autopsy in 39 flocks served by 6 veterinary investigation centres.

Forty-eight lambs of 12 different breeds or crosses were investigated. The mean age of affected lambs was 38 days; 21 lambs were aged 7 to 28 days, while only 8 were older than 2 months. Mortality in clinically affected lambs was almost 100 per cent, with no response to various treatments.

First-aid The animal needs rest, warmth, and light food. Reliable proprietary foods can be obtained for kidney disease cases. Barley water instead of plain water is often advisable. (See under NURSING.)

Treatment includes the use of antibiotics. If there is much vomiting, normal saline may be necessary.

Chronic nephritis may follow the acute form, or it may arise insidiously. One attack of nephritis is always likely to render the dog more susceptible to subsequent attacks, and chronic nephritis is common in middle-aged and old dogs. In some cases of this disease RUBBER JAW may be present. Sometimes, despite treatment, kidney failure occurs.

Kidney failure may follow either chronic interstitial nephritis (involving some degree of fibrosis), which often results from leptospiral nephritis; or from glomerular disease (glomerulonephritis). Clinically, the 2 conditions are virtually indistinguishable.

Cattle Kidney disease may also be associated with LEPTOSPIROSIS, and may be a sequel to various other infections. *Corynebacterium renale* attacks the kidneys, and abscesses of these organs are not uncommonly found in cattle. (See also pyelitis *and* pyelonephritis *below.*) Some poisons may damage the kidneys.

Symptoms in cattle include stiffness, an arched back, often the passing of small amounts of blood-stained urine, a poor appetite. Rumination may cease.

However, in non-acute cases symptoms may not be noticed, and the existence of nephritis discovered only after death. A survey carried out at a Dublin abattoir showed that of 4166 cattle, 4.2 per cent had kidneys rejected under EU export regulations. The rejection rate was 7.7, 1.7, 2.2, and 28 per cent for cows, bullocks, heifers and bulls, respec-tively; the most common reason being focal interstitial nephritis (60 per cent). Other lesions included cysts (26 per cent), pyelonephritis, pigmentation, amyloidosis, and glomerulonephritis.

Horses Nephritis may be a complication of influenza and other infections; follow contusions (arising from blows, falls) in the lumbar region; or follow feeding with mouldy or otherwise contaminated fodder. (*See also* pyelonephritis *below.*)

In the horse, symptoms of kidney disease may be somewhat vague, but in severe cases there is usually evidence of pain, stiffness in the gait, a poor appetite, often fever, and urine is passed as described above for cattle. Oedema may involve abdomen, chest, and legs.

Cats Kidney disease is, generally speaking, likely to result in a poor appetite, loss of weight, dullness, thirst. Intermittent vomiting may occur. The cat may become pot-bellied, due to ASCITES.

A cat with chronic nephritis may live to old age, seemingly still able to enjoy life. There is likely to come a time, however, when the kidneys fail, and uraemia occurs.

If a cat is losing protein in its urine, the need is for a high-protein diet; but with chronic nephritis, a low-protein diet is usually indicated. A number of specially formulated proprietary diets are available. (See PRESCRIPTION DIETS.)

B vitamins and diuretics are used in treating the nephrotic syndrome.

Other animals Causes, symptoms, and treatment (antibiotics, sometimes diuretics) are in general similar. Vomiting may occur in the pig. (See also AVIAN NEPHRITIS.)

Polycystic kidneys A congenital renal problem in which the kidney is enlarged and contains multiple fluid filled cysts. The condition, which has been recorded in pigs, is sporadic and does not usually cause illness.

Purulent nephritis, or 'suppurative nephritis', is a condition in which one or both kidneys show abscess formation. All species may be affected. It is caused by pus-producing (pyogenic) organisms, which may gain access to the kidneys either by the bloodstream – when the term 'pyaemic nephritis' is used – or by the ureters from the bladder – when the condition is pyelonephritis. Pyelitis, meaning pus in the pelvis of the kidney, is used to indicate abscess formation in the pelvis only, and generally precedes the more severe form of pyelonephritis. It may be associated with stone formation (renal calculus).

Pyelonephritis is generally preceded by an attack of inflammation of the bladder, vagina, or uterus. It is commonest in cows and mares after parturition when the genital tract has become septic, but it is seen in all females under similar circumstances. It is not so common in male animals. Generally only 1 kidney is affected, and the animal exhibits pain when turned sharply to the affected side, and tenderness when that side is handled.

Pyelitis shows symptoms that are practically the same as those of pyelonephritis, except when due to renal calculus. In such cases it causes an obscure form of colic, and small amounts of blood-stained urine are passed at frequent intervals.

Stone in the kidney A calculus or stone may sometimes form in the pelvis of the kidney as the result of the gradual deposition of salts from the urine around some particle of matter that acts as a nucleus. (See UROLITHIASIS; CALCULI.)

Parasites of the kidney include *Dioctophyma* in the dog, and occasionally *Eustrongylus gigas* in horses, dogs, and cattle; the larvae of *Strongylus vulgaris* in colts, *Stephanurus dentatus* in pigs, and the cystic stages of certain tapeworms in the ruminants. (See also DIOCTOPHYMOSIS; LEPTOSPIROSIS.)

Tumours of the kidney include carcinoma (mainly in dogs and cattle) and the usually benign nephroblastoma in pigs, puppies and calves. In cats lymphosarcoma of the kidney is common.

Hydronephrosis In this condition the kidney may enlarge, owing to an obstruction. (See HYDRONEPHROSIS.)

Injuries of the kidney are not common, owing to the great protection that the lumbar muscles provide. They may be lacerated or bruised as the result of traffic accidents in the dog. Slips or falls in the hunting field may cause similar injuries in horses. The kidney may be shattered and death from internal haemorrhage occurs, or in less severe cases the haemorrhage takes place below the capsule and the blood is passed in the urine. If only 1 kidney is affected, and provided the bleeding is not great, the other hypertrophies and acts for both.

Kilopascal (KpA)
The unit used to quantify vacuum pressure in milking machines.

Kimberley Horse Disease (Walkabout Disease)
Kimberley horse disease (walkabout disease) occurs in the Kimberley district of Western Australia, and has a seasonal incidence – January to April (i.e. 'wet season'). Horses of all ages are susceptible.

Cause Whitewood (*Atalaya hemiglauca*) taken voluntarily or fed when food is scarce.

Signs Anorexia, dullness, wasting, irritability, biting other horses, and gnawing at posts. Yawning is a marked and almost constant sign. Then muscular spasms lead to a phase of mad galloping in which the horse has no sense of direction and is uncontrollable. Gallops become more frequent but less violent, and gradually merge into the walking stage – slow, staggering gait, with low, stiff carriage of the head. The horse may walk about for hours, with a mouthful of unchewed grass protruding from its lips. (See also BIRDSVILLE DISEASE.)

'Kinky-Back'
The colloquial name for a condition in broiler chickens involving distortion of the 6th thoracic vertebra. It is the cause of lameness and sometimes paraplegia. It appears to be of hereditary origin, perhaps influenced by growth-rate.

Kirschner-Ehmer Splint
Used in treating fractures in the dog and cat. It has transverse pins which are driven into parts of a long bone on either side of the fracture, and which are then held in position by an external clamp.

'Kitchen Deaths'
Kitchen deaths in small caged birds can result from overheated utensils, particularly frying pans, which have non-stick coatings of polytetrafluoroethylene (PTFE), or from acrolein or other vapours associated with cooking oils, or from carbon monoxide poisoning from improperly ventilated heaters. PTFE fumes cause acute pneumonitis with haemorrhages and death in small caged birds (see CARBON MONOXIDE; 'FRYING PAN' DEATHS).

In 9 incidents of bird deaths involving 1 to 18 birds investigated by Penrith Veterinary Investigation Centre, 3 cases were due to PTFE poisoning, 3 to cooking oil vapours, 1 to carbon monoxide and in 2 cases there were no obvious causes found.

Kittens
The young of cats (and rabbits).

Causes of death in kittens A Glasgow veterinary-school study of the cause of death in 274 kittens showed that 55 per cent died from infectious diseases, 33 per cent from unknown causes and 5 per cent from congenital defects. Feline parvovirus caused 25 per cent of all deaths.

Klebsiella.

A genus of gram-negative bacteria. It has been suggested that *K. pneumoniae* may be an important cause of infertility in the thoroughbred mare, but see EQUINE GENITAL INFECTIONS.

Cattle The infection is occasionally the cause of mastitis and osteomyelitis; also pulmonary lesions.

Dog The infection may cause illness clinically indistinguishable from distemper, and may therefore account for some of the suspected 'breakdowns' following the use of distemper vaccines.

Sows The infection may result in acute mastitis. Both piglets and sow may die.

Klein's Disease

(see FOWL TYPHOID)

Knackers

A place for the disposal of animals unfit for human consumption, and ill or recently dead animals. Many of the tissues can be recycled, for a variety of purposes.

Knee

Knee is the name, wrongly applied, to the carpus of the horse, ox, sheep, and pig. This joint really corresponds to the human wrist and should not be called 'knee', but custom has ordained otherwise. (See JOINTS.)

Knocked-Up Shoe

Knocked-up shoe is one in which the inner branch is hammered laterally so as to increase its height but decrease its width. There is 1 nail-hole at the inside toe, and 4 or 5 along the outside branch. The shoe generally has a clip at the toe and the outside quarter, and may have a small calkin on the outside heel.

It is used for horses given to brushing, cutting, or interfering with their hind feet.

Knocked-Up Toe

A term used in racing greyhound circles to describe a type of lameness associated with the digits. It sometimes yields to rest but may require surgical treatment (even amputation of the 3rd phalanx).

Knuckling

Knuckling of fetlock simply means that the fetlock joints are kept slightly flexed forwards above the hoof, instead of remaining extended. It may result from a number of causes: genetics, positioning of the fetus in the uterus, etc.

Knuckling of the fetlocks in calves of the Jersey, Ayrshire, and Friesian breeds is an inherited defect which can sometimes be corrected by a minor surgical operation.

Occasionally foals are born with their fetlocks knuckled, but, like many other deformities of a similar nature, the condition gradually disappears as the muscles of the young animal obtain their proper control of the joints which they actuate. In older horses, the 2 chief conditions that are responsible for knuckling are: (l) thickening and contraction of the tendons or ligaments behind the cannon; and (2) chronic foot lameness, such as is produced by ringbones, navicular disease, chronic corns, etc. The horse assumes the position of partial flexion of the fetlock, apparently in order to ease the pain he feels; as the result of the relaxation of the tendons, shortening occurs, and it finally becomes impossible to straighten out the joint. (NB. For descriptive purposes the word 'flexion' here means a bending backwards of the lower section of the limb from the fetlock joint – the cannon remaining stationary. Otherwise confusion between 'flexion' and 'extension' of the fetlock might occur.)

Koala

(*Phascolarctos cinereus*) The koala bear is an arboreal, marsupial creature, a native of Australia. It is prone to chlamydial infections which can cause blindness and infertility.

Kudu, Greater (Tragelaphus Strepsiceros)

An antelope with long spiral horns. One of these creatures died in the London Zoo in 1992 from a scrapie-like spongiform encephalopathy.

Kuppfer's Cells

Phagocytic cells lining the walls of sinusoids in the liver.

Kuru

A spongiform encephalopathy of humans, described in Papua New Guinea. It was trasmitted by ritual cannibalism. Men ate the victims' muscles and heart while women and children ate the brain and other organs. 154 clinical cases occurred as a result of eating a single infected body. Although affected women did not produce affected infants, and the practice was outlawed in the 1950s, occasional cases still occur in the tribe that used to practise this ceremonial. 'Kuru' translates as 'trembling with fear'.

Kyasanur Forest Fever

Kyasanur forest fever is a disease of man and monkeys, occurring in Mysore, and resembling Omsk fever. The causal virus is transmitted by the tick *Haemaphysalis spinigera*, and believed to have been brought by birds from the former Soviet Union.

Kyphosis

Kyphosis is a curvature of the spine when the concavity of the curve is directed downwards. It is sometimes seen in tetanus, rabies, etc., and is a sign of abdominal pain in the dog.

K

L-Carnitine

A vitamin of the B complex present in meat extracts and needed for fat oxidation. In human medicine it is claimed to improve exercise tolerance, and so might have a potential use in racehorses.

L-Forms of Bacteria

Those which can survive without a true cell wall. L-forms of staphylococci and streptococci have been recovered from cases of mastitis. They are completely resistant to antibiotics such as penicillin which interfere with bacterial cell-wall formation.

Labial

Relating to the lips.

Labile

Unstable. Thermo-labile – unstable in the presence of heat.

Labium

Labium is the Latin word for lip or lip-shaped organ.

Laboratory Animals

Animals bred specifically for scientific purposes; it is illegal to use non-purpose-bred animals for scientific research. Their welfare and the conditions in which they are kept are strictly controlled by the Animals (Scientific Procedures) Act 1986 (as amended 1998); by far the largest number of such animals are mice and rats.

Laboratory Tests

Laboratory tests are widely used as an aid to diagnosis but should always be interpreted in the light of the signs presented by the animal. Many tests involve examination of samples of the blood or its cells (haematology), or plasma or serum. Other tests are based on urine, pus, peritoneal or pleural fluid. Occasionally, samples of tissues are taken for examination (biopsy). Tests may be used to determine the various biochemical constituents of the sample or to detect the presence of bacteria, viruses, fungi, mycoplasma or parasites. Samples (usually serum) may be used to detect the presence of antibodies to various infective agents.

In cattle, milk is increasingly used both to determine biological levels and to determine the herd exposure levels to infections such as bovine viral diarrhoea (BVD) and enzootic bovine leukosis (EBL). Milk samples may also be used to determine the levels of bacteria present in the herd.

Labour

(see PARTURITION)

Labrador Retriever

A popular medium-sized breed of dog with black, beige or brown coat. Progressive retinal atrophy, entropion and cataract are inherited as dominant traits; haemophilia, osteochondrotis and laryngeal paralysis may also be found.

Laburnum Poisoning

All parts of the plant, whose botanical name is *Cytisus* – root, wood, bark, leaves, flowers, and particularly the seeds in their pods – are poisonous, and all the domestic animals and birds are susceptible.

Signs The toxic agent is an alkaloid called cystine, which produces firstly excitement, then unconsciousness with incoordination of movement, and finally convulsions and death.

In the horse, when small amounts have been taken, there is little to be seen beyond a staggering gait, yawning, and a general abnormality in the behaviour of the animal. With larger doses there may be sweating, excitement, collapse, convulsions, coma and death.

In cattle and sheep, which are more resistant than the horse, the rumen becomes filled with gas, the limbs become paralysed, the pupils are dilated, the animal becomes sleepy, and later, salivation, coma, and convulsive movements follow each other. Fatal cases in these animals are not common; the symptoms may last for several days and then gradually pass off.

In the dog and pig, which vomit easily, the irritant and acrid nature of the plant causes free vomiting, and usually the animal is enabled to get rid of what has been eaten before the symptoms become acute. However, this is not always so. One dog, after 24 hours' mild diarrhoea following repeated chewing of a low-lying branch, suddenly collapsed and died. In another case, a stick, which had been cut from a laburnum tree 3 months previously, was thrown for a dog to retrieve, and caused fatal poisoning after being chewed.

First-aid Very strong black tea or coffee that has been boiled instead of infused may be given as a drench.

Labyrinth
(see EAR)

Lacombe
A lop-eared pig from Alberta, Canada. Breeding: Danish Landrace 51 per cent, Chester White 25 per cent, Berkshire 24 per cent. (The Chester White comes from Pennsylvania, and originates from 18th century imports.)

Lacrimal (Lachrymal)
Lacrimal (Lachrymal) relates to tears, to the gland which secretes these, and to the ducts of the gland.

Lachrymation This term is often used to describe an excess of tears, as a result of a blocked duct or conjunctivitis, etc.

β-Lactamase
Enzymes produced by bacteria which cause resistance to certain antibiotics (e.g. penicillins, cephalosporins) by breaking down the β-lactam ring.

Lactation
Lactation depends directly upon the fact that if the milk is not regularly removed, the secretion will cease. It reaches its maximum duration in the cow and goat which are milked by human agency for the production of milk for consumption. By this artificial method the duration of lactation and the quantities of milk have been enormously increased.

The duration of a lactation in the cow is taken to be 305 days, commencing from calving and ending when the cow ceases to be milked at least twice a day. This is in line with other European records. The period for butterfat sampling continues to be from the 4th day after calving.

To produce 9090 litres (2000 gallons) of milk, the cow must secrete over 10,700 kg (9½ tons) of milk from the mammary gland, e.g. roughly about 12 or 14 times the weight of her whole body. A remarkable British Friesian cow, Manningford Faith Jan Graceful, which died at the age of 17½ , gave a lifetime yield of 142 tonnes, 750 kg (145 tons, 14 cwt, 85 lb); and her highest 365-day yield – with her 3rd calf – was 17,409 litres (3829.5 gallons). A Jersey has, in 361 days, given over 12,120 litres (2666 gallons) (525 kg (1157.46 lb) butterfat). (See

MILK YIELD; 'LICKING SYNDROME'; MAMMARY GLAND; MILK; WEANING.)

Lactation, Artificial
The artificial induction of lactation may be brought about by means of hormones. For example, barren, anoestrus ewes have been rendered good foster-mothers to lambs by a single dose of 40 mg stilboestrol. Persistence of lactation in cows has been obtained experimentally by using bovine somatotrophin. (See also under SPAYING.)

Lactation Tetany
(see HYPOMAGNESAEMIA; ECLAMPSIA; HYPOCALCAEMIA; LAMBING SICKNESS. See also MILK FEVER; MILK TETANY)

Lactescent Serum (Plasma)
Lactescent serum (Plasma) is milky in appearance because of high levels of triglyceride. Especially if fasted, patients are at risk of developing acute pancreatitis and gastroenteritis (dogs) and skin eruptions (cats).

Lactic Acid
(See also MILK.) Excessive production of lactic acid in the rumen – such as occurs after cattle have gorged themselves with grain – is a serious condition, and is followed by absorption of fluid from the general circulation (with consequent dehydration), ruminal stasis, and often death. (See BARLEY POISONING.)

Lactic acid is produced in muscle by the breakdown of glycogen. (Oxidation of lactic acid provides energy for the recovery phase after a muscle has contracted.)

After strenuous exercise, excess of lactic acid can lead to CRAMP (see MUSCLE – Action).

Lactose
Sugar of milk. Lactose in cow's milk has a commercial value. Cows with low lactose production often have higher mastitis cell counts, a factor in deciding culling policy. (See SUGAR.)

Lagomorphs
A group of mammals that includes rabbits and hares.

Lagos Bat Virus
A rhabdovirus, carried by bats in Nigeria; it has similarities to rabies virus.

Lakeland Terrier
A small active dog whose coat resembles an Airedale's. Ununited anconeal process may be inherited.

Lakes
(see ALGAE POISONING; LEECHES)

Lamb Carcase Rejection
Lamb carcase rejection on inspection at abattoirs: causes include 'MILKSPOT LIVER'; CYSTICERCOSIS; LIVER-FLUKES.

Lamb Dysentery
Lamb dysentery is an infectious ulcerative inflammation of the small and large intestine of young lambs, usually under 10 days old, and characterised by a high mortality.

Cause *Clostridium welchei* (*C. perfringens*) type B. This organism is one of the gas gangrene group. After birth the lamb runs every risk of getting infection from its mother's udder, from the soiled wool of the hind- quarters, or from the soil itself.

Signs In the acute type nothing seems to be wrong with the lambs at night, but in the morning 2 or 3 are found dead. If symptoms appear during the day, lambs are seen to become suddenly dull and listless; they stop sucking and if forced to move, they do so stiffly. Later, the faeces become brownish-red in colour (sometimes yellow), semi-liquid, and are often tinged with bright red blood. After a few hours in this state, the lamb becomes unconscious and dies. In less acute forms, the lamb may live for 2 or 3 days.

Prevention Two methods: the newly born lamb is injected as soon after birth as possible, and not later than 12 hours, with lamb dysentery antiserum. This gives it a passive immunity enduring long enough to protect throughout the dangerous period – generally about 2 weeks. More usually, though, ewes are vaccinated using multicomponent vaccines protecting against up to 8 clostridial infections, so that the lamb will be protected by antibodies in the colostrum. The type of vaccine used depends on the infections prevailing in the area. (See also under VACCINATION.)

Lamb Survival Research
(see SHEEP BREEDING)

Lambing Difficulties
Abnormality of the fetus, or its malpresentation, accounts for a high proportion of 'difficult lambings'. The failure of the cervix to dilate is another frequent cause of difficulty, which can usually be overcome by a veterinary surgeon. (See 'RINGWOMB'; also VAGINA – Rupture.)

Lambing, Lambs
(see under SHEEP BREEDING)

Lambing Sickness in Ewes
Lambing sickness in ewes, which is also called parturient hypocalcaemia, or milk fever in ewes, is a condition similar to MILK FEVER in cows. The symptoms and treatment are the same. It may be mistaken for pregnancy toxaemia or louping-ill. (See 'MOSS ILL'.)

Lamella
(1) Concentric circles surrounding the Haversian canal in bone. (2) A small disc of glycerin jelly containing an active drug such as atropine, cocaine, homatropine, and physostigmine, for application to the eye. It is applied by inserting within the lower lid. This type of formulation has been largely replaced by eyedrops.

Lameness
Lameness consists of a departure from the normal gait, occasioned by disease or injury situated in some part of the limbs or trunk, and is usually accompanied by pain. In simple cases lameness is not difficult to diagnose; in obscure cases, however, and in those instances where more than 1 limb is affected, it may be extremely difficult for anyone, professional or otherwise, to determine where the lameness is, and to what it is due.

It is important to remember that lameness in cattle, sheep, and pigs may be the first symptom of FOOT-AND- MOUTH DISEASE.

Causes The main causes are given below, according to animal.

Cattle Foul-in-the-foot, fluorosis, laminitis, mucosal disease, and 'milk lameness'.

Lameness in cattle is of great economic importance to the dairy farmer. The pain arising from several forms of lameness can reduce a cow's milk yield to a significant extent. Economic loss can go beyond this, however, since premature culling and cost of replacement often have to be taken into· account also. A survey of 1823 herds showed that the annual incidence of lameness was about 5.5 per cent.

About 88 per cent of this lameness was due to foot lesions, with foul-in-the-foot predominating – closely followed by abscess formation at the white line, and by ulceration of the sole.

A foreign body, such as a stone or piece of broken glass, lodged between the claws of the hind feet, was a very common cause of lameness. In winter, mud at near freezing temperatures is apt to lodge there too, predisposing to foul-in-the-foot. (Institute of Research on Animal Diseases, Compton.)

Results of another survey, involving 262 farms participating in a dairy herd health and productivity service operated by the Royal (Dick) School of Veterinary Studies, University of Edinburgh, showed that 'an astonishing 25 per cent of cows were treated for lameness, and 1 per cent culled because of it, in 12 months'.

The survey showed that faulty feeding of high-yielding dairy cows often predisposed to laminitis or coronitis, resulting in chronic, often incurable, lameness. Excessive steaming up, major changes of diet at calving, heavy feeding after calving, large single cake or barley feeds, and very acid silage were predisposing causes.

Cattle housing can be a contributory factor to lameness; rough concrete surfaces can abrade the sole of the foot, as can worn slats; and bad cubicle design can also result in lameness. (See also FOOT-BATHS.)

Dairy cattle Some 25 per cent become lame every year; but for those kept in straw yards, the figure was only 8 per cent, and there were no cases of solar ulceration.

The highest incidence of the latter is found where the cows are in cubicles.

Sheep Foot-rot. (See under DIPS AND DIPPING; also FOOT-ROT OF SHEEP.)

Pigs Bush foot, foot-rot, swine erysipelas; also a biotin deficiency.

In all species, fracture of a bone may be the cause; or injuries to joints, ligaments, tendons or muscles.

Dogs (see BRACHIAL; INTERDIGITAL CYST)

Horses The following remarks refer especially to the horse, but they are to a great extent applicable to the other 4-footed animals.

Signs The most characteristic and easily seen feature of practically all forms of lameness is abnormality in the manner of nodding the head, either at the walk or at the trot. Normally, the horse's head rises and falls to the same extent at each step, and, in lesser measure, the point of the croup (i.e. the highest part of the hindquarters) follows the same course. If a horse is made to walk alongside a blank wall, the head is seen to describe a wavy line against the wall, the undulations of which are equal, provided that the rate of the gait is uniform. In

a lame horse these undulations become unequal.

Fore-limb lameness The withers of a horse which is lame in 1 of its 2 fore-legs, rise when the lame leg is on the ground, and fall when the sound leg comes to earth. This rising and falling is transferred along the rigid bar of the neck to the head. Accordingly, when a horse is lame in this way, its head is said to 'nod' heavy on the sound leg, and rise on the lame leg.

Hind-limb lameness The croup rises when the lame leg is on the ground, and falls when the sound limb is there. But the croup is connected by a rigid bar, passing over a fulcrum (the withers), with the head: it will be seen, therefore, that any rising of the croup will cause a lowering of the head, since the spinal column acts as a lever working over a fulcrum. In the horse which is lame in 1 of its hind-limbs, therefore, the head falls when the croup rises, i.e. when the lame leg is on the ground: it rises when the sound leg is on the ground. In other words, it behaves in a manner opposite to its behaviour when the lame limb is situated in front; the diagonally opposite hind-leg is indicated.

Other signs The noise made by the lame limb falling to the ground is always less than the noise made by the sound limb, for obvious reasons. The lame limb may be lifted higher than the sound one during the walk, as in cases of sand-crack at the toe (often called 'symptomatic stringhalt' when affecting a hind-limb), or, more often, it is not lifted so high (in most cases of pain in joints or in flexor tendons). On soft ground the footprint made by the lame leg is never as deep as that made by the sound leg, although this fact is not of great practical importance. In most lamenesses of the hindmost pair of limbs, the point of the haunch (external angle of the ilium) is carried higher on the same side as the lameness exists. This is most pronounced in lamenesses which involve the joints in greater pain when they are flexed. The raising of the pelvis on the same side as the lameness enables the foot to clear the ground during the stride with a lessened amount of flexion than would otherwise be the case. Finally, there may be some peculiarity of the swing of the lame limb through the air. It may be carried outward (abducted), or it may be carried too near to the other limb (adducted).

Determining the lame limb The observer should see the horse walked away from him, towards him, and then past him at right-angles.

The horse should then be trotted in the same way. If the observer watches the head carefully, he will see how it is nodding, and as soon as he gets the rhythm of the nods he should immediately commence nodding his own head at the same rate. When he is sure that he is nodding in time with the horse's head, he should at once drop his eyes to the horse's fore-feet, and determine which fore-foot comes to the ground when the nod of his head is downwards. Having decided which fore-leg corresponds with a downward nod of the horse's head, he can state that the horse is lame either on the opposite fore-leg, or else on the hind-leg of the same side.

He should now attempt to decide whether the lameness is in the anterior pair of limbs or in the posterior pair. To do this it is necessary to observe carefully in which pair of limbs there is some discrepancy in movement, either a long or a short step, a lighter noise, adduction or abduction (seen from in front and behind only), increased or diminished flexion, etc. By the aid of these rules practically all simple single-leg lameness can be determined. Where there are 2 or more limbs affected it is very much more difficult. The services of a veterinary surgeon should be obtained to diagnose the situation of the lesions and their extent and nature. (See also JOINTS; RICKETS; LAMINITIS; HORSES, BACK TROUBLES IN; LIGAMENTS; BRUCELLOSIS.)

Lamina

A thin plate or layer such as the dorsal part of the arch of the spinal vertebrae, or at the corium of the hoof.

Laminectomy

A surgical treatment for fracture of the dorsal arch of a vertebra.

Laminitis

Inflammation of the laminae of the hooves causing lameness, often severe. It can be a serious problem in the horse, less often in cattle.

Laminitis in Cattle

Laminitis has been encountered in both adult and young cattle. For many years, overfeeding with barley has been regarded as a likely cause, and the disease has been described among cattle 4½ to 6 months old in 'barley beef' units.

Excessive steaming up, a change of diet at calving, large single concentrate feeds (especially of barley), overfeeding in the early stages of lactation, and acid over-fermented silage have also been cited as causes.

Laminitis in the cow is rarely the acute disease seen in the horse, but rather a milder, more insidious condition. 'A general tenderness of all 4 feet develops, usually soon after calving. This stage may go unnoticed. It may be followed sooner or later by more clearly recognised chronic secondary foot problems such as ulceration of the sole, separation of the wall from the sole, and horizontal cracks in the wall.' Infection usually complicates such conditions.

Laminitis in Horses

This has traditionally been defined as inflammation or oedema of the sensitive laminae of the hoof. It is now considered to be a

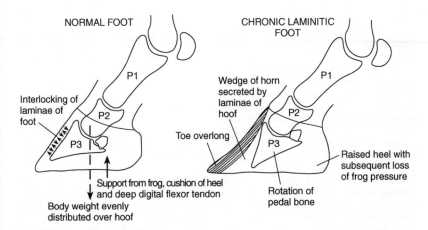

Diagnostic representation of forces involved in pedal bone rotation. (Reproduced by courtesy of the *Veterinary Record*, C. M. Colles and L. B. Jeffcott.)

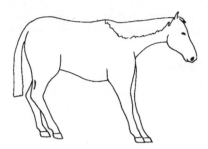

Laminitic stance – fore-legs thrust forward, hind-legs drawn under the body and weight taken on heels. (Reproduced by courtesy of the *Veterinary Record*, C. M. Colles and L. B. Jeffcott.)

transitory inflammation followed by congestion leading to breakdown of the union between sensitive and horny laminae.

Laminitis is most common in ponies, and in fat or unfit horses. Sometimes all 4 feet are affected; sometimes only the fore-feet; and occasionally only the hind-feet or 1 foot.

Causes

1. Excess carbohydrate intake ('grain overload').
2. Post-parturient metritis septicaemia.
3. Toxaemia – associated with enteritis, colitis X (exhaustion shock) and endotoxin shock.
4. Management and type – concussion in unfit horses or susceptible animal (e.g. fat pony).
5. Unilateral leg lameness putting excess strain on contra-lateral limb.
6. High-level corticosteroid administration.
7. Fatty liver syndrome.
8. Other suggested factors:
   (a) Hypothyroidism.
   (b) Allergic-type reaction to certain medication (e.g. anthelmintics, oestrogens and androgens).
   (c) High oestrogen content of pasture.

Laminitis should always be regarded as a serious disease, whether it arises secondarily during the course of a generalised illness, or whether it occurs independently of any other recognisable disease.

Intense pain results from acute laminitis, either from inflammation of the sensitive laminae or from changes in the circulation of the blood within the hoof. Prompt treatment is needed to relieve this pain, and to try to prevent permanent damage to the foot. In severe cases of laminitis, separation of the sensitive and horny laminae may occur, and any subsequent infection may put the horse's life at grave risk.

Signs Acute, subacute and chronic forms of laminitis are recognised. Symptoms, especially in acute and subacute laminitis, are both general, affecting the whole body, and local.

In acute laminitis the body temperature often rises to 40° to 41°C (104 to 106°F), breathing becomes rapid, and the pulse rate likewise (80 to 120 per minute). Pain may cause the horse to tremble, and profuse sweating may occur. Depression, a facial expression suggestive of pain felt, loss of appetite, and a reluctance to stand or move, together with an unnatural stance are other symptoms. Visible mucous membranes are often bright red, the pupils dilated.

If lying on the ground, the horse will be extremely reluctant to rise; and if standing will maintain the same position, and grunt or groan if forced to take a step.

The affected feet feel hot to the touch, especially at the coronet, and a bounding pulse in the digital arteries can be felt or even seen.

Tenderness is evident immediately any pressure is applied to the affected feet. The appearance of blood, or blood-stained exudate, at the coronary bands is usually followed by death within 24 hours or so.

Each time the affected foot is lifted from the ground, it is snatched up and held for a few moments as if contact with the ground were painful; later it may be rested out in front of the horse with the heel only on the ground. When 2 feet are affected it is always either the fore-pair or the hind-pair; diagonal feet are rarely or never attacked. If the fore-feet are involved, the horse stands with these thrust out well in front of him, resting on the heels as much as possible, while the hind-feet are brought up under the belly in order to bear as much of the body-weight as possible.

In the chronic form, which often follows the acute, laminitis presents a slowly progressive change in the shape of the foot. The toe becomes more and more elongated, the heels and the pasterns become vertical, rings appear around the coronet and move slowly downwards as the horn grows, and a bulge appears in the concavity of the sole.

The line drawings show both the stance of the horse with laminitis of the fore-feet only, and also the rotation of the pedal bone which may take place during or after the acute stage.

Treatment The underlying cause of the laminitis must be addressed and treatment will depend on the cause of the condition. Palliative measures include blocking of the digital nerves with a local anaesthetic: this gives immediate relief from pain, enables the horse to stand and walk normally, and has a beneficial effect on the blood circulation of the foot; however, care must be taken that further damage is not caused to the laminae by exercise. For the relief of pain acetylpromazine is also used, and this drug tends to reduce blood pressure. Phenylbutazone is another drug which has been used, and similarly corticosteroids. Warm or hot water applications to the feet are regarded as preferable to hosing with cold water.

Green food in small amounts is good, and a little hay should be supplied.

In chronic cases the shoeing is of great importance and special surgical shoes may be needed. (See also HOOF REPAIR.)

Lampas

A swelling of the mucous membrane of the hard palate of the horse immediately behind the arch of the incisor teeth in the upper jaw. It is often seen about the time when the permanent teeth are cutting through the gums, i.e. at 2½ , 3½, and 4½ years, and for a short time afterwards. It is erroneously thought that it is the cause of a falling-off in condition which naturally occurs when the teeth are cutting; it is really rather an effect. It was the custom to lance 'lampas' in many parts of the country; this occasions unnecessary pain and discomfort to the horse, and if the incision is made towards 1 side instead of in the middle-line there is a serious risk of wounding the palatine artery on that side.

Lampreys

Primitive fish that are parasites on other fish. There are saltwater and freshwater species, the freshwater species being larger (up to 50 cm long). They can be a problem for freshwater fish farms, particularly in the USA.

Lamziekte

Lamziekte is botulism of cattle in South Africa which occurs as an enzootic in animals on phosphorus-deficient areas of the veldt. During winter, lack of phosphorus leads grazing cattle to chew the bones of animals (often cattle) that have died, in an endeavour to take phosphorus into the body to make good the deficiency. This condition of bone-eating (osteophagia) is actually only the result of a craving for minerals. Where the animals whose skeletons are left on the veldt harboured in their alimentary canals *Clostridium botulinum*, this organism invades the carcase, and both it and its toxin are present in the decomposing remains.

Prevention The researches of Sir Arnold Theiler and the workers at Onderstepoort showed that the best means of preventing lamziekte is to feed sterilised bone- meal to cattle during the winter months in areas which are naturally deficient in phosphorus. (See BOTULISM.)

Landrace

A large white, lop-eared pig used to produce commercial hybrid breeds.

Lanolin

A type of fat found in sheep wool. It is widely used in ointments and creams.

Lantana Poisoning

Lantana poisoning of cattle and sheep has occurred in Australia and New Zealand. *L. camara* is the species commonly involved; especially the red-flowered variety. It causes light sensitisation, with exudative dermatitis of teats and vulva. Deaths have occurred.

Laparoscopy

The use of optical instruments for viewing the interior of organs such as the bladder, the interior of joints for signs of arthritis, etc., and for avian sex determination.

Laparotomy

Laparotomy means surgical opening of the abdominal cavity. The incision is either made in the middle line of the abdomen, or through one or other of the flanks.

Lapinised

This term is applied to a virus which has been attenuated by passage through rabbits. An example is afforded by lapinised swine fever vaccine.

Larkspur Poisoning

Of the several varieties of larkspur, most of which occur in America in the ranges of the West, where they cause great loss to cattle owners, only 1 species is commonly found in Britain – *Delphinium ajacis*. The seeds are the most dangerous parts of the plant, although the leaves have proved fatal when fed experimentally. Horses and sheep are not as susceptible as cattle. The active principles are 4 in number: delphine, delphisine, delphinoidine and staphisagrine, and of these the first 3 are highly poisonous.

Signs Salivation, vomiting, colicky pains, convulsions, and general paralysis.

Laryngeal Obstruction

Chronic obstruction of the larynx in cattle is characterised by difficult or painful inspiration, giving rise to 'ROARING'. The most common causes are calf diphtheria (necrobacillosis); but there is uncertainty as to the primary infective agent causing chronic laryngitis – *Fusebacterium necroforum*, for instance, is unable to penetrate intact mucous membrane.

Laryngitis

Inflammation of the larynx (see LARYNX, DISEASES OF).

Larynx

Larynx is the organ of voice, and also forms one of the parts of the air passage. It is placed just between, and slightly behind, the angles of the lower jaw. Externally it is covered by the skin, by a small amount of fibrous tissue, and sterno-thyro-hyoid muscles.

Structure The cricoid cartilage is shaped somewhat like a signet ring and connects the rest of the larynx with the 1st ring of the trachea. To its upper part are attached the arytenoids and the posterior horns of the thyroids. A crico-tracheal membrane unites it to the trachea, and a crico-thyroid membrane unites it to the thyroid cartilage. The thyroid cartilage possesses a body which in man forms the protuberance known as Adam's apple. The epiglottis lies in front of the body of the thyroid and curves forwards towards the root of the tongue; it is shaped somewhat like a pointed ovate leaf. The arytenoids are situated one on either side of the upper part of the cricoid to which they are attached. (For functions, see under VOICE.)

Larynx, Diseases of

(see also 'ROARING'; WHISTLING; COUGHING)

Laryngitis is an inflammation of the larynx, but particularly of the mucous membrane which lines its interior. It is often associated with pharyngitis or with bronchitis and tracheitis, when it is usually due to the spreading of inflammation from one of these neighbouring structures.

In the horse it may occur during influenza. (See also LATHYRISM.)

Signs In ordinary cases there is a cough, difficulty in swallowing, pain on pressure over the larynx, extension of the head to relieve pressure on the throat (a condition that is aptly described in popular terms as 'star gazing'). A wheezing or roaring sound accompanies breathing if membranes become so swollen as to interfere with respiration. A slight rise in temperature and pulse-rate accompanies the milder forms, but

when influenza is present, or if other specific diseases arise, the signs of fever are more distinct. Uncomplicated laryngitis usually lasts from a week to about a fortnight. Occasionally complications, such as roaring or whistling, follow recovery from the initial disease.

First-aid It is advisable to isolate all cases of laryngitis in a loose-box or other building, especially those arising in newly purchased animals, on account of the risk of contagious disease developing. (See NURSING.)

Wounds of the larynx are not common, owing to its comparatively sheltered position in the body, but see under DRENCHING for a danger associated with the use of a drenching gun in pigs and sheep.

Foreign Bodies

(see CHOKING)

Laryngeal Paralysis in Horses

Laryngeal paralysis in horses causes the abnormal inspiratory sound called 'roaring'.

The usual cause was for long regarded as vibration of the slackened vocal folds on one or both sides of the larynx, due to paralysis of the muscles which move the arytenoid cartilages outwards. Laryngeal paralysis is probably a hereditary condition transmitted by a simple recessive factor.

A large number of respiratory diseases may give rise to a temporary roaring due to inflammation and thickening of the mucous membranes lining the larynx. GUTTURAL POUCH DISEASE may have a permanent effect.

Treatment The traditional Hobday operation entailed encouraging the vocal fold to adhere to the wall of the larynx, out of the path of the entering stream of air, by stripping the lining membrane from a little pouch which lies between the vocal cord and the laryngeal wall. Tracheotomy is an alternative: in this, a metal tube is inserted into the trachea at a lower level than the larynx, so that air is able to enter and leave through the tube instead of through the larynx. Tracheotomy is of most use in racehorses and hunters affected with roaring, which constitutes an unsoundness.

Abnormal inspiratory noises during exercise, particularly in young horses which may have pharyngitis and laryngitis, should not be taken to indicate one-sided paralysis of the larynx. Similarly, normal respiratory sounds at exercise should not be regarded as implying soundness of the upper respiratory tract.

Laryngoplasty is sometimes used for the treatment of roaring, especially in those horses not required to perform at high speeds. The operation involves securing the arytenoid cartilage in a lateral position, using prostheses to prevent intrusion of the arytenoid cartilage and vocal cord into the lumen of the larynx.

Poisoning Four 2-year-old thoroughbreds suffered an acute gastrointestinal illness shortly after being dosed with contaminated mineral oil. Three weeks later they had developed bilateral laryngeal paralysis. Two of the horses died during severe bouts of dyspnoea 6 and 8 weeks later, and a 3rd was put down. In these horses there was a severe loss of myelinated fibres from both recurrent laryngeal nerves. The 4th horse had bilateral pharyngeal paralysis 2 years later. The acute clinical signs and delayed neurological effects were typical of ORGANOPHOSPHORUS POISONING.

Lasalocid

A coccidiostat used as a feed additive in the prevention of coccidiosis in chickens, turkeys and game birds. It must not be used in breeding or laying birds; birds may be slaughtered only after 5 days from the last administration of the drug.

Laser

An acronym for light amplification by stimulated emission of radiation.

Lasers emit beams of intense, monochromatic, non-dispersing light, and can be used as powerful sources of localised energy. They are used in ophthalmic and other surgery and may be used instead of needles in acupuncture. Operators must wear protective glasses to shield their eyes.

Lassa Fever

This disease occurs in West Africa, and is caused by an arenavirus first isolated in 1969. In man the infection is likely to prove fatal. The virus has been isolated from the rat *Mastomys natalensis*, which (possibly with other rodents) acts as a reservoir of infection.

Lateral Cartilages

Lateral cartilages are rhomboid plates of cartilage which are attached, one on either side, to angles of the 3rd phalanx (os pedis) of the foot of the horse. They extend above the coronet sufficiently to be felt distinctly at the heels and for a certain distance in front of this. In old age they often become ossified in their lower parts. When they ossify in their upper palpable margins, the name 'sidebones' is applied to the

condition. In certain cases be cartilages may become injured from treads or tramps by neighbouring horses, or from the other foot; the cartilage, being poorly supplied with blood, undergoes necrosis. (See SIDEBONES; QUITTOR; FOOT OF THE HORSE.)

Lateral Line

A structure along the sides of fish that is sensitive to movement in the water, enabling the fish to detect the presence of other fish, currents, etc.

Latex (Natural Rubber)

Hypersensitivity to this can result in contact urticaria, respiratory symptoms, and shock. The main source of the allergens is the wearing of rubber gloves during surgery. Even a vaginal examination can result in an anaphylactic reaction in atopic people.

In the rubber-growing areas of Malaysia, the ingestion of latex by cattle, e.g. from buckets left by rubber-tappers, is a 'frequent occurrence', and can be fatal.

In 1 reported case, 2 bulls consumed 9 and 14 litres, respectively, of latex from the tree *Hevea brasiliensis*. Rumenotomy brought a temporary improvement in both bulls, but they died, despite supportive treatment, 11 days after ingesting the latex.

Latex agglutination test This can be used for measuring the concentration of IgG_1 in the plasma of newborn calves. The commercial test reagent (Ab-Ag Laboratories, Ely) is prepared by coating polystyrene latex beads with antibodies against bovine IgG_1.

Lathyrism (Lathyrus Poisoning)

Lathyrism (Lathyrus Poisoning) is caused by feeding upon one of the various 'Mutter peas' – *Lathyrus sativus* principally, and *L. cicera* and *L. clymenum*, less frequently. The latter 2 samples of field peas grown in Southern Europe and North Africa, while *L. sativus* is imported from India mainly. They are poisonous to all the domesticated animals, but seem especially dangerous for horses. Many outbreaks have been recorded, and in most the percentage of deaths has been high, sometimes as much as 50 per cent of the affected.

Symptoms of poisoning may not appear until the lapse of as much as 50 days after the peas cease to be used as a food-stuff. The cause of lathyrism is the high selenium content of the plants. (See SELENIUM.)

Signs usually become visible when the animal is put to work or exercised. Typically, the chief symptoms are those of paralysis of some part of the body – usually the hind-limbs and the recurrent laryngeal nerve. This latter gives rise to the condition known as 'ROARING', and unless quickly relieved, the horse will die from asphyxia. In some instances the symptoms are so sudden in their onset that the horse drops while in harness and is unable to rise. In less severe cases there is staggering and swaying of the hindquarters, great difficulty in breathing, a fast, weak pulse, and convulsive seizures. The paroxysms may pass off in a few minutes, or the horse may collapse and die.

Treatment (See under LARYNX, DISEASES OF.) The antidote is ascorbic acid, added to the diet.

Laudanum
(see OPIUM)

Laurel (Laurus) Poisoning
The leaves of laurel shrubs and trees (family: Lauraceae) contain cyanogentic GLYCOSIDES which cause poisoning by HYDROCYANIC ACID.

Lavage
The process of washing out the stomach or the intestines. In gastric lavage, a double-way tube is passed down into the stomach either through the mouth or by way of the nose, and water or some medicinal solution poured or pumped through one channel in the tube. After a time this escapes by the other, carrying with it the contents of the stomach in small amounts. (See also ENEMA.)

Law
Law, relating to the veterinary profession and veterinary practice, scientific research, domestic pets, farm animals, wild animals, and zoos, is extensive and subject to frequent amendment. The Scottish Parliament can bring in its own Acts, and both it and the Welsh Assembly bring in their own Orders and Regulations. Parallel legislation for the different parts of the UK exists for entries identified with an asterisk (*). Later legislation may partially revoke that made previously.

Existing legislation includes the following (where appropriate, information on the topic, animal or disease covered by the legislation listed will be found under individual entries):

Abandonment of Animals Act 1960
African Swine Fever Order 1980
African Swine fever (Compensation) Order 1980

Agriculture (Miscellaneous Provisions) Act 1969; 1972.
Agriculture (Poisonous Substances) Act 1952
Animal Boarding Establishments Act 1963
Animal By-Products Order 1999; Amendment 2002*
Animal By-Products (Identification) (Amendment) Regulations 2002
Animal Gatherings (Interim Measures) (Amendment) Order 2002*; No 2 Order 2002*
Animal Health Act 1981
Animal Health Act 2002
Animal Health (Amendment) Act 1998
Animal Health and Welfare Act 1984
Animal Health Orders (Divisional Veterinary Manager Amendment) Order 1995
Animals Act 1971
Animals Act (Amendment) Regulations 1991
Animals and Animal Products (Import and Export) Regulations 2002* (Amendment 2002*)
Animals (Cruel Poisons) Act 1962
Animals, Meat and Meat Products (Examination for Residues and Maximum Residue Limits) Act 1991 (amended 1993)
Animals (Post-Import Control) Order 1995
Animals (Scientific Procedures) Act 1986, as amended 1998
Animals (Scotland) Act 1987
Animals (Third Country Imports) (Charges) Regulations 1997
Antarctic Treaty Act 1994
Antarctic (Amendment) Regulations 2002
Anthrax Order 1991 (amended 1996)
Artificial Breeding of Sheep and Goats Regulations 1993
Artificial Insemination of Cattle (Animal Health) (England & Wales) Regulations 1985 (amended 1992,1995, 2002*)
Aujeszky's Disease Order 1983
Aujeszky's Disease (Compensation for Swine) Order 1983
Authorised Officers (Meat Inspection) Regulations 1987

Badgers Act 1992
Badgers (Further Protection) Act 1991
Bovine Animals (Records, Identification and Movement) Order 1995
Bovine Embryo Collection and Transfer Regulations 1995
Bovine Spongiform Encephalopathy (No 2) Order 1996
Bovine Spongiform Encephalopathy Compensation (Amendment) Order 1997

L

Welfare of Animals (Staging Posts) Order 1998

Welfare of Animals (Transport) Order 1997

Welfare of Horses at Markets (and Other Places of Sale) Order 1990

Welfare of Livestock Regulations 1994

Wild Mammals Protection Act 1996

Wildlife and Countryside Act 1981 (variations to schedules orders 1989, 1991, 1992, 1994, 1998)

Wildlife and Countryside (Registration and Ringing of Certain Captive Birds) Regulations 1982 (amended 1982, 1994)

Wildlife and Countryside (Registration to Sell, etc. Certain Dead Wild Birds) Regulations 1982 (amended 1991)

Wild Mammals (Protection) Act 1996

Zoo Licensing Act 1981 (amended 2002)

Zoonoses Order 1988, 1989
(See also EUROPEAN UNION.)

Laxatives

SENNA, which has been recommended for pregnant sows; DIHYDROXYANTHRAQUINONE, useful in all domestic animals, including horses; EPSOM SALTS (magnesium sulphate), but of doubtful efficacy in ruminants; GLAUBER'S SALTS, but they may have ill-effects in pigs. (See also PARAFFIN – Uses.)

LD$_{50}$

Ld$_{50}$value is a statistical estimate of the number of mg of a given substance per kg of bodyweight required to kill 50 per cent of a large population of test animals. The LD value of a compound may refer to oral or parenteral administration or to application to the skin.

Lead Poisoning

Also called plumbism.

Acute form of lead poisoning

Cattle This is very common in cattle which have eaten paint, licked out discarded paint tins, licked newly painted railings, etc., or which have eaten tarpaulins. It is frequently fatal and many cattle are unnecessarily lost each year from this cause. Cows have also been fatally poisoned after licking lead-rich ash from a burnt-down shed; and after eating silage contaminated by an old battery broken up by a forage harvester; also by eating roofing material from an old railway carriage.

In another instance cows were poisoned after eating haylage made from grass in a field which had been used for clay-pigeon shooting. The haylage contained small particles of clay pigeons and lead shot. The cows in the high-yielding herd of 115 Holsteins began to lose their appetite, became dull, and had diarrhoea. A few developed stiff and swollen joints. Many became uncoordinated in their movements; also there were 25 stillbirths or abortions. Appropriate treatment brought some improvement, but 21 cows either died or had to be slaughtered.

A 24-volt lead battery was discarded but unfortunately scooped up with straw being added to a 'complete diet' in a feeder box. The result was that 55 heifers died – some rapidly, some after ataxia, head pressing, teeth grinding and convulsions.

Dogs They are sometimes poisoned through eating paint scrapings where a room is being re-decorated, or after licking out a paint tin.

Cats In one case, old lead paint was stripped by means of an electric sander, which dispersed particles of the primer so that the air soon contained a toxic amount of lead. One cat and an infant suffered lead poisoning as a result.

Pigs have been shown to be less sensitive than other farm animals. They can consume, without showing symptoms, a daily dose of lead which would rapidly kill a cow.

Geese Ten lead pellets can kill a goose.

Swans Many cases have been reported of swans dying after swallowing lead weights used by anglers.

Signs Nervous signs are an important feature of lead poisoning, and may include excitement, ataxia, blindness, paresis, and convulsions; affected animals may also show depression.

Cattle may bellow, charge around, and at intervals press their heads against a wall or other fixed object.

Abdominal pain, sometimes with constipation followed by diarrhoea, are other signs; also anaemia in chronic or subacute cases.

In horses, 'roaring' (laryngeal paralysis) may be a sign, together with carpal swelling and posterior paralysis.

Treatment The treatment of lead poisoning was revolutionised by the introduction of the chelating agent, calcium di-sodium adetate, which converts inorganic lead in the tissues into a harmless lead chelate which is excreted by the kidneys. The drug must be given intravenously.

In chronic cases, potassium iodide is given 3 or 4 times daily to hasten the elimination of the lead salt from the system. (See also CHELATING AGENTS.)

Diagnosis of lead poisoning may be made by estimating the lead content of the blood, kidneys or liver.

A differential diagnosis must take into account other possibilities such as hypomagnesaemia, encephalitis, acetonaemia, listeriosis, and poisoning by other substances.

Chronic lead poisoning has occurred as a result of flaking paintwork in dog kennels, and also in the proximity of former lead-mining sites. Four out of 5 sheepdogs, in an Australian incident, became agitated after working sheep satisfactorily for some 20 minutes. They left the work area and retreated to the underside of a vehicle or to a kennel.

The behavioural effects of lead poisoning in dogs may also include hysteria or aggressiveness.

Falcons kept in painted cages developed lead poisoning after gnawing at the bars.

Signs Chronic lead poisoning results in recurrent laryngeal nerve paralysis and paralysis of the pharynx.

Leeches

Blood-sucking aquatic annelids of the class Hirudinea, within phylum Annelida (segmented worms).

Leeches live in ponds, streams, and on damp vegetation. They have strong muscular suckers; the anterior one surrounds the mouth which, in several species, contains saw-like teeth used to pierce the skin of the host. Leeches secrete hirudin in their buccal cavity; this prevents clotting of the host's blood, on which they feed, and can cause a severe and sometimes fatal anaemia.

Leeches live in ponds, streams, and on damp vegetation.

Limnatis nilotica is found in North Africa and Southern Europe. It reaches a length of 10 cm. The ventral surface is dark; on the dorsal surface are 6 longitudinal stripes on a brownish-green background. It cannot penetrate skin, but on being taken in with water by men and animals, it attaches itself to the buccal mucous membrane. This produces, constant small haemorrhages, which sometimes cause a serious anaemia.

L. africana and species of *Haemadipsa* are active in West Africa and in the tropical forests of Asia and South America, respectively.

H. zeylanica occurs in Asia and lives on land. It is a clear brown colour with a yellow lateral stripe on each side and a greenish dorsal stripe. It has 5 pairs of eyes and 3 teeth. It lives in damp weather on the lower vegetation. These leeches are small forms, about 2.5 cm long, but are very serious pests. The bite is painless but, as they occur in such enormous numbers, very deadly. They attack all vertebrates and many different species of mammals have been killed by them through sheer loss of blood.

Two cases of infestation of dogs with *Diestecostoma mexicanum* have been reported from Honduras. In the non-fatal case, a catheter was passed through the inferior nasal meatus and a 50-ml capacity syringe containing chloroform water attached. The solution was injected slowly while the catheter was revolved. Over 70 leeches emerged after treatment.

Legionella Pneumophila

This organism, first discovered in 1976, can tolerate hot water, and is spread by aerosols of it. People, cattle, sheep, horses, pigs, goats, dogs and cats are all at risk of pneumonia caused by this infection (Legionaires disease).

Legislation

(see LAW)

Legume Poisoning

This may occur when certain legumes are fed raw, and can result in death. Both navy beans (*Phaseolus vulgaris*) and jack beans (*Canavalis ensiformis*) contain a heat-sensitive toxin which can weaken the animal's resistance to coliform and other bacteria. Heat treatment of the beans renders them safe. (See also LATHYRISM; LUPINS; POISONING.)

Leishmania

A genus of protozoon parasites. Each appears as a round or oval body with a micro- and a macro-nucleus.

Leishmaniasis

Leishmaniasis is of considerable importance in man, but not in animals other than the dog. Cutaneous leishmaniasis, or 'oriental sore', is seen in Iran, India, parts of Africa, and South America, and is caused by *Leishmania tropica*. Visceral leishmaniasis, called also kala-azar or 'dum-dum fever', occurs in the coastal countries of the Mediterranean, and is caused by *L. donovani*. (At least 5 other species, and several subspecies, are recognised.) Both forms are diagnosed by laboratory examination. A 3rd form, affecting mucous membrane of mouth

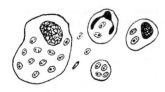

Leishmania as seen in spleen cells.

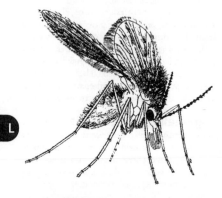

A female phlebotomine sandfly, the vector of leishmaniasis. (Reproduced with permission from *The Leishmaniasis: Report of WHO Expert Committee*, WHO Technical Report Series 701, WHO, Geneva.)

and nose, is caused by *L. brasiliensis*, and has a poor prognosis. The disease has beenrecorded in dogs returning from mainland Europe (mainly Spain) under the Pet Travel Scheme.

Signs in the dog include wasting, enlarged lymph nodes, keratitis and/or conjunctivitis, and alopecia or dermatitis. The ears are excessively waxy and the wax has a distinct and unusual smell. Dermatitis may develop.

Leishmaniasis is rarer in cats, causing skin ulcers, fistulae and enlarged lymph nodes.

Treatment The incubation period in dogs may be up to 2 years; the prognosis is not good. The treatment of choice is allopurinol at 10 to 15 mg/kg bodyweight for 6 months at least; the treatment may actually take longer, depending on the response. A cure is rare. (See FLIES – 'sandflies'.)

Prevention Housing animals between 19.00 and 07.00, when the vector (the sandfly) is most active. Fitting dogs (not cats) with a 'flea collar' impregnated with a synthetic pyrethrin may help repel the flies.

Dogs are an important source of human infection in many regions.

Lens of the Eye
(see EYE)

Lenses, Contact
Lenses, contact made of a softish hydrophilic material have been used in horses, dogs and cats with keratitis and/or penetration of the cornea. Such lenses can act more or less as a bandage for the cornea, and promote healing by reducing trauma from inflamed eyelids and so reducing pain. Ointment and eye-drops can be still used. The lens can be removed at the end of a week or so.

The effect of bright light on the retina of a racing greyhound's eye caused a lack of speed. Improvement was reported after a tinted contact lens had been fitted.

Lentiviruses
Members of this group include EQUINE INFECTIOUS ANAEMIA; MAEDI/VISNA of sheep; and CAPRINE ARTHRITIS-ENCEPHALITIS, as well as the human AIDS virus.

Lepeophtheirus
Lepeophtheirus is the sea-louse of salmonids. It is the most important disease problem for fish farming in sea lochs; the parasite literally eats the fish alive. Treatment is possible by feed medicated with azamethiphos or dichlorvos but uneaten feed attracts wild salmon to the cages. Wrasse (cleaner fish) have been suggested as a biological alternative to medication but there are doubts about the practicality. The Farm Animal Welfare Council published a report, *The Welfare of Farmed Fish*, in 1996.

Leptomeningitis
Leptomeningitis means inflammation of the inner and more delicate membranes of the brain and spinal cord.

Leptospira
This genus comprises 2 species: a pathogenic one, *L. interrogans*; and *L. biflexa*, which is found in surface water and is regarded as a saprophyte. There are numerous serotypes and subgroups. The bacteria can survive for long periods in the kidneys and, outside the body, in moist, warm conditions. Leptospires are SPIROCHAETES.

Leptospirosis
Infection with *Leptospira*.

Leptospirosis in Cattle

This is an important infection which can give rise to a generalised illness, to mastitis, or to abortion. Jaundice may be one of the symptoms and, in the case of mastitis, discoloured milk. (See MASTITIS.) The leptospires tend to localise in the kidneys. Abnormal milk is a dominant symptom. Abortion due to leptospirosis is not uncommon.

In one survey, a total of 406 cattle sera were collected at the Edinburgh abattoir from animals of 63 different herds in various parts of Scotland, the north of England and Northern Ireland, and tested against the following *Leptospira* serotypes: *icterohaemorrhagiae, canicola, pomona, bratislava, ballum, sejroe, grippotyphosa,* and *bataviae, saxaebing* and *hardjo* were included when testing the last 80 cattle sera. Of the total, 260 (64 per cent) sera had agglutinins to one or more of these 10 serotypes.

Cattle are the maintenance hosts of *L. hardjo*, which is a cause of abortion, milk drop syndrome and leptospiral MASTITIS, and also important from the public health aspect.

Leptospirosis of calves has been seen both in the UK (due to *L. icterohaemorrhagiae* and *L. canicola*) and overseas (due to other leptospires).

In Queensland an acute fever with jaundice and haemoglobinuria has been known in calves for many years. It is rapid in onset and death occurs within a few hours to 4 days after the appearance of symptoms; dullness, temperature of 40° to 41.5°C (104° to 107°F), dark red urine, pale and yellow visible mucous membranes. *L. pomona* was demonstrated in kidney sections on post-mortem examinations. Recovered calves continued to excrete leptospires for up to 3 months. Infection may occur through inhalation of droplets of infected urine splashing on concrete, or as a result of insect bites.

In the USA, where the important species are *L. pomona, L. grippotyphosa,* and *L. sejroe*, abortion is reported to be the main symptom of leptospirosis in cows. In Illinois, a survey covering over 23,000 animals showed 14 per cent to be affected.

In Kenya, outbreaks of acute illness due to infection with *L. grippotyphosa* have been reported in cattle, sheep, and goats. Jaundice is a symptom in some 30 per cent of cases, and death has followed within 12 hours of symptoms being observed. Snuffling, coughing, and holding down of the head are other symptoms. In cows, milk yield is reduced and is red in colour or otherwise abnormal. Urine varies from red to black. Temperature may rise to 40.5°C (105°F).

In Europe, *L. grippotyphosa, L. pomona* and *L. canicola* have been isolated.

Diagnosis The bacteria can be found in the aborted fetus but diagnosis is usually by detection of raised antibody levels.

Treatment Antibiotics, especially streptomycin, used at a high dosage can reduce levels of infection. Milk withdrawal requirements must be observed.

Control Vaccines are available for immunising cattle against infection by *L. interrogans* serovar *hardjo*. Two vaccinations are given 4 to 6 weeks apart with a single annual booster injection.

Wild animal hosts After an outbreak of abortion associated with leptospires in Scottish cattle, wild mammals were examined. Leptospires were isolated from 22 out of 108 rats, 3 out of 49 mice and 1 out of 3 hedgehogs; voles, mice and shrews were found to be infected on the farm where the leptospiral abortion had been diagnosed. Contamination of pastures by the urine of wild mammals may play a part in the spread of leptospirosis in cattle.

Public health aspects People working in milking parlours have become infected with leptospirosis as a result of the splashing of infected cows' urine on concrete. Inhalation of a resulting aerosol is one means of transmission. Leptospires can penetrate abraded skin and intact mucous membrane – another mode of infection.

Infection with members of the Hebdomadis serogroup has been identified as the most commonly diagnosed leptospiral infection of man in Britain. This serogroup includes *L. hardjo* and *L. sejroe*, which also cause mastitis in cows.

Two genotypes have been recognised: *hardjo bovis* and *hardjo prajitno*; the latter being less common but more pathogenic.

In one 12-month period, 72 cases of human leptospirosis, of which 7 were fatal, were confirmed in the British Isles. In 30 cases the patient's occupation was associated with farming. Nine of the patients became infected through immersion in polluted water. Illness due to Hebdomadis serogroup infection was generally less severe than that due to *L. icterohaemorrhagiae*.

L. hardjo causes an influenza-like illness which can be severe and last several weeks. In rare instances there may be meningitis, kidney failure, and death.

In New Zealand, high titres of antibodies were found in workers on farms where there was active *L. hardjo* infection of 2- and 3-year-old cattle. Conventional measures for protecting milkers from contact with infected urine appeared to be ineffective, and it was concluded that herd vaccination of cattle was the only means of protecting dairy farm workers.

Leptospirosis in Dogs

Jaundice in dogs may be caused by *Leptospira icterohaemorrhagiae*. This organism also causes jaundice (Weil's disease) in man, and illness (with or without jaundice) in a number of domestic animals, including pigs and calves. In a Glasgow survey it was found that 40 per cent of dogs had at some time been infected with *L. canicola* (the cause of Canicola fever in man), which is 2 or 3 times more common as a parasite in dogs than *L. icterohaemorrhagiae*. The parasite is the cause of much of the acute and subacute nephritis in younger dogs, especially between November and April

It was shown in a survey in the USA that of 100 rats, 55 had *Leptospira* in the kidneys, and that 23 per cent of the farm rats and 49, or 66 per cent, of the urban rats harboured *Leptospira* in those organs. (The incidence of the *Leptospira* in the rat varied with the location of the rubbish dump on which they were found. Nearly all the rats obtained in 1 area were positive.) Similar surveys in the UK have shown 37.6 per cent of rats infected.

The parasite is the cause of much of the acute and subacute nephritis in younger dogs, especially between November and April.

Signs of infection with *L. canicola* are very variable. There may be loss of appetite, depression, and fever alone, or together with marked thirst and vomiting, loss of weight, and sometimes a foul odour from the mouth. In a few cases there is jaundice. Ulceration of the tongue may occur. Collapse, coma, and death may supervene.

The symptoms first described above are related to leptospiral invasion of the bloodstream. This may be followed by invasion of, and damage to, the kidneys. This primary nephritis may be followed later by chronic interstitial nephritis, kidney failure, uraemia, and death.

Treatment Antibiotics have been used with considerable success in the early stage of *L. canicola* infection. Once the kidneys have been damaged, however, treatment is as for nephritis. In severe cases – where the 'Stuttgart' syndrome or symptoms of uraemia are evident – the animal dies, as a rule, despite all treatment. (See KIDNEYS, DISEASES OF; URAEMIA; NURSING; HEART.)

Prevention Single and multiple vaccines are available.

Most of the dogs which recover from leptospirosis excrete the organisms in the urine for long periods (sometimes 4 to 18 months). This obviously makes control of the disease difficult.

Leptospirosis in Horses

Leptospirosis in horses is usually a mild disease, though sometimes fatal in foals; but see PERIODIC OPHTHALMIA.

Leptospirosis in Pigs

Cases of leptospiral jaundice in piglets due to *Leptospira icterohaemorrhagiae* and also to *L. canicola* have been reported in the UK.

Symptoms in pigs include loss of appetite, fever, jaundice, and – in some cases – death. Pigs which have recovered excrete leptospires for some time afterwards. Indeed, infection in a herd may persist for years, with risk to human health. Sows may abort.

L. canicola can survive for 12 days in naturally infected pig kidneys kept in a refrigerator. (See CANICOLA FEVER, which farm workers may contract from pigs.)

L. pomona and *L. interrogans hardjo* may cause leptospiral abortion. *L. australia*, which in the UK has many free-living carnivore hosts, also infects pigs.

Leptospirosis in Sheep

In Britain, leptospirosis is rare in sheep, though serological surveys have shown evidence of infection. In Northern Ireland the infection was demonstrated in aborted, stillborn and weak lambs, by culture, immunofluorescence and fetal serology, from 9 out of 42 flocks investigated during the 1980 and 1981 lambing seasons. Three serogroups were implicated: Hebdomadis, Australis, and Pomona.

Clinical leptospirosis in sheep and goats in other countries has been characterised either by abortion, or by an acute, often fatal disease, with symptoms of jaundice, fever, and haemoglobinuria.

Lernea

The anchor worm. The female (only) is a parasite on fish. It attaches itself to the muscles by penetrating the skin. They may be seen round the vent. Affected fish are sluggish and grow poorly. There may be heavy mortaliy.

Lhasa Apso

A small dog with long straight hair almost covering the face. The breed originates in Tibet.

Renal cortical hypoplasia may be inherited and intervetebral disc disease may develop.

Lesion

Lesion meant originally an injury, but is now applied to all changes produced by diseases in organs or tissues.

Let-Down of Milk

(see MILKING)

Lethal Factors

(see GENETICS, HEREDITY and BREEDING)

Leucine

One of the essential amino acids.

Leuco - (Leuko-)

Leuco - (leuko-) is a prefix meaning white. 'Leuko-' is the spelling recommended by the EU.

Leucogen

The proprietary name of Britain's first genetically engineered vaccine for use against FELINE LEUKAEMIA virus (a retrovirus).

Leukaemia (Lymphosarcoma)

Leukaemia (lymphosarcoma) is a malignant disease – a form of cancer – involving lymphoid tissue especially. It occurs in all the domestic animals, in which (as opposed to man) there is commonly but not invariably no increase in the number of lymphocytes in the bloodstream (an 'aleukaemic leukaemia'). Accorddingly, lymphosarcoma is the better name.

In 1 form there may be a large tumour mass at the site of the thymus. Usually, many lymph nodes are involved, with enlargement of the spleen and infiltration of the liver. Tumours may occur in almost any organ.

Signs Enlargement of superficial or of mesenteric lymph nodes, depression, emaciation, anaemia, often diarrhoea.

In the dog, death commonly follows after 3 weeks, but the duration of illness varies from 1 to more than 60 weeks.

Leukaemia is the commonest malignant disease in the cat in Britain, and is caused by a virus. (See FELINE LEUKAEMIA.)

(For disease in cattle, see BOVINE ENZOOTIC LEUKOSIS.)

Treatment Cytotoxic drugs such as cyclophosphamide and vincristine may be used in dogs and cats. Treatment is highly specialised.

Vaccines are available for protection against feline leukaemia.

Leukocytes

Leukocytes are white cells found in the blood and lymphoid tissue. (See BLOOD; LYMPHOCYTES; INFLAMMATION; PHAGOCYTOSIS; WOUNDS; IMMUNE RESPONSE.)

Leukocytosis

Leukocytosis is a temporary increase in the number of white cells in the blood. It occurs after a feed, during pregnancy, after exertion, and when the temperature is elevated. It is seen during infections, when neutrophils will be numerous; though in some infections monocytes will be more numerous than normal for a time. In parasitic infestations and some allergic reactions, eosinophils increase in number.

Leukocytosis is seen in some cases of poisoning, e.g. by potassium chlorate, phenacetin.

The usual proportion of red cells to leukocytes in the blood of the healthy mammal is about 1000:1.

In true leukaemia there is an abnormal increase of leukocytes in the blood – some being of abnormal shape. Myeloblasts may predominate in the final stages of leukaemia. (See LEUKAEMIA.)

Leukoderma

Leukoderma means a condition of the skin and hair when areas become white as a result of injury or disease. It is seen on the backs of horses that have worn badly fitting saddles and collars, when it is called 'saddle-mark' and 'collar-mark', and after ringworm.

Leukoma

The presence of an opaque patch or spots on the surface of the cornea. (See EYE.)

Leukopenia

A condition in which the white blood cells are less numerous than normal. It occurs during the course of several diseases, e.g. swine fever, leptospirosis of cattle. (See FELINE INFECTIOUS ENTERITIS.)

Leukorrhoea

A chronic vaginal discharge, generally of a whitish or greyish colour. It is a symptom of VAGINITIS or of metritis. (See UTERUS, DISEASES OF; 'WHITES'.)

Leukosis

Multiplication of leukocyte-forming tissues; it results in leukaemia (see BOVINE ENZOOTIC LEUKOSIS; LEUKAEMIA; LEUKOSIS IN TURKEYS).

Leukosis in Turkeys

Two distinct forms of leukosis infection are recognised in the UK and have caused serious and widespread economic loss among turkey flocks.

(a) Lymphoproliferative disease (LPD) affects turkeys from 9 weeks of age and can cause a mortality of 1 per cent a week. It is characterised by sudden death of birds in good condition with gross enlargement of the spleen and tumours in the liver, lungs and elsewhere. The causative agent of LPD is suspected to be an oncovirus unrelated to recognised avian viruses of this group.

(b) Reticuloendotheliosis virus (REV) infection can be distinguished clinically from lymphoproliferative disease by the fact that it is associated with a diarrhoea which frequently affects turkeys between 8 and 10 weeks of age. This is followed by the development of tumours resulting in mortality of up to 20 per cent. The most consistent post-mortem finding has been a large leukotic liver. The causative agent is an RE virus which can be replicated in tissue culture. Viraemia develops within 2 weeks of infection and antibodies persist for the lifetime of infected birds.

Leukovirus

This genus of virus includes the Rous sarcoma virus, feline leukaemia virus and fowl sarcoma virus.

Levamisole

A broad-spectrum anthelmintic. It can be administered by injection or in the feed. Levamisole is also of value in stimulating the bodily defence mechanisms, when these have been depressed by, for example, viral infections, or by *Brucella abortus*. Any reduction of T-lymphocytes is apparently restored to normal, and phagocytosis increased, among other immuno-stimulant effects. (See ANERGY.)

In dogs, levamisole is used mainly to treat heartworm infections. Its side-effects (vomiting, diarrhoea, loss of appetite) can be reduced by giving it with or after food.

Leys, New

Highly productive pastures. Cattle grazing these are, generally speaking, more prone to hypomagnesaemia than when on permanent pasture. Clover-rich leys are also conducive to bloat, unless precautions are taken.

Lice

Two distinct families of lice are found on the domestic animals: the sucking lice and the biting lice. All the fowl lice belong to the latter family. The lice are wingless insects which undergo a direct development. The egg is laid on the body, glues itself to a hair or feather, and the young louse is, except for size, identical to the adult. There is no pupal stage, although several moults take place. The sucking lice belong to the order Siphunculata.

The biting lice belong to the order Mallophaga. The mouth parts are very different from those of the sucking lice. They cannot suck blood, and the mouth parts consist of a pair of mandibles on the ventral side of the blunt head. In this order, as in the last, all the mammalian hosts, except the horse, have their own species.

Horses Only 1 species of sucking louse is found on the horse, called *Haematopinus asini*. Two species of closely related biting lice are also found: *Damalinia equi* and *D. pilosus*. Sucking lice are more generally found at the base of the mane and tail, while the biting species are commonly on the lower parts of the body. They cause poorness of condition, itching, and loss of hair.

Cattle Sucking lice include *Haematopinus eurysternus*, *H tuberculatus*, and *Linognathus vituli*. In addition, 1 species of biting louse occurs, *Damalinia bovis*. The sucking lice are

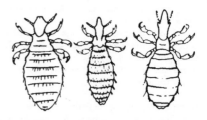

Sucking lice. × 10. (Left, *Haematopinus*; centre, *Linognathus*; right, *Solenopotus*.)

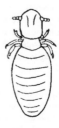

Biting louse. × 15. (*Trichodectes*.)

found mainly on the head and shoulders; the biting lice on any part of the body. They cause itchiness and scratching which may produce thickening of the skin, and cause mange to be suspected.

A 4th species of sucking louse, *Solenoptes capillatus*, is found in the UK, New Zealand, etc., but is not very common.

Sheep *Haematopinus ovillus* (on the body), *Linognathus pedalis* (on the foot), and *L. africanus* are sucking lice. *Damalinia ovis* is a biting louse.

Goats *Linognathus stenopsis* and *L. africanus*, attack the goat. Biting lice include *Damalinia caprae* and *D. limbata*.

Pigs *Haematopinus suis*, a large species causing intense pruritus, which seriously interferes with fattening. Young pigs have been known to die from the loss of blood and the extensive irritation. The lice are usually found near the ears, inside the elbows and on the breast.

Dogs and cats Important species include a sucking louse, *Linognathus setosus*, and a biting louse, *Trichodectes canis*. The latter is an intermediate host of *Dipylidium caninum*.

Poultry All the lice affecting birds are biting lice, and include *Menopon gallinae* and *Goniodes gallinae*.

Lice can cause a severe anaemia in young animals especially.

Control involves 2 applications of a suitable insecticide at a 7- to 10-day interval, repeated if necessary. Permethrin is suitable for dogs and cats.

For larger animals, sprays or dips, or ivermectin by injection, may be used. (See IVERMECTIN; BHC; FLEA COLLARS; AEROSOL; BATHS – Cats.)

Lick Granuloma

A tumour-like mass of granulation tissue on the skin of dogs which can form as a result of the incessant licking of a wound, ulcer, or even unbroken skin – in which case there may be a local neuritis causing itching of the spot, and so accounting for the licking.

Treatment An ELIZABETHAN COLLAR may be necessary to prevent the dog's access to the part. A corticosteroid may be used. In long-standing, intractable cases cryosurgery is usually the recommended treatment, but American

experience suggests that 2 or 3 applications may be necessary, but that the owner is not always willing to persevere. (For a similar condition in cats, see EOSINOPHILIC GRANULOMA.)

'Licked Beef'

'Licked beef' is that which shows greenish or yellowish tracks made by the larvae of warble-flies, with the formation of 'butcher's jelly'. This is of importance in food inspection.

'Licking Syndrome'

This is the name for a condition in which cattle tend to lick each other, or each other's urine, or the soil, in an attempt to obtain the extra salt they need, and is a sign of sodium deficiency. This occurs, in the absence of salt licks or the provision of sufficient salt in the feed, on sodium-deficient pastures which, according to ADAS surveys in the south of England, may amount to 50 per cent. A cow giving 23 litres (5 gallons) of milk loses nearly 42.5 g (1½ oz) of sodium chloride in its milk each day, and the ARC has stated that the cow has only 85 g (3 oz) of salt in her body which can safely be used to balance this loss if the supply of salt in the diet is inadequate.

Urine-drinking has been seen in yarded cows, even when given free access to salt and magnesium, in France. The habit disappeared once the herd gained access to spring pasture. Having drinking troughs placed too close together, or too few of them, in the yards led to dominant cows preventing others from approaching the sources of water and salt. (See under SALT – Salt licks; SODIUM DEFICIENCY; HAIR-BALLS; METABOLIC PROFILE TESTS.)

Lien

Lien is the Latin name for the spleen.

Life after Freezing

A lively litter of 10 albino mice, born to a brown mouse, was exhibited at the Royal Society's premises in London, in 1993. The albinos had been implanted into their surrogate mother after being, as embryos, kept for 13 weeks in liquid nitrogen at a temperature of $-196°C$.

Ligaments

Ligaments are strong bands of fibrous tissue that serve to bind together the bones forming a joint. They are cord-like in some instances, flat bands in others, and sheets in the case of the joint-capsule which surrounds a joint. (See JOINTS.)

Desmitis (inflammation) of the fetlock annular ligament was diagnosed in 30 horses which had been lame for a long time and which had chronically distended digital flexor tendon sheaths, or plantar annular ligaments. The ligament was cut longitudinally in 25 of the horses; 16 returned to full work without difficulty and 1 became sound after a 2nd operation. None of the 5 untreated horses returned to work.

Ligamentum Arteriosum

The fibrous remains of the *ductus arteriosus* of the fetus. It connects the left pulmonary artery to the arch of the aorta.

Light, Influence of

Adequate light is necessary for maximum fertility. This applies to poultry (see under NIGHT-LIGHTING), to bulls – too often kept in dark places – and to sheep, etc. (See also LIGHTING; RICKETS; VITAMINS – Vitamin D; TROPICS.)

Light Sensitisation

Light sensitisation implies a predisposing factor, such as the eating of a particular plant, which has the effect of making certain cells in the animal's body abnormally sensitive – for the time being – to light. Strong sunlight is then capable of causing serious and extensive damage, with a good deal of distress.

In Australia this trouble is frequently caused, in cattle, sheep, and pigs, through eating St John's wort. Elsewhere overseas, clover and buckwheat are often responsible. Occasional cases of light sensitisation occur even in the UK. To give an example, a British Friesian heifer was discovered in obvious distress. Over nearly all the white parts the skin was dead and had partly sloughed off. Appropriate treatment, which included temporary confinement in a darkened loose-box, was followed by a rapid recovery. Bog asphodel and rape cause light sensitisation in sheep in Britain, where pigs have also been affected (probably by St John's wort). In New Zealand, where the condition is called facial eczema, moulds have been incriminated. In Britain another plant involved is the GIANT HOGWEED.

It is the white, pigment-free skin which suffers. Thus, some breeds of livestock are never troubled with light sensitisation, while white or partly white cattle are susceptible. Similarly, grey and pie-bald horses in the USA and elsewhere are sometimes affected.

Light sensitisation is associated with disfunction of the liver, and the presence of porphyrins in the bloodstream. It also occurs in some cases of PORPHYRIA.

Lighting of Animal Buildings

Various kinds of glass substitutes have been put on the market, which are reputed to allow the ultraviolet rays of natural sunlight to pass through without appreciable absorption.

Adequate light is necessary to prevent rickets, and to ensure maximum fertility in poultry and other animals. Continuous light, however, may have harmful effects.

Artificial lighting of poultry houses is now a common practice. Red light is used in many broiler houses and in some laying houses in order to reduce cannibalism. (See also NIGHT LIGHTING.)

Lightning Strike

Cattle, sheep and horses are most often affected. (See under ELECTRIC SHOCK.)

Lignocaine

A local anaesthetic agent used to produce nerve blocks, it has also been used to treat cardiac arrhythmias.

'Limberneck'

An old, colloquial name for some of the symptoms seen in cases of botulism in poultry: a loss of power of the muscles of the neck, wings, and legs, affected birds first being dull and inactive. (See BOTULISM.)

Liming of Pastures

If this is carried out to excess it can lead to a deficiency in copper in the grazing animal and so bring about INFERTILITY. Manganese deficiency is likewise a sequel when the soil becomes too alkaline. Cattle should be kept away from downwind of liming operations, or eye inflammation (conjunctivitis and keratitis) may result.

Limousin

A pure beef breed noted for high liveweight gains, high killing-out percentages, and freedom from calving difficulties.

Lincomycin

An antibiotic effective against Gram-positive bacteria, anaerobes and mycoplasma.

Linear Assessment of Dairy Cows

(see PROGENY TESTING – Conformation)

Liner, Teat-Cup

In selecting milking machinery equipment, one should avoid any liner with a hard mouthpiece. Liners must be changed after a maximum of 2500 milkings.

Linguatula Serrata
(see MITES, PARASITIC)

Liniments (Embrocations)
Liniments (embrocations) are liquid preparations for external application (to unbroken skin), generally rubbed in, and having counter-irritant or analgesic properties. They are used for painful muscular conditions, strains and sprains.

Linognathus
A genus of sucking lice. (See LICE.)

Linseed
The flax plant (*Linum usitatissimum*). After extraction of linseed oil from the seeds, the residue is made into linseed cake for feeding to horses, cattle, and sheep.

Linseed poisoning The flax plant contains a cyanogenetic glycoside in small amounts. An enzyme in the flax can act on the glycoside, with production of hydrocyanic acid. The enzyme is not always destroyed in the process of making linseed cake. Boiling for 10 minutes destroys the enzyme and renders linseed safe. However, linseed cake should be fed dry and not made into a mash with warm water – a dangerous practice owing to the formation of hydrocyanic acid. Linseed poisoning is not common.

Lipase
A fat-splitting enzyme found in the pancreatic juice.

Lipids
Fatty substances. Simple lipids are esters of fatty acids and alcohol, and include fats (esters of fatty acids and glycerol). Compound lipids contain, in addition to fatty acid and alcohol, carbohydrate or nitrogen or phosphoric acid, for example.

'Protected lipids' are those encapsulated in a protein envelope, which is then treated with formaldehyde. Because of their high energy value, fats and oils and their fatty acids seemed worth including in cattle feed supplements; and 'protected lipids' offered the possibility of avoiding the disturbance of normal rumen metabolism likely to occur with free fats being present in the rumen.

Lipoma
Lipoma is a tumour mainly composed of fat. They are liable to arise almost anywhere in the body where there is fibrous connective tissue, but are especially common below loose skin. They are occasionally seen in the abdominal cavity, where they develop in connection with the peritoneum, and sometimes encase the bowel and obstruct its function or attain a large size. (See TUMOUR.)

Lipoprotein
A complex of cholesterol, triglycerides, phospholipids, and apoproteins. An excess of lipoprotein in the blood – hyperlipoproteinaemia – occurs in some cases of diabetes, hypothyroidism metabolic disorders and inherited disease.

Lips
Lips are musculo-membranous folds which in the horse are covered on the outside with fine hairs, among which are longer, stouter tactile hairs, while some heavy draught horses have a 'moustache' on their upper lips. On the inside, the lips are covered by mucous membrane which is continuous with that of the mouth generally.

In the horse the lips are extremely mobile, and the upper lip especially contains a very dense plexus of sensory nerves which serve tactile purposes. In the ox the lips are thick and comparatively immobile. The middle part of the upper lip between the nostrils is bare of hair and is termed the muzzle. It is provided with a large number of tiny glands which secrete a clear fluid, which keeps the part cool and moist. Within the lower lip are numbers of horny papillae; its free margin is bare, but the under part of it is covered with ordinary and tactile hairs. The sheep possesses no hairless muzzle, but has a distinct 'philtrum' instead. The lips are thin and mobile. In the pig the upper lip is thick and short and is blended with the snout or nasal disc, while the lower is thin and pointed. (See also HARE-LIP.)

Liquid Feeding
Liquid feeding of dairy cows in the parlour enables them to eat up to 6.8 kg (15 lb) of concentrates in 7 minutes.

Liquid Paraffin, Medicinal
(see under PARAFFIN for its use as a laxative).

Listerellosis
(see LISTERIOSIS)

Listeriosis
A disease caused by *Listeria monocytogenes* which attacks rodents, poultry, ruminants, pigs,

horses, dogs, and man. It causes encephalitis and abortion in cattle and sheep, and has to be differentiated from RABIES.

In cattle, the infection may be confused with rabies or poisoning. The affected animal is seen to keep aloof from the rest of the herd, and is later unable to stand without support. If walked, it usually moves in a circle. The head may be held back to one side, with salivation and a nasal discharge. Paralysis of one side of the face may occur. Some cows become violent in the terminal stages and bellow.

In an English outbreak, 12 out of 15 calves died between April and August, at 3 to 7 days old, from septicaemia. There was severe keratitis and conjunctivitis (*L. monocytogenes* is recognised as one cause of IBK), extreme dejection, and distressed breathing.

Listeria is a cause of IRITIS in cattle feeding at silage clamps. (See SILAGE.)

There is also a septicaemic form in adult cattle and sheep, which shows itself by depression, fever, weakness, and emaciation.

Pigs may have swelling of the eyelids, encephalitis, paralysis, or occasionally septicaemia.

Listeriosis is a rare cause of abortion in mares, and a common cause in other animals. It is an important cause of abortion in goats.

Infection may be spread by urine, milk, faeces, an aborted fetus, and vaginal discharges.

Listeriosis in the fowl is seen as sudden death due to myocarditis. It may occur in free-range chickens.

Good hygiene helps to prevent the disease; antibiotics may be effective in treating early cases.

(See also AVIAN LISTERIOSIS.)

Lithiasis
Lithiasis is the formation of calculi and concretions in tissues or organs. For example, cholelithiasis means the formation of calculi in the gall-bladder. (See also under CALCULI; UROLITHIASIS.)

Lithium
Lithium antimony thiomalate has been used by injection to remove multiple warts.

Lithium Poisoning
Lithium poisoning occurred in 2 dogs whose sole source of drinking water for several months was a swimming pool chlorinated with lithium hypochlorite. One dog had fits. Both had diarrhoea, became weak, and dehydrated. They recovered after being provided with fresh, uncontaminated water.

Lithontriptics
Lithontriptics are substances which are reputed to have the power of dissolving stones in the urinary system. (See HYALURONIDASE.)

Lithotomy
Lithotomy is the operation of opening the bladder for the removal of a stone.

Lithotrity
Lithotrity is an operation in which a stone in the bladder is broken into small fragments and removed by washing out the bladder with a catheter.

Litter
(see DEEP LITTER; BEDDING)

Litter, Old
Broiler chicks reared on previously used litter may, as a result of the ammonia fumes, develop a severe inflammation of eye-surfaces and eyelids. In one house, 3000 broilers were affected. The birds cannot bear to open their eyes, and appear obviously dejected. Mortality is generally low, but the trouble is a serious one for all that.

Litter Size (Pigs)
In Britain the average is between 10 and 11 born alive; mortality 0.84. Earlier figures (PIDA) showed that an average of 2.2 pigs per litter died between birth and 8 weeks old. A litter of 34 has been recorded.

Liver
A solid glandular organ lying in the anteriormost part of the abdomen close up against the diaphragm. Its colour varies from a dark red-brown in the horse to a bluish-purple in the ox and pig; it is soft to the touch though it is rather friable in consistency, and it constitutes the largest gland in the body.

Functions include the excretion of bile, the storage of glycogen and of iron, the breaking-down of old and worn-out red blood cells, and the breaking-down of toxic substances and of waste substances from the tissues of the body. From the liver, urea and uric acid find their way into the bloodstream and are excreted from the body in the urine by the kidneys. In animals except those of the horse tribe, the bile is collected in the gall-bladder and the bile-duct before passing to the small intestine, where it assists the pancreatic juice in the digestion of food after a meal.

Shape There are probably few organs which vary so much in shape as the liver, not only in different animals; but also in different individuals of the same species.

Horse It lies obliquely across the abdominal surface of the diaphragm, its highest and most posterior part being at the level of the right kidney. It possesses a strongly convex diaphragmatic surface which is moulded into the concavity of the diaphragm, and a posterior or abdominal surface which lies in contact with the stomach, duodenum, and right kidney, each of which organs forms a depression in the liver substance. It is only incompletely divided into 3 lobes in the horse. Lying mainly in the right lobe on its abdominal surface is the 'porta' of the liver, where the portal vein and hepatic artery enter and from whence the hepatic duct (bile-duct) emerges. Part of the posterior vena cava passes through the liver substance, whose blood it eventually drains. The liver is held in position by the pressure of other organs and by 6 ligaments. These are: the coronary, which attaches it to the diaphragm; the falciform, from the middle lobe to the diaphragm and abdominal floor; the round, to the umbilicus; the right lateral, to the costal part of the diaphragm; the left lateral, to the tendinous part of the diaphragm; and the hepatorenal or caudate, to the right kidney.

Cattle The liver lies mainly to the right of the middle-line through the body, and its long axis is directed downward and forward. Its diaphragmatic surface fits into the concavity of the right part of the diaphragm, and its posterior surface is very irregular. It presents impressions of the 2 main organs with which it comes into contact – the omasum and reticulum. There is only 1 distinct lobe – the caudate. There is no left lateral ligament, and the round ligament is only found in the calf. A gall-bladder is present; it is situated partly in a slight depression on the posterior surface of the liver, and partly on the abdominal wall.

Sheep The bile-duct joins the pancreatic to form a common duct instead of opening separately as in other animals.

Pigs The liver is large, very thick, and very much curved. It lies in the anterior part of the abdominal cavity, occupying the whole of the anterior hollow of the diaphragm and more to the right than to the left side of the body. It has 4 main lobes.

Dogs The liver is very large, being about 5 per cent of the whole bodyweight, and possesses 6 or 7 lobes. The gall-bladder is buried almost completely in the space between the 2 parts of the right central lobe, only a very small portion of it being visible from the outside.

Minute structure The liver is enveloped in an outer capsule of fibrous tissue with which is blended the hepatic peritoneum. The hepatic artery, portal vein, and bile-duct divide and subdivide. Between the rows of liver cells also lie fine bile capillaries which collect the bile discharged by the cells and pass it into the bile-ducts lying around the margins of the lobules. The liver cells are amongst the largest cells of the body, and each contains 1 large nucleus. With careful special staining methods there can also be seen tiny passages or canals, passing into the cells themselves; some of these communicate with the bile-duct, and others with the ultimate branches of the portal vein. After a mixed meal many of the liver cells can be seen to contain droplets of fat, and granules of glycogen (animal starch) can also be determined. In addition to the cells above described, there occur at intervals along the walls of the sinusoids in a lobule stellate cells which represent the remains of the endothelium from which the capillary-likesinusoids are developed. They are known as 'Kupfer's cells'.

Liver, Diseases of

One of the commonly known signs of liver disturbance is JAUNDICE – a yellow coloration of the visible membranes. Gallstones, which are a complication of some liver diseases, are treated under GALL-BLADDER and GALLSTONES.

Hepatitis, or inflammation of the liver, may be acute, suppurative (in which abscesses are formed), or chronic. Acute inflammation produced by viruses, bacteria or poisons (of bacterial, vegetable, animal, or mineral origin), from the intestines, and it is sometimes caused by the migration of parasites through the liver. The symptoms are pain on pressure over the abdomen, an elevation of temperature, suppression of the appetite, a disinclination to move, and often diarrhoea or constipation in the later stages. (See also CANINE VIRAL HEPATITIS.)

Chronic inflammation accompanies many diseases among animals, the commonest probably being infestation with liver-flukes, but it may also be present as a result of tuberculosis. Poisoning may be responsible. (See, for example, RAGWORT POISONING which gives rise to CIRRHOSIS.)

Signs include a gradual loss of condition, irregular appetite, a staring coat, and a general unthriftiness; often oedema.

Abscess formation is due to the entrance into the liver of pus-forming organisms, and is usually secondary to some disease, e.g. tuberculosis. In the USA liver abscesses are found in about 8 per cent of all cattle slaughtered, and they are common in 'barley beef' animals in the UK. The lesions consist of abscesses in the substance of the liver. Symptoms are vague and diagnosis is often impossible.

Fatty liver (see FATTY LIVER SYNDROME of cattle and poultry; also CEROIDOSIS)

Liver/kidney syndrome (see under this heading)

Tumours include adenoma, carcinoma, and haemangioma (see CANCER). Benign tumours may give rise to passive congestion, biliary obstruction with jaundice, or they may cause degeneration. (See under TUMOUR.)

Parasites (see LIVER-FLUKES; HYDATID DISEASE; HORSE BOTS; 'LIZARD-POISONING' IN CATS)

Rupture of the liver is by no means rare among old animals, especially dogs and cats. It may result from a blow, a kick, a traffic accident, a fall, or from violent struggling, when the liver is diseased. Even a small wound in such a vascular organ as the liver is likely to prove fatal. (See also 'MILKSPOT LIVER' of pigs and sheep.)

Rupture of the liver in lambs, aged 1 to 3 months, may be the cause of sudden death. In a survey covering a period of 12 years, the Thurso (Scotland) Veterinary Investigation Laboratory found that liver rupture in neonatal lambs from 16 farms exceeded 8 per cent. The liver surface was covered with haemorrhagic tracts made by migrating metacestodes of *Taenia hydatigena* (see TAPEWORMS).

Liver, Displacement of

A 1-year-old cat with a history of anaemia, jaundice and ascites was found to have its liver in the pericardium.

Liver-Flukes

Liver-flukes are parasitic flat worms which infest the livers of various animals, especially sheep and cattle. They may cause severe illness and even death.

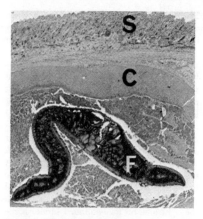

An adult liver-fluke implanted in a subcutaneous pocket in a rat. This technique showed that the rat gained thereby immunity to adult flukes without the complication of liver damage, and was part of the research carried out at the ARC's Institute for Research on Animal Diseases, Compton, into possible means of immunising cattle against liver flukes.
(S = skin; C = subcutaneous tissue; F = liver fluke)

Liver-flukes may increase the susceptibility of the host animal to *Salmonella* infection. (See SALMONELLOSIS.)

Life-history of a typical fluke The egg is usually passed to the exterior in the faeces of the host and under suitable conditions, chiefly of moisture and warmth, a small ciliated larva, called a 'miracidium', hatches from it. This larva, which is unable to feed and will die within some hours unless it finds a suitable host, gains access to the liver or some other special organ by actively penetrating the skin of an appropriate snail – usually a specific snail for any one parasite. In the snail's tissue it develops into a sac-like sporocyst which, by a process of budding from the internal lining of cells, gives rise to a number of elongated 'rediae'. Each redia is a simple, cylindrical sac-like organism which gives rise, by budding of cells, either to another generation of 'daughter rediae' or to 'cercariae'. The cercaria, which resembles a miniature tadpole in general form, leaves the snail and, after leading a free existence in water or on wet vegetation for a short time, comes to rest on grass or other objects, loses its tail and becomes encysted within a protective covering and remains in this state until it is swallowed by the final host, in which it becomes a sexually mature fluke.

Fasciola hepatica This is the common liver-fluke of sheep. (Other hosts are cattle,

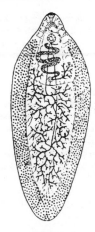

Fasciola hepatica.

goats, pigs, rabbits, hares, horses, dogs, man, beavers, elephants, and kangaroos.) It is shaped more or less like a leaf, about 2.5 cm (1 in) long, but considerable variations exist, and elongated forms are found. It has been recorded in most herbivorous animals and in man; but it is in cattle and sheep that it is of most importance. It is generally found in the bile-ducts of the liver, but may be found in other organs.

The life-history is typical, the intermediate host being various species of *Limnaea* snails. Cercariae may be swallowed with drinking water or encysted on grass.

Infestation, sometimes called 'fluke disease', results in anaemia and hepatitis.

Fasciola gigantica A parasite of cattle, sheep, and wild animals in the tropics and sub-tropics, and more pathogenic than *F. hepatica.*

Fascioloides This genus contains only 1 species, *F. magna*, the large American liver-fluke. In general anatomy, this species resembles the common liver-fluke, but differs from it in its larger size (up to 10 cm (4 in)).

Its larger size and its tendency to form cysts in the liver substance (not in the bile-ducts) make it a more formidable parasite. The cysts may become abscesses, and may be found in the spleen and lungs.

Dicrocoelium This genus is small and semi-transparent, the common species, *D. lancea-tum*, being about 1.25 cm (½ in) long. It occurs in all herbivores and in man. It is less serious a pest than *F. hepatica*. It is carried by various land snails; a second intermediate

host – the ant – is required, the ants being eaten by the grazing animal. *D. dendriticum* has similar hosts and a worldwide distribution. *D. hospes* occurs in Africa.

Clonorchis *C. sinensis* is a common fluke of carnivores, pigs, and man in Asia. It is a small form.

The first part of its life-history is on general lines, the molluscan intermediary being a species of *Bythinia*. The sporocysts give rise directly to cercariae which escape and encyst on various freshwater fish. Infection to mammals is by eating infected fish which are either uncooked or imperfectly cooked.

Closely related flukes are found in the liver of dogs in Northern Europe and North America. (See also 'SALMON POISONING' IN DOGS; 'LIZARD POISONING' IN CATS.)

Incidence of liver-flukes Although surveys have reported a higher incidence of fluke in cattle (up to 40 per cent) than in sheep (13 per cent), this is because cattle show calcification of the bile ducts following exposure to the parasite. In sheep, this calcification does not occur and so only sheep with recent infections will be recorded.

Control measures To be effective, control requires a planned campaign rather than a single battle or weapon. In the sheep, infestation does not lead to subsequent immunity, and this fact gives very little hope of an effective vaccine (similar to the irradiated huskworm larvae vaccine) ever being produced. Not until 1971 was there any drug to kill all young, immature flukes within the body, and it is these which on their mass migrations through the

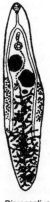

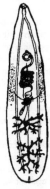

Dicrocoelium.   *Clonorchis.*

liver can damage it so severely that sudden death inevitably follows.

Triclabendazole (Fasinex) is very effective against flukes as it removes both immature and adult stages.

Other drugs used against liver-flukes include aldendazole, closantel, nitroxynil and oxycyclozanide.

In the UK, over 60 per cent of cattle and 80 per cent of sheep are kept in the main fluke areas.

While sheep farmers are mostly fully alive to the fluke problem, it is suggested that most cattle farmers are not. It has been pointed out that on farms where mixed grazing is practised, it is a waste of time and money to dose only the sheep and not the cattle.

Profit margins in beef production have been improved by a combined anti-fluke attack, using routine dosing of the cattle together with a chemical spray (Frescon) on pasture to kill the host snails. In trials, 18-month-old beef animals finished 25 to 30 days earlier than controls, giving higher profitability through savings in feed. Returns were further increased by better carcase grading.

An 8 per cent drop in milk yield has resulted from low-grade infestations in dairy cattle, and it is claimed that autumn and winter dosing of dairy cattle helps to improve, or at least maintain, milk quality levels.

A vaccine against black disease – in which spores of one of the gas-gangrene group of organisms are stimulated into activity by young flukes in the liver – can prevent deaths from the resulting toxaemia. Against the liver-flukes themselves, routine dosing is essential on all farms where they are likely to occur.

Land drainage is still high on the list of control measures.

The use of snail-killers is a recommended part of the campaign against fluke disease, but is not a snag-free method. It is easy to miss small areas inhabited by snails, and this applies even when using a knapsack sprayer – the only possible method of spraying if the land is too wet, is to take a tractor. Snail-killers can be unpleasant to work with: the cheapest is sodium pentachlorophenate. N-trityemorpholine is expensive per acre but has the advantage of being relatively harmless to stock, so that grazing need not be delayed for a fortnight as after copper sulphate dressings and pentachlorophenate. All are poisonous to fish.

Running ducks over snaily land is not among the official recommendations but it might prove of some value. A few farmers have tried it in the past. In Zambia years ago, a large-scale duck-rearing scheme was introduced in areas flooded by the River Zambesi as a method of fluke-disease and bilharzia control. Hoof-prints, where the soil is exposed, are favourite habitats of the snails. (See also under ANTS.)

Public health Watercress is the chief source of infestation. Illness is most marked during migration of immature flukes. Eosinophilia is a pointer to aid diagnosis; eggs may not appear in the faeces for 12 weeks.

Symptoms in the human patient include urticaria, jaundice, enlarged and tender liver, and eosinophilia.

Cats (see under 'LIZARD POISONING'; PANCREAS, DISEASES of IN CATS)

Liver/Kidney Syndrome of Poultry (FLKS)

Liver/kidney syndrome of poultry (FLKS) affects birds usually 2 to 3 weeks old. Symptoms may not be observed – or there may be depression for a day or two; occasionally trembling or paralysis of legs. Mortality: 1 to 5 per cent. The whole carcase may have a pink tinge. It is the result of failure of the liver to synthesise glucose. The liver is pale, swollen, and fatty. The kidneys may be very swollen. Biotin supplementation of the feed has been shown to alleviate the condition. (See also under FATTY LIVER.)

The syndrome has to be differentiated from toxic fat disease, Gumboro disease, and infectious avian nephrosis.

Livestock Production

(see BEEF CATTLE HUSBANDRY; DAIRY HERD MANAGEMENT; TROPICS; and to under PIGS and SHEEP)

'Lizard Poisoning' in Cats

This term is applied to infestation with the liver-fluke *Plarynosomum concinnum*, which has been reported from South America, the Caribbean Islands, Malaysia, the USA and, more recently, Nigeria. The life-cycle of the parasite involves a large land snail, a crustacean, and lizards, frogs, and probably other amphibians and reptiles. Symptoms in the cat include listlessness, fever, jaundice, diarrhoea, vomiting, and emaciation; but subclinical infestations also occur.

Lizards

The largest group of reptiles. These cold-blooded vertebrates, some of which are aquatic, are often kept as pets. The environment must be kept at the temperature appropriate for the particular type of lizard. It is essential to provide the diet recommended for the particular species. Most lizards require meat; crickets may provide a suitable source. Iguanas, however, are mainly, but not entirely, vegetarian. Adequate ultraviolet (UV) light must be available if normal bone development is to take place. Any lizard wih a swollen limb may have osteodystrophy, and the source of UV light should be checked and a calcium supplement provided. Chameleons and some other lizards have pigment cells (chromatophores) in their skin and can change colour to blend in with their surroundings. However, a colour change can be a sign of illness, particularly when the animal cannot blend in with its surroundings.

The water in which aquatic lizards live must be kept fresh, otherwise a build-up of aeromonas or pseudomonas organisms may occur. Conjunctivitis is not uncommon; it shows as caseous (cheesy) discharge which must be gently removed before treatment can be given. When diarrhoea occurs it is usually as a result of infestation with protozoan parasites. Skin parasites can be removed by (for example) treatment with ivermectin. The reptiles must be removed to a clean cage or tank while the original one is cleaned and treated with a suitable inseticide. Egg-binding is usually associated with a calcium deficiency but may happen if no suitable site for laying has been provided. Any heating device must be located so that the lizard does not come into contact with it.

Llamas

Long-legged, long-necked domesticated animals widely used as pack animals and for wool and hide in the South American Andes. They belong to the order Camelidae, which includes also Alpaca, Guanaco and Vicuna. They are increasingly farmed in the UK.

Importation of llamas and alpacas direct from South America into a Border Inspection Post is permitted. On arrival, each animal is examined for infectious or contagious disease. If no disease is apparent, the animals are quarantined for a month (to eliminate the possibility of foot-and-mouth disease) before going on to their destination.

Lobe

Lobe is the term applied to the larger divisions of various organs, such as the lungs, liver, and brain. The term 'lobar' is applied to structures which are connected with lobes of organs, or to diseases which have a tendency to be limited to one lobe only, such as 'lobar pneumonia'.

Lobules are divisions of a lobe. The term 'lobular' is applied to disease which occurs in a scattered irregular manner affecting lobules here and there, such as 'lobular pneumonia'.

Local Anaesthetics
(see under ANAESTHESIA; ANALGESICS)

Local Immunity
(see under IMMUNE RESPONSE; ORIFICES; SECRETORY IgA)

Lockjaw
(see TETANUS)

'Loco Weed'

The legumes oxytropis and astragalus in the USA contain toxins that cause incoordination, and extreme excitability in animals grazing them. They are also teratogenic and if consumed in sufficient quantity, abortifacient.

Loose-Boxes

Individual enclosures for accommodating an animal; also called box-stalls. The best type has well-built brick walls lined on the inside to the roof with cement-plaster finished off smooth. The floor is of cement-concrete, grooved to facilitate the draining away of fluids and to provide a foothold, and the corners are rounded off with fillets of cement. The only fittings inside are hay-rack, water-bowl, and manger – of iron, and rather larger than in the stall of a stable, so that cattle as well as horses may use them; in some cases 1 or 2 rings, to which animals may be tied, are provided. One or more windows, high up out of reach of the animals' heads, should be included, and the door should always be made in 2 halves, so that horses with respiratory diseases may stand with their heads out of the box, and so obtain a plentiful supply of fresh air. Wherever possible, loose-boxes should be built with a southerly aspect, so that the disinfectant action of sunlight may be taken full advantage of, whenever sick animals are housed in the box.

Lordosis

Lordosis is an unnatural curvature of the spine, so that the concavity of the spine is directed upwards. It is seen in tetanus, and sometimes in rabies.

Louping-Ill

Louping-ill is a paralytic disease of sheep, also called ovine encephalomyelitis; it is transmitted by *Ixodes ricinus*, the tick commonly present on hill pastures. It occurs in western Scotland, the

North of England, and the Northwest of Ireland. There is a definite seasonal incidence, most cases occurring between March and June, and between September and October; only a few sporadic cases are met with at other times of the year. All breeds of sheep are susceptible. It occurs in cattle and has been recorded as affecting pigs, horses, deer and also dogs, in which the signs are fever, nystagmus, hyperaesthesia, and sometimes a tetanus-like rigidity. In 2 cases, bitches had whelped 5 weeks previously, and eclampsia was at first suspected.

Cattle On upland grazings where ticks abound, louping-ill has become of economic importance in cattle. The animals become dull and uninterested in food, walk in an unnatural way, sometimes with their heads down, and occasionally become excited.

Pigs The first naturally occurring outbreak in pigs was reported in 1980 by the West of Scotland Agricultural College's veterinary investigation centre. Ten out of 16 piglets became severely affected with the disease when about 6 weeks old. They showed nervous symptoms, were either reluctant to move or wandered aimlessly and pressed their heads into corners. Of the 3 worst cases, 2 failed to survive transport to the VI centre, and the 3rd – being in a state of convulsions – was killed on arrival there. Of the remainder, 5 more died and 2 recovered.

Those piglets had been housed in a covered pen with a concrete run considered to be tick-proof; and the louping-ill virus was probably transmitted through the feeding of uncooked carcases of lambs which had died on the farm after showing symptoms suggestive of louping-ill.

In another outbreak, pigs 6 to 8 months old died of louping-ill after being allowed free range on tick-infested pasture.

Cause A flavivirus. This is transmitted by the bites of infected ticks (adult or nymphal). The virus primarily multiplies in the blood, and in certain cases invades the central nervous system at a later stage in the infection.

It would appear that accessory conditions favour such invasion, e.g. tick-borne fever, a disease also transmitted by *I. ricinus*.

The ticks can survive, in the absence of sheep and cattle, on deer, rabbits, hares, voles, field mice, grouse, etc., and these animals may act as host of the virus.

Signs Two forms of the disease are recognised: an acute and a subacute form. In the acute form

the symptoms may appear in from 4 to 6 days after the sheep is infested with the carrier ticks. The sheep becomes uneasy, lies down and rises frequently during the day. Its temperature ranges between 40° and 41.6°C (104° and 107°F) during the next week or 10 days, and it develops nervous symptoms. At first, it is merely more timid and more easily frightened than usual; later, the muscles of the jaws and neck begin to twitch and quiver, and there may be frothing at the mouth. It staggers when made to move rapidly or turn suddenly, and as the disease becomes firmly established it may be seen taking short spasmodic jumps, rising apparently from all 4 feet at the same time, and landing upon all 4 feet again. In this way an affected sheep can usually be easily noticed among a flock when the sheep are being driven or collected by a dog. In more advanced stages the animal becomes paralysed, unable to stand, and often has its head drawn round over its fore flank. Unconsciousness quickly appears, and the animal dies a short time afterwards.

In the subacute type the sheep is seen taking very high steps with its fore-legs; it holds its head very high, and sometimes carries it to one side (often the left); the pupils are dilated, and the expression of the sheep is one of extreme fear when caught. It may attempt to feed, but actually eats very little. Tremblings of the muscles, staggering and falling, and sometimes paralysis of one or more groups of muscles, are seen. As times goes on the sheep loses condition. If not fed by hand it dies from starvation.

Recovery from an attack confers a degree of immunity, which may last for life. (See also TICK-BORNE FEVER).

Prevention Control measures should aim at the eradication of the infecting ticks from grazing lands. This is not easy, as the tick can live under rough herbage without access to the living sheep for as long as one year. A vaccine is available and affords good protection. Cattle should be vaccinated annually; sheep and goats every 2 years.

Sheep Vaccination of ewes confers protection in their lambs. Inoculations are carried out in spring prior to the season when ticks become active.

Cattle Investigations on hill farms where louping-ill is a problem have shown that cattle play an important part in the maintenance of virus. Hill cattle as well as sheep therefore should be vaccinated, not only for their own protection, but to reduce the transfer of virus to the ticks which are the only agents passing on the infection each year.

Public health Shepherds, farmers, and slaughter-house workers – as well as veterinarians – may become infected. The main symptom is fever. Meningoencephalitis has been recorded, and has sometimes proved fatal.

Lubricants

The type of lubricant used in pellet mills and other forms of machinery for processing animal feeding-stuffs may be of the greatest importance. Lubricants containing chlorinated naphthalene compounds and used on such machines may give rise to hyperkeratosis in cattle eating the food so contaminated by the minutest quantity of lubricant.

Lucerne

A valuable leguminous plant (*Medicago sativa*) for fodder and forage. Lucerne-hay is highly valued for the feeding of horses if of good quality. (It is of little value when most of the leaf has been lost, or it is dusty or mouldy.) Lucerne is also a valuable crop for cattle, but for precautions and dangers, see BLOAT; also MUSCLES, DISEASES OF – Nutritional muscular dystrophy.

Lugol's Solution

A solution of 50 g iodine and 100 g potassium iodide in distilled water to 1000 ml. A 2 to 4 per cent dilution of the solution has been used for irrigation of the uterus in cases of bovine metritis.

Luing

A beef breed evolved by Messrs Cadzow from Beef Shorthorn and Highland cattle, and named after the island. Colour: red with a touch of gold; or roan; or white. There are a breed society and herd book.

Lumbar

Lumbar is a term used to denote either the structures in or disease affecting the loins, i.e. the region lying between the last rib and the point of the hip, from one side of the body to the other. There are lumbar vertebrae, lumbar muscles, etc.

Lumen

The space inside a tubular structure, such as an artery or intestine.

Luminal or Phenobarbitone

(see BARBITURATES)

Lumpy Jaw

(see ACTINOMYCOSIS)

'Lumpy Skin Disease'

'Lumpy skin disease' is a NOTIFIABLE DISEASE throughout the EU. It is characterised by a discharge from the eyes and nose, lameness, and salivation may be observed – depending upon the site of nodules which sometimes involve mucous membrane as well as skin.

Oedema may occur, and involve the genital organs, udder, dewlap, and limbs. Sloughing of skin may occur. Exotic cattle may die.

The disease is caused by the Neethling pox virus; and a modified sheep-pox vaccine is used for protection.

'Lumpy Skin Disease, Pseudo-'

This is characterised by the formation of raised plaques on the skin, which exude a discharge and then ulcerate; and by fever. The cause is the bovid herpesvirus 2, which also causes mamillitis of cattle.

Lumpy Wool (Wool Rot)

Lumpy wool (wool rot) is caused by a bacterium which attacks the sheep's skin during wet weather, causing irritation and the formation of a hard yellowish-white scab about 3 mm (⅛ in) thick. Healing soon occurs and the wool continues to grow carrying the hard material away from the skin as a buff or brownish zone in the wool. Severe infection may lead to loss of wool.

The bacterium causing this dermatitis is *Dermatophilus dermatonomus*. (See also DERMATOPHILUS; STREPTOTHRICOSIS.)

In America, this disease has been treated by defleecing with cyclophosphamide and the use of streptomycin and penicillin.

Lung-Flukes (Paragonimus Genus)

These flukes are plump oval forms infecting carnivores, pig and man. Generally, 2 flukes are found together in a cyst in the lungs. The presence of the flukes cause bronchitis and pleurisy. Lesions resembling tuberculosis may be developed. The flukes are found in America and Asia. Eggs are coughed up, swallowed, and passed out with the droppings. The cercariae develop in snails, and afterwards escape and encyst on freshwater crabs or crayfish. These are eaten, and the adult flukes develop in the body. Treatment with niclosamide and albendazole appears to be effective against *P. kellicotti*, which causes coughing and sneezing in cats. For the pancreatic fluke of cats, see PANCREAS, DISEASE OF.

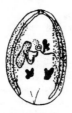

Paragonimus.

Lungworms

(see PARASITIC BRONCHITIS; ROUNDWORMS; DONKEYS)

Lungs

These 2 organs are, of course, concerned with respiration, in which carbon dioxide is exchanged for oxygen. The air breathed in is warmed before reaching the lungs via the AIR PASSAGES.

Blood is carried to the lungs by the pulmonary artery, which divides and subdivides into tiny capillaries which lie around the walls of the air cells.

Functions Apart from their main function of gaseous exchange (see AIR), the lungs can release histamine, metabolise noradrenaline, and inactivate prostaglandins. Local immune mechanisms also operate in the lungs.

Lung is composed of very highly elastic tissue which consists of multitudes of tiny sacs arranged at the terminal parts of the smallest of the bronchioles, and which collapse when the balance of pressure between the air in the sacs and on the outside of the lung surface is disturbed. Thus a lung shrinks to about one-third of its normal size when removed from the chest cavity.

Horses The lungs occupy the greater part of the thoracic cavity, and are accurately moulded to the walls of the chest and to the other organs contained within it. The right is considerably larger than the left, owing to the presence of the heart, which lies mostly to the left side of the middle plane of the cavity. In the Equidae the lung is not divided into lobes as it is in some of the other animals. The apex is that portion which occupies the most anterior part of the chest cavity, and just immediately behind it is the deep impression for the heart. Behind this again, and a little above it, is the 'root' of the lung, which consists of the blood vessels entering and leaving the lung, lymph vessels, nerves, the bronchus, and here also are situated the bronchial lymph nodes. In cross-section each

lung is somewhat triangular in shape, with one of the angles rounded. The rounded angle lies in the uppermost part of the chest, alongside the bodies of the thoracic vertebrae, and the more acute of the remaining angles lies along the floor of the chest.

Cattle The lungs are thicker and shorter than in the horse, and there is a greater disproportion in size – the right weighing about half as much again as the left. They are divided into lobes by deep fissures. The left has 3 lobes, and the right 4 or 5. The foot in each case is almost immediately above the impression for the heart. The apical lobe (i.e. the most anterior of the right lung) receives a special small bronchus from the trachea direct.

Sheep The lungs show little lobulation.

Pigs The left lung is like that of cattle, but the right lung has its apical lobe very often divided into 2 parts. Otherwise there are no great differences. Three bronchi are present, as in cattle.

Dogs The lungs are thicker than in either the horse or the ox in conformity with the more barrel-like shape of the chest. There is no cardiac impression in the left lung. Each has 3 large lobes, but the right has a small extra mediastinal lobe, and there may be 1 or more accessory lobes in either lung.

Colour In the perfectly fresh lung from a young unbled animal the colour of the lung is a bright rose-pink with a glistening surface, the pleural membrane; but in the lungs of older animals there is usually a certain amount of deposit of soot, dust, etc., which has been inhaled with the air and collected in the lymph spaces between the air cells.

Connections The lungs are firmly anchored in position by their roots to the heart and trachea, and by the pleura to a longitudinal septum running vertically from front to back, (the mediastinum) (see PLEURA). The pulmonary artery, carrying unoxygenated blood to the lungs, divides into 2 large branches after only a very short course. Each of these branches enters into the formation of the root of the lung, and there begins to divide up into a very large number of smaller vessels. These subdivide many times until the final capillaries are given off around the walls of the air-sacs. From these the blood, after oxygenation, is carried by larger and larger veins, till it eventually

Relationship of alveoli to terminations of pulmonary artery and pulmonary vein. (From John A. Clements, *Surface Tension in the Lungs.* © Scientific American, Inc. All rights reserved.)

leaves the lung by one of the several pulmonary veins. These number 6 or 7 or more, and leave the lungs by the roots. In addition to the blood carried to the lung for aeration a small bronchial artery carries blood to the lung substance for nutritive purposes. This accompanies the bronchi and splits into branches corresponding to the small bronchi and bronchioles. The lymph vessels in the root of the lungs are very numerous, and are all connected with the large bronchial glands for this part.

Minute structure The main bronchial tube, entering the lung at its root, divides into branches, which subdivide again and again, to be distributed all through the substance of the lung, till the finest tubes, known as 'bronchioles' or 'capillary bronchi', have a diameter of only about 0.25 mm. In structure, all these tubes consist of a mucous membrane surrounded by a fibrous sheath. The larger and medium bronchi have plates of cartilage in the fibrous layer, and are richly supplied with glands secreting mucus, which is poured out on to the surface of the lining membrane and serves to keep it moist. The surface of this membrane is composed of columnar epithelial cells, provided with little whip-like processes known as 'cilia', which have the double function of moving any expectoration upwards towards the throat, and of warming the air as it passes over them. The walls of the bronchial tubes are rich in fibres of elastic tissue, and immediately below the mucous membrane of the small tubes is a layer of plain muscle fibres placed circularly. To this muscular layer belongs the function of altering the lumen of the tube, and, consequently, its air-carrying capacity. It is a spasmodic contraction of the muscular layer that produces the characteristic expiratory 'cough' of true asthma.

The smallest divisions of the bronchial tubes open out into a number of dilatations, known as 'infundibula', each of which measures about 1.25 mm across, and these are covered with minute sacs, variously known as 'air-vesicles', 'air-alveoli', or 'air cells'. An air cell consists of a delicate membrane composed of flattened plate-like cells, strengthened by a wide network of elastic fibres, to which the great elasticity of the lung is due; and it is in these thin-walled air cells that the respiratory exchange of gases takes place.

The branches of the pulmonary arteries accompany the bronchial tubes to the farthest recesses of the lung, dividing like the latter into finer and finer branches, and ending in a dense network of capillaries, which lies everywhere between the air vesicles, the capillaries being so closely placed that they occupy a much greater area than the spaces between them. The air in the air vesicles is separated from the blood only by 2 most delicate membranes, the wall of the air cell and the wall of the capillary, and it is through these walls that the respiratory exchange takes place.

Lungs, Diseases of

The chief of these is PNEUMONIA. (See also under PLEURISY; EMPHYSEMA; TUBERCULOSIS; MAEDI/VISNA; CALF PNEUMONIA; EQUINE RESPIRATORY VIRUSES; ENZOOTIC PNEUMONIA OF PIGS; CONTAGIOUS BOVINE PLEURO-PNEUMONIA; PARASITIC BRONCHITIS; PULMONARY ADENOMATOSIS.)

Congestion of the lungs Accumulation of fluid, or 'congestion', is the preliminary stage of several types of acute pneumonia. It also occurs in disease of the left side of the heart. FOG FEVER of cattle is another condition in which congestion of the lungs is seen.

'Hydrostatic congestion' of a lung is apt to occur if an animal which cannot stand, lies for too long on one side. Regular turning of the animal on to its other side is a necessary nursing procedure.

Pulmonary oedema This may occur during pneumonia (some forms), in disease of the left side of the heart, and (in cattle) in FOG FEVER, and in PARASITIC BRONCHITIS of cattle and sheep.

An acute and usually rapidly fatal oedema of the lungs occurs in animals exposed to smoke in a burning building; the animal almost literally 'drowns' in its own blood serum. (Administration of oxygen can be tried if an animal has been rescued before severe lung damage has been caused.)

Poisoning by PARAQUAT and ANTU results in oedema and consolidation of the lungs. (See also DIPS AND DIPPING; ELECTROCUTION.)

Pulmonary emphysema (see FOG FEVER)

Pulmonary haemorrhage (see RACEHORSES)

Allergic alveolitis Inflammation of the alveoli of the lungs of cattle exposed to mouldy hay or straw contaminated with micro-organisms such as *Thermopolyspora polyspora*, and resembling 'FARMER'S LUNG'.

Tumours of the lung are usually of metastatic origin, i.e. they are secondary growths which have started from another centre in the body, being carried to the lung tissue either by the blood- or lymph-stream. (See CANCER.)

Gangrene of the lung may be a complication of, or a sequel to, pneumonia, and is usually fatal. It is characterised by the presence of a foul-smelling, usually rusty-red, and almost always very copious discharge from both nostrils, in addition to the other symptoms of pneumonia. It is commonest in the horse as a sequel to ordinary pneumonia, and in other animals it may occur when the pneumonia has been produced through faulty administration of drenches. (See PNEUMONIA.)

Collapse of the lung The lungs are so resilient, in consequence of the elastic fibres throughout their substance, that if air be admitted within the pleural cavities the lungs immediately collapse to about a third of their natural size. Accordingly, if the chest wall is wounded and air gains entrance through the wound (pneumothorax), the lung collapses. After the wound has healed, and provided that no complications occur, the elasticity is restored as the air is absorbed. (See PNEUMOTHORAX.)

Torsion of a lung lobe, usually the right cardiac lobe, is seen rarely in dogs and cats; it causes dyspnoea, pulmonary oedema, and death. The lobe may become twice its normal size and blackish.

Wounds of the lung are serious on account of the air admitted through the chest wall, which leads to collapse; also the haemorrhage, and the difficulty of checking it. The lung may be wounded by the end of a fractured rib pointing inwards. (See 'FLAIL-CHEST'.)

Parasites of the lungs. Liver-flukes are sometimes found in the lungs of cattle and sheep; lung-flukes attack cats, dogs, pigs, and man in the Far East and the USA. Other parasites include LUNGWORMS. (See also HEARTWORMS, for pulmonary dirofilariasis.)

Lupins, Poisoning by

Lupins of different species have often been found to cause poisoning of sheep; sometimes also of horses, cattle, and goats.

Poisoning by lupins is of 2 kinds: (1) due to alkaloids within the plant producing a nervous disease; and (2) due to infestation of the plant with a fungus which produces a toxin affecting the liver. This 2nd type of poisoning is known as lupinosis, is usually chronic, and produces loss of appetite and weight, jaundice, cirrhosis of the liver, oedema of the head, ascites and death. A few animals do recover but seldom thrive well afterwards.

In the USA great loss among sheep flocks has been occasioned by feeding on lupins by animals not accustomed to them. The alkaloids are present chiefly in the seeds.

Poisoning by the alkaloids gives rise to symptoms which include loss of appetite, laboured breathing, excitement, convulsions and death from respiratory paralysis. There is no jaundice or cirrhosis of the liver, and animals which recover are likely to do so completely.

Lupus Erythematosus

An autoimmune disease of dogs and cats which occurs in 2 forms: (1) the cutaneous or discoid form, and (2) the systemic form.

The discoid form is characterised by symmetrical lesions on face, nose, and ears. Alopecia, loss of pigment, erythema, and a scaliness may be seen. Exposure to sunlight worsens the condition.

The systemic form affects many tissues and organs. Autoantibodies against platelets, red and white blood cells may be present; with antibodies also in joints, kidney, skin, and other organs. Symptoms include bilateral polyarthritis, fever, muscle pain, enlarged lymph nodes, and sometimes nervous symptoms.

Prednisolone is used in treatment.

Luteinising Hormone (LH)

A secretion of the anterior lobe of the pituitary gland. LH controls the development of the CORPUS LUTEUM and its production of progesterone. In the male animal, LH stimulates secretion of testosterone by the testicle.

Luteolysis

Regression of a CORPUS LUTEUM. Two factors appear to be involved in luteolysis in most domestic animals – one being prostaglandin $F_2\alpha$ and the other being follicular oestrogen synthesis. It has been suggested that $PGF_2\alpha$ is the normal luteolytic compound, and that it is transferred from the non-gravid uterus to the ovary by some form of counter-current distribution between the uterine vein and ovarian artery. While the actual route for $PGF_2\alpha$ transfer is in some doubt, its physiological role is certain.

A number of procedures for inducing luteolysis in domestic animals have been used. These range from the squeezing out of an established corpus luteum by rectal palpation in cattle, to the use of oestrogens. Synthetic prostaglandins are now used.

Luxation
(see DISLOCATION)

Lyme Disease

This was first recognised in Connecticut, USA, in 1975; the vector of infection is *Ixodes* ticks on deer.

The disease occurs both in the UK and in other EU countries; in adults as well as in children.

Cause Borrelia burgdorfei. (See BORRELIA.)

Signs Blurred vision, lethargy, headaches, arthritis. In a few cases meningitis or encephalitis or myocarditis result.

Lyme disease in dogs has been reported in the UK, other EU countries, the USA and Australia.

Lymph

Lymph is a clear fluid collected from the tissues which enters the lymph vessels and thence the blood. It contains less protein than, but is otherwise similar to, the blood plasma. It also contains lymphocytes.

Lymph nourishes the tissues and returns waste products from them back into the bloodstream. There are certain tissues which are not provided with a blood supply at all, (e.g. the cornea of the eye, cartilage, horn, etc.) and in them the lymph is the only nourishing medium.

The lymph is derived in the first place from the bloodstream, of which the watery constituents exude through the fine walls of the capillaries into the tissue spaces. After meals, lymph from the small intestine may be milky in appearance due to contained fat. (See also LYMPH NODES; LYMPHOCYTE.)

The term 'lymph' was also applied to the material which collects in the vesicles of cow-pox and was used for vaccination.

Lymph Nodes

Formerly called lymph glands, these are situated on the lymphatic vessels, act as filters, and have an important role in body defence by producing lymphocytes. (See also RETICULO-ENDOTHELIAL SYSTEM; IMMUNE RESPONSE; LYMPHOCYTES; PLASMA CELLS.)

Lymphadenitis
Inflammation of lymph nodes.

Lymphadenoma
(see HODGKIN'S DISEASE)

Lymphangitis
Inflammation of the lymphatic vessels, often resulting from a streptococcal infection.

In horses 3 infective forms occur: (1) EPIZOOTIC LYMPHANGITIS (caused by a yeast); (2) ULCERATIVE LYMPHANGITIS (bacterial); and (3) GLANDERS (bacterial).

The non-infective lymphangitis used to be called Monday morning disease, often being seen in horses after a weekend of no work and a protein-rich diet.

Signs Fever, lameness in one or more legs, with enlarged and tender lymph nodes. Later, doughy swellings, which pit on pressure, may affect the whole limb.

The appetite is lost for a day or two, but the horse is usually very thirsty. Under appropriate treatment, the severity of the symptoms abates in 2 or 3 days' time, or sooner; and although lameness still persists, perhaps for as long as a week, the general appearance of the horse rapidly improves. The horse is usually able to resume work in from 10 days to a fortnight.

Recurrences are likely, resulting in some permanent thickening of the limb.

Treatment Antihistamines may be tried. Antibiotics may be necessary; also diuretics to help reduce the swelling, and phenylbutazone, or some other analgesic, to reduce the pain.

Lymphatics
Lymphatics are the vessels which convey the lymph through the body. (See LYMPH.)

Lymphocystis
A viral disease of fishes, which may give rise to whitish nodules on the cornea of the eye.

Lymphocyte
Lymphocytes in mammals are of 2 main classes: thymus-derived, called T cells; and B cells derived from bone marrow. Unlike polymorphonuclear leukocytes and monocytes, the white cells in this group have cell surface receptors for antigen, and they are not involved in phagocytosis.

T cells do not secrete antibodies and act directly on foreign cells. B cells divide rapidly to form plasma cells which secrete antibodies. (See under BLOOD; B CELLS; IMMUNE RESPONSE; RECEPTORS.)

A much-simplified scheme of the relationship between antigens and some of the lymphoid cells of the body is shown in the diagram. Natural immunity is conferred by the natural secretions of the body surfaces. If these surfaces are penetrated, scavenger cells (macrophages) attempt to engulf and destroy the antigens. Macrophages have a central role in immunity and if they are successful no further effects of antigen may be detectable. The activity of macrophages is increased if the antigen is coated with specific antibodies. Macrophages are also attracted to areas where antigen is concentrated by soluble factors secreted by certain sensitised lymphocytes.

Large granular lymphocytes are a type of T-lymphocyte, stated to have a prominent role in modulating normal immune responses, and in eliminating virus-infected and transformed cells. It has been suggested that infection of these cells by the malignant catarrhal fever agent is the essential initial step in precipitating the disease.

(See also LYMPHOKINE.)

Lymphocytic Choriomeningitis (LCM)
A viral disease of mice transmissible to human beings, in whom it may give rise to fever, headache, pain in muscles and, occasionally, death from meningoencephalitis. Dogs may act as symptomless carriers.

Lymphoid Leukosis
Lymphoid leukosis of chickens is a form of cancer caused by a retrovirus, and initially affects B-lymphocytes in the bursa of Fabricius. It metastises to the liver and spleen, which becomes swollen. The tumours are nodular and yellowish-white. The disease is spread from hen to egg and hen to hen; the incubation period is about 4 months. Lymphoid leukosis is rare in mammals.

Lymphokine
Secreted by T-lymphocytes, and formed when sensitised cells react with antigen, lymphokines can attract other lymphocytes and monocytes, modify vascular permeability and activate macrophages. In man they are believed to play an important role in the development of rheumatoid arthritis.

Lymphosarcoma
(see LEUKAEMIA; also FELINE LEUKAEMIA; BOVINE ENZOOTIC LEUKOSIS; CANCER)

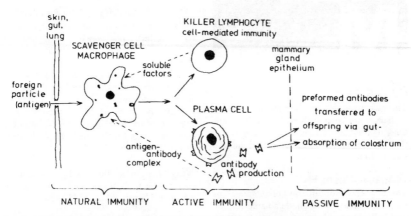

Relationships between antigen and lymphoid cells illustrating the many stages at which antigen can be destroyed. If antibodies are formed they may be passed on from mother to young.

Lysine

Lysine is a very important amino acid. Synthetic lysine is added to pig feeds (concentrates) both to improve performance and to allow the quantity of added protein to be reduced. (See AMINO ACIDS.)

Lysis

Lysis has 2 meanings: the gradual ending of a fever (as compared with crisis); and the destruction of a cell by an antibody.

Lysosomes

Lysosomes are structures within the cytoplasm of a cell which are surrounded by a membrane, contain enzymes and may carry out a digestive function for the cell, getting rid of bacteria, etc.

Lysosomal storage disease These are due to genetically determined deficiencies of specific enzymes; and are common in some breeds of dogs and cats.

An accumulation of lipofusin (granular fatty deposits), and the related pigment ceroid, is a feature of some lyosomal storage diseases. (See CEROIDOSIS.)

Lyssa

Lyssa is the name of a virus, similar but not identical to rabies, which is carried by certain European bats. The bite of a bat carrying the virus can infect man. Fatalities have been recorded in Finland and the former Czechoslovakia. In 1996, an infected bat was found in Southern England; as a result, the UK was not officially rabies free until summer 1998. Rabies vaccine will protect against lyssa virus.

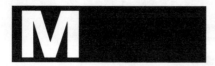

'M & B 693'

The code name given by the manufacturer May & Baker (now part of Merial) to sulphapyridine, one of the SULFONAMIDE DRUGS. It was the first sulfonamide to be introduced into the UK, in 1938.

Macaw-Worm Fly

This is a parasite of cattle and other animals in Central America. It is another name for the warble-fly *Dermarobia homini*. (See under FLIES.)

Macrocyte

Macrocyte is the term applied to an abnormally large erythrocyte especially characteristic of the blood in some forms of anaemia.

Macrophage

A former monocyte (type of white blood cell) which has migrated into the tissues and become larger. (See under BLOOD; INFECTION.)

Macules

Macules are spots or stained areas of skin or mucous membrane, usually brownish, red, or purple in colour.

'Mad Cow Disease'

(see BOVINE SPONGIFORM ENCEPHALOPATHY)

Madness in Dogs

(see RABIES; ENCEPHALITIS; MENINGITIS)

Maedi/Visna

A slowly progressive disease of sheep and goats, first recognised in 1939 in Iceland and believed to have been introduced into that country by karakul sheep imported from Germany. Iceland is now free from the disease, following 2 eradication programmes, but maedi occurs in the UK, continental Europe, North America, Africa, and Asia.

Although maedi/visna has never been recorded in Australia, a retrovirus was isolated from goats there and shown to produce antibodies indistinguishable from those produced by maedi/visna virus in goats.

Cause A lentivirus. It is usually seen in animals over 2 years old. Transmission to the lamb is often via the ewe's milk.

'Maedi' is the Icelandic word for dyspnoea, and the disease is a type of pneumonia with a very long incubation period – 1 to 3 years or even more. An early sign is dyspnoea; after physical exertion the breathing becomes very rapid and shallow. Later, breathing becomes difficult even when the animal is at rest, and death often follows.

'Visna' is a name applied to the same viral infection when the brain or spinal cord rather than the lungs are involved. Demyelination occurs.

Diagnosis can be confirmed by microscopical examination of the tissues and by isolation of the virus. There is also an ELISA test.

MAFF

MAFF is the acronym for the Ministry of Agriculture, Fisheries and Food which prior to 2001 was responsible for the control of notifiable diseases, imports of animals and welfare of animals on farms. It was replaced in 2001 by the Department of the Environment, Food and Rural Affairs (DEFRA).

Maggots

Maggots which have fed on carcases contaminated by *Clostridium botulinum* may contain a dose of toxin lethal to birds. This has caused deaths among domestic poultry, wild birds, and on game farms in the UK.

In one incident, the London Zoo lost 37 birds from botulism arising from a batch of commercially bred maggots. Maggots reared in a sterile environment are used to debride wounds.

Maggots in Sheep

In many parts of the world, certain dipterous flies may lay their eggs on the wool of sheep during summer, and the eggs hatch into maggots which either live on the surface of the skin or burrow down into the subcutaneous tissues. They cause great loss from wasting of flesh and destruction to fleeces, and sometimes result in the death of the affected sheep. The greenbottle flies (*Lucilla caesar* and *L. sericata*, in Britain, and *L. macellaria*, in both North and South America) are those responsible for this condition. (See under MYIASIS and FLIES.)

'Magic Mushroom' Poisoning

This is caused by psilocybin, a hallucinogen present in *Psilocybe semi-lanceate* and *Panaeolus foenisecii*. Consumption of the fungus by domestic animals can give rise to bizarre behaviour.

Signs In the dog, aggressiveness, ataxia, nystagmus and salivation plus a body temperature in excess of 42°C have been noted.

A normally docile pony, which had been grazing in a field where 'magic mushrooms' were growing in profusion, became aggressive.

Magnesium (Mg)

Magnesium (Mg) is a light white metal which burns in air with the production of a brilliant white flame, leaving a white powder as a residue. The salts of magnesium used as drugs are the oxide, carbonate, and sulphate. There is a heavy oxide, known as 'heavy magnesia', a light oxide called 'light magnesia', a heavy carbonate, and a light carbonate. Both the oxides and the carbonates are antacids and slightly laxative. The sulphate of magnesium is commonly called 'Epsom salts'. (For blood magnesium, see under HYPOMAGNESAEMIA.)

Uses Magnesia, whether light or heavy, is usually prescribed for foals, calves, and dogs when these require a mild antacid and laxative. The sulphate of magnesium is a saline purgative. (See under LAXATIVES.)

Calcined magnesite is used as a top-dressing for pastures in an attempt to prevent hypomagnesaemia (about 500 kg (10 cwt) per acre). For cattle, a daily dose of 50 g (2 oz) calcined magnesite is considered to be of great value in the prevention of hypomagnesaemia, but it should be fed only during the 'danger period'. This is because prolonged feeding of magnesium salts is apt to accentuate any latent phosphorus deficiency and may lead to 'milk lameness' or similar conditions.

A mixture of magnesium acetate solution and molasses has been used, being available on a free-choice basis to cattle from ball feeders placed in the field.

Magnesium oxide Too high a level in concentrate feeds for lambs and calves has led to urolithiasis. (See under URETHRAL OBSTRUCTION.)

Magnets

Magnets have been used to treat traumatic reticulitis and prevent traumatic pericarditis in cattle. (See under HEART DISEASES.)

Magnetotherapy

The use of magnetic fields to support therapy. There are claims that magnetotherapy has beneficial effects on conditions affecting the nervous and locomotor sysems and on post-surgery healing.

Maine-Anjou

A French dual-purpose breed of cattle. Colours: red and white, and roan.

Maize

(see PHYTIN; SILAGE)

Major Histocompatibility System

One of the chromosomal regions controlling immune responses.

Histocompatibility antigens are inherited through a set of genes known as the major histocompatibility complex (MHC). Every animal possesses its own unique set of histocompatibility antigens.

Class I genes code for antigens that provoke the rejection of foreign grafts. Antigens of this class are of the cell-surface type, located on all nucleated cells, and concerned with cell recognition.

Class II cell-surface antigens are located mainly on B-cells, and are concerned with regulation of the immune response.

Class III antigens are located in serum protein, and regulate complement activity. (See COMPLEMENT.)

Following the demonstration at the Animal Breeding Research Organisation, Edinburgh, of an association between MHC type in cattle and their resistance to mastitis, it was suggested that it might be possible to select for AI bulls which pass on this resistance.

Malachite Green

A dye used in the treatment of external fungal and protozoal infections of fish, and for the control of proliferative kidney disease. Only the zinc-free preparation can be used for therapy in fish.

Malacia

Softening of a part or tissue in disease, e.g. osteomalacia or softening of the bones.

Malaria

(see under MONKEYS)

'Malaria of Birds'

(see under PLASMODIUM GALLINACEUM)

Malassezia (Pityosporon)

A yeast-like fungus which sometimes produces a brownish-black deposit in dogs' ears.

Malathion

An organophosphorus insecticide which has been used for the control of external parasites in cattle and as a crop spray.

Mal De Caderas (Maladie De Caderas)

Mal de caderas (maladie de caderas) is a try-panosome disease of the horse, occurring in Brazil, Argentina, Bolivia, and Paraguay, being most serious in the latter country. It is caused by the *Trypanosoma equinum.* Suramin or quinapyramine have been used in treatment.

Mal De Playa

A form of poisoning in cattle by a plant, *Lantana camara.*

Mal Du Coit (Maladie Du Coit)

(see DOURINE)

Male Fern

The growing point of male fern (*Dryopteris felix-mas*) may attract cattle on bare pasture, and lead to poisoning. In Scotland, 61 out of 68 head of beef cattle were affected, with 45 becoming wholly blind, 10 partly blind, and 21 recumbent. All recovered within a week except for 4 cows and 4 calves, which remained completely blind. One cow was additionally recumbent and was destroyed. (See also under FERNS.)

Maleic Hydrazide

A growth-retardant used on grass verges which has caused non-fatal gastritis in small animals.

Malformation

(see DEFORMITIES)

Malignant

A progressively worsening condition.

Malignant Aphtha of Sheep

(see ORF)

Malignant Catarrhal Fever

(see BOVINE MALIGNANT CATARRHAL FEVER)

Malignant Jaundice of Dogs

(see CANINE BABESIOSIS)

Malignant Oedema

(see GAS GANGRENE)

Malignant Stomatitis

(see CALF DIPHTHERIA)

Malignant Theileriasis of Sheep and Goats

A tick-borne disease caused by the protozoan parasite *Theileria hirci*, and occurring in Eastern Europe, the Middle East, Egypt, and Sudan.

Signs include high fever, constipation, gland-ular enlargement, pale anaemic mucous mem-branes with later jaundice and death; however, the disease may be very mild in animals with some locally acquired immunity.

Mallein Test

Mallein test is a method of testing for the presence of GLANDERS in a horse.

Mamilla

Mamilla is the Latin term for the nipple.

Mamillitis Inflammation of the nipple. Bovine herpes mamillitis is a recognised disease which can also affect the skin of the udder.

Mammary Gland (Udder)

Structure

Cow The udder has 4 glands or 'quarters'. A strong septum divides the 2 right-hand glands from the 2 on the left side, but there is no such demarcation between fore and hindquarters on the same side of the body.

The structure of the gland is similar to that seen in the mare, being composed of lobes and lobules, held in position by fibrous tissue, and sending ducts down into an irregular milk sinus. This latter is large, and partly divided into compartments by folds of mucous mem-brane. From it leads 1 large lactiferous duct down the teat to its apex, which possesses a sphincter muscle of almost 10 mm in width.

Mare The mammary glands are 2 in number, situated in the inguinal region.

Ewe There are 2 mammary glands, each of which has a single teat. They are situated in the inguinal region, as in the mare and cow.

Sow The mammary glands number 12 in most sows (although a few have more), and are arranged in 2 rows reaching from just behind the level of the elbows along the abdomen to the inguinal region. As a rule, the glands which are situated towards the middle of the series are the best developed and secrete the most milk. Each teat has 2 ducts as a rule.

Bitch As in the sow, there are 2 rows of glands along the lower line of the abdomen. They are usually 10 in number, but in the smaller breeds there may only be 8, and in the larger breeds there are sometimes 12. The teats each possess from 10 to 12 tiny lactiferous ducts.

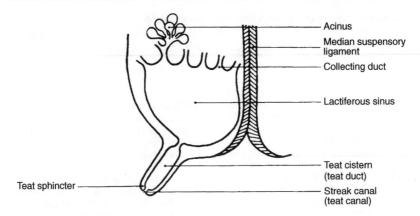

Diagram showing one-half of the cow's udder, and the median suspensory ligament which separates the 2 halves.

Secretion of milk This is a continuous process, initiated at parturition (or before) by the hormone prolactin (from the pituitary gland) and another from the thyroid. A number of other hormones may be involved, both in stimulating and in maintaining secretion of milk. Milk accumulates in the alveoli, upper channels, and milk cisterns; the rate of secretion decreases as internal udder pressure rises.

Milk 'let-down' in the cow, associated with the hormone oxytocin, is referred to under MILKING.

Colostrum is the name given to the first milk that is secreted by the udder.

(The importance of the newly born of any species of animal getting a supply of colostrum-containing first milk, soon after it is born, is explained under COLOSTRUM.)

(For other information concerning milk, see MILK.)

Conditions affecting the milk yield of cows

(1) Breed.
(2) Temperament. There is no doubt that a placid but not sluggish, alert but not highly nervous, cow makes the best milker.
(3) Health. It is, of course, necessary that a cow should be in good general health if the best results are to be obtained from her.
(4) Age. A cow in good health improves in her milk yield up to her 7th or 8th year, and remains at a high level until her 10th or 12th year. The milk of a young cow is much richer in fats and solids than that of an aged animal, so that the ideal position in a herd is to have enough young stock to counteract any possible

deficiency in those substances from the milk of the old cows.
(5) Lactation. A cow yields the greatest amount of milk between the 6th and 8th week after calving; thence she gives a smaller amount each day till about the 300th day, when she goes dry. Cows give best results when their lactation period does not exceed 8½ to 9 months, i.e. when they are dried off about 8 weeks before they are due to calve, having settled in-calf at the first. (See also PROGENY TESTING; RATIONS FOR LIVESTOCK.)

Mammary Glands, Diseases of

Mastitis, or inflammation of the udder. All the domestic animals are liable to the disease, but it is commonest in the cow, ewe, and goat. (See MASTITIS IN COWS.)

Abscess formation Antibiotics or sulpha drugs are indicated; lancing the abscess can give relief. (See ABSCESS: specific abscesses are considered under ACTINOMYCOSIS; TUBERCULOSIS.)

Tuberculosis of the udder (see TUBERCULOSIS).

Tumours include papillomas, fibro-adenomas, and adenocarcinomas. Some tumours of the bitch's mammary glands appear to be hormone-dependent and contain oestrogen receptor protein. Of 2075 malignant tumours in bitches reported by 14 veterinary schools in the USA and Canada, 1187 were histologically malignant, 557 benign, and 331 in the 'malignancy not determined' category. (W. A. Priester, National Cancer Institute, Maryland, USA.) In cats, mammary carcinoma is twice as common in the Siamese breed as in all other breeds combined. (See TUMOURS; CANCER.)

Hypertrophy of the mammary glands in the cat has been recorded both in pregnant queens and in neutered females treated with megestrol acetate for 14 months to 5 years. The condition has to be differentiated from neoplasia.

Wounds and injuries of the udder and teats are commonest in the cow and sow, owing to greater pendulousness than in other animals.

All wounds of the udder and teats are serious on account of the danger of infection and the development of mastitis.

Treatment As a first-aid treatment, wounds of the teats and udder should be washed with warm water and an antiseptic, dry sulphanilamide powder subsequently applied.

When a teat has been torn or injured so that milk escapes from the canal, it is usually difficult to get the fistula, so formed, to heal until the cow goes dry. An operation is usually necessary to obtain healing. This procedure necessitates the cow remaining dry for at least 2 months. In some cases a cow with a fistula is better turned out to grass at once, and made to rear calves until her milk-flow ceases, when she can be taken in and undergo the operation.

Eruptions on teats may be specific, such as are seen during outbreaks of foot-and-mouth disease, cowpox, malignant catarrhal fever, rinderpest, etc. (See VIRAL INFECTIONS OF COWS' TEATS.)

Many teat sores, however, are caused through 'chapping', or 'cracking', of the delicate skin of the teat. (See under MASTITIS.)

Warts on teats (see WARTS)

Teat obstructions Difficulty in milking may be caused by stricture of the sphincter, milk clots or (rarely) calculi in the teat canal; alternatively by the presence of warty growths inside the canal. The latter condition is considered under WARTS.

Manchester Terrier

A medium-sized dog with pointed face, smooth black coat and brown markings on the face and legs. The breed may develop cutaneous asthenia and Perthe's disease.

Mandelic Acid

A urinary antiseptic, effective in acid urine.

Mandible

Mandible is the bone of the lower jaw. (See under JAW.)

Mandibular Disease

(see SHOVEL BEAK)

Manganese

(Mn), a trace element, is necessary in minute quantities for a healthy diet. Insufficiency in the pasture herbage, e.g. in Devon and Cornwall, UK, may cause infertility in cattle, and deformed offspring.

In New Zealand, on one farm, 32 calves were born with very shortened limbs and enlarged joints. They had been sired by 4 bulls. Owing to a dry season, the cows had been fed large quantities of apple pulp and corn silage, both of which contained very low levels of manganese. (See TRACE ELEMENTS; 'SLIPPED TENDON'.)

Mange

A contagious skin disease caused by mites, which lay their eggs in the skin. The movement of the larvae results in intense irritation. Damage to skin, hide or fleece is caused by efforts to relieve the discomfort. There are different types of mange, each caused by a different species of mite. Sarcoptic mange occurs in man (when it is known as scabies), dogs, cats, cattle, pigs, sheep, horses, etc. Psoroptic mange in the sheep is known as SHEEP SCAB. Chorioptic mange usually affects the tail and legs. Demodectic mange (follicular or 'black' mange) is most common in dogs. Details are given below. (For causal mites, see under MITES, PARASITIC.)

Mange in cattle

Demodectic mange Fairly common but often not noticed as clinical signs are few; nodular formation in hair follicles is the main one.

Sarcoptic mange is common in Britain and North America and is the cause of 'dairyman's itch'. It is usually found on the head and neck, but may occur on any part of the body. Bulls are particularly liable to this form of mange.

Chorioptic mange is usually confined to the base of the tail, but may spread.

Psoroptic mange causes debility, failure to thrive, and reduced liveweight gain.

Psoroptic mange is an important disease of feedlot cattle in the USA, and was once the most prevalent form of cattle mange in Britain, where it is now seldom seen. In an outbreak in Britain, in a beef herd comprising 306 animals, the infected areas of skin were thickened and scabby, with blood and serum oozing from the lesions. These extended along the back and down the flanks.

Treatment Ivermectin or similar products by injection; 'pour-on' products such as fenthion and phosmet.

Mange in the horse In this host, 4 varieties of mange occur.

Sarcoptic mange In this type the parasites burrow into the epidermis and make treatment difficult. The disease commences by the hair dropping out in patches with the formation of papules and an intense continuous itching. The hair becomes thin and broken, and abrasions are present. The skin is hard and folded. Emaciation is progressive, and death may occur from exhaustion. It reaches its height in spring, and is at an ebb in late summer and autumn.

Treatment Gamma BHC is an efficient mite-killer, but its use in the UK is banned. The organophosphorus compounds, diazinon and fenchlorphos, are also effective. For the best results they should be applied by dipping or as saturating sprays, and for the sarcoptic manges particularly, 2 or more treatments may be necessary at intervals of 10 to 14 days.

Psoroptic mange Two varieties of *Psoroptes* occur on the horse, 1 in the ear and 1 on the skin. The lesions on the skin are localised at first, and usually start near the dorsal line where the hair is long. The patches are generally barer than in sarcoptic mange. The parasites bite the epidermis, but do not penetrate the skin. The serum which exudes forms a scab in which the parasites live.

Treatment is on similar lines to that for sarcoptic mange. It is important to remember the presence of parasites in the ear, and to treat this part of the body also.

Chorioptic or symbiotic mange is usually confined to the legs or root of the tail. It is not notifiable. It causes great itching, stamping, and rubbing of one leg against the other. Papules, scabs, and even ulcers may be found. Treatment is as above. Ivermectin paste, 0.2 mg/kg, in 2 doses, 2 weeks apart, has been suggested as a control measure.

Demodectic mange (*See* description under 'Mange in dogs and cats', below.)

Mange in sheep

Sarcoptic mange is usually confined to the head, and is seldom found on the woolly parts of the body. It tends to become more generalised in the goat.

Chorioptic mange, caused by *Chorioptes bovis*, occurs in horses as well as cattle and sheep, and can be serious, especially in housed sheep overseas. It is not uncommon in the UK. Of 130 sheep received from South Wales at the Central Veterinary Laboratory, 33 per cent were found infested. Lesions occur on the pasterns and in the interdigital spaces.

Psoroptic mange or 'sheep scab' is caused by *Psorotes ovis*. It occurs on all parts of the body covered with wool and in the ears. The life-cycle is typical, and can be completed in 13 to 16 days: the progress of the disease is in consequence very rapid. It is one of the worst of sheep diseases; it was formerly notifiable in Britain.

Itching is usually the first symptom of the disease, and should be investigated **at once**. The skin becomes thickened and even ulcerated; the wool becomes detached and the sheep emaciated (*see* illustration below). The itching causes the animal to rub itself against fences, and detaches the scab. This further spreads the disease, and permits secondary infections of the wound by bacteria.

Treatment is usually by means of double-dipping at an interval of about 8 to 12 days, but which depends on local circumstances. In Britain a dip sanctioned by DEFRA must be used. It should be purchased only from a reputable manufacturer and used exactly as directed. Organophosphorus dips can only be purchased by persons who have attended a course on their usage and have received an appropriate certificate to confirm this.

Prevention (see IVERMECTIN)

The 'itch-mite' of sheep *Psorergates ovis*, which occurs in Australasia, Africa, and North and South America, has not, so far, been found in Britain. This mite causes thickening of the skin and scurf formation. The growth of the wool fibre is affected and the fleece is further damaged by rubbing.

Mange in pigs

Sarcoptic mange starts on the head and gradually spreads all over the body, especially attacking the thinner skin. There is intense itching, the hair falls out, and the skin becomes covered with scab or with wart-like projections. It is found in the UK and North America.

Treatment Improved liveweight gains have followed treatment of sarcoptic mange. Amitraz, doramectin or IVERMECTIN may be effective.

Mange in dogs and cats

Sarcoptic mange in the dog generally starts on the muzzle and spreads backwards. The animal should be clipped and bathed with green soap. It may then be treated with phosmet. If the infection is generalised, treat one-half of the body, and the other half after 2 or 3 days.

Notoedric mange in cats is similar to the latter form in dogs. It is intensely irritating, affecting face, ears, and occasionally legs and external genitalia. It is now very rare in the UK.

Benzyl benzoate may prove toxic to cats and so one of the sulphur preparations or piperonyl butoxide is recommended.

Otodectic or auricular mange occurs in dogs and cats. Otodectes is the most frequent cause of irritation in the ears; it causes scratching and shaking of the ear.

The eggs and larvae are very resistant, and survive under treatments which kill the adults.

First-aid Cat-owners may be able to provide a little temporary relief by means of a few drops of olive or vegetable oil, which will help to soften waxy deposits and kill some mites. A few drops of warm, soapy water (**not** dish-washing detergent liquid) may achieve the same result. However, professional advice should be obtained without delay.

Owners should not poke around with cotton-wool wound round an orange stick or tweezers, as the wool will slip off, and the skin of the external ear canal is then likely to be abraded, or even the ear-drum punctured.

Professional treatment consists in the use of eardrops containing an effective mite-killer, plus an analgesic to reduce the irritation caused by the mites.

In neglected cases, or those complicated by bacterial or fungal infections, where a painful, suppurating condition is present, antibacterial or anti-fungal drugs must be used.

(See DEAFNESS and EARS, DISEASES OF; also HAEMATOMA.)

Demodectic mange Cigar-shaped mites invade the hair follicles, causing the hair to fall out in patches.

Demodectic mange (also known as follicular or 'black mange') is most common in dogs.

Signs Two types of demodectic mange in dogs have been described: (1) the squamous type, in which the skin becomes scaly, wrinkled and ringworm-like in appearance (and sometimes mistaken for ringworm); and (2) the pustular type in which secondary bacterial infection occurs. This is always very serious, and consti-tutes an illness as well as a mere skin disease, since the dog suffers from toxaemia. Indeed, sometimes euthanasia becomes the only humane course, especially when extensive areas of skin are involved.

Cause *Demodex canis.*

Treatment is made difficult by the fact that the mites are sometimes living at a depth difficult to reach. However, amitraz and IVERMECTIN are effective.

Diagnosis is made or confirmed by the examination of skin scrapings under a microscope.

The disease often appears in the dog when 8 to 12 months old, usually first on the head, around the eyes and nose, and on or near the feet.

Mange in goats may be caused by *D. caprae*, and characterised by palpable nodules or pustules without loss of hair. The disease usually starts on face, neck and shoulders. Ivermectin and related drugs or phosmet have proved successful in treatment.

Mange in fowls

'Depluming scabies' in fowls is caused by *Cnemidocoptes laevis*, which lives at the base of the feathers, and so irritates the fowl that it pulls them out. The stumps left may be seen to be surrounded with crusts. The affected spots and surrounding areas may be treated with IVERMECTIN.

'Scaly leg' is caused by *C. mutans*. The feet and legs become enlarged and crusted. The birds may become very lame and even lose a toe. Destruction of infected birds combined with rigorous disinfection is the most common method of eradication. If this procedure is not convenient, the scab should be removed with soap and water, the leg dried, and one of

the preparations mentioned above used. This should be repeated in 3 or 4 days.

Cage birds may suffer from this infestation. *C. pilae* causes 'scaly face' and 'tassel foot'.

Dermanyssus gallinae is the chicken mite of Europe and North America. It is whitish to red in colour. The complete life-cycle takes about 7 to 10 days.

The mite lives exclusively on blood. It is nocturnal in its habits, living in crevices during the day.

Eradication of the mite must be thorough. All wooden structures must be disinfected. A painter's blow lamp is very useful for cracks.

Affected flocks may be treated by cypermethrin, as a dilute spray.

Although primarily a parasite of fowls, this mite will attack horses and other mammals, causing much irritation, with the eruption of papules and the formation of scabs. The mite, as it feeds only at night, may be overlooked as the cause of the disease. The proximity of fowls suffering from the mite may give a clue.

Ornithonyssus sylviarum, the northern fowl mite which is also common in Britain, causes scab formation, soiling of the feathers, and thickening of the skin around the vent. In contrast to the chicken mite, this parasite remains on its host.

In Israel allergic rhinitis and bronchial asthma have been caused by this mite among poultry farmers.

Liponyssus bursa, the tropical 'fowl mite', replaces the last species in the warmer parts of the world. Unlike it, however, this species is found on the fowls and in the nest. It may feed during the day. It also lays eggs and moults on its host. The symptoms are similar.

Manioc
An ingredient of some compound animal feeds which has been found unsafe for turkeys. (See CASSAVA.)

Mannosidosis
The most widely recognised lyosomal storage disease of cattle, especially of Aberdeen Angus. It is due to a genetic deficiency of the enzyme mannosidase. Affected calves develop ataxia and become aggressive; finally, paralysis sets in.

Beta-mannosidosis, an inherited disorder of glycoprotein metabolism, has been identified in goats, and is rapidly fatal. Signs include inability to rise from a recumbent

position, carpal contractures, pastern joint hyperextension, a dome-shaped skull, and deafness.

Manure Heaps
Manure heaps are potentially a source of infection and should be fenced off. Grass growing near manure heaps may also contain pathogens and parasites. New manure should be buried under older manure; the new manure will then heat up to about 70°C, destroying most pathogens, if left for a few days. (See also SLURRY.)

Manx
A breed of cat that is without a tail, or has only a very short one. The breed originated on the Isle of Man and the Manx government maintains a breeding colony. The lack of tail is due to a dominant mutation and is seen as a depression at the end of the spinal column. There may be associated defects in vertebrae, and malfunction of the sphincter muscle. If both parents carry the mutant gene, kittens die before birth. Early deaths in kittens may be due to malformations such as fused vertebrae or spina bifida. Manx cats with a short tail are called 'stumpies'; some are born with tails and are known as 'longies'. Manx cats have longer back legs than forelegs, causing an unusual gait.

'Marble Bone Disease'
(see OSTEOPETROSIS)

Marburg Disease
(see MONKEYS)

Marek's Disease
This contagious disease of domestic poultry was first described in Austria-Hungary in 1907. It was first recorded in America in 1914, and in Britain in 1929, and spread widely. The availability of vaccines, with good hygienic practice, has greatly reduced the losses from Marek's disease, which is a neoplasm caused by a herpesvirus. Turkeys are rarely affected as they normally harbour a different herpesvirus – one that affords protection against Marek's disease. The turkey virus has been used in a vaccine for chickens.

Formerly called fowl paralysis, Marek's disease had, before the advent of vaccination against it, become the most economically important disease of poultry in many countries, in terms of fowl mortality, carcase condemnation, and lost egg production.

At least 2 forms of Marek's disease are recognised: the classical form, in which paralysis – to a varying degree – is the outstanding feature; and an acute leukosis form, in which lymphoid tumour formation is the main feature, with nervous symptoms less in evidence.

Cause A herpesvirus, which may persist for long periods in litter dust.

Signs The classical form affects birds commonly between the ages of 3 and 4 months, but cases have been recorded in broilers a little over 3 weeks old, and also in birds over a year old. It is frequently noticed that certain strains of birds are affected – in-contact birds of a different parentage remaining healthy. Affected birds may show lameness of 1 or both legs: this lameness becomes progressively worse, and general paralysis results. A common attitude for an affected bird to adopt is to lie about with 1 limb extended in front and the other extended behind. In spite of this the bird appears alert and will feed if placed beside a supply. Drooping of wings may be noted. In some cases the tip of the wing may touch the ground. Eye lesions may be seen.

In the acute form of Marek's disease, birds as young as 6 to 8 weeks may be affected. Loss of appetite and depression are noticeable; tumours can often be palpated – these involving abdominal organs, muscles, skin, and sometimes the comb. Paralysis is not the predominant characteristic of this form of the disease.

Mortality The mortality varies, but in birds 6 to 8 weeks old may exceed 20 per cent. It is difficult actually to arrive at a satisfactory figure as this disease may co-exist with others, e.g. coccidiosis, tapeworm infestations, tuberculosis, and vitamin deficiency, etc.

Control measures Vaccination at 1 day old may be repeated at 2 to 4 weeks; it provides 80 to 90 per cent protection in the case of an outbreak.

On the disease being diagnosed, all affected birds should be destroyed as soon as the first symptoms are observed. The disease is always introduced to a farm by the purchase of fresh stock, in the form of eggs, day-old chicks, or adult birds.

Careful selection of the source of fresh stock is vital in maintaining disease-fee flocks.

Both the fowl tick, *Argas persicus*, and the darkling beetle can harbour the virus of Marek's disease.

Vaccines. Freeze-dried and 'wet' cell associated vaccines are available. The latter are stored in liquid nitrogen; care is needed in handling as the ampoules may shatter or cause freeze burns. The manufacturers' instructions must be followed.

Mares, Infertility in
(see under EQUINE GENITAL INFECTIONS)

Marie's Disease
(see HYPERTROPHIC OSTEOPATHY)

Marijuana (Cannabis) Poisoning
Marijuana (cannabis) poisoning has occurred in dogs in the USA as a result of being given home-made sweet biscuits containing the drug. Symptoms include acute depression, retching or vomiting, and a staggering gait. The dogs may be ill for 36 to 48 hours, and vomiting may be frequent. Besides vomiting, muscular tremors, and weakness, 1 dog showed incontinence, ataxia, leant against objects and then sank to the floor.

Markets
Markets are covered accommodation for the sale of animals. Shelter must be provided for dairy cows in milk, calves, lambs and pigs. Animals showing any sign of disease, or which are unfit, must be put in special pens and not offered for sale. Because of the contact between animals from different sources, disease can spread rapidly. Strict regulations apply to the running of a market and the transport of animals to and from markets. The legislation involved is the Welfare of Animals at Markets Order 1990 and the Welfare of Horses and Ponies at Markets (and Other Places of Sale) Order 1990.

'Marmite Disease'
A form of dermatitis encountered in piglets 3 days old and upwards. (See 'GREASY PIG DISEASE'.)

Marrow
The soft substance that is enclosed within the cavities of the bones. Yellow marrow owes its colour to the large amount of fat contained in it, while red marrow is of a highly cellular structure. Formation of the red blood cells (erythrocytes) takes place in the marrow, as also that of the blood platelets (thrombocytes). The marrow is also the source of lymphocytes (B-cells), monocytes, and other leukocytes. (See BLOOD; BONE; also MYELOCYTE.)

Marsh Marigold Poisoning
The marsh marigold, or kingcup (*Caltha palustris*), has occasionally been the cause of

poisoning, and is similar in its effects to BUTTERCUP POISONING.

Marsupial

A mammal of an order in which the young are born in an immature state and continue their development in a maternal pouch. Examples are kangaroos and opossums in Australia.

Marteiliosis

A disease caused by *Marteillia refringens* that affects molluscs, especially oysters. It is a NOTIFIABLE DISEASE in the UK and parts of the EU.

Masham

The cross resulting from a Blackface ewe and a Wensleydale ram.

Mast Cell

Mast cell is a type of connective tissue cell. It releases histamine and heparin, which cause anaphyllaxis and atopy in cases of allergic reaction. (See under BLOOD – Basophils; also REAGINIC ANTIBODIES.)

Mast-Cell Tumours

Nodular tumours of the skin which are usually benign but may become malignant. (See also MASTOCYTOMA.)

Mastiff

A very large, light-coloured dog with short coat, folded-over ears and a broad muzzle. Hip dysplasia may be present and the breed is prone to extropion.

Mastitis

Inflammation of the udder. (See MAMMARY GLAND, DISEASES OF, for mastitis in animals other than the cow.)

Mastitis in Cows

Inflammation of the udder, involving the secreting cells of the mammary glands, or its connective tissue, or both. (*See* diagram, page 442.)

Subclinical mastitis Mastitis may be unaccompanied by obvious symptoms. This form commonly reduces milk yields by 10 per cent or so, and is consequently of great economic importance. It has been stated that approximately 1 cow in 3 in Britain is affected by subclinical mastitis.

Simple tests have been used to detect the presence of an abnormally high content of white cells in an ordinary-looking sample of milk, and so indicate the presence of mastitis.

Once it is known that it exists, bacteriological tests can be used to identify the organisms responsible and to determine the best treatments. Sometimes an excess of white cells (more than 500,000 per ml) in the milk is the result of inflammation due to trauma and not to infection. Thus the California or Whiteside Test may draw attention to a faulty milking machine or bad milking technique.

The mastitis situation in a herd can be monitored on a monthly basis by laboratories operating electronic cell counters. The table shows the ranges of white cell counts.

The graph shows the spread of mastitis in an autumn calving herd.

Mastitis tends to rise as the winter progresses and fall when the cows first go out to grass. The cell counts rise again in July and August chiefly because of the high proportion of the cows nearing the end of their lactation. Cell counts and mastitis levels fall again in September when some of the older cows are being culled and first calf heifers are coming into the herd. Mastitis levels rise again through the winter period.

Clinical mastitis should be regarded as a herd problem.

Acute Shivering may usher in the attack. Later, there is a rise in temperature; fast, full pulse; short, quick respirations; and an uneasy appearance. The animal paddles with her feet, but is usually afraid to lie on account of the pain occasioned to the udder. She refuses food, and rumination is in abeyance. When the udder is examined it is found that one (or more) quarter is swollen, tense, reddened, and very painful to the touch; the cow may stand with her hind-legs straddled apart.

'Summer mastitis' (often involving gangrene of the udder) usually occurs either in heifers or in dry cows; however, it is seen occasionally in cows just after calving. It is caused by *Actinomyces pyogenes*, often in association with other pathogenic bacteria (e.g. *Peptococcus indolicus*).

'Summer mastitis' is something of a misnomer, in that, while it is most common in July and August, it is also seen in January and February.

If the gangrene affects a large part of the quarter, or when more than one-quarter is attacked, the condition of the cow is serious in the extreme.

The animal may stand aloof from the rest of the herd, sometimes paddles with her hind feet, and is obviously in pain. On examination the

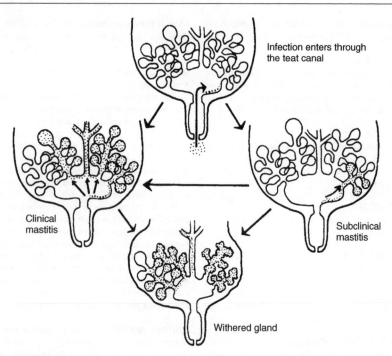

Diagram showing the relationship between the amount of mammary gland tissue involved and the form of mastitis which results.

Cell count ranges (cells/cc)	Estimate of mastitis problem	Estimate of milk production loss per cow per year
Below 250,000	Negligible	—
250,000–499,000	Slight	190 litres (42 gallons)
500,000–749,000	Average	330 litres (74 gallons)
750,000–999,000	Bad	760 litres (169 gallons)
1,000,000 and over	Very bad	885 litres (197 gallons)

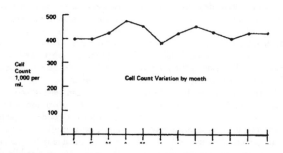

The spread of mastitis in an autumn calving herd.

trouble is soon located to the udder, where hardness – but not necessarily swelling – of a quarter is detected. Foul-smelling pus (grey, greenish-yellow, or blood-stained) is present.

Treatment Antibiotics, by injection or intramammary administration, may save the animal's life, though use of the quarter is usually lost.

Prevention The injection into the teat-canal of long-acting intramammary antibiotic prior to turning out, repeated every 3 to 6 weeks depending on the product used, during summer. (In maiden heifers and in-calf heifers, this procedure may be difficult and not always practicable. Care is needed to avoid both damage to the teat and the introduction of pathogenic bacteria.)

Give such protection against flies as is practicable.

Subacute mastitis The disease runs a course not unlike that of the acute form, but the symptoms appear much more slowly. There is a greater difficulty in milking, the first drawn milk often containing little clots and always large numbers of shed epithelial cells; later, there is a gradually increasing pain and swelling in the affected quarter, accompanied by an alteration in the colour of the milk to yellowish or yellowish-grey. The amount of milk decreases. As a rule, appetite remains normal, pulse and breathing are unaltered, and if there is any rise in the temperature it is slight.

Chronic mastitis shows little general constitutional disturbance, and an almost complete absence of pain, a slowly progressing increase in the density of the gland, a diminution in the secretion of milk, and a gradual increase in the size of the affected quarter or quarters.

Pathological changes in the udder may render any antibiotic ineffectual. One such problem is the survival within phagocytes of staphylococci, where they are protected from the lethal action of most antibiotics. (See PHAGOCYTOSIS.)

Antibiotics can more economically be used when the cow is in the dry period. Long-acting antibiotics can then be given without aggravating the problem of antibiotic residues in milk. (See under MILK – Antibiotics in milk.)

Bacterial mastitis *Staphylococcus aureus, Streptococcus agalactiae, S. uberis* and *S. dysgalactiae* are among the main organisms responsible for mastitis. However, *S. dysgalactiae* is

seldom a serious problem; *S. uberis* is more resistant.

In a survey of 5 herds, *S. uberis* was found to be the major pathogen associated with dry cow mastitis.

Coliform or 'Environmental' mastitis has become increasingly prevalent in recent years, and is common during the winter. This infection of the udder is often long-lasting, and the cow is ill with it, so that its economic effects may be greater than with streptococcal or staphylococcal mastitis. Many outbreaks have been linked with cold, wet weather; they are aggravated by damp bedding, sawdust, and muddy conditions underfoot when strip-grazing kale, etc. The above conditions would appear to favour the entry of *E. coli* through the teat-canal, but the organism may also reach the udder via the bloodstream in cattle which are scouring – often after a sudden change of diet – as a result of an active *E. coli* gut infection.

'Experimentally, severe cases of coliform mastitis can be produced only in early lactation following the stress of calving – a situation commonly prevailing in naturally occurring field cases.' (IRAD, Compton.) (See COLIFORM.)

Klebsiella spp. and *Enterobacter aerogenes* are other organisms involved in mastitic infections.

Leptospiral mastitis Leptospiral infection often causes agalactia rather than mastitis. However, in 1 outbreak in Northern Ireland, involving half a herd of 140 cows over a 2-month period, symptoms included a sudden drop in milk yield, flaccid udders with all 4 quarters affected, thickish and sometimes bloodstained milk, fever (a temperature of up to 41°C (106°F)), and quickened breathing and pulse rates. The illness in individual cows lasted from 1 to 4 days. *Leptospira hardjo* was isolated from the milk and blood of cows with clinical mastitis. (See LEPTOSPIROSIS IN CATTLE.)

Among other bacteria which may cause mastitis are *Bacillus subtilis*, which has been isolated from washing water, header tanks, and teat-cup liners; *Pseudomonas*; and *Chlamydia*. *Campylobacter jejuni* has also caused mastitis.

Mycoplasmal mastitis occurs in Britain and many other countries, and may prove resistant to antibiotics. In an outbreak in North Wales over a 5-week period, half a herd of 115 cows became infected, and 14 had to be sold for slaughter. The milk was at first brownish in colour. The mastitis was rapid in onset, producing a hard swollen quarter which was neither hot nor tender; the cows showed little sign of general illness. Unlike in other forms of mastitis, there was a rapid spread to other quarters of the udder. The first isolation of *Mycoplasma californicum* from cows with chronic, incurable mastitis in the UK was made in 1982 – 10 years after its first isolation in California. Other species include *M. bovigenitalium.*

Viral mastitis has been associated with vesicular stomatitis and infectious bovine rhinotracheitis.

Mycotic mastitis More than 25 species of fungi have been implicated. The worst of these is called *Cryptococcus neoformans* and it can cause outbreaks of mastitis severe enough to lead to cows being slaughtered.

Algal mastitis A UK outbreak of severe indurative mastitis in newly calved cows, from which *Prototheca zopfii* was isolated, has been reported. (See ALGAE.)

Man-to-cow-infections Occasionally, mastitis in cattle arises from infection by human beings. The kind of streptococci which can give rise either to a severe sore throat or to scarlet fever can result in an outbreak of mastitis in a dairy herd, and several such outbreaks have been reported in various countries. The pneumococcus, a cause of human pneumonia, has been isolated from the udders of cows with streptococcal mastitis in Essex, Bedfordshire, and other counties, the source being the cowman's throat. *Campylobacter jejuni* has also been transmitted from man to cow. (See under MILK-BORNE DISEASE for *Corynebacterium ulcerans*, etc.; see also SALMONELLOSIS.)

M

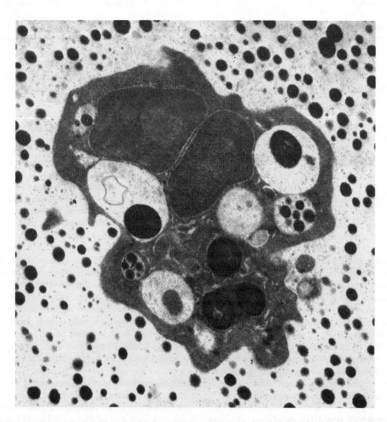

In bovine mastitis, as in other inflammations caused by micro-organisms, neutrophils, a type of white blood cell (*leukocyte*), migrate from the blood into the inflamed tissue as the first line of defence. In this electron micrograph (magnification ¥ 7000) a neutrophil or phagocyte is shown to contain five staphylococci.

The spread of infection Infection enters by way of the teat and can easily be spread from cow to cow by milkers' hands or the cups of the machine, but apparently less easily by the latter method. Udder cloths and towels are also commonly infected. It has also been shown that in an infected herd, a large proportion of sores or chaps harbour organisms, and these may be a source of infection of the udder itself in the same cow or in another. The skin of the teats and the milkers' hands may remain infected from one milking to another, and in a heavily infected herd the skin of the cows' bodies, milkers' clothes, floor, partitions, etc. become contaminated and may remain so for considerable periods.

Treatment Proper treatment depends upon a correct diagnosis and the use of suitable antibiotics in adequate dosage, introduced into the udder with aseptic precautions so as not to introduce further (and perhaps more virulent) infection. Adequate dosage is important, as otherwise strains of resistant organisms may arise. In some cases sulfanilamide may be used. (See ANTIBIOTIC RESISTANCE.)

The control of mastitis An important aid is teat-dipping. The liquid mainly used for teat-dipping is an iodophor – a type of disinfectant containing iodine but extremely mild in its effect upon the tissues. Good results can also be obtained with hypochlorite teat-dips containing 1 per cent available chlorine.

In rotary parlours with automatic cluster removal equipment and only 1 operator, teat-dipping is often impracticable and teat-spraying (probably less effective) is the only alternative.

A 2nd recommendation is the wearing by the dairyman of smooth rubber gloves, which can be dipped in disinfectant before the udder is washed. They represent a partial solution to the problem created by the fact that hands cannot be sterilised.

Warm-water sprays may be used for udder-washing, and disposable paper towels for drying. The latter obviate cross-infections from udder cloths. (See also SPONGES.)

If warm-water sprays are not available, wash the udder (if very dirty) with plain warm water first, then with an udder wash; numerous proprietary formulations are available, based on benzalkonium, cetrimide, chorhexidine, solubilised iodine, etc. If none of these is available, a 1 per cent solution of cetrimide may be used.

It is significant that in herds with a low incidence of mastitis, udder-washing is avoided in

40 per cent and practised only in 11 per cent (but see MILK – Sediment in milk).

Questions which the farmer must ask are as follows:

(1) Is the person doing the milking capable of handling the cows properly, and keen to do so?

(2) Are the vacuum gauges and cup-liners kept correctly adjusted?

(3) Is hand-stripping avoided?

(4) If a disinfectant is used, is it used at the correct strength?

(5) Are there disposable paper towels?

(6) Are there any old, chronically infected cows in the herd which do not respond to treatment and would be better disposed of?

(7) Is fly-control being practised in the milking parlour?

(8) Is attention being given to the 96-hour rule regarding the withholding of milk from a cow after calving, whether treated with antibiotics or not?

Rough inexpert milking and stripping predispose to mastitis. With machine milking, the use of a badly designed teat-cup liner, for instance, or leaving the cups on an empty quarter, may lead to trouble. (See under MILKING MACHINES for faulty use of these, leading to mastitis.) Bruising is an important predisposing cause, and for this reason cows should never be hurried, especially before milking, as the udder may be injured. This applies particularly to older cows in which the udder is large and pendulous. Chilling must be avoided, and also chapped teats (the latter should be left dry after milking). Even the smallest injuries and sores on the teats should be carefully attended to, since the germs which gain entry to these so often gain entry to the udder later.

Routine use of the strip-cup is helpful. If flecks or clots are seen in the milk, segregate the cow(s) if practicable, and – in any case – milk after the others. When a strip-cup is used, care should be taken to see that neither the handle nor the fingers become a source of infection to clean cows. Use the cup **before** the udder is washed.

Dry-cow therapy It has been shown in large-scale field experiments that the best time to treat cows to eliminate infection from the udders is during the dry period. Particularly with staphylococcal infection, there is a better chance of removing infections at this time than during lactation, and better results are achieved when cows are treated in the subclinical phase of the disease rather than during a clinical attack. Treatment during the dry period not only eliminates most of the existing infection; it also prevents most of the new infections from occurring during the dry period, including 'summer mastitis'. Another advantage is that there is no problem of milk being contaminated with antibiotic(s), provided that a cow is dry for 6 weeks or longer. It is advisable to treat **all** cows. Preparations containing cloxacillin have proved very effective. Teat-dipping of dry cows is also useful in preventing summer mastitis.

Control measures summarised.

(1) **Records** Keep all details of cell-count figures on a monthly basis and use these to monitor the incidence of mastitis in the herd. Record also details of milking-machine testing and maintenance.

(2) **Milking machines** Have machinery tested regularly and thoroughly at least once a year. At each milking check the vacuum pressures, pulsation rates, air bleeds and liners. Remember that machines are used 730 times a year and faulty machines can lead to a mastitis build-up.

(3) **Teat-dipping and hygiene** Use an effective iodophor-plus-lanolin teat-dip on each quarter as the cluster is removed. Wear smooth rubber gloves for preference; use the fore-milk cup before washing the udders with clean, running water. Use clean paper towels – not a dirty cloth – to dry the udders.

(4) **Dry-cow therapy** The farmer's veterinary surgeon will not only advise generally on mastitis control, but will also recommend the appropriate treatment at the end of lactation. This will include the infusion of a specially formulated, long-lasting antibiotic into each quarter, to destroy residues of infection and to counter new infections in the dry period.

(5) **Treatment** Clinical mastitis can occur at any time and will need prompt attention immediately by the veterinary surgeon, who can advise on the correct treatment during lactation.

(6) **Culling** Any cow which has several attacks of clinical mastitis in a lactation endangers the rest of the herd. Records of treatments and responses will identify those cows with recurring cases in 1 lactation and show which should be culled from the herd.

The cow's own protection 'Pathogens invading the mammary gland of the cow are subjected to non-specific resistance factors at 2 levels, either in the teat-canal or in the mammary gland itself. The teat-canal acts as a mechanical barrier, but in addition invading pathogens within the canal are subjected to the activity of antimicrobial fatty acids and cationic proteins. Pathogens breaching these barriers are then subjected to the defences of the mammary gland itself. In the early stages of infection there is a considerable increase in somatic cells in the milk, which is associated with an increased resistance to infection. During the early stages of the inflammatory reaction the invading pathogens are exposed to the action of neutrophils, locally produced humoral factors and proteins from the systemic circulation which pass into the mammary gland. These serum factors include the immunoglobulins, complement units and other antimicrobial proteins.' (Dr K. G. Hibbitt and Dr A. W. Hill, IRAD, Compton.)

Breeding for resistance to bovine mastitis may be possible in the future. (See MAJOR HISTOCOMPATIBILITY SYSTEM.)

Mastitis in Ewes

Common causes are *Pasteurella haemolytica*, which can produce a peracute mastitis with gangrene, and *Staphylococcus aureus*. Once the ewes are separated from their lambs, dry-cow intramammary preparations may be used as a preventive measure. It is essential to use 1 tube per teat.

Mastitis in Goats

Mastitis in goats can be a problem in humans as the milk is often unpasteurised. Potential infectious organisms include *Streptococcus zooepidemicus*, *S. pneumoniae*, *Actinobacillus equuli*, *Pasteurella haemolytica* and *Staphylococcus aureus*.

Mastitis Metritis Agalactia Syndrome (MMA)

Mastitis metritis agalactia syndrome (MMA), also known as farrowing fever, is a common problem in sows in the first 2 days after farrowing. The sow is off its food and the temperature rises; the udder may be partially or wholly swollen and painful. The piglets are restless.

Treatment involves antibiotics, possibly with anti-inflammatory agents. The piglets must be fed while the problem persists.

Mastocytoma

A type of tumour which is common in the dog and involves skin and subcutaneous tissue;

occasionally muscle. A mastocytoma may be malignant. It contains numerous MAST CELLS. In cattle this tumour is also regarded as potentially malignant.

Maternal Antibodies

Their function in protecting the offspring from infections encountered by the dam is referred to under COLOSTRUM. The immunity so produced is a temporary one, and wanes. The timing of vaccinations to induce lasting immunity is crucial (see DISTEMPER PREVENTION); for if carried out while the level of maternally derived antibody is significant, vaccination will fail. (See also MEASLES VACCINE; CANINE PARVOVIRUS.)

Mavis

Medicines Act Veterinary Information Service newsletter. Issued by the Veterinary Medicines Directorate, Woodham Lane, New Haw, Addlestone KT15 3NB.

Maxilla

(see SKULL – General arrangement of the skull)

MCG (mcg)

Microgram: 1 millionth of a gram.

Meadow-Saffron Poisoning

The meadow saffron (the autumn crocus, *Colchicum autumnale*), a common inhabitant of meadows, hedge bottoms, and woodland areas in England and Wales, is a cause of poisoning among horses and cattle. Pigs may sometimes eat the bulbous root (corm) and suffer, but sheep and goats are resistant. All parts of the plant are poisonous, both when green and when dried in hay, but the toxicity varies at different times of the year. Cases of poisoning are usually seen in the spring, when the leaves and seed-vessels are produced, and then again in summer and autumn (from August to October), when the flowers are formed.

The poison, (colchicine) is present in largest amounts in the seeds and corms; it is cumulative in its action.

Signs When only small quantities have been taken there is loss of appetite, suppression of rumination, profuse dribbling of saliva, and diarrhoea. The excretion of colchicine by the kidneys causes irritation in the urinary bladder, and induces the animal to pass urine in small amounts almost as soon as it is formed. Blood may be present in both the urine and the milk of dairy cows. Abortion is common in pregnant cows and heifers.

When large amounts have been eaten, the symptoms include ataxia and abdominal pain; death may occur in from 16 hours to 4 days.

The plant should be eradicated from pastures in the autumn when its striking pale purple crocus-like flowers can be easily seen. The bulbs should be dug out or cut with a hoe.

Meal-Feeding in Piggeries

This can result in a very dusty atmosphere under some circumstances, causing coughing and a feeling of tightness in the chest in people working there, and sometimes to a false assumption that the pigs are coughing because of enzootic pneumonia.

Measles

(see under MONKEYS; MEASLES VACCINE)

'Measles' in Beef

(see TAPEWORMS)

'Measles' in Pork

(see TAPEWORMS)

M

Measles Vaccine

An attenuated measles virus vaccine may be used in the dog to give protection against distemper. (See also under DISTEMPER.) Measles vaccine can overcome low levels of maternally derived antibodies and may be used from 5 weeks old.

Meat

(see PORCINE STRESS SYNDROME; HORSE-MEAT; DOGS' DIET, *and below*)

Meat, Dark

Meat with limited fat cover and intramuscular fat appears dark. This is seen particularly in bull carcases, and horse meat is always dark in colour. Dark cutting beef is possibly the single biggest cause of loss to beef processors. It is caused by a deficiency of glycogen in the muscles of an animal at slaughter which prevents the normal decrease in pH post-mortem. As a result there is an increase in enzyme activity; this uses up the oxygen which would normally convert the dark myoglobin into pink oxymyoglobin and the meat appears dark. It also tends to be dry because of the higher water-binding capacity of muscle protein at a higher pH. The stores of glycogen are depleted principally by muscular exhaustion and stress, and these 2 factors must be avoided in the 48 hours before slaughter in order to minimise the risk of dark cutting beef. (See also PORCINE STRESS SYNDROME.)

Long fasting times are associated with a reduction in carcase yield in pigs and an increase in the incidence of dark, firm, dry (DFD) meat.

Meat-Handlers' Occupational Hazards

Many of the infectious diseases that affect animals can be transmitted to abattoir workers and may cause illness. They include infection by beta-haemolytic streptococci, which can infect cattle, sheep, pigs and chickens. People involved in the slaughter of these animals may be exposed to ringworm and impetigo, and any cuts on their hands may become infected. (See also under ZOONOSES; *also under* specific examples such as ORF; LOUPING-ILL; TUBERCULOSIS; ANTHRAX; RABIES.)

Meat-Hygiene Regulations

Requirements for the production, inspection, cutting, storage and transport of fresh meat for domestic use and export are set out in the following legislation: The Fresh Meat (Hygiene and Inspection) Regulations 1995; The Poultry Meat, Farmed Game Meat and Rabbit Meat (Hygiene and Inspection) Regulations 1995; The Minced Meat and Meat Preparations (Hygiene) Regulations 1995; The Meat Inspection Regulations 1987 (amended 1990); The Slaughterhouses (Hygiene) Regulations 1977; The Slaughterhouses (Hygiene) and Meat Inspection (Amendment) Regulations 1991 (see also LAW).

Meat inspection in all UK licensed abattoirs is controlled by the Meat Hygiene Service, a government agency.

(See also FOOD INSPECTION.)

Meat, Knacker's

This is to be avoided for the feeding of pet animals unless sterilised. (See MEAT STERILISATION; EARS AS FOOD.) Unsterilised meat may be infested with viable hydatid cysts, or be infected with anthrax or tuberculosis. Even if it is cooked by the pet-owner before use, it may contaminate hands, cooking utensils, etc., and thereby be a danger to public health. (See also SALMONELLOSIS; E. COLI; BOTULISM; AUJESZKY'S DISEASE; HORSE-MEAT.)

Meat Scraps, Bones

These can be a source of foot-and-mouth disease or swine fever infections. (See SWILL; also under TUBERCULOSIS.)

Meat (Sterilisation) Regulations 1969

These require all knacker's meat to be sterilised before being supplied to owners of pets, kennels, etc. In 1982, new controls on the trade in meat unfit for human consumption came into force. If not sterilised, meat must be stained; likewise offal. Poultry meat is exempt. The colouring agent used is black PN or brilliant black BN.

Meatus

Meatus is a term applied to any passage or opening; e.g. the external auditory meatus is the passage from the surface to the drum of the ear.

Mebendazole

A broad-spectrum anthelmintic used in most species. Proprietary preparations include Telmin (Janssen) and Chanazole (Chanelle).

Meckel's Diverticulum

Meckel's diverticulum, of human pathology, apparently has a veterinary equivalent – a finger-like projection from the small intestine, recorded as a congenital abnormality in the dog and found in poultry.

Meconium

Faeces present in the rectum of a newborn animal. They should in all cases be discharged soon after birth. In the first milk of the dam there is a natural purgative for this purpose. (See also ILEUS.)

Mediastinum

Mediastinum is the space in the chest which lies between the 2 lungs. It contains the heart, the aorta and vena cava, the gullet, the extremity of the trachea, the thoracic duct, the phrenic nerves, and other structures of lesser importance.

Pneumomediastinum The presence of air in the mediastinum, following damage to lung alveolar tissue near its root. In other cases the trauma may be of a more serious nature – e.g. escape of air from a damaged trachea, or rupture of the oesophagus. A swelling of a dog's whole face and neck due to subcutaneous emphysema may follow pneumomediastinum, the air tracking upwards. It may take weeks before the swelling totally disappears, but the condition is seldom serious unless trachea or oesophagus are damaged.

Medicines Act 1968

The Medicines Act 1968 was designed to control many aspects of the manufacture, testing and marketing of medicines for human and animal use. In particular, its aim was to bring safety standards up to those already enforced by the leading companies. The Act required wholesalers, importers and manufacturers to obtain licences. (See also VETERINARY PRODUCTS COMMITTEE.)

The Act classifies those medicines which may be sold to the public only on a veterinary prescription (PM), and those which may be purchased from pharmacies (P) and from other outlets (GSL).

Medicines (Labelling of Medicated Animal Feeding-Stuffs) Regulations 1973

These set out the detailed particulars required on labels of containers or packages of medicated animal feeds. The Medicines (Labelling) Regulations 1976 covered the labelling of containers and packages for medicinal products.

Mediterranean Fever

A tick-borne disease of cattle and the water-buffalo, occurring in Southeast Europe, Africa, and Asia, and caused by *Theileria annulata*.

Signs Fever, loss of appetite, a discharge from eyes and nose, anaemic pallor of mucous membranes, constipation followed by diarrhoea. Survivors recover very slowly.

Mediterranean Spotted Fever

A human disease.

Cause *Rickettsia conori*, transmitted by a dog tick.

Symptoms Fever, nausea, vomiting, headache, muscle pain, and a rash.

Medulla Oblongata

That part of the brain which connects to the spinal cord (see BRAIN).

Medullary Cavity

Marrow cavity of bones.

Mega- and Megalo-

Mega- and megalo- are prefixes denoting largeness. Strictly speaking, mega indicates a multiple of 1 million times, as in megabyte.

Megabacteria

These very large bacteria cause illness and death in ostrich chicks, canaries, and budgerigars. In the latter the signs include loss of weight, difficulty in swallowing, vomiting, and diarrhoea. Sudden death may occur due to haemorrhage.

-Megaly

An abnormal enlargement, e.g. of the spleen (which may attain 4 or 5 times its normal size in, e.g., babesiosis (redwater) in sheep).

Megaoesophagus

Megaoesophagus implies usually a pathological enlargement of the oesophagus, such as may be seen in FELINE DYSAUTONOMIA and 'FLOPPY' LABRADORS.

Megestrol Acetate

The active ingredient of Ovarid (Schering-Plough); it is used in bitches as an oestrus suppressant, in cats for the treatment of miliary dermatitis (eczema), and in male cats and dogs to modify aggressive behaviour. Contra-indications are cats with diabetes or genital disease. Prolonged dosage or overdosage may adversely affect the uterus or result in hypertrophy of the cat's mammary glands. (See also OESTRUS SUPPRESSION; DIABETES.)

Meibomian Glands

These are minute sebaceous follicles situated in the eyelids: also called tarsal glands. Inflammation may develop around an eyelash, and later there may be suppuration with the formation of a stye.

Meiosis (Reduction Division)

Meiosis (reduction division) occurs during the formation of ova in the female and of spermatozoa in the male, and reduces the number of chromosomes by one-half, to the haploid number.

Melaena

The passing of dark tarry faeces, usually due to bleeding from the stomach or small intestines. The blood undergoes chemical changes as the result of the action of the digestive process, which produces large amounts of sulphide of iron.

Melanin

A dark pigment that occurs naturally in the retina, hair, skin, feathers, etc. In the skin, it protects against harmful ultraviolet radiation and is responsible for the darkening effect of suntan. It is also believed to have a role in governing the natural circadian rhythms.

Melanoma

A tumour containing the pigment MELANIN. Melanomas are potentially malignant, and not uncommon in old horses that have been grey and are turning whiter. Cimetidine has been used with some success in the treatment of such tumours.

Melanotic

Melanotic is the adjective deriving from MELANOMA.

Melatonin

Melatonin is a hormone secreted by the PINEAL BODY. It is a 'messenger' of day length by which animals recognise the seasons. Experiments in housing sheep using artificial light in winter showed that melatonin levels increased.

An implant of melatonin can be used to stimulate onset of reproductive activity and improve fertility early in the season.

Melia (Dhrek)

The fruits and leaves of this Asiatic tree, *Melia azedarach*, are poisonous to farm livestock. Abnormal gait, trembling of hind-limbs, paresis, and abdominal pain have been reported in the pig.

Melioidosis

A disease resembling glanders, caused by *Pseudomonas pseudomallei*, and occurring in rodents – occasionally in human beings and farm animals – in the tropics. Diagnosis is by complement fixation test and/or identification of the organism. Outbreaks have also occurred in Europe, in zoos. Antibiotics may be useful in treatment.

Membrana Nictitans

(see NICTATING MEMBRANE)

Membranes

(see PLACENTA; BRAIN; MENINGES; MUCOUS MEMBRANE; SEROUS MEMBRANES)

Membranous Nephropathy

A progressive disease of the kidneys of dogs and cats, affecting the glomeruli, and leading eventually (sometimes after several years) to kidney failure. Most cases in the cat are first seen when showing the nephrotic syndrome. There is persistent excretion of protein in the urine, too little protein in the blood, and subcutaneous oedema and/or ascites. (See KIDNEYS, DISEASES OF.)

Meninges

The three coverings of the brain and spinal cord: dura mater, arachnoid membrane and pia mater (see BRAIN – Structure).

Meningioma

A tumour affecting the meninges, and perhaps the commonest brain tumour in the cat.

Meningitis

Inflammation affecting the membranes covering the brain (cerebral meningitis), and spinal cord (spinal meningitis), or both (cerebrospinal meningitis). When the outer membrane is affected, the condition is called 'pachymeningitis'; when the inner membrane is it is known as 'leptomeningitis' – although clinically it is not often that these distinctions can be determined, for inflammation readily spreads from one to the other.

Causes Meningitis frequently develops in association with viral or bacterial diseases of animals, such as rabies, tuberculosis, swine erysipelas and distemper.

In lambs it may be caused by *Pasteurella haemolytica*; in pigs by *Streptococcus suis* or encephalomyocarditis virus. (See GID; TAPEWORMS.) It may be produced through an external injury which fractures the skull and allows entrance to organisms, or it may appear during the course of other head injuries in which there is no fracture. It accompanies most cases of encephalitis caused by viruses.

Signs As a rule the first signs are those of restlessness and excitement. The animal moves about in a semi-dazed fashion, and stumbles into or against fixed objects. Neighing, bellowing, squealing, and barking, apparently at nothing, may be noticed, and at times the animal exhibits a wild frenzy. After an attack of delirium or frenzy the animal becomes dull and quiet; the head hangs, the eyes stare, the expression is vacant. Other symptoms, such as turning in circles, falling over, rolling along the ground, turning forward and backward somersaults, resting the head upon any convenient fixed object, such as a loose-box door, lying curled up in an unusual attitude, etc., may be seen in some cases. Paralysis of 1 side of the body (hemiplegia), of both hind-limbs (paraplegia), or of a group of muscles is not infrequent in the smaller animals.

Treatment Absolute quiet in a dark place is advisable pending professional advice.

Dogs A form of spinal meningitis occurs in which bony tissue is laid down in the spinal canal towards the posterior part of the vertebral column. It is called 'chronic ossifying pachymeningitis' as a consequence. It mainly affects old dogs, and only causes inconvenience when severe. It may lead to complete paralysis of the hind-limbs, accompanied by incontinence of urine and faeces.

In all animals in which meningitis follows injury, the skull should be examined for fractures.

Meningocele

A congenital defect: the protrusion of meningeal membrane through an abnormal opening in the skull or spinal column.

The defect occurs in calves, foals, puppies, kittens, piglets, etc.; it is also a human abnormality.

Treatment is surgical.

In 1 case the owner of a calf stated that it was born with a 'tumour' (i.e. a meningocele) which it repeatedly damaged and caused to bleed.

On admission to the department of large-animal surgery, University of Utrecht, Netherlands, a red soft mass of tissue, which pulsated in rhythm with the heart, was seen.

The meningocele was surgically removed, under general anaesthesia, and the skin sutured.

Three months later the owner reported that the calf was doing well and showing no sign of any abnormal behaviour.

Meningoencephalitis

Inflammation of the brain and meninges. There is fever, pain and rigidity, as seen in meningitis; and muscle tremors, hyperexcitability, convulsions and paralysis, as seen in encephalitis. Most cases result from bacterial infection, including *Listeria monocytogenes*, especially in cattle and pigs, *Pasteurella multocida* in newborn calves, and streptococci in newborn piglets.

Symptoms include walking in circles, pressing the head against a wall, champing of the jaws, convulsions.

Meniscus

Meniscus is a crescentic fibro-cartilage in a joint.

Mepacrine Hydrochloride

An antimalarial drug which has been used in the treatment of coccidiosis in cattle.

Mepyramine Maleate

An antihistamine which is given by mouth, by intramuscular injection, or applied to the skin as a cream. Used in the treatment of laminitis, azoturia, urticaria, etc. (See ANTIHISTAMINES.)

Mercurochrome

An antiseptic, and a stain for spermatozoa. It is a proprietary name of a preparation of mer-bromin, and an organic compound of mercury.

Mercury (Hg)

Also known as quicksilver and hydrargyrum, it is a heavy silver-coloured liquid metal. In this form it was once used as an ingredient of ointments and even purgative powders.

The salts of mercury are of 2 varieties: mer-cur*ic* salts, which are very soluble and powerful in action; and mercurous salts, which are less soluble and act more slowly and mildly. Mercuric salts are all highly poisonous; as organic compounds less so. In strong solution they may be caustic, and in weaker solutions are irritant.

Biniodide of mercury, or red iodide of mercury, made up into an ointment, formed the base of the common 'red blister'. With this and other mercury dressings, it is essential that care be taken, for the drug may enter the system by absorption from the skin, or by the animal licking itself.

Mercury poisoning With the possible exception of calomel as a laxative, preparations of mercury have given way to safer and more effective drugs. Consequently, mercury poisoning is now far less common than it was.

However, feeding seed corn dressed with mercurial compounds has led to the death of pigs and cattle. Three out of 17 bullocks and heifers died after being given seed barley, treated with phenyl mercuric acetate, as part of their feed. The deaths were sudden; the autopsy findings multiple with extensive haemorrhages. Gastroenteritis, ataxia, and renal failure (often associated with mercury poisoning) did not occur.

Deaths of heifers from mercury poisoning occurred after the roots of cauliflower plants were dipped in mercurous chloride solution before planting. Drainage of plant trays, and perhaps also spillage of the concentrate, had contaminated the yard. (See also under SEALS for mercury poisoning in those creatures.)

In Japan, the eating of fish with a high mercury content led to an outbreak of illness, with nervous symptoms, in cats.

Acute poisoning results in vomiting, diarrhoea, and abdominal pain, with death from shock. (Cattle may show only the 1st symptom.) Stomatitis and salivation may also occur. Severe purgation occurs in the smaller animals, together with signs of acute abdominal pain. Lips and mouth may become white.

Chronic mercury poisoning (mercurialism): salivation; swelling of tongue, which bleeds readily; loosening of the teeth. Nervous signs may develop, e.g. ataxia, blindness.

First-aid Give white of egg.

Antidote A CHELATING AGENT such as dimercaprol. Absorption of mercury can be reduced by adding a binding agent such as zeolite to the diet.

A human case The mercury from a broken thermometer, spilt on a carpet, led to severe illness in a 33-month-old girl. Symptoms included loss of appetite, sensitivity to light, eczema, sweating and scaling palms. Improvement followed 2 weeks' treatment with the chelating agent, Dimaval.

Dental amalgam is another source of mercury vapour.

Mercury, Dog's

Both dog's mercury (*Mercurialis perennis*) and annual mercury (*M. annua*) are poisonous plants, especially when seed-bearing. Cows are most often affected. Animals may not show symptoms until from 7 to 10 days after the plants are first eaten.

Signs Diarrhoea. Urine is passed frequently, accompanied by painful straining, and is of a blackish or blood-red colour, as is the diarrhoea. Other signs are severe anaemia and semi-coma. Deaths have occurred.

First-aid The animal should be given strong black tea or coffee.

Mesencephalon

Mesencephalon is the mid-brain connecting the cerebral hemispheres with the pons and cerebellum.

Mesenteric Hernia

(see HERNIA)

Mesentery

Mesentery is the double layer of peritoneum which supports the small intestine.

Mesh Grafts

(see SKIN GRAFTING TRANSPLANTATION)

Mesocolon

Mesocolon is the name of the fold of peritoneum by which the large intestine is suspended from the roof of the abdomen.

Mesogenic

Of medium virulence. Often used to indicate the degree of virulence of, e.g., Newcastle disease strains.

Mesometrium

Mesometrium is the fold of peritoneum running from the roof of the abdomen to the uterus. It consists of 2 layers, between which run the blood and lymph vessels, and the nerves to the uterus, and it acts as an elastic suspensory ligament supporting the uterus in position. During pregnancy it gradually stretches under the weight of the fetal contents, but retracts again after parturition under normal conditions.

Mesosalpinx

Mesosalpinx is the suspensory ligament of the oviduct.

Mesothelioma

A tumour developing from the mesothelium covering membrane surfaces.

Mesovarium

Mesovarium is the suspensory ligament of the ovary.

Mesulphen

A parasiticide which allays itching, used in cases of sarcoptic mange.

Metabolic

Relating to metabolism.

Metabolic Profile Tests

Tests devised at IRAD, Compton, to assist management of the feeding of high-yielding dairy cows in order to achieve optimum production. They are based on the principle that imbalances between feed input and production output are reflected in abnormal concentrations of key metabolites in the blood. To be effective, metabolic profiles must take into account the age, stage of lactation, condition score and milk yield of the cow, and also the milk constituents. The diet being used, and its composition, must also be considered.

As a 1st step, 'normal values' for the main metabolites were established by analysing 2400 blood samples from 13 herds, a base continually extended over time. Then samples from herds with known production disease problems were assessed so that abnormalities in the blood could be linked to identifiable nutritional shortcomings; where appropriate, a change in diet could then be instituted to correct the problem.

Low haemoglobin levels in cows sampled at the end of winter indoor period warn of lack of iron in the diet and the need for turnout to spring pasture, or supplementation, to avoid clinical anaemia.

Low serum magnesium levels can indicate impending outbreaks of hypomagnesaemia; magnesium dietary supplements can avoid the risk. In 1 case where cows were thought to be dying from calving injuries, magnesium deficiency was the actual cause.

Used prudently, metabolic profiles can be used cost-effectively to identify deficiencies – or excesses – of blood metabolites linked to actual or potential clinical problems, which can then be corrected or avoided.

Metabolisable Energy (ME)

Metabolisable energy (ME) is defined as the available energy produced by food after deducting the energy used in the production of faeces, urine and methane. The unit of ME replaced – under metrication – the starch equivalent for calculating the composition of livestock rations. ME is measured in joules instead of calories. The ME energy requirement for maintenance of a dairy cow is about 60 million joules or 60 megajoules (MJ) per day.

Metabolism

Metabolism includes all the physical and chemical processes by which the living body is maintained, and also those by which the energy is made available for various forms of work or production. The constructive, chemical, and physical processes by which food materials are adapted for the use of the body are collectively known as 'anabolism'. The destructive processes by which energy is produced with the breaking-down of tissues into waste products is known as 'catabolism'. Basal metabolism is the term applied to the amount of energy which is necessary for carrying on the processes essential to life, such as the beating of the heart, movements of the chest in breathing, chemical activities of secreting glands, and maintenance of body-warmth. This can be estimated when an animal is placed in a state of complete rest, either by observing for a certain period the amount of heat given out from the body or by estimating the amount of oxygen which is taken in during the act of breathing and retained.

Metabolites

Any product of metabolism.

Metacarpal

This region is the part of the limb lying between the carpus and the phalanges or digits, and in the horse is commonly called the region of the 'cannon' on account of the comparatively straight tubular form of the large or 3rd metacarpal bone. There are 3 bones here, of which the central or 3rd is the largest, and the inner (2nd) and outer (4th) are rudimentary. In the ox there are 2 large metacarpals fused together; the sheep is similar; the pig has 4 separate from each other; and the dog possesses 5 bones in this region.

Metacercaria

The cyst (dormant) stage of flukes such as *Fasciola hepatica*; when ingested by an animal, the life-cycle is resumed.

Metal Detector

This instrument is put to veterinary use sometimes to confirm a tentative diagnosis of a metal foreign body in the reticulum.

Metaldehyde Poisoning

Metaldehyde poisoning has been encountered in the dog and cat following the eating of metaldehyde pellets and tablets used for killing garden slugs. Symptoms may include excitement, vomiting, muscular tetany, nystagmus in the cat, partial paralysis, and stupor. The animal should be kept quiet in the dark pending veterinary aid, when anaesthesia may be required: pentobarbitone sodium, intravenously or intraperitoneally, or diazepam, by intravenous injection.

Metaldehyde poisoning has occurred also in horses, cattle, sheep, and birds.

Cattle An estimated 0.90 kg (2 lb) of slug pellets sufficed to kill 6 calves which had broken into a store shed. In another incident, 10 suckler cows were found dead in a field. In a 3rd case, 3 out of 5 milking cows died after consuming, between them, about 9 kg (20 lb) of slug pellets.

Signs in these cows included a staggering gait, profuse salivation, scouring, partial blindness, and hyperaesthesia. Later, muscular spasms were observed.

Horses A hunter died after showing similar signs (but without diarrhoea or partial blindness) after helping itself from a pile of pellets spilled in a field and not cleared up.

Metaphase

The 2nd phase of cell division (mitosis or meiosis) in which the chromosomes are maximally contracted and the duplicate chromatids align along the midline of the cell prior to division.

Metaplasia

Metaplasia is described as 'the change of one kind of tissue into another; also the production of tissue by cells which normally produce tissue of another sort'.

Metastasis and Metastatic

Metastasis and metastatic are terms applied to the process by which a disease transfers from one organ to another. Often used in describing neoplasia, where a malignant tumour spreads to distant parts of the body, and gives rise to secondary tumours similar to the primary. Thus a sarcoma in some part of the abdomen may spread to the thorax by pieces of tumour or clusters of cells breaking away from the parent growth, and being carried by the bloodstream to the lungs, etc., and setting up new sarcomatous growths there. (See CANCER.)

Metastrongylus

A genus of nematodes which infect the lungs.

Metatarsal

Metatarsal is the name given to the bones and structures lying between the tarsus or hock and the digit of the hind-limb. It corresponds to the metacarpal region in the fore-limb, and has a somewhat similar arrangement of bones.

Methaemoglobin

Methaemoglobin is a modification of haemoglobin, the red pigment of blood – the iron being in the form of ferric rather than ferrous sulphate.

Some methaemoglobin is normally present in the blood; but various poisons can increase the amount found in blood, and sometimes in urine. Administration of large doses of certain drugs, such as acetanilide, can produce methaemoglobin and it is found also in some diseases. Chemically, methaemoglobin is the same as oxyhaemoglobin, except that it cannot part with its oxygen as readily as can the latter.

Methane (Marsh Gas)

Methane (marsh gas) has the chemical formula CH_4. Large quantities (up to 250 litres per day) may be formed in the rumen of the healthy cow. The gas is inflammable. (See SLURRY.)

Methicillin

A semi-synthetic penicillin resistant to penicillinase.

Methiocarb

A snail-killer used in agriculture. Poultry and other animals must be kept away from treated areas for at least a week.

Methionine

An amino acid containing sulphur; it is an essential part of the diet.

Methohexital

A short-acting barbiturate anaesthetic for use in cats and dogs. It is administered intravenously.

Methoprene

An insecticide used as an ingredient of flea collars for dogs and cats. It acts by preventing the young flea from developing to the adult stage.

Methoxyflurane

A volatile anaesthetic administered by inhalation; it is relatively slow in action and provides good analgesia and muscle relaxation.

Methyl

Methyl is the name of an organic radicle whose chemical formula is CH_3, and which forms the centre of a wide group of substances known as the methyl group. For example, methyl alcohol is obtained as a by-product in the manufacture of beet-sugar, or by the distillation of wood; methyl salicylate is the active constituent of oil of winter-green; methyl hydride is better known as marsh gas.

Methylated Spirit

Methylated spirit is a mixture of rectified spirit with 10 per cent by volume of wood naphtha, which renders the spirit dangerous for internal administration. (See ALCOHOL POISONING.)

Methylene Blue

Methylene blue, given intravenously at a dose of 10 mg/kg of a 4 per cent solution, is an antidote to nitrate poisoning, and also to chlorate poisoning. In cats it was formerly used as a urinary antiseptic but gave rise to Heinz-body anaemia (see under HEINZ BODIES).

Metoestrus

Metoestrus is the period in the oestrous cycle following ovulation and during which the corpus luteum develops.

Metritis

(see UTERUS, DISEASES OF)

Metrocele

A uterine hernia.

Metronidazole

A nitroimidazole drug useful against anaerobic bacterial infections, and also GIARDIASIS.

Meuse-Rhine-Ijssel (MRI)

A dual-purpose breed of cattle from the Netherlands, with good milk yields and high butterfat.

Mice

(see LYMPHOCYTIC CHORIOMENINGITIS; RODENTS). Polyoma viruses of mice and mouse hepatitis virus are other infections important in laboratory mice; also ECTROMELIA (mouse pox). (See also PETS.)

Micro-

Micro- is a prefix meaning small.

Microcephaly

Microcephaly is abnormal smallness of the head.

Microchips

In the animal field, the name is given to electronic chips about the size of rice grains that can be encoded with an identification number and implanted permanently under the skin by a veterinary surgeon. The number can be read with a special electronic scanner and lost or stolen animals thus identified. More than 150,000 pets were microchipped in the 5 years up to 1996.

The scheme has been used for identifying the animals re-homed from RSPCA centres and other animal charities.

Under the scheme, a register of the numbers of all animals 'identichipped' is held by Pet Log, a national computer database launched by the RSPCA and the Kennel Club.

Micron

Micron 0.001 mm, the unit of measurement in microscopical and bacteriological work. Its symbol is μ.

Micro-Organisms

(see BACTERIA; VIRUSES; MYCOPLASMA; RICKETTSIA; CHLAMYDIA, FUNGAL DISEASES)

Microphthalmia

An abnormal smallness of the eyes, accompanied by blindness. In piglets and calves it is believed to be associated with a vitamin A deficiency.

Microscope

The ordinary microscope with oil-immersion lens gives magnification up to 1500 diameters. (See also ELECTRON MICROSCOPE.)

Microsporum

A group of fungi responsible for ringworm.

Micturition

The act of passing urine.

Middlings

A protein supplement for cattle and pigs. (See WEATINGS.)

Midges, Biting

Species of *Culicoides* are of veterinary importance in connection with 'sweet itch' in horses, and also with the transmission of viruses to farm livestock, e.g. the virus of bluetongue, and that of epizootic haemorrhagic disease of deer.

Migram

A disease of sheep on the Romney Marsh. Symptoms include trembling and muscular incoordination. In an incident in 1983, MAFF reported that 150 out of 260 lambs collapsed while being driven to new pasture. The cause is unknown, but one line of investigation is into a possible association with blue-green algae in the dykes.

Miliary

Miliary is a term, expressive of size, applied to various disease lesions which are about the size of a millet seed – e.g. miliary tuberculosis, feline miliary dermatitis.

Milk

Composition Cow's milk is a very valuable food substance as it contains all the essential food constituents – proteins, carbohydrates, fats, and vitamins – in addition to a considerable percentage of mineral matter. The most important protein in milk is casein; this is present in a state of partial solution. Carbohydrates are represented by the milk-sugar (lactose) which is dissolved in the liquid portion of the milk. They, along with the fat which occurs as spherical globules, are heat-and energy-producing substances. The mineral matter consists, to a very large extent, of compounds of calcium and phosphorus. These substances are the essential constituents of bone.

The percentages of the main constituents of milk vary considerably. Fat and protein levels are affected not only by the diet of the animal, but also by its genetic make-up. However, the level of lactose is relatively constant (see table below).

In the young growing animal, muscle and bone are being formed rapidly. Hence the food of the young must be adequately provided with protein and mineral matter in particular. Since

M

it contains considerable quantities of both of these constituents, as well as vitamins, milk is an excellent food for growing animals; it is not however a complete one – it will not provide adequate iron in the piglet (see SOW'S MILK) or adequate magnesium in the calf.

Legal standards In Britain, under the Sale of Food and Drugs Act, milk containing less than 3 per cent of butterfat, or less than 8.5 per cent of non-fatty solids (i.e. proteins, sugar, and ash), is deemed to be not genuine (until or unless the contrary is proved) by reason of either the addition of water or the abstraction of some of the fatty or non-fatty solids. (See SOLIDS-NOT-FAT.)

The specific gravity of cow's milk varies between 1.028 and 1.032. The greater the fat content, the lower the specific gravity because fat is lighter than water and solids, bulk for bulk.

The reaction of the milk of the herbivorous animals is generally approximately neutral, while that of the carnivorous animals is acid.

Bacteria Since 1982 the total bacterial count (TBC) has been applied once weekly to samples of milk collected from each supplier. Average results over 1 month, using the Plate Count Test, determined the payment for the milk. The 'cleanest' grade, with an average number of micro-organisms of 20,000 or fewer per ml attracted a price premium; milk with more than 100,000 organisms per ml was subject to a deduction from the agreed price per ml.

Since 1996, the milk marketing organisation Milk Marque has used the more sensitive Bactoscan Test to determine milk hygienic quality. Milk is divided into 3 bands: band A, fewer than 100,000 cells per ml; band B, 101 to 500,000 cells per ml; band C, more than 500,000 cells per ml. (See also MILK-BORNE DISEASE; PASTEURISATION.)

Sediment in milk Milk containing sediment has been the subject of prosecutions under the Food and Drugs Act 1955. Milk and Dairy Regulations 1959 require that before milking is begun, all dirt on or around the flanks, tail, udder and teats of each cow shall be removed, and that the udder and teats shall be kept thoroughly clean during milking. Additionally, milking must be carried out in a good light (daylight or electric light); no dusty material may be moved during or within half an hour before milking.

In order to minimise contamination of milk during milking, the cow's udder should be sprayed or wiped with a disposable towel wrung out of water containing a disinfectant, and the hands of the milker should be thoroughly washed before the milking of each cow (preferably in water containing a disinfectant). (See MASTITIS IN COWS for recommended procedure.)

Lactic acid is produced by the action of bacteria on lactose – the result being sour milk – and is also present in sour cream and yoghurt. (See also LACTIC ACID.)

White blood cells in milk In the EU, milk may not be sold if it contains more than 400,000 cells per ml. Most milk marketing companies impose a penalty if bulk milk has a cell count of 250,000 cells per ml or more;

APPROXIMATE COMPOSITION OF MILK PRODUCTS

	Water	Proteins	Fats	Sugar	Ash
Separated milk	90.0	3.7	0.2	4.9	0.8
Skimmed milk	90.0	3.6	0.8	4.6	0.8
Butter milk	91.0	3.3	0.5	3.4	0.6
Cream (thin)	64.0	2.8	30.0	3.5	0.5
Cream (thick)	39.0	1.6	56.0	2.3	0.4
Whey	93.0	0.9	0.2	4.8	0.5

APPROXIMATE COMPOSITION OF MILK OF DIFFERENT ANIMALS

	Water	Proteins	Fats	Sugar	Ash
Mare	90.5	2.0	1.2	5.8	0.4
Cow	97.4	3.4	3.8	4.8	0.8
Ewe	81.9	5.8	6.5	4.8	0.9
Goat	84.1	4.0	6.0	5.0	0.8
Sow	84.6	6.3	4.8	3.4	0.9
(Human)	(87.4)	(2.1)	(3.8)	(6.3)	(0.3)

some have more stringent limits. High levels of white blood cells in milk are the result of sub-clinical mastitis due to (a) trauma, defective milking machine or technique; (b) infection; (c) both. (See MASTITIS IN COWS.)

Antibiotics in milk It is important that milk should not contain traces of antibiotics, which are frequently used in treating mastitis. Some people are allergic to antibiotics, and if they drink milk containing them they may suffer severe effects, e.g. a troublesome rash and a period off work. It has also been feared that the continual consumption of small quantities of antibiotic may result in people becoming sensitised, later undergoing a severe reaction when given that antibiotic by their doctor. A 3rd danger is the development of organisms resistant to antibiotics, which could possibly give rise to illness not responding to antibiotic treatment. Antibiotic residues can also affect the manufacturing processes of cheese and yoghurt.

All medicines containing antibiotics are labelled with a 'withdrawal period' which must elapse after treatment is ended before the milk can be used for human food. Unless otherwise stated, the minimum standard withdrawal period for milk is 7 days.

Chlorophenol taint Most strong-smelling disinfectants, such as those based on phenol or cresol, can cause a taint in milk, even in very low concentrations.

The disinfectants do not have to come into direct physical contact with the milk, but can be absorbed from the atmosphere by any exposed milk surface, particularly in the bulk tank. They should be stored well away from the milking parlour or dairy.

Similarly, neither creosote nor products containing phenols should be used where they may come into contact with teats and udders by indirect means, e.g. on woodwork of buildings, or in the disinfection of cubicle beds, cowsheds, loose-boxes, and collecting yards.

Plants affecting the milk A large number of plants affect milk or milk secretion in animals eating them, and very often the real cause of unusual tastes or odours in the milk is some common wild plant. Some plants give milk a characteristic taint or odour (such as garlics), and others alter its colour; some decrease the total secretion and others lessen the fat content; a few alter the colour and character of butter made from the milk; and one or two, whose poisonous principles are excreted by the

mammary gland, render the milk actually poisonous. (See BRACKEN POISONING.)

Dioxins in milk Unacceptably high levels of dioxin are occasionally found in milk.

The World Health Organisation has recommended a 'tolerable daily intake' for dioxins of 0.01 nanogrammes per kilogram of milk.

Milk, Absence of

Absence of milk in the mammary glands following parturition, is discussed under AGALACTIA, and SOW'S MILK, ABSENCE OF.

Milk Allergy in Cows

This may develop especially in the Channel Islands breeds, in cows which have become sensitised to the alpha-casein in their own milk. If milking is delayed, they may develop clinical signs of a type 1 hypersensitivity, e.g. dyspnoea, drooling of saliva, urticaria, and swollen eyelids, in an otherwise bright animal. The withdrawal of milk results in an almost immediate remission of these symptoms.

Milk-Borne Disease

Various infections may be transmitted to people through unpasteurised or defectively pasteurised milk. (See BRUCELLOSIS; SALMONELLOSIS; Q FEVER; TUBERCULOSIS.)

Over a period of 30 years, 77 per cent of 233 reported outbreaks of communicable disease attributed to milk and dairy products in England and Wales were associated with unpasteurised milk.

After compulsory pasteurisation was introduced in Scotland, outbreaks of milk-borne salmonellosis fell to 8, affecting 46 people as compared with 14 outbreaks affecting 1090 people in the previous 3 years.

Campylobacter jejuni, present in unpasteurised or incompletely unpasteurised milk, has caused outbreaks of human enteritis.

Corynebacterium ulcerans was diagnosed as the cause of sore throat in a patient from a community that drank raw milk. The source of this was a herd in which 8 cows were infected with this organism; while a 9th cow was found to be an intermittent excretor of it.

Goat's milk, if unpasteurised, may be a source of various infections transmissible to people. (See BRUCELLOSIS; Q FEVER; TOXOPLASMOSIS; TUBERCULOSIS.)

Milk Development Council

A government-backed body set up in 1995 to fund, by means of a levy on milk, research and development into milk and milk products.

Milk-Drop Syndrome

A sudden drop in milk yield in individual cows with a flaccid udder; the usual cause is *Leptospira hardjo*.

Milk Fever

Milk fever is a metabolic condition – mainly hypocalcaemia of milk cows, milk goats, and sometimes of ewes, bitches, and cats in which there is a partial or complete loss of consciousness, paralysis of the hindquarters, and sometimes paralysis of other parts.

In the hill ewe, the condition is colloquially known as 'MOSS-ILL'. Hypocalcaemia also occurs in lowland ewes.

Milk fever would appear to be one of the diseases that is to some extent traceable to artificial methods of management. It is most frequently, though not exclusively, encountered in heavy-milking cows, of the essentially dairy breeds. A few cases occur some hours before calving, but the majority take place within 3 days subsequent to parturition.

Some cases occur up to 4 weeks after calving, but, as a rule, delayed cases are mild – though they take longer to recover.

Research has suggested that the calcium-controlling 'mechanism' is a very complex one, involving all the endocrine glands and both the sympathetic and the parasympathetic nervous systems.

Blood samples have shown that as well as a shortage of calcium in the blood, there may be too little phosphorus and either too much or too little magnesium. This accounts for the differing symptoms in what is collectively called milk fever.

The level of CORTISOL in the plasma of cows during milk fever is significantly higher than in normal cows.

Signs The animal at first shows a certain amount of excitement. She paddles with her hind-feet, stares around in a somewhat fearful manner, may bellow, and if tied attempts to break loose. The pupils are dilated. After a time she staggers on her feet, loses balance, and falls to the ground. When down she may make efforts to rise, but after struggling for a time she gives up and remains quiet. In many cases a characteristic position is assumed: the cow lies on her brisket, head turned round over one shoulder (often the left), and the muzzle pointing to the stifle.

The breathing becomes deep and slow, pulse is fast but weak, the extremities of the body grow cold, the temperature falls to 4 or 5 degrees below normal, and death may follow coma.

Whereas formerly the mortality was 90 per cent or so, it has been reduced to less than 5 per cent in cases that are treated.

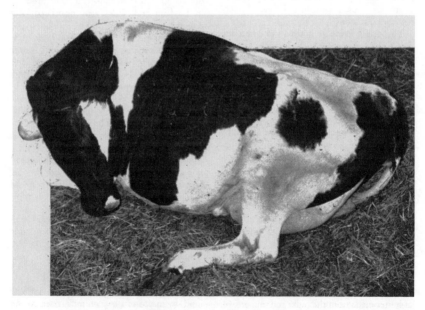

Milk fever: the characteristic posture.

Differential diagnosis In countries where rabies is present, this disease may be mistaken for milk fever – especially as the position in recumbency, with the head turned to one side, resembles the milk-fever posture.

In Britain, cases treated as milk fever but which were unresponsive to treatment with calcium borogluconate were found to be nutritional myopathy associated with low vitamin E and selenium intakes. Reluctance to move, stiffness, and recumbency were the symptoms, and some deaths occurred.

Treatment The intravenous or subcutaneous injection of calcium borogluconate solution with or without magnesium.

When a deficiency of blood phosphorus complicates milk fever, and this does not completely respond to calcium treatment, phosphorus in the form of 85 g (3 oz) of sodium acid phosphate may be given by mouth twice daily.

Prevention Milk fever has proved difficult to prevent. Reducing calcium intake in the later stages of pregnancy, followed by a boost in in-feed calcium 2 to 3 days before calving, has been suggested.

'Milk Lameness'

This is a translation of the Swedish name for a condition encountered in high-yielding dairy cattle, and characterised by hip lameness. During 1 stage they assume a characteristic posture.

Some unthriftiness and sluggishness of movement may be observed in the herd. Animals stop frequently to rest.

The cause of 'milk lameness' is a deficiency of phosphorus in the bloodstream, and – since hip lameness may have several causes – blood tests are necessary in order to confirm a diagnosis.

In a Scottish outbreak, recovery soon followed the feeding of sterilised bone-flour in small amounts. It seemed that the cows had been unable to acquire sufficient phosphorus from unsupplemented grazing.

Lameness associated with a blood-phosphorus deficiency is, of course, well known in many parts of the world – subjected either to drought or to high rainfall – where the soil or herbage is deficient in phosphorus.

Milk Ring Test

A test that has been used to determine the presence of brucellosis in dairy herds. It has largely been replaced by an ELISA test for antibodies to the disease.

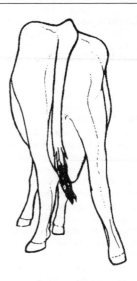

'Milk lameness': the characteristic posture.

M

'Milk Scald'

An alopecia around the muzzles of calves fed poorly mixed, or cool, milk substitute.

Milk Sinus

(see MAMMARY GLAND)

Milk Teeth

(see DENTITION)

Milk Tetany

Another name for hypomagnesaemia in the calf. It occurs at about 2 months old in suckler or veal calves and is usually caused by a predominantly milk diet.

Milk, Unpasteurised

(see MILK-BORNE DISEASE)

Milk Yield

Milk yield varies according to the breed of cow. Average annual yields are: British Holstein, 7000 kg; Friesian, 6150 kg; Guernsey, 4510 kg; and Jersey, 4325 kg. (For other figures see under LACTATION; see also STRESS.)

Milker's Nodule

Another name for PSEUDO-COWPOX (see VIRAL INFECTIONS OF COWS' TEATS).

Milking

(see also under MASTITIS; MILKING MACHINES). At milking time, the 'milk letdown' mechanism begins to operate; it is actuated by the hormone oxytocin which is secreted in the posterior pituitary gland and which is released into the bloodstream following a nervous stimulus. This stimulus may be caused by the rattling of milk pails, the placing of food in the manger, the washing of the udder, etc.

Milking Machines

Their action simulates that of the sucking calf. The teat-orifice is opened and milk withdrawn by means of a partial vacuum applied to the outside of the teat. As continuous vacuum would restrict circulation of the blood in the teat, cause pain, and inhibit milk ejection, the vacuum is applied intermittently by means of a pulsator.

The basic principles of machine milking are, in fact, vacuum and pulsation, and the way in which these are applied to the teat in the teat-cup assembly.

For maintenance of a healthy udder, what is first required is a strong stimulus to 'let-down', followed by rapid milking. As soon as the machine ceases to milk, the udder should be stripped and the machine removed. In practice, attention to this involves the herdsman not having too many units to cope with, not other tasks to perform. Automatic cluster-removal is useful here.

Milking machines can be made to milk faster by increasing the degree of vacuum, increasing the pulsator rate, or by widening the pulsator ratio. If, however, the herdsman already has more to do than he can manage, a faster milking can result only in prolonged attachment. The milking routine must be reorganised to avoid this, or mastitis will follow.

A liner with a hard mouthpiece is likely to cause trouble.

In 1 herd badly affected with mastitis, a change from slack, wide-bore liners to the narrow-bore stretched type resulted in a spectacular improvement.

Investigation has shown that the slow milker is almost invariably the cow with a small teat-orifice. If it is not practicable to cull such an animal, the milking machine pulsation ratio may, with advantage, be altered. At 60 pulsations per minute, and at 38 cm of mercury, a ratio of 4:1 (i.e. the liner being opened for 4 times as long as it is closed) will reduce milking time – especially with slow milkers – without hurting the cow, or adversely affecting the stripping yield.

Common faults in milking machines are incorrect vacuum level, or vacuum fluctuations, blocked air bleeds, unsuitable pulsation rate, and faulty liners. Such faults can lead to MASTITIS. Regular, skilled maintenance of milking machines is therefore all-important. Milking machines should be checked at least twice a year and any faults repaired at once.

During a survey among 71 farms participating in a mastitis control scheme, 95 per cent of the milking machines were found to be faulty. The importance of this is shown by another survey, of a small number of herds with a serious mastitis problem, in which cell counts were carried out before and after machine testing and adjustment. It was found that cell counts fell by about 25 per cent following the 1st annual test, and by about 15 per cent following the 2nd annual test. This shows that the correction of milking-machine faults really can achieve something worthwhile, whether measured in cow health or on farmers' profits.

Milking Parlours
(see under DAIRY HERD MANAGEMENT)

'Milkspot Liver'

'Milkspot liver' is a name given to pigs' livers showing whitish spots or streaks of fibrous tissue – the result of chronic inflammation caused by the larvae of the roundworm, *Ascaris suum*. A similar condition may occur in lambs which have been grazing fields or fodder crops to which pig slurry has been applied. On a Scottish lowland farm this led to the condemnation of 70 per cent of lambs' livers at the local abattoir in 2 successive years. (See LAMB CARCASE REJECTION.)

Migrating larvae of *Toxocara canis* may also cause 'milkspot liver' in pigs.

Milling Mistakes

The inadvertent inclusion of a medicinal compound intended for one species in feed mixed for another has caused problems. For example, lincomycin in feed for dairy cows produced severe diarrhoea, reduced milk yield, and acetonaemia. (See also MONENSIN SODIUM.)

Millipedes

Non-poisonous, many-segmented arthropods with 2 legs per segment; they may be kept as 'pets'. Those wishing to keep them should be informed about their care and nutrition, as millipedes will refuse to eat unsuitable food and may die of starvation as a result. Lesions to the integument (skin) are usually associated with problems in, shedding (dysecdysis); the condition usually clears up at the next moult. Millipedes are prone to disease caused by bacteria, fungi, or viruses. Loss of haemolymph (equivalent to blood in a mammal) due to injury may be stopped by icing sugar, Plasticine, glue, etc. In the USA *Narceus annularis* is the intermediate host of a large, 'thorn-headed' worm *Macracanthohyncus ingens*, which can cause diarrhoea (and sometimes dysentery) in dogs. Hosts of the adult worm are raccoons, black bears, skunks, foxes, and moles.

Miniature Bull Terrier
A small breed with similar characteristics to the BULL TERRIER. Lens luxation may be found in individual dogs.

Miniature Schnauzer
A small breed developed in Germany from the SCHNAUZER. With miniaturisation, certain defects have appeared. Cataract is inherited, as is von Willebrand's disease. Pulmonary stenosis and Perthe's disease may also be seen,

Mineralocorticoids
A group of hormones produced from the adrenal cortex that affect the metabolism of sodium, chloride and potassium (see ADRENAL GLANDS).

Minerals
(see under CALCIUM; COBALT; FLUOROSIS; IRON; MANGANESE; PHOSPHORUS; TRACE ELEMENTS; METABOLIC PROFILE TESTS; SELENIUM; SODIUM DEFICIENCY)

Minimal-Disease Pigs
Those reared free from certain infections. (See also SPF.)

Minimum Inhibitory Concentration
The lowest concentration of an antibiotic that inhibits the growth of a particular bacterial species.

Mink, Diseases of
These include distemper (caused by the virus of canine distemper), botulism, salmonellosis, tuberculosis, paralysis due to a vitamin B deficiency, mastitis, metritis, paragonimiasis, and transmissible mink encephalopathy. (See ALEUTIAN DISEASE.) A vaccine against botulism is available. (NB: The keeping of mink in the UK is longer lawful, except under special conditions – e.g. in zoos)

Mites, Parasitic
Parasitic mites, including mange mites (see also MANGE).

Types of mite The following genera are important. All are minute, and under favourable circumstances just visible to the naked eye.

Sarcoptes, with 1 species, *S. scabiei*, and numerous varieties. These mites live in the skin of mammals.

Cnemidocoptes, found in birds. They resemble *Sarcoptes*. *Cn. mutans* causses scalyleg. *Cn, Gallinae* is the depluming mite and *Cn. pilae* infests the cere of budgerigars

Notoedres is a genus closely allied to *Sarcoptes*, found on carnivores.

Otodectes is found in the external ear.

Psoroptes

Chorioptes (Symbiotes). One species is known – *C. equi* – with numerous varieties.

Drugs to kill them (Acaricides) A wide range of products is available, in a variety of formulations, depending on the animal to be treated and the mite causing the problem. Many are based on avermectins, pyrethrins or organophosphorus compounds (see under MANGE).

Other mites

Air sac mite (*Cytodites nudus*) is found mainly in free-range poultry and, in small numbers, does little harm. In large numbers these mites can result in weakness and loss of weight. They are said to exacerbate any respiratory condition occuring concurrently.

Cyst mite of poultry (*Laminosioptes cysticola*) is found mainly in the subcutaneous tissue of free-range, poultry turkeys, pheasants, pigeons and geese, but has been found in muscles and also in pigeon lungs. The mite does no harm to poultry but an affected carcase is rejected for human consumption on aesthetic grounds.

Harvest mites The so-called 'harvest mite' or 'chigger' is the larva of a species of *Trombidium*. It is microscopic in size, blood-red in colour, and in shape resembles a tick. The mite burrows under the skin of man, farm animals, the dog and the cat, and engorging with blood appears as a red spot in the centre of an inflamed area. In 2 or 3 days the spot becomes a blister and ultimately a scab which falls off. The spot is extremely itchy. (See HYPERSENSITIVITY.) The nymphs and adults are free-living.

Forage mites are occasionally parasites of the horse which live normally in the forage. They

M

may cause considerable damage to the skin, but are usually easily killed.

Flour mites These can cause loss of nutrients in stored animal feeds (see DIET and DIETETICS – Deterioration with storage), and can also be parasitic on animals, causing dermatitis. For such a case in horses, see FLOUR MITE INFESTATION.

Cheyletiella Two members of this genus are of some veterinary importance in Britain, viz. *C. parasitivorax* and *C. yasguri*. These mites infest dogs, cats, foxes, rabbits and hares. In the dog they are most frequently found on the nape of the neck, and down the back. Redness of the skin and intense itching may be caused – the latter symptom occurring in man also. Three dressings, at 5-day intervals, with derris or pyrethrum are recommended; for cats, selenium sulphide.

Nose mites (see CANINE NASAL MITES, *and below*)

Linguatula serrata This parasite has a flat body shaped somewhat like a tongue, but grooved. It is without appendages, apart from 2 pairs of hooks at its anterior end. The adult lives in the nasal passages of dogs, cats, and foxes, and is up to 2 cm in length.

The eggs are expelled from the nose by sneezing; they may also be swallowed and excreted in the faeces. Sheep, cattle, and rabbits swallow the eggs and become intermediate hosts.

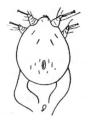

Notoedres. × 70.

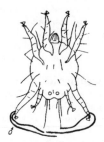

Otodectes. × 70.

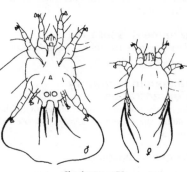

Chorioptes. × 70

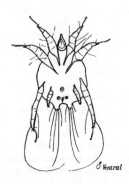

♂ Ventral

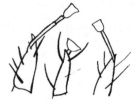

Legs of mange mites. (*Psoroptes, Chorioptes, Sarcoptes.*)

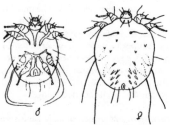

Sarcoptes. × 70.

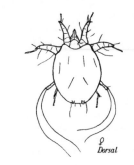

$\female$
Dorsal

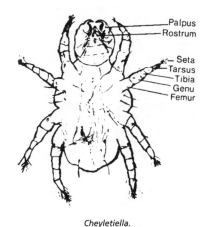

Palpus
Rostrum

Seta
Tarsus
Tibia
Genu
Femur

Cheyletiella.

After the eggs hatch in the stomach, larvae migrate to the mesenteric lymph nodes, and encyst either there or in organs such as the liver, lungs, or kidneys.

The life-cycle is completed when the final host eats viscera containing the infective nymphs.

Parasitus consanguineus. A mite which normally feeds on small arthropods, round-worms and their eggs. It is found in dung, compost, spilt grain, etc. An opportunist infestation of a recumbent cow was reported, and the white mites swarmed over a veterinary surgeon's clothing.

Cat fur mite (*Lynxacarus radooskyi*) This has a pair of flap-like appendages which enable it to cling to a hair-shaft. It causes scurfiness, especially along the cat's back, and is present in the USA, Australia, Fiji and Hawaii.

House-dust mite *Dermatophagoides pteronyssinus* can cause allergies in people and pets.

Mitochondria
Small membrane-bound cytoplasmic structures in cells; they are the main site of adenosine triphosphate (ATP) synthesis in the body (see CELLS).

Mitosis
The usual process of cell reproduction. Mitosis gives each of the new cells the same number of chromosomes as are possessed by the dividing cell, i.e. the diploid number. (Compare MEIOSIS.)

Mitral Valve
Mitral valve is the left atrioventricular valve of the heart, which is so-called because of its supposed likeness to a bishop's mitre. Disease of the mitral valve is a common condition in the dog. (See HEART DISEASES.)

Ml (ml)
Millilitre, equal to 1 cubic millimetre of fluid.

Moist Grain Storage
Moist grain storage, using propionic acid as a preservative (see MUSCLES, DISEASES OF – Nutritional muscular dystrophy).

Mokola Virus
A rhabdovirus with some similatities to rabies virus. It was first isolated from shrews in Nigeria, and has caused the deaths of cats in Zimbabwe, where rabies vaccine has been found to be ineffective. Mokola virus has also proved fatal in humans.

Molar Teeth
(see DENTITION)

Molecular Biology
The study of the structure and function of biological molecules; especially nucleic acids and proteins.

Mollities Ossium
(see OSTEOMALACIA)

Molluscicide
A snail killer. (See under LIVER-FLUKES.)

Molluscs
Formerly, veterinary interest in snails was confined to their role in the transmission of disease. Nowadays, there is a trend to keep these creatures in captivity – for food, for study, and 'as companion animals'.

Molybdenum
This trace element is commonly present in soil and pasture grasses, and is beneficial except

M

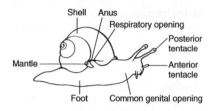

External features of the snail species *Helix pomatia*.

when it occurs in excessive amounts – such as in the 'teart soils' of central Somerset, and of small areas of Gloucestershire and Warwickshire. Here 'molybdenosis' causes scouring in ruminants, especially cattle. The scouring is worse from May until October when the grass contains most water-soluble molybdenum. Staring coats, marked loss of condition and evil-smelling faeces are observed in affected cattle. A daily dose of copper sulphate (2 g for adults and half this for young stock) obviates or remedies the trouble.

Molybdenosis may occur also as the result of aerial contamination of pasture in the vicinity of aluminium-alloy and other factories, and of oil refineries. In an outbreak near the Esso Refinery at Fawley, younger cattle showed a marked stiffness of back and legs, with great difficulty in getting to their feet and reluctance to move – in addition to diarrhoea.

If an animal is receiving extra molybdenum in its diet, it is likely to need extra copper. Levels of molybdenum which interfere with copper metabolism also inhibit the synthesis of B_{12}, the cobalt-containing vitamin, by the rumen microflora.

Monensin Sodium

Monensin sodium is licensed in the UK as a growth promoter for cattle (see ADDITIVES) and as a coccidiostat for poultry. It is produced by fermentation of a strain of *Streptomyces cinnamonensis*.

Monensin resulted in the death of 9 out of 84 beef cattle which had received 12 times the recommended dose. All the cattle lost their appetite and had diarrhoea. Autopsy findings included multiple haemorrhages and oedema of the right side of the heart.

In another incident, 9 out of 40 calves died following accidental overdosage with monensin.

Monensin toxicity has also been recorded in horses, sheep, chickens and turkeys.

Poisoning has been reported in dogs given a proprietary dog food contaminated with monensin still present in a storage bin not properly cleaned. (See also IONOPHORES.)

Mongooses

Mongooses are vectors of rabies in South Africa, Central America, West Indies, and India.

Monilia

A group of yeast-like organisms.

Moniliasis

Moniliasis is a disease due to the yeast-like fungus *Candida albicans*. In humans it follows, in some cases, the use of certain antibiotics.

The disease occurs in turkeys and fowls, and in other domestic animals. It including dogs and cattle must be borne in mind when using antibiotics. A high temperature, loss of weight, and oedema of the lungs may result.

Nystatin has been used – successfully, it is claimed – in the treatment of turkeys with moniliasis.

Monkeys

Monkeys belong to the order Primata which includes about 200 species, ranging in size from the tree shrew, weighing about 100 g, to the gorilla, weighing up to 275 kg.

Two sub-orders are recognised: New World monkeys (catarrhines); and Old World monkeys (platyrrhines), apes, and man.

Monkeys, Anaesthetising

Ketamine is recommended.

Monkeys, Diseases of

These include:

(1) Infection with herpes simian B virus. This is easily transmitted to people bitten by monkeys (or perhaps to people merely handling monkeys with B virus lesions); it is of the greatest importance, as an encephalitis or encephalomyelitis is produced in man, with death as the usual outcome. This infection should be suspected in monkeys showing vesicles on the lips, tongue, inside of the cheeks, or on the body. The vesicles burst and give rise to ulcers and scab formation. Occasionally, affected monkeys have conjunctivitis and a thick discharge from the nose.

(2) Tuberculosis. This is generally the miliary form, due to the human type of tubercle bacillus. Symptoms include: loss of weight, of appetite, dullness; sometimes cough and rapid breathing. Monkeys may be tuberculin-tested by injecting mammalian tuberculin into an eyelid. The result is noted by the presence or absence of swelling after 72 hours.

(3) Pneumonia (unconnected with tuberculosis). A monkey that is coughing and sneezing can be assumed to be seriously ill. Death from

pneumonia can occur within 24 hours, and affect a high proportion of any group of monkeys.

(4) Dysentery due to *Shigella* organisms. This is a common cause of death among laboratory monkeys.

(5) Phycomycosis.

(6) Marburg disease, which can be fatal in both monkeys and man, has been seen in laboratory workers in contact with blood and tissues of Vervet monkeys. Symptoms: headache, fever, muscular pain, prostration, diarrhoea and vomiting, with epistaxis and vomiting of blood.

(7) Rabies.

(8) Monkey pox. This is an apparently rare disease of monkeys. The virus was first isolated in 1958 in a monkey colony in the Statens Seruminstitut, Copenhagen. Cases of presumed monkey pox (resembling human smallpox) in man occurred in Africa in 1970. Since the worldwide eradication of smallpox, monkey pox has become the most important orthopox virus infection of man. Yet, despite a recent increase in the number of cases reported, human monkey pox remains 'a rare sporadic disease'.

(9) YELLOW FEVER.

(10) Measles. This was reported in 1975 in 11 colobus monkeys imported into the UK. No rash was seen; symptoms comprised a nasal discharge, conjunctivitis, cough, facial oedema, and pneumonia. All died. Diagnosis was by laboratory tests.

(11) Malaria. Fulciparum malaria has occurred in owl monkeys.

(12) *Yersinia enterocolitica* infection. (See also KYASANUR FOREST FEVER.)

(13) Leptospirosis.

(14) Simian sarcoma virus.

(15) Toxoplasmosis.

(16) Infectious hepatitis.

(17) Jaundice and blindness (temporary) have been caused by lead poisoning as a result of cage bars being painted with lead-containing paint. A chelating agent was used with success.

(18) Cases have occurred of laboratory workers contracting viral haemorrhagic disease caused by an Ebola-related filovirus and by simian haemorrhagic fever in monkeys imported from the Philippines. (See also PETS.)

Monkshood Poisoning
(see ACONITE)

Monochloroacetate Poisoning
Monochloroacetate poisoning has occurred in cattle, sheep, and other animals. Sodium monochloroacetate is a contact herbicide.

Monoclonal Antibodies
Identical immunoglobulin molecules produced by a single clone of plasma cells (see GENETIC ENGINEERING).

Monocyte
A type of white blood cell. (See under BLOOD.)

Monocytosis
(*see* 'PULLET DISEASE')

Monogenetic Flukes
Parasites that infest the gills of freshwater fish; they belong to the groups Gyrodactylus and Dactylogyrus. In the EU *Gyrodactylus solaris* infestation is a NOTIFIABLE DISEASE and there are restrictions on the movement of fish out of areas where this parasite has been detected.

Monoplegia
Monoplegia means PARALYSIS of a single limb, or part.

Monorchid
This term is commonly used by dog-breeders to mean an animal in which only 1 testicle has descended into the scrotum. Such an animal is correctly called a unilateral cryptorchid, the term 'monorchid' being reserved for the animal with a single testicle (a far rarer condition).

Under Kennel Club rules, a dog which has not both testicles in the scrotum cannot be entered for show; but there is as yet no ban on the registration of dogs sired by a cryptorchid.

Cryptorchidism is an inherited condition (though it has been claimed that feeding rats on a biotin-deficient diet caused their testicles to return to the abdomen after 2 or 3 weeks), but the precise mechanisms of inheritance has not yet been determined.

Monosaccharide
Monosaccharide, or simple sugar, is a sugar having no more than 6 carbon atoms in the molecule. Among monosaccharides are fructose, glucose, galactose, levulose, etc. Monosaccharides have been termed the 'building blocks' of carbohydrates.

Monotocous
Normally producing only 1 offspring at birth, like cattle and horses, as compared with a litter of, for example, puppies.

Monster (Teras)
Severely malformed young are occasionally born to all species (teratogenesis). The cause may be genetic, or disease; or it may follow

consumption of toxic substances. Haemolytic disease, for example, is responsible for abnormal piglets. (See also under TERATOMA; BULL-DOG CALVES; GENETICS, HEREDITY AND BREEDING – Genetic defects).

'Moon Blindness'
(see PERIODIC OPHTHALMIA)

Moraxella
Small rod-shaped bacteria found in pairs. Outbreaks of conjunctivitis and keratitis are often associated with *M. Bovis* (formerly *Haemophilus bovis*) infection. (See under EYE, DISEASES OF.)

Morbidity
Morbidity is the condition of having a disease. Proportional morbidity is the incidence of disease in a flock or herd, e.g. 'morbidity is 60 per cent' in a given group of animals with reference to a particular disease.

Morbilliviruses
These include the viruses of canine distemper, rinderpest, *peste de petits ruminants*, and human measles. (See also SEAL.)

Morbillivirus in Horses
Morbillivirus in horses caused a severe disease outbreak, with transmission to man, in Queensland. Deaths occurred in both species. The clinical signs were severe respiratory distress, panting, high temperature, stiffness and frothy nasal discharge. If the horse survived for 2 days, there were cyanosis and oedema.

The virus is believed to have come from fruit bats; a bat miscarriage was found on the pasture grazed by the horses and the virus isolated from it. A survey found the virus in the reproductive tract of 3 species of fruit bat and 12 to 15 per cent had antibodies to the virus.

Morel's Disease
This affects sheep and is caused by a Gram-positive micrococcus. The disease bears some resemblance to caseous lymphadenitis, with abscesses in subcutaneous tissue and intramuscular fascia, and has been reported in France and Kenya.

Morlam
A strain of sheep bred at Beltsville, USA. The best ewes have given 6 lambs in 2 years, lambs being born in September, May and January – an 8-month breeding cycle.

Morning Glory
Plants of the *Ipomoea* spp. are common in most warm climates. They are grown for their attractive flowers and spread as a weed in some areas. Some varieties produce seeds containing the hallucinogen, lysergic acid. The pink or reddish flowered *Ipomoea muelleri* is said to have caused losses of up to 7000 sheep on some sheep stations in Western Australia. There is a loss of condition, and after a time forced exercise gives rise to a swaying, uncoordinated gait, and knuckling of the hind-feet, with panting when the animal is driven a few yards.

Morphine
Morphine is the chief alkaloid of opium. Widely used in human medicine, it is the standard against which other analgesics are measured. In animals, it is used mainly for the relief of severe pain in dogs. In the horse and cat, morphine may produce great excitement and is contra-indicated.

Mortar Eating
Mortar eating by cattle may be regarded as an indication of a mineral-deficient diet. The animals are probably seeking calcium and magnesium.

Mortierella
A genus of fungi. *M. wolfii* is the most frequent cause of mycotic abortion in cattle in New Zealand. It has been isolated in the UK from cases of abortion; rarely, from mastitis; and from the diseased liver of a calf.

Morula
In the cow, some 5 days after fertilisation of the egg, the embryo comprises a minute spherical group of 30 to 60 cells, inside a transparent shell. This is known as the morula because of its mulberry-like appearance.

Mosaic
An animal having 1 or more cell populations with different KARYOTYPES which have originated from a single zygote as a result of mutation or mitotic loss, etc. (See CYTOGENETICS.)

Mosaicism
(see under ERYTHROCYTE MOSAICISM)

Mosquitoes
(see under FLIES)

'Moss-Ill'
A colloquial name for hypocalcaemia (see under MILK FEVER) in hill ewes. It is seen mainly in the mature ewe, and during the weeks preceding and following lambing. It often follows within 12 to 48 hours of a move to fresh pasture.

Signs Stilted gait, abnormally high carriage of the head, muscular tremors (particularly of the lips in the early stages), recumbency, coma.

Treatment Calcium borogluconate by subcutaneous or intravenous injection.

Moth Balls

(see NAPHTHALENE POISONING)

Moths, Parasitic

In tropical Africa, Asia, and America, a small moth (*Arcyophora longivalvis*) feeds on the secretions of the eyes of cattle; its long proboscis is able to reach under the cow's 3rd eyelid (nictitating membrane). After sunset these moths fly out from their daytime woodland cover and alight on cows' faces. Several moths may be seen feeding from the same eye at the same time, and they are apparently attracted to eyes which are already inflamed. During the daytime the cattle's eyes are visited also by numerous flies, which transmit bacteria, worms, and other infective agents causing eye disease. As a result of their feeding habits, the proboscis of the moth becomes contaminated and transmits infection to other cattle.

A. patricula also frequents eyes, as do some African hawk moths. Their hosts include elephants, horses, pigs, cattle, and man.

In Malaya, Hans Banziger found blood-feeding moths. Some of these take blood from wounds already inflicted, or they take surplus blood left on the skin surface by mosquitoes. Banziger also found what one might call a vampire moth – *Colpe eustrigata* – which can, with its proboscis, penetrate human or animal skin in order to obtain blood.

Motor

Motor is a term applied to those nerves and tracts in the brain and spinal cord that have to do with the impulses which pass from the higher nerve-centres to the muscles causing movement. (See NERVES.)

Mouldy Food

(see DIET – Palatability; also MYCOTOXICOSIS). Mouldy hay or straw can lead to FARMERS' LUNG, and to abortion in cattle. (See ASPERGILLO-SIS; also SWEET VERNAL GRASS.)

'Mountain Sickness'

A disease of cattle kept at high altitudes in North and South America. Local cattle are affected to an extent of only 1 per cent or so; recovery is unusual. Death occurs from congestive heart failure, after symptoms of depression,

oedema of the brisket, and distressed breathing on light exertion. There may also be pulsation of the jugular vein.

Mouse

(see MICE; RODENTS)

Mouth, Diseases of

The mouth is one of the few internal cavities which can be examined by direct vision, so that its examination affords valuable evidence in some cases of disease (e.g. in anaemia, jaundice, cyanosis, and see TONGUE).

Inflammation of the mouth is known as stomatitis, and that of the gums as gingivitis.

Conditions of the mouth As a rule the symptoms that lead one to suspect that the mouth is diseased are as follows: salivation and difficulty in feeding in all animals; 'quidding' in the horse; smacking of the lips, in cattle particularly; rubbing the mouth along the edge of the trough, floor, etc., or pawing at it with the front feet, and much working of the jaws. Dogs may occasionally hold their mouths open, especially when a piece of bone or other substance becomes fixed between the teeth, and this symptom is also present in rabies. (See also FELINE CALICIVIRUS; FELINE STOMATITIS; RANULA.)

Deformities of the mouth occasionally occur in all animals. (See CLEFT PALATE. Jaw deformities are referred to under TEETH, DISEASES OF and, in the case of cattle, under ACTINOMYCOSIS.)

Ulceration The presence of ulcers in the mouth may be associated with foot-and-mouth disease, swine vesicular disease, mucosal disease of cattle, cattle plague (rinderpest), blue-tongue; and sometimes with orf in sheep, feline enteritis, and kidney failure/leptospirosis in dogs.

In calf diphtheria, a whitish false membrane may cover part of the inside of the mouth. 'BROWN MOUTH' may be accompanied by necrosis. A bluish discoloration may be seen after asphyxia or in blue-tongue.

Gingivitis The gums may become inflamed (and often ulcerated) as a result of the diseases mentioned above, of cutting teeth, diseased teeth, and the deposition of tartar in the dog and cat. Actinobacillosis gives rise to abscesses on the gums and tongue, lining of the cheeks, etc. (See also FELINE GINGIVITIS.)

Tumours in the mouth are sometimes seen. Warty growths, scattered over the mucous membrane of the whole of the cavity of the mouth, are not uncommon in young dogs. In addition to papillomas, fibromas, squamous cell carcinomas and malignant melanomas may occur. (See also EPULIS, a non-malignant gum tumour often difficult to remove.)

In one series of cases, oral tumours were removed from 100 dogs by mandibulectomy or maxillectomy. For basal cell carcinomas and squamous cell carcinomas, these techniques gave 1-year survival rates of 100 per cent and 84 per cent, respectively. However, the prognosis for sarcomas was not so good: the tumours recurred in 32 per cent of cases and metastases developed in 27 per cent of cases; the 1-year survival rates for fibrosarcomas, osteosarcomas and malignant melanomas were 50 per cent, 42 per cent and 0 per cent, respectively.

High-energy ionizing radiation gives good penetration of bone, and may be used for tumours of the mouth which are not practicable to treat by surgical excision.

Wounds and injuries In the majority of cases, mouth wounds do not prove serious after any foreign bodies have been removed, for the whole cavity is so well supplied with blood vessels that healing is always rapid. Haemorrhage may be alarming at first, but, unless a larger artery has been severed, it soon ceases. Large tears in the mucous membrane, or in the skin of the lips or cheeks, should be sutured. Antiseptic mouth washes should be applied afterwards. When the wounding has been severe, an animal will often refuse to eat solid food, and may require to be fed on liquids for a few days. Plenty of water should always be provided for drinking purposes. (See also under TONGUE; SALIVATION; TEETH.)

Movement of Cattle
(see IDENTIFICATION OF CATTLE)

Movement of Goats
(see MOVEMENT OF SHEEP AND GOATS)

Movement of Pigs
Movement of pigs is controlled by the Pig (Records, Identification and Movement) Order 1995. All owners of pigs must inform the Divisional Veterinary Manager, MAFF, of their holding. Records of pig movement, including identification marks, must be kept for 3 years. Pigs moved to slaughter need have only a temporary mark ('slap mark') but those moved between holdings or exported must have permanent markings, including the herd identification number. Pigs must not be moved between markets or collecting centres. When pigs are moved to another farm, none may be moved off those premises for 20 days following. If pigs are fed waste food, they can only be moved to other premises under the same ownership, or to a slaughterhouse. A licence to move pigs is filled in by the owner and a copy must be kept for inspection by a local authority officer.

Movement of Sheep and Goats
Records must be kept of all sheep and goat movements to or from the premises on which they are kept; the destination of the animals must be noted. Each flock or herd is allocated an identification number. In addition, all sheep and goats born on a holding must be individually identified with an eartag or tattoo within 1 year of birth, or before they are moved, whichever is earlier. The Sheep and Goats (Records, Identification and Movement) Order 1996, as amended, gives details of the requirements.

Moxidectin
Moxidectin is effective both as an anthelmintic and against ectoparasites in sheep and cattle. It can be administered orally, by injection, or as a 'pour-on'.

MRD (Multifocal Retinal Detachment)
An inherited condition in some breeds of dogs that can cause serious eye problems. About 4 per cent of golden retrievers examined under a scheme run jointly by the British Veterinary Association, the Kennel Club and the International Sheep Dog Society were found to be affected.

MRI
Magnetic resonance imaging (see NUCLEAR MAGNETIC RESONANCE).

MRL (Maximim Residue Level)
The maximum permitted level of a medicine in a food animal's body at slaughter. The MRLs are set by EU regulation. (See also WITHDRAWAL PERIOD.)

Mucilage
Mucilage is an aqueous solution of a gum such as acacia or tragacanth. It is used as a demulcent and to suspend insoluble ingredients in oral medicines.

Mucin
(see MUCUS)

Mucometra (Hydrometra)

An uncommon condition in cats in which the uterus becomes filled with mucin-containing fluid. It is usually discovered at hysterectomy, but can be diagnosed in advanced cases by an ultrasound scan.

Mucopolysacchariomis VI

A rare genetic defect which causes facial deformity, skin nodules and clouding of the cornea. It is caused by lack of an enzyme which breaks down mucopolysaccharides.

A feline case was treated at Colorado State University, using bone marrow from a healthy female Siamese cat, transplanted into a crippled 2-year-old male cat with the same parents but from a different litter.

The transplant was successful, and the recipient's appearance and condition much improved.

Mucopurulent

Containing a mixture of mucus and pus.

Mucormycosis

Infection with *Rhizopus microsporus* is a cause of death of piglets under a fortnight old. The organism has been isolated from stomach ulcers in piglets which, before death, showed symptoms of vomiting and scouring. In many cases moniliasis was also present. Abortion in cattle has been attributed to mucormycosis.

Mucosal Disease

(see BOVINE VIRAL DIARRHOEA)

Mucous Membrane

Mucous membrane lines many hollow organs; the air passages; the whole of the alimentary canal and the ducts of the glands which open into it; the urinary passages; and the genital passages. (See MUCUS; BRUSH BORDER; IMMUNE RESPONSE.)

Mucus

Mucus is the slimy secretion derived from mucous membranes, such as those lining the nose, air passages, stomach, intestines, etc. Mucus is composed of a substance called mucin, water, and cells cast off from the surface of the membrane, white blood cells, particles of dust, etc.

Under normal circumstances the surface of a mucous membrane is lubricated by only a small quantity of mucus. Excessive mucus secretion is the familiar accompaniment of nasal catarrh.

Mucus Agglutination Test

This is used in the diagnosis of *Vibrio fetus* infection in cattle. (See under CAMPYLOBACTER INFECTIONS.)

Mud, Muddy Gateways

(see 'POACHING')

Mud Fever

Common name for an infection, particularly of the featherings of the legs, of horses and goats. The cause is *Dermatophilus congolensis.*

'Mulberry Heart'

A disease caused by vitamin E and selenium deficiency which is usually fatal in pigs. It is a faulty diet for the pregnant sow which can lead to mulberry heart being caused in the newborn piglet; whereas after weaning, the cause is usually lack of vitamin E and selenium supplements in the weaner/grower ration. The disease is mainly one of pigs between 3 and 4 months old.

The main thing to note about the disease is that it is preventable.

Symptoms include lack of appetite, and shivering – especially of shoulders and hindquarters. The fore-legs may be splayed in an effort to maintain balance, and the snout may be rested on the ground. A sitting-dog posture may be assumed. Black spots on buttocks, ears, etc., may be seen on many pigs in the herd. Temperature is subnormal. Distressed breathing may be observed. Death usually follows within 12 hours of the onset of symptoms. Occasional survivors are usually blind and unsteady on their legs. (See also under HEART DISEASES.)

Post-mortem findings include oedema of the pericardium and epicardial haemorrhages, which give rise to the characteristic 'mulberry' appearance.

Mule

The common definition of a mule is the sterile offspring of a jack donkey and a mare. However, scientifically authenticated reports from both China and the USA have supported ancient folklore – to the effect that a female mule is sometimes fertile.

A 4-year-old fertile female mule which appeared to have inherited a mixture of both horse and donkey chromosomes was therefore technically a chimera rather than a hybrid. This mule, mated to a jack donkey, produced a colt foal. This, on karyotyping, proved chromosomally to be a mule. There are also authenticated (by Texas A & M College) cases of a female mule mated to a stallion producing a colt foal with the characteristics of its sire, and which itself sired horse-like offspring.

In the context of sheep, 'mule' is a most imprecise term; indeed, it is a colloquial expression varying according to period, locality, and changes in breeding policy.

The following crosses have all been referred to as a 'mule': Border Leicester ram × Blackface ewe; Border Leicester or Hexham/Leicester ram × Swaledale or Swaledale/Blackface ewe; Blueface Leicester ram × Swaledale or Blackface ewe (though this cross is now known as the North Country mule).

Mule is also the term used for a cross between a British finch (bullfinch, greenfinch and goldfinch) and the domestic canary: e.g., a bullfinch-canary mule.

Mule's Operation

This involves the removal of a fold of skin from the crutch of Merino sheep and is carried out by Australian shepherds for the control of blowfly strike. Mulesing is a synonym.

Multiple Suckling

(see under NURSE COWS)

Multiple Vaccines

(see under VACCINATION)

Mummification of Fetus

Mummification of the fetus sometimes occurs after resorption of fluid from the placenta and fetus following the death of the latter. It is not uncommon in dairy cattle. In sows, it has been reported following Aujeszky's disease and swine erysipelas. In ewes, it may be associated with toxoplasmosis and enzootic abortion. A mummified fetus, remaining in the uterus for longer than the normal gestation period, will lower a cow's productivity. (Cloprestonol can be used to abort the mummified fetus in many instances.) Mummification may also occur in the bitch and cat.

Mumps

Mumps is another name for parotiditis or inflammation of the parotid glands at the base of the ears and at the back of the angle of the lower jaw. (See PAROTIDITIS.)

Antibodies against the human mumps virus have been detected in the blood serum of dogs.

A survey revealed that 38 out of 209 apparently healthy country dogs in Pennsylvania, USA, had at some time been exposed to human mumps infection. Mumps has also been confirmed, rarely, in dogs in the UK. Symptoms include loss of appetite, depression, and greatly enlarged and painful submaxillary lymph nodes.

Munchkin

A dwarf breed of cat originating from the USA. Dwarfism has been bred into munchkins, which have very short legs. They find it difficul to climb and jump, rendering them vulnerable to attack by dogs and other cats.

'Munga'

The African name for the grain of the bulrush millet, *Pennisetum typhoides*. The grain, when parasiticised with ergot, has caused agalactia in sows without other symptoms. A heavy piglet mortality resulted.

Murine Typhus

A disease of rodents caused by a rickettsia, which is transmissible to people, in whom it has been known to cause death in some cases.

Murmur

A sound on auscultation indicating heart or vascular problems (see HEART).

Murrain

An obsolete name formerly applied to a number of diseases affecting domestic animals such as anthrax, foot-and-mouth disease, etc.

Murray Grey

An Australian beef breed, originating from a roan Shorthorn cow and an Angus bull. A first consignment of 50 reached the UK in 1973. The breed is noted for its size, docility, and easy calving.

Murray Valley Encephalitis

Caused by a mosquito-borne flavivirus, this disease occurs in Australia and New Guinea. It affects wild birds. In children it may cause fever, vomiting and encephalitis, sometimes with a high mortality.

Muscle

Muscular tissue is divided into 3 great classes: *voluntary muscle, involuntary muscle* and *cardiac muscle*. Of these, the 1st only is consciously (i.e. voluntarily) controlled, the 2 latter working automatically (involuntarily). Voluntary muscle is often called 'striped' or 'striated', because under the microscope each muscle fibre shows very distinct cross-striping, while involuntary muscle does not, and is consequently often called 'unstriped', 'non-striated', or 'plain'. Cardiac muscle is striated in an imperfect manner, is not under the conscious control of the brain, and has a specialised arrangement of its fibres.

Structure of muscle Voluntary muscle forms the chief clothing of the skeleton, and is the red flesh forming beef, mutton, pork, etc., of the food animals. The voluntary muscles are arranged over the body, the majority of them being attached to some part of the bony or cartilaginous skeleton, and are called 'skeletal muscles'. The muscle is attached at each end by a tendon to part of the skeleton, which it operates, in effect, as a system of levers.

Each muscle is enclosed in a sheath of fibrous tissue, known as the 'fascia' or 'epimysium', and from this, partitions of fibrous tissue, known as 'perimysium', run into the substance of the muscle, dividing it into small bundles of 'fibres'. A muscle fibre is about 0.05 mm (1/500th inch) thick, and of varying length. Each is enclosed in an elastic sheath known as the sarcolemma. If the fibre is cut across and examined by the microscope, it is seen to be further divided into 'fibrils'. Within the sarcolemma lie numerous nuclei belonging to the muscle fibre, which was originally developed from a single cell. To the sarcolemma, at either end, is attached a minute bundle of fibrous tissue fibres, which unite the muscle fibre to its neighbour or to one of the connective tissue partitions in the muscle; by means of these connections the fibre produces its effect upon contracting. The sarcolemma is pierced by a nerve fibre, which breaks up upon the surface of the muscle fibre into a complicated 'end-plate', and by this means each muscle fibre is brought under the guidance of the central nervous system, and the discharge of energy which produces muscular contraction is controlled.

Between the pillar-like muscle fibres run many capillary blood vessels. They are so placed that the contractions of the muscle fibres empty them of blood, and thus the active muscle is ensured of a continually changing blood supply. None of these capillaries, however, pierces the sarcolemma surrounding the fibres, so that the blood does not come into direct contact with the fibrils themselves. They are nourished by the lymph which exudes from the capillaries and bathes the outside of the sarcolemma, passing into the fibrils by a process of osmosis. The lymph circulation is also automatically varied, as required, by the muscular contractions. Between the muscle fibres, and enveloped in a sheath of connective tissue, lie here and there special structures known as 'muscle spindles'.

Involuntary muscle forms the greater part of the walls of the hollow organs of the body, such as stomach, intestines, bladder, etc., and the walls of the blood vessels, ducts from glands, the uterus and Fallopian tubes, the urethra, ureters, the iris and ciliary muscle of the eye, the 'dartos' tunic of the scrotum, and is associated with the skin and hair follicles. The fibres are smaller than those of voluntary muscle. Each is pointed at the ends, has usually 1 oval nucleus in the centre, and a delicate sheath of sarcolemma enveloping it. The fibres are grouped in bundles, much as are the striped fibres, but they adhere to one another by a cementing material, not by tendon bundles found in voluntary muscle.

Cardiac muscle is a specialised form of involuntary muscle in which the fibres are provided with numbers of projections, each of which is united to a similar projection from an adjacent cell, so that the whole forms an intricate network or mesh of fibres instead of an arrangement of bundles. Each fibre possesses a large nucleus which is more or less central in position.

Development of muscle All the muscles of the developing animal arise from the central layer (mesoblast) of the embryo, each fibre taking origin from a single cell. Later on in life muscles have the power both of increasing in size – as the result of use, e.g. in racehorses and greyhounds and other animals that are trained to be fit – and of healing themselves after parts of them have been destroyed by injury or removed surgically. This occurs by development of cells called myoblasts in the same way as muscle is formed in the growing embryo. Unstriped muscle as well as striped muscle can take part in this increase in size, as witness the development of the muscular wall of the uterus during pregnancy. In this case not only do the numbers of muscle fibres increase, but each becomes 3 or 4 times its previous size. The fully pregnant uterus increases its weight about 20 times what it is when empty, and in the course of a month to 6 weeks after parturition decreases again in weight and size.

Action of muscle A nerve impulse originates in some part of the brain or spinal cord, either as the result of volition or as a reflex, and passes down the fibres of the motor nerve to the muscle, where a series of complex chemical reactions occur. The source of energy for muscular contraction is adenosine triphosphate (ATP). When this is split into adenosine diphosphate (ADP) and phosphoric acid, energy becomes available. For subsequent resynthesis of ATP from ADP, creatine phosphate (CP) is converted to creatine plus phosphoric acid – oxygen from the bloodstream being required. (These are but 2 of many complex reactions, involving several enzymes.) (See also LACTIC ACID.)

During strenuous exercise, more oxygen may be needed than is readily available, leading to the so-called 'oxygen debt', which results in panting. This 'oxygen debt' can be partly offset as the muscle makes use of another chemical reaction, involving the conversion of glycogen to lactic acid.

Fatigue The accumulation of this acid in the muscles causes the stiffness of fatigue, which has been defined as 'a decrease in capacity for work caused by work itself'. In large quantities, lactic acid in the muscles can lead to CRAMP.

After exercise, lactic acid is either eliminated as carbon dioxide and water, or converted in the liver back to glycogen.

The importance of a sufficient period of rest for animals which have been called upon for great exertion, such as in hunting or racing, is obvious.

Muscle tonus is the state of partial contraction of a muscle by virtue of which it is ready for work at all times. Tonus is specially evident in the plain muscle fibres present in the walls of the arteries, and it is owing to tonus that such striking and rapid changes in the amount of the blood in a part can occur. If the inhibitory fibres (called 'vasodilators') in the arteries are activated, an immediate increase of blood takes place; while if the stimulating fibres (called 'vasoconstrictors') are acted upon, the muscle fibres in the walls contract, the calibre of the vessels is decreased, and the blood supply is lessened.

Condition is that remarkable state into which horses and other animals can be brought by care in feeding, general management, and carefully regulated work, which is the highest pitch of perfection to which muscles can attain. It is a potential quality not possessed by all animals, and, even when attained, does not last for long periods. In the process of training it is possible by excessive enthusiasm to produce a condition of 'staleness', in which speed or staying-power diminishes, but recovery from which follows a period of rest. Condition consists in a gradual education of the muscles of the skeleton, of the heart and respiratory organs particularly, as well as of the body generally, so that they will sustain fatigue with greater and greater facility.

All superfluous fat is removed from the body; the volume of the muscles is increased, and their elasticity, tone, responsiveness to stimuli, power of contraction, and blood supply are heightened; the respiratory system is made to accommodate itself to the oxygenation of vastly greater amounts of blood in a shorter space of time than normally; the heart muscle – the main pump of the circulation – hypertrophies, and the walls of the smaller arteries – the secondary pumps of the circulatory system – are keyed up to the highest state of responsiveness to local requirements. In the production of all this lies the art of the trainer.

Equine and canine athletes The speed and stamina of the thoroughbred and the greyhound are due to the fact that both animal species can increase, during exercise, their packed cell volumes to between 60 and 70 per cent. Together with large increases in the heart's output, the result is much larger increases in effective blood flow to the muscles than occurs in humans. In the fit thoroughbred, resting heart rates of 25 to 30 beats per minute can be increased to between 240 and 250; and in the greyhound, heart rates below 100 can be increased to 300 beats per minute. Both species also have large hearts for their bodyweight. Approximately 57 per cent of the greyhound's liveweight is due to muscle, as compared with 40 per cent for most other mammals.

Muscles

Muscles, which are collectively and popularly known as the 'flesh' of an animal, comprise the voluntary muscles, and amount to over one-third the weight of the whole body in an average animal of ordinary condition. The total number of voluntary muscles is over 700 in the horse, and more than this in some of the other domesticated animals, so that they cannot all be described here. Each voluntary muscle is named, its blood and nerve supplies are mentioned, and its shape, relations, and actions are considered in works on comparative anatomy, to which reference must be made for further details.

Generally speaking, muscles which cause a joint to bend are called 'flexors'; those which straighten a bent joint are 'extensors'; one which carries a limb further away from the middle line of the body than previously is an 'abductor'; one which has the opposite action is an 'adductor'; and one which causes a segment of a limb to revolve is a 'rotator', or 'supinator', or a 'pronator', according to its position. A sphincter is usually involuntary, but a few are voluntary; they cause a contraction of the ring-like opening which they circumscribe. Many muscles have an insertion distant from their fleshy part (called the 'fleshy belly') by means of a tendon which is composed of fibrous tissue strands.

Muscles, Diseases of

Atrophy, or wasting, of muscles may occur as the result of inaction, diminished blood supply, or nerve injuries, as well as from malnutrition.

Inflammation of muscle, or myositis, may arise as the result of injury through kicks, blows, falls, etc. It also frequently arises as the result of a sprain or strain in the limbs. Occasionally it may be associated with partial or complete rupture.

Signs The part affected usually becomes swollen and is painful on manipulation. The muscles affected are held relaxed, and if in a limb, the foot is rested. When handled, they contract and become hard to the touch, and upon occasion they may crackle or be oedematous. When resulting from external injury there is usually some sign of this on the covering skin, but when due to strain no external lesions may be seen. Occasionally, after injury, an abscess may develop in the affected muscle, but much more frequently there is HAEMATOMA.

Atrophic myositis This has been described in the dog. The cause is unknown, but possibly damage to the 5th nerve due to over-extension of the temporo-mandibular joint.

Signs Inability to eat solid food or to lap, atrophy of the jaw muscles, very little voluntary movement of the jaws, and resistance to any attempt to force the jaws apart. With careful nursing, recovery takes place naturally in a high proportion of cases after 3 to 6 months. (See also 'STIFF-LIMBED LAMBS'.)

Eosinophilic myositis A disease of dogs, especially Alsatians, in which there is hardening of the muscles of mastication and of the temporal muscles. The dog assumes a foxy appearance. The nictitating membrane is in evidence. There may be tonsillitis. The cause is unknown; the outlook grave. Diagnosis may be confirmed by blood smear.

Ischaemic contracture A disease of muscles due to failure of their arterial supply. There is necrosis and the muscle is replaced by fibrous

tissue which contracts or shortens. The condition has been reported in the dog.

Nutritional muscular dystrophy This is most common in beef cattle, but is occasionally seen in dairy cattle also. In calves and lambs it is often called 'white muscle disease'. Muscular dystrophy also occurs in foals and pigs. It may prove fatal.

Cause Animal feeds deficient in selenium (a trace element) or vitamin E, between which there is a complex relationship. Crops grown on selenium-deficient land may give rise to nutritional muscular dystrophy unless concentrates are fed as well or unless the diet is supplemented with vitamin E. This vitamin is sometimes adversely affected by the use of propionic acid as a preservative in the storage of moist barley.

A vitamin E deficiency may also be brought about by giving cod-liver oil in conjunction with rations low in vitamin E, such as dried skim milk powder, for research has shown that the inclusion of cod-liver oil in the diet leads to a striking increase in the animals' requirements of vitamin E. The disease may also be associated with poor-quality food, such as the mainly turnip and oat straw diet fed to pregnant cows during the winter in Scotland. Deterioration of food in storage, and especially of those containing unsaturated fatty acids, may be associated with the condition.

High rates of application of fertilisers containing sulphates may inhibit absorption of selenium from the soil by plants, which in turn can lead to a deficiency in grazing animals. Lucerne, clover, and beans all contain an unidentified antagonist to vitamin E: another point to bear in mind when considering supplementing the diet.

Signs Muscular dystrophy takes 3 forms, as far as symptoms are concerned. The most dramatic form occurs when the heart muscle is involved – causing a heart attack which is usually followed by death within minutes or hours.

When the muscles of the back and legs are affected, the animal prefers to remain lying down, rises with difficulty, and walks slowly and stiffly. The 3rd form is seen when the chest muscles are affected. Exaggerated compensatory movements are then made by unaffected muscles in order to maintain breathing.

The more severely affected cattle may pass dark reddish-brown urine, resulting from the presence in it of myoglobin. This symptom accounts for another name for the condition – 'paralytic myoglobinuria'.

M

Prevention Give the cow and calf vitamin E, or alternatively plenty of good-quality silage.

Selenium supplements are useful; but care must be taken not to add them excessively to feed. There have been many cases of poisoning due to over-dosage in farmers' home-mixes. (See CONCENTRATES.)

Back muscle necrosis (*see under* this heading for a disease of pigs)

Muscular rheumatism is a form of myositis which attacks dogs and pigs especially, although horses and cattle are also affected. Certain animals seem to have a susceptibility to this trouble.

Causes include exposure to cold, draughts, and dampness, insufficient protection against changes in the weather, standing for long periods in rainy weather, and insufficiency of bedding (especially in piggeries and kennels).

The affected muscles are found tense and quivering, and manipulation of them causes such excruciating agony that the smaller animals often scream with the pain when the parts are handled, and the larger animals may grunt or moan. Sometimes voluntary movements in the part of the animal itself excite the same distress. The muscles of the neck, shoulders, and abdominal wall are those most often affected in all animals; the muscles of the lower jaw are frequently affected in dogs; and the condition may attack almost any of the muscles of the body. When the loins are affected the condition is called 'lumbago', and when the croup and thigh are involved it is known as 'sciatica'.

Massage of the affected muscles with some mild liniment, such as soap liniment, hot applications, exercise, and warmth are necessary outwardly, and internally salicylates or phenylbutazone may be given.

Cramp of the muscles is common in animals that are not in a fit condition when they are worked or exercised. (See under CRAMP; also SCOTTIE CRAMP.) PARASITES are sometimes encountered in the muscles (see TRICHINOSIS; GIARDIASIS).

Tumours are occasionally found.

Shivering, stringhalt For these 2 muscular diseases of horses, *see under* those headings. (See also MYASTHENIA; MYOTONIA; MYOGLOBINURIA.)

Muscular Dystrophy
(see MUSCLES, DISEASES OF)

Muscle Relaxants
Muscle relaxants are drugs which produce relaxation or paralysis in voluntary muscle, such as does curare. They are used to facilitate such procedures as inserting a breathing tube into the trachea (endotracheal intubation). They may be used in conjunction with a general anaesthetic, thereby enabling a lower dose of anaesthetic to be used and reducing side-effects. The use of muscle relaxants, however, requires special skills and equipment.

Mushroom Poisoning
This occurs following the eating of mushrooms containing the alkaloid muscarine. It occasionally happens in dogs; the signs include vomiting, diarrhoea and collapse.

'Mushy Chick' Disease
(see OMPHALITIS OF BIRDS)

Mussel, Freshwater
The larvae (glochidia) of the mussel are parasites of fish gills and may be seen as white specks (cysts) on the gill. Unless present in large numbers they do little harm. The freshwater fish, bitterling, may be parasitised in this way but the female lays her eggs in mussels for protection.

Mustard Poisoning
English mustard consists of the dried ripe seeds of *Brassica nigra* and *B. alba* ground together. The seeds contain toxic compounds (isothiocyanates) in non-toxic form. They also contain the enzyme myrosinase which, in the presence of cold or lukewarm water, converts the glycosides into the volatile oil to which the action of the mustard is due. Cattle have died as a result of white mustard seed being swept off the floor of a barn on to pasture. Symptoms included walking backwards and in circles, profuse salivation, and curvature of the spine. Acute gastroenteritis also occurs.

Musth (RUT)
A period of great sexual excitement in male Asian elephants, which become very aggressive during the autumn.

Musty Food
Musty food should not be used for animals' food. It is very unpalatable, and a small quantity can spoil a large amount of food. It is not easily digested, and may lead to serious digestive upsets. There is also a risk of ASPERGILLOSIS. (See MOULDY FOOD.)

Mutation

A permanent change in the characteristics of bacteria or viruses. This is the usually implied, though not exact, meaning. (See also GENETICS.)

Mutilation

This term is used in a veterinary sense as meaning any operation affecting the sensitive tissue or bone structure of an animal other than for therapeutic purposes. (See FARM ANIMAL WELFARE COUNCIL.)

Muting Of Dogs

This involves a surgical operation under general anaesthesia, when the vocal cords are completely excised. It was performed during the 1939–45 war on army dogs. Although considered ethically undesirable, it may be the only alternative to euthanasia where complaints have been made about a dog's excessive barking.

Mutter-Pea Poisoning

(see LATHYRISM)

Mutualism

Mutualism is the association of 2 species as a mutually beneficial partnership. See also SYNERGISM.

Muzzle, Tape

(see under RESTRAINT – Dogs)

Myalgia

Pain in a muscle.

Myasthenia Gravis

A disease of muscles seen in dogs and cats, and occurring in both a congenital and an acquired form.

The former, less common, has been diagnosed in puppies from 6 to 8 weeks old and showing muscular weakness exacerbated by exercise.

The acquired form is regarded as an immune-mediated disease in which there is an impairment of neuromuscular transmission.

Apart from the muscular weakness, there may be difficulty in swallowing, vomiting, urinary incontinence, and depression. (See also MEGAOESOPHAGUS.) Diagnosis can be made with the aid of neostigmine, given orally, which often gives relief within the hour. Neostigmine is also used for treatment, which may need to be prolonged.

Mycobacterium

A genus of acid-fast, Gram-positive, non-motile bacteria in the form of slender rods. Species include: *M. tuberculosis, M. johnei, M. leprae* (the cause of leprosy); and *M. intracellular* and *M. xenopi*, both of which may cause a tuberculoid infection, resembling avian TB in pigs, chickens, mice. *M. phlei* is the timothy-grass bacillus.

In cats *M. bovis* has been reported to have caused respiratory, alimentary, and joint involvement.

Mycoplasma

An infective agent distinct from bacteria as well as from viruses. In size they resemble a large virus and they are filterable, but they can be cultured on artificial media. *Mycoplasma dispar* is a major component in the disease of cuffing pneumonia in calves and *M. hypneumoniae* is responsible for enzootic pneumonia in pigs. Polyserositis in piglets occurs with *M. hyorhinis* and multiple joint arthritis in pigs over 10 weeks old is due to *M. hyosynoviae*.

M. mycoides was isolated from cattle with pleuro-pneumonia in 1898; *M. agalactiae* from goats in 1923. Since then, other species have been isolated from humans and dogs but so far no strain has been found in rabbits. This makes them ideal for raising hyperimmune sera for diagnostic purposes since there are no antibodies to 'native' mycoplasmas to interfere with the resultant use of the serum.

In avian species, *M gallisepticum* is a serious complicating infection in chickens; it is a primary pathogen in turkeys and pheasants. Clinically, some birds will have a swelling on one or both sides of the head; more commonly, air sacculititis is present. Infection is transmitted vertically via the eggs. The number of infected eggs in a batch is small but the disease spreads rapidly among young chicks and poults in the hatcher and during the initial weeks of life. Treatment is by antibiotics such as tetracycline, spiramycin, tylosin or spectinomycin. Eradication programmes in both chickens and turkeys have been successful but birds free from infection must be kept away from infected birds. *M. meleagridis* is a pathogen of the turkey and is transmitted venereally. It causes a transient respiratory condition before settling in the genital tract, especially that of the male (stag); it can cause leg problems in commercial turkeys. *M. meleagridis* is more difficult to eradicate than other species. It is resistant to antibiotics and, as most turkeys are now produced by artificial insemination, an infected male used for artifical insemination can quickly wreck an eradication programme; the percentage of infected eggs is very high compared with *M. gallisepticum*. *M. iowae* is also present in turkeys

M

and causes decreased hatchability. *M. iowae* infection is usually detectable only in flocks that have been freed from the other mycoplasmas. Eradication is difficult but not impossible. *M. synoviae* affects chickens and turkeys, causing tenosynovitis. It may be treated by high doses of tetracyclines. The method of spread is unclear; even biting insects have been suggested as possible vectors.

In goats *M. mycoides* causes contagious caprine pleuropneumonia, as well as septicaemia and mastitis.

M. bovis, first isolated in the USA in 1962, has caused severe respiratory disease in the UK. It also causes mastitis.

M. canadense was first reported in the UK in 1978, and causes abortion in cattle; and *M. californicum* causes mastitis.

In many parts of the world, even where contagious bovine pleuropneumonia has been eradicated, mycoplasmal diseases are of considerable economic importance. They include mastitis, arthritis, bone disease, and keratitis. In cattle, *M. bovigenitalium* is a cause of abortion and mastitis.

M. hyosynoviae has caused lameness in pigs. The pigs frequently adopted adopt a 'dog-sitting' posture; and develop areas of hyperaemia on the hams.

Mycoplasmas are also important as contaminants of cell cultures used for vaccine production. (See also under KENNEL COUGH.)

Mycoplasmosis

A mycoplasma infection. (See MYCOPLASMA; CONTAGIOUS BOVINE PLEUROPNEUMONIA; VULVO-VAGINITIS; ENZOOTIC PNEUMONIA OF PIGS; SINUSITIS; INFECTIOUS BRONCHITIS OF POULTRY; MASTITIS.)

Mycosis, Mycotic Infections

Mycosis, mycotic infections are diseases due to the growth of fungi in the body. Among the commonest are ringworm, sporotrichosis, aspergillosis. Mycotic mastitis is important in dairy cattle and 26 or more species of fungi are involved. (See also RHINOSPORIDIOSIS; FUNGAL DISEASES; SPORIDESMIN.)

Mycotoxicosis

Poisoning by toxins produced by fungi. (For examples of such toxins, see ERGOT OF RYE; AFLATOXINS; OCHRATOXIN A; ZEARALENONE; SPORIDESMIN; T_2 TOXIN; FUSARIUM; PENITREMA; and under FESCUE, RYEGRASS.)

When, in farm animals, a change of feed leads to depressed output, or to symptoms of illness, poisoning by fungal toxins may be suspected. However, when analysed most suspect rations are found to contain fungal toxins in amounts too small for chemical detection.

Nevertheless, there is no doubt that occasional outbreaks of aflatoxicosis, ergotism, and zearalenone (F_2) intoxication do occur in the UK.

In one outbreak, 2 cows became dull and feverish, with bleeding from mouth and eyelids, and died within 48 hours. Other cows became ill, some with diarrhoea. About 60 members of this Friesian herd had bleeding eczema-like lesions of both black and white skin of udder and abdomen. A 3rd cow died later and 2 had to be slaughtered. The final tentative diagnosis was fungal poisoning, after examination of mouldy barley (containing many potentially poisonous fungi) which formed 87 per cent of a supplementary concentrate ration. Similar haemorrhages and deaths from this cause have been reported in the USA.

Mydriasis

An excessive dilation of the pupil of the eye. Drugs which are given when dilation is required for diagnostic purposes are called 'mydriatics'. (See also ATROPINE.)

Myelin

Myelin is the white fat-like substance forming a sheath round myelinated nerve fibres.

Myelitis

Myelitis is a condition in which destructive changes occur in the spinal cord. It usually follows upon viral infections. Paralysis of a muscle or of groups of muscles may occur; there may be twitchings or spasms of muscles; the penis may hang from the prepuce, the bladder and rectum become unable to retain their contents, and finally a form of paraplegia often occurs. The paralysis may gradually pass forwards; the sensation is lost in the skin of the loins, then of the back, and later the fore-legs become unable to support the weight of the body. Occasionally the condition disappears spontaneously, but the majority of cases end fatally. (See also OSTEOMYELITIS.)

Myelocyte

A bone-marrow cell, from which white cells (basophils, neutrophils and eosinophils) of the blood are produced. They are found in the blood in certain forms of leukaemia.

Myelography

Radiography of the spinal cord, using a contrast medium. (See SPINAL CORD, DISEASES OF.)

Myeloid

Cells similar to those found in bone marrow. (See LEUKOSIS COMPLEX.)

Myeloma

A tumour of the bone-marrow cells (see under GENETIC ENGINEERING).

Myeloproliperative Diseases

These develop as the result of the abnormal proliferation of bone-marrow cells, both within and outside the medullary cavity of bones.

Signs Fever, weight loss, anaemia. A veterinary examination will reveal enlargement of both spleen and liver.

In cats the feline leukaemia virus (FeLV) is often a complicating factor.

Myiasis

Also known as fly strike, as in sheep blowfly myiasis, it is the presence of larvae of dipterous flies in tissues and organs of the living animal, and the tissue destruction and disorders resulting therefrom. The condition may occur in cats. (See FLIES and 'STRIKE'; also UITPEULOOG.) Cyromazine, administered as a 'pour-on' treatment, is used to protect sheep against the blowfly.

Myocarditis

(see HEART DISEASES MYOCARDIUM)

Myocardium

The heart muscle. Disease of this can lead to congestive heart failure, which is characterised by congestion of the veins, with a tendency towards liver enlargement and ascites. It results from pathological changes in the heart muscle rather than from disease of the coronary artery or heart valves, and is seen in the giant breeds of dogs, e.g. Great Dane, Irish Wolfhound. Symptoms include loss of appetite, lethargy, accelerated heartbeat, irregular pulse and, in the later stages, ascites. Death occurs within days or weeks. Dilation of auricles and ventricles is seen at autopsy.

Myocarditis, or inflammation of the heart muscle, is referred to under HEART DISEASES, but it should be added that epidemics of myocarditis have been seen in puppies 5 to 16 weeks old in Britain, Australia, and the USA. Spaniels, boxer crosses, Alsatians, Scottish terriers and poodles are breeds in which sudden death has occurred – puppies dropping dead a moment after eating or playing, no premonitory symptoms having been noticed. (See CANINE PARVOVIRUS INFECTION.)

In cattle, for the effect of nutritional muscular dystrophy, see under MUSCLES, DISEASES OF.

Myoclonia Congenita

(see TREMBLING of pigs)

Myoclonus

(see CANINE DISTEMPER; EPILEPSY.)

Myodystrophia of Lambs

(see 'STIFF-LIMBED LAMBS')

Myoglobinuria

The presence of muscle pigment in urine. It occurs in azoturia. In cattle, for example, it occurs during muscular dystrophy. (See EQUINE MYOGLOBINURIA; MUSCLES, DISEASES OF.)

Myoma

Myoma is a tumour which consists almost totally of muscular tissue. They are rare in animals, and when encountered are generally found in the wall of the uterus.

Myopathy

Non-inflammatory degeneration of muscles, such as may occur in muscular dystrophy.

Myosin

A contractile protein present in muscle, along with actin. Their interaction is controlled by calcium.

Myosis

Myosis means an unusual narrowing of the pupil.

Myositis

Myositis means inflammation of a muscle. (See MUSCLES, DISEASES OF.)

Myotics

Myotics are drugs which contract the pupil of the eye, such as eserine and opium.

Myotonia

A difficulty or delay in muscle relaxation after muscular effort; also a type of muscular dystrophy. Myotonia was the diagnosis in a case involving a 9-month-old cavalier King Charles spaniel, which could not withdraw its tongue into its mouth. The tongue protruded from the left side of its mouth. Eating and drinking were rendered difficult. It was considered that the condition was not inherited in this case. Replacement of muscle fibres by fat was the main finding.

Mysoline

An anti-convulsant drug used in the treatment of epilepsy. A side-effect of this drug may be thirst, polyuria resulting in urinary incontinence, in the dog.

Myxoedema

A thickening and degradation of the skin that occurs in hypothyroidism; seen mainly in pigs and dogs (see THYROID, DISEASES OF).

Myxoma

Myxoma is a tumour consisting of imperfect connective tissue, set in a mucoid ground substance. (See TUMOURS.)

Myxomatosis, Infectious

A disease of rabbits caused by a virus. Hares are occasionally affected also. The disease has a very high mortality rate when introduced into a country, but later the virus may become less potent or the survivors more resistant. Myxomatosis appeared in wild rabbits in Kent and Sussex in October 1953, and spread rapidly throughout most of Britain. Symptoms include conjunctivitis, 'gummed' eyelids, swelling of the nose and muzzle, and of the mucous membrane of the vulva and anus. Orchitis is caused in the male. Emaciation, fever, and death follow. The disease is transmitted by the rabbit flea and, mechanically, by thistles. A vaccine is available.

Myxovirus

(see VIRUSES)

M

Nagana

Nagana is an unscientific but convenient name for trypanosomiasis transmitted by tsetse flies (*Glossina* spp.) in Africa. The trypanosomes involved are Trypanosoma vivax, T. uniforme, T. congolense, T. brucei, T. simiae, and T. suis. (See TRYPANOSOMES.) The symptoms of nagana include anaemia, intermittent fever, and (except in pigs, in which the disease may be very acute) a slow, progressive emaciation. In both horses and dogs the eyes may be affected, as shown by corneal opacity. Horses often have oedema affecting the limbs and abdomen. Cattle may abort.

The drug quinapyramine is used (among others) in treatment.

The kudu, hyena, and bush-buck, as well as other wild animals, act as reservoirs of the infection.

Nail Binding

(see INJURIES FROM SHOEING)

Nails (Claws)

A claw contains a matrix with blood vessels, nerves, etc., from which it grows and is nourished. Lying within the matrix is the bone of the terminal phalanx of the digit, which gives the nail its characteristic form in the different animals. When not in use in the carnivora, nails are retracted by ligaments in an upwards direction; this is more marked in cats, where the nail may almost disappear, than in dogs.

Nails, Diseases of

The nails of cats and dogs sometimes become torn or broken through fighting or accidents. Sometimes only the tip is injured, and the matrix higher up is undamaged; in such cases a fine pellicle of horn covers the tip until such time as the horn has grown down from above, and the whole nail is not shed. In other cases infection occurs, causing great tenderness of the part.

Ingrowing nails occur upon the 'dew claws', on the insides of the paws of dogs. These more or less rudimentary digits do not touch the ground, and are consequently not subjected to wear from friction. The nails grow, and owing to their curve eventually penetrate the soft pad behind them. Where actual penetration has occurred, the nail should be cut short and an antiseptic dressing applied. It is customary for owners of sporting and other dogs to have the dew claws removed during puppyhood to avoid future trouble of this nature. Amputation of dew claws can be carried out in the adult under anaesthesia.

Onychomycosis, or a fungal infection of the claws, is a not uncommon condition in cats, and is of public-health importance as a reservoir of ringworm transmissible to children. (See RINGWORM.)

Nairobi Sheep Disease

Nairobi sheep disease is an acute infectious fever of sheep and goats, caused by a bunyavirus, and occurring in eastern and southern Africa. The virus is transmitted by the tick *Rhipicephalus appendiculatus.*

Signs Imported sheep usually show an acute febrile disturbance within 5 or 6 days after being infected by the ticks. This lasts for up to 9 days and then a fall in temperature occurs and other clinical symptoms appear. Death may take place a day or two later, or a further rise in temperature may be shown, death or recovery following. There is rapidity and difficulty in breathing, a mucopurulent nasal discharge and green watery diarrhoea, which may contain mucus or blood. The genital organs of ewes are swollen and congested, and abortion may occur in pregnant ewes.

Immunity In the great majority of cases, recovery confers a strong and lasting immunity. This is also possessed by sheep in areas where the infection is endemic.

Nanogram (ng)

A unit of weight equivalent to 1000 micrograms µ 1000 micrograms equal 1 milligram (mg).

Nanometre (nm)

A unit of linear measurement used in e.g. virology. One nm equals one millionth of a millimetre.

Naphthalene Poisoning

Naphthalene poisoning might arise from the ingestion of moth-balls. In the dog, it has been shown experimentally to give rise to haemolytic anaemia. (In children, poisoning from moth-balls gives rise to 'port-wine coloured' urine.) Another symptom is cataract. Chlorinated naphthalenes have been identified as one cause of HYPERKERATOSIS in cattle; and tear stains may be a symptom of this type of poisoning.

Narcolepsy

Narcolepsy is a sudden collapse into deep sleep. It has been recorded in dogs, and may be partly genetic in origin. A case was recorded in the UK in a 3-year-old Corgi which sometimes collapsed when taken for his first walk of the day, or offered food. Often yawning and a vacant expression would precede a sudden drop from a standing position to a sitting one or a lying one. No excitement, salivation, or convulsions were seen, and at other times the dog was active and mentally alert; he was easily aroused after he had collapsed. Electro-encephalograms supported the diagnosis. The condition has also been recorded in daschunds, dobermanns, labradors and poodles.

Nares

Nares is the Latin word for the nostrils.

Nasal Bot Fly (Oestrus Ovis) Larvae

Nasal Bot Fly (Oestrus Ovis) Larvae are serious parasites of sheep. (See under FLIES.)

Nasal Disorders

(see NOSE & NASAL PASSAGES, DISEASES OF)

Naso-Oesophageal Tubes

Narrow tubes inserted through the nose into the stomach. They are tolerated by many, if not most, cats, and can be used to provide nutritional support via liquid foods for a week or two. The use of small-diameter tubes does not prevent voluntary intake of food.

Naso-Pharynx

The upper part of the throat lying posterior to the nasal cavity.

Natamycin

An antibiotic used for the treatment of ringworm in cattle and horses. Application can be made with a knapsack sprayer. (See RINGWORM.)

National Scrapie Plan

A long-term UK plan which aims to reduce and, eventually, eradicate the number of sheep not genetically resistant to scrapie and other transmissible spongiform encephalopathies. Under the scheme, sheep are individually identified by electronic tag, and blood-tested to establish whether they are susceptible or resistant to scrapie. Sheep identified as susceptible

must not be bred from. Under DEFRA proposals in 2003, farmers with confirmed scrapie cases on their farms will have their flocks genotyped so that the more susceptible sheep can be identified and removed, or the whole flock disposed of.

National Office of Animal Health (NOAH)

Founded in 1986, to represent those UK companies which manufacture animal-health products licensed under the Medicines Act. Address: 3 Crossfield Chambers, Gladbeck Way, Enfield, Middlesex EN2 7HF. Publications include: *The Safe Storage & Handling of Animal Medicines; Poisoning in Veterinary Practice.*

National Pet Register

This provides a service for reuniting lost pets with their owners, and also for third-party liability. Address: Heydon, Royston, Herts. SG8 8PN.

Nature

Oedema of the udder (see under OEDEMA).

Navel-Ill

(see JOINT-ILL)

Navicular Bone

Navicular bone is the popular name for the sesamoid of the 3rd phalanx of the horse. It is a little boat-shaped bone, developed just above the deep flexor tendon, and serves, as do all sesamoid bones, to minimise friction where the tendon passes round a corner of another bone. It enters into the formation of the 'coffin-joint', between the 2nd and 3rd phalanges of the digit. It is of great importance in deep punctured wounds of the foot when these are situated towards the heels, for, when damaged, its surface becomes inflamed, the inflammation spreads to the coffin-joint and may produce incurable lameness.

Navicular Disease

Navicular disease is a chronic condition of inflammation affecting the horse's navicular bone and its associated structures. The fore-feet are usually both attacked, though the condition may arise in only one of these, or in the hind-feet (rarely). Ulceration of the cartilage first, and later of the bone on the surface over which the deep flexor tendon plays, may sometimes be seen at autopsy.

Causes These are still a matter of hypothesis rather than certainty, and controversy persists.

Some authors have referred to increased vascularisation of the navicular bone; others suggest that ischaemia may be responsible, leading to pain and, if at least 2 of the distal arteries are occluded, to chronic lameness. In horses lame as a result of navicular disease, occlusion of the main artery and progressive arterial thrombosis are frequent, with a resulting area of ischaemic necrosis and cavitation of the navicular bone.

Another view is that the disease is not caused primarily by ischaemia and subsequent necrosis, but is a consequence of bone remodelling due to altered pressure from the deep flexor tendon and increased load on the caudal part of the foot – the condition not being irreversible unless secondary lesions such as adhesions and bony spurs have developed. Special shoeing to alter the load on the navicular bone is recommended.

Signs Navicular disease usually develops so slowly that the owner has considerable difficulty in remembering exactly when the first symptoms were noticed. In fact, little or no importance may be attached to the almost characteristic 'pointing' of one or both fore-feet, because 'he has always done that'. 'Pointing' consists of resting the affected foot (or feet) by placing it a short distance in advance of the other when standing in harness or in the stable. When both feet are affected, each is alternately pointed. Later, the horse may go lame or be tender on his feet at times, but with a rest he generally becomes sound again. As the disease advances, he may either start off in the mornings stiff and become better with exercise as he warms to his work, or may become lame as the day goes on. Sooner or later, however, there comes a time when he will go permanently 'pottery', or 'groggy'. The length of the stride decreases and there is difficulty in advancing the feet, so it looks as if the shoulder is the seat of the lesion. When made to turn, the horse pivots round on the fore-feet instead of lifting them, and when made to back, drags the toes. If the shoe of such a horse is examined it is usually found to be more worn at the toes than at the heels. In fact a 'groggy' horse may wear his shoes quite thin at the toes before the heels show much sign of wear at all. In the final stages the horse becomes distinctly lame and unfit for work. When observed in the stable he is noticed to be continually shifting from one foot on to the other, and the resting foot is placed well out in front.

Treatment must aim at the relief of pain and improvement of the local blood circulation. The vasodilator isoxuprine or a formulation of warfarin may be added to the feed of horses; the dosage of warfarin requires great care – with overdosage there is a danger of haemorrhage. Warfarin treatment has been reported effective in about 75 per cent of cases of navicular disease.

Before the advent of drug therapy it was customary to perform the operation of neurectomy, which consists of a section of the plantar or median nerve of the limb. In a favourable case, following operation, the horse becomes apparently sound, although the diseased condition is still at work in the bone. No pain is felt, and the horse is fit for light work at slow paces. The feet require constant attention to ensure that no stones, nails, etc. lodge in the hoof, for even when these inflict serious damage the horse still goes sound, not feeling the pain.

Navy Beans
Navy beans may cause death if fed raw. (See LEGUME POISONING.)

Near East Encephalitis
An alphavirus infection of horses and donkeys; less frequently of cattle and sheep. Convulsions/paralysis may follow fever and precede death. (See EQUINE ENCEPHALITIS; BORNA DISEASE.)

Neck
In animals, the neck is that part of the body connecting the head with the trunk. It contains the trachea, oesophagus, blood vessels, the spinal cord and cervical vertebrae. Both the mouse and giraffe have 7 cervical vertebrae, as do most mammals.

The weight of the head is supported by the powerful *ligamentum nuchae*, which takes the strain off the muscles, thereby avoiding fatigue. In the horse the ligament extends from the spines of the withers to the posterior of the occipital bone of the SKULL.

Necrobacillosis
Damage of an organ, or tissue, caused by *Fusobacterium necrophorum*. The necrotic area has a characteristic rotting odour.

Necropsy
Examination of a dead body (see AUTOPSY).

Necrosis
Death of cells or of a limited portion of tissue.

Necrosis (Bacillary) or Necrobacillosis
(see CALF DIPHTHERIA)

Necrotic Enteritis

A subacute or chronic enteritis which follows a more severe episode caused by infection with *Salmonella* spp. or *Campylobacter sputorum* var. *mucosalis*. A condition of unweaned and older pigs, characterised by scouring and loss of condition.

The lesions are in the caecum and ileum. (See also under ILEUM.)

Cold, damp, dirty surroundings appear to predispose to necrotic enteritis. (See PORCINE INTESTINAL ADENOMATOSIS.)

Necrotic Enteritis in Chickens

A disease of chickens characterised by unthriftiness and diarrhoea caused by *Clostridium perfringens* (*welchii*) type C. There is usually a concurrent defect in nutrition. The disease has been reported in most European and North American countries, and in Australia.

Necrotic Stomatitis

A serious infection of the inside of the mouth and the tongue, seen in calves; it may also be found in reptiles. (See CALF DIPHTHERIA.)

Negri Bodies

Negri bodies are comparatively large, rounded bodies in the brain cells of animals infected with rabies. Their presence can be demonstrated by staining with Seller's stain, among others. The cerebral cortex, Ammon's horn, and the Purkinje cells of the cerebellum are the main sites to examine. The diagnosis of rabies once depended upon the demonstration of Negri bodies in the affected animal. (See RABIES.)

Neisseria

Spherical, Gram-negative bacteria, some of which are associated with eye infections.

Nematocide

A drug that destroys nematodes.

Nematode

Nematode is a general term applied to the parasitic *Nemathelminthes*, which include the round-worms, as distinct from the *Platyhelminthes*, or flatworms. (See WORMS.)

'Nematode Poisoning'

In the USA, larvae of *Anguina agrostis* on Chewing's fescue in immature hay caused an outbreak of poisoning in cattle. Symptoms included knuckling of the fetlocks, head tucked between the fore-legs, recumbency, convulsions, and death.

Nematodiriasis

Infestation of the intestine or abomasum of ruminants by *Nematodirus* species. It is endemic in some parts of the UK. Disease develops suddenly and leads to dullness and loss of condition, with black diarrhoea and dehydration; in lambs, death may follow in a few days.

Prevention As the eggs can survive over winter, the life-cycle can be broken by not using the same lambing ground in successive seasons. Routine dosing of lambs in susceptible areas can be effective.

Nematodirus

Parasitic worms of, particularly, lambs; also sheep and calves. *N. battus* infection is transferred from one season's lambs to the next as large numbers of eggs are deposited on pasture. Development of the eggs occurs only after exposure to cold and moisture. (See WORMS.)

Nembutal

(see PENTOBARBITONE SODIUM)

Neoarsphenamine

A drug effective against BLACKHEAD OF TURKEYS. It has been largely superseded by dimetridazole and nifursol.

Neomycin

An aminoglycoside antibiotic obtained from *Streptomyces fradiae*. It must not be given by injection, owing to resulting kidney damage. Its action closely resembles that of streptomycin. It is used, sometimes in combination with other medicaments, in a number of veterinary formulations. A topical spray of this antibiotic has caused profound deafness in children. (See DEAFNESS.)

Neonatal

Neonatal diseases are those of the newborn.

Neoplasm

Neoplasm means literally 'a new growth', and is applied to tumours in general.

Neospora Caninum

This parasite was discovered in Norway in 1984, and later recognised in Sweden, the USA, Australia, and the UK in 1990.

Cause A protozoan, named as above, and resembling *Toxoplasma gondii*. Congenital infection occurs in cattle, dogs, and cats.

Signs Infected animals may develop ataxia, a fleeting paralysis, and nystagmus. Meningitis appears in some cases. The parasite may also be found in aborted ovine fetuses.

Neoteny
The retention of juvenile activities and appearance into adulthood. It is the basis of popularity of some breeds of dog that remain as playful as puppies throughout their life. The extreme example is an amphibian, the axolotl or Mexican walking fish, which rarely matures to the adult stage.

Nephrectomy
Nephrectomy is the name given to the operation by which one of the kidneys is removed. (See KIDNEY, DISEASES OF.)

Nephritis
Inflammation of the kidneys (see KIDNEY, DISEASES OF; LEPTOSPIROSIS).

Nephrolithiasis
The presence of a stone (calculus) in the pelvis of the kidney.

Nephron
The structural unit of the kidney (see KIDNEYS).

Nephroptosis
'Floating kidney' – abnormal positioning of the kidney (see KIDNEY, DISEASES OF).

Nephrosis
This is a disease of the kidneys, involving damage to the tubules. It leads to albuminuria and often to oedema. (See also KIDNEY, DISEASES OF.)

Nephrosis, Infectious Avian
A disease of chickens. (See GUMBORO DISEASE; INFECTIOUS BURSAL DISEASE.)

Nephrotic Syndrome
(see NEPHROSIS)

Nephrotomy
Surgical incision into a kidney.

Nerve Block
Anaesthesia of a nerve or nerves supplying part of the body to assist diagnosis or treatment. Often used in diagnosing the cause of lameness in the horse.

Nerves
The nerves are fibre-like tissues that convey impulses ('messages') between the central nervous system and other parts of the body. The basic unit of the nervous system is the neuron, a cell with at least 1 projection. Bipolar neurons have 1 long projection, the axon, and 1 short branching projection, the dendrite. A typical neuron (multipolar) has several dendrites but usually only 1 axon (nerve fibre).

Dendrites conduct nerve impulses towards the nerve cell; axons conduct away from it.

A synapse is a point or area where 1 neuron is able to make contact with another; the contact being between the axon of 1 neuron and a dendrite of another neuron, or between the axon of 1 neuron and the cell of another neuron. Any neuron may connect with axons or dendrites of several other neurons.

Nerve fibres may be myelinated (enclosed in a sheath) or unmyelinated (see MYELIN). Some nerve fibres (axons) convey impulses to brain or spinal cord from skin or sense organ, and are termed sensory or afferent. Their impulses are passed, through connecting links or interneurons, to motor or efferent nerves from brain or spinal cord (*but see* spinal reflex under SPINAL CORD – Functions).

Nerve impulses are dependent upon the permeability of cell membranes. There is a potential difference of about 70 to 80 millivolts between the inside and the outside of an axon – the inside being the negative. This is owing to the fact that in a resting state the cell membrane is permeable to $K(+)$ and $Cl(-)$ ions, but not to $Na(+)$ ions. Stimulation of the nerve results in the membrane becoming permeable to the sodium ions, which flow in causing the inside of the axon to carry a positive electrical charge instead of a negative one. A so-called depolarisation wave is set up, 'self-perpetuating', along 1 neuron after another. A single nerve fibre can send about 1000 separate impulses per second.

ACETYLCHOLINE is released by somatic (muscle) nerve fibres at synapses between neurons on either side of ganglia, and also at the junction of motor nerve endings and voluntary (striated) muscle. Acetylcholine is released also at synapses by parasympathetic nerve fibres. NORADRENALIN is released at synapses of sympathetic nerve fibres, and at their junction with smooth (unstriated) involuntary muscle fibres.

Nerves, Injuries to
Continued or repeated severe pressure upon a nerve trunk may be sufficient to damage it and result in paralysis; severe bruising in which a nerve is driven against a bone with considerable force may produce paralysis or inflammation of the nerve; a nerve may be severed along with

other tissues in a deep wound; fracture of a bone, such as the 1st rib, may produce rupture of any nerves that lie upon or near to it; and other accidents may also involve the nerves of the part. A nerve may sometimes be injured at its origin before it leaves the brain or spinal cord by haemorrhage. (See also under IMMUNISATION.)

Signs Sometimes, it is not until after a wound has healed that the injury to the nerve becomes obvious. In 'radial paralysis', or in other cases where large and important motor nerves have been damaged, the resulting paralysis of the muscles they supply is seen at once. (See RADIAL PARALYSIS.) Atrophy of muscles results.

(See FACIAL PARALYSIS for another example of a nerve injury.)

A tumour, such as a neurofibrosarcoma or (in the cat) a lymphosarcoma, may press upon or infiltrate the brachial plexus causing progressive lameness and pain. (See BRACHIAL.) Another tumour is a NEUROMA.

If a nerve is cut, the distal part degenerates. This is called Wallerian degeneration.

Neuritis (*see under* this heading)

Nervous System
(see CENTRAL NERVOUS SYSTEM)

Nervous System, Diseases of
(see BRAIN, DISEASES OF; ENCEPHALITIS; BOTULISM; CHOREA; DISTEMPER; CANINE VIRAL HEPATITIS; TETANUS; RABIES; SPINAL CORD; LISTERIOSIS; etc.)

Nettle-Rash
(see URTICARIA)

Neurectomy
Neurectomy is an operation in which part of a nerve is excised. The operation is sometimes performed to give relief from incurable lameness in the horse, but only a few months' work may be gained.

Neurilemma
Neurilemma is the thin membranous covering of nerve fibres.

Neuritis
Inflammation affecting nerves or their sheaths. It is often accompanied by pain (neuralgia), sometimes by spastic paralysis. Causes include viral infections, allergies, malnutrition, and poisoning, as well as physical injuries. (See NEUROMA; NERVES, INJURIES TO; and under IMMUNISATION.)

Neuroglia
A fine web of tissue and branching cells which supports the nerve fibres and cells of the nervous system.

Neuroleptanalgesia
A state of combined sedation and analgesia. It is used for carrying out minor surgical procedures where full anaesthesia is not required. A combination of a sedative, e.g. acepromazine, and a powerful analgesic, e.g. pethidine, is used.

Neuroma
A tumour connected with a nerve, and very painful.

Neuron
Neuron is a single unit of the nervous system, consisting of 1 nerve cell, with all its processes. (*See* illustration and also NERVES.)

Neurotropic Virus
Neurotropic virus is one which shows a predilection for becoming localised in, and fixing itself to, nerve tissues. The best known of these is that of rabies. Rabies virus enters the body through torn nerve fibres at the seat of an

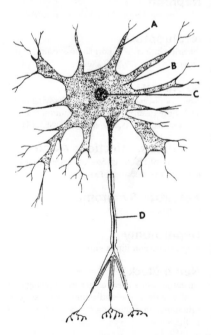

A typical neuron: A – dentrites, B – nerve cell body, C – nucleus, and D – axon. (After Francis, *Introduction to Human Anatomy*, courtesy of C. V. Mosby Co.)

injury, such as a bite, and, growing along them, eventually reaches the spinal cord and brain. Other neurotropic viruses are those of louping-ill in sheep, and Borna disease in horses and cattle.

Neutering
(see CASTRATION and SPAYING; also VASECTOMY)

Neutrons
Elementary particles with approximately the same mass as a proton. The latter has been defined as a stable, positively charged elementary particle found in atomic nuclei in numbers equal to its atomic number.

Neutropenia
A reduced number of neutrophil granular leukocytes in the blood.

(In human medicine, most cases are attributed to the direct toxic effect of certain antibiotics, e.g. penicillin and the cephalosporins, or to immune-mediated mechanisms. With this type of blood dyscrasia patients are at serious risk of an overwhelming infection.)

Neutrophil
A type of white blood cell which can migrate into the tissues and engulf bacteria, etc. (See under BLOOD; ABSCESS.)

New Forest Disease (Infectious Bovine Keratitis)
A painful eye condition which can lead to blindness if neglected. (See EYE, DISEASES OF.)

New Forest Fly
A blood-sucking fly, found in many parts of Britain. *Hippobosca equina* attacks horses and cattle. It deposits larvae (not eggs) in the soil. When disturbed, it makes a characteristic sideways movement. (See FLIES.)

Newcastle Disease
An infectious, febrile notifiable disease of chickens, turkeys, ducks, pigeons and wild birds. Globally, it is the most economically important disease of livestock. Aviary birds, particularly finches (canaries, etc.), may be infected by wind spread. Waterfowl can be infected but clinical disease is rare. In humans, conjunctivitis is the main clinical sign, but people working with infected birds may develop an influenza-like illness.

Cause Paramyxovirus.

Signs The first sign noticed in laying birds may be a drop in egg yield with the production of pale, misshapen and/or soft-shelled eggs. According to the virus strain, infected birds develop respiratory or nervous signs; it is rare to find both together. Severe breathing difficulties develop in birds affected with the respiratory strain. In the nervous form, torticollis, paralysis of the wings or legs and impaction of the intestine are features. In mild cases, the main clinical sign may be diarrhoea, usually black. Mortality varies. Egg production may recover, but not to its former level.

Control Live and inactivated vaccines are used. Vaccination regimes can vary according to local circumstances and must be established on the basis of veterinary advice; the manufacturer may need to be consulted. Live vaccines include the Hitchner B1; they are administered in the drinking water, by beak-dipping, by eye-dropper or by aerosol spray. The manufacturer's directions must be strictly followed in each case. The inactivated vaccine is used for secondary vaccination after primary immunisation with live vaccine. It is administered intramuscularly into the thigh muscle or subcutaneously into the back of the neck.

It should always be assumed that, in the vicinity of an outbreak, every flock to be vaccinated is incubating the disease. The incubation period is around 21 days and it takes 10 to 14 days to build up an immunity.

Newfoundland
A large breed of dog developed in Canada to rescue people from rivers and the sea; it is a powerful swimmer. It is long-haired and usually black or brown. Hip dysplasia, aortic stenosis, ununited anconeal process and osteochondritis may be inherited.

'Newmarket Cough'
(see EQUINE INFLUENZA; COUGH)

Niacin (Nicotinic Acid)
One of the vitamin B group, present in most animal feeds, and produced in the digestive system from tryptophan. With maize feeding, a niacin deficiency may occur. It has been suggested that niacin supplements benefit dairy cows, as synthesis of the vitamin in the rumen may not be sufficient, which was formerly thought to be the case. In dogs a niacin deficiency causes 'BLACK TONGUE'. (See SHEEPDOGS; VITAMINS.)

Nicking
This is defined in the Docking and Nicking of Horses Act 1949 as 'the deliberate severing of

any tendon or muscle in the tail of a horse'. The practice is illegal.

Nicotine Poisoning

Nicotine poisoning has killed cattle dressed with nicotine against warbles, and may also arise from the old practice by shepherds of dosing their flocks with tobacco against parasitic worms. Poisoning has also been reported in poultry when perches have been painted with nicotine sulphate to try to control red mite (*Dermanyssus galinae*).

Nicotinic Acid

One of the vitamin B group present naturally in the body and convertible to NIACIN.

Nictitating Membrane

The '3rd eyelid', or haw, consists of a plate of cartilage covered with conjunctiva, and having lymphatic tissue and the Harderian gland. Often pigmented, the membrane is always prominent in breeds of dogs such as the bloodhound and St Bernard. In other breeds of dog, and in the cat, its protrusion across part of the eye may indicate general debility if bilateral; other causes include the presence of a foreign body, ulceration, a nerve injury, or occasionally a tumour.

'Night Blindness'

'Night blindness' is seen in vitamin A deficiency and early progressive retinal atrophy (see EYE, DISEASES OF).

NIGHT LIGHTING

Night lighting is commonly practised in poultry houses, using 40-watt lamps to give a 14-hour day, or 1500-watt lamps for three 20-second exposures a night. The object is increased egg production during the winter months, and the effect is due not merely to the provision of extra feeding-time, but also to the influence of light indirectly on the ovaries. However, an investigation carried out in conjunction with the ADAS into eye abnormalities in turkey breeding flocks, leading to blindness, showed that the cause was continuous artificial light. Seventy per cent of poults showed symptoms after 5 weeks of this, and it was proved that it was the continuity and not the intensity of the light which was doing the damage.

NIGHTSHADE POISONING

The nightshades comprise garden or black nightshade (*Solanum nigrum*), woody nightshade or bittersweet (*S. dulcamara*), and deadly nightshade or belladonna (*Atropa belladonna*).

(See GARDEN NIGHTSHADE POISONING; BITTERSWEET; and ATROPINE POISONING).

Nigroid Bodies

Nigroid bodies are black or brown irregular outgrowths from the edges of the iris of the horse's eye. (See IRIS.)

Nipah Virus

Nipah virus is responsible for a disease of pigs in tropical areas. It causes fever, nervous signs, respiratory difficulties and abortions. An outbreak of encephalitis among pig farmers in Malaysia, caused by the virus, resulted in the slaughter of 1.1 million pigs (out of a total pig population of 2.4 million) on 956 farms in an effort to control the outreak. Only 796 pig farms remained. Of 256 people who suffered from encephalitis, 105 died. The infection is thought to have originated in flying foxes.

Nipple-Drinkers

Nipple-drinkers are popular in pig and poultry enterprises as they supply water on demand without using troughs, and avoiding the possiblity of drinking water being fouled. Similar drinkers are available for use by dogs in kennels. Animals may have to be taught how to use them.

Nipples

Infection and necrosis of sows' nipples are not uncommonly caused by *Fusiformis netrophorus*, and may lead to the death of piglets from starvation. (See also MAMILLA – Mamillitis.)

Nit

Egg of louse or other parasitic insect.

Nitrite Poisoning

Poisoning as a result of eating plants with a high potassium nitrate content is common in some of the western parts of the USA. The nitrate is reduced to nitrite by substances within the plant under certain climatic conditions, and when such a plant is eaten the nitrite is rapidly absorbed from the digestive system and converts haemoglobin into methaemoglobin. This is incapable of giving up its oxygen to the tissues and as a result the animal dies.

Sodium nitrite is used for curing meat and has found its way into swill, causing fatal poisoning in pigs. The main symptoms observed were vomiting, squealing, and distressed breathing. Nitrite poisoning has also occurred, in piggeries with poor ventilation, from condensation dripping down. It may arise, too, in grazing animals where nitrogenous fertilisers have been spread during dry weather, or before rain has had time to wash it all in. This could be called nitrate poisoning, but the nitrate itself has a fairly low toxicity, being converted into the poisonous nitrite. The nitrate content of heavily fertilised plants may increase the animal's intake of nitrates.

Treatment consists of methylene blue intravenously, and ascorbic acid. (See NITROSAMINES.)

Signs include abdominal pain, sometimes diarrhoea, weakness and ataxia, dyspnoea, rapid heart action and, especially, cyanosis. The mucous membranes appear brown, due to the presence of methaemoglobin. Convulsions, coma, and death may follow.

In a case reported by the State Veterinary Service, acute poisoning was seen in 13 cows after they had been brought into a shed. An hour or two later, 2 were dead, 2 were dying and 9 were very distressed, showing dyspnoea, salivation, cramping pains and head-pressing. Their blood was dark brown. The local hospital was asked to make up a 4 per cent solution of methylene blue, which they did within 15 minutes. When each cow was injected intravenously with 500 ml, the response was dramatic and reminiscent of that seen in the successful treatment of milk fever with calcium. Sequelae of this event were abortion in 2 of the cows and a change in temperament, normally quiet cows becoming wild. The source of the nitrate was believed to be straw bedding contaminated with fertiliser from broken bags.

Fatal nitrite poisoning of pigs has occurred following the use, for drinking purposes, of rainwater containing decaying organic matter.

Nitrites

Nitrites are salts which, in excess, convert haemoglobin into methaemoglobin, and may cause death from lack of oxygen. (See NITRITE POISONING; NITROSAMINES.)

Nitrofurans

A group of drugs developed in the USA during the 1940s, and including nitrofurazone, furazolidone, and nitrofurantoin (for urinary tract infections). They are effective against a wide range of bacteria, including Gram-negative; some against protozoa and fungi. It is thought that they interfere with the carbohydrate metabolism of micro-organisms. The use of furazolidone and nitrofurantoin for medicines in food-producing animals is prohibited in the EU.

Nitrogen

(see AIR). For liquid nitrogen see CRYOSURGERY; ARTIFICIAL INSEMINATION; LIFE AFTER FREEZING.

Nitrogen dioxide

A reddish-brown heavy gas with an offensive odour. This is formed by oxidation, on exposure to air, from the colourless nitric oxide. The latter appears to be the chief oxide of nitrogen produced in the early stages of silage-making.

Emissions of this gas from silage clamps have caused human illness and the death of farm animals.

Signs Dyspnoea, cyanosis, muscular weakness and, in piglets, vomiting.

Nitrophenide Poisoning

Nitrophenide poisoning, characterised by paralysis, has occurred in pigs fed medicated meal intended for poultry and containing nitrophenide as a treatment for coccidiosis.

Nitrosamines

They are very powerful chemical carcinogens. They cause cancer of specific organs irrespective of the route of administration. Some nitrosamines can be formed from nitrite and secondary amine or amide in the acid stomach contents of animals. Nitrites used as food preservatives, and high levels of nitrates in drinking water, can be carcinogens.

Nitroscanate

A general anthelmintic for use in dogs. It acts against both tapeworms and roundworms.

Nitrothiazole

The drug 2-amino-5-nitrothiazole is effective in controlling blackhead in turkeys (by preventive medication).

Nitrous Oxide

This anaesthetic is not much used in veterinary practice but, where it is, there is a need for good ventilation, as it interferes with vitamin B metabolism and, in a pregnant anaesthetist, may bring about a miscarriage.

Nitroxynil

Nitroxynil, a fasciolicide, is used by injection for the treatment of fluke in cattle and sheep and, given by mouth, against gapeworm in birds. Animals must not be slaughtered for meat until 30 days after administration.

NOAH

(see NATIONAL OFFICE OF ANIMAL HEALTH)

Nocardiosis

Infection with *Nocardia asteroides* in cattle, dogs, cats, and man. It is a saprophytic inhabitant of the soil and belongs to the genus *Actinomycetes*. It was formerly classified as a fungus but is now regarded as a bacterium. It has occasionally been isolated from the udders of cows affected with mastitis, and has been reported as the cause of 'incurable mastitis' in an outbreak on a Texas farm. Involvement of the liver and mesentery, with marked loss of condition, thirst, and some diarrhoea – calling for euthanasia – has been recorded in the dog in Britain. Pleuropneumonia, occasionally also a skin infection, may result from *Nocardia* in dogs and cats.

Node

(see LYMPH NODES)

Nodular Panniculitis

An inflammatory reaction involving subcutaneous fat, and characterised by nodules which burst. Abscesses and sloughing may occur. (See AUTO-IMMUNE DISEASE, of which the above is an example, occurring in dogs.)

Noise

(see STRESS)

Noradrenalin

A hormone secreted by the adrenal gland medulla. It causes increased heart rate, and constricts the blood vessels, causing a rise in blood pressure. (See NERVES.)

Normal Saline (Physiological Saline)

Normal saline (Physiological saline) is a solution of sodium chloride in sterile distilled water, which is isotonic with the strength of this salt in the bloodstream – that is, about 0.9 per cent for mammals. (See also DEHYDRATION; DEXTRAN.)

Normoblast

Normoblast is a red blood cell which still contains the remnant of a nucleus.

Northern Fowl Mite

This can infect canaries as well as poultry, and has caused allergic reactions in poultry-keepers in Israel. (See MITES.)

Norwegian Scabies

This is a form of sarcoptic mange. The skin becomes red, the hair falls out in patches, and there is intense pruritus.

Nose and Nasal Passages

The 'nose' of an animal, which is more often termed the 'muzzle', or 'snout', according to the species, serves 3 important functions. It forms the outermost end of the respiratory passage; it is the organ of smell; and it contains some of the end-organs of the sense of touch.

Horses Externally, the rims of the nostrils are built up on a basis of cartilages covered over by a fold of delicate skin possessing long tactile hairs. The cartilages are not complete laterally, thereby allowing the nostrils to become greatly distended during occasions of emergency. Situated at the upper and outer part of each nostril there is a pouch-like sac which opens into the nostril at one end, but is blind at the other. This is often called the 'false nostril'. Lying just within the entrance to the nasal passages about an inch or so inside each nostril is the lowermost opening of the lacrimal duct carrying tears secreted by the lacrimal gland of the eye.

Internally, each nostril, and the nasal passage to which it gives access, is completely divided from the other by the septum of the nose and its associated structures. This is composed partly by the vomer bone, and partly by a wall of cartilage which is continuous with the cartilages of the nostrils. The walls of each passage are lined by mucous membrane which is reflected on to the two turbinated scroll-like bones that are found in the passage; this membrane, being well supplied with blood, and being continually moist from the secretion of its mucin glands, serves to warm and moisten the incoming air before it passes to the lungs, and to extract the larger particles of dust, soot, etc., that the air picks up, by causing them to adhere to its sticky surface. The entrance to the air sinuses of the skull leads out from the posterior part of each passage, the mucous membrane lining the sinuses being continuous with that of the nose. (See SINUSES OF THE SKULL.) The end-organs of the sense of smell are scattered throughout the nasal mucous membrane in the upper parts particularly. The olfactory nerves from the brain, which pass out of the cranial cavity into that of the nose by way of the ethmoid bone, are distributed to these end-organs. Posteriorly, the nasal passages lead into the pharynx.

Cattle The nostrils, situated on either side of the broad expanse of moist hairless muzzle, are smaller and thicker than in the horse. No false nostril is present, and the opening of the lacrimal duct is not visible.

Nose and Nasal Passages, Diseases of

Catarrh Inflammation of the nostrils is called RHINITIS, and may accompany ordinary catarrhal inflammation of the nasal passages such as occurs in cases of distemper in the dog, of other febrile illnesses. The symptoms often resemble those of a human 'cold in the head', with a discharge from the nostrils which is at first clear and colourless, later becoming thick and yellowish-green. Horses and cattle often snort and shake their heads; dogs sneeze. Conjunctivitis may accompany the nasal catarrh.

In horses, the presence of ulcers in the mucous membrane with a punched-out appearance may indicate GLANDERS. For a specific condition in the pig, *see* ATROPHIC RHINITIS.

Parasites, such as larvae of the sheep-nostril fly, *Linguatula,* or leeches in dog or cat, may cause a discharge from one or both nostrils.

A discharge from 1 nostril only may in the dog, for example, indicate the presence of a FOREIGN BODY such as a grass awn; or there may be a fungal infection (e.g. ASPERGILLOSIS) which may follow local injury or tumour formation. Another possible cause is an abscess at the root of a tooth, with pus collecting in the maxillary sinus and escaping through the nasomaxillary opening.

Treatment Nasal catarrh should be considered contagious. The animal should be isolated accordingly, and attention paid to comfort, ventilation, and suitability of food, as discussed under NURSING OF SICK ANIMALS. Symptoms of other diseases must be looked for, especially when the temperature is high, and a professional diagnosis should be obtained. The nostrils should be kept moist and pliable by rubbing small quantities of Vaseline around their rims daily, after sponging away discharges.

Diseased conditions of the turbinated bones or of the molar teeth call for surgical measures for their correction; parasites in the nasal cavities must be expelled (see MITES); and if other foreign bodies are present they must be removed.

Haemorrhage from the nostrils may be due to injuries which cause tearing or laceration of the mucous membrane; it may occur during violent exertion, such as racing or hunting with horses not in maximum condition; it may be associated with ulceration, congestion, tumour formation, or other diseased condition of the nasal mucous membrane; it may be due to

fracture of a horn core in cattle and sheep, the blood entering the nose from the sinuses of the skull; in horses it may be seen in GUTTURAL POUCH DISEASE; and see 'BLEEDER HORSES'.

When the haemorrhage is only slight, little more than keeping the animal quiet, and applying douches of cold water to the bridge of the nose, will be required. A thin trickle of blood coming from 1 nostril only can be disregarded, as it will generally cease of its own accord. When the bleeding is very profuse, and there may be danger of collapse, more drastic measures are needed. Where only 1 nostril is affected it should be plugged with swabs of cotton-wool enclosed in gauze, and so arranged that some of the gauze is left outside the nostril to allow of removal some hours afterwards. In horses, care must be taken not to confuse nose bleeding with pulmonary bleeding. Severe bleeding from both nostrils requires veterinary intervention; both nostrils may need to be plugged after first having performed a tracheotomy.

Tumours include polyps, especially in the cat; and adenocarcinoma in dogs and other animals.

Among other conditions in which the nose or the nasal passages are affected may be mentioned: fungal infections, TUMOURS, mucosal disease, malignant catarrh, GLANDERS, URTICARIA, PURPURA HAEMORRHAGICA, STRANGLES, and INFLUENZA. (See also INFECTIOUS NASAL GRANULOMATA IN CATTLE; RHINOSPORIDIOSIS; RHINOTRACHEITIS, INFECTIOUS BOVINE.)

Nosocomial

Hospital-acquired. Human nosocomial infections, usually associated with medical or surgical interventions, affect about 5 to 6 per cent of hospital patients, i.e. about 2 million people in the USA alone, resulting in some 6 million excess hospital bed-days. About 1 per cent of the victims die.

Nostril

(see NOSE)

Nostril Flies (Oestridae)

Nostril flies (oestridae) are members of the class of 2-winged flies, whose larvae are parasitic in the nasal cavities, and in the air sinuses of the skull, of sheep. (See under FLIES.)

Notifiable Diseases

Notifiable diseases are those which, when they occur upon farm premises, must be notified to the Divisional Veterinary Office of the State Veterinary Service of the Department of the

Environment, Food and Agriculture (DEFRA). The list of notifiable diseases is amended from time to time and usually applies to all member states of the European Union. Those which are notifiable in the UK but not in all other member states are identified by an asterisk in the list below.

African horse sickness
African swine fever
American foul brood (bees)
Anthrax
Aujeszky's disease*
Avian influenza
Bluetongue
Bonamiasis (in shellfish)*
Bovine spongiform encephalopathy (BSE)
Brucella melitensis
Brucellosis (bovine)
Cattle plague (rinderpest)
Classical swine fever
Contagious agalactia
Contagious bovine pleuropneumonia
Contagious epididymitis
Contagious equine metritis
Dourine
Enzootic bovine leukosis
Epizootic haemorrhagic virus disease (deer)
Epizootic lymphangitis
Equine infectious anaemia
Equine viral arteritis
Equine viral encephalomyelitis (Eastern, Western and Venezuelan)
European foul brood (bees)
Foot-and-mouth disease
Furunculosis (fish)
Glanders and farcy
Goat pox
Gyrodactylosis caused by *Gyrodactylus solaris**
Haplosporidiosis (in fish)
Infectious haematopoetic necrosis (in fish)
Infectious salmon anaemia*
Iridovirosis (in fish)
Lumpy skin disease
Marteiliosis (in shellfish)*
Mikrocytosis (in fish)
Newcastle disease
Paramyxovirus in pigeons
Perkinosis
Peste des petits ruminants
Rabies
Rift Valley fever
Scrapie
Sheep pox
Spring viraemia of carp*
Swine vesicular disease (SVD)

Teschen disease
Tuberculosis (bovine)
Tuberculosis (deer)
Varroasis (in bees)
Vesicular stomatitis
Viral haemorrhagic septicaemia (in fish)*
Warble fly (bovine)*

The following are notifiable diseases in the whole of Ireland (north and south):

Brucellosis, in ruminating animals and swine
Caprine viral arthritis-encephalitis
Caseous lymphadenitis
Enzootic abortion of ewes
Fowl typhoid
Infectious bovine rhinotracheitis
Johne's disease
Maedi/visna
Mycoplasmal (infectious) synovitis
Mycoplasmosis (*M. gallisepticum* or *M, melea gridis*)
Parasitic mange of horses
Porcine epidemic diarrhoea (coronavirus)
Porcine respiratory and reproductive syndrome (PPRS; Blue ear disease)
Pullorum disease
Pulmonary adenomatosis
Psittacosis
Salmonellosis
Transmissible gastroenteritis of pigs
Tuberulosis in ruminating animals
Turkey rhinotracheitis

In Northern Ireland only:

Duck plague
Fowl pox
Infectious laryngotracheitis
Trichinosis
Vesicular exanthema
In the Republic of Ireland only:
Avian yersiniosis
Campylobacteriosis

(See under DISEASES OF ANIMALS ACTS – Diseases of Fish Act 1937 (as amended 1983), Diseases of Fish (Control) Regulations1994 and the Fish Health Regulations 1997 for duties and responsibilities of animal-owners.)

Notoedric Mange
(see under MITES)

Nsaids

Nsaids is an acronym for Non-Steroidal, Analgesic, anti-Inflammatory Drugs. They are very widely used in the control of post-operative pain, arthritis, joint pain, and inflammatory oedema; also as anti-inflammatory agents where pain may not be an issue and steroids are best avoided. Flunixin, paracetamol, phenylbutazone, ketoprofen, and aspirin are examples of NSAIDs. They may be administered orally or by injection according to type and formulation. There are restrictions on the use of most NSAIDs in horses competing under Jockey Club, etc., rules.

Nuclear Magnetic Resonance (NMR)

Also known as magnetic resonance imaging (MRI), this is a hazard-free, non-invasive technique for generating images of internal sections of the body. The system works by utilising the differing absorption of radio waves by atoms in the body when exposed to a magnetic field. The amount of absorption is measured and the data used to generate a computer image.

Nuclear Medicine

Involves the use of radio-isotopes for diagnosis and therapy. (See RADIO-ISOTOPES.)

Nuclear Weapons

(see under RADIOACTIVE FALL-OUT)

Nucleic Acids

(see DNA and RIBONUCLEIC ACID.)

Nuclein

Nuclein is a protein substance containing phosphorus derived from the nuclei of cells.

Nucleotides

(see RADIO-ISOTOPES)

Nucleus

The central body in a cell which controls its activities. (See CELLS.)

Nursing of Sick Animals

The advent of qualified professional VETERINARY NURSES has been of great benefit to practising veterinary surgeons, especially those engaged in small-animal practice, and to their patients; and has facilitated measures for intensive care.

Nursing of small animals at home If your dog or cat has an infectious disease, nursing will have to be undertaken at home, since veterinary hospitals usually cannot accept such cases owing to the risk to other patients.

In other cases, after initial veterinary treatment, it is often preferable to have the animal at home for nursing. There is likely to be less stress for your pet when it is not sent or kept away from its familiar surroundings.

A dog or cat which is ill, or recovering from an operation or accident, tends to seek solitude and require peace. Continual fussing and interference, however well-meant, are to be avoided. (This is something which has to be impressed on children.)

Fresh air, warmth, and an absence of bright lights and noise (such as those emanating from a TV set) are desirable. A patient with eye inflammation, tetanus, or some other nervous system disorder needs protection from bright light.

In many cases, it is helpful to put down old newspaper, which can be burnt after use. If a dog cannot go outside, a box of earth or ashes, or the material sold for cat trays, may be useful too. An extra sanitary tray will be needed for an ill cat under these circumstances.

Constipation may be a problem. A little of the oil from a tin of sardines may be taken voluntarily. (Remember that a cat straining ineffectually over a litter tray may be trying to pass urine and not faeces.)

Temperature-taking often forms a part of animal nursing. Buy a clinical thermometer with a stout, stubby end, and lubricate the latter before passing it into the rectum. Cooking oil will serve for this purpose.

An improvised jacket, with holes for the front legs, is useful in cases of bronchitis or pneumonia.

Never omit to wipe away the discharges from the eyes and nose of an ill animal.

It is sometimes difficult to keep an ill dog or cat clean. Any hair or fur which becomes soiled should be cut away, and the part washed.

Feeding

Prescription diets are specially formulated for use in assisting the treatment of specific canine and feline disorders. They are available in canned and dry form, as prescribed by veterinary surgeons; see DIET AND DIETETICS. Human invalid foods (e.g. Complan) are often useful.

Do not force solid foods on a sick animal which, if suffering from a digestive upset, is usually better off without solid food for a day or two. (See also under VOMITING.) Variety is important in feeding the sick.

During convalescence the animal may be tempted to eat by offering small quantities of warmed proprietary food or meat jelly, minced liver or rabbit, or sardine.

Nursing of horses The affected horse should be removed from its stall in the stable and placed in isolation. It should have plenty of bedding, be provided with clean water, and if the weather is cold it should be clothed with a rug. In cases where the horse is unable to stand, a specially thick straw be should be given, and one or two bags filled with straw, or bales of hay, are useful to prop it up in an upright position on the breast. Horses that are down must be turned over on to the other side twice or thrice daily. The rectum and bladder may require evacuation artificially, if it does not occur naturally. If bed sores appear, they should be dressed twice daily with surgical spirit, and more bedding should be supplied. In respiratory diseases the most important factor in nursing is the adequate provision of fresh air. Small feeds should be offered several times daily, and when a horse refuses one type of food it should be offered another. Whenever the breathing is faster than normal drenching should be avoided.

Nursing of cattle Isolate in a loose-box. Calves should be shut alone in a pen. The same conditions as to bedding, clothing, water, ventilation, etc., apply to cattle as to horses. Patient kindly treatment, the avoidance of all unnecessary fuss and haste, and a gentle firmness are essential.

A sick cow which refuses hay from a new ley will often eat hay from old pasture. Molasses may add palatability to food otherwise rejected; so may a little salt.

Nutrition, Faulty

Nutrition, faulty can lead to disease and losses of farm animals. Examples are nutritional muscular dystrophy (see under MUSCLES, DISEASES OF); blindness as a result of vitamin A deficiency (see EYE, DISEASES OF); poisoning by excessive fluorides in the diet (see FLUOROSIS); and an all-muscle meat diet can lead to CANINE and FELINE JUVENILE OSTEODYSTROPHY. (See also 'CAT, ANGRY' POSTURE.)

Nutritional Myopathy

A condition resulting from a deficiency of vitamin E or selenium. (See MUSCLES, DISEASES OF; PARALYTIC MYOGLOBINURIA; SUDDEN DEATH.)

Nuttallia

Nuttallia is the name given to a genus of piroplasms which cause biliary fever in horses in many parts of the world. There are 2 forms involved – *Babesia* (*Nuttallia*) *equi*, which is the smaller and more important, and *B.* (*Nuttallia*) *caballi*. Each is transmitted by one or more ticks. (See BABESIA – Babesiosis.)

Nux Vomica

Nux vomica is the seed of the *Strychnos nuxvomica*, an East Indian tree. It has intensely bitter taste. The medicinal properties are due to 2 alkaloids – strychnine and brucine, which the plant contains. Brucine has an action similar to, though much weaker than, strychnine. (See under STRYCHNINE.)

Nyctalopia or Night-Blindness
(see EYE, DISEASES OF)

Nymphomania

A condition in which a female animal is (or behaves as if) in constant oestrus. It is associated with pathological changes, often of a cystic nature, in the ovaries. Hormone treatment may be tried under veterinary advice; or removing the ovaries by surgical measures, as early as possible after the erotic symptoms have made their appearance. (See OVARIES, DISEASES OF; HORMONE THERAPY.)

Nystagmus

Nystagmus is a condition in which the eyeballs show constant fine jerky movements of an involuntary nature.

Oak Poisoning

Both the acorns and the leaves of the oak (*Quercus* spp.) may be dangerous when eaten by stock, but the leaves are usually harmless unless eaten in large quantities. It is when there is a scarcity of food in pastures towards the end of very dry summers that symptoms of poisoning occur. The animals most affected are young store cattle.

In a Northumberland outbreak, however, in a herd of 40 Galloways, 6 cows died and 4 aborted. A taste for oak buds was acquired early in the year when trees were felled and keep was scarce. Felling went on until September, when symptoms (fever and scouring with blood-stained faeces) were first shown after one cow had aborted and died.

Horses have been poisoned through eating either oak leaves or acorns.

It is well known that both pigs and sheep can eat acorns in small quantities without ill-effects.

Signs Ruminants that have eaten many acorns become dull, cease feeding, lie groaning, and appear to be in considerable pain. At first, there is severe constipation accompanied by straining and colicky pains, cessation of rumination, weakness of the pulse, and a temperature below normal. Later, small amounts of inky-black faeces are passed, and a blood-stained diarrhoea sets in. Great prostration is seen, and the animals die in from 3 to 7 days when large amounts have been eaten. In chronic cases there is always great loss of flesh, and death does not take place till weeks or months after the beginning of the symptoms.

Horses may not show signs of pain. The poisoned animal becomes weak and dull, has a subnormal temperature, may discharge food and saliva from its nostrils, show head-pressing, have mouth ulcers, have reddish-brown urine, ataxia and convulsions.

Autopsy findings include a uraemic smell from the carcase, oedema and haemorrhages, and kidney lesions.

Treatment Cattle should be given long hay. The animals should be made comfortable, with plenty of bedding provided. During convalescence, the animals require liberal feeding to make up the loss of flesh they have sustained.

Oats
(see CEREALS; DIET; and HORSES, FEEDING OF)

Obesity

Obesity is an important condition in the dog and cat, and may arise from overfeeding, an unsuitable diet, or from a hormone imbalance. Obesity is often associated with, and may predispose to, heart disease, arthritis, and some skin and respiratory disorders, as well as intolerance of heat. Old dogs need less carbohydrate and more protein in the diet. Overfeeding a pet can actually constitute an offence under the Protection of Animals Act 1911 by causing unnecessary suffering.

Obstetrics
(see PARTURITION, DRUG-INDUCED; CALVING)

Occiput

Occiput is the uppermost posterior part of the head where it meets the neck. The occipital bone lies in the part of the skull which forms the occiput, and can be felt as a hard bony plate in most animals. Some of the neck muscles are attached to the occipital bone, and the powerful ligamentum nuchae, which is the main supporting structure of the head and neck, is inserted into the prominence that can be felt between the ears.

Occupational Hazards
(see SHEPHERDS; ORF; PIGS, TRANSMISSIBLE DISEASES OF; MEAT-HANDLERS; ZOONOSES IN UK VETERINARIANS; NITROGEN DIOXIDE; SPOROTRICHOSIS; SALMONELLOSIS; BUBONIC PLAGUE)

Ochratoxin A

Ochratoxin A is a fungal toxin sometimes found in stored feeds and originating from *Penicillium viridicatum*, for example. Poisoning in pigs may result in thirst, enlarged kidneys, and polyuria. (See MYCOTOXICOSIS.)

Odontoma

Odontoma is a tumour arising in tissues which normally produce teeth. They are encountered in horses and cattle in association with the roots (usually) of teeth, where either they may appear as rounded or irregular masses attached to an otherwise normal tooth (sometimes making extraction extremely difficult), or they may occur as large, irregular, solid masses replacing the greater part of a normal tooth and causing a swelling on the side of the jaw. They are usually extremely dense and difficult to cut.

A so-called 'temporal odontoma' is a tumour, not uncommon in horses, about the size of a bantam's egg occurring in connection with the temporal bones. These tumours generally have an opening to the surface of the skin just below, or just in front of, the base of the ear. They contain 1 or 2 large, or many (sometimes over 100) small, imperfectly formed teeth enclosed in a single fibrous capsule.

Oedema

Oedema is an accumulation of exudate in one or more of the body cavities, or beneath the skin.

A normal, physiological form of oedema affecting the region of the mammary glands occurs in cows and mares shortly before parturition, and disappears within a day or two afterwards.

Otherwise, oedema is a pathological condition. When affecting tissue spaces immediately below the skin, it is usually due to a local disturbance of circulation or it may arise through weak heart action, and is not uncommon following debilitating diseases or in old age. Oedema of the lungs occurs in an animal exposed to smoke in a burning building, parasitic bronchitis and as the result of an allergy (e.g. milk allergy, and POTATO POISONING). Oedema involving the brisket or under the jaw may be a sign of severe liver-fluke infestation in sheep or cattle. (See also PARAQUAT.)

Oedema affecting the abdomen is also known as ascites and may give rise to a visible swelling or 'pot-bellied' appearance. It is seen in cases of tuberculosis in the dog and cat especially, and may also result from disease of heart, liver or kidneys; it sometimes accompanies diabetes. It may be associated with parasites such as liver-flukes.

Excessive fluid in the chest is also known as hydrothorax, which may be associated with e.g. chronic pleurisy.

Oedema is a symptom rather than a disease, and accordingly treatment must be directed at the cause. If due to parasites, the appropriate parasiticide must be used. A heart condition may be responsible and need appropriate treatment with digoxin or diuretics, or both. 'Tapping' the chest, i.e. aspiration of the fluid, may be indicated but will not alone effect a permanent improvement. If tuberculosis is diagnosed, immediate destruction on public-health grounds is called for. (See also BOWEL OEDEMA.)

Oedema, Malignant

(see GAS GANGRENE)

Oesophageal Groove

Also known as the reticular groove, it is part of the gastric groove which in the ruminant has 3 parts. The other 2 are the omasal and obamasal grooves.

Oesophagostomiasis

Infestation with *Oeso-phagostomum* worms. In calves, there is a reduced intake of food for several weeks, anaemia, and diarrhoea. In goats, peritonitis has been recorded in India. In pigs, these worms may be important in the causation of NECROTIC ENTERITIS. Third-stage larvae of these (and also *Ostertagia*) worms have been found clinging to psychodid flies cultured from pig faeces. Larvae have also been recovered from flies caught near a field in which pigs were grazing. It is possible that rats may also transmit larvae from farm to farm. (See also THIN SOW SYNDROME and under ROUNDWORMS.)

Oesophagotomy

A surgical operation involving incision of the oesophagus for removal of a foreign body, etc.

Oesophagus

Passage from throat to stomach. Food passes down from the mouth to the stomach by the process of PERISTALSIS.

Oesophagus, diseases of

In the tropics, stricture of the oesophagus in dogs and cats is caused by *Spirocerca lupi* larvae.

Stricture has also followed anaesthesia in cats; the suggested cause is a reflux of gastric fluid causing oesophagitis. Signs may appear some days after anaesthesia.

A balloon oesophageal dilator has been used to relieve some cases of stricture. (See also under CHOKING.)

Oestradiol and Oestrone (Estradiol and Estrone)

Oestradiol and oestrone (estradiol and estrone) are hormones secreted by the ovary (interstitial cells and graafian follicles) which bring about oestrus and, in late pregnancy, stimulate development of the mammary gland. The early conceptus synthesises oestrogens. In dairy cattle these are secreted in the whey fraction of the milk as oestrone sulphate. (See PREGNANCY DIAGNOSIS.)

Oestrin (Estrin)

Oestrogen (see HORMONES).

Oestriol (Estriol)

A hormone used to treat urinary incontinence in spayed bitches. It must not be used in intact bitches, nor if signs of polydipsia are present.

Oestrogens (Estrogens)

Hormones, either of natural origin or prepared synthetically, which have the effect of inducing oestrus. (See under HORMONES.) Pasture oestrogens may cause infertility and sometimes abortion. (See INFERTILITY and HORMONES IN MEAT PRODUCTION; also under OESTRADIOL.)

Oestrus (Estrus)

'Season', or 'heat', is the period during which the female shows desire for the male, and during which oestrogens from the Graafian follicle are circulating in the bloodstream. Oestrus precedes, or may coincide with, ovulation – rupture of the follicle and release of the ovum which passes into the top of the Fallopian tube. (See OVULATION; PHEROMONE.)

The oestrous cycles in animals vary in different species and in different breeds, and to some extent in different individuals.

Mare The mare is a polyoestrous animal with a breeding season during spring and summer. In the British Isles most mares first show normal oestrous cycles in mid-April; the frequency of ovulation is greatest in late July, and oestrous cyclical activity is at its lowest in early February.

During the oestral period the mare behaves unusually. She may become irritable or sluggish, and is easily tired. Her appetite is capricious and she may lean against the stall partition when in the stable. If her flanks are accidentally touched she may squeal or kick. The clitoris is frequently raised and there is usually a discharge of some amount of mucus from the vulva. Urine may be passed at frequent intervals. She shows a strong desire for the society of the male – even occasionally for that of the usually scorned gelding. Occasionally hysteria may be seen when the animal becomes quite unmanageable.

Cow The oestrous cycle is controlled by complex interactions among higher brain centres, the hypothalamus, anterior pituitary gland, ovary and uterus. Higher brain centres mediate responses to light, temperature, pheromones, and other stimuli which exert their effects through the central nervous system. The most important hormone, in regulating the oestrous cycle, is gonadotrophin-releasing hormone (GnRH).

The cow mounts her fellows or stands to be mounted by them. She may bellow and race about with tail raised, or break out of a field in search of a bull. In other instances, signs are so slight as to be missed by the herdsman. (See OESTRUS (ESTRUS), DETECTION OF, IN COWS.) Both cows and heifers in milk usually give less milk during the oestral period than in the intervals. (See CALVING EARLIER; INFERTILITY.)

Goat Rapid side-to-side and up-and-down tail movements may be seen; the animal is restless

OESTRUS

Animal	Time of year	Periodicity of oestrus	Duration	First occurrence after parturition
Mare	Feb. to July	21 days (14 to 28 days or more)	2 to 8 days	3 to 12 days; service on 9th day often successful
Cow	All year; most intense midsummer or more)	20 days (16 to 24 days	4 to 24 hours	30 to 60 days*
Ewe	End of Aug. till Jan., depending on breed and district	16 to 17 days (10 to 21 days)	1 to 2 days	†
Sow	Oct. to Nov. and Apr. to June	21 days (15 to 30 days)	1 to 3 days	8 weeks after farrowing, or 1 week after weaning of litter
Bitch	Usually Dec. to Feb., and in spring	Once only during each period	9 to 18 days	‡
Cat	Jan. onwards for 8 to 10 months (if unmated) oestrus may recur every 2 or 3 weeks		7 to 14 days	

*In the cow that is suckling a calf it is seldom that oestrus occurs until after weaning, when its appearance is somewhat variable, but often on 3rd to 12th day.

†With the exception of ewes of the Dorset Horn breed, which comes into season twice a year, and can rear two crops of lambs per year, sheep only show season in the autumn. It depends upon the breed as to how soon the rams may be put out with the flock. Generally speaking, the more low-lying the district and the milder the climate the earlier the ewes come into season; thus Suffolks are served from August till the end of September, and lamb from January till March. Mountain breeds are served from November till January, and lamb in April, May, and June.

‡The bitch usually comes in season twice a year, but great variation takes places with the smaller toy breeds. Bitches of the Basenji breed (and a few individuals of other breeds) have only one heat period per year.

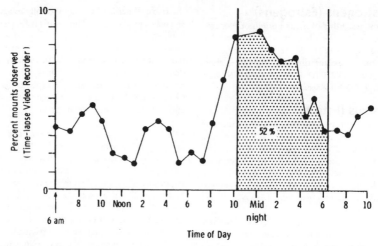

Oestrus in the cow. Mounting activity over 24 hours. Composition of 2880 cow-days. (36 adult Holsten cattle.) (With acknowledgements to Dr J. Frank Hurnik, University of Guelph, Canada, and to Dr D. B. Harker.)

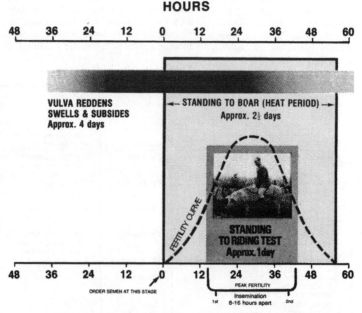

A guide to insemination time in the sow. (With acknowledgements to the MLC.)

and bleats. Oestrus occurs every 19 to 21 days during the autumn, and lasts 12 to 48 hours.

Sow The sow becomes torpid and lazy, and when asked to move often grunts in a peculiar whining manner. If housed with others she behaves like the cow – mounting or being mounted. The vulva is usually distinctly swollen, and there is sometimes a blood-stained discharge. Oestrus in the sow lasts up to 60 hours and ovulation begins at 34 to 50 hours after its onset, the process taking up to 5 hours. The sow

THE SEXUAL CYCLE

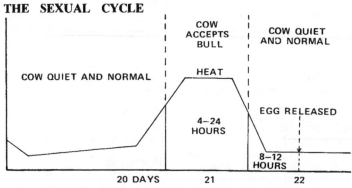

(With acknowledgements to the East of Scotland College of Agriculture.)

will accept service between 15 and 35 hours after the onset of oestrus, with the optimum at 25 to 35 hours.

Bitch She wanders away from home unless confined, and the odour of her blood-stained vaginal discharge attracts male followers. As bleeding from the vulva is slight in some bitches, especially at their 1st oestrus, owners should watch for swelling of the vulva. During the 7 to 9 days of pro-oestrus, the bitch will flirt with a dog but not accept him. Usually it is only during the last week of heat that the bitch will accept the dog, usually between the 10th and 12th days.

Cat The signs may suggest pain and/or a strong desire to have her back and flanks rubbed or scratched. She will roll over and over on carpet or floor, rub herself against furniture, etc., and utter little pleased mews.

The 1st oestrus may be expected between the ages of 6 and 8 months: however, it may occur as early as 3½ months, or occasionally be delayed until the queen is about a year old.

Oestrus (Estrus), Detection of, in Cows

Especially in winter, detection of oestrus is not as easy as might be thought. Studies in the USA suggest that where cows are watched 4-hourly round the clock, the efficiency of heat-detection should be around 95 per cent, but in a herd where cows are seen only twice a day, the percentage is likely to drop to around 74 per cent.

Other studies suggest that those figures may be over-optimistic, however; in Britain, the rate may be as low as 55 per cent on some farms.

The main sign of oestrus in a heifer or cow is standing still to be ridden by others ('bulling').

Part of the problem is that while 'bulling' lasts 12 hours on average, it may last only 1 hour; and as to the timing, 50 per cent of the displays occur at night. Moreover some cows may stand only once in 20 minutes; others will stand only for favourites; and some aggressive cows mount other cattle at a crowded trough in order to induce them to move aside to create a space.

Sometimes a cow is seen to mount another from the front. This is valuable evidence of oestrus, but it is important to remember that it is the riding cow which is bulling, not the one underneath.

The importance of pinpointing heat dates cannot be overemphasised. Only by record-keeping is it possible to identify animals that are not coming in heat at the normal time, in addition to those which are cycling (coming in heat) irregularly. Delay in seeking veterinary advice may lead to delay in conception.

As an aid to herd management, a VASECTOMISED bull may be used, or a heat-detection device may be placed on a cow's back, liberating a dye when she is mounted. Applying paint to the tail which is rubbed off by mounting is also useful.

Oestrus (Estrus), Suppression of

Bitches and cats may be prevented from coming 'on heat' by oral dosing with the synthetic equivalent of the naturally occurring hormone, progesterone; MEGESTROL ACETATE (Ovarid) is an example. Synthetic progestogens are also used to lessen aggressive behaviour in dogs and spraying in cats.

Some progestogens can cause pathological changes in the uterus, particularly if used for prolonged periods. They may induce abnormal levels of growth hormone, suppress cortisol levels, and possibly increase the risk of mammary tumours.

Offal

The practice of incorporating offal – animal organs – in cattle feeds was banned in 1988 because of the risk of transmitting BOVINE SPONGIFORM ENCEPHALOPATHY.

Offals Middlings

A high-protein feed supplement for cattle (see WEATINGS).

Office International Des Epizooties (OIE)

Office International Des Epizooties (OIE) was set up in 1924 following the realisation that joint action between countries was necessary to control contagious animal diseases. It determines the animal health standards for international trade, advises the veterinary services in member countries, and aims to work towards the eradication of the most dangerous animal and zoonotic diseases. The membership comprises 144 countries and international organisations such as the UN's Food and Agriculture Organisation and the World Health Organisation.

Oie

(see OFFICE INTERNATIONAL DES EPIZOOTIES)

Old English Sheepdog

Its very shaggy, grey and white coat is the distinguishing feature of this large dog. Wobbler syndrome (cervical spondylolithesis) and cataract may be inherited. Hip dysplasia, deafness and osteochondritis dessicans may also be found in the breed.

Oilfield Hazards, Poisoning

In the USA about 500 cases of suspected poisoning by oilfield wastes are investigated each year at the Oklahoma animal disease diagnostic laboratory.

Hazards arise from the ingestion by cattle of petroleum hydrocarbons, salt water, heavy metals, chemicals stored on site, and rubbish such as discarded soda bags. A quantity of lead-based pipe-jointing material is used, and also chemicals to treat the mud which lubricates the drilling bit.

Signs of poisoning include weight loss and unthriftiness. A differential diagnosis has to take into account the possibility of internal parasites, faulty nutrition or other causes of debility; but standard analytical methods make it relatively easy to detect the ingested poisons.

The presence of petroleum in lung tissue and in rumen contents is frequently confirmed. Liver and kidney lesions may be found.

Oils

Oils are divided into fixed oils, which are of the nature of liquid fats, and are derived by expression from nuts, seeds, etc.; and volatile or essential oils, which are obtained by distillation. Examples are the oils of aniseed, cajaput, eucalyptus, peppermint, and turpentine. (See also PARAFFIN.)

Oilseed Rape

Horses grazing in fields adjacent to this crop are at risk of developing respiratory disease.

Oldenburg

A breed of sheep native to the Hamburg Marshes, Germany. Fleece weights up to 6.35 kg (14 lb) and high lambing percentages are claimed.

Olfactory

Relating to the sense of smell.

Olfactory Nerve (Nerve of Smell)

Olfactory nerve (nerve of smell) is the 1st of the cranial nerves.

Oliguria

A diminution in the amount of URINE excreted.

Olive Pomace

A by-product of the olive-oil industry that has been used to replace wheat bran in cattle diets and barley in sheep diets. Pre-treatment with sodium hydroxide helps to delignify the product and improve palatability.

Ollulanus

(see CATS, WORMS IN)

Omasum ('Many-Plies')

Omasum ('many-plies') is the name given to the 3rd stomach of ruminants. It is situated on the right side of the abdomen at a higher level than the 4th stomach and between this latter and the 2nd stomach, with both of which it communicates. From its inner surface project large numbers of leaves or folia, each of which possesses roughened surfaces. In the centre of each folium is a band of muscle-fibres which produces a rasping movement of the leaf when it contracts. One leaf rubs against those on either side of it, and large particles of food material are ground down between the rough surfaces, preparatory to further digestion in the succeeding parts of the alimentary canal.

Studies at the ARC's National Institute for Research in Dairying have shown 'massive exchanges of water and solutes in the omasum of the steer. The organ appears to be the main site of magnesium absorption, and it is probably here that the cause of clinical hypomagnesaemia should be sought'.

Omentum

Omentum is a fold of peritoneum which passes from the stomach to some other organ. There are several such folds, but the most important is that which passes to the terminal part of the large colon and the beginning of the small colon, and which is called the great omentum. This does not run direct to the colon from the stomach, but forms a loose sac occupying the spaces between other organs in the abdomen. In health, there is always a considerable amount of fat deposited in the folds of the great omentum, and this, in the ox, sheep, and pig, forms part of the suet of commerce.

In the dog, the great omentum lies between the abdominal organs and the lower abdominal wall, and acts as a kind of protective bed which supports the intestines, etc.

Omphalitis
'Navel-ill'.

Omphalitis of Birds

Infection of the yolk sack, by bacteria found in the alimentary canal and on the skin of the hen, or in the nostril of hatchery workers. It can cause high mortality of embryos and chicks. The bacteria may be relatively non-pathogenic elsewhere than in the yolk where, having a rich medium in which to grow, they cause serious disease. This can take the form of 'mushy chick disease' in birds under 10 days old, or true omphalitis. Sending birds out from a hatchery before the navels have completely closed is also a risk.

Omphalophlebitis

Omphalophlebitis means inflammation of the umbilical vein. It occurs in young animals and is commonly present in the early stages of 'navel-ill'.

Omsk Fever

The cause of this is related to the RUSSIAN SPRING-SUMMER VIRUS, but is more serious in its effects and is spread by the tick *Dermacentor pictus*.

Onchocerciasis

Infestation with worms belonging to the class Onchocerca. (See ROUNDWORMS.)

Oncogene

A gene associated with tumour formation. (See CANCER.)

The determination of the protein encoded by the *ras* oncogene has helped to explain how genes of this kind cause cancer.

The *ras* protein is part of the system on the cell surface that transmits signals from growth factors in the interior of the cell. In its mutated, oncogenetically coded form, the signal is locked in the 'on' position, so causing unrestrained growth.

Oncogenic

Giving rise to tumour formation.

Oncology

The study of tumours.

Oncornaviruses

Oncornaviruses are those which give rise to tumours, e.g. the feline leukaemia virus; the Rous sarcoma virus. (See CANCER; RETROVIRUS.)

Ondiri Disease

An infection of cattle and sheep by *Cytoecetes ondiri*; signs are fever and small haemorrhages of the mucous membranes (see BOVINE INFECTIOUS PETECHIAL FEVER).

Onion Poisoning

The toxic effects of onions have been seen in cattle, sheep, horses and dogs.

The toxic principle is a pungent volatile oil, n-propyl disulphide. This gives rise to Heinz bodies, and red blood cells which contain them are removed by the reticulo-endothelial system; giving rise to anaemia.

Signs Inappetence, tachycardia, staggering, jaundice, haemoglobinuria, collapse, and sometimes death.

'Ontario Encephalitis'

A disease of piglets, as young as 4 to 7 days, ending in a fatal encephalitis and caused by a virus. (See ENCEPHALOMYELITIS, VIRAL, OF PIGS.)

Onychetomy

De-clawing.

Onychia

Onychia is an inflammation affecting the nails or claws of animals. (See NAILS, DISEASES OF.)

Onychomycosis

Infection of the claw with a fungus. In cats, *Microsporum canis* infection is not uncommon. (See RINGWORM.)

Oocyte

An immature ovum.

Oophorectomy
(see SPAYING)

Oophoritis
Oophoritis is another name for ovaritis or inflammation of an ovary.

Open Joints
(see JOINTS, DISEASE OF)

'Opening the Heels'
'Opening the heels' means the cutting of the horn at the angles of the heels of the horse's foot, by which the continuity between the horn of the wall and of the bar on either side of the foot is destroyed. It is performed by some farriers and owners in the hope that it will allow the heels to expand and so produce a 'fine open foot'. Actually, the operation results in an interference with the shock-absorptive mechanism of the foot, and eventually produces contraction of the heels. It is by no means to be recommended. (See FOOT OF THE HORSE.)

Ophthalmia
Ophthalmia means inflammation of the whole of the structures of the eye, but is sometimes restricted to mean keratitis. Contagious ophthalmia is caused by *Rickettsia conjunctivae* in sheep, and by *Moraxella bovis* in cattle. Verminous ophthalmia also occurs in cattle. (See EYES, DISEASES OF.)

Ophthalmoscope
Ophthalmoscope is an instrument used for the examination of the back of the eye.

Opioids
Endogenous opioids in the central nervous system, the encephalins and endorphins, are able to modify the perception of pain.

Opisthotonos
Opisthotonos is the position assumed by the backbone during one of the convulsive seizures of tetanus, and also sometimes seen during epileptiform convulsions and strychnine poisoning. The spinal column is markedly arched with the concavity facing upwards away from the lower parts of the body, so that the head is drawn backwards, and the tail and hind-parts of the body pulled forwards. The condition is due to the spasmodic contraction of the powerful muscles lying above the vertebral column.

Opium
Opium is the dried milky juice of the unripe seed-capsules of the white Indian poppy, *Papaver somniferum*. Good opium should contain about 10 per cent of morphine, the chief alkaloid and active principle. It also contains other alkaloids, the most important of which are codeine, narcotine, thebaine, papaverine, apomorphine.

The preparations of opium used in veterinary medicine are now virtually nil, but have included the following: (1) Powdered opium, which is the dried juice powdered, contains about 9.5 to 10.5 per cent morphine. (2) Tincture of opium, or laudanum, consists of the powder treated with distilled water and alcohol, and contains about 1 per cent of morphine. (3) Opium extracts, 1 dry of 20 per cent morphine, and 1 liquid of 3 per cent morphine, as well as a fluid extract which contains about 5 per cent morphine. (4) Compound tincture of camphor, or paregoric. (5) Compound ipecacuanha powder, or Dover's powder, contains 10 per cent of opium. (6) Gall and opium ointment, containing 7.5 per cent of opium, is used as an astringent ointment. (7) Compound tincture of morphine and chloroform which contained morphine, chloroform, dilute prussic acid, as well as Indian hemp and capsicum, is similar to the proprietary mixtures which are called chlorodyne. Morphine, codeine, apomorphine, heroin, and dionin are also preparations from or derivatives of opium. (See MORPHINE.)

Opsonins
Substances present in blood serum which facilitate the engulfment of bacteria (and other foreign proteins) by certain white cells. (See PHAGOCYTOSIS.)

Optic Nerve
Optic nerve is the 2nd cranial nerve running from the eye to the base of the brain. It conveys the sensations of light that are received by the retina, and registers them in the optic centres of the brain. (See EYE, VISION.)

Orbit
Orbit is the eye socket.

Orbital Gland
(see HARDERIAN GLAND and EYE, DISEASES OF)

Orbiviruses
These cause African horse sickness, blue-tongue, and a haemorrhagic disease of deer.

Orchards
Animals grazing in orchards may run the risk of poisoning if fruit-trees have recently been sprayed with insecticides or fungicides. Orchards, like paddocks, sometimes become a reservoir of

parasitic worm larvae. (See PADDOCKS; also ALCOHOL POISONING.)

Orchitis

Inflammation of the TESTICLE.

Oregon Muscle Disease

A condition in turkeys and chickens in which the inner breast (deep pectoral) muscles become necrotic and greenish. The cause is possibly an inherited abnormality affecting the blood vessels.

Orf

A disease of sheep, cattle, and goats which has a very wide distribution and many names. Among its numerous designations are the following: 'ulcerative stomatitis', 'contagious pustular dermatitis'; 'contagious ecthyma'; 'necrobacillosis of sheep'.

Orf is enzootic in the Border counties of England and Scotland, but outbreaks may arise in any county in Britain, as well as in Germany, France, Austria, the USA, and other sheep countries.

The disease attacks sheep of all ages, sexes, and breeds, and kept under all conditions of management. It frequently attacks lambs just before or after weaning, or after docking or castration, and from them it may spread to the teats of the ewes. In other cases it is common among gimmers until they are 1 year old.

Causes Essentially, a parapoxvirus; but secondarily *Fusiformis necrophorus* (*Fusobacterium*). The virus is needed to produce pox-like lesions first, which the necrosis organism then invades.

Signs In the milder form of the disease, vesicles, followed by ulcers, appear on the lips – especially at the corners of the mouth. Sometimes healing takes place uneventfully; in other cases verrucose masses form and persist. The animal loses weight.

In the severe form the inside of the mouth becomes involved in most cases, and in addition other parts of the body such as the vulva and the skin of the face, legs, tail, etc. A greyish-black crust often appears which, if removed, leaves a raw, angry-looking surface.

Sheep with lesions on the head frequently rub their muzzles on their fore-feet, or scratch at their heads with their hind-feet. In this way the feet and legs often become affected. Abscesses may form in the region of the coronet. The sheep becomes extremely lame, so much so that it is frequently unable to put the affected leg to the ground, and hobbles about on 3 legs. If both fore-feet are affected – which is commonly the case – the animal may be observed feeding from a kneeling position. In severe cases the horn separates from the sensitive structures below, large quantities of foul-smelling thick pus are produced, and the hoof may be shed. The space between the claws, and the parts around the front and sides of the coronets, are the commonest situations of the lesions.

Less commonly the external genitals of both male and female are affected. (See also PENIS AND PREPUCE – Balanoposthitis.)

After 550 apparently healthy 5-month-old lambs had been transported over a period of 23 hours, a severe outbreak developed and 10 per cent of the lambs died. The outbreak was attributed to spread of the virus from an affected animal in the confined space inside the truck.

Treatment As soon as a case of orf appears among a flock of sheep, it should be isolated at once. Isolated sheep that are already affected usually do best when they can be shut up indoors, given hand-feeding, and provided with clean dry litter. A dressing is applied over the raw ulcerated area and around its margin. Crystal violet is very suitable as a dressing, and antibiotics are useful in treatment. Cryosurgery may be helpful.

On farms previously heavily infected, and where orf was very common on the feet, passing the whole of the sheep through a foot-bath at 3-weekly intervals has resulted in a complete disappearance of the disease. (See FOOT-BATHS FOR SHEEP.)

Orf is well recognised as an occupational hazard of shepherds.

Control A modified live vaccine is available; it is applied by scarifications. The resulting scabs can be a source of infection when they detach.

Orf in the dog Outbreaks of orf in hounds and sheepdogs are not unknown. They are characterised by circular areas of acute inflammation, with a moist appearance, ulceration and scab formation.

Public health In one 5-year period there were 344 laboratory reports of patients with orf lesions in Britain. Contact with live sheep or lambs was reported 142 times. In 49 cases the people affected were abattoir workers, butchers, or domestic meat-handlers. The possible source in 36 patients (including 13 milkers) was contact with cows or calves. Sixteen patients were farmers; 7 were veterinary surgeons or veterinary students. (Communicable Disease Surveillance Centre.)

Severe mouth lesions have been successfully treated by DIATHERMY and CRYOSURGERY.

Organelles

Specialised structures within a CELL.

Organic Diseases

Organic diseases, as distinct from 'functional diseases', are those in which some actual alteration in structure takes place, as the direct result of which faulty action of the organ or tissue concerned follows.

Organochlorine Poisoning

(see CHLORINATED HYDROCARBONS)

Organophosphorus Poisoning

This may arise from contamination of crops, or other food material, with organophosphorus insecticides such as dimethoate, schradan, parathion or dimefox, or by skin contact or inhalation.

Signs are varied but include salivation, muscle tremors, slow heartbeat, constricted pupils, swaying gait, and recumbency.

For a case of laryngeal paralysis arising from organophosphorus poisoning of racehorses, see under LARYNX, DISEASES OF.

Treatment Atropine sulphate given intravenously or intramuscularly, and repeated in 30 minutes. Barbiturates may be needed to control excitement. Oxygen for distressed breathing, and gastric lavage are recommended in the human subject. In the latter, PAM has been recommended as an antidote to parathion and other insecticides in this group – in conjunction with atropine.

Protective clothing must be worn when dipping sheep in organophosphorus dips; only properly trained operatives may use sheep dips (see DIPS AND DIPPING).

Orifices, Immunity at

Defence mechanisms, directed against the invasion of pathogenic bacteria, exist in the natural orifices of the body. For example, research at IRAD, Compton, led to the isolation of a number of cationic proteins from the keratin of the teat-canal's lining, and these have been shown to inhibit the growth of mastitis strains of staphylococci and streptococci. These proteins, which are soluble in distilled water and carry a positive electrical charge, were shown to inhibit the growth of 2 strains of *Staphylococcus aureus* and 1 strain of *Streptococcus agalactiae*. The proteins in very low concentration caused a 50 per cent mortality in test bacterial cultures.

The secretions of the uterine cervix of the cow during oestrus also contain cationic proteins which possess antibacterial activity against staphylococci. In the laboratory these proteins were shown also to inhibit growth of *Brucella abortus*.

The anionic proteins from the cervical mucus, however, showed no inhibitory action on the bacteria. This difference 'suggested that the killing of the bacteria was preceded by an electrovalent binding of the positively charged cationic protein on to the negatively charged surface of the bacteria', and this has proved to be the case.

Antibacterial cationic proteins have also been isolated from cells normally present in cow's milk, and research has shown that synthesis of these proteins can be stimulated. Induction of a mild sterile mastitis by the injection of *E. coli* endotoxin through the teat-canal led to increased numbers of neutrophils in the milk from which was extracted cationic proteins with a higher antibacterial activity.

Ornamental Fish

Ornamental fish are widely kept in the UK. The species vary considerably and, therefore, so do their environmental requirements. A general rule is that when changing water, not all the old water should be removed; about a third should be left (unless advised otherwise in certain circumstances, such as where a disease is present). There is evidence that fish may secrete, in the mucous covering their skin, substances with antibiotic activity. Beneficial bacteria will also have become established in the water and enough should be left to re-establish numbers in the tank.

Stress is a factor in most diseases of fish. Imported fish can undergo considerable stress during catching and transport before reaching the hobbyist. Ulceration of the skin is not uncommon in goldfish and koi; the bacteria responsible vary. As with farmed fish, protozoal infestations by *Ichthyophthirius* (white spot), *Trichonodina, Costia, Chilodonella, Scyphidia,* etc, can occur. Gill flukes may also present a problem: *Sapreolegnia* is usually a complicating infection.

When fish are kept in ponds, great care must be taken to prevent spindrift from garden chemicals contaminating the water.

Ornithosis

The name formerly given to *Chlamydophila psittaci* infection in birds other than those of the parrot family. *C. psittaci* infections in all birds are now designated as psittacosis. (See CHLAMYDIA AND CHLAMYDOPHILA.)

Orthopox Viruses

This genus contains those pox viruses genetically and antigenetically related to smallpox virus. (*See* table under VIRUSES.)

OS

The Latin word for a bone. Examples: *Os cordis*, a bone (1 of 2) present in the hearts of cattle; *Os penis* in the dog.

Ossification

Ossification means the formation of bone tissue. In early life the bones are represented by cartilage or fibrous tissue, and in these, centres appear in which the cells undergo a change and lime salts are deposited. This process proceeds until the areas or centres meet each other, and the tissue is wholly converted into bone. When a fracture occurs, the bone unites by ossification of the blood-clot which forms between the broken ends of the bone. (See FRACTURES.) In old age, ossification takes place in parts where normally there are cartilages found, such as in the larynx, in the rib-cartilages, in the scapular cartilages, etc., and these parts lose their normal elasticity and become easily broken. (See SIDEBONES.)

Osteitis (Ostitis)

Inflammation of bone (see BONE, DISEASES OF).

Osteoarthritis (Osteoarthrosis)

Inflammation/degeneration of the bone at a joint. In human medicine, the name 'osteoarthrosis' is now preferred, emphasising the view that this is a degenerative rather than an inflammatory disease. The primary disturbance is usually regarded as occurring in articular cartilage, and as resulting from a combination of ageing and mechanical factors. An alternative hypothesis is that the disease originates in the synovial lining cells (see ARTHRITIS).

Osteoblasts

Cells which assist in the formation of bone. (See also OSTEOCLASTS.)

Osteochondritis

Inflammation of bone and cartilage. (See HIP DYSPLASIA IN DOGS.) *O. dissecans* is characterised by separation of a piece of articular cartilage which, together with a small piece of underlying bone, forms a loose body within a joint (*see below*).

Osteochondritis Dissecans

Osteochondritis dissecans is a disturbance in the endochondral ossification (conversion of cartilage into bone) affecting the growth plates and the articular cartilage. It is an inherited trait in some dog breeds but rapid growth in any animal may cause the condition. Clinical signs include lameness and abnormal gait. There is pain around the affected joints. The stifle and hock may be more severely affected as they bear greater weight. Rest, and perhaps surgery, may be required.

Osteochondrosis

Abnormal differentiation of cartilage. It is similar in some respects to OSTEOCHONDRITIS, and may be a more accurate description in cases where there is no inflammatory response to the changes in bone and cartilage. There may be necrosis of bone and separation of splinters or flaps of articular cartilage. A hereditary basis for the condition has been recorded in man, horse, dog, and pig. In pigs, as many as 80 per cent can show lesions at slaughter.

In young horses, the most frequently diagnosed conditions are *O. dissecans* and a subchondral bone cyst. These are 2 separate entities, though often bracketed together under the osteochondrosis syndrome. Severe lameness may be caused by the former, and surgical treatment needed.

Osteoclasts

Cells which aid the breakdown or resorption of excess bony tissue, laid down following fractures, as part of the repair process. (See also OSTEOBLASTS.)

Osteodystrophia Fibrosa

A degenerative condition of bone resulting from over-activity of the parathyroid gland. Affected animals show lameness, pain, incoordination, paralysis, curvature of the spine, fractures and constipation. Diagnosis is confirmed by X-ray. Treatment is by giving mineral supplements; steroids and sex hormones have also been used.

Osteodystrophic Diseases

Osteodystrophic diseases are conditions in which the metabolism of the bone is upset. This may be caused by mineral deficiencies or imbalances in the diet or pasture.

Osteogenesis Imperfecta

A failure of bone to develop properly in young animals. Animals show incoordination, and pain at the joints; they may be prone to greenstick or complete fractures. Rest is necessary; anti-inflammatory medication will relieve the pain.

Osteomalacia

Osteomalacia is the equivalent of rickets occurring in the adult animal. The bones become softened as the result of the loss by absorption of the salts they contain. The cause of the disease is obscure, but it appears to be more common in pregnant females than in other animals, and it may be associated with a deficiency of vitamin D and/or phosphates. (See VITAMINS.)

The most serious feature is the deformity which occurs in the softened bones, owing either to the weight of the body or to the pull of the muscles upon them. When the deformity is located in the pelvis of the dam, great difficulty is often experienced at the birth of the young animal, and fractures of this part are not unknown.

Treatment Vitamin D and good nourishing food with an adequate phosphate content.

Osteomyelitis

Inflammation and infection of the bone marrow. It is sometimes a complication of atrophic rhinitis of pigs and of actinomycosis of cattle. (See BONE, DISEASES OF.)

Osteopenia

A reduction in the body's bone tissue.

Osteopetrosis ('Marble Bone' Disease)

Osteopetrosis ('marble bone' disease) is characterised clinically by thickening of the legs of poultry (*see* illustration, below). On postmortem examination, involvement of other bones is seen. The cause is a virus of the avian leucosis group.

Osteophagia

Osteophagia means bone-eating, and is a symptom shown by sheep and cattle in certain parts of South Africa where soil and herbage are deficient in phosphorus and sometimes in calcium. (See LAMZIEKTE.)

Deer living wild in forests where there is a similar deficiency, as in many parts of the Scottish Highlands, exhibit osteophagia by chewing and actually eating portions of shed antlers. Sheep exhibit similar tendencies in the same areas.

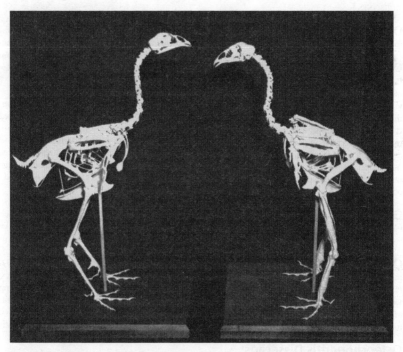

Two chicken skeletons at the Regional Poultry Research Laboratory at East Lansing, Michigan. One (left) is the skeleton of a 216-day-old normal White Leghorn cockerel. The other is the skeleton of a 202-day-old White Leghorn cockerel affected with osteopetrosis, a disease that causes an enlargement and hardening of the bones. (With acknowledgements to USDA, photograph by Madeleine Osborne.)

Osteoporosis

Osteoporosis is a rarefying condition of bones which lose much of their mineral matter and become fragile. It can occur in young animals through deficiency of protein in the diet, and in older animals through lack of exercise. In old animals appropriate sex hormones may be given; in younger ones the diet must be checked. Extra thiamine (vitamin B₁) may be useful.

Osteosarcoma

A malignant cancer of the bone. Some large breeds of dog appear to have a predisposition towards the disease.

Ostertagiasis

Infestation with species of *Ostertagia* worms, which produce gastroenteritis. It is seen in calves and lambs. This is an important disease in Ireland. (See WORMS, FARM TREATMENT AGAINST.)

Ostrich (*Struthio Camelus*)

Ostriches, once farmed extensively for their tail feathers, are now farmed mainly for their meat, which is low in cholesterol, although – the feathers, leather and eggs are also marketed.

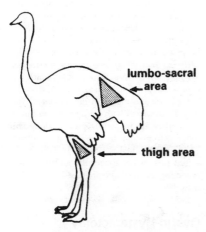

Darting sites suggested for ostriches.

An adult male may be up to 2.75 m (9 ft) tall, and weigh 135 kg (300 lb). Ostriches can be dangerous and have been known to disembowel people when angry. That is why 2 areas of the drawing have been shaded – to indicate sites for the administration of IMMOBILON by means of a PROJECTILE SYRINGE.

Ostriches cannot fly, but they can run extremely fast.

Ostriches are included under the Dangerous Wild Animals Act. In the UK, the melon-sized eggs are usually used for hatching only.

Diseases Among infectious conditions that have been reported are the following:

Newcastle disease in the ostrich usually affects the nervous system. Avian influenza can cause severe mortality, particularly among young birds. Ostriches are susceptible to fowl pox; vaccination is recommended where this disease is prevalent. *Clostridium perfingens* type C can be a problem; vaccination should also cover other types of this organism. *Clostridium chauvoei* has been implicated in a condition resulting in partial paralysis and inability to urinate. Unusually for birds, ostriches are susceptible to anthrax; they can also be infected with avian tuberculosis, *E. coli*, salmonella and klebsiella, among other micro-organisms. Aspergillosis and candidiasis have been reported. *Houttuynia struthionis* is a tapeworm specific to the ostrich, imported into the UK with birds from Namibia. Nematodes specific to the ostrich include the wireworm *Libyostrongylus douglassi* (not in the UK as at 2004), *Codiostomum struthionis* and *Dicheilonema spirularium*. Feather lice are usually of the species *Struthioleupiris struthionis* and quill mites of the *Pterolichidiae* may be found. Occasionally ticks (*Ambyloma*, *Hyalomma* or *Rhipicephalus* can be present. Borna disease has affected ostriches, causing paresis.

Otitis

Otitis means inflammation of the ear. (See EAR, DISEASES OF.)

Otodectes

Mites which cause ear mange in dogs and cats. (See MITES.)

Otorrhoea

Otorrhoea means a discharge from the ear. (See EAR, DISEASES OF.)

Otterhound

A large dog with pendulous ears and a long, oily coat. It is liable to an inherited disorder of the blood platelets.

'Oulou Fato'

A form of rabies occurring among dogs in parts of Africa, and probably Asia also. People are rarely bitten, epidemics are uncommon; infected dogs may show either no symptoms, or transient symptoms followed by recovery. Repeated attacks prove fatal, however.

Ovarid
(see MEGESTROL ACETATE; OESTRUS, SUPPRESSION OF)

Ovaries

The female reproductive organs. They are suspended in a fold of peritoneum from the roof of the abdomen, called the 'mesovarium'. In the mare they are situated in the abdomen, lying a little below and behind the kidneys, usually in contact with the muscles of the lumbar region. Each possesses a groove which gives the organ a shape not unlike a bean, and which is called the *ovulation fossa*. It is into this groove that the ripe ova escape from the ovary, and it is the only part covered by germinal epithelium in the mare. In the cow the ovaries are oval in outline and possess no fossa. Each is situated about half-way up the shaft of the ilium of the corresponding side of the body. The ovaries of the sow are usually situated in a position similar to those of the cow, but their position changes somewhat after breeding has occurred. They are studded over the surface with irregular prominences, so that the organs present a mulberry-like appearance, and are enclosed in a 'purse' of peritoneum. In the bitch the ovaries are situated in close proximity to, if not in actual contact with, the kidneys of the respective sides.

Structure Each ovary is composed of a stroma of dense fibrous tissue in whose spaces are numerous blood vessels, especially towards the centre. On the surface of the organ is a layer of germinal epithelium from which arise the Graafian follicles. These vary very much in size: when young they are microscopic, and lie immediately under the outer surface, but as they grow older they become more and more deeply situated, and finally, as ripening occurs, they once more come to the surface. Growth or ripening of a follicle occurs following stimulation of the ovary by the follicle-stimulating hormone (FSH) from the pituitary gland. The follicle produces, also as the result of FSH, oestrogens which prepare the uterus, Fallopian tubes and vagina for the other processes of reproduction. In a ripening Graafian follicle there is 1 (rarely 2) of the essential female germ cells, called an ovum. This is situated at the pinnacle of a mass of cells which project inwards from the inner surface of the follicle, and which is known as the cumulus.

Function When the follicle is ripe, a process known as ovulation occurs, in which the outer surface wall of the follicle ruptures and liberates the contained ovum, which escapes from the ovary. The ovum is caught by the oviduct, and either fertilised or passed on through the female system to the outside. The cavity of the Graafian follicle fills up afterwards with spindle-shaped cells, under the influence of the luteinising hormone (LH) from the pituitary. LH becomes more plentiful as FSH becomes less so, and the structure is called the CORPUS LUTEUM or yellow body.

If an ovum is fertilised, resulting in pregnancy, the corpus luteum persists and secretes progesterone, a hormone necessary for the maintenance of pregnancy.

If the animal does not become pregnant, the corpus luteum breaks down and disappears. (Occasionally, however, it fails to do so, and may then cause infertility, especially in the dairy cow .) (See also under CYSTS and below for cystic ovaries – leading often to NYMPHOMANIA.) (See also OESTRUS and diagram under UTERUS.)

Ovaries, Diseases of

In cystic degeneration, large cavernous cysts appear in the substance of the organ, and fill with fluid. For a time there are no definite symptoms shown, but after the cysts attain considerable size the animal begins to exhibit signs of fretfulness and excitability. As time goes on these symptoms increase in violence until in the mare, in which the condition is quite common, it usually becomes dangerous to work her. Upon the slightest provocation, and often with no provocation at all, the mare starts to kick. After her bout of kicking is over she resumes her normal behaviour, but another attack may come on at any time afterwards.

Cysts are also met with in cows where they may be associated with sterility, and in bitches where they are frequently present along with tumour formation in the mammary glands. They are recognised as a cause of sterility in gilts – heat periods being irregular and the clitoris becoming enlarged. Hypoplasia of the ovaries may also occur.

(See NYMPHOMANIA; also under INFERTILITY.)

Ovario-Hysterectomy

Surgical operation for removal of the uterus and ovaries. This is carried out in the dog and cat in cases of pyometra, and following dystokia where a recurrence is feared. It is the usual technique for spaying, especially of cats to prevent the birth of unwanted kittens. (See also SPAYING.)

Ovariotomy

Surgical operation for removal of a diseased ovary. (See also SPAYING.)

Overgrown Foot

Overgrown Foot is one in which the horn of the wall all the way round has continued to grow downwards and outwards, without any compensatory wear along its lower edge. A horse with overgrown feet which may arise either from overlong periods between successive shoeings, or from living on marshy land where the unshod foot gets no wear, is unable to walk correctly. The frog does not reach the ground, the toe is too long, and the heels are too high, so that the normal anti-concussion mechanism of the foot is thrown out of action. The condition predisposes to the occurrence of sprains and contractions of tendons, upright pasterns, and splitting of the horn, with the production of sandcracks as a consequence. Horses' feet that are shod should have the shoes removed at least once a month, and the growth since the last shoeing should be removed by rasping the lower edge of the wall. Young colts, running out at grass, should have their feet properly reduced at least once during every 2 months or so. Overgrown foot is of importance in cattle and sheep, and in animals confined in zoos.

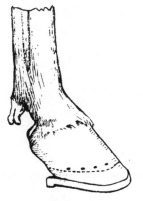

Overgrown hoof, showing how much should be cut away at the next shoeing.

Overlying

Overlying by the sow is one cause of PIGLET MORTALITY and can be prevented by the use of farrowing crates, rails, and the roundhouse. It should be remembered, however, that an ill piglet is more likely to be crushed by the sow than a healthy one; and it has been shown that after 1 hour in an environmental temperature of 1.6° to 4.4°C (35° to 40°F) a piglet becomes comatose. (See under ROUNDHOUSE for an effective means of preventing overlying.)

Over-Reaching

A problem seen in horses when the toe of a hind leg strikes the back of the front leg on the same side. The injury caused is called an 'over-reach' or 'strike'. It usually occurs when the animal is travelling at a gallop; it is also seen in trotters and when jumping of rising ground. Special shoes, designed to hasten the breakover of the front feet and delay that of the hind, may prevent the problem.

Overstocking

The term refers to an excess of grazing animals on a given acreage of pasture. (See STOCKING RATES.) It is also used to describe the practice of leaving a cow unmilked in order to increase the size of the udder and impress potential buyers. It causes great distress to the animal and is illegal under the Welfare of Animals in Markets Order 1990. Both the owner of the cow and the operators of the market can be prosecuted if such a cow is exposed for sale.

Oviduct

(see FALLOPIAN TUBES; SALPINGITIS; EGG-BOUND; PROLAPSE OF OVIDUCT)

Ovine Encephalomyelitis

(see LOUPING-ILL)

Ovine Enzootic Abortion

(see ABORTION, ENZOOTIC, OF EWES)

Ovine Epididimytis

Ovine epididimytis caused by *Brucella ovis* is a NOTIFIABLE DISEASE throughout the EU. It is of considerable importance in Australia and New Zealand. (See RAM; BRUCELLOSIS.)

Ovine Interdigital Dermatitis (OID)

This has been described in foot-rot free flocks in Australia, and is caused by *Fusiformis necrophorus*. (See also SCALD and SCAD.)

Ovine Keratoconjunctivitis (OKC)

The name for a group of infectious eye diseases of sheep. (See also EYE, DISEASES OF.)

Ovulation

In the mare, cow, ewe, sow, and bitch, ovulation has no relation to coitus; whereas in the cat, ferret and rabbit it is coitus that determines the onset of ovulation. (See under OVARIES and OESTRUS.)

Ovum

Ovum is an egg cell. (See EMBRYOLOGY; OVARY; TRANSPLANTATION.)

Oxfendazole

An anthelmintic of the benzimidazole group.

Oxygen

(see OZONE; AIR; RESPIRATION)

Cylinders of oxygen are essential items of equipment for anaesthesia. They are fitted with a pressure gauge and a reducing valve. A flowmeter is incorporated in the anaesthetic circuit. (See ANAESTHESIA.)

Oxygen is used in the treatment of animals rescued from burning buildings and suffering from the effects of smoke inhalation.

Hyperbaric oxygen is that used at high pressures (e.g. 3 atmospheres) for the treatment of carbon monoxide poisoning; and it has also been used for gas gangrene in a dog.

Oxygen embolism is a potential danger when hydrogen peroxide is syringed into a deep wound.

Oxygen Debt

(see MUSCLE – Action of muscles)

Oxytetracycline

An antibiotic. (See TETRACYCLINES.)

Oxytocin

A hormone, secreted by the posterior pituitary gland, and also by the corpus luteum, which actuates the 'milk let-down' mechanism; and also stimulates contraction of the muscles of the uterus in late pregnancy.

Oxyuris

Oxyuris is another name for the thread worm, which possesses a long finely-tapered tail. (See ROUNDWORMS.)

Ozaena

Ozaena is a chronic inflammatory disease of the nasal passages. (See NOSE, DISEASES OF.)

Ozone

The chemically highly reactive allotropic form of oxygen, (O_3). As a constituent of the upper atmosphere it forms a layer which protects people from excessive exposure to ultraviolet radiation from the sun. Ozone may be the main constituent of smog.

It has been described as the most hazardous of all the gaseous air pollutants because of its long-term association in laboratory animals with emphysema, lung cancer, accelerated ageing, increased neonatal deaths, decreased litter size, teratogenesis, and jaw anomalies. In animals exposed to ozone the mortality from lung infections is increased.

O

Pacemaker

An electronic device implanted under the skin of the chest which stimulates the heartbeat.

Pacemakers have been successfully implanted into dogs which show an impaired conduction of the impulse that regulates the heartbeat, so that a lack of coordination between the beating of the atria and that of the ventricles occurs.

Following repeated episodes of loss of consciousness, which heart medication failed to obviate, a 2-year-old dachshund in Switzerland had a pacemaker electrode inserted into the right ventricle of its heart via the jugular vein. The batteries were inserted between abdominal muscles. Local irritation from the battery implant was stated to be slight. Two years later the heart had given no further trouble.

A pacemaker was inserted in a pregnant mare at the Royal Veterinary College. The mare foaled normally and she and the foal fared well.

Pacheco's Disease

Pacheco's disease is caused by a herpesvirus which is present in South American psittacines (parrots, parakeets). In the wild it does not appear to cause any harm. In aviaries, however, sudden onset of disease and death may occur, with up to 100 per cent mortality. The birds become weak and have diarrhoea. Post-mortem examination shows necrosis of the liver and spleen.

Pachymeningitis

Inflammation of the dura mater of the brain and spinal cord. (See MENINGITIS.)

Pacinian Corpuscles

(see under TOUCH, SKIN)

Packed Cell Volume

(see under BLOOD – Composition)

Paddocks

These often become reservoirs of parasitic worm larvae – a point for animal-owners to bear in mind. Paddocks need 'resting' for 12 months, or grazing by a different species of animal, periodically.

Pain

(For relief of pain, see ANALGESICS; ANAESTHESIA.) Animals which are natural hunters (predators) may cry out when suffering pain. Species which are, or were, normally hunted may not do so because it would reveal that they are injured or hiding. Thus, because an animal does not cry out, or show signs of restlessness, it should not be assumed that it is free from pain. The clinical signs of pain can differ from species to species. Pain can be a cause of aggressiveness. The effect of pain can last longer than the pain itself: it has been shown that as long as a month after foot pain has been corrected in cattle, cows still behave as if in pain, as the animal's body has not returned to normal. In sheep, this can last even longer. As a result, bodily condition and milk production may not return to normal until some time after the animal has made an apparent recovery.

Paint

(see HOUSE DECORATING, POISONING; LEAD POISONING, CAGE AND AVIARY BIRDS, DISEASES OF)

Palatability

(see under DIET AND DIETETICS)

Palate

Palate is the partition between the cavity of the mouth below, and that of the nose above. It consists of the hard palate and the soft palate. The hard palate is formed by the bony floor of the nasal cavity covered with dense mucous membrane, which is crossed by transverse ridges in all the domesticated animals. These ridges assist the tongue to carry the food back to the throat. The hard palate stretches back a little beyond the last molar teeth in animals, and ends by becoming continuous with the soft palate. This latter is formed by muscles covered with mucous membrane, and in the horse acts as a sort of curtain between the cavity of the mouth and that of the pharynx. Material brought up from the stomach must pass out by way of the nostrils. In racehorses, distressed breathing may arise as the result of inflammation or partial paralysis of the soft palate, which may be linked with paresis or paralysis of the vocal cords. Partial resection of the soft palate has been carried out as treatment for this latter condition. (See GUTTURAL POUCH DISEASE.)

Prolonged soft palate is a recognised inherited abnormality of the short-nosed breeds of dogs, e.g. boxers, bulldogs, Pekingese, pugs, cocker spaniels. It makes breathing difficult at times, with snoring or even loss of consciousness resulting. An operation to correct the condition is often very successful.

Severe injury to the hard palate is not uncommonly seen in cats which have fallen from a height, and suturing may be required.

Pale Soft Exudative Muscle (PSE)
(see PORCINE STRESS SYNDROME)

Palo Santo Trees
The leaves, fruit, and seeds cause poisoning in cattle in South America. Signs include tympany, depression, and convulsions.

Palpebral
Relating to the eyelids.

Pan-
Pan- is a prefix meaning all or completely.

Pancreas
Pancreas is partly an endocrine gland, producing hormones; and partly an exocrine gland, producing the pancreatic juice for digestive purposes.

The pancreas is situated in the abdomen, a little in front of the level of the kidneys and a little below them. When fresh it has a reddish-cream colour.

The pancreatic juice is secreted into the small intestine to meet the food which has undergone partial digestion in the stomach. The juice contains alkaline salts and at least 9 enzymes: e.g. trypsin, which carries on the digestion of proteins already begun in the stomach; amylase, which converts starches into sugars; and lipase, which breaks up fats; as well as a substance that curdles milk. (See DIGESTION, ABSORPTION and ASSIMILATION – Intestinal digestion.)

The pancreas also has groups of cells, the islets of Langerhans. (See INSULIN; DIABETES MELLITUS; GLUCAGON; HORMONES.) Here alpha-cells produce glucagon, and beta-cells, insulin.

Pancreas, Diseases of
These include DIABETES MELLITUS, inflammation, suppuration, atrophy, tumour formation, etc. (See INSULINOMA.)

Acute pancreatitis occurs in obese dogs, more rarely in cats. Signs include abdominal tenderness or pain. Hyperglycaemia and shock may follow. Treatment includes witholding food, and intravenous fluid therapy to maintain the balance of fluid and electrolyte.

Exocrine pancreatic insufficiency in dogs has 3 main causes: congenital hypoplasia,

degenerative pancreatic atrophy, and chronic pancreatitis. Signs include a ravenous appetite, loss of weight, fatty faeces, and a dry scurfy coat. Treatment includes supplementation of the diet with pancreatin as oral powder or granules. Cimetidine may be used in addition in severe cases.

Parasites which may be found in the pancreatic ducts include *Toxocara canis* and, in cats in America, the pancreatic fluke *Eurytrema procyonis*. The latter may interfere with the gland's exocrine function to a great extent. Fenbendazole is effective against the fluke.

Pancreatin
A preparation of the exocrine part of the pancreas used to treat pancreatic deficiency in dogs and cats.

Pancreatitis
(see PANCREAS, DISEASES OF)

Pancytopenia
A reduction in the number of red cells, white cells, and platelets in the blood; usually due to a bone-marrow dyscrasia.

Panhypopituitarism
A condition caused by development failure of the pituitary gland, destruction of the pituitary tissue or a cyst or tumour in the gland. In puppies, the milk teeth and puppy coat are retained for longer than normal and the animals are stunted. There may be alopecia with skin pigmentation. The gonads may be abnormally small. Polydipsia and polyuria may develop; affected animals may be aggressive. Treatment will depend on the cause.

Panleucopenia
Feline infectious enteritis.

Panniculitis
(see under NODULAR PANNICULITIS)

Pannus
(see EYE, DISEASES AND INJURIES OF)

Panosteitis
A condition in which an entire bone is inflamed.

Pansteatitis
(see STEATITIS)

Pantothenic Acid
(see VITAMINS – Vitamin B)

Papain

An enzyme extracted from the pawpaw (custard apple) and used to tenderise meat.

Papilla

A small projection.

Papilloma

A wart (see WARTS; PAPILLOMA; VIRUS GROUP; also VIRAL INFECTIONS; TUMOUR). In some animal species a papilloma may, through the action of sunlight, lead to a squamous cell carcinoma.

Papilloma Virus Group

Papilloma virus group includes viruses infecting cattle, sheep, goats, horses, dogs, rabbits, etc.

Papillomatosis

The development of multiple WARTS.

Papule

A pimple.

Para-

Para- is a prefix meaning near, aside from, or beyond.

Paracentesis

The technique of puncturing a body cavity, e.g. the abdomen, with a hollow needle or by means of a trocar and cannula in order to extract fluid; or to obtain a sample of tisse for a biopsy.

Paracetamol (Acetaminophen)

An analgesic. It should not be given to cats, in which it is toxic. Symptoms include cyanosis and facial oedema. Acetylcysteine, given orally, is an antidote.

Paraffin

Paraffin is the general term used to designate a series of saturated hydrocarbons. The higher members of the series are solid at ordinary temperatures, some being hard and others soft. Lower in the scale comes petroleum, which is liquid at ordinary temperatures. Naphtha, petroleum spirit, and hydramyl are members of the series lower still, which are very volatile bodies, and finally lowest comes methane or marsh-gas.

Uses Internally, only medicinal liquid paraffin is used; it is a gentle laxative, but has the disadvantage that it is liable to become tolerated by the system and lose its effect when given continually as a routine laxative. It should not be given regularly as it prevents the absorption of vitamin D and may cause rickets. Externally, the hard and soft paraffins are used in the preparation of various ointments and lubricants.

Parafilaria

A genus of filarial worms. *P. bovicola* causes serious skin lesions in cattle in several parts of the world. (See FILARIASIS.)

Paragle Fly

(see under FLIES)

Paragonimiasis

Infestation with LUNG FLUKES of *Paragonimus* species in dogs, cats, foxes, mink.

Parainfluenza 3 Virus

Infection with this is widespread in sheep in the UK; the virus is also a cause of CALF PNEUMONIA and of respiratory diseases in the horse. (See EQUINE RESPIRATORY VIRUSES.) Parainfluenza 5 infects the dog, and may be associated with KENNEL COUGH. (See also INFLUENZA.)

Parakeratosis

The name applied to a scaly, elephant-like skin. The condition has been seen in pigs suffering from a zinc deficiency. It occurs in pigs fed dry meal *ad lib*, and gradually clears up when a change to wet feeding is made. It often begins with a red pimply condition of the skin on the flanks, abdomen, etc. Thin, dry yellowish or greyish scales may be seen on the skin, which later becomes thickened. It responds to small doses of zinc sulphate. (See CALCIUM SUPPLEMENTS.)

Inherited parakeratosis has been reported in calves of Friesian descent, and although a zinc supplement proved successful in treating the encrusted skin of head, neck and limbs, the lesions returned after cessation of the supplement.

Paraldehyde

A narcotic. It is used in some slug pellets and poisoning in domestic pets can follow ingestion.

Paralysis

Paralysis, in its widest sense, may mean loss of nerve control over any of the bodily functions, loss of sensation, and loss of the special senses, but the term is usually restricted to mean loss of muscular action due to interference with the nervous system. When muscular power is merely weakened, without being lost completely, the word 'paresis' is often used.

Various terms are used to indicate paralysis distributed in different ways. (See HEMIPLEGIA; PARAPLEGIA; QUADRIPLEGIA.)

Paralysis should be regarded as a symptom rather than as a disease by itself.

Varieties

Cerebral paralysis: conditions resulting from brain lesions, such as encephalitis, tumour formation, fracture of the skull with depression of a portion of bone, haemorrhage, etc., are accompanied by severe general or local paralysis, either of the whole body (when death usually follows very rapidly), or of one side (hemiplegia).

Paralysed limbs when examined are found to be flaccid, with the muscles totally relaxed, and passive movements are not resisted. Sensations of pain may be felt, however, and an indication that sensation is not destroyed is shown by raising the head, or struggling with the sound limbs when a pinprick is made in a paralysed part.

In cases of cerebral haemorrhage, the seizure is sudden; in encephalitis there is usually some co-existing disease, such as influenza or distemper, and the brain symptoms develop as a complication – or the encephalitis may be the result of a primary viral infection, such as equine encephalitis or rabies. With fracture and depression there is an immediate loss of power, just as when an animal is stunned.

Spinal paralysis or paraplegia is most often due to fracture of, or severe injury to, the vertebrae. (See PARAPLEGIA.)

In complete paralysis death usually takes place within 12 to 48 hours after the injury. (See SPINE AND SPINAL CORD, DISEASES AND INJURIES OF; and, for horses, under COMENY'S INFECTIOUS PARALYSIS OF HORSES and EQUINE VIRAL RHINO PNEUMONITIS.)

Peripheral paralysis: there is usually some injury to a nerve trunk, or lesion of the nerve-endings in the muscle fibres. (See SUPRASCAPULAR PARALYSIS; RADIAL PARALYSIS.)

Brachial paralysis results from road accidents, collisions, or stake wounds. Gluteal paralysis is very uncommon: wasting of the muscles of one hindquarter and a tendency to carry the limb out to one side occur. 'Paralysis of the sciatic nerve' causes a loss of power in all the muscles of the thigh except those situated above and to the front of the stifle joint, i.e. the quadratus group. The limb hangs loosely and the animal jerks it forward when attempting to walk; although the stifle is advanced, the hock and

the fetlock remain flexed and the front of the foot comes to the ground.

When there is severe injury to the side of the thigh from a fall, kick, or other similar cause, paralysis of the external popliteal nerve (common peroneal) may occur, resulting in an inability to extend the foot or flex the hock. When the horse is made to walk, the limb is drawn out backwards into a position resembling that seen in dislocation of the stifle, but the fetlock is flexed instead of being fully extended. The limb is then carried a short distance forward and the foot comes to rest upon the ground on its anterior face instead of on the sole. In 'crural paralysis' (paralysis of the femoral nerve) the quadriceps muscles above the stifle, which normally extend that joint, are paralysed. When weight is put upon the limb the stifle sinks to the level of the hock or below it, all joints are flexed, and there is a peculiar drop of the hindquarter on the same side. (See also PARAPLEGIA.)

Paralysis in the dog (see also DISTEMPER; BOTULISM; THROMBOSIS; SPINE, DISEASES OF; TICK PARALYSIS; LEAD POISONING; RABIES; RACOONS; ORGANOPHOSPHORUS POISONING)

Aid A wheeled trolley which supports the hindquarters can be an alternative to euthanasia for some paraplegic dogs.

Paralytic Myoglobinuria

(see MUSCLES, DISEASES OF – Nutritional muscular dystrophy)

Paraminobenzoic Acid

A growth factor produced in bacteria which is blocked by certain antibacterials, such as sulphonamides.

Paramphistomiasis

A disease caused by RUMEN FLUKES of the genus *Paramphistomum*.

Paramyxoviruses

An important group of disease-causing viruses. Parainfluenzavirus, morbillivirus and pneumovirus are the 3 genera of paramyxovirus. (See Paramyxovirus parainfluenza 3 virus in the table under EQUINE RESPIRATORY VIRUSES.) Two paramyxoviruses infecting dogs are the canine distemper virus (a mobillivirus), and canine parainfluenza virus/SV5. (See also PIGEONS and NEWCASTLE DISEASE.)

Paraphimosis

A constriction preventing the penis from being withdrawn into the prepuce. This is not uncommon in the dog, and is serious, for gangrene may occur unless relief is afforded. As a first-aid measure, swab the penis with ice-cold water. Surgical interference under anaesthesia may be necessary. The use of hyaluronidase in normal saline, by injection, has been recommended.

For paraphimosis in horses and cattle see under PENIS AND PREPUCE, ABNORMALITIES AND LESIONS.

Paraplegia

PARALYSIS of the hindlegs. It may be accompanied by paralysis of the muscles which control the passage of urine and faeces to the outside. It is seen following accidents involving injury to the spine – frequently in the dog knocked down by a car – and may also be associated with 'disc' lesions. A rare cause is thrombosis of the femoral arteries. In the dog, this may occur suddenly – the animal playing one minute, and collapsing with a yelp the next. Absence of pulse in the femoral arteries assists a diagnosis. (See also under THROMBOSIS; COMENY'S INFECTIOUS PARALYSIS OF HORSES.)

Parapox Viruses

Apart from those affecting domestic animals (see table under VIRUSES), a parapox virus carried by grey squirrels, but apparently harmless to them, has had a devastating effect on the native red squirrel. A parapox virus is also though to be the cause of high mortality in British frogs in certain parts of Britain.

Paraquat

This herbicide has caused fatal poisoning in man, usually through accidental ingestion of the undiluted concentrate; an emetic is now included. Poisoning in the dog gives rise to lung oedema, congestion and consolidation; also kidney damage. Three cases, and the outcomes, are reported below.

Paraquat was detected in the urine of 2 out of 5 dogs showing acute respiratory distress, leading to cyanosis after 4 days' illness. Three of the dogs died, and euthanasia was resorted to with the others.

In New South Wales, a dog died and a cat recovered (partially if not completely); the latter animal had been seen eating grass from a lawn of which the weedy areas had been treated with undiluted Gramoxone (20 per cent paraquat). In both animals vomiting was a symptom, as well as distressed breathing.

Cyanocobalamin has been suggested as an antidote for small animals, though it is generally held that no effective antidote exists. However, complete recovery was achieved for a dog taken to the University of Dublin's veterinary clinic, with a history of weakness, and rapid breathing over the previous 6 hours.

The animal's condition deteriorated, despite intensive treatment. Nursed at home, the patient was seen at the clinic daily. On the 15th day came improvement: although the dog was still breathing through its mouth, respirations were down to 120 per minute. It was 7 weeks before they had come down to 60.

P

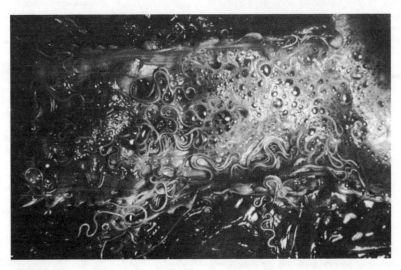

Adult worms in the air passages of a calf's lungs. In a heavily infected animal several thousand lungworms may be present.

The patience and perseverance of both owner and clinic staff were rewarded, for when seen again 6 and then 18 months later, the dog was well and fully active again.

Parasites and Immunity

Parasite antigens are a potent stimulus for antiparasite antibodies of the IgE class (see IMMUNOGLOBULINS), and parasite infection can potentiate a pre-existing IgE response to an unrelated antigen.

Examples of the effect of parasitism on the immune response are given under CANCER and ALLERGY.

Parasitic Bronchitis

This occurs in cattle, sheep and goats; on account of the husky cough produced, the disease is commonly called 'husk' or 'hoose' in the UK.

Although of greater economic importance in calves, nevertheless the cost of an outbreak in a dairy herd may be very high – not so much as a result of deaths (which do occur in adult cattle) but on account of reduced milk yields and the need for extra feed. Marshy land and mild, wet weather both favour the parasites, as does overstocking.

Cause In cattle the lungworm *Dictyocaulus viviparus* is the important species (see ROUND-WORMS; also illustration, page 513). Parasitic bronchitis normally affects cattle in their first grazing season. Affected animals experience a drop in the saturation level of oxygen in their blood to 70 per cent even before clinical signs become apparent. In clinical cases the percentage may be reduced to 30.

Workers at Glasgow University defined infection with the parasite into 5 phases: penetration, pre-patent, patent, post-patent, and reinfection. In all but the first phase, oedema and emphysema are found .

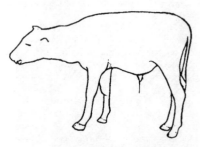

In a case of parasitic bronchitis, the neck is held extended and there may be continual coughing and/or distressed breathing.

Spread of the worm larvae is assisted by their rocket-like propulsion by the fungus *Pilobolus*, which is found in faecal deposits on pasture. The worm larvae are projected along with the fungal spores, often between 10.00 and mid-day.

Signs The characteristic husky cough is a symptom in the milder cases, but in acute cases may be absent, with the main symptom being dyspnoea (laboured breathing). In calves, death may occur from actual suffocation due to masses of worms obstructing the air passages, or it may result from general debility or pneumonia. In adult cattle pneumonia develops, with *Actinomyces pyogenes* acting as a secondary invader. Oedema of the lungs may occur, and cause death.

Prevention and treatment Live oral vaccines are available. A number of ANTHELMINTICS, including albendazole, iver-mectin and fenbendazole, may be used to treat infected cattle. Some anthelmintics are available in bolus form. If the animal is exposed to infection while the anthelmintic bolus is active, the animal will develop immunity without showing signs of the disease (see under WORMS, FARM TREATMENT AGAINST).

Parasitic Disease, Nature of

Parasitic diseases are caused by organisms that live within an animal (endoparasites) or on its surface (ectoparasites). Endoparasites include worms and flukes; ectoparasites include fleas, mites and ticks. Disease is seldom caused by one or a few parasitic organisms, but as a rule depends on mass infestations. There are exceptions to this, however, as a single *Ascaris* may obstruct the bile-duct with fatal results. Parasites, with few exceptions, do not spend all their lives in the animal body, but always need to spend a certain proportion of their life-cycle outside the host. They may cause damage to the host in the following ways:

(1) By abstraction of nourishment properly belonging to the host, e.g. many of the intestinal worms;

(2) By mechanical obstruction of passages or compression of organs, e.g. gapes (in chickens) and hydatid;

(3) By feeding on the tissues of the host, e.g. blood-sucking worms or flies;

(4) By production of toxins with varying effects;

(5) By actual traumatic damage, e.g. by piercing and destroying skin (ticks, mites, flies, etc.), by depositing eggs in the tissues

(lung-worms), by migrations of larvae (*Ascaris* and *Trichinella*), by clinging to surfaces by means of sharp hooks (tapeworms), and in many other ways;

(6) By facilitating the entrance of bacteria, e.g. stomach worms in pigs allow the entrance of *Fusiformis necrophorus* (the necrosis bacillus);

(7) By transmitting diseases for which they act as intermediate hosts, e.g. ticks and babesiosis;

(8) By causing inflammatory or neoplastic reactions in the invaded tissues, e.g. pneumonia, gastritis, and fluke adenomata in the liver.

These are only some of the more obvious methods of injuring the host. Apart from the loss due to actual deaths, the depreciation in value of hides, meat, milk, and work is enormous, and, although less spectacular than a bacterial epizootic, the loss is more constant, and in the aggregate even greater than the loss due to bacterial diseases. (See BRAIN DISEASES – Parasites, for parasites which migrate to the brain.)

Parasitic Gastroenteritis of Cattle

This is an insidious and economically important disease, and the cause of death in many calves and yearlings. It is known that the output of worm eggs in the faeces does not bear any constant relation to the number of worms present. It rises to an early peak and then declines, and is not a reliable guide to the degree of infestation.

Cause Infestation with various species of ROUNDWORMS.

Signs A gradual loss of condition; a harsh, staring coat; sometimes, but not always, scouring; pale mucous membranes; progressive weakness and emaciation. In adult cattle, which acquire a high degree of resistance (only broken down when under-feeding, chilling, pregnancy, or massive contamination of pasture occurs), no symptoms may normally be shown, but nevertheless the animal's efficiency is lowered.

Treatment Dosing with an appropriate anthelmintic should not be delayed until the stock are weak.

Prevention Calves should be dosed once with an anthelmintic in mid-July and moved to pasture which has not been grazed that season by other cattle. Dose again in the autumn.

(See WORMS, FARM TREATMENT AGAINST; PASTURE, 'CLEAN'.)

Parasitic Gastroenteritis of Sheep

It is likely that outbreaks in early lambs in March and April are the result of over-wintered larvae. In 1 experiment, worm-free lambs were turned on to a pasture – 'rested' during the winter – in the spring and became infested with 12 species of gastrointestinal worms.

Lambs may also be infected by eggs in the dung of ewes at lambing, when a periparturient rise occurs.

Treatment and prevention Routine use of, e.g., Tetramisole. (See WORMS, FARM TREATMENT AGAINST; PASTURE, 'CLEAN'.)

Parasitic Tracheobronchitis
(see TRACHEAL WORMS)

Parasitism
Parasitism is the association of 2 organisms, 1 of which (the parasite) benefits by nourishing itself at the expense of the other (the host) but without normally destroying it.

The following types of parasitic relations are recognised: 1 (a) ectoparasites, which live on the host; and (b) endoparasites, which live within the body of the host; 2 (a) accidental parasites, which are normally free-living animals but may live for a certain period in a host; (b) facultative parasites, which are able to exist free or as parasites, e.g. blowfly larvae; and (c) obligatory parasites, which are completely adapted to a parasitic type of life and must live in or on a host, e.g. most parasitic worms; 3 (a) temporary or transitory parasites, which pass a definite phase or phases in their life-history as parasites and during which time the parasitism is obligatory and continuous, e.g. botflies, ticks; (b) permanent parasites, which always live for the greater part of their life as parasites, e.g. lice, tapeworms, coccidia, etc.; and (c) periodic, occasional, or intermittent parasites, which only visit the host for short periods to obtain food, e.g. blood-sucking flies, fleas; 4 (a) erratic parasites, which occur in an organ that is not their normal habitat, e.g. *Fasciola hepatica* in the lungs; (b) incidental parasites, which, exceptionally, occur in an animal that is not their normal host; they are incidental only in this first host, e.g. *Dipylidium caninum* is incidental in man; and (c) specific parasites, which occur in a particular species of host or group of hosts, e.g. *D. caninum* is specific for dogs and cats.

PARASITES and PARASITOLOGY

Parasympathetic Nervous System

The parasympathetic nervous system is 1 division of the autonomic nervous system; the other division being the sympathetic. (See AUTONOMIC NERVOUS SYSTEM; CENTRAL NERVOUS SYSTEM.)

Parathion

Parathion is chemically diethyl-*para*-nitrophenyl-thiophosphate and is used for agricultural purposes to destroy aphis and red spider. In man and domestic animals it is a cumulative poison which readily enters the system through inhalation, by the mouth or by absorption through the skin. Animals should not be allowed to graze under trees sprayed with parathion for at least 3 weeks. In man, symptoms of poisoning include headache, vomiting, and a feeling of tightness in the chest. Later there is sweating, salivation, muscular twitching, distressed breathing and coma. (See ORGANOPHOSPHORUS POISONING.)

In animals, copious salivation and lachrymation, twitching, and increased intestinal movement are shown. Cattle are apparently tolerant of parathion, being able to break it down chemically.

The danger of spray drift, and the risk to dogs and cats wandering in sprayed areas, are obvious.

SOME OF THE EFFECTS OF PARATHYROID HORMONE AND CALCITONIN, THE 2 MAJOR HORMONES CONTROLLING THE REGULATION OF BLOOD CALCIUM

	Parathyroid hormone	Calcitonin
Mode of action	Separates fast and slow components Increases cell membrane permeability Activates adenyl cyclase enzyme systems	Uncertain
Effect on kidney	Increases P excretion by decreasing tubular reabsorption Decreases Ca excretion by increasing tubular reabsorption Increases Na excretion by decreasing tubular reabsorption	Increases Ca, P, Na, and K excretion Decreases Mg excretion
Effect on intestine	Increases Ca, P and Mg absorption	? Decreases P absorption Decreases volume and acidity of gastric juice
Effect on bone	Increases resorption Stimulates osteoclast and osteocyte activity Inhibits formation Suppresses osteoblast activity	Inhibits resorption
Resultant effect on blood calcium	Elevated	Diminished

(With acknowledgements to Professor D. Bennett and to The Veterinary Record.)

Parathyroid Glands

Parathyroid glands are small structures situated either wholly within, or upon the surface of, the thyroid gland. Their secretion, the parathyroid hormone, is important in the control of the level of blood calcium. Insufficiency of this hormone leads to muscular twitchings or tremors or, in more severe cases, to convulsions. (See TETANY.) The hormone also controls phosphate excretion via the urine. (See table.)

Hyperparathyroidism in dogs. Of 21 dogs with primary hyperparathyroidism, 20 had a parathyroid adenoma and 1 had a parathyroid carcinoma. The most common clinical signs were polydipsia/ polyuria, listlessness, muscular weakness and inappetence. The only consistent biochemical abnormality was persistent hypercalcaemia (12.1 to 19.6 mg/100 ml). The external parathyroid tumours, found in 9 of the 19 dogs which underwent surgery, were easily removed; internal parathyroid tumours were removed by thyroidectomy.

Primary hyperparathyroidism in a cat
A 12-year-old cat showed clinical signs of lethargy, reluctance to move and pain along the back. Radiological examination revealed multifocal lesions, particularly in the skeleton. There was bilateral parathyroid hyperplasia but no evidence of neoplastic change. Histological examination revealed that a large proportion of bone had been resorbed and replaced by fibrous connective tissue and that osteoclasts were numerous. It is suggested that hyperparathyroidism should be considered in the differential diagnosis of conditions involving skeletal pain and lethargy in the cat.

Paratuberculosis

A synonym for JOHNE'S DISEASE.

Paratyphoid

Infection with any species of salmonella; a synonym for SALMONELLOSIS.

Parenchyma

Parenchyma is a term used for the functional cells of an organ, as opposed to its supporting, connective tissue (interstitial) cells. In a gland the parenchyma is the mass of secreting cells; in the lung, similarly, the parenchyma comprises the cells concerned with respiration, not the fibrous supporting tissue.

Parenteral

Administration of a medicinal substance other than via the digestive system, e.g. by injection.

Paresis

A state of slight or temporary PARALYSIS, also called 'fleeting paralysis'. (See MILK FEVER; MUSCLES, DISEASES OF – Nutritional muscular dystrophy; LEAD POISONING; GUTTURAL POUCH DISEASE.)

Parietal

Parietal is the term applied to anything pertaining to the wall of a cavity, e.g. parietal pleura, the part of the pleural membrane which lines the wall of chest.

Paronychia

Paronychia is inflammation near to the nail. (See RINGWORM.)

Parotid Gland

Parotid gland is one of the salivary glands. It is situated just below and behind the ear on either side, in the space between the angle of the jaw and the muscles of the neck. From its base commences a duct, the parotid duct, or Stenson's duct, which in the horse runs within the border of the mandible for a distance, and then turns round its rim to the side of the face in company with the external maxillary artery and vein, and ends by opening into the mouth opposite the anterior part of the 3rd upper cheek tooth; in other animals it runs straight across the face instead of along the lower jaw bone.

The SALIVARY GLANDS are composed of collections of secreting acini held together loosely by a certain amount of fibrous tissue, but they do not possess a distinct capsule.

Parovarium

Parovarium is the name of rudimentary structures situated near the ovary, which are the remnants of the Wolffian bodies. The name Paroophoron is also used. These structures are often the seat of cysts in the young adult. (See OVARIES, DISEASES OF.)

Parrots

(see PSITTACOSIS; also BIRD IMPORT CONTROLS and PACHECO'S DISEASE)

Parthenogenesis

Asexual reproduction, in which the ovum develops into an embryo without fertilisation by a spermatozoon.This is a common method of reproduction among invertebrate animals, particularly insects, including ants and bees.

Partridges

(see GAME BIRDS, MORTALITY)

Parturient Paresis

(see MILK FEVER and 'DOWNER COW' SYNDROME)

Parturition

Parturition is the expulsion of the fetus (and its membranes) from the uterus through the maternal passages by natural forces, and in such a state of development that, in domesticated animals at least, though not in the marsupials, the fetus is capable of independent life. The process is called 'foaling' in the mare, 'calving' in the cow, 'lambing' in the ewe, 'kidding' in the goat, 'farrowing' in the sow, and 'whelping' in the bitch. It is more likely to proceed successfully without than with human interference in the great majority of cases. (See CALVING, DIFFICULT for information on traction.)

Stages in parturition Although the act is really a continuous one, it is customary to divide it into 4 stages: (1) Preliminary stage; (2) Dilatation of the cervix stage; (3) Expulsion of the fetus stage; (4) Expulsion of the membranes stage.

(1) *Preliminary stage* may occupy some hours or even days. The udder swells, becomes hard and tender, and a clear waxy fluid material oozes from the teats or may be expelled by pressure of the hand. The external genitals become swollen, enlarged, and their lining is reddened. A vaginal secretion appears. The abdomen drops and becomes pendulous. The quarters droop and the muscles and ligaments of the pelvis slacken. The animal separates itself from its fellows if at pasture; if at liberty, it seeks a remote or an inaccessible place in which to bring forth its young, and some, such as the sow, bitch, and cat, prepare a bed or nest.

(2) *Dilatation of the cervix stage* merges with the preceding. Restlessness is evident. The mare paces around the loose-box (often with tail raised) – perhaps lying down and rising again several times. Sweating occurs under the mane and tail, and soon over most of the body.

During the 2nd stage of labour, the mare is usually lying down on her side, and in some cases will show symptoms of COLIC, i.e. kicking at the belly, turning and gazing at her flanks, or wandering round in an aimless fashion. Meanwhile the labour pains have been getting more and more powerful and the intervals between them shorter. The pulse is quickened, and the breathing rapid. When a pain has passed the animal calms down and remains so till the next takes place. After a variable time – from about 1/2 to 3 hours – the 'water-bag' appears at the vulva. It is tense and hard during a pain, but becomes slack and flaccid in the intervals. It is found to be empty at first, but the fore-feet of the young animal can be felt in it later. At this time the cervix is fully dilated, and the 3rd stage follows without any appreciable break in the sequence of events.

(3) Expulsion of the fetus stage In this stage the severity of the pains is greatest, and the auxiliary muscles of the abdomen assist in the contractions. The animal may remain standing, may lie down in the recumbent position, or may alternately lie and stand. The back is arched, the chest expanded, and the muscles of the abdomen become board-hard with each labour pain. The animal may groan, or squeal or even scream with each effort. Frequently the rectum forcibly discharges its contents and the urinary bladder does likewise. At each contraction the 'water-bag' protrudes farther and farther from the vulva until it finally ruptures in its most dependant part. There is a rush of fluid from the uterus to the outside and the animal has a period of ease. Then fore-feet, and the muzzle lying behind and over them, appear at the vulva, forming a kind of cone which dilates the softer tissues of the genital canal. In the larger animals the feet come first, but in the carnivora, where the head is large, the head precedes the fore-feet, which are tucked against the young animal's chest and sides. When the head has cleared the vulva there is usually another pause, which allows the tissues to become accustomed to the great distension, and prepares them for the still greater distension and strain that is soon to follow. The thorax and shoulders are now in the pelvis of the dam, and are driven slowly through it by the most powerful and painful of the contractions that occur during the process. As this part of the fetus reaches the outlet of the pelvis there is generally a more energetic and painful effort than all the others – which pushes the fetal trunk to the outside. This culminating effort may cause the bitch or cat to cry out.

Sometimes the foal's umbilical cord does not rupture, in which case the mare will usually gnaw through it, and so liberate the foal. It sometimes happens that a foal is born completely enveloped in its membranes; in such instances, unless assistance is at hand to free the foal, it will be rapidly suffocated.

In cows the umbilical cord is much shorter and it ruptures before the hind legs of the calf have passed to the outside. Owing to the cotyledonary attachment of the placenta the membranes are seldom born along with the calf.

the smaller animals, especially in the sow, bitch, and cat, the young are frequently born in their membranes, and these are licked away and cleared from the young by the dam, the umbilical cord being broken or bitten through in the process.

(4) Expulsion of the membranes stage, or the 'delivery of the afterbirth', may occur with, immediately following, or not for some considerable time after, the production of the young in an animal.

Very soon after the young animal is born the uterus contracts and becomes smaller – a process known as 'involution' – so that its capacity is decreased. The attachment between the membranes and the mucosa of the uterus is loosened and the placenta is separated from the uterus. These contractions also serve to push out the membranes through the wide open cervix.

With the mare, owing to the diffuse and not very intimate adherence between the uterine mucous membrane and the placental membrane, the separation and the discharge of the envelopes are soon accomplished. In fact, if these are retained for more than a very few hours (4 or 6 or so), serious results are probable, but retention of the membranes is rare in the healthy mare.

In the cow, the attachment is limited to the surfaces of the cotyledons and is very close, and where the shrinkage in the uterine wall (i.e. involution) does not tend greatly to upset the intimacy of the adhesion, the calf is not born in its membranes, and retention of these is more common. They are generally discharged within a few hours of the birth of the calf, but the time varies.

Animals which produce more than 1 young at a time generally discharge the membranes of each at the same time as or soon after it is born, with the exception of the last of the litter, whose membranes are occasionally retained in the extremity of 1 horn of the uterus.

In animals that are really uniparous (i.e. produce only 1 fetus at a birth but which have been modified by breeding so that they often produce 2 or more young, such as the sheep and goat) the membranes of the 1st twin come away with the 2nd, and those of the 2nd are expelled after it has been born.

Early discharge of the membranes is desirable, because as long as they remain in position they are likely sources of infection to the uterus, and they prevent that organ from returning to normal. After they have been evacuated the involution of the uterus becomes more and more complete, until in a few days it has shrunk to less than half its former size. It never decreases to its original virgin size.

The mare should have been housed in the 'foaling-box' for a month or so previously, so that she shall feel quite at home (see PREGNANCY AND GESTATION – Care of the dam during pregnancy), and the ventilation, warmth, bedding, cleanliness, etc., should be as near an approach to the ideal as circumstances will allow. If possible, the cow should calve in a separate loose-box. Ewes lamb out in the open and do quite well, but if the weather is cold or stormy, or if the ground is very wet, it is better to provide a 'lambing-pen', especially with Lowland breeds which have not the same hardiness as the mountain varieties. Sows should on all occasions have a pen to themselves, for if other pigs are present the little pigs will most probably be eaten as soon as they are born.

When the birth process has begun, the attendant may need to soothe and quieten the dam if she becomes very excited, but beyond this the prospective mother should be left alone for some time. If all is going well, the 'water-bag' will soon appear and later burst. No hard-and-fast rule can be laid down, but if the fore-legs and nose of the fetus do not appear within 10 to 20 minutes in the mare, and in double that period in the cow, a simple examination should be made by the attendant to ensure that the presentation is a normal one. After washing hands and arms in mild antiseptic, such as Dettol or Cetrimide solutions, and thoroughly lubricating them with a vaginal lubricant, the hand should be gently inserted into the posterior genital passage to explore by touch whatever presents itself. The 2 fore-feet should be distinguishable in that part of the passage that lies lowermost when the dam is standing. Above them and slightly behind, the nose and mouth should be felt. These structures are often covered with fetal membrane, but in a normal case can be located. In such cases as this, nothing further need be done in the meantime; the dam will probably produce her young quite normally, and any attempts at assistance will only irritate and perhaps exhaust her.

It may happen, however, that 1 or both of the fore-legs or the nose cannot at first be found. On introducing the arms still further these parts can sometimes be discovered, and, by gentle pulling or readjustment, can be brought into the normal position. Before the process of parturition has advanced very far, abnormal positions of the fetus can be comparatively easily corrected, and serious trouble from subsequent jamming may be avoided. If all efforts at correction prove futile, a veterinary surgeon should be called in.

Upon comparatively rare occasions none of the foremost positions of the body can be felt, but the 2 hind-feet or legs (distinguishable by the difference between knees and hocks), and perhaps the tail of the young animal, are discovered. This is a posterior presentation, and as the head is the last part of the fetus that will be born, respiration cannot begin until birth is complete, and the risk of suffocation is great. Accordingly, it is necessary to attempt to hurry the whole process and a veterinary surgeon should be called.

Attention to offspring As soon as the young animal is born and free from the maternal passages, it is absolutely essential to ascertain that the fetal membranes are not obstructing its mouth or nostrils. It generally gives 1 or 2 spasmodic gasps or struggles, and then begins to breathe. Each respiration is shallow and weak at first, but in a very few minutes the breathing settles down to the normal.

Suspended animation Occasionally, foals and calves are born in a state of suspended animation, and ARTIFICIAL RESPIRATION will be needed.

The umbilical cord This is best not interfered with. In the foal, early severance of the cord can lead to the loss of 1000 to 1500 ml of placental fetal blood, whereas under 'natural' conditions the amount concerned is probably well under 200 ml. The well-being of the animal is better served when it is allowed to retain the blood, as would usually be the case under natural conditions. The umbilical cord has a point at which it will rupture normally, generally by movement of the mare, after a period during which mother and foal rest. Since haemorrhage from either end of the severed cord is then extremely rare, the cord should require no human attention after a normal birth. The natural sealing of the umbilical cord provides an effective barrier against both bleeding and infection.

The Animal Health Trust's Equine Research Centre has commented: 'It is difficult to imagine a worse procedure than leaving a substantial "meaty" mass of umbilical cord at the navel as happens so commonly after cutting the cord with scissors. This provides an ideal medium for the passage of micro-organisms whose entrance to the abdominal portions of the umbilical vein and arteries are not hindered in any way by the

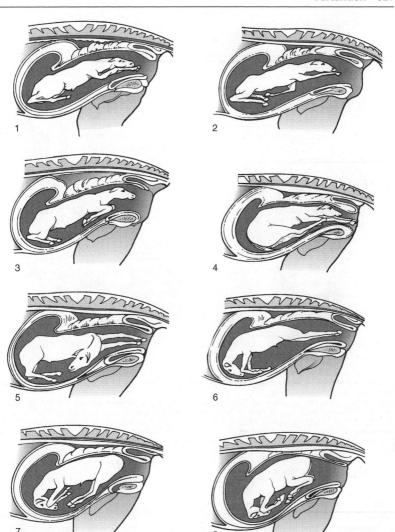

Different varieties of presentations of the foal.

1. Normal anterior presentation – nose and both fore-feet in passage.

2. Anterior presentation with 1 fore-limb retained completely. This should be brought forward by hand, or by passing rope round flexure of knee.

3. Anterior presentation with both fore-limbs retained at the knees, corrected as in No. 2.

4. 'Dog-sitting' presentation – nose and all 4 limbs presenting. The 2 fore-limbs should be corded and the hind-limbs repelled or pushed back.

5. Anterior presentation with head and neck retained. Delivery may often be effected by traction on fore-limbs in foal, the head being pressed into the soft abdomen. In calf, owing to the short neck, this is not usually possible. Where possible, fore-limbs should be corded, pushed back, and the head brought round by the hand or, in difficult cases, by hooks and cords.

6. Posterior presentation. Successful delivery often possible if the birth is speeded up by traction to avoid suffocation (see text).

7. 'Breech presentation'. Delivery difficult, foal nearly always dead. Cords in front of the foal's stifles and round buttocks may be applied if mare is large and foal is small, but usually necessitates amputation of 1 or both hind-limbs.

8. 'Thigh and croup presentation'. Cord round hocks may be successful in converting this into an ordinary posterior presentation. Quarters must be firmly pushed back after hocks are corded.

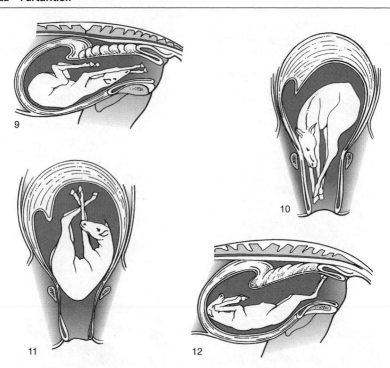

9. 'Upside-down' anterior presentation. Occasionally delivery may be effected without adjustment, but assistance is always necessary. Removal of 1 or both fore-limbs, with or without head and neck, often essential.

10. Ventral transverse presentation. This and No. 11 are the 2 worst positions in which foal can lie. Each case must be treated differently. Fore- or hind-limbs may be pushed back or brought forwards according as they lie back in the passage or advanced. Removal of the foal in portions, a limb at a time, is often necessary.

11. Dorsal transverse presentation. Foal usually requires to be disected and each half removed separately.

12. 'Upside down posterior presentation'. Delivery may be possible as soon as limbs have been adjusted, or amputation or version may be carried out.

"sterile" piece of tape so frequently used to "tie off" the stump. Almost as undesirable a procedure is the application of strong antiseptics (notably iodine), destructive as they are to tissue with which they come in contact.'

Other advice If a young mare, for instance, does not at once begin to dry and cleanse her foal, a little salt rubbed over its coat may induce her to do so. Should the mother refuse to perform this office, the offspring must be dried with a towel, cloth, wisp of hay, etc., so far as is possible.

Suckling The first suck is of great importance. Within about half an hour the young of the domesticated animals are usually able to stand on their feet – although they are shaky at first – and as soon as they master this feat they make endeavours to reach the teat. The first milk contains a natural laxative, and it is essential that the newly born should obtain some of this as soon as possible. Colostrum – the first milk – promotes a secretion from the intestinal glands and stimulates peristalsis, so that the debris and black, gummy, faecal material (called 'meconium') that has been lying in the bowels of the foal is evacuated and the way prepared for the digestion of food. When a dam dies before the foal obtains any colostrum, it is necessary to supply colostrum provided by another animal or a substitute such as melted butter and milk.

Attention to the dam Where parturition has been easy and normal, the dam rapidly recovers from her trying experience, and may be up on to her feet within a few minutes of the discharge of the fetus. It is usually better to allow her to remain lying as long as she wishes while attention is being paid to her offspring. It is good practice to offer a drink of warm barley-water or thin oatmeal gruel containing a table-spoonful of common table-salt, as soon after the act as convenient. Her system has undergone a considerable shock, and has lost quantities of fluid which should be replaced. The larger animals may require a rug if the weather is at all cold. After 3 to 6 hours or thereabouts, a pailful of bran mash and a little hay should be given.

When the dam is very exhausted by her labour it is necessary to administer stimulants. If the birth of the young was difficult, and when the passages have been exposed to considerable strain by assisted labour, hot (but not scalding) fomentations may be applied to the external genital organs. Afterwards the parts must be covered with a warm and dry blanket, to prevent any chilling. The loose-box must be warm yet well ventilated, and the dam should be encouraged to rest as much as possible.

Subsequent management No oats or concentrated food-stuff should be given to the dam for the first 2 days after parturition; her rations should consist of water, bran mashes, and hay or green food given 3 times daily. After that time a gradually increasing amount of crushed oats and cut hay or chaff may be added to the mash daily, until at the end of a week or 10 days she is back on to her usual diet. Gentle exercise is as necessary for the foal or calf as it is for their dams, and if the weather is suitable the dam and her progeny should be allowed out on to a sheltered meadow for an hour or so twice daily, after the first 3 or 4 days following the birth of the young. This period is gradually increased until in 2 weeks' time the pair may be left out from 9.00 a.m. till 5.00 p.m., or even may be allowed to sleep out all night if the weather permits. In this connection it should be remembered that cold dry nights are much less harmful than those that are wet or foggy. Young animals of all species withstand dry cold very much better than wet cold, and it is inadvisable to allow foals or calves less than a month old to sleep out on a wet or marshy meadow. A useful method is to erect a covered-in shed in a corner of the meadow, containing a feeding-trough and well littered with straw, into which both dam and her offspring may retire whenever they wish. The amount of hand feeding which the dam receives must be judged according to circumstances. If the grass is rich and well forward, 1 feed of oats and hay may be sufficient after the first 3 or 4 weeks, but it is always better to err on the safe side and keep the dam in good general condition, for much of the subsequent quality of the offspring depends upon the start in life that it receives through its mother's milk, and if she herself is in poor condition her milk will be inferior.

Parturition, Drug-Induced

Prostaglandins are frequently used to induce parturition in pigs, and sometimes in other livestock, so that it occurs at a planned date. It is a technique also used in some cases of debility of the dam in late pregnancy, where there is some abnormality associated with the pregnancy, to avoid dystokia in the cross-breeding of dairy cows for beef production.

Parvovirus

This has been associated with infertility in the sow, and is a cause of mummified fetuses and small litter size. (See VIRUSES – Classification table; CANINE PARVOVIRUS (CPV); and FELINE INFECTIOUS ENTERITIS.)

Human parvovirus infection This is most common in children, and is associated with a rash and fever; and sometimes pain in the joints.

Pas

Pas is the abbreviation for para-aminosalicylic acid, a drug which has been used in the treatment of tuberculosis in zoo animals.

Passage

Passage (pronounced as in the French) is a term meaning the passing of a strain of organisms through a series of animals to decrease virulence. For example, passage of cattle plague virus through goats is done to reduce its virulence for cattle, and is a technique used in the production of cattle plague vaccine.

Pastern

The name given to the 1st (long) and 2nd (short) phalanges of the fore-limb, and to the joint so formed.

Pasteurella

A genus of bacteria, which are small, ovoid, Gram-negative, bipolar staining. Both non-motile and motile species occur, and they are aerobic or facultatively anaerobic. For the diseases they cause, see following entries.

Pasteurellosis in Cats

(see YERSINIOSIS and BUBONIC PLAGUE; see BITES for human infection with *Pasteurella multocida*, formerly known as *P. septica*).

The cat harbours *P. multocida* as one of its bacterial flora.

Pasteurellosis in Cattle

This includes HAEMORRHAGIC SEPTICAEMIA of cattle and buffaloes in the tropics; 'SHIPPING FEVER' ('Transit fever') of the American feedlots and elsewhere; and other pneumonias occurring in Europe.

In calves, *Pasteurella haemolytica* serotype A1 may be the primary pathogen. Serotype A2 and *P. multocida* may also be isolated. Both bacteria are normal inhabitants of the upper resiratory tract. Under stress, or infection by viruses, the bacteria multiply rapidly, causing disease. Symptoms include a nasal discharge, a respiratory rate of 60 to 100 per minute, and a temperature of up to 41.6°C (107°F).

(See CALF PNEUMONIA for viruses which may be involved, and for synergism between Pasteurella and Mycoplasma.)

The pneumonia is fibrinous in type, and this is seen also in older cattle – *P haemolytica* or *P. multocida* often being found in large numbers.

Pasteurellosis in Ducks

Caused by *Pasteurella anatipestifer*, this is a disease of considerable economic importance in ducklings, with a mortality sometimes as high as 70 per cent. Less acutely infected birds may shake their heads or draw their heads close to their bodies. Sulfadimidine has been used in treatment. See also FOWL CHOLERA.

P Pasteurellosis in Man

Pasteurella multocida is a commensal organism in the mouth and naso-pharynx of many animals. In humans, superficial infections of the skin and mucous membranes, such as corneal, oral or leg ulcers and infections of compound fractures, conjunctivitis or sinusitis and panophthalmitis may result from animal bites or scratches. In these infections *P. multocida* is likely to have been acquired when saliva from the animal contacted injured tissue. Pasteurella organisms may also invade the body via the respiratory system or, less commonly, via the alimentary tract and skin lesions. The most commonly seen internal infections of *P. multocida* are associated with chronic obstructive lung disease. A 3rd category of infection is suggested: septicaemia and bacteraemia in patients with chronic disease, especially chronic liver disease. *P. multocida* may result from handling raw poultry carcases. Small domestic pets may be carriers of *P. multocida*. Internal infections may derive from farm animals; in one study, 27 of 37 patients with internal infection lived on farms. Other *Pasteurella* species that affect animals rarely occur in man.

In the UK during one 10-year period there were reports of 3699 cases of human pasteurellosis. Eighty-six per cent of these were skin infections; two-thirds due to dog bites; a quarter due to cat bites. In a small proportion of cases meningitis and septicaemia were complicating factors.

Pasteurellosis in Pigs

Bronchial pneumonia, sometimes with pleuritis and pericarditis, is the commonest symptom; *P. multocida* is the usual cause but clinical pasteurellosis may be a complication of mycoplasmal pneumonia.

Signs There is fever, and the animals maybe seen struggling for breath, with frothing in the mouth. Death may follow.

Treatment and control Antibiotics should be given; antiserum is effective if the causal bacteria is known. Vaccination with a combined *A. pyogenes*, *P. haemolytica*, *P. multocida* and staphylococcus vaccine (Pastacidin; Hoechst) is used for control where there is a known risk of pasteurellosis.

Pasteurellosis in Sheep

Pasteurellosis in sheep is caused occasionally by *Pasteurella multicocida* but far more commonly by *P. haemolytica*, and subclinical infection may develop into pneumonia if parainfluenza III virus is present too.

P. haemolytica biotype A causes enzootic pneumonia; while biotype T is mainly associated with septicaemia. Both may be isolated from cases of arthritis. *P. haemolytica* also causes mastitis in ewes, and meningitis – especially in lambs.

Young sheep are liable to die from the acute septicaemic form, while older ones show a slower type of the disease, in which the pneumonic lesions predominate.

Signs The acute cases are ushered in by high temperature, great dullness and nervous depression, difficult respirations, muscular tremors, followed by rapid collapse and death within 3 days.

In the less acute cases, similar but slightly milder symptoms occur. These are accompanied by a discharge from the eyes and nose, loss of appetite and absence of rumination, with signs of pneumonia or pleurisy.

Diagnosis The acute form may be confused with anthrax or braxy.

Immunisation Vaccines containing several strains of *P. haemolytica* are available; also a combined clostridial and pasteurella vaccine. A serum has also been prepared. (See also PNEUMONIA IN SHEEP.)

Pasteurisation of Milk

High temperature pasteurisation

consists of heating the milk for 10 to 20 minutes at a temperature of 75°C (167°F). This is sufficient to render harmless the germs of enteric and scarlet fever and diphtheria, and also bacteria which give rise to summer diarrhoea in children. It also affords a considerable measure of protection against tuberculosis.

Low temperature pasteurisation

consists of maintaining the milk for at least half an hour at a temperature between 63° and 65°C (145° and 150°F). This has the effect of considerably reducing the number of bacteria contained in the milk and greatly delaying souring and similar changes. This procedure is sufficient for the sale of milk as 'pasteurised milk' in England. (See also ULTRA HIGH TEMPERATURE TREATMENT OF MILK.)

Unpasteurised milk (see MILK-BORNE DISEASE)

Pasture, 'Clean'

Pasture that has not been grazed by the same species for some time. The actual period varies with the parasites involved, climate and other factors. Criteria for clean pasture vary with the time of year. In spring, it is pasture not grazed by the same species in the previous grazing season – that is, a new ley, an area grazed by another species or used for conservation. In the summer, clean pasture is defined as an area not grazed by that species the same year up to mid-June, for sheep, and mid-July for cattle. However, pasture rarely becomes completely free from parasites.

Professor James Armour and colleagues at the University of Glasgow veterinary school found clinical parasitic bronchitis ('husk'), due to the lungworm *Dictyocaulus viviparus*, and gastroenteritis due to *Osertagia ostertagi*, in young cattle grazing aftermath pasture in late summer. Calves on pasture lightly infested with *Ostertagia* 'were effectively treated with an anthelmintic and transferred to a silage aftermath in late July. A marked increase in 3rd-stage larvae numbers on the aftermath occurred within the first week, and clinical signs of type I ostertagiasis were observed 4 weeks later.

'In both instances the aftermath pastures had not been grazed since the previous autumn, and the interval between entry to the aftermath and clinical or other evidence of infection precluded the possibility of the calves being responsible for cycling of the infection.'

Such findings suggested the existence of a reservoir of infective larvae in the soil persisting from previous grazing seasons. 'Preliminary observations on core samples of soil from permanent cattle pastures in the Glasgow area revealed that *Ostertagia* 3rd-stage larvae were regularly present, and lungworm 3rd-stage larvae occasionally present,' over a 12-month period from August to July.

Research in the USA showed that if *Ostertagia* eggs are buried to a depth of 12.5 cm under pasture, or beneath 15 cm of soil in the laboratory, 3rd-stage larvae develop and migrate vertically through the soil. However, the good husbandry rule of keeping young stock off pasture previously grazed in the same season by adult stock is, obviously, still worth applying as a means of avoiding even worse outbreaks.

Pasture, Contamination of

This may occur in the vicinity of smelting works (see under FACTORY CHIMNEYS), or as the result of droplets of chemical sprays being carried by the wind to adjoining fields. (For a list of chemical sprays, see under WEEDKILLERS and INSECTICIDES.) Contamination may also occur as the result of atomic fall-out. (See RADIOACTIVE FALL-OUT.) Bacterial contamination can result from organsims that are able to exist for long periods outside the animal body. Examples are bovine tuberculosis (at least 4 months), Johne's disease (at least a year), anthrax (at least 30 years) and clostridial spores. Resting pasture for 3 weeks provides a measure of control of foot-rot, the organism responsible being unable to survive for more than a fortnight. For contamination by worm larvae, see PARASITIC BRONCHITIS; GASTROENTERITIS; PASTURE, 'CLEAN'. For contamination by organic irrigation see under SLURRY. (See also BASIC SLAG; FERTILISERS).

The average cow defecates about 12 times daily and each pat weighs about 2.5 kg (5½ lb); in a 180-day grazing season, she will put about 5 tons of faeces (containing about 680 kg (1500 lb) dry matter) on to the pasture. (See DAIRY HERD MANAGEMENT.) (For contamination by slurry applications, see SLURRY and 'MILKSPOT LIVER'; also SOIL-CONTAMINATED HERBAGE.)

Contamination of pasture may occur during flooding and, in a sense, when ticks are left behind by a batch of cattle infected with piroplasms; the ticks then infect other cattle put on to that land (see RED-WATER FEVER).

Pasture Management

Pasture management is of the greatest importance in relation to diseases such as BLOAT, HYPOMAG-NESAEMIA, PARASITIC GASTROEN-TERITIS and PARASITIC BRONCHITIS. (See also under DEEP-ROOTING PLANTS, TOPPING, and WILTING.) Controlled grazing is effected by means of an electric fence. (See STRIP-GRAZING and PADDOCKS.)

It is important that heavy application of nitrogenous and potash fertilisers to grassland should be made at the right time, or animals grazing there will be exposed to a greatly increased risk of hypomagnesaemia. (See also HOOF-PRINTS.)

The sudden (and harmful) change of diet which may occur when stock are turned out in the spring, or brought off pasture into yards for the winter, are discussed below.

In spring, it is a mistake to turn calves straight out on to grass. This means a sudden change from protein-poor food to the rich protein of the early bite, and the resulting effect upon the rumen will set them back. It is wise to get them out before there is much grass for a few hours each day; let them have hay and shelter at night to protect them from sudden changes of weather. Hypomagnesaemia, too, is far less likely under these circumstances.

Before yarding cattle in the autumn, it is wise to make a gradual change from sugar-poor autumn pasture to things like roots, and to accustom them to concentrates. Otherwise digestive upsets are very likely to occur.

It should be borne in mind that *Trichostrongylus axei* is a parasite common to cattle, sheep, goats, and horses, and grazing one species of animal after another in a field could give rise to a very heavy contamination with this one parasite.

Prompt removal of faeces from pasture has been found effective in reducing the worm burden, and practicable where acreage is small, labour cheap, or racehorses are concerned.

Use of goats in sheep grazing systems.

Goats prefer to graze plant species not readily eaten by sheep; also, given the choice, goats will discriminate against plant species such as clover which are important and beneficial in sheep production systems. The introduction of goats can benefit the sheep stock by helping to prevent the degeneration of the improved areas and by keeping the indigenous vegetation in a more productive and nutritious state, while at the same time not competing with the sheep for the more valuable plant species. (Hill Farm Research Organisation.)

Other aspects of pasture management are referred to under the following: PASTURE, CONTAMINATION OF; BRACKEN POISONING; RAGWORT POISONING; DIGITALIS POISONING; WORMS, FARM TREATMENT AGAINST; EXPOSURE; STRESS; 'POACHING'; BEEF CATTLE HUSBANDRY IN BRITAIN; SHEEP BREEDING AND MANAGEMENT; SILAGE; FOG FEVER; HAY; STOCKING RATES; TOPPING OF PASTURES.

Grass varieties Plant breeding for improved pastures is in its infancy as compared with that for the agronomically less complex arable crops.

Yield (whether annual or seasonal) is only 1 of 4 criteria useful in judging a new variety of herbage. Its persistency, palatability and nutritive value are important criteria, too; a high-yielding variety may be contraindicated if animals lose weight on it, as they do with 1 variety of *Phalaris*. The effect which the system of grassland management has, and how varieties will stand up to a given system, must also be considered. For example, with regular defoliation, perennial rye grass yields more than Italian rye grass; whereas with infrequent cutting, Italian rye grass yields more.

For systems of farming at high production, consideration should be given to a species like tall fescue, whose biological potential is known to be very high, and whose reaction to intensive systems of defoliation is favourable.

Horses Pasture grasses and herbs recommended by the Animal Health Trust for horses are classified as under:

Desirable species
Perennial Rye grasses, Sceempter, Melle, Petra, Midas S.23 and S.321, Timothy S.50 and S.48, Cocksfoot S.143, Crested Dogstail, Wild White Clover, Dandelion, Ribgrass, Chicory, Yarrow, Burnet, Sainfoin.

Probably useful (turf species which are also palatable)
Tall Fescue Alta, Canadian Creeping Red Fescue, Smooth Stalked Meadow Grass, Rough Stalked Meadow Grass.

Best excluded
Perennial Rye grass S.24, Creeping Red Fescue, Brown Top, Meadow Foxtail, Red Clover.

Patella

Patella is the bone that lies at the front of the 'stifle joint', and is called the 'knee-cap'. It lies in the tendon of the large extensor muscles of the joint, just above and in front of the true femorotibial joint. It is roughly pyramidal in the horse, with the apex of the pyramid pointing downwards. It is dislocation of the patella that constitutes the condition known as 'slipped stifle'. (See BONE.)

Dislocation of the patella (patellar luxation) may occur as an inherited abnormality in certain breeds of dogs, e.g. Boston terriers, boxers, bulldogs, cairn terriers, chihuahuas, wire fox terriers, griffons, Pekingese, Maltese, papillons, Pomeranians, poodles, Labradors, Scotch terriers, King Charles spaniels.

Indications for surgery of the canine stifle are congenital medial luxation and rupture of the anterior cruciate ligament.

Congenital patellar luxation occurs also in cats, rendering them unable to walk normally or jump.

Patent Ductus Arteriosus

An abnormality in which the ductus arteriosus, between the aorta and the pulmonary artery, fails to close at or shortly after birth. This condition has been recognised in the puppy, and gives rise to a characteristic murmur on auscultation; and also in cattle and cats. (See LIGAMENTUM ARTERIOSUM.)

Pathetic Nerve

The trochlear nerve. It is the 4th nerve arising from the brain and controlling the superior oblique muscle of the eye.

Pathogenic

Disease-producing.

Pathognomonic

Pathognomonic is a term applied to those signs or symptoms of a particular disease which are characteristic of that disease, and on whose presence or absence the diagnosis depends.

Peas, Mutter

(see LATHYRISM)

'Peat Scours'

'Peat scours' is a name given in Australasia and Canada to MOLYBDENUM poisoning in grazing cattle.

Peck Order

This is the equivalent in poultry of the order of precedence described under BUNT ORDER.

Pedal Bone

Pedal bone, or coffin bone, is the bone enclosed within the hoof of the horse

Pediculosis

Pediculosis is infestation with lice.

Pekingese

A toy dog originating from China. It has long straight hair, snub nose and pendulous ears. Its shape predisposes the breed to cleft palate, inguinal hernia, intravertebral disc disease, Perthe's disease, and retrognathia (underdeveloped lower jaw). Distichiasis and patellar luxation may be inherited.

Pellagra

(see 'BLACK TONGUE')

Pellets

(see CUBES)

Pelvis

Pelvis is the posterior girdle of bones by which the 2 hind-limbs are attached to the rest of the skeleton. It is composed of 2 ilia, 2 pubes, and 2 ischia, united together by fusion into a basin-shaped whole (see BONE). Strictly speaking, it includes the sacrum and the coccygeal vertebrae. The 2 'haunch bones' are the external angles of the ilia; the 'croup' is composed of the internal angles of these bones along with the spines of the sacrum; and the 'points of the buttocks' are the tuberosities of the two ischia. The pelvis is spoken of as having an 'inlet', formed by the brim of the pubes, and an 'outlet' posteriorly. In the living animal the outlet is occupied by the soft tissues forming the perineal region, except for the anus in the male and the anus and vulva in the female. The deep notch between the sacrum and the haunch bone is closed by the sacrosciatic ligaments, upon which lie the gluteal muscles which give the quarters their shape. The pelvis varies in the 2 sexes: in the female it is broader from side to side, and deeper from above downwards, than in the male; this difference being chiefly necessary to allow of the act of parturition.

The contents of the pelvis are the rectum and urinary bladder in both sexes (except in the dog, where the urinary bladder is abdominal in position). In the male there is in addition the prostate gland and the seminal vesicles around the neck of the bladder and the beginning of the urethra; while the female pelvis contains the vagina, uterus, their appendages, and perhaps the ovaries.

Pemphigus

An autoimmune disease of dogs also seen in cats and horses. It can take various forms: in *Pemphigus vulgaris*, lesions affect the mucous membrane lining the mouth, and the junction with the lips, giving rise to ulcers. Sometimes the pads of the feet are affected. *P. erythematosis* is characterised by crusty lesions on and around the nose, and elsewhere on the face.

In *P. vegetans,* alopecia and pruritus follow pustules which ulcerate on the body and extremities.

Treatment is with corticosteroids; cytotoxic drugs are also used. The prognosis in severe cases is not good.

-Penia

A suffix meaning too few, less than normal. (See LEUKOPENIA for an example.)

Penicillin

The first of the antibiotics, discovered by Sir Alexander Fleming in 1929. Benzyl penicillin (penicillin G) was the original preparation to be introduced for clinical use and remains widely effective against Gram-positive bacteria. It is the sodium or potassium salt of the antimicrobial acids produced when the moulds *Penicillium notatum* or *Chrysogenum* (or related species) are grown under suitable conditions.

Purified penicillin salts occur as a white crystalline powder, readily soluble in water.

Following injection into the animal body, penicillin is rapidly absorbed and diffused in the bloodstream throughout the body, being excreted by the kidneys. It is non-poisonous even in large doses (although allergic reactions are not uncommon) and is effective against:

Staphylococci, causing local pyogenic inflammation as primary or secondary infections.

Haemolytic streptococci, usually causing localised infections either primary or secondary.

Streptococcus equi, causing strangles in horses.

S. agalactiae, causing mastitis in cattle.

Bacillus anthracis, causing anthrax.

Clostridium chauvoei, causing blackleg in cattle.

Corynebacterium renale, causing pyelonephritis in cattle.

Erysipelotrix rhusiopathiae, causing swine erysipelas.

Actinomyces bovis, causing actinomycoses.

Leptospira canicola, causing leptospirosis in dogs.

Penicillin is of value in the treatment of wounds and for the prevention of sepsis in surgery.

It is of great importance that penicillin should be used in full doses; otherwise there is a risk of strains of bacteria resistant to penicillin being developed. The dosage for systemic administration is 10 mg/kg bodyweight.

'The long-established benzyl penicillin has the following shortcomings: (1) It is unstable in acids, and therefore cannot be given orally. This consideration, however, is of little importance in the veterinary field. (2) Organisms which produce penicillinase, and these are not uncommon, are resistant to benzyl penicillin. (3) It is active against only a narrow range of organisms. Semi-synthetic penicillins were developed to overcome these drawbacks. Firstly, Phenethicillin potassium was developed as a penicillin stable in acids and which is an improvement on the older acid-stable penicillin Phenoxymethylpenicillin, because after oral administration it gives twice as high a level in the blood. It is slightly resistant to penicillinase and is used in the veterinary field mainly in the treatment of mastitis involving susceptible strains of streptococci and staphylococci. Secondly, Methicillin; the main feature of methicillin is that it is resistant to penicillinase; it can, however, be given only parenterally. Methicillin should never be used in the treatment of infections caused by organisms susceptible to benzyl penicillin, since it is much less potent and may give rise to strains of organisms which show a penicillin resistance which is not due to the production of penicillinase. Moreover, methicillin actually stimulates the production of penicillinase. Thirdly, Cloxacillin; this penicillin is resistant to penicillinase, is stable in acids, but induces the production of penicillinase. Fourthly, Ampicillin: this is a most important introduction, because it is a penicillin active against both Gram-positive and Gram-negative organisms. It is useful particularly in the treatment of tetracycline-resistant coliforms, strains of *Proteus* and *Pseudomonas, Salmonellae, Shigellae,* and *Pasteurellae.* It is not resistant to penicillinase, and is acid stable.

'Benethamine penicillin is a long-acting preparation, given by intramuscular injection as an insoluble suspension from which benzyl penicillin is slowly released. Benzathine penicillin has the same properties as benethamine penicillin, but is acid stable and can therefore be given by mouth to dogs and cats.

'While these long-acting preparations of penicillin eliminate the necessity for frequent administration, they do, however, present the risk of inducing resistant strains because they must by their nature provide a lower level of penicillin in the tissues for a long period after their administration has terminated. This feature should be borne in mind when using them.' (Professor F. Alexander.)

Penicillin in Milk
(see PENICILLIN, SENSITIVITY TO)

Penicillin, Sensitivity to
People handling penicillin suffer a risk of sensitisation, shown by skin lesions. There is danger in the use of milk containing penicillin (e.g. milk from quarters of the udder treated for mastitis), especially in people sensitised to penicillin. Extremely severe skin lesions, and accompanying illness, have been caused in this way among farmers and others. (See also under MILK – Antibiotics in milk.) Hypersensitivity to penicillins has been recorded also in cattle and other animals, including cats.

Penicillinase (Beta-Lactamase)
A penicillin-destroying enzyme produced by certain bacteria, including strains of *E. coli*. Its activity is blocked by clavulanic acid which is added to some semi-synthetic penicillins to make them effective against such bacteria.

Penis
Penis is attached by roots (crura) to the ischial arch of the pelvis. From the roots extends the body of the penis along the interior of which runs the urethra, for the passage of urine and semen. Erection of the penis depends upon the increased flow of blood into the spongy, erectile tissue in the body of the penis, and simultaneous decrease in relative outflow from the veins, partly as a result of contraction of the ischiocavernosus muscles. The bull, ram and boar each have a sigmoid or S-shaped curve in the penis. On erection this curve is straightened. The penis increases in length but not much in girth. In the stallion and dog, in which the penis is straight, erection brings an increase in girth to a greater extent. The os penis in the dog is a grooved bone within the glans penis, which is the terminal portion of the penis (except in the boar). The shape of the glans differs in the other species as regards shape. The penis of the cat is a frequent site of urethral obstruction owing to its very small diameter. Sand-like deposit, a calculus, plug of organic and crystalline deposit, or a grass seed may cause blockage. In some cases manipulation of the penis may allow the passage of urine; otherwise the use of a catheter may be tried. (See UROLITHIASIS; FELINE UROLOGICAL SYNDROME.)

Penis and Prepuce, Abnormalities and Lesions
These include the following conditions:

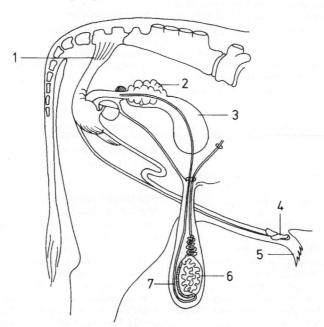

Genitalia of the bull: 1, muscles which controls penis; 2, vesicles which store semen; 3, bladder; 4, penis; 5, sheath which covers penis; 6, testicle; 7, epididymis.

Necrosis of the prepuce has been recorded in pigs kept in poor hygienic conditions. There is no indication that the condition causes pain or distress.

Phimosis A narrowing of the orifice of the prepuce, preventing normal protrusion of the penis. Congenital phimosis is occasionally seen in dogs, cats, and horses. It can be corrected surgically.

Paraphimosis A condition in which the penis cannot be retracted into the prepuce. This is not uncommon in the dog, and is potentially serious unless quickly relieved, owing to interference with the circulation. As a first-aid measure, swabbing the penis with ice-cold water may prove helpful.

Prolapse of the penis due to paralysis is seen in bulls which have rabies, and also as a chronic condition in Zebu cattle (*Bos indicus*) and occasionally in breeds of UK origin.

Horses Prolapse of the penis may follow use of acepromazine (to effect relaxation of the retractor muscles so that swabbing can be undertaken for contagious equine metritis). In 6 cases involving protrusion, oedema, and paresis of the penis, 4 of the horses had received acepromazine with etorphine hydrochloride, and 2 had received the former drug along with others.

After such drugs have been used, it is important to check that retraction of the penis is taking place as the effects of medication wear off. If not, treatment should be started without delay.

Priapism A persistent erection of the penis unassociated with sexual stimulation. (See also PRIAPISM.)

Balanitis Inflammation of the glans penis – the cap-shaped spongy tissue at the end of the penis, normally covered by the foreskin.

Posthitis Inflammation of the prepuce.

Balanoposthitis A viral infection affecting both the penis and the prepuce. One example is an enzootic form, called 'pizzle rot' or 'sheath rot', of sheep (especially merinos) in Australia. *Corynebacterium renale* is the primary cause.

A herpesvirus also causes balanoposthitis in cattle and sheep.

An infectious balanoposthitis (also known as 'ulcerative dermatosis') of sheep may affect not only the penis, prepuce and vulva but also the face, feet and legs; this has to be differentiated from ORF. It occurs in Europe and South Africa. In lambs mortality may be up to 30 per cent.

Tumours of the penis include WARTS (papillomas) and also, in dogs, infective granulomas. (See VENEREAL TUMOURS.)

Traumatic lesions include injury to the penis from a kick by the cow or mare at service, or when a bull proves too heavy for a heifer. There is usually an accompanying haematoma. Trauma may also result in adhesions at the sigmoid flexure. In dogs a fracture of the os penis may occur as the result of being hit by a car.

Spiral deviation of the penis occurs in bulls. Service is prevented. (In the USA deviation of the penis is sometimes deliberately produced surgically in teaser bulls.)

Penitrem A

A mycotoxin. It was isolated from mouldy cream cheese from a refrigerator given to a dog which became very ill with ataxia, muscular tremors, and opisthotonos. The mould was identified as *Penicillium crustosum*.

Pentastomiasis

Infection with the nymphs of the pentastomid *Armillifer armillatus*, the adults of which infest snakes in Africa and Asia.

The disease has been recognised in man, dog and cat.

Signs Abdominal or thoracic oedema.

Infection occurs through drinking water contaminated by the eggs, or eating a snake.

Diagnosis In human medicine this is based on the radiographic appearance of calcified nymphs.

Pentobarbitone Sodium (Pentobarbital)

(Sodium ethyl/methylbutyl barbiturate). A white crystalline powder, soluble in water, and used for its narcotic and anaesthetic effects.

First used as a general anaesthetic in veterinary surgery in America in 1931. A proprietary name is Nembutal.

Pentobarbitone has been used to produce anaesthesia in all the domestic animals including the fowl, but it is not recommended for horses, calves, or sheep. For anaesthesia in the dog and cat, however, pentobarbitone is very extensively employed, and is usually given by the intravenous route – a method which permits of varying depths of anaesthesia being obtained and the avoidance of overdosage. The drug may also be given by intra-peritoneal injection or by mouth; narcosis being then slower in onset (8 to 20 minutes), and occasionally preceded by some degree of excitement, while the dose has to be an estimate calculated on the basis of bodyweight.

Deep anaesthesia with pentobarbitone may last for an hour, being followed by 2 to 7 hours of narcosis. (See ANAESTHESIA, GENERAL; EUTHANASIA.)

Pepsin

Pepsin is an enzyme found in the gastric juice which digests proteins.

Peptides

Peptides are composed of 2 or more amino acids, and represent an intermediate stage in the digestion of protein.

Polypeptides are proteins composed of several amino-acids linked by the peptide grouping CH– CO–NH–CH.

Synthetic polypeptides have potential uses as vaccines, e.g. against foot-and-mouth disease.

Peptococcus Indolicus

A Gram-positive bacterium which is sometimes a complicating factor in CASEOUS LYMPHADENITIS of sheep and summer mastitis in cattle (see MASTITIS IN COWS, 'SUMMER MASTITIS').

Perforation

Perforation is one of the serious dangers attached to the presence of ulcerating conditions in the stomach and bowels. When a perforation of one of these hollow organs takes place in the peritoneal cavity, multitudes of bacteria, much ingesta, mucus, and other putrescible materials escape and set up PERITONITIS. The immediate signs are a collapse of the patient, with, later, collections of gas or fluids in the abdominal cavity. It is not uncommon to observe vomiting in the horse when the stomach ruptures and the contents escape into the abdominal cavity; this is one of the very rare times when the horse is seen to vomit, and it is important accordingly.

Performance Testing

A method of comparing strains or breeds of, e.g. beef cattle, by studying liveweight gains over a stated period with given rations. (See also PROGENY TESTING.)

Peri-

Peri- is a prefix meaning round, or about. Examples: PERICARDIUM; perianal abscess.

Pericarditis

Inflammation of the pericardium. Traumatic pericarditis is common in cattle as a result of swallowing pieces of wire, nails, etc. (See also HEART DISEASES.)

Pericardium

Pericardium is the smooth lubricating membrane which surrounds the heart. (See also HEART DISEASES.)

Perineum

Perineum is the region lying between the anus and the genital organs in the male, and lying between the anus and the mammary region in the female of the horse, ox, sheep, goat, and pig. In bitches and cats the female genital organs lie lower than in other animals, and in them the perineum lies between the anus and the vulva. Rupture of the perineum sometimes occurs in the cow at calving, when the fetus over-distends the vulva. Suturing, under local anaesthesia, is usually required.

Periodic Ophthalmia

Specific ophthalmia, or 'moon blindness', is a condition of the eyes of horses, due to inflammation of the uveal tract (especially of the iris and ciliary body) which is characterised by a tendency to recur.

Causes These are still in doubt, but it is known that leptospirosis is one. Some 2 to 8 months after acute leptospirosis, periodic ophthalmia appears in up to 45 per cent of the horses affected. Leptospires have been isolated from eye lesions over long periods.

Signs In the 1st stage a horse is found one morning with the eyelids on one side half-closed; tears run from the eye down the face, and any effort to examine the eye is resented. Bright light is avoided, and the eyeball appears sunken in the socket. This period of inflammation may last up to 10 days, after which it gradually disappears and the eye returns to practically its normal appearance. Repeated attacks are apt to occur. Total blindness may follow and/or lesions of the retina. Periodic ophthalmia is common in Europe, the USA, and Asia.

Periodontal
(see TEETH, DISEASES OF)

Periople
(see FOOT OF THE HORSE)

Periosteum
Periosteum is the membrane surrounding a bone. The growth of a bone in its thickness is due to the action of the cells of this membrane forming fibrous tissue in which lime salts are deposited. (See BONE.)

Periostitis
Periostitis means inflammation on the surface of a bone affecting the periosteum. (See BONE, DISEASES OF.)

Periparturient
Used to describe any condition occurring shortly before or shortly after birth.

Peristalsis
Peristalsis is the succession of involuntary muscular contractions which propel ingested food along the alimentary canal. (See INTESTINES.)

Peritoneum
Peritoneum is the membrane lining the abdominal cavity, and forming a covering for the organs contained in it. That part lining the walls of the cavity is called the 'parietal' peritoneum, and that part covering the viscera is known as the 'visceral' peritoneum. Between the 2 parts is a film of lubricating liquid.

Peritonitis
Inflammation of the PERITONEUM. It may be either localised or diffused.

Acute peritonitis

Causes The direct cause of acute peritonitis is nearly always the invasion of the membrane by micro-organisms. It occurs through a wound in the abdominal wall, in the stomach or intestines, uterus, bladder, etc., or through the spreading of inflammatory conditions from one or other of these parts. It may follow castration, when the infection gains entrance by the inguinal canal. Peritonitis may occur during the course of anthrax, acute tuberculosis, etc.

Signs These include restlessness and signs of distress and pain. Horses and cattle usually remain standing, but the smaller animals lie almost continually. The temperature is raised by 5° to 10°C (3° to 6°F), and the pulse is quick,

small, and wiry. Faeces and urine are usually retained and lead to further complication, and vomiting in dogs is common. Pressure over the sides of the abdomen is painful; the animal usually 'boards' the muscles of the abdomen, and may groan or grunt. As the disease progresses, fluid may be thrown out into the cavity in great quantities, leading to ASCITES. (See OEDEMA and PARACENTESIS.)

Treatment Operative treatment and drainage may be undertaken.

Antibiotics and/or sulfa drugs may be given by injection. Hot fomentations to the abdomen relieve the acute pain. The prognosis is seldom good.

Chronic peritonbitis

Causes Slowly-forming abscesses in the liver, tuberculous lesions in the peritoneal cavity, foreign bodies in the reticulum, etc.

Signs There may be slight attacks of pain at times, but very often it is only after death that the condition is discovered. Ascites and a gradual loss of condition may be seen.

Treatment This will vary according to the nature of the infection or of adhesions. (See ANTIBIOTIC.)

Permethrin
A synthetic pyrethroid (derivative of pyrethrum) used as an insecticide. Excessive applications to cats can induce hyperaesthesia, with excitement, a staggering gait, muscular twitching, and occasional collapse (see INSECTICIDES; FLIES – Fly control measures).

Peroneal
Relating to the fibula.

Perosis
(see under 'SLIPPED TENDON')

Perruque Antlers
Perruque antlers describes a defect in antler growth in red deer where the antlers form clumps close to the head.. In severe cases, the animal has the appearance of wearing a judge's wig, hence the name.

Perthe's Disease
This name is given to a deformed condition of the head of the femur in the dog. The animal is noticed to be lame. The condition may clear up spontaneously within 6 months, but during

that time drugs to relieve pain are indicated. It is sometimes called Von Perthe's disease.

Pervious Urachus

Pervious Urachus is a failure on the part of the umbilicus to close at or before birth. In the condition, which is also popularly called 'leaky navel', there is a continual dribbling of urine and serum from the navel.

Before birth the urinary bladder is in direct communication with the fluid in the allantoic sac, and the fetal urine which is formed escapes into this sac, thus preventing over-distension of the bladder. Immediately before the young animal is born, this communication is narrowed down to only a very small passage, and at birth either it is already closed, or it has practically ceased to function as a means of escape for the urine. With the tying of the umbilical cord – or with the shrinkage that follows exposure of this structure to the air – the urachus, which hitherto has connected the bladder with the outside of the animal's body, becomes quite impervious in the normal animal, and the urine now escapes by the urethra or natural passage to the outside. In pervious urachus this closure does not take place, and there is a continual dribble from the region of the umbilicus. The fluid tends to blister the skin of the surrounding area, and causes considerable discomfort, besides being very unsightly. Surgical treatment is necessary.

Pessaries

Pessaries, or vaginal suppositories, are a means of administering drugs into the uterus. The medicaments are formulated in a base, traditionally of cocoa butter or gelatine, so that they may gradually liquefy and liberate their active substances. In some instances pessaries are made with dry powders of the active ingredients filled into gelatine capsules.

Peste Des Petits Ruminants (PPR)

A highly contagious disease of sheep and goats; similar to rinderpest, it causes high mortality. The cause is a paromyxovirus. It is a NOTIFIABLE DISEASEthroughout the EU.

Signs A foul oculo-nasal discharge, diarrhoea, severe stomatitis and bronchopneumonia.

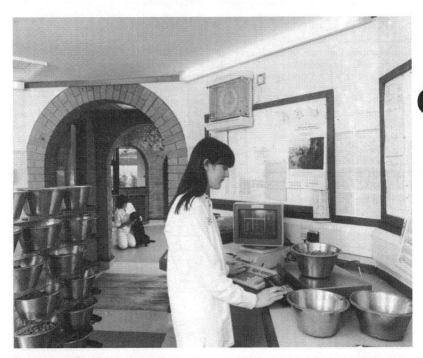

Pet food being prepared at the Waltham Centre for Pet Nutrition, research facility for a major pet-foods manufacturer. Products are developed and tested to ensure that dogs and cats obtain complete and balanced nutrition from these foods.

Pestivirus

(see BOVINE VIRAL DIARRHOEA; BORDER DISEASE OF SHEEP; SWINE FEVER; EQUINE VIRAL ARTERITIS)

Pet Animals Act 1971

Pet Animals Act 1971 covers the licensing of pet shops, and the conditions under which animals are kept there and offered for sale.

Pet Bereavement Support Service

A counselling service for people whose pets have died is operated jointly by the animal charities Blue Cross and Society for Companion Animal Studies. The telephone helpline is open between 08.30 and 17.00; the number is 0800 0966606.

Petlog

A UK national scheme for identifying pets by microchipping. The Petlog Reunification Service helps to trace lost microchipped animals and reunite them with their owners.

Pet Foods

Pet foods come under the Feeding Stuffs (Sampling and Analysis) Regulations 1982. The Feeding Stuffs Regulations 2000 list the special diets which are permitted. Together, these regulations satisfy the requirements of the appropriate EU directives. (See also DIET and DIETETICS; DOGS' DIET; CAT FOODS, etc.)

P Pet Travel Scheme (PETS)

An arrangement by which cats and dogs may travel to and from European Union countries, Norway, Australia, New Zealand, Japan, and certain islands in the Atlantic and the Caribbean without having to go into quarantine. This was made possible under the Pet Travel Scheme (Pilot Arrangements) Order 1999 (as subsequently amended). Strict conditions apply: the animals must have been identity microchipped, vaccinated against rabies at least 6 months previously and have their blood levels of rabies-immunity tested by a DEFRA-approved laboratory before being allowed to travel. In the case of dogs, vaccination against distemper is obligatory. Most countries also require an export health certificate before a pet will be allowed to enter. Prior to arrival in Britain, the animals must have been wormed, especially against the tapeworm *Echinococcus multilocularis,* and have been treated for the presence of ticks. Failure to observe those requirements will lead to the animal being quarantined. In the first 3 years of the scheme, 136,500 dogs and cats entered Britain without being quarantined. In 2003 alone, there were 48,329 dogs and 5838 cats.

Companies operating the scheme have to provide trained staff to deal with checking animals and make available adequate facilities for handling them.

Details are available from PETS Helpline, telephone 0870 2411710; fax 020 7904 6834; e-mail pets@ahvg.defra.gov.uk or from the DEFRA website at www.defra.gov.uk/animalh/quarantine.

Petechiae

Petechiae are small spots on the surface of an organ or the skin, generally red or purple in colour and resembling flea-bites. They may be minute areas of inflammation or they may be small haemorrhages. (Petechial fever is another name for PURPURA HAEMORRHAGICA.)

Pethidine

An analgesic (pain reliever) used for dogs and cats. It may also be used in rabbits and rodents and for the relief of the pain of colic in horses.

Petri Dish

A shallow circular glass dish with lid in which bacteria are grown on a solid medium.

Pets, Children's and Exotic

For information on the breeding, care, diseases and treatment of mice, rats, rabbits, hamsters, guinea pigs, gerbils, reptiles, fish, birds, and monkeys, the reader is referred to the British Small Animal Veterinary Association's *Manual of the Care and Treatment of Children's and Exotic Pets.* (See also under CAGE AND AVIARY BIRDS, DISEASES OF; MONKEYS; HAMSTERS; GUINEA-PIG; AMERICAN BOX TORTOISES; TORTOISES; PIGS – Foreign breeds; CHINCHILLA; also ANAESTHESIA, GENERAL.

Peyer's Patches

Peyer's patches are lymph follicles on the small intestine; they appear as raised oval areas in mucous and submucous areas. In sheep they have a function analogous to that of the bursa of Fabricius in birds. An investigation of jejunal Peyer's patches (JPP) and ileocecal Peyer's patches (IPP) showed that, in JPPs, there are big interfollicular T-cell areas, but IPPs contained mainly B-lymphocytes. Germinal centres of JPPs had about 40 per cent IgM positive cells and, in IPPs, about 80 per cent of these cells were present. (Larsen, H. J. & Landsverk, T. *Research in Veterinary Science,* **40**, 105.) (See also under INTESTINES.)

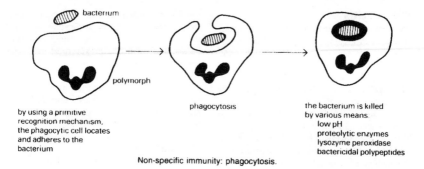

by using a primitive recognition mechanism, the phagocytic cell locates and adheres to the bacterium

phagocytosis

the bacterium is killed by various means.
low pH
proteolytic enzymes
lysozyme peroxidase
bactericidal polypeptides

Non-specific immunity: phagocytosis.

pH

A symbol used to express acidity or alkalinity – pH7 being neutral, a higher figure being alkaline and a lower figure being acid.

Phage

(see BACTERIOPHAGES)

Phagocytosis

Phagocytosis is the process by which the attacks of bacteria upon the living body are repelled and the bacteria destroyed through the activity of the white blood cells other than lymphocytes. Bacteria coated with antibodies are phagocytosed more efficiently. (See BLOOD; IMMUNE RESPONSE; INFECTION– Blood cells which counter infection; ABSCESS; INFLAMMATION.)

Many bacteria may be able to survive within phagocytes in mammary tissue, where staphylococci are protected from the lethal action of most antibiotics used in treating bovine mastitis. The situation may then arise where the staphylococci live longer than the phagocytes, so that when the latter die and disintegrate, the staphylococci are released, with potential for further mastitis-production.

Phalanx

Phalanx is the name given to each of the main bones below the metacarpal and metatarsal regions. There are 3 in each limb in the horse, 6 in the ox, 12 in the pig, and 14 in the dog. In general each of the digits possesses 3 phalanges, but the first digit in each foot of the dog has only 2 (as in the thumb and great toe of man). The horse has now only 1 functional digit left in each of its limbs.

'Phalaris Staggers'

A condition seen in Australia and New Zealand among cattle and sheep grazing on pasture dominated by *Phalaris tuberosa*. Cattle may show stiffness of the hocks and dragging of the hind-legs. Similar symptoms are shown in sheep, with the addition of excitability, muscular tremors, and head nodding in the early stages. Phalaris is believed to contain a specific nervous-system poison which is normally destroyed in the digestive passage of the animal; but, where there is a deficiency in cobalt, the destruction of the poison is impeded and the symptoms occur. Provision of oral cobalt seems to stimulate the growth of organisms in the digestive system which in turn destroy the toxin.

Phantom Pregnancy

(see PSEUDO-PREGNANCY; also 'CLOUDBURST')

Pharmacokinetics

The study of the movement of drugs within the body, including absorption, distribution, and excretion. (For an example see LUNGS – Functions.)

Pharmacology

The science of drugs, and especially of their actions in the body.

Pharmacopœia

Pharmacopœia is an official publication dealing with the recognised drugs and giving their doses, preparations, sources, and tests. Most countries have a pharmacopœia of their own, that of Britain being known as the *Pharmacopœia Britannica*, or often called the 'BP' or the *Pharmacopoeia Europa* (denoted by 'Ph Eur' after the name. In the USA the official publication is the *United States Pharmacopeia*, often called the 'USAP'.

The *British Pharmacopœia* (*Veterinary*), published by the British Pharmacopoeia Commission, provides standards for drugs and medicines for veterinary use.

Pharyngitis

Pharyngitis means inflammation of the pharynx. It often accompanies catarrhal inflammation in adjoining areas, viral infections, and tonsillitis.

Pharynx

Pharynx is an irregularly funnel-shaped passage situated at the back of the mouth, common to both the respiratory and the digestive passages. It acts as the crossroads between these systems. Into its upper part open the 2 'posterior nares', by which air enters and leaves the nasal passages during respiration. Below is the opening from the mouth, known as the 'fauces'; while lower still is the entrance to the larynx – the 'glottis'. Situated most posteriorly is the beginning of the oesophagus, and on either side are the openings of the Eustachian tubes, communicating with the middle ear. (See EAR.)

The walls of the pharynx are composed of muscles which are the active agents of swallowing, along with a sheet of fibrous tissue known as the pharyngeal aponeurosis. On the inside they are lined with mucous membrane which is continuous with that of the several cavities which open into it.

Pharyngeal injuries In a study of 65 dogs treated for penetrating wounds of the pharynx, the following findings were noted. Recent wounds resulted in dysphagia, pain, pyrexia and local cellulitis; longstanding wounds led to discharging sinuses of the head, neck or cranial thoracic region. Pieces of wood were removed from 37 dogs, and they recovered. No foreign body was found in 18 dogs whose clinical signs resolved after treatment of the wounds. Four dogs died shortly after the injury from major oesophageal tears which resulted in mediastinal contamination. In 6 dogs the discharging sinuses persisted, although no foreign body was recovered at surgery.

Pheasants

(see GAME BIRDS, MORTALITY)

Phenobarbitone (Phenobarbital)

A sedative; used in dogs and cats for the treatment of epilepsy. In large doses it is used for euthanasia; administered intravenously, it produces smooth and rapid loss of consciousness.

Phenol (Carbolic Acid)

A tar derivative, related to the cresols and, like them, used in disinfectant preparations, but not suitable (1) where animals may come into contact with them, as absorption through the skin – leading to poisoning – readily occurs, and (2) in the proximity of milk. (See MILK – Chlorophenol taint.)

Phenol is a corrosive poison when swallowed, giving rise to shock, convulsions and death; cats especially may be fatally poisoned as a result of absorption of phenol compounds through the skin.

First-aid consists in the administration of milk and raw white of egg. The skin (in cases where the phenol or cresol compounds have come into contact with it) should be washed with soap and water.

Phenolphthalein

Phenolphthalein is a substance used as an indicator in the testing of urine, gastric juice, etc., being colourless in an acid and a brilliant red in an alkaline medium. It is also sometimes given to dogs as a mild purgative.

Phenolsulphone-phthalein has been used as a test for the excretory powers of the kidneys; a known amount is injected into a muscle and the urine is tested by comparison of its colour with that of known standards during the next few hours. Phenoltetrachlor-phthalein is a coal-tar derivative used to estimate the functional power of the liver.

Phenothiazine

A pale greenish-grey powder which darkens on exposure to light and is practically insoluble in water. In the body it is oxidised to colourless compounds which are excreted in the urine, and on exposure to air are converted to a red dye.

Phenothiazine is an anthelmintic, at one time widely used in farm animals against a variety of parasitic roundworms; but it has been superseded by more modern drugs. (See WORMS, FARM TREATMENT AGAINST.)

Phenotype

In heredity this refers to all the individuals showing the same characters. The term can also mean the individual resulting from the reaction between genotype and environment.

Phenylalanine

One of the essential amino acids.

Phenylbutazone

An NSAID analgesic for the relief of pain associated with inflammation of joints and muscles. It apparently acts as an analgesic by reducing the synthesis of prostaglandins and to some extent via the central nervous system, while its anti-inflammatory effects have been attributed to reduced capillary permeability. Phenylbutazone can be given orally or intravenously. It is often used for chronic arthritis and associated bone disease. Withdrawal of the drug before a horse competes in international events is necessary. As the drug can be detected at very low levels, the withdrawal period can be lengthy.

Phenylephrine

A drug used in the investigation and treatment of PTOSIS. It is also used as a mydriatic in dogs (see MYDRIASIS).

Phenytoin Sodium

An anti-convulsant drug used in the treatment of epilepsy.

Pheromone

A substance produced by glands in the body of an animal which is detected by another individual via the vomeronasal (Jacobson's) organ. Pheromones can have a potent effect on the animal detecting them. The most obvious example in companion animals is the distance over which a male dog can detect a bitch in heat.

The normal mating process in pigs is much influenced by pheromones; the sexes must be able to smell each other before being introduced.

In some cases, the substance has a different effect. In pregnant mice the odour of a strange male will cause fetal resorption. Some pheromone preparations are available commercially. Feline pheromone is sold as a spray to stop urine-spraying, scratching of furniture, for calming a cat during transport, and to counteract stress. A canine pheromone product is claimed to calm anxious dogs.

Phimosis

A narrowing of the prepucial orifice, preventing normal protrusion of the penis (see under PENIS AND PREPUCE, ABNORMALITIES AND LESIONS).

Phlebitis

Inflammation of a vein. Most cases seen in animals arise following intravenous injections or catheters, or inflammation of the umbilical vein (omphalophlebitis).

Phocine Distemper

This is the name given to distemper in members of the family *Phocidae* – mainly seals. The cause is believed to be a mobillivirus. Outbreaks caused a high death-rate among seals in European waters in 1988; the disease returned with equally devastating effect in 2002. Seals have been vaccinated against distemper, but handling wild animals can cause severe stress which can iself upset the immune mechanism. There is also the problem of the substantial layer of subcutaneous fat in seals: injection into fat will not provoke an immune response. There is evidence that the virus has also caused outbreaks of distemper in farmed mink and in dogs.

Pholedrine Sulphate

A drug which raises the blood pressure, and is used in cases of heart failure after pneumonia or bronchitis and shock.

Phosgene

This gas, first produced experimentally by John Davy in 1812 by the combination of carbon monoxide with chlorine in the presence of sunlight, has the formula $COCl_2$. Phosgene has a characteristic smell of musty hay, and is 10 times more toxic than chlorine. The gas in the presence of water is converted into carbon dioxide and hydrochloric acid, and it is the latter which damages the lung tissues, giving rise to pulmonary oedema. Horses usually die between the 7th and 24th hour following exposure to the gas. Birds are highly susceptible. The gas may be liberated from chloroform, carbon tetrachloride, and paint-strippers in the presence of heat. Still-births and heavy piglet losses followed the feeding in the USA of mouldy, weevily grain which had been fumigated with a mixture containing carbon tetrachloride.

Phosmet

An organophosphorus liquid parasiticide.

Phosphates

Phosphates are salts of phosphoric acid, and as this substance is contained in many articles of food, in bone, the nuclei of cells, as well as in the nervous system, quantities are continually excreted in the urine.

Phosphorescence

Phosphorescence of meat is a luminous condition due to the organism *Photobacterium phosphorescens*. The meat is apparently unchanged during the daytime, but in the dark it glows with a yellowish light. Fish, especially herring, show this condition normally, but sausages, pork and occasionally beef may also exhibit the phenomenon.

Phosphorus

Phosphorus itself is not used in medicine, but is usually given in the form of one or other of the glycerophosphates, or hypophosphites of sodium, potassium, calcium, magnesium, or iron. Preparations are used with calcium and dextrose in the treatment of MILK FEVER.

Phosphorus Deficiency

This is seen in RICKETS; 'MILK LAMENESS'; POST-PARTURIENT HAEMOGLOBINURIA; and may complicate MILK FEVER. (See also INFERTILITY.)

Phosphorus Poisoning

Phosphorus poisoning may occur in the dog and cat, either through puppies eating matches, or from animals gaining access to rat poison made with phosphorus.

Signs When an animal has been poisoned by phosphorus there is acute abdominal pain, vomiting, intense thirst, diarrhoea, and great dullness. The material vomited may be green in colour and is often luminous in the darkness. Collapse rapidly follows, and the animal dies in a few hours. Where less has been taken, death may not occur for 2 or 3 days.

First-aid An emetic should be given at once, as soon as the symptoms appear, Washing-soda crystals (sodium carbonate), salt (sodium chloride) or mustard placed at the back of the tongue are effective emetics. Sulphate of copper (bluestone), in solution, may be given: this induces vomiting, gets rid of the majority of the phosphorus, and renders inert what remains. In 15 minutes another dose dissolved in water as before should be given, and this should be repeated every quarter of an hour till 4 doses have been given. In all cases, white of egg, milk, oils, and fatty substances must be avoided; these dissolve the phosphorus and render it able to be absorbed with greater rapidity. (See also ORGANOPHOSPHORUS POISONING, which arises from contaminations with certain farm chemicals.)

Phrenic Nerve

This arises from the 5th, 6th, and 7th cervical spinal nerves, passes through the thoracic cavity, and ramifies in the muscular part of the diaphragm.

Phthiriasis

Infestation with lice of the genus *Phthirus*.

Phycomycosis

A group of fungal infections by species of *Absidia*, *Mucor*, *Rhizopus*, etc., which affects the lymph nodes and may give rise to loss of weight and tumour-like (granulomatous) swellings. It may affect the lungs and intestines. A monkey died from systemic phycomycosis in the UK after loss of appetite, depression, and laboured breathing.

Phylloerythrin

A substance formed in the rumen from chlorophyll by bacterial digestion. Some is absorbed and excreted in the bile, but when the liver is damaged in any way the phylloerythrin may reach the peripheral circulation and give rise to LIGHT SENSITISATION.

Physiotherapy

In the UK, some veterinary practices use the services of qualified physiotherapists for the treatment of selected cases of disease in animals.

Physis

A synonym for EPIPHYSIS (see also BONE, DISEASES OF).

Physitis

Inflammation or disease of the growth plate (see EPIPHYSITIS).

Physostigmine

Physostigmine is an anticholinesterase. Eye drops containing physostigmine sulphate are used to contract the pupil and lessen intra-ocular pressure. Alternated with atropine, it has been used for adhesions of the iris, following iritis. It is prepared from the ripe seeds of *Physostigma venenosum*, a tree from West Africa.

Phytin

A substance present in oatmeal, maize meal (and in other cereals) that binds to phosphorus, making it unavailable to animals. As a result, calcification of bone is disturbed and ricketts may result. Phytase is added to many diets to break down phytin and remove this risk.

Pia Mater

Pia mater is the membrane that closely invests the brain and spinal cord. (See BRAIN; SPINAL CORD.)

Pica

Depraved appetite. It is often the result of a deficiency in the diet such as lack of fibre or salt, or inadequate trace elements such as phosphorus or copper. (For causes, see under APPETITE.)

Picornavirus

A member of the Picornaviridae family which includes apthovirus, responsible for foot-and-mouth disease; rhinovirus, responsible for respiratory diseases in cattle and sheep; and enterovirus, which causes poliomyelitis in pigs and chickens (see FELINE CALICIVIRUS; VIRUSES).

Picrotoxin

Used in veterinary medicine principally as an antidote to barbiturate poisoning.

Piétrain

This Belgian breed of pig dates from about 1920, but the Breed Society was formed in the 1950s. There is uncertainty as to the origins of the Piétrain, but it is thought that it stems from old native stock crossed with English breeds such as the Berkshire, Tamworth, and Wessex, and with the French breed Bayeux. There is still some lack of uniformity within the breed, but a constant feature is the extreme development of the hams – perhaps the result of a mutation such as is believed to have occurred in a strain of Devon cattle.

The Piétrain is white with large black spots. It is a pork pig which gives high killing-out and lean-meat percentages, but it is slow growing and has, in comparison with Large Whites and Landrace, a somewhat high food conversion ratio.

The boars attain a weight of between 250 and 295 kg (550 and 650 lb), sows 272 kg (600 lb). The sows are usually quiet and docile. Litter-size is smaller than that expected in the UK. Pale-muscle disease and heart failure are by no means rare in this breed, of which there are now many in the UK. (See PORCINE STRESS SYNDROME.)

Pig Carcases, Rejection of

Analysis of the causes of rejection of carcases and viscera among 1.3 million pigs slaughtered in 7 abattoirs showed that 2556 (0.2 per cent) whole carcases and parts of 25,583 (2.0 per cent) carcases were rejected. The principal causes of rejection of whole carcases were pneumonia, pleurisy, peritonitis and fever; for parts of carcases, abscesses and arthritis. The main reasons for rejection of liver, heart and lungs were 'milk spot', pericarditis and pneumonia, respectively. The variation between abattoirs in the amount of meat and viscera rejected was very large and economically significant.

Pig, External Parasites of the

Half the bacon pigs examined at an abattoir were found to have external parasites – mange mites, lice, or forage mites; and a survey made at the department of veterinary medicine, University of Edinburgh, suggested that 20 per cent of pedigree pigs and piggeries in Britain are infested with sarcoptic mange mites.

The itchiness and scurfiness of many infested pigs are attributed to the results of dry feeding or of a zinc deficiency, but pig breeders would be wise not to be in too much of a hurry to make this assumption.

A proper investigation by a veterinary surgeon would not merely pay for itself, but could effect a big saving; for mange can have an important effect upon food conversion ratios. Moreover, mange can actually kill piglets – and lead to stunting of others which do not succumb.

It is recommended that, once buildings have been cleared of the infestation, each new intake of pigs should be treated with an ectoparasitide. (See also IVERMECTIN.)

Pig Management and Disease

From a veterinary viewpoint, outdoor pig rearing has advantages: namely, fresh air, exercise, and the availability of grass (and soil) which can minimise any deficiencies of vitamins or trace elements. (The outdoor piglet will not need iron injections to avert anaemia, but may still need a vitamin A supplement in autumn and winter.)

The disadvantages are that, especially in the bleaker parts of the country, piglets in arks on grassland may not thrive during the winter; also, where sows and their litters share an enclosure, there may be some savaging by sows of other sows' piglets. The system is suitable only where there is light soil on free-draining land.

Straw-bale 'houses' have much to be said for them. They provide excellent insulation and hence warmth, and can be burnt after use – which obviates the need for disinfection.

Fattening pigs, if properly fed indoors, make better liveweight gains than those outside. They are, however, utterly dependent upon the feed provided, having no opportunity to graze or scavenge. Should the feed be deficient in trace elements or vitamins, their health will suffer.

Pregnant sows thrive best when allowed free access to grassland and the opportunity for exercise, but see PADDOCKS for the danger of contamination of pasture by parasitic worm larvae, unless precautions are taken.

Housing Pig housing, varying from simple wooden huts and arks to costly and elaborate controlled-environment buildings, naturally has an important bearing on health. The type and quality of building materials can be as important as the design of the building. Abrasive concrete can lead to injuries and abscesses, resulting in lameness. (See CONCRETE.)

Straw bedding is the ideal from a health angle. It can keep the pigs warmer, improve liveweight gains, obviate boredom (a possible cause of tail-biting), and reduce stress. (See BEDDING AND BEDDING MATERIALS.)

Recommended temperatures for pigs are given under HOUSING OF ANIMALS. With controlled-environment buildings, precautions must be taken against the effects of power-cuts: it is useful to have a tractor-pto generator for such emergencies. These may arise during both winter and summer, and be due not to a power-cut but to fuses blowing in the building itself. In one case, fuses blew during a thunderstorm, and fail-safe ventilators failed to operate, with the result that 500 pigs inside that building died of heat-stroke. (DEFRA veterinary investigation service report.)

As pigs are particularly susceptible to the effects of water deprivation, precautions must be taken to ensure that water pipes do not freeze, and that the levers of automatic drinkers are not too stiff for piglets to manage. (See under WATER AND WATERING OF ANIMALS for other dangers).

Feeding stalls prevent greedy and aggressive sows from obtaining more than their fair share of feed, leaving others undernourished. However, confinement of sows in stalls (other than for feeding only) deprives the animals of any opportunity for the slightest exercise, and they are unable to move away to escape any cold draughts. Stress results (see THIN SOW SYNDROME).

Stress (which reduces bodily resistance to infection) may also occur at times when pigs are moved from one building to another, or when litters are first mixed. Accordingly, the use of farrowing-to-finish pens has been advocated.

However, relatively few fatteners breed their own pigs. Bought-in pigs are best kept away from other stock on the farm for 3 or 4 weeks. Young pigs are said to do better at this period if they are kept as far away from their dung as possible, and this is one reason why slatted floors and floor feeding rarely work at this stage.

A popular way of achieving good accommodation at this time is to provide a simple covered straw yard allowing about 3 m² (10 sq ft) per pig of total area preferably with part of the area 'kennelled' to give a warm sleeping area. If the latter is raised and dark it will usually be kept clean, and the dung placed in the lighter and lower strawed area. Suitable-sized groups are of 25 to 30 weaners and a lean-to yard will be as cheap a method of housing as any, particularly with ad lib feeding from large hoppers.

For the farmer who cannot use straw or other bedding, there are a number of designs of kennel-type pens with covered or uncovered yards where the muck can be readily cleared away, with tractor or squeegee, or with a hose to wash it down a drain. An essential of this system is to have pigs in small and separated groups perhaps no more than 20 to a pen.

After the conditioning period, the usual practice is to finish the pigs under more intensive conditions. This often involves keeping pigs in litter-less pens, and there is little doubt that this is the type of environment that can be conducive to tail-biting and cannibalism.

Ventilation – at pig level – becomes all the more important in such circumstances. Railed or Weldmesh pen fronts or sides are often preferred as they allow a much better circulation of air in a low-roofed building in particular. Their advantages do not stop there. Many farmers find that it is difficult to get the younger pig dunging in the passage rather than in the pen: a sure help is a gate of Weldmesh or of bars, as a new group will appear to follow the habits of its older companions on the other side of the gate.

It is good practice to have separate sections or units which can be cleaned and disinfected between batches.

The age for weaning piglets is usually 5 to 7 weeks. Where for any reason the sow is not wanted for breeding again immediately, the period of suckling may be extended by an additional week or two. In countries with a severe winter climate, where only spring litters are satisfactory and where consequently only 1 litter per year is bred, the last course is that normally followed. (For early weaning, see under WEANING.)

It is not normally advisable to put pigs into the finishing house until they are at least 32 kg in weight, and most feeders continue the weaner-pool system until this weight is reached.

Feeding Many unsatisfactory results are directly attributable to badly balanced rations. (See CONCENTRATES.)

The growing pig needs a diet that provides the amino acids required to build body proteins as well as vitamins. These (particularly A, D and E) are best added as a special preparation according to the manufacturers' recommendations. (See ADDITIVES; RATIONS FOR LIVESTOCK; COPPER; SOW'S MILK.)

Floor feeding has been shown to have a link with vices. If pens are dirty and the food goes on top of this muck, a scouring, uncomfortable pig can be the result – and it does not seem to take long for the other pigs to set about the weakened individual. Also if ventilation is bad, the dust from meal fed on the floor can appear to induce coughing and fractiousness.

A virtually automatic system of liquid feeding via pipelines is not uncommon in large, modern piggeries. Dry meal may be delivered from hoppers in pre-arranged quantities and at set intervals by means of a time-switch. It has been shown that dry-fed pigs take 10 days longer to reach bacon-weight and 90 g (0.21b) more food for each 450 g (1 lb) liveweight gain, as compared with wet feeding.

Good results have been obtained by feeding moist barley from a Harvestore tower silo.

A method practised at Harper Adams College is for weaners to be brought into the fattening house at 8 weeks old, and there they have free access to meal from self-feeders. At 45 kg (100 lb) liveweight, the ad lib feeding ceases, and the pigs are trough-fed daily. Water is run into the trough (from a conveniently placed tap) and the meal is placed on top, being mixed with the water by the pigs themselves. They are given as much as they will clean up in 20 minutes, subject to a limit of 3 kg (7 lb) per head per day. (See RATIONS FOR LIVESTOCK.)

Aspects of pig husbandry having a bearing on health and disease problems, and of economic importance to the farmer, are given under the following headings: ADDITIVES; ARTIFICIAL INSEMINATION; BEDDING AND BEDDING MATERIALS; BUNT ORDER; CASTRATION; CONTROLLED BREEDING; CONTROLLED ENVIRONMENT HOUSING; COPPER; COPPER POISONING BY; CREEP-FEEDING; DIET; DISINFECTANTS; DRENCHING; DRESSED SEED CORN; DRIED GRASS; FARROWING CRATES; FARROWING RATES; FLIES – Fly control measures; GENETICS; HEAT-STROKE; HOUSING; INFERTILITY; INJECTIONS; INTENSIVE LIVESTOCK PRODUCTION; LAMENESS; LIGHTING; MEAL FEEDING; MUMMIFICATION OF FETUS; NIPPLES; NITRITE POISONING; NOTIFIABLE DISEASES; OESTRUS; OVERLYING; PARASITES; PIGLET ANAEMIA; PIGLET MORTALITY; POISONING; RATIONS; ROUNDHOUSE; SALT POISONING; SENNA; SLURRY; SOW STALLS; SOW'S MILK; STILLBORN PIGS; STRESS; SWILL; TAIL-BITING; THIN SOW SYNDROME; TRACE ELEMENTS; TROPICS; VENTILATION; VITAMINS; WATER; WEANING; WHEY; WORMS, FARM TREATMENT AGAINST.

Pig-Meal, Surplus

Pig breeders who rear cattle and sheep should be wary of feeding surplus pig-meal to those animals unless it is definitely known that the meal does **not** contain a copper supplement. Sheep are very easily poisoned by repeated dosage of a copper supplement well tolerated by pigs, and the death of a heifer was reported after 5 months of supplementary feeding on pig-meal. Conversely, poultry meal medicated with nitrophenide against coccidiosis should never be fed to pigs. It has caused paralysis.

Pig Pox
(see under POX)

Pigeon Pox

A highly contagious viral disease with high morbidity but low mortality. Visible signs are sores around the mouth and eyes. It is caused by a paramoxyvirus and controlled by routine vaccination. Birds over 5 weeks old are vaccinated, all birds in a loft being vaccinated a the same time. Thereafter, the birds are vaccinated annually, between 30 September and 31 December – that is, out of the racing season. The vaccine is administered by removing 6 to 8 feathers and brushing the vaccine onto the skin so that it enters the plucked follicles. The manufacturer's directions must be followed.

Pigeons

Pigeons in cities may constitute a hazard to public health, since many are infected with ornithosis. Some harbour salmonellae, and *Cryptococcus neoformans* has been isolated from pigeon droppings. Grain soaked in the narcotic chloralose has been successfully tried as bait; loss of consciousness begins 10 minutes or so after eating the bait.

Dieldrin is highly poisonous to pigeons. (See also under GAME BIRDS, MORTALITY.)

Racing pigeons in Europe have suffered outbreaks of a highly contagious viral disease causing high morbidity but low mortality. The virus belongs to the avian paramyxovirus sero group 1. The clinical signs include watery droppings, polydipsia and neurologic signs ranging from ataxia and tremor of the head and neck, to torticollis varying from slight head tilt to carriage of the head upside down. The most important differential diagnosis is salmonellosis. Adult pigeons should be vaccinated after moulting and before breeding and young pigeons should be vaccinated 4 weeks before racing.

Live Newcastle disease vaccine stimulates a rapid, but short-lived, immunity.

Ornithosis occurs in young racing pigeons, the symptoms including diarrhoea, conjunctivitis, and nasal discharge. (See CHLAMYDIA.)

Pigeon pox is associated with vesicles around the beak and eyes, and with hard growths – which, if on the feet, may cause lameness.

'Canker' may give rise to a 70 per cent mortality; it is caused by *Trichomonas gallinae* which affects the liver and alimentary canal.

Salmonellosis is often fatal in recently hatched birds, and in adults may cause diarrhoea, distressed breathing, swollen joints, lameness, dropped wing, and loss of weight.

Parasitic worms, especially capillaria, may cause huddling, loss of weight and anaemia.

Pigeons imported into the UK must be vaccinated against paramyxoviruses within 24 hours of their arrival. Four weeks later they must receive a 2nd dose of vaccine, and remain in quarantine for a further week.

Piglet Anaemia
A common cause of pre-weaning losses among housed pigs.

Cause The disease is associated with a deficiency of iron, and is aggravated by cold and damp. (A deficiency of copper and cobalt may sometimes also occur.)

Signs Dullness, a pale whitish skin, scouring, and sometimes exaggerated heartbeats.

Treatment Turn sow and litter out to grass. Give an iron and copper preparation sold for the purpose.

Prevention If outdoor rearing is not desired, give a suitable iron preparation (with cobalt and copper, preferably) at 7 days of age. (A solution made by dissolving 25 g (2oz) of commercial iron pyro-phosphate in 500 ml (1 pint) of water is effective; a quarter of a teaspoonful being given daily for 4 or 5 days.) Place a fresh turf in the farrowing house. Acute iron poisoning, often leading to death within 24 hours, sometimes follows the injection or oral dosing of normally used iron preparations. To prevent this it is advisable to wait until the piglets are a week old, when this danger is reduced; it is also wise to ensure that gilts' rations contain adequate vitamin E.

The intramuscular injections of iron dextran to prevent piglet anaemia are sometimes followed by ham abscesses – the result of broken-off needles or failure to clean the skin adequately before making the injection.

Unweaned piglets eat a significant amount of their dam's dung, and if the sow's diet is supplemented with 2000 mg iron per kg dry matter, it is possible to prevent piglet anaemia; the dung will then contain enough iron to protect the piglets.

Supplements of calcium carbonate fed to fattening pigs from weaning onwards can cause iron deficiency, shown by reduction in blood haemoglobin concentrations and rates of liveweight gain. This effect is especially marked in litters with low weaning weights, probably because their reserves of iron are generally lower. Iron injections or dosing at weaning will overcome these harmful effects.

A secondary anaemia, due to blood-sucking lice, must be borne in mind.

Piglet Mortality
Causes include Aujeszky's disease, 'baby pig' disease, piglet anaemia, haemolytic disease, leptospiral jaundice, *E. coli* infections, streptococcal meningitis, swine erysipelas, swine fever, trembling, enzootic pneumonia, Glasser's disease, Talfan disease, atrophic rhinitis, and transmissible gastro-enteritis (TGE); also overlying by the sow. (See also under ILEUM for another form of enteritis and BOWEL, OEDEMA OF THE; DYSENTERY; GASTRIC ULCERS; MUCORMYCOSIS; LISTERIOSIS; HEART DISEASES – Pericarditis; DERMATOSIS VEGETANS; SPLAYLEG, CONGENITAL.) *Chlamydia psittaci* is another cause of piglet mortality. A list of diseases which affects pigs usually after weaning is given under PIGS, DISEASES OF.

Pigmentation, Loss of
This mostly affects Siamese cats. Eyelids, foot-pads, etc., are altered, with resultant exclusion from cat shows. The causes are various, including hereditable factors.

PIGS, transmissible diseases of
Occupational hazards of people handling pigs include: erysipeloid (the human form of swine erysipelas infection); PORCINE STREPTOCOCCAL MENINGITIS; SWINE VESICULAR DISEASE, which has been transmitted to laboratory workers, but there appear to be few, if any, reports of farm workers becoming ill; and LEPTOSPIROSIS IN PIGS.

Pigs
As seen by research workers, pigs are the fastest growing of the domestic animals, prone to heart troubles and disease of the arteries, and greatly affected in body by mental stress.

Domesticated pigs are believed to be the descendants of the native European wild pig

(*Sus scrofa*), with probably an admixture of the blood of the closely related Asiatic species (*S. vitatus*).

During the 18th and early 19th centuries there were introduced into Britain considerable numbers of pigs belonging to a markedly different type, which originated at a very early date in China and Southwest Asia. This type, variously known as the Siamese or Chinese, and given the specific designation of *S. indicus*, was of smaller size than the native stock; and was short-legged and round-bodied, with a short dished snout and a coat of soft hair. Its most marked economic characteristics were early maturity and a tendency towards rapid fattening. At the same time it was both less hardy and less prolific than the native type. The Chinese type was not long preserved in a pure state in Britain, but was widely employed for crossing with the native sorts, and it seems certain that all of our modern breeds have been influenced to a greater or lesser extent by the infusion of this Eastern blood. The influence is most clearly to be seen in the smaller and earlier maturing breeds such as the Middle White and the Berkshire, while it is least apparent in breeds such as the Tamworth and Wessex.

British breeds of pigs include 10 main breeds:

White breeds
Large White
Middle White
Welsh
British Landrace

Black and black-and-white breeds
Large Black
Wessex Saddleback
Gloucester Old Spots
Berkshire
Red
Tamworth

Most favoured crosses
Large White × Landrace; Large White or Landrace × LA/LW; Duroc × LW/LA.

Chinese Meishan pigs can rear an average of 14 to 16 piglets, compared with 10 to 12 from Western breeds. Meishans reach sexual maturity when 3 months old.

Foreign breeds Pigs imported into the UK for commercial use and breeding trials, crossing purposes, etc., include Duroc, Hampshire, Lacombe, Piétrain, Poland, and China.

The Vietnamese pot-bellied pig and the kuni-kuni are popular as pets, and have been imported for that purpose. They are subject to the Movement and Sale of Pigs Order 1975.

Leading hybrids include the Camborough female and the Cotswold.

Breeding (see GENETICS – Heritability of certain traits).

Boars may be used for breeding at from 7 to 9 months according to size and development. Oestrus occurs, in females that are in good thriving condition, at all seasons of the year, except when the animal is pregnant or nursing. The period of gestation is about 16 weeks; the time allowed for nursing varies from 7 to 12 weeks, and oestrus generally recurs within 10 days, and very commonly on the 3rd or 4th day, after the litter is weaned. The whole breeding cycle is thus completed in 24 to 28 weeks, and it is possible to arrange for sows to produce 2 litters a year regularly throughout their breeding life. Some pig farmers, by means of early weaning, managed to obtain 3 litters in little over a year; but early weaning, and so-called 'piglet batteries', are sometimes accompanied by unacceptable losses. The normal breeding life is 5 or 6 years, but exceptionally good breeders are sometimes kept much longer, and 12 years or more is not unknown.

Pigs, Diseases of
(see AGALACTIA; ANAEMIA; ANTHRAX; AUJESZKY'S DISEASE; CLOSTRIDIAL ENTERITIS; ENCEPHALOMYELITIS, VIRAL, OF PIGS; ENZOOTIC PNEUMONIA OF PIGS; EPERYTHROZOON PARVUM; GASTRIC ULCERS; HAEMOLYTIC DISEASE (see under HAEMOLYTIC; PARVUM; HEAT-STROKE; LEPTOSPIROSIS; LISTERIOSIS; MANGE; MASTITIS; MENINGOENCEPHALITIS; 'MULBERRY HEART'; NECROTIC ENTERITIS; BOWEL, OEDEMA OF THE; PERICARDITIS; POST-PARTURIENT FEVER OF SOWS, PYELONEPHRITIS; RHEUMATISM; RHINITIS, ATROPHIC; SALMONELLOSIS; SWINE DYSENTERY; SWINE ERYSIPELAS; SWINE FEVER; SWINE FEVER, AFRICAN; SWINE INFLUENZA; TAIL-BITING; TALFAN DISEASE; TESCHEN DISEASE; TOXOPLASMOSIS; TRANSMISSIBLE GASTRO-ENTERITIS; TRICHINOSIS; TUBERCULOSIS. See also BACK MUSCLE NECROSIS; 'BLUE-EAR' DISEASE; FOOT-ROT; GLASSER'S DISEASE; 'GREASY PIG DISEASE'; HAEMORRHAGIC GASTROENTERITIS; LOUPING-ILL; OESOPHAGOSTOMIASIS; PITYRIASIS; PNEUMONIA; PORCINE INTESTINAL ADENOMATOSIS; PORCINE STREPTOCOCCAL MENINGITIS; PORCINE ULCERATIVE SPIROCHAETOSIS; SWINE

VESICULAR DISEASE; VOMITING AND WASTING SYNDROME; WORMS, FARM TREATMENT AGAINST and headings under PORCINE.

For causes of death among unweaned pigs, see list of diseases, etc., given under PIGLET MORTALITY. See also PIG CARCASES, REJECTION OF.)

Pigs, names given according to age, sex, etc.

The naming of pigs at various times in their life, and according to their age, sex, etc., varies in different areas; the following gives the most usual names:

Store pig – a pig between the time of weaning and being fattened.

Hog (barrow in the USA) – a male pig after being castrated.

Stag, steg, or seg – a male castrated late in life.

Gilt or yelt – a female intended for breeding purposes, and up to the time that she has her 1st litter.

Boar, bran, or hogg – an uncastrated male.

Sow – a breeding female after the 1st litter.

Pigs, Sale of

In the UK this is subject to the Pigs (Records, Identification and Movement) Order 1996. Pigs moved on to a premises must not be subject to further transport to other premises for 21 days, except for slaughter. The farmer is responsible for the necessary certification.

Pigs, Sedation of

Sedation is useful to prevent fighting after the mixture of litters or re-grouping of pigs; to 'cure' fighting after it has broken out; to make the aggressive sow accept her litter; to facilitate castration, nose-ringing, detusking, etc. Among drugs used for this purpose is azaperone, which is administered by intramuscular injection.

Precaution There is a risk of damaging the sciatic nerve when making intramuscular injections into the hind-legs of pigs; it is therefore advisable to inject into the neck muscles, just behind the ear.

Case histories Within 1 to 8 weeks of an injection of an antibiotic into the ham of 1 hind-leg of 180 4-week-old piglets, 150 had developed paralysis of that leg. In another group of 380 5-week-old piglets, 30 per cent had become paralysed within 10 days, and 30 per cent had died from complications such as septicaemia and pneumonia – 'probably due to necrosis of the foot'.

Pigs, Transport of

The use of containers for the transport of pigs can reduce the risk of infection being carried on to a purchaser's farm. One crate can hold a complete litter group, and keep the pigs from coming into contact with the sides and floor of the lorry – which are often not properly cleaned and which can seldom or never be sterilised.

Pilobolus

A fungus often present in bovine faeces on pasture, it acts as a disperser of lungworm larvae, by means of a 'rocket-like' effect caused when the fungal spores are dispersed.

Pilocarpine

A cholinergic alkaloid used in ophthalmic treatments to constrict the pupil and to reduce intra-ocular pressure in cases of glaucoma.

Pilus

Another name for bacterial FIMBRIAE. For sex pilus, see under PLASMIDS.

Pin Bone (Tuber Ischii)

The rearmost (caudal) projection on the floor of the pelvis.

Pineal Body

Pineal body is a small structure situated in a deep recess of the mid-brain. It occupies a position similar to the third eye in certain reptiles. The pineal body is often regarded as an endocrine gland, concerned with growth. It is the source of melatonin, and it has an inhibitory action on the gonads.

'Pining' (Pine)

A term formerly used to describe any progressive loss of condition in sheep, but nowadays – together with 'vinquish' – usually reserved for copper or cobalt deficiency. This occurs in many parts of the world, is known as bush sickness in New Zealand, and has been reported in areas of Scotland, Northumberland, Devon, and North Wales, where tracts of land are cobalt deficient. (See under COPPER and COBALT.)

'Pink-Eye'

'Pink-eye' is the colloquial name for infectious keratitis of cattle caused by _Moraxella (Haemophilus) bovis_; and also for equine viral arteritis.

'Pink Tooth'

The colloquial name for congenital PORPHYRIA in South Africa.

Pinna

The major part of the external ear, supported by the conchal cartilage.

Piperazine Compounds

Piperazine compounds are used in the treatment of roundworm infestations in dogs and cats; also in pigs, poultry, and horses. They are of low toxicity and can be given in wet or dry food.

Piroplasms

Piroplasms are protozoon parasites of the red-blood cells and the cause of numerous tick-transmitted diseases. They include *Babesia* and *Theileria*. (See BABESIOSIS.)

Pitangueiras

A breed of cattle; Red Poll and Guzera (itself originally a Red Poll Brahman) developed in Brazil with Red Poll semen from the UK.

Pitch Poisoning

This has occurred with fatal results in pigs after eating clay pigeons, and after contact with tarred walls and floors of pig pens. The symptoms are inappetence, depression, weakness, jaundice, and anaemia.

Pitohui

An orange and black songbird, of attractive appearance but possessing a venom powerful enough to kill a mouse within minutes. An inhabitant of New Guinea, this bird has a sharp beak and claws. The venom is present in the bird's feathers, skin, and flesh. The birds sometimes attack people.

Pituitary Gland

Pituitary gland is a small oval body up to 2.5 cm (1 in) in diameter, attached to the base of the brain and situated in a depression in the upper surface of the sphenoid bone called the *Sella turcica*. The gland is connected to the hypothalamus.

The anterior lobe produces several hormones. One of these, the growth hormone somatotrophin (STH), has an important effect on protein metabolism. Lack of this hormone causes or contributes to dwarfism. STH controls body growth, including fetal growth in pregnant females.

Adrenocorticotrophin (ACTH) stimulates the cortex of the adrenal gland. Thyroid-stimulating hormone (TSH) stimulates the thyroid.

Pituitary gonad-stimulating hormones include luteinising hormone (LH), follicle-stimulating hormone (FSH), and prolactin which is associated with lactation. (For the functions of LH and FSH see under LUTEINISING HORMONE and FOLLICLE-STIMULATING HORMONE, respectively.)

When hypertrophied in the young, the gland causes gigantism, in which a great increase in size occurs. Hypertrophy or increased function in adults results in acromegaly, in which there is a sudden growth of extremities of the body. If it atrophies, growth ceases, and a condition of infantilism results. In this there is a pronounced lack of development of ovaries and testes and of secondary sex characters, together with deposition of fat, and a general sluggishness and lack of development. In the male there is a tendency towards reversion to female characteristics, but the opposite effect in the female is not observed. Anterior lobe extract is used to correct such atrophic conditions. (See also TWINNING, ARTIFICIAL.)

The posterior lobe secretes 2 important hormones:

(1) vasopressin, which is also known as the antidiuretic hormone (ADH), being concerned with water loss from the body; lack of ADH gives rise to diabetes insipidus; (2) oxytocin acts on the muscular wall of the uterus causing contraction, e.g. during birth; it also acts on the mammary gland and is sometimes known as the 'let-down hormone' in connection with the release of milk.

Pituitary tumours

Pituitary tumours in 8 dogs were found to be carcinomas in 2 of them, and adenomas in 5.

Signs Lethargy, pacing, circling, head-pressing, and partial paralysis affecting all 4 limbs.

Death occurred in from 2 weeks to 13 months.

Pituitrin

An extract prepared from the posterior lobe of the pituitary gland, and containing 2 distinct fractions: one affecting the blood vessels and the other, the uterine muscle. These fractions are named the 'pressor' and 'oxytocic' principles, respectively. In human and veterinary medicine the purified oxytocin fractions are prepared as a separate product. (See HORMONES; ENDOCRINE GLANDS; OXYTOCIN.)

Pityriasis

Pityriasis is a bran-like eruption 3 to 4 cm in diameter that appears on the surface of the skin. In animals, it is found only in pigs; the cause is not known. *Pityriasis rosea* was recorded in 72 out of 120 litters sired by a Landrace boar. Lesions resembled ringworm, were red, and lasted 10 weeks.

'Pizzle Rot'

A disease mainly of merino sheep in Australia. (See under BALANITIS.)

Placenta

PLACENTA is the technical name for the afterbirth. Strictly speaking, placenta means the medium by means of which the mother nourishes the fetus.

Structure It is composed of 3 fetal membranes:

(1) The chorion, which is the outermost, is a strong fibrous membrane, the outer surface of which is closely moulded to the inner surface of the uterus. The chorion has villi, which are vascular projections inserted into the crypts of the uterine mucous membrane.

(2) The allantois is the middle membrane. It develops early in embryonic life as an outgrowth from the hindgut, and insinuates itself between the other 2 membranes. That part of the allantois remaining inside the abdominal cavity of the fetus forms the urinary bladder in after-life, and, until the time of birth, is in direct communication with the extra-fetal portion by means of the urachus – that part passing through the umbilicus. Fluid secreted by the kidneys of the fetus and passing to the urinary bladder gains exit to the allantoic cavity, which is outside the fetus, until just before the time of birth, when the passage is closed.

(3) The amnion, which is continuous with the skin at the umbilicus (navel), and completely encloses the fetus but is separated from actual contact with it by the amniotic fluid, or the 'liquor of the amnion', which in the mare measures about 5 or 6 litres (9 to 10½ pints).

This 'liquor amnii' forms a kind of hydrostatic bed in which the fetus floats, and serves to protect it from injury, shocks, extremes of temperature, allows free though limited movements, and guards the uterus of the dam from the spasmodic fetal convulsions which, late in pregnancy, are often vigorous and even violent.

At birth it helps to dilate the cervical canal of the uterus and the posterior genital passages, forms part of the 'waterbag', and, on bursting, lubricates the maternal passages. (See PARTURITION.)

The membranes should be discharged from the uterus with or soon after the young animal, but it is not uncommon to find their expulsion delayed for a variable time, depending upon the species and the individual. Immediately after the birth of the young animal the uterus contracts to a size smaller than when pregnant, with the result that the attachment between fetal envelopes and maternal uterus is severed to a greater or lesser extent. Afterpains follow, similar to those of normal labour, but less severe, with the object of expelling the membranes.

In the mare, with a scattered and slight attachment, the afterbirth separates rapidly and is soon expelled; indeed, not infrequently the foal is born still enveloped in, or attached to, its membranes. These appear as a complicated mass of pinkish-grey tissue, plentifully supplied with blood, and often possessing little bladder-like pockets of amniotic or allantoic fluid.

If in 6 hours the placenta has not been discharged naturally, measures should be taken to effect its prompt removal, for the mare is very susceptible to metritis.

In the cow, where the attachment is cotyledonary, the fetal membranes may be expelled at any time during the first 6 hours after calving, or not for 1 or 2 days, without any serious consequences. Retention occurs frequently.

In those animals which normally produce multiple offspring at a birth – ewe, sow, bitch, and cat – as each fetus is born the corresponding membranous envelope either accompanies or else immediately follows it. The exception to this otherwise almost invariable rule is in the case of the last fetus to be born, that fetus which occupied the extremity of one or other horn of the uterus; the envelopes of this, the youngest member of the family, are sometimes retained, and may occasion a mild or severe metritis, until such time as they are expelled.

The bitch, cat, sow, cow, and even the mare eat the membranes.

Retained placenta is one of the undesirable sequels of parturition. Retention of the fetal membranes is commonest in the cow. Normally, the membranes should be expelled in from half an hour to 4 or 5 hours after the birth of the calf, but owing to the intricate cotyledonary attachment in cattle, they are often retained for long periods. (See PARTURITION.)

Signs A portion of the fetal membranes hangs from the lips of the vulva attached to what remains inside the cavity of the uterus. The exposed portion may measure only a few inches, or be a large mass reaching to the cow's hocks. In some cases there is no membrane visible externally, but there is an odour of decomposition evident.

During the first day after calving the membranes in an ordinary uncomplicated case are fresh, slimy, and pinkish in colour. There is no objectionable smell, and the cow is not distressed. After the second day the external portions undergo decomposition; the colour becomes greyish; an offensive chocolate-coloured discharge makes its appearance and soils the hindquarters and tail of the cow. She stands with her back arched, frequently switches her tail and paddles with the hind-feet.

Masses of semi-dissolved membrane, looking like pieces of wet cobweb, are passed out at intervals, and can be found behind the cow along with quantities of greyish foul-smelling discharge; the mucous membrane of the vagina is inflamed, and the cow resents having her hindquarters examined.

It is certainly not advisable that a mass of decomposing fleshy material should be allowed to hang from a cow's uterus for a longer time than is absolutely necessary, but too hasty attempts at removal may be followed by infertility or even death.

In modern practice, hormone injections have largely displaced manual removal, with its attendant risks. Manual removal consists of introducing the hand and arm, protected in sterile disposable plastic sleeve-length gloves; if these are not available, the hand and arm must be cleansed as far as possible by thorough washing in an antiseptic solution, and a subsequent rinsing in strong salt and water. The membranes should not be removed until they can be displaced without difficulty, and without distress to the cow. Each cotyledon is grasped as it is reached, and the adherent membrane is peeled off from its surface with the fingers and thumb. At the same time gentle traction should be exerted upon the protruded membranes from the outside.

After removal it may be advisable to douche out the uterus with a suitable antiseptic solution, and to give prophylactic antibiotics (see UTERUS, DISEASES OF – The cow).

In the sow and bitch the membranes that are liable to be retained are those belonging to the fetus that is born last, which occupied the extremity of one or other of the horns of the uterus, but the condition is rare in each of these animals.

It is most advisable that owners of animals which have retained their afterbirth after parturition should seek veterinary advice.

Plague

(see CATTLE PLAGUE; AVIAN INFLUENZA (FOWL PLAGUE); BUBONIC PLAGUE)

Plant Juice

At grass-drying plants, when mechanically de-watering forage before drying, a rich green juice is expressed. The juice represents a source of protein concentrate comparable with fish meal in value.

From 6 tons of fresh material, such as lucerne or grass, 2.5 tons of this plant juice is squeezed out. However, using plant juice presents some problems, as it is very unstable, due to enzyme action. It must be heated to about 85°C (185°F) to stabilise the protein, and some chemical preservative is also added.

The easiest way to use the juice is to include it in liquid pig feed.

Plantar

At the back of the hind-limb.

Plantar Cushion

Plantar cushion is the dense fibro-fatty rubber-like structure which lies immediately above the frog in the foot of the horse, and is one of its most important anti-concussion or shock-absorbing mechanisms. (See FOOT OF THE HORSE.)

Plasma

Plasma is the fluid portion of the blood.

Plasma Cells

Larger than lymphocytes, with dark-staining granules in the nucleus, plasma cells are found in the lymph nodes, and are concerned with antibody production. (See diagram under LYMPHOCYTE.)

Plasma Substitutes

(see DEXTRAN; GELATIN, SUCCINYLATED)

Plasmids

Plasmids are genetic structures which many species of bacteria possess in addition to their chromosomes, and which, like the chromosomes, determine the inheritance of various properties. Since plasmids are not essential to cell growth, the cell may gain or lose them without lethal effect. Some plasmids can unite with chromosomes: these are called episomes. All episomes are plasmids but not all plasmids are episomes.

Plasmids have been defined as 'circular lengths of DNA which behave as viruses with a restricted range of host bacteria, and which are replicated in step with the organism'. (See also GENETIC ENGINEERING.)

Infectious (self-transmissible) plasmids are found in Gram-negative rods. In addition to genes coding for specific properties (e.g. R-determinants coding for antibiotic resistance), these plasmids also possess other genes which code for the production of sex pili by which conjugation with a recipient cell is made possible. Non-transmissible plasmids, also found in Gram-negative rods, lack the genes necessary for self-transfer; for these plasmids to be transferred the cell must first be infected with a sex-factor from another cell.

In Gram-positive organisms, plasmids may be transduced from one cell to another by bacteriophages.

Plasmodium Gallinaceum

A parasite which causes bird malaria in poultry. *P. durae* causes death in turkey poults.

Malaria of birds is a group of almost worldwide infections which include *Haemoproteus* and *Leucocytozoon* as well as *Plasmodium.*

Plaster Casts

(see SPLINTING MATERIALS)

Plastic Bags or Sheeting

Cattle have died following ingestion of plastic bags discarded on grazing land. In some instances the material is digested and does not cause an obstruction.

Plastic 'Bones'

A fractured scaphoid in the right hind-leg of a racing greyhound has been successfully replaced by a plastic replica of a scaphoid bone. For a further use of plastics, see under HOOF REPAIR.

Plate Culture

The growing of bacteria in a medium contained in a Petri dish, a covered, shallow, circular glass dish which gives a large surface area.

Platelets (Thrombocytes)

Platelets (Thrombocytes) are described under BLOOD.

Plating

Plating is the cultivation of bacteria on flat plates (Petri dishes) containing nutrient material. The term is also applied in surgery to the method of securing union of fractured bones by screwing to the sides of the fragments narrow metal plates which hold them firmly together whilst union is taking place.

Pleura

Pleura is the membrane which covers the external surfaces of the lungs and lines the inside of the chest walls. (See LUNGS.)

Pleural Cavity

In normal healthy animals this is merely a potential cavity, since between the pleura lining the chest and the pleura covering the lungs there is usually a thin film of fluid. Surface tension holds the one surface to the other.

Pleurisy (Pleuritis)

Inflammation of the PLEURA, which may occur as a complication of pneumonia, of 'shipping fever' in cattle, and in cases of tuberculosis and other infections; occasionally from a chest wound.

Friction between the inflamed surfaces gives rise to pain each time the animal breathes, and the breathing is changed in character – i.e. there is minimal movement of the chest walls, and extra effort by the abdominal muscles, which appear to be doing all the work. The line of the rib cartilages often stands out prominently, giving rise to what has been called the 'pleuritic ridge'. Other symptoms include fever, dullness, and what is often described as a 'hacking' cough; sometimes a rasping sound due to friction may be heard.

After 12 to 48 hours the painful stage of pleurisy may be followed by an effusion of fluid. Removal of this fluid becomes necessary if respiration is seriously impaired by it.

Sometimes the fluid is purulent, a condition known as 'empyema'. Sometimes there is very little effusion, and the condition remains one of 'dry pleurisy'.

A complication of pleurisy is that adhesions sometimes occur, and persist, between the parietal and visceral pleura. (See also PLEURODYNIA; PLEURO-PNEUMONIA.)

Treatment Pleurisy is one of those conditions in which professional advice is highly desirable in the early stages, and reliance should not be placed on first-aid. It may be necessary to withdraw fluid from the chest, to administer an appropriate antibiotic; and it is important to establish the presence or absence of tuberculosis. (See also NURSING.)

Pleurodynia

Pleurodynia means a painful condition of the chest wall. It is a symptom of PLEURISY; it may be due to fractures of the ribs; it is sometimes seen in tumours affecting the chest wall, and it is commonly recognised by pressing the fingers into the spaces between the ribs.

Pleuro-Pneumonia

Pleuro-pneumonia is a combination of PLEURISY with a PNEUMONIA. Acute pneumonia is often accompanied by some amount of pleurisy, which is largely responsible for the painfulness which accompanies pneumonia. (See also CONTAGIOUS BOVINE PLEURO-PNEUMONIA.)

Plexus

Plexus is a network of nerves or vessels, e.g. the brachial and sacral plexuses of nerves and the choroid plexus of veins within the brain.

Plumbism

Plumbism is another name for chronic lead poisoning. (See LEAD POISONING.)

PML

Pharmacy and merchants' list: a category of veterinary medicines which may be sold to the public only through pharmacies; and to farmers or others 'maintaining animals in the course of their business' through pharmacies or agricultural merchants. Horse and pony owners may obtain PML horse wormers from pharmacies, agricultural merchants or registered saddlers.

PMS

Pregnant mare's serum, a source of gonadotrophin.

PMWS

(see POST-WEANING MULTISYSTEMIC WASTING SYNDROME)

Pneumocystis Pneumonia

Pneumocystis pneumonia, one of the most serious diseases of human AIDS patients, has been found in dogs, cats, rodents, and primates.

Pneumogastric nerve

Another name for VAGUS NERVE.

Pneumomycosis

A fungal infection of the lungs.

Pneumonia

Pneumonia may be defined as inflammation of lung tissue.

Pneumonias have been classified in various ways, e.g. according to the area or tissue involved, or according to lesions, or causes.

Lobar pneumonia is that in which a whole lobe is involved; in lobular pneumonia the inflammation is less localised and more patchy. Broncho-pneumonia is that in which the inflammation is concentrated in and around the bronchioles leading from the bronchi. Pleuro-pneumonia, as the name suggests, involves the pleural membranes as well as the lung itself. Interstitial pneumonia affects the fibrous supporting tissue of the lung rather than the parenchyma though consolidation of the latter can then occur. (See also LUNGS, DISEASES OF for lesions.)

Pneumonia, which can be acute or chronic, may – as mentioned above – also be classified according to causes, e.g. viral, mycoplasmal, bacterial, mycotic, parasitic and non-infective. It must be borne in mind, however, that infections may be mixed and changing. (See RESPIRATORY DISEASE IN PIGS for an explanatory diagram.)

Pneumonia may arise from a primary viral infection, with complications caused by secondary bacterial invaders, as in canine distemper. Some viruses and bacteria depend upon each other, as explained under SYNERGISM. The infection may be a very mixed one, e.g. in ENZOOTIC PNEUMONIA OF PIGS. Bacterial pneumonia may be acute, e.g. KLEBSIELLA infection, or of a chronic suppurative type, e.g. TUBERCULOSIS.

The main effect of pneumonia, whether through the presence of exudate in the bronchioles and alveoli, or destruction of areas of lung by abscess formation or consolidation or hepatisation, is that the normal exchange of carbon dioxide for oxygen is impaired and impeded. The animal has to struggle for breath to obtain sufficient oxygen.

Signs With less oxygen available to the red blood cells (and hence to the organs and tissues) at the normal respiratory rate, the animal accordingly needs to breathe faster. This increased respiratory rate (tachypnoea) is therefore a main symptom. The breathing may also become laboured and painful (dyspnoea). Fever is usually present, with accompanying dullness and loss of appetite (but see under CALF PNEUMONIA for an exception to this). There is often a cough, though this is not an invariable or attention-catching symptom.

Viral pneumonia In cattle, most cases of viral pneumonia, uncomplicated by secondary bacterial infection, show areas of collapse in the lungs, emphysema of the apical lobes, some in the cardiac lobes but little in the diaphragmatic lobes, with little or no exudate. An acute pneumonia may develop in some cases of infectious bovine rhinotracheitis. (See RHINOTRACHEITIS.) Bovine syncytial virus is another important pathogen, causing coughing, oedema of the lungs, consolidation and emphysema. (See also CALF PNEUMONIA.) In horses, pneumonia in young foals may be caused by equine herpesvirus 1. (See also SWINE PLAGUE.)

Mycoplasmal pneumonia An example of this is fully described under CONTAGIOUS BOVINE PLEURO-PNEUMONIA – a disease not normally present in the UK. *Mycoplasma bovis* and *M. dispar* are primary pathogens in the UK. The latter may cause CALF PNEUMONIA of a mild type except for the harsh cough. (See also under MYCOPLASMA.)

Bacterial pneumonia Bacterial toxins may have an important additional effect in this. In cattle, *Pasteurella haemolytica* can be a primary cause of pneumonia, typically producing much exudate as well as a secondary invader. In horses *Corynebacterium equi* causes a suppurative bronchopneumonia in foals, and in adult horses a suppurative pneumonia may also occur during the course of strangles.

   Streptococcus pneumoniae and *Staphylococcus aureus* are other important secondary invaders of damaged lungs.

Parasitic pneumonia This may be an extension of PARASITIC BRONCHITIS in calves, caused by the lungworm *Dictyocaulus viviparus.* Autopsy findings include dark red consolidation of some lung lobes. In pigs, lungworms (*Metastrongylus*) are also a cause of pneumonia.

Mycotic (fungal) pneumonia is caused by *Aspergillus* species, and also by *Candida albicans.* (See MONILIASIS.) The latter may be associated with oedema of the lungs, in both mammals and birds, and may follow the use of certain antibiotics. (See also PHYCOMYCOSIS.)

Allergic pneumonia (see 'FARMER'S LUNG' which affects cattle also)

Non-infective pneumonia can result from the action of certain poisons, e.g. PARAQUAT, ANTU, and phenolic sheep dips (see DIPS), as well as from aspiration pneumonia. The latter may result from milk 'going the wrong way' in bucket-fed calves, and also from medicines administered to animals by stomach tube passed in error into the trachea instead of the oesophagus (fortunately a rare occurrence!). Aspiration of vomit is another example.

   Non-infective pneumonia quickly becomes infective, as micro-organisms take advantage of the inflamed mucous membranes. The animal becomes suddenly dull, uninterested in food, feverish, and may show signs of chest pain. Death can be expected within 72 hours, and autopsy findings may include areas of necrosis and abscess formation.

Treatment of pneumonia Separate affected animals, provide good-quality feed in a well-ventilated environment, free from draughts, and good bedding. Appropriate antibiotics, sulfa drugs, and trimethoprim may all be of service. Heart stimulants, the administration of oxygen, and possibly diuretics in the case of oedema, may be indicated. Anti-inflammatory drugs, e.g. flunixin, may help in the acute stage. The one golden rule in the treatment of pneumonia in all animals is: 'Do not drench.' Medicines should be administered by injection, in the food, or perhaps as an electuary. (See also NURSING.)

Pneumonia in Calves
(see CALF PNEUMONIA)

Pneumonia in Cats
Bronchopneumonia can be a complication of feline viral rhinotracheitis in young cats.

   In older cats tuberculosis is still sometimes a cause of disease of the lungs, though with nearly all milk now pasteurised in EU countries, feline TB is no longer at all common. It can, however, result from a cat eating TB-infected prey.

   A granulomatous pneumonia is caused, rarely, by *Corynebacterium equi.* Theoretically, a stable cat would be more prone to it.

Pneumonia in Horses
In a USA study, anaerobic bacteria were isolated from pleural fluid or tracheobronchial aspirates obtained from 21 of 46 horses with bronchopneumonia. *Bacteriodes oralis* and *B. melaninogenicus* were the species most commonly isolated (9 and 5 horses, respectively). Other *Bacteriodes* species were cultured from 12 animals and *Clostridium* species from 8. A putrid odour was associated with the pleural fluid and/ or breath of nearly two-thirds of the horses from which anaerobes were isolated. The prognosis was significantly poorer in cases with anaerobic infections; 14 of the 21 horses involved either died or were euthanased. (See also under FOALS, DISEASES OF).

   Another cause is *Corynebacterium equi*, which can also infect cats.

Pneumonia in Pigs
Actinobacillus (Haemophilus) pleuropneumoniae is a major cause of pneumonia in pigs. (See RESPIRATORY DISEASE IN PIGS.)

   For the most common form of pneumonia in pigs, see under ENZOOTIC PNEUMONIA. (See also SWINE PLAGUE.)

Pneumonia in Sheep

In Britain, pneumonia caused by *Pasteurella haemolytica* has become more frequent. This organism commonly lives in normal sheep, and causes disease only when the animal's resistance is weakened by bad weather, transport from one farm to another, movement from a poor to a richer pasture, or perhaps by a virus. In some outbreaks, where the disease takes an acute form, a sheep which seemed healthy enough in the evening may be found dead in the morning. Usually, however, the shepherd sees depressed-looking animals with drooping ears, breathing rather quickly and having a discharge from eyes and nostrils, and a cough. Death often occurs within a day or two. The last sheep to be involved in the outbreak tend to linger for several weeks, looking very tucked-up in the meantime, with a cough and fast breathing. Antisera and vaccines are available for treatment and prevention.

Another cause of pneumonia in sheep is *Chlamydia psittaci*. (See also HAEMORRHAGIC SEPTICAEMIA, which occurs in the tropics; PARAINFLUENZA 3 VIRUS; MAEDI/VISNA.)

Pneumothorax

Pneumothorax is a condition in which air has gained access to the pleural cavity through a wound in the chest wall. (See LUNGS, DISEASES AND INJURIES OF.)

Pneumothorax is not uncommon in the dog which has fallen out of a window, or been run over or hit by a car. Distressed breathing and cyanosis are, following an accident, suggestive of pneumothorax.

Mild cases may be accompanied by mild symptoms, and spontaneous recovery may occur. Severe cases may die. Treatment includes aspiration of the air from the pleural cavity. (See also LUNGS, DISEASES OF – Collapse.)

Simple pneumothorax In such cases, the condition may be caused by sudden non-penetrating trauma to the chest wall which momentarily raises the intrathoracic pressure. If this occurs against a closed glottis, then alveolar tissue may rupture. In many cases the leak will be small, but in others, sufficient air will enter the pleural cavity to cause marked dyspnoea.

Open pneumothorax is caused by a penetrating wound of the chest wall, resulting in an immediate and total collapse of the lung. Air can be heard entering the chest wound at each respiratory effort. There is severe dyspnoea.

Tension pneumothorax may develop following an open pneumothorax, or when a small bronchus ruptures, and air accumulates in the pleural space during inspiration but is not expelled during expiration. The mediastinum is apt to be displaced from the midline, partially collapsing the remaining functional lung.

Pneumovirus

A cause of rhinotracheitis in turkeys and chickens. An ELISA test is available for diagnosis.

'Poaching'

Land becoming muddy and broken up by the feet of animals. Especially on heavy land, with high stocking rates, wet weather can bring serious poaching problems. (See DAIRY HERD MANAGEMENT.) At gateways, deep mud (in winter often at near-freezing temperatures) can lead to foul-in-the-foot and mastitis.

Pododermatitis

(see FOUL-IN-THE-FOOT)

Poikilocyte

Poikilocyte is a malformed red blood cell found in the blood in various types of anaemia.

Poikilothermic

'Cold-blooded'. The rate of metabolism of such an animal varies with its environmental temperature.

Pointer

A medium-sized, slim dog with long neck and pointed tail; used as a gun dog. Entropion and ununited anoconeal process are inheritable, as may be calcinosis circumscripta.

Poisoning

Most cases result from the poison being swallowed. In a few instances poison may be taken in through a wound of the skin, or even through the unbroken skin, e.g. phenol preparations. Malicious poisoning is most frequently carried out against dogs and cats, although horses and ruminants also sometimes suffer.

The use of poison to control vermin – rabbits, foxes, rats, mice, etc. – is a hazard, for when the poisoned bait is accessible to domesticated animals, cases of poisoning may result. It should be remembered that the exposure of such poison above ground constitutes an offence.

The constituents of common and commercial rat-poisons are mentioned under RODENTS – Rodenticides.

Many cases of poisoning result from the careless use of sheep-dips, paints, weed-killers and insecticides, which, in powder, paste, or solution, are left about in places to which animals have access. Cattle are notoriously inquisitive, and will lick at anything they find, sometimes with fatal consequences.

It is perhaps not widely enough realised that cattle seem to like the taste of lead paint – 1 heifer helped herself to a whole pint of it – and that very small quantities spattered on the ground can kill several beasts. Even the contents of old, discarded paint tins can be lethal. In one instance, children found such tins and scraped out the residue on to pasture, killing 5 yearlings. In another instance, cattle licked out old paint tins on a rubbish dump in a pit to which they found their way. A recently painted fence is also a danger.

Thirsty cattle will drink almost anything: diesel oil and a copper-containing spray liquid have each caused death in these circumstances. Salt poisoning is certainly no myth, and pigs should never be kept short of drinking water.

Some insecticides, such as TEPP and Parathion, are totally unsuitable for use on livestock. Fatal poisoning of a herd of cattle sprayed with TEPP has been reported from Texas. A farmer in Ireland used aldrin as an orf-dressing, and killed 105 out of 107 lambs. Fatal poisoning of cattle has also occurred through the application to their backs of a carbolic-acid-arsenic preparation against flies. (See also HERBICIDES; WEEDKILLERS.)

Near factories and chemical works, grass, etc., may become impregnated with fluorine compounds, copper, lead or other metals, and lead to chronic poisoning of any animals grazing nearby. The same thing applies in orchards after spraying of fruit-trees. Pasture may be contaminated by spray-drift or dusting operations, particularly from the air, and the chemicals used may cause poisoning. This applies also to other treated green crops which animals may eat. DDT and BHC and other insecticides (used in home and garden) of the CHLORINATED HYDROCARBON group may poison birds, cats and dogs. (See also ORGANOPHOSPHORUS POISONING; FARM CHEMICALS; FLUOROSIS.)

The use of pitch (the poisonous ingredient of clay-pigeons) or coal tar on the walls and floors of piggeries is a cause of poisoning. Some wood preservatives cause hyperkeratosis.

Poisoning may result from indiscretion on the part of owners or attendants in the use of patent or other animal medicines, or from the administration to animals of tablets, etc.

intended for human use, e.g. paracetamol, caffeine.

Dogs and cats may also be poisoned by gaining access to unsecured medicines (pills, tablets, etc.) intended for human use. For home and garden hazards to pet animals (including cage birds), see under CARBON MONOXIDE; 'FRYING PAN' DEATHS; ANTIFREEZE; CREOSOTE; LEAD POISONING; METALDEHYDE; BHC POISONING; BENZOIC ACID POISONING; WARFARIN; DDT; HOUSE PLANTS; HOUSE DECORATING. If one considers dogs out for walks, one should add DIELDRIN; PARAQUAT; FARM CHEMICALS. As regards dog and cat foods, poisoning has resulted from biscuit meal made from corn dressed with dieldrin, from stored food contaminated by rats' urine containing warfarin, from aflatoxins, and from horse-meat containing barbiturates or choral hydrate. In the cat, food containing benzoic acid as a preservative has caused poisoning.

Fodder poisoning Excess of fodder beet may cause scouring in both pigs and cattle, and the after-effects may be serious. In sows just farrowed, the milk supply may almost disappear. Beet tops have caused the deaths of cattle when given unwilted, and even when wilted they should be strictly rationed. Kale and rape poisoning can occur in cattle and sheep; these must be used sparingly and not constitute an animal's sole diet, and hay in particular is necessary in addition. Deaths have occurred in horses and cattle restricted to rye-grass pasture. Sheep have been fatally poisoned by feeding them surplus pig-meal containing a copper supplement; a heifer likewise. Pigs have been poisoned by giving them medicated meal intended for poultry and containing nitrophenide against coccidiosis. Which all goes to show that medicated feeds are by no means always interchangeable between different species of livestock, since there are genetic differences between them as regards susceptibility to poisoning, depending in part upon possession or absence of some enzyme which can readily detoxify the poison. (See GROUNDNUT MEAL.)

The use of surplus seed corn for pig-feeding has led to fatal poisoning – the mercury dressing having been overlooked! (See DIELDRIN for poisoning from seed dressings, and FLOOR SWEEPINGS; also MONENSIN SODIUM.)

Hay contaminated with foxgloves or ragwort is a source of fatal poisoning. Silage contaminated with ragwort has similarly caused death. Silage contaminated with hexoestrol has caused abortion. (See under HORMONES IN MEAT PRODUCTION.)

Poisonous plants growing in pastures, in swampy or marshy places, in the bottoms of hedges, on waste land and in shrubberies and gardens, are other very common sources of poisoning. In the early spring, when grass is scarce, and when herbivorous animals are let out for the first time after wintering indoors, the tender succulent growths attract them, often with serious consequences. Similar results may be seen during a very dry summer when grass is parched. Ragwort and bracken are the most common causes of plant poisoning in cattle; in sheep, bracken can cause night blindness and neoplasia as well as true poisoning. (See BRACKEN.)

Clippings from shrubs, especially from yew, rhododendrons, aconite, boxwood, lupins, laurel, laburnum, etc., should never be thrown 'over the hedge', because in some of these the toxic substances are most active when the clippings have begun to wither, and animals are very prone to eat them in this condition. It is a safe rule to regard all garden trimmings as unsafe for animals, with the exception of vegetables, such as cabbages and turnips. (See under ACONITE; BITTERSWEET; FOXGLOVE; HEMLOCK; LABURNUM; POTATO; RAGWORT; WATER DROPWORT; YEW; LOCOWEED, etc.)

Signs The symptoms of each of the more common poisonous agents are given under their respective headings.

It must be emphasised that the symptoms of some illnesses are the same as those of some poisons, and vice versa. For example, not only vomiting and diarrhoea but also cramp, fever, rapid breathing, convulsions, hysteria, jaundice, salivation, blindness, and deafness are common to both. A professional diagnosis is therefore important.

Irritant poisons produce acute abdominal pain, vomiting (when possible), purging, rapidly developing general collapse, and often unconsciousness, perhaps preceded by convulsions.

Narcotics produce excitement at first, unsteady movements, interference with sight; and later, stupor and unconsciousness appear; coma, with or without spasmodic or convulsive movements, supervenes, and death occurs in many cases.

Narcotic irritants produce symptoms of irritation in the first place, and later, delirium, convulsions, and coma.

As a general rule poisoning should be suspected when an animal becomes suddenly ill, soon after feeding; when put out to pasture for the first time in the season after dipping; or when a change of food has recently taken place. Newly purchased animal feeds may be followed by an outbreak of illness, and such results point to the inclusion of some harmful substance. Fungal poisoning may occur as a result of mouldy barley, etc.

First-aid In suggesting simple first-aid measures, it should be emphasised that they necessarily differ from – and are likely to be less effective than – those the veterinary surgeon will take. It should be realised, too, that against some poisons there are no effective antidotes.

Where it is suspected that poisoning has arisen from use of some proprietary product, take the container (or the label from it) to your veterinarian (or write down the name of the manufacturer and product) so that he or she may ascertain the chemical ingredients and, if necessary, consult the manufacturer as to the recommended antidote.

If it is suspected that poisoning may have resulted from a skin dressing, wash this off with warm soapy water to prevent further absorption. (See CARBOLIC ACID POISONING.)

Where a poison is believed to have been taken by mouth, give an emetic. However, emetics should be avoided if strong acids or alkalis are involved.

Emetics which may be safely used are: for pigs, a dessertspoonful of mustard in a cupful of water; for dogs, a strong salt solution (ordinary household salt), or a crystal of washing soda; for cats, the latter.

To hinder absorption in the horse, ox, or sheep, strong black tea or coffee which has been boiled may be given. These, all of which contain tannic acid or tannates, are useful against vegetable poisons.

To counteract the effects of irritants, use demulcents (olive oil, milk, milk and eggs, or liquid paraffin). Yellow phosphorus is an exception to this rule; oily substances favour its absorption and must be avoided; copper sulphate should be given instead. Against narcotics, stimulants are needed, e.g. strong coffee or black tea, given by the mouth as a first-aid measure.

Advice on poisons In the UK, veterinary surgeons may obtain information and advice concerning poisonous compounds, and their antidotes, if any, from the National Poisons Information Service, Avonley Road, London SE14 5ER.

Confirmation of poisoning No matter how strong circumstantial evidence seems to be, it is always essential that a post-mortem examination be made, and that necessary samples of the stomach contents, portions of the liver and perhaps other organs, should be submitted to a qualitative and quantitative chemical examination by an analyst, before a suspected case of poisoning can be considered to be definitely proved. The necessity for this procedure is obvious when legal proceedings are contemplated.

Poisoning by Salmonella
(see SALMONELLOSIS)

Poland China
A breed of pig from Ohio, USA. Colouring is black with 6 white points (feet, tip of noise, and tail). Rapid growth and good meat production are characteristics of the breed.

Polioencephalomalacia
(see CEREBROCORTICAL NECROSIS)

Poliomyelitis of Pigs
This disease is distinct from that of human beings and is possibly identical with TALFAN DISEASE.

Poll
The region lying between the ears and a little behind them.

'Poll Evil'
'Poll Evil' is an old, colloquial name sometimes incorrectly applied to any swelling in the POLL region, but which should be reserved for a sinus following infection of some of the deeper tissues and giving rise to pus-formation. It may result from an injury which displaces a chip of bone from the atlas. Apart from this, and its situation, 'poll evil' resembles fistulous withers.

Causes Self-inflicted injuries such as striking the poll against the top of a doorway, or falling backwards with the poll striking the ground; blows, such as from a whip-handle; bridle pressure.

Fusiformis necrophorus has been associated with some cases and may have gained entrance through damaged skin. It has been suggested that some cases may arise through infection without injury. *Brucella abortus* and the worm *Onchocerca reticulata* have each been found, and the former is now known to account for some cases of fistulous withers.

Signs A painful swelling on one or both sides with, after a time, the appearance of one or more orifices exuding pus. The animal resents the part being touched and, if the *ligamentum nuchae* is involved, avoids downward movement of the head.

First-aid measures include the use of a poultice and the placing of food at a level which the animal can reach without pain.

Treatment may necessitate the removal of any dead tissue and the surgical enlargement of any openings to allow free drainage. Antibiotics may be used to overcome the infection.

Polled
Inherited hornlessness of an animal belonging to a normally horned breed, e.g. Hereford cattle. (See SCUR.)

Pollen
Pollen of oilseed rape has been linked to obstructive lung disease seen in horses at pasture. Clenbuterol is recommended for treatment.

Polyarthritis
Inflammation of several joints occurring simultaneously, as in 'JOINT-ILL'. In pigs a common cause is *Erysipelothrix rhusiopathiae*; streptococci and staphylococci may also be involved. The disease is seen also in lambs, calves, and foals.

Polycythaemia
A marked increase in the number of red blood cells. This disorder is seen, rarely, in dogs and cats.

Polydactyly
A congenital defect in which an animal has an extra digit. Cattle, horses (rarely), dogs and cats may be affected.

Polydipsia
Polydipsia is excessive thirst.

Polymelia
A developmental disorder resulting in an extra limb or limbs.

Polymorph
Polymorph is a name applied to certain white cells of the blood which have a nucleus of varied shape. (See BLOOD.)

Polyneuritis

Polyneuritis means an inflammation of nerves or their sheaths occurring in different parts of the body at the same time. (See NEURITIS.)

Polyoestrous

Polyoestrous animals are those which have several oestrus cycles per year – the converse being monoestrous.

Polyp

Polyp is a tumour which is attached by a stalk to the surface from which it springs. The term only applies to the shape of the growth and has nothing to do with its structure or to its nature. Most polyps are benign, but some may become malignant. They are generally of fibrous tissue in the centre covered with the type of local epithelium. In animals, the common situations where they are found are: in the nostrils; in the vagina, where they sometimes interfere with successful copulation; and in the interior of the bladder.

Polyphagia

Excessive ingestion of food. While it is a common attribute of animals, it can in companion animals lead to obesity, and mask metabolic disease.

Polyploidy

The presence of multiples of the haploid number of chromosomes greater than the diploid number, e.g. triploidy, tetraploidy.

Polyradiculoneuritis, Idiopathic

A disease of dogs, and occasionally cats, affecting nerves.

Signs Weakness of the hind-legs, followed by paralysis of them within a few days. The fore-legs then become involved. Hyperaesthesia of all legs occurs. Body temperature remains normal.

Muscle wasting occurs. Recovery is gradual. In one case a puppy was able to walk again after 4 weeks; but complete recovery took over 6 months.

Polysaccharides

(see SUGAR)

Polytocous

Producing several offspring at birth, i.e. a litter.

Polyuria

Polyuria is a condition in which a much greater amount of urine is passed than is usual.

Polyuria is also a symptom of diabetes, and it occurs in certain forms of inflammation of the kidneys, especially in the early stages of pyelonephritis affecting cows after calving, when infection has travelled into the bladder, up the ureters, and so into the kidney. (See INCONTINENCE; KIDNEY, DISEASES OF; URINE; STRESS.)

Polyvalent Vaccine

One prepared from cultures of several strains of the same bacterial or viral species or from different species. A single polyvalent vaccine can now protect against as many as 8 diseases.

Pom

(see PRESCRIPTION-ONLY MEDICINES)

Pomeranian

A small alert dog with tail carried over the back, pointed ears and prominent eyes. Patellar luxation is inheritable and patent ductus arteriosus may be present.

Ponds

Salmonella typhimurium was isolated from marl ponds on a farm where the dairy herd had a reduced milk yield, fever and dysentery. Fencing off the ponds to prevent access by the cattle stopped the outbreak immediately. (See also LEECHES, ALGAE POISONING, COCCIDIOSIS, JOHNE'S DISEASE, BOTULISM.)

Ponies

(see under HORSES, FEEDING OF)

Pons (Pons Varolii)

Pons (Pons Varolii) is the so-called 'bridge of the brain'. It is situated at the base of the brain in front of the medulla, and behind the cerebral peduncles, and appears as a bulbous swelling not unlike a small curved artichoke. It is mainly composed of strands of fibres which link up different parts of the brain.

Poodle

A breed of dog originating in Germany (in spite of being known as a French poodle) where it was used as a gun dog for retrieving game, especially that which had fallen in water. The characteristic clip of its curly black coat was designed to streamline the dog as it swam. The topknot of the head and the tip of the tail were to show the hunter the position of the dog in the water; the hair left round the leg joints was to protect them against underwater objects they might strike. There are 3 types: standard, miniature and toy. The standard was the original and is less liable to defects than the others. Toy and miniature poodles are prone to Perthe's disease, patent ductus arteriosus and progressive retinal atrophy. Distichiasis may be inherited. Cleft palate is found in toys. Miniature poodles are prone to epilepsy, epiphyseal dysplasia, patellar luxation and glaucoma.

Popliteal

Popliteal refers to a region that lies behind the stifle joint, and to the vessels, lymph glands, nerves, etc., lying in this region. It is protected laterally by the biceps femoris, posteriorly by the semitendinosus and the gastrocnemius, and internally by the gracilis and semitendinosus tendon; consequently it is seldom that its vessels or nerves are injured.

Porcine Coronavirus Infection

This has become enzootic in the UK and in some other EU countries. The virus has a close antigenic relationship with transmissible gastroenteritis virus and is a cause of a non-severe pneumonia.

Porcine Cytomegalovirus (PCMV)

Porcine cytomegalovirus (PCMV) is a name for inclusion-body rhinitis virus, which can produce rhinitis and pneumonia in pigs.

Porcine Dermatosis and Nephropathy Syndrome (PDNS)

A condition of young pigs (10 to 16 weeks) in which red-brown circular lesions and haemorrhages appear under the skin of the ears, face, flanks and limbs. Often only a few animals are affected but many of those die, sometimes suddenly after lesions develop. The lesions may be caused by an antigen-antibody reaction; porcine intestinal circovirus type 2 has been isolated from cases. The condition was first identified in Chile in 1976 and in England in 1987.

Porcine Encephalomyelitis

Also called TALFAN DISEASE and TESCHEN DISEASE.

Porcine Enterovirus England/72

Porcine Enterovirus England/72 is the cause of SWINE VESICULAR DISEASE.

Porcine Intestinal Adenomatosis (PIA)

Porcine Intestinal Adenomatosis (PIA) is the most common form of proliferative enteropathy, a serious economic problem for pig farmers. The signs include poor growth and chronic diarrhoea or acute haemorrhagic diarrhoea, sometimes with perforation of the intestine, and death. Growing and finishing pigs are usually affected, although it can occur in adult pigs. Many cases may not be noticed, and failure to make satisfactory weight gains may be the only indication of the disease. The cause is the bacterium *Lawsonia intracellularis*.

Salinomycin or zinc bacitracin in the feed have been reported to improve weight gain and general condition.

(See also Proliferative haemorrhagic enteropathy *under* HAEMORRHAGIC GASTROENTERITIS OF PIGS.)

Porcine Parvovirus

This can be a cause of fetal death and mummification, if infection occurs during the first half of the gestation period. An inactivated vaccine is available.

Porcine Reproductive Respiratory Disease (PRRS)

(see 'BLUE-EAR' DISEASE OF PIGS)

Porcine Respiratory Coronavirus Infection (PRCV)

(see under RESPIRATORY DISEASE IN PIGS)

Porcine Streptococcal Meningitis

This was first recognised in fattening pigs in the UK in 1975 (though in unweaned pigs in 1954).

Streptococcus suis type I causes meningitis as a complication of septicaemia in the unweaned piglet. Symptoms include fever, loss of appetite, a tendency for the piglets to bury themselves in the litter, stiffness, and an unsteady gait. The ears may be drawn back and held close to the side of the head. An inability to rise and paddling movements of the hind-legs precede death in many instances. Some pigs recover; others die from septicaemia associated with arthritis or pneumonia.

Streptococcus suis type II affected pigs mainly in the age bracket 4 to 8 weeks, but pigs up to 16 weeks can be involved.

The death of a large pig in excellent condition is often the first sign of the disease. If symptoms are observed, they are similar to those already described for the unweaned pig. In untreated cases the illness is usually brief and fatal.

This streptococcal meningitis is 'primarily associated with the mixing and moving of young weaned pigs', and may affect from less than 1 per cent to over 50 per cent of pigs, depending on management factors, etc. Poor ventilation favours a higher incidence, which is seen more in imperfectly managed controlled-environment buildings than in old or converted fattening houses.

Control measures So far vaccination has not been very successful. Accordingly, control measures can be aimed at either eradicating the infection on the farm or, if this is considered impracticable, minimising losses. If weaners are being bought from different suppliers, it may be possible to discover which is the source of infection. On some farms, buildings could be emptied, disinfected, and restocked – avoiding buying from anyone known or suspected of having the disease on the premises. If carrier sows can be identified, they should be culled.

Penicillin or broad spectrum antibiotics may be used for treatment.

Public health People working with pigs should be warned of the risk to them, even though it is a small one.

Streptococcus suis type II was isolated from a case of meningitis in an abattoir worker by the public health laboratory, Cambridge. Seven of 10 cases of streptococcal meningitis occurring in the Netherlands were associated with infection with the porcine streptococcus group R. The other 3 isolates were similar but lacked the R antigen. All streptococci fell into the bacterial species provisionally named *S. subacidus*. Nine of the 10 patients had contact with pigs, while the other person liked to eat raw meat. One of the affected people died of the disease.

Porcine Stress Syndrome (PSS)

A group of symptoms, due to a single gene, occurring in some breeds of pigs, notably Dutch Piétrain, Belgian Landrace, German Landrace, and French Piétrain. Under stress, death from heart failure may occur suddenly. The syndrome is associated with pale watery meat (pale soft exudative muscle (PSE)). The anaesthetic halothane can be used for on-farm testing of pigs to discover whether they are susceptible. A selective breeding programme has eliminated this gene from some strains of pig.

Porcine Ulcerative Spirochaetosis

An infection believed to be present in the UK, and reported also in the USA, Australia, and New Zealand. Experimentally, injection of the spirochaetes has led to foot-rot, schirrhous cord, and ulceration of the skin.

Porcupine Quills

In some areas of the USA and Canada, dogs require treatment as a result of rash encounters with porcupines. The North American porcupine uses its tail as a means of defence, leaving behind numerous quills; while if the dog attempts to bite a porcupine, the result may be a mouthful of quills, which stick in the tongue and cheeks.

In the UK, free-living porcupines (Asiatic and African species) in both Devon and Staffordshire are, like mink and coypu, escapers, and have bred since gaining their freedom.

Removal of quills must be a very painful process, for they are barbed. American veterinary authorities nevertheless recommend that the owner should, if the dog will allow it, remove quills as soon as possible as a first-aid measure, especially from the tongue and over the chest and abdomen, as deep penetration may occur with possible fatal injury involving internal organs. Quill removal should be completed under a general anaesthetic by a veterinary surgeon.

If there is delay, some quills will have disappeared from sight and, as they are not revealed by X-rays, no veterinary surgeon could guarantee 100 per cent removal. Some quills may work themselves out through the skin in due course. One dog died after penetration of the pericardium by quills.

Porker

In Britain, porkers weigh 40 to 67 kg (90 to 190 lb) (liveweight). Baconers are 101 kg (220 lb). 'Heavy hog' weight is 102 kg (225 lb) and above.

Porphyria

A condition in which porphyrins accumulate in the tissues or are excreted in the urine. The clinical signs vary in different species but include discoloration of bone, teeth and urine, and photosensitivity. The condition may be inherited or acquired. (See BONE, DISEASES OF, and HEXACHLOROBENZENE; also under ALUMINIUM TOXICITY with reference to the rat.)

Portal Vein

Portal vein carries to the liver the blood that has been circulating in many of the abdominal organs. It is unique among the large veins of the body in that on entering the liver it breaks up into a capillary network, instead of passing its blood into one of the larger veins to be carried back to the heart. It is formed by the confluence of the anterior and posterior mesenteric with the splenic vein in the horse, and by the union of the gastric and mesenteric radicles in the ox; from a point behind the pancreas and below the vena cava, it runs forwards, downwards, and a little to the right, to reach the porta of the liver. Here it divides and subdivides in the manner usual with an artery. (See LIVER for further course, and DIGESTION.)

The blood that is carried to the liver by the portal vein is that which has been circulating in the stomach, nearly the whole of the intestines, the pancreas, and the spleen.

Portosystemic Shunt
An abnormality of the blood circulation system, resulting in blood from the heart bypassing the liver and entering the general circulation. The condition has been seen in cats, dogs, and a foal.

Posological
Relating to dosage.

Posthitis
(see PENIS AND PREPUCE)

Post-Mortem Examination
(see under AUTOPSY)

Post-Partum
Following parturition.

Post-Parturient Fever of Sows
Post-parturient fever of sows occurs, as a rule, 2 or 3 days after a normal farrowing. The animal goes off her food, is slightly feverish, and apt to resent suckling by her piglets. The udder is hard, the hardness beginning at the rear and extending forward. A watery or white discharge from the vagina is not invariably present. The uterus may not be involved at all. Treatment by antibiotics is successful if begun early. (See also UTERUS, DISEASES OF.)

Post-Parturient Haemoglobinuria
This disease is seen in high-yielding dairy cows in North America, 2 to 4 weeks after calving. A deficiency of phosphorus in the diet and/or consumption of rations containing cruciferous plants or beet products are among the causes. Mortality may reach 50 per cent. In New Zealand it is associated with copper deficiency, and mortality is low.

Signs These are sudden in onset and include red-coloured urine, loss of appetite, and weakness. Faeces are firm. Breathing may be laboured. Death may occur within a few days.

Treatment A suitable phosphate preparation intravenously, or bone-meal by mouth. Blood transfusion may be indicated in severe cases. (See also under KALE.)

Potash Fertilisers
Potash fertilisers are best not applied to pasture land in the spring shortly before grazing, owing to the increased risk of HYPOMAGNESAEMIA.

Potassium (K)
Potassium (K) is a metal which, on account of its great affinity for other substances, is not found in a pure state in nature.

Potassium is a mineral element essential for the body. It helps to control the osmotic pressure of the fluid within cells. Its content in body fluids is controlled by the kidneys. (See also under ALDOSTERONE, and PURGATION.)

Potassium salts are used in human and animal medicine, but as their action depends in general not upon the metallic radicle, but upon the particular acid with which each is combined, their uses vary greatly and are described elsewhere. Thus, for the action and uses of potassium iodide, see IODIDES.

All salts of potassium are supposed to have a depressing action on the nervous system and on the heart, but in ordinary doses this effect is so slight as to be of no practical importance. The corresponding sodium salts can be used if preferred. For intravenous injections, however, potassium salts must not be used as they are liable to be rapidly fatal; sodium salts must be used instead.

Potassium chloride, given intravenously, has caused accidental deaths (when mistakenly used instead of sodium chloride).

Potassium deficiency This was diagnosed in 6 cats at the College of Veterinary Medicine, Colorado. They all showed an acute onset of weakness, loss of weight, a reluctance to walk, a stiff stilted gait. Their necks were bent downwards, and palpation was painful.

Treatment Lactated Ringer's solution supplemented with potassium chloride by intravenous or subcutaneous injection; with further K supplementation by palatable elixirs. All recovered.

Post-Weaning Multisystemic Wasting Syndrome (PMWS)

A condition in young pigs in which there is failure to thrive. It was first recorded in Canada in 1991 and appeared in Britain in 1999. Seen in pigs 6 to 14 weeks old, signs are variable and slow in onset. There is wasting and depression; affected pigs often look pale or jaundiced and have diarrhoea; conjuctivitis may be seen as well as respiratory signs. Sometimes sudden death is the only sign. Morbidity is 3 per cent to 50 per cent and up to 80 per cent of affected animals die. It is seen more often in wet, mild conditions, may be triggered by stress, and may be complicated by other infections. Attention to such factors assists in reducing the problem.

Potato Poisoning

Both the haulms and the tops contain varying quantities of solanine, an alkaloid, which is present to a dangerous extent in green and sprouting potatoes. The haulms are most dangerous just after flowering.When boiled, the alkaloid is dissolved out in the water, and does no harm.

There is some evidence that solanine alkaloids can cause deformities in litters of piglets born to sows fed on green or sprouting potatoes.

Rotting or mouldy potatoes have also caused poisoning.

Signs Pigs have shown loss of appetite, dullness, exhaustion, watery diarrhoea, low temperature, and coma.

Cases on the continent of Europe have exhibited peculiar skin lesions. They occurred after the green haulms had been eaten by cattle, and consisted of eczematous ulcerated areas occurring on the scrotum of the male and the udder of the female. In addition, there were ulcers in the mouths of some animals, and blisters about the hind-limbs which suggested foot-and-mouth disease, except that considerable quantities of pus were produced.

The most constant symptoms appear to be loss of appetite, prostration or interference with movement, a weak pulse, and a low or subnormal temperature.

In North America, sweet potato (*Ipomea batatas*) poisoning may cause acute respiratory distress in cattle fed mouldy tubers – the fungus (*Fusarium solani*) causing toxin production by the potato itself.

Potentiate

To increase the effectiveness of 2 drugs by administering them together.

Potomac Horse Fever

This occurs in the USA, and has a seasonal incidence (May to October).

Cause Ehrlichia sennetsu or *E. risticii.*

Signs In addition to fever there may be acute diarrhoea, sometimes abortion, leukopenia. The clinical signs are said to be similar to those of EQUINE INFECTIOUS ANAEMIA.

The vectors are mainly black flies of *Simulium* species.

The infection has been detected in farm cats.

Poult

A young turkey or pheasant.

Poult Enteritis and Mortality Syndrome (PEMS)

A complex viral infection of young turkeys involving a coronavirus, an astrovirus, several groups of rotavirus and other viral agents. The multiviral nature of the infection causes high mortality (up to 80 per cent). The litter gives off a sickly-sweet odour. The syndrome has a detrimental effect on the immune system.

Poultices and Fomentations

Poultices and fomentations are useful in all stages of inflammation to soothe pain and promote resolution, or in the late stages, when pus is forming, to hasten the formation of an abscess.

Poultices include a mixture of kaolin and glycerin, made into a paste, incorporated with an antiseptic and applied hot upon a piece of gauze or cotton-wool to the part.

Hot fomentations are usually made by cooling boiling water down to a temperature that can be easily borne by the bare elbow, wringing a piece of flannel or blanket out of the water, and applying it to the part.

Poultry and Poultry Keeping

These have, so far as large-scale production is concerned, undergone great changes in recent decades. Many of the older breeds and strains of poultry have given way to more efficient hybrids – a form of genetic selection, in effect. Increasingly, intensive production of layers or broilers in controlled-environment houses has been practised. Formulation of poultry foods for optimum production has advanced, too, and well-balanced proprietary compounds are extensively used.

Hybrids The following have done well in Britain: Double-A1, Babcock 300, CH20,

Honegger, Shaver 288, Sykes 3, SW20, Thornber 606, Sterling White Link.

Large-scale production Information will be found under CONTROLLED-ENVIRONMENT HOUSING; HOUSING OF ANIMALS; BROILERS; INTENSIVE LIVESTOCK PRODUCTION; BATTERY SYSTEM; NIGHT LIGHTING; CANNIBALISM; DEEP LITTER, EGG YIELD.

Hen yards are nowadays preferred to large pens for birds kept intensively, and are often adapted from old bullock yards. Protection from cold winds and rain is necessary. The high cost of straw is sometimes a disadvantage.

Free range The keeping of poultry in open fields, where they can move freely and supplement their rations by foraging is once again popular. Cabins, to which the hens have free access, are provided for shelter. 'Free range' eggs attract a premium price.

Housing Competitive broiler and egg production has led to the use of specially constructed, controlled-environment buildings in which temperature, ventilation, etc., are maintained at optimum levels. The main features are described under CONTROLLED ENVIRONMENT HOUSING and HOUSING OF ANIMALS.

What follows relates to non-intensive housing where high capital expenditure is not possible or desirable.

Height A very high house is apt to be cold and draughty, while a very low one is difficult to ventilate and troublesome to clean. From 200 to 215 cm (6 ft 6 in to 7 ft) at the highest point to 175 to 195 cm (4 ft 6 in or 5 ft) at the lowest should be allowed.

Ventilation There must be good top ventilation. The amount to be given depends a good deal upon the situation and exposure. Houses of the open-fronted type may prove to be too draughty for exposed wind-swept districts. For such places a pitched roof is rather to be preferred to a lean-to. Dampness in a house may be due to faulty ventilation.

Light The maximum amount of light and sunshine should be aimed at. Fowls will not shelter during the day in a dark house. Additional windows should be placed a few centimetres/inches above the level of the floor, if possible at the east and west sides. This means that the floor will always be light, and the birds

will always be encouraged to scratch for grain buried in the litter. (See also NIGHT LIGHTING.)

Litter The floor should be covered to a depth of 30 cm (1 foot) or more with clean dry litter, such as straw. (See DEEP LITTER.)

Perches These should measure 5 cm² (2 in by 2 in) and have the edges on the upper surface smoothed off. They should be all on one level about 75 cm (2 ft 6 in) from the floor, and made to drop into sockets. About 15 or 20 cm (6 or 8 in) below the perches should be placed a removable dropping board. This keeps the floor clean and prevents upward draughts. They must be cleaned regularly, and lightly sprinkled with sand or peat moss litter.

Nests are best placed on the same sides as the windows, so that the light does not shine directly into them.

Houses should be regularly cleaned and sprayed with disinfectant from time to time.

Runs Fresh clean ground is very necessary. If birds remain too long in one place the ground becomes foul, and the egg-yield and the birds' health soon suffer. Where space permits (as on farms) the birds may be kept on free range in portable houses. When the ground round the house becomes dirty, the house may be removed to another place. In this way the fowls always have clean land.

Hatching and rearing The time to begin hatching depends on the breed, the strain, and the poultry-keeper's requirements. Quick-maturing breeds, such as Leghorn, Ancona, and good laying strains of White Wyandottes, Rhode Island Reds, and Light Sussex, will, if properly fed and managed, lay at 5 or 5½ months, so that if pullets are wanted to lay in October, chickens should be hatched in March or April. It is generally considered that birds hatched early in the year have more natural vitality and mature more rapidly than those hatched later. Against this must be the fact that in very cold weather and in exposed districts the percentage of fertility may be low in the first 2 months of the year, and there may be heavy mortality in the rearing of the chickens unless adequate protection can be given. June or even July chicks may be brought on to lay if they are well fed. As soon as the days begin to get short, these late-hatched chicks should be fed by lamplight, otherwise they are not getting sufficient food to make their full growth. Where only a few chickens are to be raised, or where very special eggs are to be set, the hen is to be preferred to the incubator.

Silkies make excellent sitters and mothers. They are small eaters, their eggs are of fair size, they lay a small batch, and then go broody almost irrespective of the season. A silkie hen can cover from 6 to 8 ordinary eggs.

Brooders Bottled gas is much used nowadays for heating brooders, and has advantages over paraffin burners. Infra-red heating, especially the dull-emitter kind, is popular where reliable electricity supplies are available, and enables the chicks to be readily observed.

Rearing houses These should be well ventilated but free from floor draughts, well lit by windows, and spacious enough. Allow 15 cm² (6 sq in) per chick up to a month old.

Drinking water (see under CHICKS) must be constantly available.

Trough space About 2 metres (6 ft) of trough space per 100 chicks should be provided until the birds are 3 weeks old; 3 m (10 ft) per 100 chicks at from 3 to 6 weeks old; 3.5 m (12 ft) at from 6 to 12 weeks old; 5 m (16 ft) at from 12 to 16 weeks old, and 6 m (20 ft) thereafter.

Bought-in stock If buyers insist on 'Accredited' stock, they can be almost certain of avoiding trouble from pullorum disease (bacillary white diarrhoea) and from fowl typhoid.

When chicks are bought as day-olds, mortality should not exceed 3 per cent by the third week. Losses exceeding 5 per cent indicate the need for an investigation; and several dead chicks should be sent to a laboratory for a post-mortem examination.

Chick feeding There is no longer support for the old idea that chicks must not be fed for the first 48 hours. It is better to feed day-olds on arrival (otherwise they pick at their bedding) and to allow them ample cold water. Feeding appliances must be of a good design and not placed in a dark spot where chicks may fail to find them.

Proprietary crumbs, or mash or meal, may be fed. Limestone grit and oyster shell should **not** be given with these. (See under GRIT FOR POULTRY.) Day-olds do not need this unless they are to be fed on grain or to be put on grass when very young. Grain should not be fed ad lib, but rather as a twice-daily scratch feed, until chicks are a month old.

Dirt, dampness, and overcrowding are the chickens' worst enemies. Coops and brooders should be moved constantly, so that the chickens have fresh clean ground to run on. After the birds have been removed from the rearing ground, the land should be dressed with burnt lime at the rate of 2030 kg (40 cwt) to the acre. The cockerels should be separated from the pullets as soon as it is possible to differentiate them. The pullets need plenty of space both in their houses and in their runs. It is best to get them into their winter quarters by August or September and not move them again, as changes of all kinds are apt to check laying. As a preventive of soft-shelled eggs, 2 per cent steamed bone-flour or bone-meal may be added to the mash. Pullets should begin to lay in October or November if hatched in good time. Trap-nesting should be adopted wherever it is possible, as it is important to find out the winter records of the pullets. A good winter record (for 4 months) is from 30 to 40 eggs, but birds of good strain, properly managed and fed, will produce up to 70 or 80 eggs. A good flock average for the year is 180, but there are, of course, instances of birds producing up to 300 eggs in their first year.

Feeding Where fowls have access to good grass runs, and especially where these contain a fair proportion of clover, they can themselves correct any faults in a badly balanced ration, but birds on earth runs, or kept purely on the intensive system, are entirely at the mercy of the poultry-keepers, and their diet must be carefully considered. An excess or deficiency of any one substance in the ration may cause derangement of the digestive system of the bird, and so may affect egg-production. Birds, especially those kept in confinement, often suffer from a deficiency of some sort. Modern carefully formulated proprietary foods have been developed to obviate all known deficiencies in housed birds.

The amount which a fowl will eat must depend on the breed, the condition of the bird, whether she is laying or not, and the conditions under which she is kept. The bird's appetite is the best guide, but a rough rule is to allow about 60 g (2 oz) of grain and 60 to 70 g (2 to 2½ oz) of mash per bird per day. For a grain food, a mixture of 2 parts oats and 1 part cracked maize may be recommended. The grain should be lightly buried in the litter, so that the birds have to work for it. The mash may be fed either wet once a day, or dry in hoppers, so that the fowls can help themselves. (See under RATIONS.)

Poultry, Diseases of

(see under ASPERGILLOSIS; AVIAN INFECTIOUS ENCEPHALOMYELITIS; AVIAN LISTERIOSIS; AVIAN TUBERCULOSIS; BUMBLE-FOOT; 'CAGE LAYER FATIGUE'; COCCIDIOSIS; 'CRAZY CHICK DISEASE'; E. COLI; EGG-BOUND; FAVUS; FOWL CHOLERA; FOWL PARALYSIS; FOWL TYPHOID; GAPES; MONILIASIS; NEWCASTLE DISEASE; OMPHALITIS; 'PULLET DISEASE'; PULLORUM DISEASE; SALMONELLOSIS; SLIPPED TENDON; SYNOVITIS; TOXIC FAT SYNDROME; GUMBORO; BRONCHITIS; NEPHROSIS; LIVER/KIDNEY SYNDROME; MAREK'S DISEASE.)

Poultry-Keepers

The occupational hazards of people looking after poultry include: allergy to the northern chicken mite (see MITES); conjunctivitis and/or an influenza-like illness from NEWCASTLE DISEASE virus. See also VENT GLEET; AVIAN TUBERCULOSIS; SALMONELLOSIS.

Poultry Waste, Dried

This has been fed to beef cattle as part of their diet, especially in the USA. The product is very variable in its content – droppings being the main ingredient; litter, feathers, broken eggs may also be present. From a veterinary point of view there may be dangers – high levels of copper or arsenic, for example, used in broiler diets; also high calcium carbonate levels. Crude protein content may vary from 15 to 35 per cent, crude fibre 12 to 35 per cent.

Feeding beef cattle with large quantities of this waste product has, in Israel, caused sudden deaths from heart failure. It was found that the broilers had been receiving a coccidiostat, either maduramycin or salinomycin. 'Some ionophores are well recognised as having a cardiotoxic potential in certain species'.

Ensiled poultry litter, fed to cattle, proved to be a source of *Clostridium botulinum*, and caused botulism.

Producers intentionally or inadvertently feeding poultry carcase material to livestock on their premises commit an offence under the Disease of Animals (Waste Food) Order 1973.

The World Health Organisation has pointed out that the feeding of poultry manure introduces the risk that people may acquire zoonoses, such as salmonellosis from cattle products, and that there is a danger of drugs and other chemicals fed to poultry accumulating as residues in cattle.

Pox

The best known pox diseases, caused by orthopox viruses, are cowpox (vaccinia) and smallpox (variola). The latter disease was eradicated on a world-wide basis, the World Health Organisation announced, in 1980. However, the other pox diseases are transmissible to human beings.

Some of the pox diseases are mild, whereas in others there may be a high fever, and even a high mortality.

These pox diseases are all contagious, and characterised by skin lesions. Typically they begin with small red spots followed by papules. Exudate causes these to become vesicles, and pus forms, so that the vesicles become pustules. These either burst or become desiccated, and the larger ones may leave a pock mark which can be a deep lesion with permanent scarring.

Mucous membranes may be affected as well as skin. (In horses lesions may occur in the mouth; and in canaries lesions may be found only in the trachea.)

Public health Human cases of cowpox are reported only rarely, and may be severe. However, mild or subclinical infections may occur, and the possibility of person-to-person infection has been suggested.

Cowpox is now a rare disease in the UK. In the days of hand milking it was spread from cow to cow by that means (and also sometimes by milkers recently vaccinated against smallpox). Lesions appear on the teats and skin of the udder mainly, but the lips and perineal region may be affected too. Cowpox is usually a mild disease, with slight fever, reduced appetite and milk yield. Cowpox is transmissible to people, horses, dogs, sheep and goats. It was diagnosed in cats for the first time in the UK in 1978, but see 'Cat-pox' below, as a different virus may be involved.

Pseudo-cowpox (parapox) is a common disease of cattle, and affects man also. The papules tend to be larger than with cowpox. A mild disease.

Cat-pox This name has come to be preferred to 'cowpox in cats', since evidence for the cow's involvement is questionable, and there is a greater likelihood that the infection comes from some small wild animal.

The pock may appear at the site of a bite, and several cases have occurred in cats known to be keen hunters. The siting of pocks on the lips or at the base of the claws further supports the idea that the infection comes from cats' prey.

Previously it was thought that cat-pox was not transmissible from cat to cat, but evidence from the Netherlands indicates that it can be, and that cat-to-human infection may also occur.

Cat-pox appears to be patchy in its geographical distribution, and not common.

Lesions in the cat vary from no more than a scabby condition along the back, in mild cases, to small red glistening areas of skin covered by scabs. White pus may be present. The paws become ulcerated in some cases; also lips and eyelids.

Buffalo-pox is a mild disease but one of economic importance. Similar to cowpox, it is caused by an orthopox virus distinct from vaccinia virus. (The latter can also cause pox in buffaloes.)

Camel-pox is usually a mild disease, except in young camels in which a generalised form may prove fatal. Facial oedema and lip lesions occur in adult camels.

Sheep-pox This is the most serious of the poxes affecting farm or domestic animals. Infection can occur through inhalation, direct contact, and probably the bites of insects.

Symptoms include high fever, perhaps dyspnoea, salivation as a result of mouth lesions, a discharge from eyes and nose. Skin lesions follow in a day or two, and may cause intense irritation or pain, leading to self-mutilation. Areas of skin may slough off, leaving deep ulcers. In peracute cases the mortality may be as high as 80 per cent; in mild cases a figure of 5 per cent is to be expected. White nodules may be found in many organs at autopsy.

In the UK sheep-pox is a NOTIFIABLE disease, and compulsory slaughter is the policy in the event of its introduction.

Goat-pox In the tropics goats may suffer from stone pox or goat dermatitis, the symptoms of which are similar to those of sheep-pox – mortality varying from less than 10 per cent to over 50 per cent.

Ordinary goat-pox, which occurs in most parts of the world, is relatively mild, and if death occurs it is usually the result of a secondary bacterial pneumonia.

Horse-pox is usually a mild disease. Lesions may appear on the back of the pastern, hollow of the heels, and be confused with grease; or may involve the lips, mouth, nostrils, vulva. A painful stomatitis, with loss of appetite and salivation, may occur. Recovery may take 2 to 4 weeks. However, in a few cases lesions may

affect much of the body; the horse becomes debilitated and young ones may die.

Swine-pox is usually mild. Lice may possibly spread the infection. (Cowpox may also appear in pigs.)

Monkey-pox (see under MONKEYS)

Pox in birds (see FOWL POX; PIGEON POX)

PPR
(see PESTE DES PETITS RUMINANTS)

Precardial (Precordial Region)
Precardial (Precordial Region) is the region of the chest cavity that lies in front of the heart.

Precipitins
Precipitating antibodies, e.g. to *Micropolyspora faeni* in 'farmer's lung'.

Predetermined Sex of Calves
Research at the Babraham Institute in collaboration with the United States Department of Agriculture and Animal Biotechnology, Cambridge ('Mastercalf') led to a technique for separating the X- and Y-carrying sperm of bulls.

The technique is based upon the fact that sperm carrying the X chromosome, which results in heifer calves, have about 4 per cent more genetic material (DNA) than the male-determining Y-carrying sperm.

The sperm are stained with a fluorescent dye and separated by passage through a laser beam, using a specially modified flow cytometer/cell sorter.

Prednisolone
A CORTICOSTEROID which is used in treating inflammatory and allergic disorders. It can cause immunosuppression and exacerbate the effects of worm infestations (e.g. *Filaroides hirthi*, feline heartworms), and viral diseases such as cat-pox (see under POX). (See CORTICOSTEROIDS for reference to the treatment of rheumatoid arthritis and other diseases.)

Pregnancy and Gestation
The uterus, the ovaries, and the whole of the tissues of the mother are influenced directly or indirectly during pregnancy, but the gross changes exhibited, with certain exceptions, subside quickly after the birth of the young. The minor alterations which persist throughout life, such as increased size of the mammary glands, enlargement of the uterus, and of the whole of the genital canal, are not generally obvious

P

PERIODS OF GESTATION

Animal	Average period		Shortest period young born alive	Longest period young born alive
	Months (calendar)	Days		
Mare	11	340	340	414
Ass	12¼	374	365	385
Cow	9	283 or 284	200	439
Ewe and goat (merinos)	5	144 to 150 (150)	135	160
Sow	—	114	110	130
Bitch	—	58–63	55	76
Cat	—	55–63	—	—

PERIODS OF DEVELOPMENT DURING PREGNANCY

State of pregnancy		Mare	Cow	Ewe and goat	Sow	Bitch
I	Duration of period	14 days	14 days	14 days	14 days	10 days
	Length of fetus	Ovum 2 mm	Ovum 2 mm	Ovum 1.25 to 1.5 mm	Ovum 1.25 to 1.5 mm	Ovum 1.25 to 1.5 mm
	Stages in development	Fertilised ovum has reached uterus from oviduct				
II	Duration	3 to 4 weeks	3 to 4 weeks	3 to 4 weeks	3 to 4 weeks	10 days to 3 weeks
	Length of fetus	12.5 mm	8 mm	3 mm	12.5 mm	3 mm
	Stages	Traces of fetus appear; head, body and limbs are discernible by end of this period				
III	Duration	5 to 8 weeks	5 to 8 weeks	5 to 7 weeks	4 to 6 weeks	3 to 4 weeks
	Length of fetus	55 mm	45 mm	32 mm	45 mm	25 mm
	Stages	First indications of hoofs and claws visible as little pale elevations at ends of digits				
IV	Duration	9 to 13 weeks	9 to 12 weeks	7 to 9 weeks	6 to 8 weeks	5th week
	Length of fetus	150 mm	140 mm	90 mm	75 mm	64 mm
	Stages	Stomach well defined in foal, pig and puppy; differentiation of four stomachs in ruminants at end of this period				
V	Duration	14 to 22 weeks	13 to 20 weeks	10 to 13 weeks	8 to 10 weeks	6th week
	Length of fetus	33 cm	30.5 cm	15.25 cm	12.5 cm	90 mm
	Stages	Large tactile hairs appear on lips, upper eye-lids, and above eye. Teats visible in female fetuses				
VI	Duration	23 to 24 weeks	21 to 32 weeks	13 to 18 weeks	11 to 15 weeks	7 to 8 weeks
	Length of fetus	68.5 cm	60 cm	35.5 cm	18 cm	12.5 cm
	Stages	Eye-lashes well developed. A few hairs appear on tail, head and extremities of limbs				
VII	Duration	35 to 48 weeks	33 to 40 weeks	19 to 21 weeks	15 to 17 weeks	9th week (8th in cat)
	Length	107 cm	91 cm	46 cm	230–300 cm	15–20 cm (kitten 13 cm)
	Stages	Fetus attains full size. Body becomes gradually covered with hair, hoofs and claws complete, but soft				

except after repeated breeding, and in from 4 to 6 weeks the dam has returned to normal to all intents and purposes, always excepting the flow of milk in the mammary glands. In most uniparous animals – producing 1 young at a time – the horn of the uterus which becomes pregnant greatly enlarges and becomes straightened out so as to be practically continuous with the body of the uterus, and the non-pregnant horn appears as a small appendage projecting from its side; in the multiparous animals, however, both horns usually carry a share of the number of the young, and both are consequently nearly alike in size.

As the organ gradually increases in size to accommodate its contents, the broad ligament, which supports it from the roof of the abdomen, increases in length and strength to allow the uterus to move further and further forward and downward in each animal, so that eventually it may occupy the greater part of the abdominal cavity. At the same time there is a very great increase in the muscular coat of the uterus.

Duration of pregnancy This varies greatly in different species and to some extent in different individuals. Male fetuses are carried longer than females. Debility, weakness, or illness in the dam shortens the duration of pregnancy. (See table.)

A prolonged gestation period in ewes has been reported on occasion. In an incident in western Scotland, gestation periods extended up to 8 months; unless relieved of their fetuses surgically, the ewes usually died. Long hairy coats, skeletal deformities, and extensive liquefaction of the central nervous system were characteristic of the fetuses. The cause is unknown, but could be a toxic plant.

A similar syndrome occurs in southwest Africa, associated with feeding on the shrub *Salsola tuberculata* var. *tomentosa*; and in the USA prolonged pregnancy in ewes has been linked to the plant *Veratum californicum*.

Signs of pregnancy When well advanced, the typical signs of pregnancy are sufficiently known to the majority of livestock owners, and require no mention here; but in the earlier stages they are not always so clear, and for the first few weeks in the larger animal it is often difficult to diagnose pregnancy by clinical signs. The chief changes and differences to be looked for are as follows:

Cessation of oestrus: in the majority of cases, but not in all animals, the female exhibits no desire for the male after conception occurs. There are many instances, however, when service is allowed until late on in pregnancy, and there may be all the usual signs of oestrus evident on each occasion. In such cases abortion of the fetus may occur, or no harm may result. When the bull refuses to serve a cow which is apparently in season it may be taken as a strong sign that she is pregnant.

Alteration in temperament: vicious, troublesome, or easily excited mares generally become very much more tractable and quiet after conception, whereas if they are served and do not conceive they are frequently more intractable than previously. The same signs are sometimes seen in the cow.

Fattening tendency: in the sheep and the cow particularly, condition markedly improves during the first few weeks of pregnancy, but during the latter stages when the abdomen has increased in size the opposite effect is seen in all animals.

Easily induced fatigue: in the later stages, pregnant animals almost always show an increased desire to rest as much as possible.

Enlargement of the abdomen: this occurs in every direction, and is a most important sign of pregnancy; it occurs at about the same rate as the rate of development of the young, which is greatest towards the end of the period. The abdomen descends or 'drops'; the flanks become hollow; the spine appears more prominent, and its line tends to become flat or even concave in the thoracic and lumbar region; the muscles of the quarters appear to fall in, making the haunches and the root of the tail appear more prominent; and the pelvis tilts into a more vertical position.

Enlargement of the mammary glands: this commences very soon in pregnancy in those animals which are bearing young for the first time. The glands become larger, and firmer, and more prominent.

Increase in weight: this is of course, a sine qua non of normal pregnancy in a healthy, well-nourished animal. (See PREGNANCY DIAGNOSIS.)

Care of the dam during pregnancy In all species of animals, exercise (or work) is essential if the vigour of the dam is to be retained, and if her circulatory, digestive, muscular, and nervous systems are to be maintained in a fit state for the strains they will have to withstand at parturition. Food is of great importance: no sudden changes in the ration should be made. It is better to give an extra feed each day rather then unduly to increase the quantities given at each feed. This avoids excessive distension of stomach and intestines which may lead to nausea and indigestion.

Mares should be treated as usual until the time that the abdomen begins to increase in size.

During the last month an extra feed per day should be given, and if clover (or, better, lucerne) hay is available it should be given in preference to other kinds of hay. Lucerne, being rich in lime and magnesium salts, provides a plentiful supply of these for the mare's milk, as well as for the developing foal. During this last month it is well to allow the mare to sleep in the foaling-box, so that she may become accustomed to it, and settle better. The box should have previously been thoroughly cleaned out, its walls scrubbed with boiling water containing a suitable disinfectant, especially where joint-ill exists upon a farm. Where the climate is mild, mares may, with great advantage, be allowed to foal out of doors. The foal is often born during the night.

Food given should be gently laxative; for this purpose the addition of pulped roots, carrots, bran, or treacle to the food is good. (For further information see under PARTURITION.)

Cows are usually allowed to calve in a loose-box. (See under STEAMING-UP.)

Ewes may be either kept out on the hill, or brought down to lower land, and housed in a lambing-pen during the last week or so of pregnancy, but otherwise little special attention is necessary. Chasing by dogs, crowding through gateways, and all other forms of rough treatment are to be avoided. Care is needed when catching. Heavy in-lamb ewes should not be turned up to have their feet dressed.

Sows greatly benefit from having access to an old pasture or paddock, where they will not be disturbed by other animals, and where they may take as much exercise as they desire. But at night they should have a clean, warm, dry bed to sleep on. Pregnant sows are best fed individually or in twos: otherwise some sows get more than their fair share, while others suffer from under-feeding. Wet, cold floors and cold, draughty premises predispose to mastitis and agalactia.

Bitches must be given regular exercise, and after the first month extra meals of protein-rich food, including a little liver once a week. An improvised whelping box is useful. (See also SUPERFETATION; BREEDING OF DOGS; PARTURITION; PREGNANCY DIAGNOSIS.)

Pregnancy Complications

In the mare these include twin foals (see ABORTION) and PREPUBIC TENDON RUPTURE. (See also PREGNANCY ECTOPIC; MUMMIFICATION OF FETUS; SUPERFETATION.)

Pregnancy Diagnosis

As well as traditional techniques such as rectal or abdominal palpation, confirmatory tests for pregnancy are widely used. There are 2 types: those relying on the detection of hormones in blood, urine or milk; and those depending on visualisation of the fetus by ultrasound scanning instruments.

Farm animals In cattle, rectal palpation is widely used. It may be carried out 5 or 6 weeks after insemination in cows and by 5 weeks in the heifer. Among more sophisticated tests is that for PROGESTERONE, based on a radioimmuno-assay technique for the detection of progesterone in a sample of milk. The milk sample is taken 24 days after the last insemination.

A test based on the measurement of oestrone sulphate in milk uses a milk sample taken 15 weeks or more after insemination.

An enzyme method of milk pregnancy testing, using do-it-youself kits, is available; the test takes about 45 minutes.

Real-time ultrasonic scanning is widely used for the early detection of pregnancy. The technique, which requires special equipment, is applicable to most species.

Bitch Pregnancy cannot be diagnosed in the early stages. From 24 to 32 days is the best time for abdominal palpation; after 35 days pregnancy may be difficult to recognise by this means, though occasionally posterior fetuses can be felt at 45 to 55 days (when the fetal skeleton can be palpated). Auscultation of fetal hearts in the final week of pregnancy will differentiate pregnancy from pyometra and show that the fetuses are alive. Pregnancy has to be differentiated also from pseudo-pregnancy, ascites, adiposity, and diabetes mellitus.

Eighty-two bitches were examined for pregnancy using several different techniques. Abdominal palpation 26 to 35 days after mating was 82 per cent accurate in detecting bitches that would whelp, and 73 per cent accurate in identifying those that would not do so. A-mode ultrasound was best used 32 to 62 days after mating, and was 90 per cent and 83 per cent accurate in diagnosing pregnancy and non-pregnancy respectively. The better of the 2 ultrasound instruments used was 85 and 100 per cent accurate in detecting pregnancy in the periods 36 to 42 days and 43 days to term respectively. It was completely accurate in detecting bitches which were not pregnant.

Mares An ultrasonic scanner is often used for pregnancy diagnosis in mares. It is possible to detect the presence of a developing fetus with great accuracy as early as 14 days after conception, and this technique is particularly useful in the diagnosis of twin pregnancies.

Pregnancy, Ectopic

The presence of a fetus (or more than one) inside the abdomen but outside the uterus. Many cases occur as the result of trauma, e.g. in a dog or cat struck by a car. The uterus is torn and the fetus becomes dislodged and undergoes mummification. The latter also occurs when a fertilised egg has 'gone the wrong way'; i.e. instead of taking the normal route down the Fallopian tube to the corresponding horn of the uterus, it develops outside the uterus.

Pregnancy Examination

Pregnancy examination of cattle, when carried out by means of rectal palpation, requires expert knowledge not only of anatomy but also of physiology and pathology. It is not always a simple matter and an accurate diagnosis is not achieved every time. The dangers of attempts by herdsmen and other untrained people to carry out such an examination include: rupture of the heart of the embryo calf; perforation of the rectum; and abortion due to malhandling of the ovaries. In the mare, rectal palpation is a common method of pregnancy diagnosis. (See also PREGNANCY AND GESTATION – Signs of pregnancy; PREGNANCY DIAGNOSIS.)

Pregnancy, False
(see PSEUDO-PREGNANCY and 'CLOUDBURST')

Pregnancy, Termination of
Termination of pregnancy following misalliance of a bitch may be achieved with oestradiol benzoate, used with 4 to 7 days of mating. In cattle, termination using prostaglandins may be undertaken up to 150 days gestation. Abortion also occurs from a variety of causes. (See RESORPTION; MUMMIFICATION OF FETUS; PARTURITION, DRUG-INDUCED; CLOPROSTENOL.)

Pregnancy Toxaemia in Ewes
An acute metabolic disorder occurring during the last few weeks of pregnancy; perhaps more accurately, a number of disorders – one of which may be acetonaemia.

Causes In the more typical outbreaks, ewes are generally in good bodily condition, are carrying twins or triplets *in utero*, or have a particularly large single lamb. They are on good rich grazing, seldom getting much exercise. Bad weather, e.g. a fall of snow, has often occurred previous to the outbreak. It has been claimed that the disease can be produced experimentally by a short period of starvation during advanced pregnancy, and that ewes which become fat during the first 3 months of pregnancy are especially susceptible.

Signs The first symptoms are incoordination of movement, the animal lagging behind others when driven, stepping high, and often staggering and falling. In another hour or 2 the ewe lies down and can only be induced to rise with difficulty. She stands swaying and will fall or lie down again almost immediately. In general appearance she is dull, hangs her head, her eyes appear to be staring – owing to widely dilated pupils – and breathing is laboured or stertorous. Fluid may be copiously discharged from the nostrils. Acetonaemia may be present, giving rise to the characteristic odour from breath and urine. A comatose condition develops. Death occurs within 1 to 6 days.

Prevention It has been recommended that after the pre-tupping flush, ewes should be kept in store condition for the first 3 months of pregnancy.

Treatment Ewes should be dosed at once with glycerine 150 ml (2 tablespoonfuls) in water; or glucose, 60 g in 300 ml (2 oz in ½ pint) warm water; or, preferably, glucose solution may be given intravenously. A number of ready made-up proprietary products, most based on the glucose precursor propylene glycol, are available. (See ACETONAEMIA.)

Pregnant Mare's Serum
(see PMSG under CONTROLLED BREEDING – Synchronisation in ewes; HORMONES).

Premature Birth
(see ABORTION and PARTURITION, and the table under PREGNANCY)

Premedication
Use of a drug or drugs before administration of a general anaesthetic. An analgesic will relieve pain in an animal awaiting surgery, and a tranquilliser will relieve anxiety and facilitate handling. Both effects may be obtained by the same drug. (See ANALGESICS; TRANQUILLISERS.)

Premilking
(see under PREPARTUM MILKING)

Premunition
Premunition is a term used in relation to the type of resistance shown by animals against severe illness caused by infection. Animals which are premunised are infected with a micro-organism but are not affected by it.

The term has often been used in veterinary medicine in relation to trypanosomiasis. Cattle which are premunised will not succumb to trypanomiasis although infected by trypanosomes. There are 2 types of premunition recognised: (1) natural premunition, which occurs inside or in close proximity to a fly-belt, where trypamomiasis is endemic; and (2) artificial premunition, which results from the administration of a substerilising dose of a trypanocidal drug. Unfortunately, it seems very probable that, at least in the majority of cases, natural premunition only gives protection against 1 local strain of trypanosomes, and cattle which are thus premunised against a local strain may succumb when exposed to infection with a different strain of the same species; if, for instance, they are moved out of one fly-belt to another. The occurrence of intercurrent diseases of other varieties may also lead to a breakdown in premunition. Similarly, artificial premunition can only be relied upon to protect against a single strain. (See also TSETSE FLY.)

Prepartum Milking

Milking a heifer or cow a few days before the birth of her calf. Where this is practised, the calf when born must be provided with colostrum from another cow.

Prepotency

The ability of one parent, in greater degree than the other, to transmit a characteristic (e.g. high milk yield) to the offspring.

Prepubic Tendon, Rupture of

A possible complication of pregnancy, especially in heavy mares. Diagnosis is difficult but the condition should be suspected whenever ventral oedema occurs suddenly in late gestation, and is associated with considerable pain (due to the trauma). The condition is usually fatal, and may be a cause of sudden death.

Prepuce

The fold of skin covering the end of the penis. Crystals on the hairs here in the calf are seen in some cases of UROLITHIASIS. (See also PENIS AND PREPUCE, ABNORMALITIES AND LESIONS.)

Presbyopia

Presbyopia is the term used to indicate the changes that normally affect the eye in old age, quite apart from any disease. The most important of these changes is a diminution of the natural elasticity of the lens of the eye, resulting in an impaired power of focusing objects near at hand.

Prescription Diets

Specially formulated dog and cat foods designed to assist the treatment of certain metabolic and functional disorders. Available in both dry and moist form, from veterinary surgeons.

Prescription-only Medicines (POM)

Medicines that may be supplied only on the prescription of a doctor, veterinary surgeon or dentist. Under the terms of the MEDICINES ACT 1968, veterinary surgeons in the UK may supply prescription-only medicines only for animals or herds under their care, and not to the public at large.

Presentation

(see under PARTURITION)

Pressor

Pressor is the term applied to anything that increases the activity of a function, e.g. a pressor nerve or pressor drug. Producing a rise in blood pressure is its most common meaning.

Prevalence

This is defined as the number of cases of disease or infection existing at any given time in relation to the unit of population in which they occur. It is a static measure as compared with the dynamic measure, INCIDENCE.

Preventive Veterinary Medicine

This is the keynote of modern veterinary practice, and is of increasing importance in these days of intensive livestock husbandry and of very large units. (See HEALTH SCHEMES FOR FARM ANIMALS.)

Priapism

Persistent erection of the penis. Cases of priapism in horses, with protrusion, oedema and paresis of the penis, have been recorded after neuroleptanalgesia and anaesthesia using acepromazine with etorphine chloride and other anaesthetic agents. It is recommended that following the use of neuroleptic drugs a check should always be made to ensure that penile retraction is taking place as the effects of the drug wear off. If not, treatment should be started without delay. (See also PENIS; PENIS AND PREPUCE, ABNORMALITIES AND LESIONS.)

Primary Mosaicism

Primary mosaicism is a sequel to fertilisation of an ovum by spermatozoa derived from the same zygote but having different chromosomes. (See ERYTHROCYTE MOSAICISM; GENETIC ENGINEERING.) Secondary mosaicism occurs in the FREEMARTIN.

Primates

These include about 200 species, ranging in size from the tree-shrew, weighing about 100 g, to the gorilla, weighing up to 275 kg.

Two suborders are recognised: New World monkeys; and Old World monkeys, apes, and man.

Prions

Prions are proteins found in the brain which are, apparently, self-replicating. In mice, experimentally removing the gene responsible for producing prions resulted in their being totally resistant to spongiform encephalopathies. (See BOVINE SPONGIFORM ENCEPHALOPATHY; FELINE SPONGIFORM ENCEPHALOPATHY; SCRAPIE.)

Privet Poisoning

Privet poisoning is very rare, and occurs only when horses and cattle have free access to privet hedges, or break into gardens and shrubberies containing this common ornamental shrub. Privet (*Ligustrum vulgare*) contains a glucoside (ligustrin), which causes loss of power in the hind-legs, dilated pupils, slightly injected mucous membranes, and death in 36 to 48 hours.

Probang

A rod of flexible material designed to aid removal of foreign bodies from the oesophagus. (See CHOKING.)

Probiotics

Preparations containing live micro-organisms such as lactobacilli and yeasts; yoghurt is an example. They are used in some animal-feed supplements to act as growth-promoters. Probiotics are believed to act by preventing colonisation of the gut by pathogenic organisms.

Procaine Hydrochloride

Procaine hydrochloride is used in solution as a local anaesthetic, and for EPIDURAL ANAESTHESIA. It is, generally speaking, as effective as cocaine (except for anaesthetising the cornea, for which cocaine is preferable) but far less toxic and safer to use, besides not coming under the Controlled Drugs Regulations; it is a prescription-only medicine. It is often combined with adrenaline, in order to lessen haemorrhage during minor surgery.

Toxicity Excessive amounts of procaine hydrochloride cause stimulation of the central nervous system. In the horse, 5 mg per lb bodyweight gives rise to nervousness (tossing of the head, twitching of the ears, stamping of the feet, snorting, or neighing), while muscular incoordination and convulsion follows larger doses. In the dog, 20 mg per lb causes salivation and vomiting, with muscular tremors and incoordination.

Procaine penicillin The procaine salt of penicillin is often used, the concentration of penicillin in the blood remaining for a longer period, and the injection being less painful.

However, procaine penicillin G can sometimes cause a febrile reaction in pigs. The toxicity can be potentiated by swine erysipelas.

Proctitis

Irritation situated about the anus. It is a sign of the presence of parasitic worms in almost all animals.

Prodromal

Prodromal is a term applied to symptoms of a disease which are among the first seen, but which are not necessarily characteristic.

'Production Disease'

A name suggested to embrace all the syndromes formerly classified as metabolic disease. It has been used particularly in connection with intensive farm husbandry, because high production is frequently expected on diets which are not always suitable for the purpose.

GENERAL CHARACTERISTICS		No.	%
Size	Large	21	38
	Medium	34	60
	Small	1	2
Temperament	Quiet	54	96
	Nervous	2	4
Ease of Milking	Satisfactory	55	98
	Hard	—	—
	Too easy	1	2

Proestrus

The 1st phase of the oestrous cycle, when the ovary is producing hormones which bring about enlargement of uterus, oviducts, and vagina, and when the ovarian follicle containing the ovum is also increasing in size. (See OESTRUS.)

Progeny Testing

A method of assessing the value of, e.g. a bull as a sire, by examining the milk yield, etc., figures for an unselected sample of his daughters. Dam:daughter comparisons may show whether a high-yielding cow can transmit her capability to her progeny, but these comparisons are valid only under identical systems of feeding and management.

Conformation Selection of proven bulls for use as artificial insemination sires depends not only on the production figures of the daughters, but also on an assessment of (as many as possible) daughters.

Qualities of commercial importance taken into account are size, temperament, ease of milking – plus appearance, dairy character, udder, legs, feet, etc. Gradings are Excellent, Very Good, Good Plus, Good, Fair and Poor.

Below is shown a summary for a particular bull which had 56 daughters inspected by a type assessment panel. It will be noted that all but 2 of his daughters were quiet, and over half of them were in the top 3 ratings. The score of 107 indicates that the fore udder was the best point when compared with the national average.

Width of rear udders

very narrow   very wide
    (1)   8   (9)

Rear legs (side)

very straight   very sickle
    (1)   5   (9)

Angularity

very thick/round   very angular/sharp
    (1)   7   (9)

The progeny group illustrated in the diagram would have very high rear udders, legs about midway between very straight and very sickle, and would be rather sharper, cleaner cut animals than average, though not excessively so. (MMB.)

Linear assessment This is widely used in the USA and Canada, and in the UK. It does away with the idea of scoring against an ideal, makes no attempt to define good or bad, but simply describes where, between the biological extremes for agreed traits, an individual animal comes.

The linear system identifies the point between the extremes at which an animal is felt to come by describing it numerically in the range 1 to 9. Since the total number of single biological traits is very large, the most important ones have to be selected to keep the total a manageable one.

Name	Product, or other name
Altrenogest	Regumate
Delmadinone	Tardak
Megestrol acetate	Ovarid
Medroxyproges- terone acetate	MAP (Methyl acetoxy progesterone), Perlutex. Promone, Veramix
Fluorogestone (Flugestone) acetate	Cronogest
Norgestomet	*in* Crestar
NB. The list is not comprehensive	

A common set of 16 traits was agreed following discussions with the British Friesian Cattle Society and the Associated AI Centres. The traits are: stature, chest width, body depth, angularity, rump angle, rump width, rear legs (side view), rear legs (rear view), foot angle, fore udder attachment, rear udder attachment, udder support, udder depth, teat placement (rear view), teat placement (side view), teat length.

Other traits which need recording, such as weak pasterns, teats not plumb, or high pelvis, can be dealt with by means of a list of miscellaneous characteristics.

Progesterone

A sex hormone from the *corpus luteum* and (in the pregnant animal) the placenta which prepares the reproductive tract for pregnancy. It inhibits follicle-stimulating hormone (FSH) and action of oxytocin. (See under ENDOCRINE GLANDS.)

Progestogens

These drugs are used in CONTROLLED BREEDING and have a progesterone-like action. A progestogen is administered over a period of time so that the established oestrous cycle is arrested at the point at which all *corpora lutea* have regressed. The removal of the progestogen then allows the continuance of reproductive activity. Examples of progestogens are:

Their use can sometimes lead to diabetes in dogs and cats.

Proglottis

A segment, of an adult tapeworm, capable of reproduction.

Progressive Retinal Atrophy (PRA)

Degenerative diseases of the eye leading commonly to night blindness and ultimately total loss of vision. In the UK there is a joint scheme operated by the British Vet-erinary Association and the Kennel Club to reduce the incidence of this disease in any breed of dog; certificates are issued to dog-owners. (See EYE, DISEASES OF.) The disease also occurs in some breeds of cats.

The genetic defect responsible for causing the disease in Irish setters has been identified by US and UK researchers, and could provide a means for eliminating the condition from the breed.

Projectile Syringe

Fired from a cross-bow, gun or blowpipe, this instrument is useful for immobilising and/or anaesthetising wild animals. The use of dart guns is, in the UK, restricted under section 5 of the Firearms Act 1968.

Blowpipes and dart guns are short range – up to 36 m (40 yards) only. They use a compressed air discharge system to shoot a small hypodermic syringe loaded with the appropriate drug. They facilitate the treatment of dangerous or unapproachable animals with safety. They are often used to administer antibiotics, vaccines, and so are not purely for anaesthetics.

Projectile Vomiting
This term is used when the vomitus is thrown some distance (up to a metre) from the body – a symptom of pyloric stenosis in the dog.

Prolactin
A hormone associated with lactation and secreted by the PITUITARY GLAND. Also called leuteotropic hormone or leuteotropin.

Prolan
An old name for chorionic gonadotrophin.

Prolapse
Prolapse means the slipping down of some organ or structure. The term is applied to the displacements of the rectum and female generative organs, which result in their appearance to the outside.

The best plan is to seek professional assistance at once. (See UTERUS, DISEASES OF; RECTUM, DISEASES OF.)

Prolapse of Oviduct
This condition is fairly frequently encountered in fowls, particularly in birds which have been laying heavily. It is nearly always associated with some aberration from normal of the cloaca or oviduct, irritation resulting and causing the bird to strain. Occasionally it is seen after an endeavour to pass a large or malformed egg, yolk concretion, etc., and in cases known as 'egg bound'. It is also sometimes met with in cases of vent gleet. The prolapsed oviduct appears as a dark red swelling protruding from the vent. Other birds are attracted by the swelling and peck at it, frequently leading to evisceration and death. Treatment consists in removing the affected bird from the flock. The prolapse should be washed with warm water containing a mild antiseptic, and then gently pressed back into the abdominal cavity after first removing the egg or other foreign body, if the presence of such can be detected. It greatly aids return to have the bird held head downwards by an assistant.

Proliferative Enteropathy (PE)
An infectious intestinal disease of pigs associated with *Lawsonia intracellularis*. There may be diarrhoea but no specific clinical signs.

Proliferative Haemorrhagic Enteropathy in Pigs
(see HAEMORRHAGIC GASTROENTERITIS).

Proliferative Kidney Disease
A disease mainly of fingerling salmonids; affected fish show abdominal swellings and any stress will result in death. The cause is unknown. At post-mortem exmination, fluid is found in the abdominal cavity and the kidneys and spleen appear grey and swollen.

Prolonged soft Palate
An inherited abnormality of dogs. (See under PALATE.)

Promazine Hydrochloride
An effective sedative and prenarcotic, administered to the dog by intravenous or intramuscular injection.

Pro-Oestrus
A period in the oestrus cycle when the Graafian follicles are increasing in size (see OVARIES) and the female reproductive organs are being prepared for possible pregnancy.

Prophylaxis
Prophylaxis means any treatment that is adopted with a view to preventing disease.

Propionate, Sodium
A bacteriostatic and fungicide which has been recommended in the treatment of obstinate infections of the conjunctiva and cornea.

Propionic Acid
(see MUSCLES, DISEASES OF – Nutritional muscular dystrophy).

Propofol
One of a group of alkyl phenols, propofol (Rapinovet; Schering-Plough) is useful as an intravenous anaesthetic for dogs and cats, as well as for minor surgical procedures and caesarian section. Recovery from it is quiet and rapid – an advantage when the patient has to be returned to the owner's care with the minimum delay.

Propylene Glycol
Propylene Glycol is used in the treatment of acetonaemia in cattle and pregnancy toxaemia in sheep. It is often formulated with minerals.

Prostaglandins
A group of hormone-like compounds which can cause contraction of the uterus, lower blood pressure, have an effect on platelets, and lower body temperature.

Prostaglandin $F_{2\alpha}$ or its analogues cloprostenol, dinoprost, luprostiol and tiaprost, are used in veterinary practice to bring about regression of the *corpus luteum* for control of oestrus or to induce abortion or parturition.

A code of practice relating to the use of prostaglandins in cattle and pigs has been agreed by the RCVS and the BVA. Care must be taken when handling prostaglandin products to avoid skin contact and self-injection. Asthmatics and women of child-bearing age are particularly at risk.

Prostaglandins can cause local ischaemia at the intramuscular injection site, followed by diffuse swelling and emphysema.

In one case, sloughing of skin and muscle occurred, and *Clostridium chauvoei* was isolated from the exudate. The mare became recumbent, and euthanasia was decided upon.

(See CONTROLLED BREEDING; PYOMETRA; RETAINED PLACENTA. See also UTERUS, DISEASES OF – Chronic metritis.)

Prostate Gland

Prostate gland is one of the accessory sexual glands that lies at the neck of the bladder in the male animal, and partly surrounds the urethra at that point. Hyperplasia is an enlargement of the prostate and is seen in older animals. When greatly enlarged, not only does it interfere with urination, but it may also obstruct the passage of faeces. Affected animals will show constipation, and eventually tenesmus with the production of ribbon-like faeces. The condition can cause perineal hernia. Oestrogens are used in treatment but castration may have to be carried out.

Apart from this gradually occurring hyperplasia of the gland in dogs over 5 years old, enlargement may be due to an acute infection, when evidence of pain (with arched back and a stiff-legged gait) may be added to the symptoms. Cancer of the prostate is not rare in the dog; cysts sometimes occur. (See also BRUCELLOSIS.)

Prostatitis

Inflammation of the prostate ocurring as a result of infection ascending the urethra. Affected animals are anorexic, show malaise and may vomit. There is severe abdomnal pain with arching of the back. Urination will be difficult and painful. Antibiotics, oestrogens, smooth muscle relaxants and castration have been used in treatment, but in chronic cases the prognosis for improvement is not good.

Prosthesis

An artificial replacement of a part of the body.

Protection of Animals Act 1911. (Protection of Animals [Scotland] Act 1912)

These are the Acts under which actions for cruelty to animals are taken in Britain. Both have been amended subsequently. The Acts make it an offence to carry out an act, or to do something, that results in a domestic or captive animal suffering unecessarily. either by deliberate cruelty or neglect.

Protection of Animals (Anaesthetics) Act 1964

(see under ANAESTHESIA)

Protein Calories

A measure of the nutritional value of a food, not of a requirement by the animal.

Protein Concentrates

Products specifically designed for further mixing with planned proportions of cereals and other feeding-stuffs, either on the farm or by a feed-stuff compounder.

Protein Equivalent

This provides the measure of the value of a feeding-stuff, taking into account the protein content plus the non-protein nitrogen content, capable of being converted into protein by the animal's digestive system. It is expressed as a percentage. For example, the protein equivalent of linseed cake is 25 per cent; i.e. 100 kg of the cake is equivalent to 25 kg of protein and potential protein. The protein equivalent of grass silage is about 2 per cent; that of kale, 1.3 per cent.

Protein, Hydrolised

A mixture of amino acids and simple polypeptides prepared by enzyme digestion of whole muscle. A valuable source of protein used in cases of shock, malnutrition, convalescence, fevers, chronic nephritis, etc. It may be given by mouth or injection.

Protein Shock

A reaction following parenteral administration of a protein. (See ANAPHYLACTIC SHOCK.)

Proteins

Proteins are complex chemical compounds containing nitrogen, carbon, hydrogen and oxygen, found in every body tissue and living cell. Proteins are formed from (and convertible to) amino acids. (See DIET.)

Proteoglycans

Proteins which are combined with a carbohydrate.

Protetamphos

A compound used as a sheep dip, and also for fly strike and control of keds, ticks and lice.

Proteus
A genus of bacteria. *Proteus* species are common pathogens affecting the urinary system of the dog and generalised infections of duck.

Prothrombin
A substance formed in the liver with the assistance of vitamin K, and essential for the clotting of blood.

Protoplasm
(see CELL)

Protothecosis
Poisoning by a colourless alga, prototheca; possibly a mutant form of chlorella, a green alga. (See MASTITIS.)

Protozoa
Single-celled organisms.

Proven Sire
Proven Sire is one having an adequate number of measured progeny. (See PROGENY TESTING.)

Proventriculus
The true, glandular stomach of birds. In it digestion is effected by hydrochloric acid and enzymes. (See diagram below.)

Proventricular
region of the horse's, and pig's, stomach is near the oesophagus.

Proximal
Proximal is a term of comparison applied to structures which are nearer the centre of the body or the median line, as opposed to more 'distal' structures.

PrP
A protein found on the surface of neurons (nerve cells) and involved in the development of transmissible spongiform encephalopathies, including BOVINE SPONGIFORM ENCEPHALOPATHY.

Pruritus
Pruritus is the symptom of itching which is a prominent feature of most parasitic skin diseases, and of Aujeszky's disease and scrapie. (In human medicine, an iron deficiency is recognised as one cause of pruritus.)

Pruritus, Pyrexia, Haemorrhagic Syndrome
A syndrome recorded mainly in dairy cows fed large amounts of silage, often after use of a silage additive. The signs vary but include fever and persistent skin lesions which sometimes result in self-mutilation and haemorrhages. The

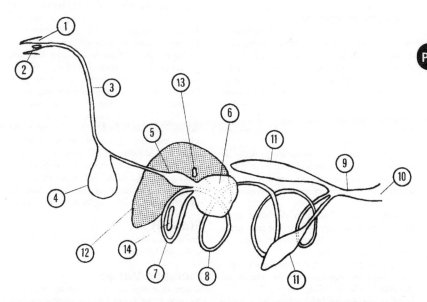

Proventriculus. Its position in the digestive tract of the fowl is indicated (5). Other numbers indicate beak and tongue (1 and 2); oesophagus (3); crop (4); gizzard (6); duodenum (7); small intestine (8); large intestine (9); cloaca (10); caeca (11); liver (12); gall bladder (13); pancreas (14). (Reproduced with permission from the *UFAW Handbook on Care and Management of Farm Animals*, Churchill Livingstone.)

outcome is often fatal. It has also been reported in cattle fed on citrus pulp which was mouldy and contained citrinin.

Prussic Acid
(see HYDROCYANIC ACID)

Psammoma
Psammoma is a small hard tumour of the brain.

Pseudo-Cowpox
Caused by a parapox virus, this infection is characterised by inflammation of the teats of cows, and of the hands of milkers.

Pseudomonas
A genus of bacteria. *P. pyocyanea* is a motile, Gram-negative rod, 1.5 to 3 μ long. It flourishes in suppurating wounds, and has been found in cases of otitis in the dog. It has also been reported as causing outbreaks of disease in turkey poults and other birds as well as in sheep.

Chronic mastitis, with diarrhoea and wasting resembling Johne's disease, has been caused in cows by *P. aeruginosa*. This organism, often found in non-mains water supplies, is thought likely to be increasingly involved in mastitis in cattle. It appears to have an increased incidence during August, September and October. (See WOUNDS; also MELIOIDOSIS.)

Pseudo-Pregnancy
Pseudo-pregnancy is a condition commonly seen in the bitch, but probably occurring in all breeding female animals to a lesser degree. In it the physical signs of pregnancy are exhibited in the absence of fetus or fetuses. The abdomen increases in size, the uterus becomes swollen and turgid, its walls are thickened, and in extreme cases mammary development may occur and milk may be secreted. The bitch may actually make a bed.

In time, since no fetuses are present, the organs and tissues return to their normal state without the occurrence of parturition; heat returns, and successful breeding may occur subsequently.

The condition has been described as an intensification and prolongation of metoestrus. The essential feature is persistence of the *corpora lutea* in the ovaries.

The condition can – where necessary – be treated by injection of the appropriate hormone.

In a review of 442 cases of pseudo-pregnancy in a total of 142 bitches, 19 had only 1 pseudo-pregnancy, 31 had 2, 54 had 3, and 39 had 4 or more pseudo-pregnancies.

In another reported series, a total of 81 per cent of pseudo-pregnancies responded to treatment with bromocriptine, and 80 per cent of the behavioural or psychological problems were resolved.

(See REPRODUCTION; BREEDING; 'CLOUD-BURST'.)

Pseudo-Rabies
A name occasionally used for AUJESZKY'S DISEASE.

Pseudo-Tuberculosis
(see YERSINIOSIS; CASEOUS LYMPHADENITIS)

Psittacines
Parrots, parrakeets, cockatiels, budgerigars and other members of the order Psittaciformes.

Psittacosis ('Parrot Fever')
A NOTIFIABLE DISEASE in the UK. It causes severe respiratory illness in man and birds of the parrot family (psittacines), including budgerigars and cockatiels. It is caused by *Chlamydia psittaci*. (See CHLAMYDIA; ORNITHOSIS.)

Psoas
Psoas is the name of 2 muscles, psoas major and psoas minor, which lie along the roof of the abdomen immediately beneath the last 2 or 3 thoracic and the whole of the lumbar vertebrae, and stretch into the pelvis. The psoas minor is inserted in the psoas tuberele of the ilium, and the psoas major runs to the inner or lesser trochanter of the femur in common with the iliacus muscle. The action of these muscles is to bend the pelvis on the rest of the trunk, or if those of one side of the body are acting alone, to bend the posterior part of the trunk towards that side. The act of crouching preparatory to kicking is accomplished by these muscles and others, and they are largely concerned in the movements of galloping. Disease or injury, such as a severe sprain, is shown by a difficulty in walking both forwards and backwards, by a crouching appearance of the back, and by extreme difficulty in rising from the ground.

Psoriasis
Psoriasis is a chronic inflammatory skin disease with scurf formation.

Psoroptic Mange
A type of mange caused by various species of *Psoroptes* mites. It can affect most animals, and causes sheep scab, ear mange in horses and widespread skin lesions in cattle. (See under MANGE.)

Ptosis

The drooping of the upper eyelid, due to paralysis of the oculomotor nerve. It is seen in the horse after accidents involving the head; and also in GUTTURAL POUCH DISEASE. A case of ptosis in a bird was treated by the topical application of phenylephrine, which rapidly resolved the condition.

Ptyalin

Ptyalin is the name of the enzyme contained in the saliva, by which starchy food-stuffs are changed into sugars, and so prepared for absorption.

Ptyalism

The overproduction of saliva. It may be the first clinical sign of eplepsy in dogs.

Puberty

Ewes, sows, and bitches may mate when only 6 or 7 months old; mares reach puberty at from 15 to 18 months old; heifers from 7 to 15 months old. In the cat oestrus may occur as early as 3½ months, or occasionally be delayed until the queen is about a year old. In the male, puberty commonly occurs at an age of 10 to 12 months, but here again there may be considerable variation. Some toms may reach puberty as early as 6 months, while others do not mate until their 2nd spring.

Pubis

Pubis is the bone that forms the lower anterior parts of the pelvis. The pubes of right and left sides meet each other at the 'symphysis of the pubes', which in old age is no longer a separable union, bony fusion having taken place.

Public Health

(see MILK; FOOD INSPECTION; ANTIBIOTIC RESISTANCE; and information given under the main animal diseases communicable to people. See also ZOONOSES)

Puffer Fish

(see TOADFISH)

Pug

A small dog with large rounded head, prominent eyes, smooth coat and tail arched over the back. It is suceptible to Perthe's disease but other inherited defects are not common.

'Pullet Disease'

A transmissible enteritis of pullets and turkey poults, first described in the USA in 1951. (See also VISCERAL GOUT.)

Signs Loss of appetite, diarrhoea with watery or whitish evacuations and, sometimes, darkening of the comb. Birds appear drowsy. About 10 per cent die. The cause is a REOVIRUS.

Pullorum Disease of Chicks (Bacillary White Diarrhoea)

Pullorum Disease of Chicks (Bacillary White Diarrhoea) has been virtually eradicated in the UK. It is an acute, infectious, and fatal disease of chicks, causing much loss during the first 2 weeks of life. Adult fowls, especially laying hens, act as carriers and transmit infection through their eggs to the chick before hatching. They may also spread infection in their droppings.

Cause *Salmonella pullorum*, which is found in the ovary and oviduct of carrier hens – birds which themselves contracted the disease when young, but which survived.

Signs Lameness, with swelling of the hocks, is characteristic of chronic pullorum disease.

Prevention This can be achieved by testing all birds, eggs from which are to be used for hatching, by an agglutination test.

Pulmonary Adenomatosis (Jaagsiekte)

Pulmonary adenomatosis (jaagsiekte) is caused by a retrovirus, often in association with a herpesvirus (see HERPESVIRUSES) and is a contagious neoplasm of the lung of adult sheep. First recognised in South Africa, it occurs also in the UK, Iceland, and the USA. In Britain, one East Anglian farmer lost 50 out of 200 half-bred ewes from jaagsiekte.

Pulmonary Diseases

(see LUNGS, DISEASES OF)

Pulpy Kidney Disease

Pulpy kidney disease attacks lambs between about 3 and 18 weeks of age, particularly those which are thriving. The disease has been seen in lambs under a week old; its occurrence is widespread.

Cause *Clostridium welchii* type D.

Signs As a rule the affected lambs are found dead without having previously been noticed ailing. Usually the lambs in the best condition are the first to be affected. The loss may be very heavy, especially with the larger earlier maturing breeds. The liver usually shows haemorrhagic spots on its surface.

Prevention It is recommended that immunity be maintained by autumn vaccination, with a second dose of vaccine in the spring, preferably about 10 days before lambing – unless the ewes are to be moved to a better pasture prior to lambing, when the second dose should be given before the move is made. These 2 doses should protect the ewe through the spring months and allow her to pass to the lamb via the colostrum sufficient antibodies to protect it for the first 8 to 12 weeks of life. That temporary immunity in the lamb should be converted to an active one by the use of vaccine.

Pulse

The forcing of blood from the heart into the arteries of the systemic circulation causes a pulsation (regular expansion and relaxation) in them. The beating of the heart drives blood out from the left ventricle into an already full aorta, in which it is imprisoned by the closing of the aortic semilunar valves. To accommodate this extra blood the aorta dilates, and the blood already in it moves onwards throughout the vessel, and through the larger branches arising from it. The wave of dilatation also travels along the course taken by the blood, and is therefore distributed along all the larger arterial trunks. If the fingers are placed over any of these latter, which lie near the surface, a periodic thrill or 'pulse' can be felt, occurring at a regular frequency according to the species; in the horse, it is about 35 to 45 times per minute.

The pulse-rate varies according to the state of the animal's health, being faster in fevers, and slower and weaker in debilitating non-febrile diseases; according to the age of the animal (faster in the very young and very old); according to the climate; according to bodily condition; and under other circumstances. During and immediately after exercise it is greatly increased, but in health it subsides rapidly subsequently. During sleep and unconsciousness it is slower.

The normal pulse-rates of the domesticated animals at rest are as follows:

	Per minute
Horse	36 to 42
Ox	45 to 50
Sheep ⎫ Pig ⎭	70 to 80
Dog	90 to 100
Cat	110 to 120

and of certain other animals as follows:

	Per minute
Elephant	25 to 28
Camel	28 to 32
Buffalo	40 to 45
Reindeer	60 to 65
Mouse	130 to 150

Roughly speaking, the smaller the animal, the faster the pulse. The same principle applies to animals of one species but of different sizes or of different breeds: e.g. the pulse of the Shire stallion is usually about 35 per minute, while that of the Shetland pony is 45 or more. These facts must be taken into account when counting the pulse of any given animal. (See also under HEART.)

Pupil
(see EYE)

Puppies, Newborn, Infection in
(see FADING; TOXOCARA)

Purgation
Evacuation of the bowel following administration of a cathartic medicine. It must be applied, if at all, with moderation. Excessive purgation involves dangers which include potassium depletion.

Purgatives
This is the age of LAXATIVES rather than purgatives. The old drastic purgatives are obsolete; they tended to make the patient's condition worse.

Purpura Haemorrhagica
Purpura haemorrhagica often occurs in a horse recovering from a respiratory infection such as influenza or strangles; Streptococcus equi is frequently involved. The disease is characterised by oedema of the head and also of the lower parts of the body. There may be kidney lesions.

Signs appear suddenly; often overnight. Swellings, very often the same on each side of the body, are found on the limbs, the breast, the eyelids, and almost always about the muzzle and nostrils. These swellings may be diffuse from the first, or they may begin as isolated circumscribed flat prominences which coalesce in the course of a day or more; when pressed with the point of the thumb, a little pit remains afterwards for some moments. Petechial haemorrhages are present in the nostrils (from which a bloodstained discharge is often seen) and on any mucous membrane.

The horse is dull, loses its appetite, moves stiffly and with difficulty, and if the swellings of the nostril are large, shows rapid and laboured breathing. Swollen lips may prevent a horse from feeding or drinking; swollen eyelids may hinder or prevent vision; and a swollen sheath in the male may make the act of micturition difficult. The temperature usually remains between 39° and 40°C (102° and 104°F); the pulse is soft, feeble, generally rapid, and may be very irregular.

The percentage of recoveries is not large in well-marked cases, and even where death does not occur, complete recovery takes a long time with relapses common. It is said that cases showing nervous complications always end fatally, and the same may be said of those with pneumonia.

Treatment The most careful nursing and feeding are essential in all cases of purpura. (See NURSING OF SICK ANIMALS.) Good results often follow the intravenous injection of an antihistamine.

After apparent recovery the horse must have a long period of convalescence.

Pus

This thick, often yellowish fluid, found in abscesses and sinuses, and on the surfaces of ulcers and inflamed areas where the skin is broken, comprises blood serum, bacteria, white blood cells, and damaged tissue cells. (See ABSCESS; STREPTODORNASE; PHAGOCYTOSIS.)

'Pushing Disease'

A colloquial name for poisoning of cattle by 'Staggers weed' (*Matricaria nigellaefolia*) in South Africa.

Pustule

Pustule means a small collection of pus occurring in the skin, or immediately below it. (See ABSCESS.) 'Malignant pustule' is the name applied to the form that anthrax most commonly takes when it affects the human being.

Putty

Eating of this can result in lead poisoning. A discarded drum of putty thrown into a field led to 12 bullocks dying within 24 hours, and a further 40 requiring treatment. (VI Service report).

Pyaemia

The presence of pus in the bloodstream.

Pyelitis

Pyelitis means a condition of pus-formation in the kidney which produces pus in the urine. It is due to inflammation of the part called the 'pelvis of the kidney', which is connected with the ureter. The condition is commonest among cows after calving, when infection has reached the bladder, invaded the ureters, and has arrived at the pelvis of the kidney.

Pyelonephritis

This term is used when both the pelvis and much of the rest of the kidney are involved, as described under PYELITIS.

Contagious bovine pyelonephritis is a specific infection of cattle caused by *Corynebacterium renale*, giving rise to inflammation and suppuration in kidneys, ureters and bladder. As a rule, only 1 cow in a herd is attacked though others may be carriers. The passage of bloodstained urine and abdominal pain are symptoms. Penicillin is useful in treatment. Otherwise, death may occur (sometimes after several weeks).

In the pig, an infectious pyelonephritis is caused by *C. suis*. It is a common cause of death or culling.

Pyloric Stenosis

This occurs as a rare congenital defect in the dog. Only liquid food can pass into the stomach. Projectile vomiting is a symptom. The defect can be corrected by means of surgery. (See PYLORUS.)

Pylorospasm

Pylorospasm means spasm of the pyloric portion of the stomach. This interferes with the passage of food in a normal, gentle fashion into the intestine, and causes distress from half an hour to 3 hours after feeding. It is associated with severe disorders of digestion.

Pylorus

Pylorus is the name of the lower opening of the true stomach. Exit of food from the stomach is controlled by a strong ring of muscular tissue called the 'sphincter of the pylorus', which opens under nervous activity and allows escape of small amounts of partly digested food material into the small intestine. (See STOMACH; DIGESTION.)

Pyo-

Pyo- is a prefix attached to the names of various diseases to indicate the presence of pus or the formation of abscesses.

Pyoderma

A pustular condition of the skin. In dogs allergic skin disease is regarded as predisposing to infection by staphylococci.

Pyogenic

Pyogenic is a term applied to those bacteria which cause the formation of pus, and so lead to the production of abscesses.

Pyometra

A collection of pus in the uterus: a condition not uncommon in maiden bitches, and occurring in all species. (See UTERUS, DISEASES OF.)

Pyorrhoea

Inflammation of the gums, in which suppuration is produced and ultimately interference with the integrity of the teeth. It is a common condition in aged dogs and cats. (See TARTAR.)

Pyosalpinx

Distension of a Fallopian tube with pus.

Pyothorax

The presence of pus within the chest. It may be a sequel to pneumonia, or to a penetrating wound of the chest, perhaps a bite. This is a fairly common condition in the cat, which is likely to rest on its brisket, be disinclined to move, and to have laboured breathing. Cyanosis may be present. Tenderness of the chest is another symptom. The temperature may be 37°C (98.6°F). In many cases the condition develops very rapidly in the cat, death occurring before treatment has been obtained. Treatment involves aspiration of the pus, and the introduction of an antibiotic. In cats, however, the mortality despite treatment may be 50 per cent.

Pyramidal Disease

An exostosis affecting the pyramidal process (extensor process) of the 3rd phalanx of the horse's foot. It is usually found in association with low ringbone. (See RING-BONES.)

Pyrenean Mountain Dog

One of the largest breeds of dog, powerfully built with a thick, usually white, coat. Haemophilia may be inherited and the breed is disposed to osteochondritis dissecans and hip dysplasia.

Pyrethroids

Synthetic equivalents of some of the active principles of pyrethrum flowers are useful and potent insecticides.

Commercial preparations are widely available (See FLIES – Control.)

Pyrexia

(see FEVER)

Pyridine

Pyridine is an alkaloidal substance derived from coal-tar, tobacco, etc. It is added to methylated spirit in order to render this unpleasant to drink.

Pyridoxine

Vitamin B6.

Pyrrolizidine Alkaloids

These cause poisoning in animals which have eaten ragwort. (See RAGWORT POISONING.)

Pyruvic Acid

An organic acid which is an intermediate product in carbohydrate and protein metabolism. Excessive quantities accumulate in the bloodstream in cases of vitamin Bl deficiency.

Pyuria

Pus in the urine produced by suppuration in some part of the urinary tract. (See URINE.)

Q Fever

A disease first recognised in Australia in 1935, and now known to have a worldwide distribution, Q fever is an infection of man, cattle, sheep, goats, fowls, and rodents. In Iran, serological evidence of Q fever has been found also in horses and camels.

Cause A rickettsia, *Coxiella burnetii*, which is resistant to heat and drying, and can be transmitted by ticks. Human infection can be acquired from these, from inhalation, and from drinking unpasteurised, infected milk; as well as from handling or coming into contact with the fetal membranes, faeces or urine of infected animals.

Signs In farm animals, many Q fever infections may be present without obvious symptoms. However, the rickettsia is a cause of abortion, and less often of pneumonia.

Incidence In the UK a preliminary survey showed that 2581 farms in England, 553 in Wales, and 240 in Scotland were infected. It has been found possible to isolate the parasite from 13,600-litre (3000-gallon) milk tankers.

In a survey, sera from cattle and sheep in the northeast of Scotland were tested for antibodies to *C. burnetii*. Approximately 1 per cent of 4880 cattle had antibodies to the organism. These potentially infected cattle were distributed throughout the area. Two flocks of sheep were tested; in one flock, 30 per cent of sheep had antibodies, while the other was negative. The flock with the high prevalence of *C. burnetii* antibodies appeared to be associated with an outbreak of human Q fever on that farm.

Treatment Most antibiotics are rickettsiostatic rather than rickettsiocidal; tetracycline has been used effectively. However, the organism can remain dormant for long periods inside the host's body cells.

Public health Acute Q fever may involve the liver and heart (with resultant myocarditis). Mild cases may resemble food poisoning or influenza with headaches. Chronic Q fever occurs.

Q fever in snakes Many snakes imported into the USA are infested with ticks, which transmitted Q fever to dockside workers handling a shipment of Ball pythons.

Q fever from contaminated clothing This was the presumed cause of 16 out of 32 employees at a truck- repair plant becoming ill with the disease. Serological tests on a cat were positive for *C. burnetii*. The cat was fed at home by one of the workers at the plant.

Quadriceps

Quadriceps means having 4 heads, and is the collective name applied to the powerful muscles situated above the stifle-joint. These are medial and lateral vasti, and the rectus femoris; the 4th muscle (vastus intermedius) in the horse is so blended with the medial vastus that it has lost its autonomy.

Quadriplegia

Paralysis of all 4 limbs. (See PARALYSIS; TICK PARALYSIS; RACOONS; CURARE.)

Quail

Small, rapidly maturing game birds included as poultry in British legislation. Females start to lay eggs at 5 to 6 weeks of age; the first eggs laid are usually infertile, but thereafter high fertility can be obtained. Males are sexually active at 5 weeks. Among the diseases they may suffer are: botulism, lymphoid leukosis, Marek's disease, Newcastle disease, pasteurellosis, mycoplasmosis, salmonellosis, quail disease (ulcerative enteritis), quail bronchitis and coccidiosis.

Quail Bronchitis

A highly contagious viral infection. Signs appear in all susceptible birds within 3 to 7 days of infection having been spotted in individuals. Clinical signs are very severe respiratory distress with 100 per cent morbidity and mortality from 10 per cent to 100 per cent.

Quail Disease (Ulcerative enteritis of quail)

A severe bacterial infection caused by *Corynebacterium perdicum*. Birds may die suddenly without showing clinical signs; these birds are usually in good condition with feed in their crop. Birds less acutely affected are listless, huddling with eyes partly closed and with ruffled feathers. Emaciation develops witin a week. Survivors become immune. Streptomycin, chloromycetin and bacitracin have been used in treatment. Effective control of other diseases will help to reduce the severity of quail disease.

Quarantine

The imposition of measures for preventing the spread of infectious disease by which an animal or animals, which have come from potentially infected countries or areas, are kept separate from indigenous animals until their disease-free status is confirmed (or otherwise).

The regulations dealing with quarantine of animals are altered from time to time, and so information on the matter is best obtained direct from the government department that deals with livestock in a particular country.

The length of quarantine depends on the disease whose entry is being prevented. For rabies it is 6 months (except in the case of dogs and cats from specified countries, for which new regulations apply); for foot-and-mouth and Newcastle disease it is 30 to 35 days. It is a sensible precaution that new stock introduced to farms, zoos, etc. should be kept separate until it is certain that they have not brought in new diseases or virulent strains, even if this is not required by law.

(See RABIES; IMPORTING/EXPORTING ANIMALS; NOTIFIABLE DISEASES; PET TRAVEL SCHEME; PIGEONS.)

Quarter Horse

(see AMERICAN QUARTER HORSE)

Quaternary Ammonium Compounds

Quaternary ammonium compounds are used as antiseptics, and have found widespread application in dairy hygiene. Cetrimide – or cetyl trimethyl ammonium bromide – is an example. It is used in 0.1 per cent solution for washing cows' udders, teats, and milkers' hands, being effective against *Streptococcus agalactiae*. In higher concentrations it acts as a detergent. Such compounds are readily neutralised by organic matter and should only be used on visibly clean surfaces. (See also CETRIMIDE; HIBITANE.)

Queen

A female cat.

Queensland Itch

This is caused by sensitisation to bites of the midge *Culicoides robertsi*. The lesions resemble those of mange or eczema, and are seen usually along the animal's back. Antihistamines are useful in treatment. The condition is regarded as an allergic dermatitis, and is similar to 'sweet itch'. (See under FLIES.)

Quey

A heifer.

Quidding (Cudding)

Quidding (cudding) is the name given to that condition in horses, depending upon injuries to the mouth or diseases of the teeth, in which food is taken into the mouth, chewed repeatedly, and then expelled on to the floor of the stall or into the manger. It may result from the teeth being too sharp, irregular in height, uneven in alignment, or from permanent teeth pushing the temporaries out from the gums; it may also arise when the gums, cheeks, or tongue have been injured or are diseased. Paralysis of the throat, or some other condition which causes inability to swallow, can cause quidding. (See MOUTH, DISEASES OF; TEETH, DISEASES OF.)

Quinine

Quinine is an alkaloid obtained from the bark of various species of cinchona trees in South America. The bark contains 4 alkaloids, of which quinine is the most active and important, the others being quinidine, cinchonine, and cinchonidine.

Quinine is usually used in the form of one of its salts, i.e. sulphate, hydrochloride, or hydrobromate of qui-nine.

Action. Quinine causes a lowering of temperature in fevers. In man, it is used for the relief of malaria.

Uses These have dwindled. Before the advent of the sulfa drugs and antibiotics it was much used in influenza, distemper, and similar conditions. It is sometimes given as an intramuscular injection. Owing to its very bitter taste it is seldom that it will be taken in the food.

Toxicity The dog is very susceptible to quinine and may become blind at plasma concentrations readily tolerated by man.

Quittor

Quittor is a condition of the 'lateral' cartilages of the horse's foot, in which suppuration occurs, with pus escaping from an opening in the region of the coronet. This, and the bulbs of the heels, are swollen and painful. The cause is an injury to the cartilage or to infection, or both. There is usually some degree of lameness. Antibiotics are used in treatment.

R Factor
(see PLASMIDS)

Rabbit Fur Mite
This may be picked up by dogs and rabbit-keepers, and cause intense irritation. (See CHEYLETIELLA PARASITIVORAX.)

Rabbit Haemorrhagic Disease
Rabbit haemorrhagic disease is widespread throughout the UK and the rest of Europe. The disease, caused by a calicivirus, originated in China and may have been imported into Europe in rabbit meat. Cases are not known in rabbits under 4 months, at which age liver metabolism changes. This makes it a serious problem for breeders when a doe dies, leaving an orphan litter. Clinical signs are often transient: difficulty in breathing, or a short squeal followed immediately by the rabbit falling over, is often accompanied by sudden death. Animals surviving the acute stage develop jaundice and die after a few weeks. Haemorrhage from the nostrils and/or anus may be seen. Prevention is by vaccination.

Rabbit Rings
The British Rabbit Council issues 100,000 metal rings each year in the UK to members to use in identifying rabbits, but advises that the rings should be removed from rabbits sold or given away as pets. 'Injury can occur if bedding material becomes trapped between ring and leg,' or if the ring has become – with the rabbit's growth – too tight, with the risk of causing necrosis. Should that occur, surgical intervention or euthanasia will be needed.

'Rabbit Syphilis'
'Rabbit syphilis' is caused by a spirochaete, *Treponema cuniculi* (which does not affect humans). It is a venereal disease characterised by the appearance of nodules and superficial ulcers covered with thin, moist, scaly crusts and oedematous swellings of the surrounding tissues mainly in the region of the genitalia (hence the colloquial name, 'vent disease') and also sometimes in the region of the nose.

Rabbits
Breeds of domesticated rabbits used for table purposes include the New Zealand white, the California, and the Dutch rabbit. (See also PETS, CHILDREN'S AND EXOTIC.)

Handling When lifting a rabbit, a fold of skin over the shoulder and back should be grasped with one hand, while the other supports the rump. A rabbit should not be lifted by its ears. Struggling while being inexpertly handled can lead to fractures of limbs. A startled rabbit may leap and fracture the spine.

Diseases include APPENDICITIS; ATROPHIC RHINITIS; COCCIDIOSIS; HYDROMETRA (the accumulation of watery fluid in the uterus); IMPACTION of colon or stomach (often the result of insufficient hay being provided); LISTERIOSIS; MASTITIS; METRITIS; MYXOMATOSIS; PASTEUREL-LOSIS; PNEUMONIA; RABBIT HAEMORRHAGIC DISEASE; 'RABBIT SYPHILIS'; SALMONELLOSIS; SCHMORL'S DISEASE; TOXOPLASMOSIS; TUBERCU-LOSIS; TYZZER'S DISEASE; YERSINIOSIS.

Pasteurella multocida causes a pneumonia which may be acute and fatal in rabbits under 12 weeks old. It may cause also middle-ear disease with a loss of balance, circling, and head held to one side, epiphora, and also 'snuffles' in which there is a discharge from eyes and nose and sneezing.

Rabbits act as hosts of the liver-fluke of sheep, and of the cystic stages of some tape-worms, e.g. *Taenia pisiformis, T. serialis.*

Rabbits have been used experimentally as incubators for sheep's eggs.

A hermaphrodite rabbit served several females and sired more than 250 young of both sexes. In the next breeding season the rabbit, which was housed in isolation, became pregnant and delivered 7 healthy young of both sexes.

Pregnancy diagnosis An ELISA test is available for this purpose. It can also differentiate between pseudo-pregnancy and pregnancy, and detect rabbits about to ovulate.

Anaesthesia A wide range of anaesthetics is suitable for use in rabbits. Halothane and other inhalation anaesthetics are suitable and convenient to administer. Premedication with atropine (50 micrograms per kg by hypodermic or intramuscular injection) or acepromazine (1 mg per kg intramuscularly) is advisable half an hour earlier. Alfaxalone/alfadolone (Saffan) is one of several injectable anaesthetics recommended for surgery. Oxygen should be ready to hand.

The Veterinary Formulary, published by the BVA/Royal Pharmaceutical Society, gives comprehensive details of anaesthetics and analgesics suitable for rabbits and small rodents.

Rabies

The Latin word for madness, it is a specific inoculable contagious disease of virtually all mammals, including man; and occasionally it occurs in birds, e.g. domestic poultry and vultures. It is characterised by nervous derangement, often by a change in temperament, with paralysis occurring in the final – and sometimes in the intermediate – stages.

Foxes and cattle are both highly susceptible to infection.

Rabies occurs in all continents with the exception of Australasia and Antarctica. In Turkey, dogs remain the principal vectors; in a few countries in Europe cats attack more people than do dogs. In Asia and South America dogs are still the most important vectors, but in many countries wild animals provide a reservoir of infection, and infect dogs and cats and farm animals – which in turn may infect man, who is an incidental host of the disease. (*See table of vectors.*)

Public health Rabies is virtually always fatal in the human being, and there is danger not only from being bitten by rabid animals, but also from contamination by their saliva of wounds, cut fingers, eyes, etc. Scratches may convey infection as well as bites.

People have died from rabies following attacks by rabid dogs, cats, foxes, wolves, badgers, skunks, racoons, mongooses, bats, rodents, etc.

Pet animals, such as rabbits, may be bitten by rabid animals and themselves become rabid; and it has sometimes happened that wild or exotic animals (originating in countries where rabies is endemic) were bought as pets while in the incubation stage of rabies, with unfortunate results.

In the UK as in most other countries, rabies is a NOTIFIABLE DISEASE, and must be reported

Rabies in wild animals – principal vectors in various regions	
Europe	Foxes, roe-deer, badgers, martens
Asia	Wolves, jackals, bats, mongooses
North America	Foxes, skunks, coyotes, bats
Central America	Bats
South America and Trinidad	Vampire bats

to DEFRA or to the police. Bitten persons should seek medical advice immediately.

Cause A Lyssavirus (one of the Rhabdovirus group). When it is injected into the tissues, either naturally (from a bite) or artificially, the virus passes along the nerves and reaches the central nervous system. The time elapsing between infection and onset of symptoms varies greatly with the location of the bite, its severity, and – no doubt – the quantity of virus in the saliva. In the most rapidly developing cases the symptoms may be shown as early as the 9th day after being bitten, and at the other extreme, cases have appeared several months after the incident. It is owing to this fact that the 6-months period of quarantine insisted upon in Britain is something of a compromise. The average incubation periods in dogs, sheep, and swine are from 15 to 60 days; in horses and cattle, from 30 to 80 days. In young animals the period of incubation is shorter than in adults.

Signs

Dog There are 2 distinct forms of rabies in the dog – the 'furious' and the 'dumb'; but these are in reality 2 stages only. It is customary to consider 3 stages of typical symptoms.

(1) Melancholy. The prodromal dull stage is often not noticed, or, if it is, only scant attention is paid to it. The habits of the dog change. It becomes morose and sulky, indifferent to authority, disregards its usual playthings or companions, shows a tendency to hide in dark corners, and may appear itchy or irritable as regards its skin. Noisy, boisterous animals become quiet and dull, while animals that are normally of a gentle, quiet disposition may become excitable. After 2 or 3 days of such behaviour the next stage is reached.

(2) Excitement. The symptoms described above become exaggerated, and there is a tendency towards violence. The dog pays no attention to either cajoling or threatening. It becomes easily excited and very uncertain in its behaviour. Food is either disregarded completely or eaten with haste. Vomiting is a not uncommon symptom. A fear of water is **not** a symptom to expect in the rabid dog, which will often drink or attempt to do so even when partly paralysed. After a time the appetite becomes deranged. The dog refuses its ordinary food, but eats straw, stones, wood, coal, carpet, pieces of sacking, etc., with great avidity. If the animal is shut up in a kennel, it persists continually in its efforts to escape. Should it be released or should it escape, it almost invariably runs away

from home. It may wander for long distances. In its travels it bites and snaps at objects which it encounters, real or imaginary, animate or inanimate. Some rabid dogs bite several people. The tone of voice is altered.

The face has a vacant stare, the eyes are fixed and expressionless, and the pupils are dilated. This stage lasts from 2 to 4 days, unless the dog's strength gives out sooner, and the next stage appears.

(3) Paralysis. The characteristics of the last stage in the train of symptoms of rabies are those of paralysis, especially of the lower jaw and the hindquarters. The dog begins to stagger in its gait, and finally falls. It may manage to regain its feet when stimulated, but soon falls again. The lower jaw drops, the tongue lolls out of the mouth, and there is great salivation. The muscles of the throat and larynx are soon involved in the progressive paralysis.

The dumb form of rabies consists of this paralytic stage – the stage of excitation having been omitted. The dumb form is the more common in the dog: barking ceases – hence the name. Vomiting may suggest merely a digestive upset. Protrusion of the nictitating membrane partly across the eye, together with a dropped jaw, i.e. partly opened mouth which can be closed by gently raising the lower jaw by means of a stick, are highly suggestive of rabies.

In parts of Africa and Asia, the classical form of rabies in dogs (described above) is replaced by a form called (in Africa) 'OULOU FATO'.

Cat In this animal the furious form is more common than in the dog. The aggressive stage is most marked, the cat attacking other animals and man with great vigour, and attempting to injure their faces with teeth or claws. Sometimes the rabid cat will at first show extra affection. The course of the disease is usually shorter than in the dog.

It is worth mentioning that occasionally dogs and cats die from rabies without any observed symptoms. They may be found dead or dying. It is not unknown for a cat to be found lying in a field or garden unable to walk but still able to bite.

Cattle These animals are usually affected through having been bitten by a rabid fox or dog. The stage of excitement is short and the dumb stage most evident. Affected cattle behave in an unusual manner; they may stamp or bellow, salivate from the mouth, break loose, and may do much damage. Rumination and milk production cease, muscular quiverings are seen, sexual excitement is noticed, and there is a great loss of condition. Exhaustion soon follows and paralysis sets in. Death occurs within 2 to 6 days or more after the commencement of the condition.

Rabies may be mistaken for hypomagnesaemia, milk fever, botulism, anaplasmosis, listeriosis, lead poisoning, choking, etc.

In Central and South America, cattle are infected with rabies by vampire bats, and may show long streaks of blood on their shoulders, necks and backs.

Sheep, goats and swine The sheep and the goat are affected in a manner similar to cattle, but the stage of excitement is shorter or absent, and the dumb paralytic stage is more often noticed. Pigs become excitable; they may squeal and show muscular spasms before paralysis ensues.

Horse The furious form is common but the animal may appear calm between bouts of aggressiveness. Dumb forms also occur and may be mistaken for colic, paresis or encephalitis from other causes. Signs may include a facial twitch, biting of woodwork or self-mutilation, head-tossing, frequent whinnying, abnormal posture, apparent lameness, ataxia, paralysis of hindquarters. The horse may continue to eat and drink until shortly before death. The tone of voice may be altered.

Diagnosis The routine examination for Negri bodies has now in most countries been superseded by the fluorescent antibody test, with confirmation by mouse inoculation if necessary. (If a dog which bit someone is still alive after 10 days, it **cannot** be assumed that the dog is not rabid.)

Differentiation between laboratory and street rabies virus, between rabies vaccine virus and street virus, and between rabies virus and rabies-like viruses (e.g. Mokola, Lagos bat, and Duvenhage viruses) is possible by laboratory tests based on differentiation of monoclonal antibodies.

Prevention Prevention of the disease in man and animals stems from the research of Louis Pasteur in the 1880s. He discovered the process of attenuation, by which the virulence of a micro-organism is reduced but not its ability to produce antibodies against disease. Pasteur achieved this by infecting rabbits with rabies from a dog. Although this was fatal to the rabbits, dogs survived infection with the rabbit virus. Tissue from the spinal cord of an infected rabbit was then used to prepare a vaccine.

His triumph came in 1885 when the vaccine saved the lives of 2 badly bitten boys.

In the intervening years many modifications have been made, and new techniques developed, to make rabies vaccines which would be safe and free from dangerous side-effects, and so could be used to immunise people and animals against rabies ('pre-exposure' – vaccination), as well as provide 'post-exposure' treatment of those bitten by rabid animals.

The table shows examples of vaccines prepared from tissue culture cells. The last one, the Merieux, was developed by the Merieux Institute of France using a technique pioneered at the Wistar Institute of Philadelphia. Only 1 ml doses are required, and 2 injections (apart from any booster doses). (See also VERO CELLS.)

In the UK, 2 vaccines approved for use in dogs and cats: Rabisin rabies vaccine (Merial) containing inactivated GS-57 Wistar virus strain; and Nobivac Rabies (Intervet) prepared from virus grown on cell-line tissue culture.

Mass vaccination of dogs is carried out in many countries as a control measure; and in Central and South America, cattle on ranches are vaccinated against vampire-bat-transmitted rabies. In France and other countries of Europe, hundreds of thousands of cattle are vaccinated against rabies (often a combined rabies/foot-and-mouth disease inoculation).

It must be remembered, however, that no vaccines are 100 per cent effective, that certificates of vaccination can be forged, and that consequently it is still essential to control the import of animals, whether vaccinated or not, and to enforce quarantine measures where appropriate.

Control of rabies in Britain From 1902 until 1918, no cases occurred in the British Isles; but in that year infected dogs were smuggled from the Continent, and the disease obtained a fresh hold for a period of little more than 3 years. Britain had been free since then, but in 1969 a dog released from quarantine 10 days earlier showed symptoms of rabies and bit 2 people at Camberley, Surrey; a 2nd case occurred in 1970. In 1965 there was a case in a recently imported leopard in quarantine at Edinburgh Zoo. In Britain, in 1969, the danger of allowing the importation of rabies-susceptible exotic animals, for sale as pets or for research, was officially recognised, and the quarantine regulations amended to include monkeys, mongooses, etc.

Following strong pressure to replace quarantine for pet dogs with a vaccination/identification policy, a government committee was set up in 1997 to examine the issue. The committee recommended that a strict scheme of medical examination, rabies vaccination and veterinary certification should replace the compulsory quarantine regulations for dogs and cats. The recommendation was accepted and an arrangement introduced in 2000 under which dogs and cats may travel to and from the UK and specified countries without quarantine under the PET TRAVEL SCHEME. (See also IMPORTING/EXPORTING ANIMALS.)

Other points to note: (1) the saliva is sometimes infective before symptoms of rabies appear – a hazard for a person licked; (2) farmers have died through mistaking rabies for 'choking' and, with abraded fingers, examining their cow's mouths; (3) non-typical cases of rabies are not uncommon; (4) a dog may bite a small child or household pet and promptly run away – rabies not being suspected, though running away is in itself a canine symptom; (5) the virus may be present in semen, as well as in milk, tears, faeces, and urine; and (6) subclinical rabies, and a 'carrier' state, have long been recognised in Africa (see 'OULOU FATO') and in Asia.

Vaccination of foxes has been an outstanding success in controlling the disease in Western Europe. Currently Britain, Andorra, Ireland,

Examples of rabies vaccines prepared from tissue culture cells		
Live virus: ERA	Cells used: Pig kidney	Cats, dogs, cattle and other animals
HEP-Flury	Dog kidney	Cats, dogs, and cattle
Inactivated: Fixed	Hamster kidney	Cats, dogs, cattle and other animals
	Hamster embryo	Cats, dogs, horses, cattle and sheep

Italy, Netherlands, Norway, Sweden, Denmark, Greece, Spain and Portugal are all rabies-free. There are still black spots in Germany, while there are enzootic areas in Poland and Turkey. The oral vaccine is genetically engineered on vaccinia virus so that the antigen to rabies is absorbed from the intestine. The vaccine is put into fish-flavoured capsules scattered from helicopters. In the areas so treated, up to 93 per cent of foxes, stoats, weasels, polecats and badgers caught and bloodsampled have been found to have taken up the vaccine.

Rabies (Control) Order 1974

This gives powers to deal with an outbreak of rabies outside quarantine premises. In a declared infected area, an order may be made for the destruction of foxes and other wild mammals, and for access to land for this purpose. Fences or other types of barrier may be erected to restrict movement of animals into or out of an area while such destruction is in progress.

Orders may be made for compulsory vaccination, confinement, and control of domestic animals, including strays. Anyone knowing or suspecting that an animal has rabies must notify that suspicion to the police. Deaths of animals in an infected area must also be notified, and the authorities can take over ownership of carcases and determine the means of their disposal. This is because it is essential to confirm a diagnosis of rabies, so that precautions can be taken concerning in-contact animals and human beings. The order can override a dog-owner's reluctance or refusal to part with the body of a dead pet or working dog.

The Rabies (Importation of Mammals) Order 1974 prohibits the landing of susceptible mammals in Britain unless from Ireland, Isle of Man, or the Channel Islands. Any animal brought in from elsewhere has to undergo a period of quarantine. Imported animals are vaccinated while in quarantine as a precaution against a quarantined animal developing the disease. Those animals not a threat to human health (ruminants, pigs and horses) do not go into quarantine for rabies but may be quarantined for other diseases. Control under the Order is exercised on the transport of imported susceptible animals within Britain.

If an animal is landed at a port or airport not authorised to receive such animals, that constitutes an illegal landing even if the circumstances are outside anyone's control (e.g. if an airport is fogbound).

Under a 1984 amendment order, animals which have not been in contact with another animal (e.g. have been on an oil rig) are permitted to be landed in Britain. A similar relaxation applies to animals belonging to the police, Customs & Excise and H.M. Forces, if the animal has been abroad but under the constant control of a trained handler while outside Britain. (See also PET TRAVEL SCHEME (PETS).)

Rabies-Related Viruses

These include *Duvenhage virus*, the cause in fruit-eating bats of a disease very similar to rabies; the *Mokola virus*, which has been isolated from shrews, and causes nervous symptoms in man; the *Lagos bat virus*; the *Nigerian horse virus* and *Lyssa virus*.

Raccoons

Raccoons are, in Canada and the USA, among the wildlife creatures which sometimes transmit rabies.

A dog bitten by a (non-rabid) raccoon may become paralysed in all 4 limbs (quadriplegia).

Racehorses

Every year between 1400 and 1600 thoroughbred mares go to stud in the UK. About 67 per cent of them foal successfully, and for every 1000 mares covered, 270 or so of the resulting progeny finally appear on the racecourse. Temperament, unsoundness, or sale abroad account for the non-appearance of more in the UK.

An epidemiological study of wastage among racehorses has been conducted among 6 stables, 5 of which were in Newmarket. The basis of the survey was the inability of horses to take part in cantering exercise as a result of injury or disease. The greatest number of days lost to training was caused by lameness (67.5 per cent) and respiratory problems (20.5 per cent). Conditions of the foot (19 per cent), muscle (18 per cent), carpus (14 per cent), fetlock joints (14 per cent), tendons (10 per cent) and sore shins (9 per cent) were the major reasons for training days being lost in 198 cases in which a positive diagnosis of the site of lameness was made.

Pulmonary haemorrhage In horses which show blood at their nostrils after exercise such as racing, the blood does not come from the nasal cavity but from the lungs. Endoscopic examination showed an incidence of 42 per cent in a group of horses with only 15 per cent showing blood at the nostrils. Affected horses might appear distressed, with dilated pupils.

Exercise-induced pulmonary haemorrhage was observed in 23 of 49 endoscopic examinations after high-speed training, in 9 of 37 examinations after cantering, and in 1 of 17 after

walking or trotting; it was not possible to predict its occurrence. Mucoid or mucopurulent
exudate was observed in 60 of 118 examinations
and the amount increased after exercise.

Pulmonary haemorrhage was diagnosed by
endoscopic examination in 255 2-year-old quar-
terhorses after racing. Only 9 (3.5 per cent) of
the animals had visible epistaxis.

Fatal pulmonary haemorrhage occurred in a
racehorse which panicked as the aircraft in which
it was travelling landed.

(See HORSES, BREEDS OF; HORSES; EXERCISING
HORSES; etc.)

Rachitis
(see RICKETS)

Radial Paralysis ('Dropped Elbow')

Radial paralysis ('dropped elbow') is commonest in horses and dogs, though it may be seen in
any animal.

Causes Probably the majority of cases are due
to a fracture of the 1st rib on the same side of
the body, the broken ends of the rib lacerating
the nerve-fibres as they pass the rib, or pressing
against them. In other cases the origin of the
paralysis seems to be situated in the end-plates
of the nerve-fibres where they are distributed to
the muscles, and in some cases a neuritis involving the radial nerve, or a tumour pressing upon
it at some part of its course, is responsible for
producing the condition.

Signs In a typical case the horse stands with the
elbow dropped lower than normally, and with
the knee, elbow, and fetlock joints flexed. Little
or no pain is felt, unless there is a fractured rib,
or some inflammatory condition which has
caused the paralysis. The limb is held in the
position assumed at the commencement of a
stride, but the animal is incapable of advancing
it far in front of the sound limb. No weight is
borne upon the leg, the muscles are flaccid and
soft, and if the horse is made to move forward
either it does so by hopping off and on to the
sound fore-limb, or it may fall forwards. If the
hand be forcibly pressed against the knee, so
that the limb is restored to its natural upright
position, the horse is able to bear weight upon it
and may lift the other limb from the ground,
but as soon as the pressure is released, the joints
fall forward again. Sometimes the toe is rested
upon the ground, but at other times the horse
stands with the wall of the foot in contact with
the ground. In cases that are not so severe, the
flat of the foot may rest on the ground, and the

limb can be advanced forwards to a considerable
extent.

Treatment The majority of such cases as these
will recover in a few weeks. Patience on the part
of the owner is essential.

Radiation, Exposure to

The 1986 Chernobyl nuclear power-station dis-
aster in the former USSR led to controls being
imposed on the movement and slaughter of
sheep in parts of Scotland, Cumbria, and Wales,
after between 1000 and 4000 Becquerels/kg of
caesium-137 had been detected in lambs.
Similar controls were applied in other countries
affected by the fallout. The ban temporarily
affected about 2 million sheep and lambs in
some 500 flocks.

The Atomic Energy Authority stated that
10,000 Bq/kg represents a health risk.

However, the contamination figures exceeded, in 9 cases, the internationally recommended
action levels for radiocaesium of 1000 Bq/kg.
The highest figure was 4000.

'Although the physical half-life of radiocaesium is 30 years, its biological half-life is much
shorter. In an adult animal, the half-life is estimated at between 30 and 100 days, but for lamb
it would be between 25 and 50 days.' (MAFF)

(See also RADIOACTIVE IODINE; RADIOACTIVE
STRONTIUM.)

Annual human exposure Of the average
UK citizen's annual exposure to radioactive discharges, only 0.1 per cent comes from the nuclear
power industry, according to the Radiological
Protection Board.

For radiation exposure associated with veterinary practice, see RADIOISOTOPES and X-RAYS.

Carbon-14 is among internal sources of natural radiation, and is present in the human
body to the extent of about 2000 Bq.

Radiation, Protection against

Regulations governing the use of X-ray equipment, and the precautions to be taken by those
handling it, are very strict. Details are given
in the Health and Safety at Work Act. (See under
X-RAYS.)

A concise guide to the Health and Safety at
Work Act 1974 can be obtained from HSE
Books, PO Box 1999, Sudbury, Suffolk COI0
6FS.

Radiation Sickness

Dogs exposed to radiation following a nuclear
explosion will vomit as a result of gastroenteritis, become dull and lose their appetite. This

may return after a day or two, but leucopenia develops, and may be followed by haemorrhage or septicaemia.

Radioactive Caesium

High levels of caesium 137 were found in areas of Wales and Scotland following the nuclear power-station explosion at Chernobyl in 1986. Certain flocks of sheep were affected by the fall-out and the meat declared unfit for human consumption for some time.

Antidote A ferric-cyano-ferrate (AFCF), in the form of a dark blue powder, can bind radiocaesium both *in vitro* and in the gastrointestinal tract of animals very effectively, preventing the isotope from being absorbed and secreted into the milk or transferred to the meat of cows, etc. The addition of only 3 g AFCF per day to the diet of lactating cows reduced the radiocaesium content of their milk by between 80 and 90 per cent, and of their meat by 78 per cent.

The radiocaesium content of the meat from sheep fed 1 g AFCF per day or of calves or pigs fed 2 g AFCF per day was reduced by approximately 90 per cent. The compound was given official clearance as a feed additive against radiocaesium in Germany.

Radioactive Discharges

Of the average UK citizen's annual exposure, only 0.1 per cent comes from the nuclear power industry, according to the Radiological Protection Board.

Around 90 per cent comes from natural sources, principally radon gas released from building materials.

For radiation associated with veterinary practice, see RADIOISOTOPES and X-RAYS.

Radioactive Fall-Out

Radioactive fall-out, following the explosion of nuclear bombs, etc., or accidents at atomic plant, may be dangerous to farm livestock on account of the radioactive iodine and strontium released. After an accident at Windscale, radioactive iodine alone contaminated pasture in the area. (See also RADIATION, EXPOSURE TO; RADIATION SICKNESS; RADIOACTIVE IODINE.)

Radioactive Iodine

Cattle grazing pasture contaminated by fall-out pick up 10 times as much radioactive iodine as do people in the same locality, according to American reports. Much is excreted in the milk, and much concentrated in the thyroid glands.

Feeding-stuffs or pasture contaminated by fall-out containing radioactive iodine and strontium may give rise to illness in cattle. Digestive organs may be damaged, changes in the blood occur, and deaths follow within a month or so, after a period of dullness and scouring. (See RADIOACTIVE STRONTIUM.)

Radioactive Strontium

Whereas the half-life of radioactive iodine is a matter of days, that of strontium is 30 years. Following the grazing of contaminated pasture or the eating of other contaminated feed, radioactive strontium is excreted in the milk, but much of it enters the bones and is liable to set up cancer many years afterwards.

The UK average ratio of strontium-90 to calcium in milk was 2.8 picocuries per gram of calcium in 1975, compared with 3.3 picocuries per gram in the previous year; this result is about one-tenth of the maximum reached in 1964. The average concentration of caesium-137 (7 picocuries/litre) was about four-fifths of the value in 1974 and less than one-twentieth of the 1964 maximum. (AFRC.)

Radio-Frequency Treatment
(see under CANCER – Treatment)

Radiography
(see under X-RAYS)

Radioimmune Assay

A method of measuring antigen or antibody concentration by means of radioactively labelled reagents (see RADIOISOTOPES).

Radioisotopes

A radioisotope is a form of an element that undergoes decay while emitting radiation. Artificial radioisotopes (radiopharmaceuticals) are widely used in diagnosis and in human medicine. Nuclear medicine involves the use of unsealed radioisotopes for diagnosis and therapy. For example, in bone scanning, the most commonly used radiopharmaceutical is methylene diphosphonate, labelled with Technetium 99 mm (Tc-99). With a half-life of only 6 hours, high doses can be given for a low radiation burden, permitting high resolution pictures to be obtained.

Radio 'Pills' (Telemetering Capsules)

Radio 'pills' (telemetering capsules) have been developed for research purposes. A radio transmitter, the size of an ordinary drug capsule, can give information concerning pressure, temperature or pH within an organ.

Radius

The inner of the 2 bones of the fore-limb. In the horse and ox particularly, the radius forms the main bone of this part, the ulna being much smaller and not taking part in weight-bearing. (See BONE.)

Radon

A colourless gas produced by the disintegration of radium. It is found naturally in low concentrations in certain areas, e.g. parts of Cornwall, where it has given rise to public-health concerns (see under RADIOACTIVE).

Ragdoll

A breed of cat originating in the USA, so called because it tends to 'flop' if carried. They have a high pain threshold and, if involved in a fight, could continue long after a normal cat would have stopped. As a result, it could sustain serious injuries even if it won the fight.

Ragwort Poisoning

Ragwort poisoning causes losses among cattle and sheep in Great Britain, Canada, and New Zealand. It is the cause of the 'Pictou cattle disease of Canada', and of 'Molteno cattle disease' in South Africa. The plant (*Senecio jacobaea*, or sp.) is very often fed off by sheep when it becomes too plentiful in grass land. In the UK fatal poisoning has followed the giving of hay contaminated with ragwort – death occurring many weeks after the last mouthful. The death of 28 head of cattle was caused 2 to 4 months after feeding ragwort-contaminated silage. Acute ragwort poisoning may also occur, causing death in 5 to 10 days with symptoms of dullness, abdominal pain, and sometimes jaundice.

Ragwort contains PYRROLIZIDENE ALKALOIDS, which produce cirrhosis of the liver, inflammation of the 4th stomach, and other lesions.

In grazing horses, ragwort will be eaten only if other food is not available but may be ingested in hay or silage. In the UK after a mild, damp winter, when the plant grows earlier in the year than usual, and is sprouting among the grasses, horses may eat it.

Chronic liver damage may result, with acute signs apparent when the cirrhosis becomes advanced.

Milk from a cow which has eaten ragwort may be dangerous to children, causing liver damage.

Signs include loss of appetite and of condition, constipation, sometimes jaundice. Cattle may strain and later become excited and violent; horses may become drowsy, with a staggering gait. Secondary gastric impaction and rupture in horses has been reported.

Treatment There is no specific antidote, but methionine has been reported to be helpful. (See LIVER, DISEASES OF.)

Diagnosis A liver biopsy may be helpful in the diagnosis of chronic ragwort poisoning in horses – 'probably the most common cause of chronic hepatic pathology in horses in the UK'.

'Rain Scald'

An old name for *Dermatophilus* infection in horses subjected to prolonged wetting. Lesions occur on withers, shoulders, and rump. For appearance of the lesions, see under GREASY HEEL, and DERMATOPHILUS.

Rainfall

Rainfall may influence outbreaks of HYPOMAG-NESAEMIA; BLOAT; FOOT-AND-MOUTH DISEASE.

Rales (Moist Sounds)

Rales (moist sounds) are sounds heard by auscultation of the chest during various diseases. They are divided into 2 main classes: (1) crepitant or vesicular rales, which are heard in the 1st stages of pneumonia, and are sharp, fine, crackling noises noticed during inspiration only; and (2) mucous rales, which are heard during expiration as well as during inspiration and may be described as bubbling or gurgling sounds.

Ram Epididymitis

This is a disease of economic importance in most of the sheep-farming areas of the world, including Australia and Mediterranean Europe, but not the UK. The cause is *Brucella ovis*. Diagnosis by clinical means (palpation, mainly) is not very satisfactory. Laboratory tests to confirm the organism confirm the diagnosis. Vaccination and culling are methods of control, but vaccination is not free from problems.

Contagious epididymitis is a NOTIFIABLE DISEASE throughout the EU.

Rancidity

Rancidity of cod-liver oil or other fish oils, etc., can be extremely dangerous. Rancid mash may bring about deficiencies of vitamins A, D, and E, with acute digestive disorders and death in chicks. Growing and adult birds may also suffer losses from this cause; with osteomalacia, and decreased egg production. (See also under VITAMIN E.)

Rangoon Beans
(see JAVA BEAN POISONING)

Ranula
Ranula is a swelling which sometimes appears below the free portion of the dog's tongue. It is caused by a collection of saliva in one of the small ducts that carry saliva from the glands below the tongue, or further back, into the mouth, and when of some size a ranula may cause considerable interference with feeding. It is treated by incision or excision, and is usually not serious.

Rape Poisoning
Rape poisoning occurs in animals which are not given hay or other food in addition to rape. Poisoning can be extremely serious, especially in sheep.

Signs include dullness, red-coloured urine, and blindness. In one outbreak reported by the Reading VI Centre, 36 out of 360 sheep died from rape poisoning.

A form of light sensitisation called 'rape scald' occurs in sheep on rape. Swelling of the head occurs, there is irritation leading to rubbing, the ears may suffer damage. Jaundice may occur.

Rapeseed Cake
A compressed 'cake' of rapeseed is used as a cattle feed. The oil is first removed and the cake may be processed to remove any toxicity.

Rapeseed Oil
This has been shown experimentally to be toxic to the hearts of rats. The degree of toxicity varies according to the erucic acid content of the oil, and perhaps to closely related monoethylenic acids (e.g. cetoleic and nervonic). It is apparently the breakdown of erucic acid in the myocardium and skeletal muscles which produces the damaging effects. The use of the oil in margarine manufacture and as a substitute for more expensive olive oil has led to anxiety over the effects on the human heart.

Rapeseed meal fed to poultry may depress growth and egg yield, and cause hypertrophy of the thyroid gland, liver haemorrhage, abnormalities of the skeleton, and a fishy taint in the eggs. The liver haemorrhages resemble those associated with the 'fatty liver/haemorrhagic syndrome'. Rapeseeds of low toxicity, such as the Canadian variety canola, have now been bred.

Raphe
Raphe means a ridge or furrow between the halves of an organ.

Rarefaction of Bone
A decrease in the mineral content.

Rat and Mouse Poisons
(see under RODENTS)

Rat-Bite Fever
This is a disease recognised in man and caused, following the bite of a rat (or, sometimes, dog, cat, mouse, weasel, or squirrel), by infection with *Spirillum minus* or *Streptobacillus moniliformis*. In addition to fever there may be an extensive rash.

Rations for Livestock

Dairy cattle

Winter rationing The home-grown foods available naturally vary from farm to farm. Farm-mixed rations often make good use of barley. Proprietary compound feeding-stuffs are well balanced and formulated to contain all necessary ingredients such as vitamins, trace elements, etc., and are nowadays extensively used. Proprietary barley balancers and straw balancers are also much used. (See also under WINTER DIET.)

Rations: theoretical basis for calculation Traditionally, it is customary to regard the ration as being composed of 2 parts: (1) the 'maintenance' part, which provides the material for all vital activities and makes good the normal wear and tear of the body without causing increase or decrease in liveweight; and (2) the 'production' part, which supplies the materials used for increase in body size, fat production, growth of the fetus, and milk production.

ADAS Advisory Paper No. 11, *Nutrient Allowances and Composition of Feeding-Stuffs for Ruminants*, contains 2 valuable sets of information: firstly, what different classes and weights of ruminant stock need for maintenance and production; and secondly, the analyses of a wide variety of feeds.

Maintenance and 4.5 litre (1 gallon) rations for cows of Friesian breed or similar:

		kg (lb)
(a)	Hay	8 (18)
	Brewer's grains	4.5 (10)
	Dried sugar beet pulp	1.8 (4)
(b)	Hay	8 (18)
	Dried sugar beet pulp	1.8 (4)
	Silage	23 (50)

with parlour-fed concentrates, 1.5 kg (3H lb) per 4.5 litres (1 gallon), for both (a) and (b).

Maintenance plus 9 litres (2 gallons):
Ryegrass/lucerne haylage   ad lib

Brewer's grains plus minerals   7 kg (15 lb)

with every 1.8 kg (4 lb) hammer-milled maize fed in parlour for every additional 4.5 litres (1 gallon).

Summer rationing Grass is the standard summer food for cattle. On a good, well-managed pasture – where over-stocking is avoided – young, leafy grass will supply enough protein for high yielders, but they will require additional carbohydrate. This may be supplied in the form of cereals, e.g. 1.8 kg (4 lb) for each 4.5 litres (1 gallon) of milk over about 20 litres (4H gallons) produced per day.

It has been recommended that in April, cows grazing young, leafy grass 10 to 15 cm (4 to 6 inches) high for 4 hours daily, should receive 3 kg (7 lb) hay and cereals (plus a mineral mixture) at the rate of 1.8 kg (4 lb) for each 4.5 litres (1 gallon) over 13.5 litres (3 gallons). In May, with unrestricted grazing of grass 20 or 25 cm (8 or 10 inches) long at the pre-flowering stage, the hay is discontinued; the cereal ration remaining as before. In June and July, with grass at the flowering stage, the cows receive balanced concentrates for yields over 11 litres (2½ gallons) (June), then over 9 litres (2 gallons). In

August, grazing aftermath (or green fodder during a drought), the cows receive concentrates for each 4.5 litres (1 gallon) over the first 4.5 litres (1 gallon). In September, with young aftermath or maiden seeds, there is a hay ration of 3 kg (7 lb) (or 13 kg (28 lb) kale) plus concentrates for yields over 9 litres (2 gallons) per day.

More sophisticated calculations for feed requirements are based on the metabolisable energy requirements of specific herds or even animals. Calculations take into account the amount of energy required for maintaining condition; the quantity of milk produced; and the stage of pregnancy. For growing cattle, rations are calculated based on the maintenance requirement plus the daily liveweight gain.

Beef cattle (see table re suckler cows, and under BEEF)

Calves (see CALF-REARING)

Pigs

Creep feed	Per cent
Barley meal	40
Flaked maize	30
White fish-meal	15
Wheatings	15

Rations for suckler cows					
	Autumn calvers			**Spring calvers**	
	Blue-Grey	Hereford × Friesian		Blue-Grey	Hereford × Friesian
	(kg per day)			(kg per day)	
Calving to mating			*Mid-pregnancy to calving*		
1. Grass silage			1. Grass silage	20	20
(25% DM, 60D)	27	27	Mineralised barley	0.5	0.5
Mineralised barley	1.25	2	2. Hay	6	7
2. Hay (57D) 35%	8	10	Protein concentrate	0.5	0.5
protein concentrate	1.75	1.75	3. Barley straw	7	7
			Protein concentrate	1.5	1.75
Mating to turnout			*Calving to turnout*		
1. Grass silage	25	27	1. Grass silage	25	27
Mineralised barley	0.5	0.5	Mineralised barley	1	1
2. Hay	7	8	2. Hay	8	8.5
Protein concentrate	0.75	0.75	Protein concentrate	1	1
During this period cows can lose about 0.5 kg per day so that condition falls by about ¹/₂ score to turnout.			3. Barley straw	7	7
			Protein concentrate	2.75	3.25
Mid-pregnancy to calving					
	grazing	grazing		grazing	grazing

Breeders and growers*	Per cent
Barley meal	70
White fish-meal	10
Wheatings	10
Ground maize	10

Fatteners*	Per cent
Barley meal	75
Soya bean-meal	5
Wheatings	20

*Plus mineral and vitamin supplements.

Sheep (see under SHEEP, and FLUSHING OF EWES)

Horses (see under HORSES, FEEDING OF)

Poultry

Chicks to 12 weeks	Per cent
Maize meal	23
Ground barley	10
Ground oats	10
Ground wheat	20
Wheat bran	13
Grass meal	5
White fish-meal	10
Soya bean-meal	5
Dried yeast	1.5
Ground limestone	1
Salt mixture	0.5

(10 parts of common salt, 1 of manganese sulphate)

Vitamin pre-mix	1

Layers/growers' mash	
(Balancer for grain)	Per cent
Ground wheat	30
Ground barley	25
Wheat middlings	8
Wheat bran	5
Grass meal	8
White fish-meal	3
Meat and bone-meal	3
Soya bean-meal	10
Ground limestone	3
Steamed bone-flour	2.5
Salt mixture	0.5
Vitamin pre-mix	2

Rats

Rats are important from a veterinary point of view as carriers of infection to cattle, pigs, dogs, etc. Examples of rat-borne diseases are: Aujeszky's, leptospirosis, salmonellosis, ringworm, trichinosis, and foot-and-mouth. (See also PETS; RODENTS.)

RBC

Red blood cells.

RBV

Relative breeding value (see PROGENY TESTING).

Reaginic Antibodies

These are immunoglobulins which become fixed to mast cells and, in the presence of antigen, cause the release of histamine (and other compounds) giving rise to allergic reaction. (See ALLERGY; ASTHMA.) They react with antigens produced by parasitic worms.

Receptors

These are or contain antibody molecules, occur on the surface of lymphocytes, and enable specific antigens to be recognised. (See under IMMUNE RESPONSE; BLOOD.)

Physiological receptors include those for enzymes, and for hormones.

Recessives

(see GENETICS)

Recombinant DNA Technology

A process by which genes from one organism are transferred – usually by a modified bacterium or virus – to another to reproduce a desirable characteristic. For example, some vaccines are made by modifying a virus so that its virulence is removed but its antigenic potential – its ability to confer immunity – remains. Similarly, bacteria have been modified so that they produce human insulin. The possibility for using the technique to synthesize biological medicines not currently commercially available, or to improve plant breeds to enhance food yields, is likely to become increasingly important.

Plants may also be modified so that desirable characteristics such as resistance to disease are 'bred' into them.

Recovery Quilts

Recovery quilts for cats and dogs have been developed. Marketed as Flectabed, the quilts contain Flectalon, a special fibre developed for emergency blankets. It is stated that the product reflects back 95 per cent of the infra-red heat lost by the body. Details from Flectabed, 17a Moor Street, Chepstow, Gwent BP6 5DB.

Rectum

The posterior end of the intestine. It commences on a level with the anterior opening of the pelvis and extends to the anus, passing through the upper part of the pelvic cavity. In most of the domesticated animals it possesses a dilatation, known as the 'ampulla', which serves to collect the faeces that are slowly passed into it from the colon, and holds them until time and circumstances are convenient for their evacuation to the outside. (See INTESTINE.)

Rectum, Diseases of

With the exception of the dog, the domestic animals are comparatively free from disease of this part of the alimentary system.

Impaction This occurs mainly in dogs (and to a lesser extent in cats) when pieces of bone, string, and other foreign materials form with the faeces a hard mass. The affected animal attempts to pass faeces, but after considerable efforts fails to do so. If the impacted material contains spicules of bone or other hard material, every effort at defaecation causes the animal to cry out with the pain.

Removal of the offending matter is effected by the administration of an enema of glycerine, oil, or soapy water, and the introduction of the gloved finger. Hard masses are broken up and taken away in portions if too large to remove whole. A mild laxative should be given by the mouth after the impacted material has been cleared from the rectum, and the dog should receive a soft semi-fluid diet for some days afterwards.

Inflammation of the rectum may follow impaction, or it may commence as the result of an injury. The animal frequently strains, and the owner may surmise that it is constipated, but exploration reveals the absence of faeces.

Abscesses, tumours and ulcers may also affect the rectum, but they are not common. (See also under ANUS.)

Prolapse of the rectum may occur in any animal, but is especially common in the smaller animals. A portion of the gut is protruded from the anus to an extent of a few inches. It appears as a tumorous swelling of a bright-red appearance, cold to the touch, and usually covered with mucus or faecal material. There is usually some straining when the condition is of recent origin, but after a time the animal appears to become used to the protrusion of the piece of bowel, and only strains when it is handled or when attempts are made to return it. Anaesthesia or analgesia will be needed. It may be gently bathed with warm water containing common salt in solution (5 per cent) while awaiting assistance. An operation, in which the rectum is sutured to some part of the abdominal roof, is sometimes necessary to prevent its recurrence after replacement. Prolapsed rectum is not uncommon in the horse. Sometimes it may be easily returned by placing the neck of a quart bottle within the central depression that is always present, and pressing slowly and cautiously in a forward direction.

In some instances amputation of the protruded portion becomes necessary, especially if it has been outside for some considerable time and has become gangrenous.

Recumbency

In a veterinary sense, this means not merely lying down but also a failure to get up. (See 'DOWNER COW' SYNDROME.) In animals in dorsal recumbency during anaesthesia, pressure of viscera on the posterior VENA CAVA may result in hypotension. In rare cases, this has been followed by spinal cord necrosis, leading to paralysis of a horse's hind-legs, necessitating euthanasia. It has been suggested that a slightly oblique dorsal recumbency is advisable.

Anaesthetised horses, when positioned in left lateral recumbency, showed least muscle or nerve injuries when lying on a water mattress. Foam rubber was 'far from satisfactory'.

Recurrent Laryngeal Nerve

Recurrent laryngeal nerve is a branch of the vagus nerve which leaves the latter at different points on the right and left sides of the body. On the right side it leaves the parent nerve opposite the 2nd rib, curves inwards round the subclavian or the costo-cervical artery, and runs up the neck on the lower surface of the trachea and below the carotid of the same side. In the case of the left, the branch leaves the vagus where that nerve crosses the arch of the aorta, winds inwards around the concavity of the aortic arch, and runs up the neck in a position similar to that of the right side. Both nerves supply the muscles of the larynx which are concerned in the production of voice and in maintaining the glottis open during ordinary and forced respiration.

'Redfoot'

A condition seen in newborn lambs, in which the sensitive laminae of the feet become exposed owing to detachment of the overlying horn. The cause is unknown, no treatment effective, and the lambs soon die.

Red Squill

Preparations of the dried ground bulbs of the sea onion *Urginea maritima* are used for poisoning rodents, baits being made up to contain 10 per cent red squill. Domestic animals refrain from eating such preparations owing to the smell and taste. Symptoms of poisoning include profuse vomiting in the pig but not in the cat, excitement, muscular incoordination, and convulsions. Poisoning in rodents by red squill may be agonising and prolonged. Its use in the UK is banned.

Red Urine

Causes of red discoloration of the urine include: haematuria – blood in the urine, which settles out on standing; haemoglobinuria – the breakdown of red blood cells, in which urine does not change colour on standing; and pigments. The coloration is usually a sign of disease: pyelonephritis and cystitis cause haematuria; red-water fever, leptospirosis, infection with *Clostridium haemolyticum*, kale and rape poisoning, copper poisoning, and the drinking of very large quantities of water all result in haemoglobinuria. Azoturia results in breakdown of muscles to produce myoglobin-urea, a brown-red coloration. Dosing with phenothiazine produces a red pigment.

Red-Water

Also called bacillary haemoglobinuria, or ictero-haemoglobinuria, in the USA it occurs in California, Colorado, Idaho, Louisiana, Montana, Nevada, Oregon, Texas, and Utah. *Clostridium haemolyticum* is the cause. (See also TEXAS FEVER, the American red-water fever.)

Red-Water Fever

In the British Isles, babe siosis or piroplasmosis (see under BABESIA), to give red-water fever its proper names, is a disease of cattle and sheep,

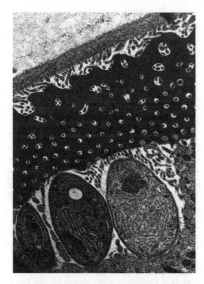

An electron microscope picture showing three profiles of *Babesia divergens* – the cause of red-water fever – inside the egg of a tick. (With acknowledgements to IRAD, Compton.)

due to the presence in the blood of a protozoon parasite which attacks the red blood cells, destroying their envelopes and liberating haemoglobin, which is excreted by the kidneys and colours the urine reddish or blackish. It occurs mainly in the south and west of England, in the north and west of Scotland, and practically all over Ireland, but it is also seen at times in districts that are not included in these areas. It is common in low-lying, rough-pastured, and moorland districts, where ticks, which harbour and transmit the parasite, can find abundant shelter and suitable breeding places. Cattle are usually attacked from the age of about 6 months upwards, but young calves are practically immune. One attack gives a degree of immunity, and cattle that have been bred upon infected farms, and from infected cattle, are more resistant than those brought from a clean district. It is more prevalent in the spring and autumn months, since the ticks are then at their maximum activity.

Cause *Babesia (Piroplasma) divergens.* This is transmitted by the common tick *Ixodes ricinus*, and occasionally by *Haemophysalis punctata.* (See under BABESIA and TICKS; also MUSCLES, DISEASES OF; MYOGLOBINURIA.)

Signs Two varieties of the disease are recognised: an acute and a mild form.

The acute type is sudden in its onset and frequently fatal. The animal becomes very dull and depressed, separates itself from the rest of the herd, moves slowly or not at all, grunts, groans, arches its back, salivates freely, grinds its teeth, and often staggers and falls. The coat becomes hard and staring, the skin is dry and often hide-bound, and there is almost always a profuse, watery, violent 'pipe stem' diarrhoea, due to spasms of the anal sphincter. The temperature rises to as high as 40.5° to 41.5° C (105° to 107°F), the pulse is fast and weak (often 100 per minute), and the respirations are laboured, blow-ing, and rapid (80 to 100 per minute). The visi-ble mucous membranes are pale. After a few days the animal's distress becomes less acute, and the most alarming symptoms subside. The signs of fever, however, are still evident, and the cow is still in a serious condition. The urine usually shows some degree of coloration, which varies from a clear reddish claret to a deep dark brown or black – almost like stout.

The duration of acute attacks varies, but it is seldom that the high temperature lasts for more than a week. Death may take place in from 3 to 5 days, or later on, when it is usually due to exhaustion.

In the mild type the urine is not usually highly coloured; there is only slight dullness and loss of appetite. The animals are ill for a week or 10 days, and the only marked sequel is anaemia.

There are irregular forms of red-water met with at times, in which the general symptoms are similar to these seen in the typical acute attack, but the urine does not become discoloured. Many of these cases end fatally.

Treatment Imidocarb (Imizol). For use under prescription only. A single dose of 1 ml per 100 kg bodyweight for treatment, or 2.5 ml per 100 kg bodyweight for prevention; the dose must be given subcutaneously. Cattle must not be slaughtered for human consumption for 90 days after administration, and milk from treated animals must be withheld for 21 days. Veterinary surgeons who prescribe Imizol are advised that:

1. Full records of product administration to identifiable animals must be maintained, and that it is the duty of the farmer to keep a careful record of all administration of the product, as required by the Animals and Fresh Meat (Examination for Residues) Regulations 1988.

2. The local DVM must be notified of the address of the farm where treatment is to take place.

3. Farmers should be informed that they must notify the local DVM when treated animals go for slaughter for human consumption or when milk from treated animals is intended for human consumption.

Any suspected adverse reactions, including evidence of lack of efficacy, should be reported to the Veterinary Medicines Directorate, New Haw, Weybridge, Surrey, immediately.

Ticks should be removed, either by hand-picking or by spraying with a suitable parasiticide. (See TICKS, CONTROL OF.)

The few piroplasms taken into the bloodstream, when young cattle are bitten by infected ticks, tend not to multiply but to give rise to a useful degree of immunity. This may wane if the piroplasms die, so that the animal becomes susceptible again. Immunity may likewise break down if the animal becomes ill from some other cause.

Control Measures involve tick control, and not mixing cattle from red-water areas with susceptible cattle. Even then there are risks.

Twenty deaths occurred when local cattle were placed on sea marsh land in Lincolnshire that had previously been used for fattening imported Irish steers which were carriers of

B. divergens. Cornish cattle brought to a farm in Sussex set up a focus of infection because infected ticks became established in the new habitat. And Simmental, Charolais and other European breeds are imported into Britain with no screening for blood parasites.

Red Worms

The common name for strongyles. These can cause severe anaemia, unthriftiness, and debility. (See under FOALS, DISEASES OF; also under EQUINE VERMINOUS ARTERITIS; HORSES, WORMS IN.) Benzimidazoles, ivermectins and thiabendazole are useful drugs for the removal of red worms. (See also ROUNDWORMS.)

Reduplication

Reduplication is a term applied to a duplication of the normal heart-sounds as heard by auscultation. There are heard a 1st and a 2nd sound in a normal heartbeat, and in the above condition one or both of these may be doubled. It is found in certain diseases of the heart, such as obstruction of the valve between the auricle and ventricle on the left side of the organ (the mitral valve).

Reflex Action

Reflex action is one of the simplest forms of activity of the nervous system. For the mechanism, see NERVES.

Superficial reflexes are well instanced in the sudden shivering movement that is seen when a fly or other insect settles upon the skin of a horse, particularly in the region of the back of the shoulder.

Visceral reflexes are those connected with various organs, such as the narrowing of the pupil when the eye is exposed to a bright light. (See SPINAL CORD.)

Regional Anaesthesia

This consists in the anaesthetisation of a region of the body by means of a local anaesthetic solution injected either into the connective tissue surrounding a sensory nerve trunk or into the spinal canal. (See EPIDURAL ANAESTHESIA, ANALGESICS.) The most common example of perineurial injection is plantar block in the horse.

Register of Veterinary Surgeons

The Register of Veterinary Surgeons lists veterinary surgeons who can practise in the UK. It may be consulted in some public libraries or is obtainable from the Royal College of Veterinary Surgeons, Belgravia House, 62–64 Horseferry Road, London SW1P 2AF.

Rehydration

The restoration of the correct levels of water and electrolytes in animals suffering from DEHYDRATION.

Reindeer (Rangifer Tarandus)

Both in northern Europe and North America these animals are of economic importance. Parasites include WARBLES. Subcutaneous injections of ivermectin are recommended for prevention of infestation and treatment.

Relapse

A relapse occasionally occurs when antibiotic or sulfa drug treatment of an infectious disease is stopped – the infection having been suppressed but the animal's powers of resistance not having been stimulated to establish a sufficient degree of immunity. Some forms of lameness are particularly liable to relapses, especially those associated with sprains of tendons or ligaments.

Relative Breeding Value

(see PROGENY TESTING)

'Remote Injection' Method

(see PROJECTILE SYRINGE)

Renal

Relating to the kidney.

Renin

An enzyme, secreted by the kidneys, which may control the secretion of the hormone aldosterone by the adrenal glands.

Reovirus

The name derives from the words 'respiratory enteric orphan virus'. Reoviruses have double-stranded ribonucleic acid (RNA), and will replicate and produce changes in cells of cattle, pigs, dogs, cats, rabbits, monkeys, and man. Reovirus in poultry is often seen as tenosynovitis. The tendon sheaths, synovial membrane and the myocardium are all affected. Vaccination is possible but attention to hygiene is also essential for effective control. Only flocks known to be free from the infection should be selected for producing hatching eggs. (See also CALF PNEUMONIA.)

Repair

Repair of tissue after injury is described under WOUNDS; for the repair of special tissues, see under BONE, MUSCLE, NERVE, etc. (See also HOOF REPAIR WITH PLASTICS.)

Reproduction

Ovulation At OVULATION the Graafian follicle bursts, and the ovum is expelled by the rush of the escaping fluid. The cavity of the Graafian follicle becomes filled with special cells to form the corpus luteum, and the ovum begins its career as an absolute entity. In normal circumstances the fimbriated and dilated funnel-shaped end of the Fallopian tube, or oviduct, is applied to the point at which a follicle will burst, so that upon escape of its ovum this latter may be caught and retained. The dilated end of the oviduct is usually known as the vestibule, and it is in this part that the sperm usually meets the ovum and fertilises it. (See also under OVARIES.)

Coitus The act of copulation. As mentioned under OESTRUS, service by the male is only allowed during the period of oestrus by the females of the majority of species of higher animals. At other times there is little or no desire exhibited by the male, and all attentions are resented by the female. Artificial methods of domestication have to some extent modified the frequency and duration of oestrus, so that the domestic animals sheltered under the protection of man breed more frequently than do the majority of wild animals of similar species.

During a single ejaculation of an adult vigorous stallion about 80,000,000 sperms are released. As soon as the sperms are free in the uterus or vagina, they travel towards wherever the ovum is situated. This they accomplish partly by a kind of wriggling movement of their tail, which drives them onwards always in the same direction. They are attracted to the ovum by 'chemotaxis'.

Fertilisation Somewhere in the oviduct, generally in its vestibule but not necessarily so, the spermatozoa arrive in the region of the waiting ovum. More than one sperm may penetrate the wall of the ovum, but except in rare instances (giving rise to PRIMARY MOSAICISM) only one sperm fertilises the ovum.

The sperm, having penetrated the ovum, loses its tail, which is no longer required, and lies within the protoplasm of the ovum. The nucleus of the ovum and that of the head of the sperm now fuse, each contributing half the number of chromosomes that are to be found present in nearly all the cells of the future young animal. The fused body is known as the segmentation nucleus, and from it, when it begins to divide, all the body cells of the embryo are formed. The process of the formation of the young embryo is

R

considered under EMBRYOLOGY. (See also TESTI-CLE; OVARIES; OESTRUS; BREEDING OF ANIMALS; PREGNANCY; PARTURITION; PARTHENOGENESIS.

Reproductive Organs
(see diagrams under UTERUS and PENIS)

Reptiles
A class of animal which includes tortoises, lizards and snakes. They tend to favour warm places when they are ill. Reptile housing should be heated at all times, but a range of heat should be available in different areas, within the normal limits for the species, so that they can choose which suits them best. Under no circumstances must they be allowed to come into direct contact with the heat source. Many species require ultraviolet light, otherwise bone rarefaction (weakening) may occur; expert advice must be sought before buying such a pet. (See also PETS.)

Resection
Resection is an operation in which a part of some organ is removed – as, for example, the resection of a piece of dead bone, or resection of a part of the intestine which is diseased; resection of a rib in thoracotomy; aural resection done to overcome chronic disease of a dog's ear.

Resistance Transferability
(see under PLASMIDS; ANTIBIOTIC RESISTANCE)

Resistant Strains
This phrase is commonly used of bacteria which are not sensitive to antibiotics, or of insects which are not killed by an insecticide.

R Resorption
Mummification. Resorption of the fetus occurs, e.g. in heifers receiving a high calcium and low phosphorus diet. In sows, mummification can be a feature of Aujeszky's disease, 'blue-ear' disease (PRRS), and both African and classical swine fever. With the banning of sow stalls and the need to find alternatives, it has been reported that the level of mummification tends to be higher in dry sows kept in straw yards. The reason is not clear, but bullying has been suggested as a cause. (See MUMMIFICATION.)

Respiration
(see also NOSE AND NASAL PASSAGES; LUNGS)

Mechanism of respiration For the structure of the respiratory apparatus see NOSE AND NASAL PASSAGES; LUNGS, etc.

Inspiration is due to muscular effort which enlarges the chest in all 3 dimensions, so that the lungs have to expand in order to fill up the vacuum that would otherwise be left; and since, although the lungs are not fixed to the chest wall, surface tension between the pleura lining the chest and the pleura covering the lungs, has much the same effect.

In most vertebrates, except birds, the lungs are not normally attached to the walls of the chest, but are rather suspended in them from their 'roots', so that there is no direct pull upon the lungs when the chest cavity increases in size. The vertical diameter of the chest is increased during inspiration through the downward tilting of the sternum. This movement is best seen in the dog when it is out of breath; at other times, and in other animals, it is so slight that it escapes detection. The transverse dimension of the chest increases when any 1 of the ribs behind the first 2 or 3 are forcibly pulled forward by muscular action. Each rib only moves a small amount, but the mass effect of the series is considerable. The muscles which bring about these changes in ordinary inspiration are the diaphragm, the intercostal muscles which are situated in two layers between each rib and its two neighbours, and possibly the levators of the ribs, and the serratus muscles.

When the chest expands, the lungs expand too; but initially the quantity of air within them remains the same. Accordingly, the pressure falls, leading to an inflow of air.

	Inspired air	Expired air
	Per cent	Per cent
Nitrogen	79.04	79.04
Oxygen	20.93	16.02
Carbon dioxide	0.03	4.38

Expiration is in ordinary circumstances merely an elastic recoil, the diaphragm moving forward and the ribs settling back into their original positions, partly through muscular action, and partly through the elasticity of their cartilages. It occupies a slightly longer period of time than does inspiration.

Nervous control Respiration is usually an automatic act under the control of the respiratory centre in the medulla oblongata.

Although the respiratory centre is itself capable of carrying on respiration, it is in its turn liable to be controlled by the higher conscious centres. This is seen particularly well in human beings, where it is possible to 'hold the breath', or inhibit respiration for considerable periods (when diving underwater, for example).

Rate of respiration The speed of the respiration varies with many internal and external factors. It is faster during fevers, after violent exercise, or even after mild exercise (though it soon returns to normal upon cessation); during powerful emotions, such as fear, anger, sexual excitement, etc.; during very cold or very hot weather; when the body condition is very fat, or when radiation is obstructed, through too thick a covering of wool, fur, etc., or too much clothing. (See also ANAEMIA.)

It is slower than normal during resting, either when merely lying or when sleeping; and in cases of unconsciousness.

The normal rates in adult domesticated animals are as follows:

In each case, the larger the particular animal, the slower it breathes, other things being equal. For instance, a Shetland pony respires about 12 times per minute, while a shire stallion respires only 8 times; also, the young of any species breathe faster than do adults; and females breathe faster than males – especially during pregnancy.

When this air is taken into the lungs its composition is altered, so that upon leaving the lungs its CO_2 content is about 4 per cent greater and its oxygen content about 4 per cent less.

Quantity of air The lungs do not by any means completely empty themselves at each expiration and refill at each inspiration. What is left after maximum expiration is called the residual volume. The volume of air exchanged during normal breathing (i.e. passing in and out of the nose) is the tidal volume – about 5 litres in the horse. The volume of air in the airways leading to the alveoli of the lungs is the anatomical dead space. Air available for the supply of oxygen in the lungs is the tidal volume minus the anatomical dead space.

Irregular forms of respiration Apart from mere changes in rate and force, the respiration is modified in various ways under certain conditions. Coughing is a series of violent expirations, during each of which the larynx is at first closed until the pressure of air in the lungs and lower passages is considerably raised, and then suddenly opened, so that the contained air is released under pressure and rushes to the outside; its object is to expel some irritating object from the air passages. Sneezing is a single sudden expiration, which differs from coughing in that the sudden rush of air is directed by the

soft palate up into the nose in order to expel some source of irritation from the nasal chambers. It is particularly well exhibited by the dog.

Yawning is a deep slow inspiration followed by a short expiration, the air being taken in by the open mouth as well as by the nose. Hiccough is due to a sudden spasmodic contraction of the diaphragm, along with a sudden closing of the larynx, producing a sound not unlike a very loud heartbeat. Hyperpnoea is a term applied to the slightly increased frequency and depth of respiration occurring during gentle exercise, or from some mild stimulus to the respiratory centre. Dyspnoea means that there is distinct distress in breathing, due to a more powerful stimulus to the respiratory centre, and is usually characterised by convulsive movements of the chest and diaphragm. It is frequently the forerunner of asphyxia. Apnoea is seen when there is a hyperoxygenation of the tissues, and consequently no further immediate demands for oxygen. It consists of a complete cessation of the respiratory movements without the exhibition of any distress. It is artificially produced in human beings when a diver takes 10 or 12 deep breaths before entering the water, where he must hold his breath. It is not commonly seen in the domestic animals, but the seal and other diving animals have developed the power of inducing apnoea to a marked extent. (See also under ASTHMA; LARYNGEAL PARALYSIS; VOICE; TACHYPNOEA.)

Respiratory Difficulty, Failure

(see under BREATHLESSNESS; ANAEMIA; OEDEMA; ASPHYXIA; BRONCHITIS; PNEUMONIA; FOG FEVER; ANAESTHETICS.) Many poisons bring about respiratory failure, e.g. chloroform, hydrocyanic acid, paraquat.

Respiratory Disease in Pigs

Pigs are susceptible to a number of respiratory problems; the most common being the following (see also under main dictionary entries).

Atrophic rhinitis This is generally agreed to be the result of bacterial infection with *Bordetella bronchiseptica* followed by toxigenic strains of *Pasteurella multocida*, leading to progressive atrophy of the turbinate bones (see RHINITIS); a vaccine is available. A few cases are caused by cytomegalovirus (inclusion body rhinitis).

Enzootic pneumonia is a common problem, particularly in growing pigs; affected animals have a dry cough, reduced weight gain and poor feed conversion efficiency. The cause is *Mycoplasma hyopneumoniae*.

R

Pleuro-pneumonia of pigs is a rapid onset respiratory disease resulting in dyspnoea and, often, death in acute cases. Less severely affected animals have a variety of subclinical problems. The cause is *Actinobacillus pleuro-pneumoniae*. Often seen following other disease problems, pleuro-pneumonia can affect only some of the animals in a herd, causing high temperatures, laboured breathing with, often, a bloody frothy discharge from the nose. Early antibiotic treatment can effect a recovery; tetracyclines, lincomycin and ceftiofur are among drugs used. Vaccines are available for control.

Swine influenza can sweep through a pig unit, causing a variety of respiratory signs and sometimes precipitating other respiratory diseases. Little can be done to control the spread of infection, but the pigs recover after 4 to 6 days; subsequent immunity lasts about 3 months.

Porcine respiratory reproductive disease (PRRS) ('blue-ear' disease) results in variable signs, but affected animals may have respiratory difficulties; it often exacerbates any underlying respiratory diseases, such as pneumonias.

Porcine respiratory-coronavirus infection (PRCV) Outbreaks are often relatively mild, but other respiratory problems may result. Coughing, sneezing or dyspnoea can occur.

Ascarids Infection with *Ascaris suum* can result in coughing during the migratory stage of the larvae.

Aujeszky's disease sometimes causes respiratory signs such as sneezing, coughing and nasal discharge, occasionally with dyspnoea. Vaccines are available (in Ireland).

Lungworm Infection with *Metastrongylus apri* is usually only a problem in outdoor pigs; signs are often limited.

Not all the factors involved in respiratory disease are infections: management factors play their part, too. Space allowance per pig, number of pigs per group, effects of mixing and crowding, temperature, humidity, nutrition, age and genetic status of the pigs all exert their effects. (See also under ATROPHIC RHINITIS.)

Respiratory Stimulants

Respiratory stimulants are used to promote breathing in the newborn and to relieve respiratory depression associated with, for example, general anaesthesia. They include doxapram (Dopram V), cropropamide and crotethamide (Respirot), and etamiphylline (Dalophylline).

Respiratory Syncytial Virus

Respiratory syncytial virus was first isolated from chimpanzees showing 'cold-like' signs; since the mid-1950s it has been detected in clinical cases of respiratory disease in man, cattle, sheep, goats, and horses. It is a cause of acute bronchiolitis and alveolitis.

Restraint

In order to examine an animal thoroughly for signs of injury or disease, in order to carry out inoculations, or even to administer an anaesthetic, some form of restraint is often necessary.

The introduction of effective tranquillisers and sedatives facilitated the handling of horses, cattle and small animals, and may assist or replace the use of several means of restraint described below. (See also TRANQUILLISERS; XYLAZINE; ANALGESIA.)

The following methods should not be used indiscriminately upon any and every animal. A method that is sufficient to restrain one animal may prove aggravating to another; e.g. while the common twitch may serve for a heavy draught gelding, it is likely to cause a thoroughbred stallion to be more restive than ever. A person who finds it necessary to employ some means of restraint should first of all consider the temperament, age, breed, and, if possible, the individual characteristics of the animal, as well as the purpose of the restraint, before deciding upon what methods will be employed. Firm gentleness, a kindly spoken word, and a hand-pat, with a little coaxing or urging, will very often allay an animal's fears, but there are those of a temperament which will not respond to gentleness; it is to those particularly that such methods as described here are applicable.

Horses The usual halter, head-stall, or bridle is generally sufficient to control broken horses that are to be handled or examined without the infliction of pain. In some cases it may be necessary to tie the animal to a ring in the wall or manger, or to the heel-posts, but it is better in such cases to take a couple of turns round the ring and have a man hold the end of the rope. For measures which involve handling of the hind-parts of the body, it is usually advisable to have one of the fore-feet picked up and held (preferably that upon the same side of the body as the operator is to work).

For greater control a TWITCH may be applied. (See also TRANQUILLISERS; ANAESTHETICS.)

Cattle A cattle CRUSH; either of a commercial pattern or one constructed of timber by farm labour, is useful; a gate may be hinged to a wall and closed so as to act as a crush for inoculations, etc. (See also VETERINARY FACILITIES ON THE FARM.)

A halter is also useful in cattle, as in horses.

In the case of comparatively quiet cattle, milk cows, etc., it will generally suffice if an assistant takes the animal by the nose. The thumb and middle finger of one hand are inserted into the respective nostrils, and the nasal septum is pinched between them. It is important that the stockman's fingers do not block up the airway.

The other hand may be placed under the jaw. In this position the majority of adult quiet cattle can be easily held. For bulls and those cattle that are more difficult to control it is usual to use a pair of bull-holders ('bull-dogs'; 'bull-tongs'); or if the animal is already rung (with a copper or aluminium ring), to attach a rope or bull-leader to the ring in the nose. For drenching purposes it is necessary to keep the head and neck in as straight a line as possible to obviate the risk of choking. If an assistant is needed he should stand on the opposite side of the beast and take the horns in his hands so that he may tilt the head upwards and at the same time keep the head and neck straight out. A pair of bull-holders may be inserted into the nostrils, and have a rope attached to them which is passed over a beam and the head pulled up.

For lifting a hind-leg, a pole, broom handle, etc., may be placed in front of that hock and behind and above the other. Two helpers take hold of ends of the pole and pull the leg upwards and backwards, at the same time steadying the animal's balance by leaning against its thighs with their shoulders. For the fore-feet it is usual to pass a rope around the cannon or above the heels and over the back to the opposite side, where it is held by an assistant. (See also TRANQUILLISERS.)

Sheep For most purposes the sheep may be turned up into a position in which it sits upon its rump, by placing the left hand round under the neck from the near side, and the right hand over the back to seize the wool of the abdomen, lifting the animal's fore-end off the ground and twisting its hind-legs from under it. In this position its feet may be dressed, its fleece may be examined, etc. It is not advisable to turn in-lamb ewes, due to the possibility of harming them or the fetus; they may be held against a wall or fence by an assistant while their feet, etc., are being dressed. Sheep stocks are sometimes used, or modern shearing tables.

Pigs The adult pig is proverbially a difficult animal to handle and restrain, especially when the handling involves pain or discomfort, but piglets are easily held by the hind-legs with the hands, while the knees grip the dependent head. With large sows and boars it is wise to remember that they are apt to be vicious with strangers, and to use a shield of wood or a hurdle to prevent a rush by the angry animal.

A method of securing a large pig is to drive it into a corner and pen it there with a door, gate, or heavy hurdle carried by 2 helpers, and held so that the pig has no room to turn while a noose is dropped over its head and pulled tight round its jaws, and another is secured to a hind-leg above the hock. The ends of these ropes are then passed round a post or a rail in the fence and pulled tight when the pig is released from its corner.

Dogs and cats These animals are usually more easily restrained than some of the larger animals because of their intimate association with man, but there are certain animals that present difficulty when angry or excited. A kind word and a caress will often be necessary to gain the animal's confidence before attempting to examine it, and, wherever possible, severe methods of restraint should be avoided except as a last resort. The human voice often exercises a degree of control over an excitable animal, and there are certain people who appear to possess the faculty of immediately gaining almost any dog's confidence and of being able to do anything with it.

However, it is always wise in any case of doubt to take no risks. The safest way of dealing with a dog is to muzzle it first. A tape muzzle may be applied; this is simply a piece of tape or a bandage about 118 cm (3 ft) long whose middle is wound round the dog's nose, the ends being crossed under the jaw and tied round the neck or on to the collar. With bulldogs, and those with a short face and a pug nose, it is better to tie the tape round the jaws, finishing with the end above the nose, tying them together there, and then passing the ends back to the collar.

Cats can be rolled in a sack or towel. With cats it is important to prevent them from using their claws, which inflict injuries more often than do the teeth. (See also under TRANQUILLISERS; ANAESTHETICS.)

Resuscitation

A basic method of pulmonary resuscitation with expired air, using a device portable and simple enough for emergency use by herdsmen and shepherds, is in use on farms. The device consists of a mouthpiece, non-return valve, flange, and mouth tube. (See ARTIFICIAL RESPIRATION; RESPIRATORY STIMULANTS; ACUPUNCTURE.)

Retention of Afterbirth
(see PLACENTA – Retained)

Reticulocytes
The penultimate stage in the formation of red blood cells. Reticulocytes are numerous in the blood only in anaemic conditions and indicate an effort of the blood-forming tissues to restore the red blood cell count to normal levels.

Reticulo-Endothelial System
This consists of macrophages, special cells present in the liver, spleen, lymph nodes and bone marrow. The system has a number of functions including the regulation of immune responses (see under ANTIBODY). It also removes disintegrating red cells from the blood.

Reticulum
The 2nd stomach of ruminants.

Retina
The innermost layer of the eye; it includes the light-sensitive rods and cones which transmit impulses to the optic nerve. Detachment of, or haemorrhage into, the retina is a cause of sudden blindness in dogs. It is often due to hypertension, the long-term effects of which may be hypertrophy of the left ventricle of the heart and kidney failure. (See EYE and EYE, DISEASES AND INJURIES OF.)

Retinoblastoma
A type of tumour which occurs on the RETINA.

Retro-
Retro- is a prefix signifying behind or turned backwards.

Retropharyngeal Abscess
Retropharyngeal abscess is the name given to an abscess occurring at the back of the throat in the region behind the pharynx. Such abscesses generally make swallowing difficult or impossible until they burst, which they frequently do into the cavity of the pharynx, whence the pus is swallowed. (See STRANGLES.)

Retrovirus
A member of the Retroviridiae, the family of viruses which includes the lentiviruses and the oncornaviruses. Retroviruses are naturally occurring gene transfer organisms. When the virus infects a cell, it is uncoated; the viral RNA is transcribed into DNA and this DNA integrates into one of the cell's chromosomes. This property could be used to produce disease-resistant transgenic animals. Certain viral groups appear to need the presence of a receptor on the cell membrane in order to gain access into the cell. Retroviruses are enveloped viruses and carry a glycoprotein on their surface; a specific interaction with this glycoprotein and the cellular receptor is a prerequisite for infection. Immunodeficiency viruses of humans, cats, cattle and primates are retroviruses.

(See table under VIRUSES; also GENETIC ENGINEERING.)

Rhabdomyolosis
Rhabdomyolosis, also called azoturia, is a breaking down of skeletal muscle in consequence of which the urine contains myoglobin. (See EQUINE MYOGLOBINURIA.)

Rhabdovirus
A group of bullet-shaped viruses which includes the rabies virus and that of vesicular stomatitis. Several rhabdoviruses are associated with disease conditions in fish.

Rhea
Ostrich-like flightless bird, native to South America. Smaller than ostrich, about 120 cm (4 ft) tall, and has 3 toes.

Rheumatism
A general term indicating a painful condition of muscles, tendons, joints, bones, or nerves; it is generally less common in animals than in humans.

Rheumatism is seen in dogs, pigs, and horses most commonly, but it can affect all of the domesticated animals. Young animals are most often attacked by the acute type, especially young pigs and puppies, and adults by the muscular form and by chronic or particular rheumatism.

For the muscular type see under MUSCLES, DISEASES OF.

Treatment There is no absolute specific, although certain drugs have enjoyed a great reputation in the alleviation of this disease, especially salicylates. Phenylbutazone has been used with reported success. (See also CORTISONE.)

Rheumatoid Arthritis
This may occur in the dog from the age of about 2 years upwards, and in cats.

Signs are at first vague; the dog appears depressed, often with a poor appetite and some degree of fever, but with no lameness. This appears later, sometimes involving several joints simultaneously, sometimes affecting one limb and then shifting to another. There may be crepitus when the limb is moved.

Diagnosis depends for confirmation upon radiography and on laboratory tests.

(See also AUTO-IMMUNE DISEASE.)

Rhinitis

Inflammation of the NOSE.

Rhinitis, Atrophic

This has been defined as the product of a severe persistent inflammatory reaction in the nasal mucosa of a growing, and therefore very young, pig, and as such is non-specific with regard to aetiology.

The generally accepted view is that in the first 2 or 3 months of life, the rapidly growing nasal structures are extremely liable to attack by infectious agents – but quite often, recovery from these is complete. In herds with severe disease, however, the condition may progress to give rise to the marked displacement or atrophy of the turbinate bones and also to an associated pneumonia.

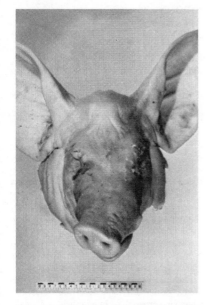

Distortion of the pig's snout as a result of atrophic rhinitis. (With acknowledgements to Professor R. H. C. Penny and the Royal Veterinary College.)

Causes *Bordetella bronchiseptica, Pasteurella multocida* and *Pseudomonas aeruginosa*, as well as inclusion-body rhinitis virus, may all be involved at some stage. Respiratory disease in the pig is a changing, developing process with many agents and factors involved; rhinitis and pneumonia often occur together.

From other sources it is known that *B. bronchiseptica* secretes a substance which inhibits the deposition or transfer of calcium salts in the infected tissues. Accordingly the bones may fail to ossify properly or may become weak and liable to distortion.

The disease in a severe form may occur only when there is a double infection with *B. bronchiseptica* and *P. multocida.*

Signs The acute form is to be found in piglets 2 or 3 weeks old, when there is no deformity of the snout to be seen and not always an overflow of tears. Sneezing is perhaps the most common symptom. The eyelids may be puffy, and sometimes the piglet has a copious discharge from its nose and breathes through its mouth. The disease can be so mild that symptoms pass unnoticed, or so severe that death occurs within a week. In some outbreaks the mortality is 10 per cent or more, and survivors suffer a growth check from the disease which continues in the subacute form.

Incidence Examination of the snouts from 2701 pork, bacon and heavy pigs killed at 5 abattoirs in England and Scotland during March to July 1974 revealed obvious atrophy of the turbinate bones in over 44 per cent and severe atrophy in over 17 per cent of the snouts examined.

Prevention Inactivated vaccines prepared from *B. bronchiseptica* and *P. multocida* are available.

Rhinopneumonitis

(see EQUINE VIRAL RHINOPNEUMONITIS)

Rhinosporidiosis

A chronic disease of the nasal mucous membrane, and associated with polyp formation leading to difficulty in breathing, caused by a fungus *Rhinosporidia seberi.* The disease occurs in cattle and horses, in the USA, South America, Australia, and India.

Rhinotracheitis, Infectious Bovine (IBR)

A disease of cattle recognised in the USA in 1951.

Cause The bovine herpesvirus 1, which can produce disease of the respiratory, reproductive, nervous and digestive systems.

Signs In America the disease is usually severe in feedlot cattle, but mild in dairy/range cattle. In Britain outbreaks of severe IBR occurred in 1978–9, causing heavy losses on some farms, with reduced milk yield, loss of appetite, fever (up to 42°C (108°F)), laboured breathing, a discharge from eyes and nose, and sometimes drooling of saliva. Reproductive disorders such as vulvo-vaginitis and orchitis have also occurred in Britain. In America abortion has followed natural infection or vaccination against IBR.

IBR is sometimes associated with a fatal pneumonia. The disease may closely resemble mucosal disease, with which at one time it was thought to be possibly identical, and also malignant catarrh.

At least one strain of the virus is neurotropic and has caused encephalitis in calves in Australia and elsewhere.

Control Live vaccines are available; depending on the product, they are given by intranasal application or by intramuscular injection.

Rhinovirus
This genus of viruses have RNA as their nucleic acid and include equine rhinovirus. They can cause upper respiratory tract infections.

Rhodesian Ridgeback
A very large, tan or redcoated dog with the unique characteristic of a strip of hair running from tail to nose along the back opposite to the normal lie of the rest of the coat. This may account for the breed being prone to sebaceous cysts in that region and to dermoid sinus. Wobbler syndrome (cervical spondylothesis) is inheritable; achalasia may also develop.

Rhodococcus
(see CORYNEBACTERIUM)

Rhododendron Poisoning
Rhododendron poisoning is not common. There are about 20 varieties which have been recorded as causing poisoning in sheep, cattle, goats, and even man. The shrubs contain a glycoside called andromedotoxin, which is the only poison capable of making ruminants vomit.

Poisoning may occur when sheep are brought in to graze former amenity land on an estate. In one outbreak, lambs were turned into a crop of rape bordered by rhododendrons, before having had time to adjust to the new diet. Fifty out of

300 lambs were found weak and salivating; 2 were attempting to vomit; 6 were recumbent; and 3 dead.

Weak tea may be helpful in countering the effects; the tannin acts as an antidote.

Rhonchi (Dry Sounds)
Rhonchi (dry sounds) sometimes referred to as 'dry rales'; continuous sounds heard during breathing by auscultation of the chest, when there is some obstruction of the bronchi. (See also RALES.)

Rhoncus
An abnormal sound detectable by means of a stethoscope and indicating chronic inflammation of a bronchial tube.

Riboflavin
(see under VITAMIN)

Ribonucleic Acid
A substance related to DNA, RNA includes the sugar ribose combined with nucleic acid. It appears to be concerned with protein synthesis within the cell. (See CELLS.) In some experiments it has been shown that RNA from malignant cells will cause normal cells *in vitro* to show characteristics of malignancy; and the converse is possible. (See VIRUSES; CANCER; GENETIC ENGINEERING.)

Ribosomes
Ribosomes are granules containing RNA. (See CELLS.)

Ribs
Ribs are the long bones which together form the cage of the thorax. Their numbers vary in the different animals, according to how many thoracic or dorsal vertebrae are present, as follows: horse, 18 pairs; ox, 13 pairs; pig, 14 or 15 pairs; dog, 13 pairs. In any of these animals an extra rib (often called a 'floating rib' because it possesses little or no cartilage to unite it to the costal arch) may be present on one or both sides of the body. The first 8 of these in the horse and ox, the first 7 in the pig, and the first 9 in the dog, have cartilages which are united to the sternum, and are called sternal ribs, while those further back in the series in each case have cartilages which do not reach the sternum, but form an arch by overlapping each other, and are known as asternal ribs. (See STERNUM.)

Each rib possesses a 'head', by which it is joined to the anterior part of the vertebra to which it corresponds in number, and to the posterior part of that immediately in front, and this is succeeded by a 'neck'; a short distance further down the shaft is a 'tubercle', which articulates with the transverse process of the vertebra to which it corresponds. The rest of the rib is composed of a long, curved, flat shaft, whose curve varies according to the position of the rib in the chest, being greatest about the middle of the series, and also according to the animal to which it belongs. Posterior to each runs the intercostal nerve and blood vessels which are situated in a little groove along the borders of each rib. In life the ribs are attached to each other by the intercostal muscles to form the continuous wall of the chest. (See BONES.)

Ricinus Communis
The plant from which castor oil is obtained.

Rickets (Rachitis)
Rickets (rachitis) is a deficiency disease of young animals characterised by a tendency towards the formation of enlarged extremities of the long bones, and a bending of their shafts. Dogs, pigs, lambs, foals, and calves are all affected, the first 2 more frequently than the other species of domesticated animals. It has also been encountered in intensively managed poultry establishments where chicks are deprived of sunlight.

Cause Rickets may be caused by a deficiency of either vitamin D or phosphorus, or in some cases both of these.

Absence of sunlight is a contributory cause and animals kept in dark buildings, especially if inadequately fed, are prone to rickets.

Often a diet consisting largely of oatmeal or maize meal, such as is commonly the lot of sheepdogs, results in rickets. (See PHYTIN.)

Signs The typical changes consist of the development of bony swellings upon the ends of the long bones of the limbs, where they meet other bones to form joints, and the production of swellings at the point where a rib joins its rib cartilage, i.e. along each side of the chest about two-thirds the way down from the spine. In puppies, there is also a tendency for the shafts of the long limb to bend in an outward direction under the influence of the weight of the body.

Treatment A vitamin D supplement is recommended or fresh COD-LIVER OIL. (See also OSTEOMALACIA.)

Rickettsia
The generic name for a group of minute Gram-negative bacteria. They will not grow in ordinary culture media, and their metabolic requirements are more akin to those of the filterable viruses.

They are distinguished from chlamydia and other bacteria by being found in the cytoplasm of arthropods such as ticks, lice, mites and fleas. (For rickettsial infections in cattle, see TICK-BORNE FEVER; Q FEVER. For tropical diseases caused by rickettsiae, see BOVINE PETECHIAL FEVER; HEARTWATER; see also ROCKY MOUNTAIN FEVER.)

Rickettsial Pox
A mild form of mite typhus transmitted to people by the mouse mite *Allodermanyosus sanguineus*, and caused by *Rickettsia akari*.

Rida
A disease of sheep involving the nervous system, similar to SCRAPIE, in Iceland.

Rideal-Walker Coefficient
Expresses the comparative efficiency of antiseptics, as based on the Rideal-Walker Test, taking carbolic acid as unity. It does not take into account the influence of body fluids upon the efficiency or otherwise of the antiseptic.

Riding Establishments Act 1963
The Riding Establishments Act 1963 sets out the standards which riding schools and similar establishments must meet to obtain a licence to operate. It empowers local authorities to select a veterinary surgeon to inspect, and report upon, a riding establishment. The decision on whether to grant a licence is based on that report. Points taken into consideration include the competence of the owner, the suitability of the accommodation, the supply of food, water and bedding, the availability of veterinary treatment, and satisfactory provisions for evacuation of horses in case of fire. Prosecution may follow if the terms of the Act, or licence, are broken.

Rifampicin
This bactericidal antibiotic has proved effective against some bacteria resistant to other antibiotics. It is sometimes used in combination with erythromycin.

Rift Valley Fever (Enzootic Hepatitis)
A disease of sheep, cattle, buffaloes, goats, camels, horses, donkeys, and man, occurring in Africa. Until 1973 it had not been recorded in northern Africa, but in that year it reached the Sudan, and then Egypt, where major epizootics occurred in 1977–8. In 1982 WHO stated that this disease might be of greater concern outside Africa than in many of the countries where it is endemic; and expressed anxiety over its possible

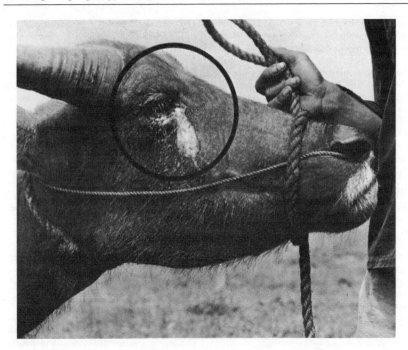

Rinderpest. This buffalo is showing what is usually the first symptom of the disease – a discharge from the eyes. (Unations.)

spread to Mediterranean and Middle East countries unprepared for it. Rift Valley fever is a NOTIFIABLE DISEASE throughout the EU.

Cause A bunyavirus, transmitted by mosquitoes. The virus causes necrosis of liver cells; also abortion.

Signs The disease is seen at its most acute in young lambs, which die within a few hours. Fever, vomiting, ataxia, and death within a day or two may occur in older lambs, calves, and occasionally adult sheep. Mild or subclinical infections also occur in adult animals. Abortion accounts for much economic loss; also a temporary halt in lactation.

Prevention A live vaccine made from the attenuated Smithburn strain of the virus was WHO approved in 1983.

Public health The human illness is like an acute attack of influenza, and sometimes there is also an encephalitis lasting 5 to 15 days, which may prove fatal. Jaundice may occur in another fatal form of the disease. Impairment of vision may be permanent as a result of inflammation of the retina.

The 1977–8 outbreaks in Egypt involved over 200,000 human cases, with nearly 600 deaths, and about 800 cases of eye disease and encephalitis, respectively.

Rig, Ridgling (Cryptorchid)
A male animal in which one or both testes do not descend into the scrotum from the abdomen at the usual time. (See also under CRYPTORCHID; MONORCHID; GELDING.)

Rigor Mortis
Temporary stiffening of the muscles several hours after death (e.g. 4 to 8 hours in the pig carcase). It is associated with the breakdown in the muscles of adenosine triphosphate (ATP), which also occurs when muscles contract during life.

Rigors
Shivering fits. When prolonged, rigors may be the warning sign of the approach of some disease or fever.

Rima
Rima is a term meaning a crack or fissure, applied to any narrow natural opening, e.g. rima glottidis, the space between the vocal cords.

Rinderpest (Cattle Plague)

Rinderpest (cattle plague) is an acute, specific, inoculable, and febrile disease of cattle, characterised by an ulcerative inflammation of mucous membranes, especially those of the alimentary tract. It is caused by a paramyxovirus. It is a NOTIFIABLE DISEASE throughout the EU.

This disease ravaged Europe intermittently for 15 centuries. In France, a very severe outbreak resulted in the government establishing the first veterinary college at Alfort in the late 18th century. Following the Great Exhibition of 1851, the UK adopted a free trade policy and rinderpest entered the country with cattle from the Baltic states. This prompted the British government to set up the Cattle Plague Department of the Privy Council, which was the forerunner of the State Veterinary Service. The last case in Britain was in 1877.

One of the most serious threats to world food-supplies, cattle plague – like foot-and-mouth disease – is caused by a virus, but one far more deadly. Indeed, when cattle plague strikes a herd, 9 out of 10 animals may die – a catastrophe which is not infrequently followed by famine – and the total loss of food and draught animals (cattle and buffaloes) from this cause is immense.

A global rinderpest eradication programme was set up by the FAO in the 1990s with the aim of eradicating the disease by 2010. By 2003, the only remaining focuses of infection were in Somalia and northern Kenya, and the goal was in sight. However, constant vigilance is needed to ensure that the infection does not spread to other countries.

Susceptibility Cattle are by far the most susceptible animals. Eland and bush pig are known to contract rinderpest, and ailing wild game may carry infection to healthy cattle. Sheep and goats occasionally become infected; and the disease may exist subclinically in sheep and goats for a time, with consequent risk of an outbreak among unvaccinated cattle.

Most pigs show only a mild fever, with some depression and anorexia; they could, therefore, act as a means of transfer of virus from contaminated meat to cattle. There is evidence that Asiatic pigs are more susceptible than those of European origin to infection with rinderpest virus, and they have long been known to be affected naturally in Indo-China. Horses are immune.

Incubation period 3 to 9 days.

Signs include fever, dullness, and loss of appetite. Soon the nasal mucosa becomes red and gives off a watery discharge which then becomes mucoid. The mouth is found to be pasty and inflamed.

Ulcers occur in front of the incisor teeth, on the gums, inside the cheeks, on the borders of the tongue, and in front of the dental pad. The epithelium comes off in bran-like scales, leaving a ragged surface. This feature of the ulcers is important as one of the distinguishing characters from the ulcers found in foot-and-mouth disease.

Constipation gives place to diarrhoea of a fetid nature, and much straining takes place. The diarrhoea is followed by dysentery. The anus becomes dilated and the mucous membrane of the rectum is exposed, appearing dark, or purple. The affected animal becomes very weak and emaciated.

In milking-cows the milk falls off. Pregnant cows usually abort at the height of the disease. The lungs are affected only in chronic cases, as a rule.

Course and duration The disease is usually acute, lasting 4 to 10 days. Outbreaks of a more chronic type do occur in some countries: these produce a greater number of recoveries. In new outbreaks of cattle plague, death may claim up to 90 per cent of the victims, while at other times the death-rate may be as low as 20 per cent.

Prevention Several vaccines are available. In continents other than Asia and Africa, quarantine measures are relied upon to exclude the disease from countries. In the event of an outbreak, immediate slaughter of all infected or in-contact cattle, sheep, goats, or other ruminants must be carried out, and all movement of stock prohibited in a given area.

Duration of immunity Cattle were immunised with a single dose of a rinderpest cell culture vaccine and maintained in a rinderpest-free environment for 6 to 11 years. They were then challenged by either parenteral or intranasal inoculation of virulent virus or by contact exposure to reacting cattle. None of the vaccinates reacted clinically and a rinderpest viraemia was never detected.

Cross-immunity Infection of dogs with the rinderpest virus apparently confers immunity against distemper.

Ring-Bones

A term used for any bony exostosis affecting the interphalangeal joints of the horse's foot, or indeed any bony enlargement in the same region: (1) high ring-bone, where the pastern joint (i.e. between the long and short pastern bones) is the seat of the disease; (2) low ring-bone, where the deposit occurs round the coffin-joint, between the short pastern bone and the coffin-bone; and (3) false ring-bone, where the enlargement occurs upon the shaft of one of the bones and does not involve the edges of a joint surface (though it may do so later). From the point of view of etymology it would appear that the term 'ring-bone' should be restricted to conditions in which a partial or complete ring of bone is formed round one or other of the joints, and that all other bony enlargements affecting the surface of the shaft of the bones, but not involving the edges of the joint surfaces, should be called exostoses. Difficulty arises, however, when examining a horse's foot, in determining exactly whether the joint surfaces are affected, or are likely to become affected, in any particular given case.

Causes Injury, inflammation of the periosteum or of the bone – sometimes following infection, possibly a vitamin D deficiency.

Signs In the early stages nothing more than a fleeting lameness is seen. Eventually the horse will go lame all day if it is worked, or becomes too lame to take out of the stable. After a time one or other of the joints becomes enlarged, and the cause of the lameness becomes obvious. It is only in the case of high ring-bones (around the pastern joint) that the exostosis can be felt; when the lower (coffin) joint is affected there is at first no outward visible or palpable sign; but after a time the hoof alters in shape, becomes distinctly bulged or 'buttressed' at the coronet. This latter effect is due to the fact that in low ring-bone the extensor or pyramidal process of the coffin-bone is usually involved, and the deposit of bone upon it pushes the coronet, and the wall which grows from it, in an outward direction ('pyramidal disease'). At times the alteration in the outline of the hoof is not by any means regular; it may be bulged at any point from one heel to the other, denoting a deposit of bone wherever there is a bulge.

In 'true ring-bone' the joint that is affected almost always ends by becoming stiff (ankylosed), owing to fusion between its complementary bones and obliteration of the joint having occurred. In this state the horse may become fairly sound, because the pain occasioned by movement at the joint has disappeared, but the gait will always be stiff.

Treatment Prolonged rest in a loose-box or, preferably, at grass is indicated. More harm than good results when blistering is carried out. Corticosteroids may be used.

Ring Vaccination

A disease-control process by which susceptible animals in a prescribed area surrounding an outbreak are vaccinated. It is used, for example, in the control of foot-and-mouth disease where there is no slaughter and eradication policy. Vaccination is begun at the perimeter of the areas, progressing inwards towards the centre. For success, diagnosis, typing of virus and the vaccination itself must all be speedy.

Ringer's Solution

Ringer's solution consists of sodium chloride, 9 grams; calcium chloride, 0.25 g; potassium chloride, 0.42 g per litre.

'Ringwomb'

This is the colloquial name for a condition which sometimes complicates lambing, and is due to failure of the cervix to dilate. Usually, the *os uteri* will admit 1 or 2 fingers, which can feel what seems like a firm ring.

The shepherd may recognise the condition on seeing a small portion of fetal membrane protruding from the vulva. The ewe remains in good health (but does not lamb) until death and decomposition of the fetus occur.

Manual dilation of the cervix is practised by some veterinary surgeons. Should this prove impossible, Caesarean operation is the only alternative. (See UTERUS and PARTURITION.)

Ringworm

A contagious skin disease caused by the growth of certain fungi, which live either upon the surface of the skin or in the hairs of the areas affected. Ringworm may affect any of the domesticated animals, but it is probably commonest in young store cattle when they are enclosed in buildings during winter, and in pet cats and kittens. Dogs and horses are also frequently affected, but the disease is not often seen in the sheep and pig in the UK.

Ringworm and favus in the domesticated animals are caused by parasitic fungi which belong to the family Gymnoascidae.

Lesions generally Ringworm appears in the form of patches of dry, raised, crusty skin, from the surface of which the hairs have fallen and upon the surface of which there are scales or scabs. The patches are often more or less circular, but in bad cases large irregular areas may be produced, which result from the coalescence of adjacent areas. Favus is a type of ringworm

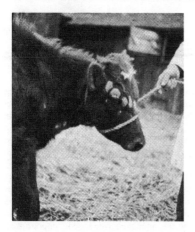

Ringworm.

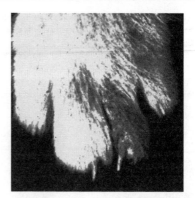

A bare scaly patch on a kitten's toe due to ringworm.

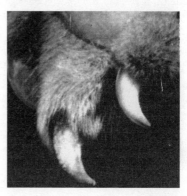

The roughened appearance of an infected claw. *Microsporum canis* Bodin was responsible.

in which the lesions have cup-shaped depressions which bear some similarity to a honeycomb, from which they get their name (*favus*, honeycomb). Favus affects the dog and cat, the mouse and rat, rabbits sometimes, and fowls occasionally.

Horses Ringworm may be due to parasites belonging to the genera *Trichophyton* or *Microsporum*. In cases due to the former, the first affected areas are usually confined to the head, neck, withers, and sometimes to the root of the tail. The hair becomes matted in patches about the size of a large coin, and in the centre of each patch appears a bare area from which the hair has fallen off; this gradually extends until the whole area is denuded. The skin becomes raised and scurfy, and greyish-white crusts are formed; at times there may be grey or yellow scales adherent to begin with, but becoming detached later. There is usually little or no itchiness, except when due to *T. mentagrophytes*.

When the horse is affected with ringworm due to *Microsporum* parasites, practically any part of the body may be attacked.

Cattle Ringworm is nearly always due to *T. verrucosum* infection. It is very common among young animals in autumn, winter, and early spring, especially if they are kept indoors. The head and neck are most often affected, especially the eyelids, lips, ears, and above the jaws, but it may occur anywhere on the body. The lesion begins as a raised ring-like patch on which the hairs stand erect. In a day or so the hairs fall off, and the surface of the skin becomes covered with masses of scales heaped up into a greyish-white or greyish-yellow crust. The areas are usually very numerous and often

become confluent, so that large areas become bare of hair and present roughened, crusty, hard, dry surfaces with a tendency towards pronounced wrinkling of the skin around and between them. Where calves are extensively affected with ringworm there is always a good deal of loss of condition and itchiness.

Sheep When they are affected the fleece becomes matted, and falls out in circular patches over the shoulders, neck, and chest. *T. verrucosum* is one cause. Control is by isolating affected animals and disinfecting troughs, etc.

Dogs Ringworm may be caused by one of 4 genera: *Trichophyton, Microsporum, Oidmella,* or *Oospora,* the last-named causing favus. The lesions produced by the first three of these are very similar in all respects to those seen in horses and cattle. In favus caused by *Oospora canina* the lesion appears as a raised circular patch upon whose surface there is a pale yellow

R

crust with little depressions (honeycomb) scattered through it. The skin in such cases is often very much thickened.

Hedgehogs Caused by *T. erinacei*, this infection may cause lesions on the face of dogs where the skin has been damaged by the hedgehog's spines.

Cats Ringworm is of 3 kinds: due to *Trichophyton, Microsporum* and *Achorion*, the latter producing favus. When due to the first two of these, the symptoms and lesions are similar to those seen in other animals. (See ONYCHOMYCOSIS.)

Cats become infected from mice with mouse favus (*A. quickeanum* or *A. arlongi*), although it may also be due to *A. schoenleinii* – the favus of man. The lesions are chiefly confined to the fore-paws and the head and the neck, though they may spread to other parts of the body. Itchiness is usually absent. The areas affected vary in size from that of a pin's head up to a 5p piece or so, and are not always regular in outline. The skin is thickened and the edges are raised. When newly formed, the covering crust is yellow and soft to the touch, but when old it is grey and powdery. The characteristic cup-shaped depressions are seen in most cases, but when affecting the claws they may be absent.

Ringworm due to *M. canis* Bodin is of public-health importance. It is often overlooked by owners, but children are readily affected.

Cats, especially Persians and other longhairs, may be 'carriers' of ringworm fungus. In a survey involving 200 selected cats seen at a veterinary clinic, none of them showed any sign of ringworm. Fur samples taken with a brush showed that 39 per cent of the 200 were carrying spores of ringworm fungi. (In 72 samples the spores were those of *M. canis*.) A survey in England of fur samples taken at 4 cat shows revealed that, overall, 35 per cent of longhairs were carrying *M. canis* spores.

Decontamination of households is important for human health after ringworm has been diagnosed. Hypochlorite, benzalkonium chloride, and glutaraldehyde-based compounds are recommended.

Favus in the fowl, due to *T. gallinae*, affects the comb, wattles, and other parts of the fowl's head.

If the condition spreads down to feathered parts, the feathers become dry, brittle, and break off at the surface of the skin, leaving large bare areas. There is always a most disagreeable odour from fowl favus.

Treatment Oral administration of griseofulvin is by far the simplest method. Cattle and

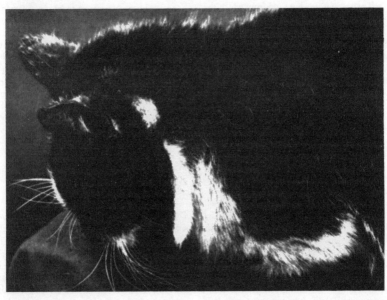

Ringworm in the cat: whitish, scaly lesion can be seen to the right of the ear, above the white fur.

horses can be given a supplemented feed. This makes possible group treatment, and avoids handling of infected animals – thus reducing the risk of infection being transferred to man. However, it is inadvisable not to use griseofulvin in pregnant animals. In a cat which could not tolerate griseofulvin, a thiabendazole (see ANTHELMINTICS) dip was successfully used.

Natamycin and enilconazone which are used as a wash or spray can be applied to infected cattle and horses with a knapsack sprayer. Ketaconazole, applied as a shampoo, may be used to treat dogs.

Otherwise, treatment consists, in the first place, of removing the hair from around the lesions, collecting it and burning it. There are many suitable dressings to choose from: e.g. gentian violet solution; undecylenate ointment; and copper naphthenate lotion, which has given rapid and good results in the treatment of ringworm in cattle. A vaccine for use in cattle is available.

Dressing should be carried out twice a week for a fortnight for cattle and horses, and by then most of the fungus will be killed. The cases should not be considered cured until there is a level crop of new hair over each of the areas. For the smaller animals it is better to use the dressing once every 2nd day.

In all instances it is very important to remember that ringworm spreads from the centre outwards, and edges and margins of the areas should be especially well dressed.

Vaccination of calves against *T. verrucosum* involves 2 intramuscular doses, 10 to 14 days apart.

In Russia the vaccination of racehorses, and other horses taking part in competitive events, is compulsory.

Public health Ringworm is readily transmissible to human beings, so precautions such as hand-washing and disinfection after contact with known infected animals should not be neglected. Dettol is useful for these purposes.

Diagnosis Microscopic examination or culture methods. (See also WOOD'S LAMP.)

RNA
(see RIBONUCLEIC ACID)

Road Accidents
Dogs and cats struck by cars may suffer chest injuries in addition to limb injuries. (See FRACTURES; ACCIDENTS; DIAPHRAGMATOCELE; HYDROTHORAX; PNEUMOTHORAX.)

Roaming
Roaming is a behavioural habit in certain male dogs and cats. If the animal does not respond to training from an animal behaviourist, it may be castrated – although there is no guaranteee that this will stop the habit.

'Roaring' in Horses
An abnormal sound made when the horse breathes in; the usual cause has for long been regarded as vibration of the slackened vocal folds on one or both sides of the larynx, due to paralysis of the muscles which move the arytenoid cartilages outwards. (For treatment and further details, see LARYNX, DISEASES OF – Laryngeal paralysis.)

Rock Salt
(see SALT – Salt licks)

Rocky Mountain Fever
Also called Rocky Mountain spotted fever, this is a disease of man caused by *Rickettsia rickettsii*. Wild animals provide a reservoir of infection.

Rocky Mountain fever affects human beings usually between March and July. The onset of fever is sudden, and in 2 to 5 days a rash appears over the whole body, including the palms of the hands. The rash changes to a sort of mottling – petechiae, scattered over the skin, which gives the condition its name of 'spotted fever'. The infection is transmitted by ticks, especially *Dermacentor andersoni,* the Rocky Mountain wood tick.

Dogs The infection causes fever, abdominal pain, depression, loss of appetite, nystagmus, with sometimes conjunctivitis and petechial haemorrhages in the mouth. Oedema of a limb(s) is common, and the scrotum and prepuce may be similarly affected. Over 30 cases are confirmed serologically each year, with many more being diagnosed, in Long Island, New York.

Diagnosis is most reliably confirmed by the immunofluorescent test. Treatment is by antibiotics, e.g. tetracycline.

Precautions There is a risk to veterinarians taking a blood sample or carrying out a post-mortem examination, as the rickettsia is present in the blood during the acute phase.

Rodent Ulcer
In human medicine this term is reserved for carcinoma of the skin, but is sometimes misapplied by animal-owners to EOSINOPHILIC GRANULOMA or LICK GRANULOMA.

Rodents

Rats and mice are important from a veterinary point of view on account of the diseases which they may transmit to domestic animals. For examples, see AUJESZKY'S DISEASE; SALMONELLOSIS; LEPTOSPIROSIS; RINGWORM; FOOT-AND-MOUTH DISEASE. In countries where the disease is present, rodents may transmit RABIES.

Zoonoses Members of the family Muridae (Old World rats and mice) can infect man with plague, tularaemia, listeriosis, pseudotuberculosis, erysipelas, leptospirosis, brucellosis, melioidosis, murine typhus, Q fever, scrub typhus and other rickettsioses, histoplasmosis, lymphocytic choriomeningitis, Lassa fever, rabies and other viral infections, Asian schistosomiasis, Chagas disease, rat-bite fever, and HANTAvirus.

Rodenticides In the UK brodifacoum was cleared by MAFF (for indoor use only) in 1984; and difenacoum had also been scrutinised under the Pesticides Safety Precautions Scheme. (No incidents linking barn owl deaths with these two rodenticides had been reported in the UK.)

A calciferol preparation, Rodin C (Rentokil) – claimed to be effective against warfarin-resistant rats – had earlier received MAFF approval. (See also WARFARIN.) ALPHACHLORALOSE is used for the same purpose.

A rodenticide containing vitamin D_1 caused the death of 2 dogs.

Signs Weakness, anorexia, vomiting and passing blood.

Accidental poisoning of domestic animals has occurred from some of the above, and also from others banned in the UK, e.g. RED SQUILL; THALLIUM; ANTU; THIOUREA; PHOSPHORUS; FLUOROACETATE; barium salts; zinc phosphide; STRYCHNINE.

Romagnola

An Italian breed of cattle, white in colour, and reared for beef. Romagnolas have been imported into the UK.

Rompun

Proprietary name for XYLAZINE.

Rose Bengal Plate Test

A simple and quick screening test used in the diagnosis of brucellosis in cattle. Sera giving positive results may then be tested by means of the Serum Agglutination Test and Complement Fixation Test.

Rostral

Towards the nose or front end of the body.

Rostral teeth are the incisors and canines.

Rotavirus

So-called because of its resemblance to a wheel. Responsible for causing diarrhoea in the young of many species – children, foals, calves and piglets. It has been shown that, in piglets, only the pig and calf rotaviruses cause diarrhoea, although the human and foal rotaviruses can replicate in the pig.

Research at the Moredun Institute led to a method of diagnosis based on the direct detection of the viral nucleic acid, which comprises 11 molecules of double-stranded DNA. This method is 'rapid and as sensitive as ELISA'.

A vaccine Rotavec K99 (Schering-Plough) was introduced in 1986, following research at Moredun, to protect calves against rotavirus (and also K99 *E. coli*). The vaccine is used to immunise cows in late pregnancy, producing enhanced antibody levels in the colostrum; this is given to calves at the rate of 2.5 to 3.5 litres daily for the first 2 weeks of life.

Rotenone

The insecticidal principle of derris root. Rotenone is highly poisonous to fish and is used deliberately for removing coarse fish from enclosed waters before establishing trout fisheries.

Rothera's Test

A test for ketones in milk or urine; a modified version requires the following reagent: ammonium sulphate, 100 g; anhydrous sodium carbonate, 50 g; sodium nitroprusside, 3 g.

If the bottom half-inch of a test-tube is filled with this powder, and a little of the fluid to be tested runs down the side of the tube, a red colour will develop after 3 or 4 minutes if ketones are present, as with acetonaemia.

Roughage

By this is meant food of a bulky and fibrous nature, such as hay and straw. These have a low water-content, and are in a sense the opposite of succulents, e.g. kale, silage. (See also DIET AND DIETETICS – Fibre.)

Rottweiler

A large powerful breed developed as a guard dog in Germany. The breed is prone to deafness and retinal dysplasia; hip dysplasia may also be a problem.

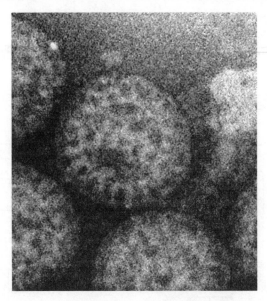

The rotavirus. (By courtesy of the AFRC.)

Rough Collie

A rough-coated medium-sized dog with an elongated face and nose, orginally developed as a sheep-dog. The breed is prone to cleft palate, corneal dystrophy, deafness, epilepsy and umbilical hernia. Central progressive retinal atrophy is a dominant trait; collie-eye anomaly is a recessive trait. Patent ductus arteriosus may be inherited, as may neutropenia.

Rouleaux

Rouleaux is the term applied to the columns into which red blood cells collect as seen under the microscope. The appearance somewhat resembles a pile of stacked coins.

Round Heart Disease

In chickens, this occurs only on some types of deep litter. The cause is not known, but litter from affected houses can transmit the disease to healthy chickens. Sudden death occurs; on post-mortem examination, the heart is firm, bright pink in colour, barrel shaped and with a dimple at the apex. Replacement of the litter stops mortality.

In turkeys, the disease is more common in the small white strains. It causes sudden death in birds in apparently good condition. There appears to be a genetic factor.

Roundhouse

A type of circular farrowing pen devised in New Zealand. It consists of a circle of hardboard, about 2.4 m (8 feet) in diameter and 1.2 m (4 feet) high, bolted to a light iron framework and fitted with an internal creep rail. A smaller circle, about 1 m (3 feet) in diameter, made partly of hardboard and partly of tubular rails, is fitted eccentrically within the larger one, and the whole is fastened with bolts to the concrete floor of the piggery. The smaller circle, which is warmed by an infra-red lamp, acts as a creep for the piglets, while the sow is kept in the space between the 2 circles. Because of the shape of this space, the sow invariably lies in the same position, with her udder towards the piglet's creep. This gives the piglets the maximum degree of safety.

Roundworms (Nematoda)

Most nematodes lay eggs, but some produce living larvae. The life-history may be direct or indirect, i.e. an intermediate host may be necessary.

Nematodes can be the cause of anaemia, wasting, gastroenteritis, bronchitis and pneumonia, aneurism, convulsions and blockage of the intestine. Some are of public health importance. (See TRICHINOSIS; TOXOCARA.)

Horses

1. **Stomach** Two species of *Habronema* (*H. muscae* and *H. microstoma*), and *Drascheia megastoma*, inhabit the stomach of Equidae in various parts of the world.

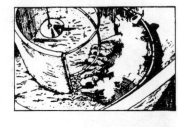

The New Zealand pen: a drawing showing the position which the sow voluntarily assumes, and, below, a plan for the pen's construction. (See entry for Roundhouse.)

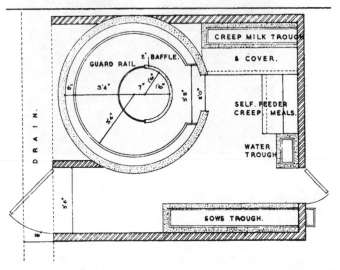

The worm larvae are passed in the horse's faeces; swallowed by maggots, and continue through the pupal and adult stages of the stable-fly or house-fly; finally the larvae become located in the fly's proboscis. When the fly settles near a horse's mouth, the larvae enter it, and reach the stomach. However, if the horse has a wound, some of the larvae will be attracted to that, and give rise to the cutaneous or orbital form of habronemiasis, 'summer sores' or 'bursati'.

Habronemiasis is common in the tropics and subtropics, but has also been seen in the UK. Hard nodules or granulomas may form on the skin or at the inner canthus of the eye.

D. megastoma forms nodules, in which it lives, in the stomach. *Habronema* worms may penetrate the gastric mucosa and become embedded causing gastritis, thirst, colic and pica.

Trichostrongylus axei, seldom more than 8 mm long, also causes gastritis. This worm also inhabits the duodenum.

2. **Small intestine** *Parascaris equorum* is the common large roundworm of the horse. The female may be up to 50 cm long. Pica, colic and unthriftiness may result from heavy infections, which may also lead to partial blockage of the intestine.

The larvae, which migrate to the lungs after hatching in the stomach, are capable of causing a catarrhal bronchitis or broncho-pneumonia; and possibly some damage to the liver also, during their migration through that organ.

Strongyloides westeri is another worm found in the duodenum, and a cause of diarrhoea in foals. This and other worms of this genus may also cause broncho-pneumonia.

3. **Caecum and colon** *Strongylus*. Three species are important.

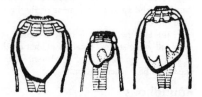

Strongylus (head). (Left to right) *S. edentatus,*
S. vulgaris, S. equinus.

S. (Delafontia) vulgaris is a cause of verminous arteritis, or thrombosis, affecting the cranial mesenteric artery. (See EQUINE VERMINOUS ARTERITIS.)

S. (Alfortia) edentatus produces nodules in the peritoneum. If very numerous, the larvae may cause peritonitis, bleeding, and anaemia. After 2 or 3 months they return to the large intestine and become adult worms.

S. equinus. The larvae of this large worm also produce nodules in the caecum and colon, and later migrate to the liver and pancreas.

Oxyuris equi. The female worm comes to the end of the rectum to deposit its eggs, which are ejected as a yellowish or greenish mass surrounding the anus. Resulting pruritus can lead to emaciation in severe cases, and more usually to unsightly bare patches on the tail and hindquarters.

4. Lungs *Dictyocaulus arnfieldi* is the cause of a verminous bronchitis which may be recognised by a cough and, if the worms are numerous, by loss of appetite and emaciation.

'Demonstration of the presence of larvae in the faeces is sufficient to confirm the presence of infection in donkeys, but even if respiratory symptoms are present, this finding should not be allowed to obscure the more likely possibility that other causal agents are involved. Diagnosis of infection in horses may be very difficult. Recovery of larvae from faeces will identify the "silent carriers" but most horses have very low larval output and several examinations may be necessary. Most cases of clinical disease, in horses, are seen during the prepatent phase and larvae will not therefore be present in the faeces. Most infected horses, although showing respiratory signs, do not develop patent infections. It is therefore important not to exclude lungworm as a possibility just because it is not possible to recover larvae from the faeces. Naturally acquired infections are known in which larvae were not recovered from horses with clinical respiratory signs extending for more than a year. Complete recovery followed specific lungworm therapy. While an association with donkeys is added circumstantial evidence on which diagnosis can be based, infection may be transmitted from horse to horse in the absence of a donkey contact. This frequently occurs on thoroughbred studs.'

The efficacy of orally administered ivermectin against induced *D. arnfieldi* infection was evaluated in a controlled study comprising 12 yearling ponies. Treatment with ivermectin paste, orally once, was 100 per cent effective against both adult and immature or inhibited stages of the horse lungworm.

5. Connective tissue *Onchocerca. O. reticulata* is found in the horse, especially in tendons. It is common near the suspensory ligament, but is also reported in the withers. They may cause no symptoms, or may induce hypertrophy of the tendon or may cause fistulous withers. *O. cervicalis* occurs in the *ligamentum nuchae* of equines, and is often associated with poll-evil.

6. Skin *Parafilaria multi-papillosa* (*Filaria haemor-rhagica*) is found in intermuscular tissue or under the skin. The female worms penetrate the latter to lay their eggs on the surface, where hard nodules subsequently develop, and these open and bleed.

Haematobia flies in Russia, and *Drosophila* in tropical regions, transmit the worm larvae.

7. Nervous system The larvae of *Setaria equina* invade the central nervous system of horses in Asia, causing epizootic cerebrospinal nematodiasis. This is characterised by paralysis, and the disease may prove fatal.

The adult worm, milky-white, lives in the peritoneal cavity. Transmission is by mosquitoes.

8. Eyes *Thelazia lachrymalis* causes conjunctivis (and sometimes keratitis too). (See EYEWORMS.)

Cattle, sheep and goats

1. Oesophagus and stomach *Gongylonema.* Two species occur in ruminants and 1 in pigs. They are found just below the epithelium in the thoracic third of the oesophagus. The intermediate hosts are various species of dung-beetles.

Haemonchus contortus. This is the large stomach worm or 'barber's pole' worm of ruminants, so-called because of the female's spiral red and white stripes. The male is red. It is a trichostrongyle, with a length of about 30 mm and the thickness of a pin. It is a voracious blood-sucker, and inhabits the abomasum. It can cause serious anaemia and unthriftiness, especially in lambs.

H. placei is another of several species.

Ostertagia worms, which are of considerable economic importance, are peculiar in that while most infective larvae living in the abomasum moult twice to become adults, some – especially perhaps those ingested by the calf during late summer and autumn – moult only once and remain as 4th-stage larvae in a dormant state. These dormant larvae are unaffected by many anthelmintics but are usually, though not always, susceptible to ivermectin, fenbendazole and albendazole. Later they develop into adults causing a winter outbreak of gastroenteritis. Calves should therefore be dosed in September and moved to 'clean' pasture.

Also known as the small brown stomach worm, *Ostertagia* cause severe irritation of the mucous membrane by the formation of nodules. Infested animals may lose weight, scour, and become anaemic.

2. Small intestine *Ascaris vitulorum.* This large round worm of cattle is generally of little importance, but it may be a frequent and fatal parasite of calves in certain localities.

Nematodirus. This is a common trichostrongyle genus found in large numbers in the small intestine of sheep. It is a very slender form under 2.5 cm long. In recent years nematodirus infestation has caused severe losses.

The infestation is a 'lamb-to-lamb' one, and can be avoided – where practicable – by confining lambs to pasture which carried no lambs in the previous 2 seasons. *Nematodirus* species found in Britain are *N. filicollis, N. helvetianus, N. spathiges,* and *N. battus. N. helvetianus* and *N. battus* are parasites of calves. (See PASTURE, CONTAMINATION OF.)

Cooperia species are important. They are usually present in association with other species of worms, e.g. *Ostertagia, Trichostrongylus.* They seldom cause anaemia, but are responsible for weight loss and scouring. *Trichostrongylus* worms are very small (only 2 to 7 mm long) and inhabit the abomasum and duodenum.

Bunestomum (hookworms) live in the small intestine. The larvae may either enter their host via the mouth or penetrate the skin. They suck blood and accordingly cause anaemia and sometimes oedema under the throat. (See HOOKWORMS.)

Oesophagostomum. This is a genus of strongyle worms related to the horse forms, and found in ruminants and pigs. They are about 2.5 cm long. They are the cause of nodular disease of the intestine ('pimply gut'). If present in small numbers, the only result is to render the intestine unfit for sausage skins. If in large numbers, the symptoms are anaemia, emaciation, diarrhoea, and oedema. The disease in this case often has a fatal termination.

Trichuris. This genus of whip-worm occurs in the caecum of various animals, but is usually of little importance. The worms have very slender

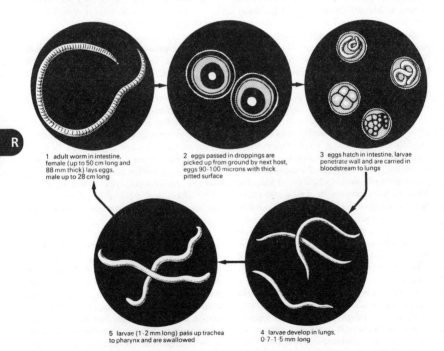

1 adult worm in intestine, female (up to 50 cm long and 88 mm thick) lays eggs, male up to 28 cm long

2 eggs passed in droppings are picked up from ground by next host, eggs 90-100 microns with thick pitted surface

3 eggs hatch in intestine, larvae penetrate wall and are carried in bloodstream to lungs

5 larvae (1-2 mm long) pass up trachea to pharynx and are swallowed

4 larvae develop in lungs. 0·7-1·5 mm long

Life-cycle of the large roundworm of the horse, *Parascaris equorum.* (Reproduced with permission from H. T. B. Hall, *Diseases and Parasites of Livestock in the Tropics,* Longman.)

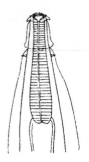

Oesophagostomum (head-end).

necks with stoutish bodies. The necks are threaded through the mucous membrane of their host.

They may cause inflammation at the point of insertion of the head and may admit bacteria.

Strongyloides worms are found in the small intestine, often deep in the mucosa. Scouring is caused in heavy infestations. The worm larvae can enter the body via the skin.

3. Lungs *Dictyocaulus.* Three species are known in cattle, but only 1 is important – *D. viviparus,* which causes a form of bronchitis. The male is about 4 cm long and the female about 7 cm. Eggs hatch in the lung, and the larvae climbing up the trachea are swallowed, passing to the exterior with the faeces. After moulting twice, they reach the resistant infective stage, and can live thus on pasture through the winter. When swallowed, they continue their development.

The signs and treatment are described under PARASITIC BRONCHITIS.

Parasitic bronchitis ('husk') Several species of roundworm occur in sheep and goats.

Dictyocaulus filaria is the largest and most common species. The male is about 5 cm long and the female 8 cm. The infective stage is reached in about 10 days. Apparently lambs can be infected prenatally. This worm is cosmopolitan in its distribution. Its life-history is direct.

The symptoms are those of a verminous bronchitis, sometimes complicated by bacterial infection, but otherwise similar to those in cattle.

Protostrongylus (Synthetocaulus) rufescens is a red and much smaller form. The male is about 2 cm and the female 3 cm long. It is found mainly in Europe. These worms live in the bronchioles and in the pulmonary parenchyma, and cause a verminous lobular pneumonia. The eggs cause a diffuse nodular pneumonia. Cough

is less prominent than in the above form, but breathing is difficult.

4. Connective tissues *Onchocerca.* Several species occur in cattle in various parts of the world. They are the cause of 'worm nodules'.

The nodules are found mainly in the brisket, but also occur in the flank and forequarters. They appear to cause little harm to their host, but as the capsule is a product of inflammation, beef containing worm nodules is condemned, and in Australia they have caused considerable loss in the export trade.

Dracunculus. Only 1 species of this worm is found in the domestic animals, *D. medinensis,* the 'guinea worm'. It is found in India, Africa, and South America. The female is of considerable length, but is generally recovered from the host in small pieces. It is milky white in colour, smooth and without markings. Nearly the whole of the worm is occupied by the uterus, packed with coiled-up embryos. The worm occupies a subcuticular site, as a rule in the extremities, with the head-end projecting to the exterior. The larvae are released by a prolapse of the uterus through the cuticle of the worm. They escape into the water, and are swallowed by a cyclops in which they develop. The cyclops is in due course swallowed in the drinking water by a suitable host – practically any of the domestic animals will do – and larvae are released by the digestive juices and proceed to their adult habitats. The worm may give rise to local abscesses, and sometimes affects the feet of dogs.

5. Eye *Thelazia.* (See EYEWORMS.)

Pigs

1. Stomach The most important worm here is *Hyostrongylus rubidus.* Its life-cycle is direct. (See also THIN SOW SYNDROME.) The latter may sometimes be due to various species of *Oesophagostomum* worms. (See OESOPHAGOSTOMIASIS.)

2. Small intestine *Ascaris suum.* This worm is a very common parasite of pigs in all countries.

The eggs have a remarkable vitality, and have been kept alive for as long as 5 years. The egg, in a few weeks after passing to the ground, develops an embryo, but this does not hatch until the egg is swallowed. When this happens, the larva, which is about 0.25 mm long, bores through the intestine, reaches the bloodstream, and is carried through the liver and heart to the lungs. Here it remains for some days, but it finally climbs up the

R

trachea and is swallowed. The larva which leaves the lung has grown to about 2.5 mm in length. In the intestine it continues its development, taking about 2½ months to do so.

In passing through the lungs a certain amount of bleeding is caused, and if the larvae are numerous, pneumonia results. During this period the animal shows the symptoms known as 'thumps'. If it survives the lung symptoms, it often fails to grow properly and remains small and stunted.

Macrocantorhynchus hirudinaceus is found in the small intestine of pigs. It is a whitish worm, the male being 5 to 10 cm long, while the female is 20 to 35 cm long. The neck is thin and the posterior region stout. The intermediate stages are found in beetles.

The parasite may cause a catarrhal enteritis or even actual perforation with peritonitis.

Trichuris suis, the pig whip-worm, causes mainly subclinical disease in temperate climates, but in the tropics it may cause dysentery, anaemia, and even death. In the Americas up to 85 per cent of pigs may be infested; in some areas of the UK, from 75 per cent. *Trichuris* occurs in the caecum.

Treatment in the pig includes oxibendazole, fenbendzole and thiophanate.

3. **Lungs** In pigs 2 species are common, both belonging to the genus *Metastrongylus*. The male is about 2 cm and the female about 4 cm long. Both species are common in Europe and America, and may occur in the same pig. They cause a verminous bronchitis and sometimes pneumonia. Young animals are more susceptible and may die from it. Both species are carried by earthworms.

4. **Muscles** *Trichinella spiralis*. This is a small worm found in the intestine. The female produces living larvae (0.1 to 0.16 mm long) which migrate through the mucosa, reach the bloodstream, and are carried to various muscles. Here they pass into a cystic stage (the cyst being formed by the host), in which they remain until they are swallowed by some flesh-eating host or until they calcify and degenerate. In the intestine of the new host they reach sexual maturity and produce a new lot of larvae, which in turn migrate to the muscles.

The normal hosts are carnivores (dogs and cats). Rodents may be infected, and rats can be a source of infection to pigs. Man may be infected from the pig. (See under TRICHINOSIS.)

5. **Kidney** *Stephanurus dentatus* is a thickish worm of fair size, the male being nearly 3 cm long and the female a little larger. It is found as a rule in the kidney fat of pigs, but also occurs in the liver and other locations in these animals and in ruminants. It is found in America and Australia, and is responsible for considerable damage. Its life-cycle is similar to that of the hookworms. Thiabendazole, fenbendazole and ivermerctin have proved effective in controlling this parasite.

Dogs and cats

1. **Oesophagus** *Spirocerca lupi* is found in nodules in the oesophagus and, less frequently, the stomach of the dog, in all hot countries and in Europe.

It is a reddish worm. The male is 3 to 5 cm long. The intermediate hosts are various beetles and cockroaches.

The disease is often undiagnosed during life, but in countries where it is common the presence of the worm may be suspected from a frequent cough followed by repeated vomiting. Death from exhaustion may result.

Damage to the carotid artery by *S. lupi* worms (3 in each of 2 nodules attached to the oesophagus) led to the death in the UK of an Alsatian from internal haemorrhage. This parasite appears also to be closely associated with sarcoma of the oseophagus.

2. **Stomach** A microscopic gastric nematode of cats, *Ollulanus tricuspis*, has been found in the Americas, Australasia, and Europe. The worm causes unthriftiness and vomiting in kittens.

3. **Small intestine**

Ascarids include several species that occur in dogs and cats. In cats the species seem to be *Ascaris tubaeforme* and *A. braziliense*.

Hookworms in dogs Two species of hookworm are found in dogs: *Ancylostoma caninum* and *Uncinaria stenocephala*. The latter is found in Britain. These are smallish worms, about 2.5 cm long, found in the small intestine.

Eggs are passed to the exterior in the faeces and hatch in the soil or water. After several moults, the resulting larva becomes infective, and is able to gain access to the host either in the food or by penetrating the unbroken skin. It enters the bloodstream and is carried to the lungs. It then passes up the trachea and is swallowed. It completes its development in the small intestine, where it becomes mature.

4. **Caecum** The whip-worm *Trichuris vulpis* occurs in the UK, and gives rise to diarrhoea/dysentery, loss of condition and a harsh, staring coat.

5. **Heart** *Dirofilaria*. There are 2 species occurring in dogs and cats. *D. immitis* occurs in the heart of the dog and occasionally the cat. The female may reach a length of 30 cm, but the male is little more than half this size. It is found in Asia and, of recent years, in Britain. The embryos are hatched in the body of the female, and the young larvae, passed into the bloodstream, are sucked up by a mosquito in which they develop. After a certain period they escape from the fly, when it attacks another dog, and entering the blood are carried to the heart, where they complete their development.

The worms interfere to a greater or lesser extent with the circulation. No symptoms may be shown; or the dog may suddenly die. Other symptoms include anaemia, respiratory troubles, ascites, etc. Various complications may be due to emboli, such as cough, dyspnoea, etc. Diagnosis is by demonstration of the microfilaria in the blood.

Another heartworm of the dog is *Angiostrongylus vasorum*, which has, as intermediate hosts, slugs and snails. This worm, which has caused an outbreak of infestation in kennels in Ireland, lives in the pulmonary artery and the right ventricle of the heart. Symptoms include malaise, stiffness on running, and subcutaneous swellings (due to suppression of normal blood clotting by the parasites). Some lung damage may be caused; likewise anaemia.

(See also under HEARTWORMS.)

6. **Kidney** *Dioctophyme renale*. The kidney worm of dogs and wild carnivores is very large, reaching 1 m in length, and is a blood-red colour. It is found in Europe and the USA. It occurs in the pelvis of the kidney, and occasionally destroys the kidney tissue, to leave only the wall as a cyst filled with a purulent fluid. The other kidney usually shows a compensatory hypertrophy. It is occasionally found in the bladder. Infestation follows the eating of raw fish.

The worm's eggs are barrel-shaped and may be seen in the urine, under the microscope.

7. **Bladder** In the UK the bladder-worm *Capillaria plica* is rare, and seldom gives rise to obvious symptoms. A severe infestation can lead to inflammation of the bladder and a mucoid discharge from vagina or prepuce. In cats cystitis may, rarely, be caused by *C. feliscati*.

8. **Trachea** *Oslerus (Filaroides) osleri* occurs in the UK and gives rise to a sporadic but persistent cough, especially on exercise or if the dog is excited. Retching may be caused. Severe infestation can give rise to emaciation despite a fair appetite, laboured breathing, sleeping standing, and death in young dogs. For control, thiabendazole has given promising results.

Another tracheal worm, *Capillaria aerophilia*, seldom gives rise to obvious symptoms.

9. **Lungs** A minute worm lives in the lungs of cats in Britain and elsewhere in Europe and America. It may cause a fatal form of parasitic pneumonia. The parasite (*Aelurostrongylus abstrusus*) is transmitted to cats by mice. In Africa, *Bronchostrongylus subcrenatus* is found.

Lung lesions found at the autopsy of 5 out of a batch of 20 beagles were due to *Filaroides* species, 'probably *F. milksi* rather than *F. hirthi*'. The lungs had the appearance of being peppered with black spots. Signs of larval migration were seen microscopically in the liver, mesenteric lymph nodes, and gastrointestinal tract.

Poultry Roundworms more commonly occur in free-range systems where it is also difficult to ensure that all birds can be treated. There may be no obvious clinical signs but breeding flocks (chickens and turkeys) often show reduced hatchability.

Public health aspects (see under TOXOCARA)

Rous Sarcoma of Chickens
This is produced by a virus. (See under CANCER.)

Royal Army Veterinary Corps (RAVC)
It has a long and honourable history. An Army Veterinary Service was established in 1796; this became the Army Veterinary Corps in 1906, the title of 'Royal' being bestowed in 1918.

A History of the RAVC 1796–1919 was compiled by Major-General Sir Frederick Smith KCMG, CB, a former Director-General, Army Veterinary Services, and published by Baillière, Tindall & Cox. A 2nd volume, by Brigadier J. Clabby, was published in 1963 by J. A. Allen & Co.

Royal College of Veterinary Surgeons (RCVS)
Belgravia House, 62–64 Horseferry Road, London SW1P 2 AF. The governing body of the veterinary profession in the UK. (See also REGISTER.)

-Rrhaphy

-Rrhaphy is a suffix meaning an operation in which some opening or tear is closed by stitches.

Rubarth's Disease (Hepatitis Contagiosa Canis)

This is named after the Swedish scientist Rubarth who, in 1947, described for the first time a disease in dogs which he called, on account of its contagious nature and the damage caused to the liver, *Hepatitis contagiosa canis*. This is now commonly known as CANINE VIRAL HEPATITIS. He regarded this disease, on the basis of the microscopical findings, as identical with fox encephalitis, which had been known in America for some 17 years previously.

Rubber Bands

These sometimes get, or are put, on to the legs of cats (and possibly dogs), where they may remain unnoticed until the continual pressure has destroyed the skin beneath the band and caused damage to the underlying structures. Gangrene or loss of use of the limb results.

A successful prosecution has followed the application of rubber bands to cows' teats in the UK.

Rubber rings have been used for castration of lambs and calves, and for the docking of lambs. (See ELASTRATOR, etc.)

'Rubber Jaw'

A condition seen in the dog in some cases of chronic nephritis. It may be associated with enlargement of the parathyroid glands. Softening of the bones of the skull, particularly the jaw, occurs, and in a severely affected part the bone can be cut with a scalpel. There is resorption of bone and its replacement by vascular fibrous tissue. 'Rubber jaw' is not, of course, seen in all cases of chronic nephritis, though some changes may be detected microscopically.

Rumen

The 1st stomach of ruminants. It lies on the left side of the body, occupying the whole of the left side of the abdomen and even stretching across the median plane of the body to the right side. It is a capacious sac which is subdivided into an upper or dorsal sac and a lower or ventral sac, each of which has a blind sac, at its posterior extremity. These divisions are defined by the presence of grooves on the outside of the organ and by pillars or ridges internally. The whole organ is lined by mucous membrane which possesses a papillated, stratified, squamous epithelium containing no digestive glands, but mucus-secreting glands are present in large numbers. Its entrance is through the oesophagus, and its exit is into the reticulum or 2nd stomach through the rumeno-reticular orifice.

Coarse, partially chewed food is stored and churned in the rumen until such time as the animal finds circumstances convenient for rumination. When this occurs, little balls of food are regurgitated through the oesophagus into the mouth, and are subjected to a second, more thorough mastication. Each bolus is chewed 30 to 60 times and mixed with copious amounts of saliva, to be swallowed and passed onwards into other parts of the compound stomach.

In rare instances, the rumen may be situated on the right-hand side.

Rumen Flukes

Belonging to the genus *Paramphistomum*, these are found in both the tropics and North America.

Conical in shape, round in cross-section, they inhabit not only the rumen but also the reticulum, and – when immature – the duodenum. They are also found occasionally in the bile ducts and urinary bladder.

Little damage is caused to the rumen, but in young animals a severe enteritis is the important aspect of the disease, resulting in diarrhoea, unthriftiness, anaemia, and sometimes death.

Paramphistomum flukes have a life-history similar to that of the common liver-fluke *Fasciola hepatica*; several species of snails being the intermediate hosts.

Rumen, Ulceration of

In calves, ulcers in the rumen may be associated with lesions of the liver caused by *Bacteroides* (*Fusiformis necrophorus*), or with BVD infection. (See also STOMACH, DISEASES OF.)

Rumenotomy

Opening the rumen via the left upper flank for the purpose of emptying the contents.

Ruminal Digestion

In the rumen, bacteria break down the cellulose (which forms the structural materials of plants), and starch by means of enzymes, and convert them into fatty acids. The bacteria fall a prey to the protozoa which, besides digesting starch, thus perform the useful task of converting plant protein into animal protein. This becomes available to the cow when the protozoa are, in their turn, destroyed further down the digestive tract and themselves digested.

A sample taken from the rumen, at the Hannah Research Institute, contained 100 million protozoa and 5 million bacteria (giving some idea of the proportion of the two). Examples of protozoa included *Entodiniomorph* species, which feed on plant material, bacteria, and each other; and *Holotrich* species, which ferment soluble sugars from plants and feed on bacteria. (See also under, DIET AND DIETETICS – Fibre; LACTIC ACID.)

Ruminal Tympany
(see BLOAT)

Rumination ('Cudding')
Rumination ('cudding') is the process whereby food taken into the stomachs of ruminants is returned to the mouth, subjected to a second, more thorough chewing, and is again swallowed.

The act occurs at intervals of from 6 to 8 hours, and occupies a longer or shorter time according to the nature of the food and the amount taken at the last meal. It usually commences about half an hour after feeding ceases, and probably continues until all the coarser constituents have been re-chewed, or at least until the animal is disturbed. This fact is of considerable importance practically; cattle and sheep should be allowed at least 2 hours' rest after feeding before they are subjected to any severe exertion. Disregard of this is a fruitful contributory cause of stomach disorders in both cattle and sheep. (See also under RUMEN.)

The act of regurgitation appears to be in reality a complex one, but it may be briefly summarised as follows:

(1) The tension of the oesophagus relaxes, partly by dilatation, and partly through an inspiratory movement of the diaphragm (the glottis being temporarily closed), which reduces pressure in the thorax.

(2) The rumen and the reticulum powerfully contract and squeeze upon their contents.

(3) The abdominal muscles contract and raise the intra-abdominal pressure.

The direct result is that ingested foodstuffs are forced from the area of high pressure (i.e. the rumen and reticulum) through the open oesophagus into an area of lower pressure (i.e. into the thoracic portion of the oesophagus). When a small quantity, sufficient to form a bolus or 'cud', has entered the oesophagus, the lips of the oesophageal groove and the muscles in the vicinity close the terminal part of the oesophagus, and there commences an antiperistaltic movement which conveys the 'cud' upwards past the closed glottis, underneath the soft palate, and so into the mouth. Excess fluid is immediately squeezed from the mass and swallowed, and chewing movements commence at once. Each bolus is chewed 30 to 60 times according to its consistency, size, and to the nature of its constituents; coarse straw or hay fodder requiring the longest time. The chewing occupies from 30 to 90 seconds, and then the bolus is rolled up by the dorsum of the tongue and again swallowed. In from 3 to 6 seconds another bolus has reached the mouth, and so the process is continued.

'Run-back'
This must be avoided by means of back fences. (See under STRIP GRAZING.)

Runch
(see CHARLOCK POISONING)

'Runners'
This is an old, popular term for hounds unable to gallop properly. 'Runners' are usually recognised as such when they return to hunt kennels at about 7 months old after being walked; and they are then often culled from the pack. Technically, the condition is known as osteochondrosis of the spine. Symptoms include poor muscular development in the spinal region, poor bodily condition, an unnatural gait, and often inability to jump a fence successfully negotiated by the rest of the pack. Some curvature and rigidity of the spine may also be observed. It seems that this is, in part at least, an inherited defect of foxhounds.

The term is also applied to young budgerigars affected by French moult.

Runt Pigs
Runt pigs can be reared in special nursing units designed for runts and excess piglets in a litter. Runt pigs and underweight babies have similar biochemical and physiological abnormalities.

Runting and Stunting Syndrome
A condition of economic importance in poultry production. Clinical signs include pallor of the skin, decreased skeletal density, lameness, late development of plumage, distortion and bending of quills or primary feathers and orange-coloured mucus in the droppings, along with particles of undigested food. The problem

occurs sporadically and tends to last for abou a year on the farm before any improvement is seen. Retroviruses, enteroviruses and other viral agents, as well as anaerobic bacteria, have all been suspected as the cause. Disappearance of the syndrome over much of the USA coincided with the use of reovirus vaccines.

Rupture

Rupture is a popular name for HERNIA. The term is also applied to the tearing across of a muscle, tendon, ligament, artery, nerve, etc. Rupture of the aorta is a cause of death in male turkeys at 5 to 22 weeks old.

Russian Gad-Fly

(*Rhinoestrus purpureus.*) This attacks horses in Europe and North Africa.

Russian Spring-Summer Virus

Russian spring-summer virus causes an encephalitis of man and goat, caused by a virus and transmitted by the tick *Ixodes ricinus* in Russia, Poland, the Czech Republic and Slovakia.

Rye-Grass

Rye-grass poisoning has caused the death of cattle and horses restricted to grazing rye-grass pasture (*Lolium perenne*). In New Zealand and Australia, a fungus present on the rye-grass may cause facial eczema. A staggering gait – and convulsions – may occur in cattle and sheep on rye-grass pasture giving rise to the colloquial name 'rye-grass staggers'. In a UK outbreak in sheep, they had 'a rocking-horse gait, and when chased fell down and trembled violently'. (Veterinary Investigation Service report.) Fungal toxins are the cause of 'rye-grass staggers' in both the UK and New Zealand. The rye grass is infected with a seed-borne enfophytic fungus, *Acremonium lolii*, containing the alkaloid loitrem B. (See also CEREBROCORTICAL NECROSIS.)

R

Sabulous
Gritty, sandy.

Sacks
Sacks may be a means of passing infection from one farm to another, for when empty they are put to many uses. Poisoning has occurred through contamination of feeding-stuffs by sacks previously used for sheep-dip. For these reasons, non-returnable paper sacks have advantages over jute sacks.

Sacrum
The part of the spinal column lying between the lumbar region and the tail. It consists of 5 vertebrae in the horse and ox, 4 in the sheep and pig, and 3 in the dog and cat, fused together in each case. It is roughly triangular in shape in all animals, and forms the roof of the pelvic cavity, lying midway between the 2 'points of the hip' or 'haunch bones'.

Saddle-Sores
Saddle-sores are formed through uneven pressure upon the back by some part of the saddle. They may be found in the middle line, immediately over the upper ends of the spinous processes; they may occur on either side of the middle line where the fore-arch of the saddle-tree presses; or they may be found just behind the elbow, when they are caused by badly fastened girths, and are often called 'girthgalls'.

The injuries consist of raw areas from which the hair has been rubbed or chafed off and, later, ulcers. Alternatively, patches of the skin, varying in size from 2.5 cm in diameter to almost 7 cm, may become hard and leathery, pus being formed underneath. These are known as 'sitfasts'.

Treatment Attention must first of all be paid to the saddles. They should fit evenly all over the back, and the stuffing or padding should be adequate to protect the skin from pressure by the rigid framework of the saddle-tree. The hollow of the arch of the saddle should never press upon the middle line of the back, and the girth should never be fastened with the skin folded under it. Rest from work will be necessary. (See ULCER; WOUNDS.)

Sagittal
A structure or section running transversely across the trunk or a limb.

Sainfoin
(*Onobrychis sativa*) A leguminous forage crop which fixes its own nitrogen; it contains tannins, so its rumen protein degradability is low (this means that the protein is used more efficiently); and it does not cause bloat. Voluntary intake by animals is high – intakes of sainfoin can be 25 per cent higher than that of ryegrass. Furthermore, it is drought-resistant.

Unfortunately, sainfoin does not grow as well as bred strains of grasses, clovers and lucerne; 30 per cent less yield than lucerne is quoted.

St John's Wort
This plant, *Hypericum perforatum*, which may be present in hay, does not lose its poisonous character when dried. It causes LIGHT SENSITISATION in cattle, sheep, and pigs, especially in Australia.

St Louis Encephalitis
Transmitted by mosquitoes, and caused by a flavivirus, this disease occurs in North and South America, affecting wild birds, bats, horses and man (in which it may cause encephalitis and death in the elderly, although only fever in other people).

Salicylic Acid and Salicylates
Originally derived from the willow (genus *Salix*), salicylic acid and its salts have long been used in pain relief. ASPIRIN, which is acetylsalicylic acid, largely replaced the other salicylates as pain relievers (see ANALGESICS), and has been given in fevers. It must be used with extreme caution in cats, which metabolise aspirin very slowly. A standard 250 mg tablet given daily to a cat may prove fatal in 12 days.

Salicylate poisoning has occurred in young animals following overdosage. Symptoms include depression, loss of appetite and vomiting. Treatment involves the use of an emetic or gastric lavage and respiratory stimulants.

Saline
(see under NORMAL SALINE)

Salinomycin
An IONOPHORE used as a coccidiostat in chickens, and also (outside the UK) as a growth-promoting feed additive for pigs. Its use had to be phased out within the EU by January 2006.

Salinomycin poisoning Four hundred point-of-lay turkeys died within a week after the introduction of a diet containing 50 ppm salinomycin.

In horses the signs of poisoning are eyelid-swelling, anorexia, colic, weakness, ataxia.

Salivary Glands

Salivary glands include the parotid gland, lying in the space below the ear and behind the border of the lower jaw; the submaxillary gland, lying just within the angle of the lower jaw, under the lower part of the parotid; and the sublingual gland, which lies at the side of the root of the tongue. Each of these glands is paired, so that actually there are 6 glands, not all of which function at the same time.

Salivary Glands, Diseases of

Calculi and tumours may occur. In rabies, the salivary glands must become infected before transmission of the virus to another host can occur through a bite. (See also MUMPS.) A foreign body, such as a grass seed, may cause an obstruction to one of the ducts, particularly in the dog.

Salivary-gland tumours in dogs and cats are rare. The majority of 138 tumours in dogs (81) and cats (57) involved animals of 10 years of age or more, were malignant and of epithelial origin (84 per cent). Local recurrence after excision occurs frequently, and metastasis to regional lymph nodes and beyond is common.

Salivation

'Foaming at the mouth', to use a colloquial but apt expression, is seen in the dog, e.g. in an epileptic or other fit. (See FITS.) 'Drooling of saliva' is seen in the dog with a bone wedged across the roof of its mouth, or in a cat with a needle embedded in its tongue – or in cases of RABIES in all species.

Salivation is a symptom of CHOKING, of almost any painful condition of the mouth or tongue, and of poisoning (e.g. by benzoic acid in the cat), arsenic, lead, phosphorus and organophosphorus compounds; see also TOAD.

Salivation is also an important symptom of FOOT-AND-MOUTH DISEASE, and of other diseases and conditions mentioned under MOUTH.

Salmincola

Parasites on the gills of salmonid fish which affect respiration. Affected fish show reduced growth and delayed sexual maturity.

'Salmon Poisoning' in Dogs

'Salmon poisoning' in dogs occurs on the Pacific coast of the USA, and is the result of eating salmon or trout infested with the fluke *Troglotrema salmincola*, containing a rickettsia. The latter, *Neorickettsia helminthoeca*, produces a haemorrhagic gastroenteritis which is usually fatal unless antibiotics are used in time.

Salmonellosis

Infection with organisms of the salmonella group is of importance from 2 distinct aspects: (1) food poisoning in man; and (2) disease in domestic animals.

Salmonella poisoning – routes of infection (see diagram)

In cattle and calves Salmonellosis and brucellosis have 4 points in common – both diseases are important from the public health point of view; both can lead to abortion in cattle, to a carrier state likely to perpetuate infection on the farm, and to considerable financial loss to the farmer.

While the salmonella group of bacteria includes more than 1000 different serotypes, the 2 of most importance to the dairy farmer are *Salmonella dublin* and *S. typhimurium*. Either can produce acute or subacute illness in adult cattle and in calves.

S. typhimurium infection is of greater public-health importance, and is a notorious cause of outbreaks of food poisoning in man. *S. typhimurium* type 204C has been a major source of problems in calves bought from markets and is highly resistant to antibiotics. An outbreak of this same infection involved more than 200 cows on a single farm, and led to the death or slaughter of 29 of them.

S. typhimurium 104 also has a relatively high resistance to antibiotics. It can result in severe illness and deaths in small groups of cows or calves; it is the second most common salmonella in food poisoning.

S. dublin infection may be associated with abortion, sometimes without any other symptoms being observed. Animals which recover may excrete the organisms for years. Besides this carrier state, which may keep infection on the farm, there is also a latent carrier state in which the organism remains dormant within the animal until it is subjected to some stress or superimposed disease, when excretion of the organism occurs and fellow members of the herd become infected.

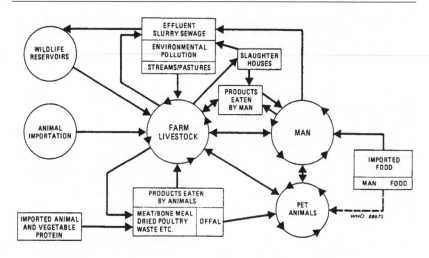

Salmonella poisoning – routes of infection. (With acknowledgements to World Health Organisation, Technical Report No. 774.)

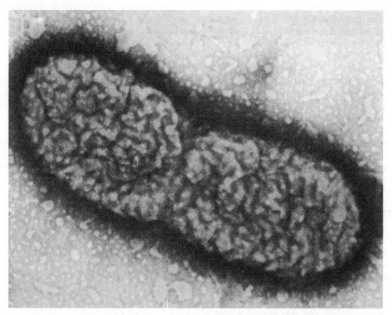

An electron-micrograph of *Salmonella dublin*. (Magnification × 50,000.) (Reproduced by courtesy of the Department of Veterinary Preventive Medicine. University of Liverpool.)

Signs The 2 infections are usually very similar and can be distinguished only by laboratory tests. In the acute form of the disease, the cow becomes dull, feverish, goes off her food, and the milk yield suddenly drops. Scouring is usually severe, and the animal may pass blood and even shreds of mucous membrane from the intestine. Death may occur within a week. If treatment is delayed, mortality may rise to 70 per cent or so; whereas early treatment can bring the death rate down to 10 per cent. In animals which recover, scouring may persist for a fortnight, and it may be several weeks before the cow is fit again.

The subacute form in adult cattle runs a milder course and, indeed, the infection may exist without any symptoms being shown. A latent infection may become an overt one following stress of any kind or when another disease becomes superimposed – sometimes masking the symptoms of salmonellosis itself. A liver-fluke infestation may be a precipitating factor.

Salmonellosis may run through 8 calves out of a batch of 10, and kill 4 of them. Some calves collapse and die without ever scouring; others become very emaciated as a result of persistent scouring. Pneumonia, arthritis, and jaundice may be among the complications; occasionally the brain is involved, giving rise to nervous symptoms.

S. typhimurium infection seldom persists from one season to another on any particular farm because there are fewer 'carrier' animals than there are with *S. dublin*; it is often brought on to the farm by calves bought in from markets and suffering from the effects of stress, rough travelling conditions, lack of food or a change of diet. The infection occurs in many species of animal including, as the name suggests, mice.

S. dublin infection arises mostly from other cattle. It can be spread from farm to farm via slurry and streams. Infection may enter even a closed herd if it is grazing flooded pasture land.

Lack of shelter, overcrowding, dirty surroundings, and faulty feeding have all been implicated in outbreaks. In adult cattle, the fortnight after calving is regarded as a danger period, especially where the calving has been a difficult one.

S. dublin can survive in slurry for at least 12 weeks.

It is also known that salmonella organisms can survive for 6 months or so in dung and litter, and *S. dublin* can survive for up to 307 days, if not longer, on dung splashes on a wall, so that thorough cleaning and disinfection of buildings are necessary, and reliance must not be placed on a simple 'resting period' between batches of calves.

Salmonella organisms may be present in domestic sewage, and river pollution from this source has led to outbreaks of salmonellosis in cattle.

Preventive measures include trying to keep rats and mice off cattle feed, avoiding pig and poultry effluent for organic irrigation, having piped drinking water for cattle, and not buying in through markets or dealers but rather from farms with a known health record. The earlier housing of cattle in the autumn may help, and it is important not to neglect liver-fluke infestation which can sometimes act as a 'trigger' to outbreaks of salmonellosis in which the infection was hitherto latent.

Treatment Drugs used include antibiotics, potentiated sulfonamides and sulfadimidine. A range of vaccines and antisera-vaccine combined preparations is available for prophylaxis and therapy. They usually contain *E. coli*, *Pasteurella* and *S. typhimurium* and *S. dublin* strains.

In sheep *S. typhimurium* has caused diarrhoea and abortion. *S. agona* has caused abortion, death of ewes from septicaemia, death of lambs within a week of birth, and sometimes diarrhoea. *S. dublin* is likewise a cause of abortion and diarrhoea.

One outbreak in an upland sheep flock was characterised by rapid spread and heavy mortality in ewes and young lambs. Clinical signs included diarrhoea and abortion. Abomasitis (inflammation of the abomasum) was the most striking and consistent post-mortem lesion. Vaccination was the only control method that was apparently successful. Infection also occurred in the cattle, farm personnel, and a dog.

(See also ABORTION – Ewes.)

In pigs The term 'salmonellosis' is now usually reserved for a severe septicaemia. *S. cholerae suis* causes this; symptoms include fever, huddling together, purple discoloration of ears, unsteady gait, and sometimes scouring. The

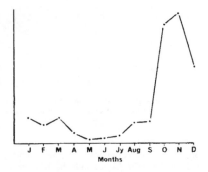

Seasonal incidence of salmonellosis. (With acknowledgements to the *British Veterinary Journal*.)

same organism may give rise to a chronic infection with scouring. The organism can infect man.

Infection with *S. dublin* sometimes occurs in pigs, and may give rise to dysentery.

More common is infection with *S. typhimurium*. This causes fever, scouring, vomiting, and unsteady gait – usually in younger pigs than the first-named organism. Sulfadimidine has proved useful in treatment.

In horses *S. typhimurium* has caused serious outbreaks of illness in young horses. Horses may also be symptomless carriers of this infection. In 1976 an outbreak of *S. newport* infection caused the death of many horses in the UK. (See also FOALS, DISEASES OF.) Outside the UK, *S. abortus equi* is a cause of abortion in mares.

Stress, associated with the hospitalisation of horses, is said to have led to acute enteritis, often from *S. senftenberg*.

In dogs Illness may be mild, with fever and malaise; or there may be severe gastroenteritis and death. Many salmonella serotypes infect dogs. It is possible for a dog to become a symptomless carrier of *S. typhimurium* and to infect man.

Feeding raw offal to dogs had been suspected as an important source of salmonellosis in Berlin. Accordingly, 408 samples of edible offal (liver, lungs, heart, bovine rumen, and porcine oesophagus) were examined bacteriologically. It was found that 231 samples (57 per cent) were infected with salmonella. *S. typhimurium* was the most prevalent of 24 serotypes.

In cats Infection with *S. enteritidis* and *S. typhimurium* may be set up following the catching of infected rats and mice. For this reason cats should not be allowed to lie on uncovered food-stuffs. Cats may also become infected through eating contaminated meat.

In poultry As a specific disease, salmonellosis is rare except in broilers, although it is involved in numerous other disease conditions. Over 50 members of the salmonella group have been isolated from poultry in the UK, and several have caused outbreaks of disease in broiler plants. (See PULLORUM DISEASE; FOWL TYPHOID.)

Arthritis, due to a variant strain of *S. pullorum*, gives rise to a mortality of 5 per cent or so, as a rule, but in one outbreak 200 deaths occurred in a 1000-bird unit. Apart from lameness and swelling of the foot and hock joints, symptoms include poor feathering and under-

development. Death can be expected between the ages of 10 days and 5 weeks.

It was found that survivors did not react to a blood test carried out with standard *S. pullorum* antigen, but reacted strongly to antigen prepared from the variant strain. This probably accounts for carrier birds having remained undetected in the past.

During a 5-year period, birds in 144 flocks in Sweden were given cultures of caecal contents as a means of controlling salmonella infection by the competitive exclusion technique. In all, 2.86 million birds were treated and it was concluded that this treatment was associated with a reduction in salmonella infections. No adverse effects were reported.

Salmonellae will remain alive for periods of up to 6 months or more in dung and litter. Therefore such material should be stacked so that heating occurs; no animals should have access to the heap.

As mice may play a significant role in maintaining *S. enteritidis* infection in flocks, rodent control and disinfection of housing may be effective in dealing with the problem.

A vaccine prepared from *S. enteritidis* phage type 4 is available (Salenvac; Intervet).

In ducks Salmonella species sometimes cause a high mortality in ducklings. Fatal cases of human food poisoning have occurred as a result of infected ducks' eggs.

In geese *S. typhimuriam* may be found in goslings, affecting only the eye; the vitreous body is totally destroyed.

Public health As already mentioned, salmonellosis is an important cause of food-poisoning in man, often leading to serious illness. Numerous instances linking food-processing with outbreaks have been investigated. *S. seftenberg* has been linked with isolates from human beings and a poultry processing plant. *S. kiambu* and *S. enteritidis* were isolated from frozen turkeys from the same batch which caused 64 cases of illness in people. *S. panama* and *S. brandenburg* were similarly isolated from abattoirs/processing plants and human beings.

S. agona is a public-health problem in the USA, the UK, the Netherlands, and Israel. In each country the original source of the infection was Peruvian fish meal used in animal feeds. It has been demonstrated that animal feeds can play an important role in the transmission of salmonellosis to man.

Unpasteurised milk is another source of human salmonellosis. A 65-year-old woman was infected in this way, and was ill with diarrhoea and meningitis. After her death a brain abscess was found. Both the latter and meningitis are 'rare complications of salmonellosis in man'. Seventeen other people were ill with salmonellosis from drinking the unpasteurised milk.

Viable salmonellae were found in the meat fraction of domestic refuse from 120 houses. This source could provide a reservoir of infection accessible to wild animals. Tipping should be carefully controlled, and refuse covered immediately.

The protective gloves, worn by a veterinary surgeon while calving a cow, unfortunately burst. Within 48 hours numerous non-pruritic papules had appeared over both arms, especially the upper arm, where the gown cuffs had chafed the skin. The papules developed into pustules which burst and resolved in approximately 10 days without treatment. No other symptoms were observed.

A pustule was swabbed and a pure growth of *Salmonella* species was recovered.

(See also under SAUSAGE.)

Saloliths

These are CALCULI, found mainly in STENSON'S DUCT of horses.

Salpingitis

Salpingitis is inflammation in the Fallopian tubes or oviducts, sometimes the cause of sterility in cattle. (See INFERTILITY.)

Salt

A chemical substance in which a metal is substituted for the hydrogen of an acid.

Sodium chloride (common salt) (NaCl) is an essential ingredient of body fluids.
Sodium depletion results, ultimately, in circulatory collapse.

Salt is an appetiser, and commonly incorporated in animal feeds in carefully measured proportions. Ruminants will avidly consume salt; any excess is harmlessly excreted in the urine and faeces.

Salt licks It has been suggested that a 500-kg (10-cwt) cow needs 30 g (1 oz) of salt a day for maintenance and a further 3.5 g (⅛ oz) for 4.5 litres (1 gallon) of milk produced. Therefore, a 3200-litre (700-gallon) cow requires about 14 kg (30 lb) of salt yearly.

On some pastures, or under some systems of management, cattle may not obtain sufficient salt. To obviate this danger, salt licks are commonly provided. In some salt licks traces of iodine are incorporated, together with other trace elements such as copper, manganese, cobalt, and magnesium. (See 'LICKING SYNDROME'.)

Salt Poisoning

Salt poisoning has been reported in both pigs and poultry. It is essential that pigs are not kept short of water, or given food that is too salted.

An outbreak, reported from Scotland, involved piglets aged 6 weeks brought indoors from field arks at weaning. A proprietary meal was fed dry. The water bowls in the house were not very accessible, and some of the piglets were not strong enough to depress the levers. Two days after being housed, 23 out of the 32 piglets were showing symptoms of salt poisoning, and some died.

Signs Often a number of pigs are found dead without signs having been observed, the remainder being weak and very thirsty. Vomiting and diarrhoea may occur. (For other signs, see under MENINGOENCEPHALITIS.)

In poultry, adult birds show excessive thirst and diarrhoea, with sometimes cyanosis of the wattles, somnolence, and sudden death. In young birds gasping and ascites may occur.

Samoyed

A medium-sized breed of dog characterised by thick straight cream or white hair. Like the chow-chow, they tend to be 'one-person' dogs. Haemophilia has been recorded; pulmonic stenosis may be inherited.

Sand

Horses on the seashore or along tidal mud flats learn that the sand contains salt, and may lick up large quantities of it in their endeavour to get the salt. The signs set up are chiefly those of COLIC with impaction.

Cattle feeding on the seashore take in quantities of sand, which in some cases may be so great as to hinder the movements of the rumen (where the sand always collects), and, by upsetting digestion, may cause unthriftiness and even emaciation.

Sand Tampan (Ornithodorus Savignyl)

(see TICKS – Family Argasidae)

Sandcrack

Sandcrack is a pathological condition affecting horses' feet, in which a deep fissure or crack forms at some part of the wall of the hoof, extending downwards from the coronet, and usually involving the whole of the thickness of the wall.

Causes Anything which interferes with the proper nutrition of the horn at the coronet predisposes to sandcrack, the actual splitting of the horn occurring as the result of the strains put upon the foot. Treads on the inside of the coronet, occasioned by hurried turning when at work, are frequent causes in the fore-feet, and continual pressure on the coronary matrix by the 2nd phalanx, especially when the toes have been allowed to grow too long, appears to be the commonest cause in the hind-feet. A predisposition to sandcrack may be inherited.

With all cases it is advisable to place the animal under veterinary care. (See HOOF REPAIR.)

'Sandflies'
(see under FLIES)

Sanguineous
Sanguineous means containing blood.

Santa Gertrudi
This breed of cattle are ⅝ Shorthorn and ⅜ Brahman in origin.

Saponins
These are natural detergents, present in some plants such as corncockle and soapwort. Saponins contain a sugar and a steroid-like compound, and with water form a lather. Poisoning by them results in gastroenteritis. The central nervous system may also be affected, with consequent paralysis. Saponins break down red blood cells. In the USA the leaves and nuts of the tung tree, grown for the sake of its oil, can cause fatal poisoning.

Saprolegnia
A fungus that can infect fish. It is sometimes found as a secondary infection to another condition such as ulcerative dermal necrosis in salmonids, and autumn aeromonad disease in adult brown trout. The infection can be controlled by bathing the fish in zinc-free malachite green but the healing process is prolonged. In a salmon hatchery, it is important to remove dead and infertile eggs as these can be invaded by the fungus and passed on to healthy eggs.

Sarco-
Sarco- is a prefix signifying flesh or fleshy.

Sarcolemma
The membrane covering each voluntary (striated) muscle fibre.

Sarcocystis
A genus of protozoal, coccidian parasites having a 2-host life-cycle. Carnivorous animals such as dogs, cats and foxes ingest the cysts when eating infected flesh of cattle, sheep, pigs and horses. Human infection also occurs, and sarcocystis is a zoonosis (see ZOONOSIS).

While the cysts in the intermediate host's muscles may not have any serious effect upon health, the second-generation schizonts are certainly harmful – damaging the endothelium of blood vessels, and causing serious illness in many cases.

Signs Cattle showed loss of appetite, fever, anaemia, and wasting, after ingesting sporocysts from canine faeces, and some cattle died within 33 days. Sarcocystosis has also killed sheep. In horses, signs of central nervous system damage may be seen, as well as signs of muscle inflammation, resulting in lameness.

Prevalence In Europe 61 per cent of slaughtered cattle have been found to be infected. In Germany a prevalence rate of 5 per cent in pigs has been recorded.

Human sarcocystosis may give rise to abdominal pain, diarrhoea, fever, tachycardia, and an increased respiratory rate.

'Sarcoid'
A tumour which resembles histologically a sarcoma (see CANCER), but which is regressive in character, disappearing within a matter of months. It has the appearance of a reddish button, raised about 0.30 mm (⅛ in) above the surrounding skin. It affects the dog.

A fibroma-like sarcoid is perhaps the most common tumour of equines, especially older ones, occurring on limbs or head. Believed to be caused by a virus, the equine sarcoid commonly ulcerates and recurs following surgery. Cryosurgery may be tried, or a BCG vaccine; the latter may be more successful in donkeys. A guarded prognosis should be given.

Bovine papillomavirus is involved in the process by which sarcoids develop from normal equine fibrous tissue.

Sarcoma
(see CANCER)

Sarcoptes
Sarcoptes are members of a class of parasitic acari, which cause MANGE in animals and man.

Sarcoptic mange occurs in cattle, horses, sheep, pigs, and dogs – also in man, when it is called scabies – and is caused by the parasitic mite *S. scabei.* (See MANGE.) Cats are only very rarely infected.

Sarcosporidia, Sarcosporidiosis
(see SARCOCYSTIS)

Sars
A form of AVIAN INFLUENZA that is transmissible to man, often with fatal results. Outbreaks occured in several Far Eastern countries in 2004; many poultry flocks were destroyed in an attempt to prevent the disease from spreading. Fears that migrating wild fowl would carry the SARS virus to Western Europe led ??? consider preventive measures.

Sausage
Discarded portions of sausage, or sausage-skin, can be a source of infection when fed, unboiled, to pigs, etc. Foot-and-mouth disease has been transmitted in this way. African swine fever and swine fever could similarly be spread by this means. (See SWILL.)

The incidence of salmonella-contamination of pork and beef and pork sausages taken from a large factory during the course of production was 65 and 55 per cent respectively. The salmonella serotypes isolated (in descending order of incidence) included *Salmonella derby, S. dublin, S. newport, S. stanley, S. typhimurium, S. heidelberg, S. infantis* and *S. agona.*

Savaging of Litters by Sows
Various causes of this have been suggested, including: an inherited tendency; absence of any straw for nesting purposes; a painful udder; insufficient time to have become used to her farrowing quarters; and fright resulting from the use of a farrowing crate. (See PIGS, SEDATION OF.)

Sawdust
(see under BEDDING and MASTITIS)

Sawflies
Four-winged insects which have a saw-like ovipositor. The larvae can cause poisoning if swallowed.

Sawfly poisoning This affects both sheep and goats.

Cause The larvae of the birch sawfly (*Arge pullata*).

Signs Depression, anorexia, muscular incoordination with a difficulty in rising to their feet.

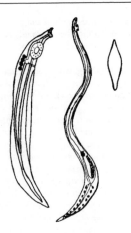

Schistosoma, o, μ, and egg.

Autopsy Findings Liver necrosis, petechial haemorrhages, and sometimes degeneration of the kidney tubules.

Scabies
A common name for sarcoptic mange. (See under MANGE – Sarcoptic mange.)

'Scad'
A colloquial name for a transitory lameness, in sheep, which may follow frost. (See 'SCALD'.)

'Scald'
Inflammation between the digits of young sheep resulting from infection by *Bacteroides nodosus*; it causes acute lameness. Its onset is said to be associated with frosts and frosty. Recovery may occur spontaneously under dry conditions. The term is vague, however, and has been used to include the non-progressive 'benign' form of foot-rot. It has to be differentiated from foot-and-mouth disease. (See also 'SCAD'; OVINE INTERDIGITAL DERMATITIS.)

Scalds
(see BURNS)

'Scaly Leg'
(see MANGE – Mange in fowls)

Scanner, Body
A device utilising computer tomography to produce an image of a section of the whole body. (See X-RAYS.)

Scanning
(see RADIOISOTOPES)

Scaphoid

The name given in human anatomy to a small bone present in the carpus and tarsus. In the racing greyhound, fracture of the right hind scaphoid is a common accident. Treatment has included the removal of bone fragments and the successful insertion of a plastic 'scaphoid'.

Scapula

The scapula is the shoulder blade – the large, triangular, flat bone that lies on the outside of the front of the chest, to which are attached many of the muscles that unite the fore-limb to the trunk.

Scheduled Diseases

(see under NOTIFIABLE DISEASES)

Schistosomiasis

Infestation with *Schistosoma* worms or flukes, which are also known as bilharzia worms. They inhabit the portal and mesenteric veins mostly, one species preferring veins of the urinary bladder, and another the veins of the nose. Cattle and sheep and virtually all domestic animals, and man, may become infested.

Several species have been reported from mammals in India, Africa, and Europe. *S. bovis* may cause anaemia, emaciation and death of cattle in Africa, or the infestation may be subclinical. In India *S. nasalis* may produce a nasal discharge and difficulty in breathing, with sometimes the formation of a granuloma. In the Far East *S. japonicum* occurs in water-buffalo and infests man, in which the disease is very serious.

The life-cycle differs from the typical case, in that the free cercaria may pierce the skin of its host instead of being swallowed.

The sexes are separate, and are usually found with the female lying in a groove formed by the incurved edges of the male.

Control Provision of clean drinking water and treatment of pasture with molluscicides such as copper sulphate to kill the intermediate host will reduce infection. However, such measures are rarely practicable in affected areas. Drugs such as praziquantel may be effective in treatment.

Schistosomus Reflexus

A deformity of the bovine fetus, in which the spine is bent, so that head and tail curve towards each other, causing dystokia. Fetal intestine may be visible at the vulva, or located in the vagina.

Schmorl's Disease

Schmorl's disease is a disease of rabbits, involving areas of necrosis of skin or mucous membrane, and caused by *Bacteroides necrophorus* (often after the animal's resistance has been lowered by some other pathogen).

Schnauzer

A German breed of dog with wiry coat that forms characteristic eyebrows, mouth and chin whiskers. There are miniature, standard and giant forms. The standard has fewer defects than the miniature, which is predisposed to cataracts and progressive retinal atrophy.

Schradan

An organophosphorus insecticide used in agriculture and a potential danger to farm livestock. (See also PARATHION.) Symptoms of poisoning may include vomiting, lachrymation, salivation, straining, twitching, distressed breathing, and coma.

Sciatica

Sciatica means pain connected with the sciatic nerve which runs down the thigh.

Scintigraphy

The application of nuclear medicine to the diagnosis of bone pathology and lameness. It has applications for dogs and horses. (See NUCLEAR MEDICINE.)

Scirrhous Cord

Scirrhous cord is a condition in which there is a chronic fibrous enlargement of the cut end of the spermatic cord following castration. In most cases the castration wound does not completely heal, but a small sinus discharging a thick white pus persists. The discharge may cease later, but the swelling of the cord goes on increasing slowly in size, until eventually it may be nearly as large as a man's head. In extreme cases the swelling extends upwards through the inguinal canal and into the abdomen and a mass weighing as much as 45 kg (100 lb) has occasionally been encountered in the horse on postmortem examination. Treatment is entirely surgical.

Scirrhus

Scirrhus is a term applied to a growth or to other hard fibrous conditions of various organs.

Sclera (Sclerotic Coat)

Sclera (sclerotic coat) is the outermost hard fibrous coat of the EYE.

Scleritis

Scleritis means inflammation of the sclerotic coat of the eye.

Scleroderma

(see CHANCRE)

Sclerosis

Sclerosis means hardening of tissues.

Scolecobasidium

A soil-dwelling fungus which may infect salmonids, causing swelling of the skin and, if it penetrates the body, in the kidney.

Scoliosis

Lateral curvature of the spine.

Scombiotoxic Poisoning

Scombiotoxic poisoning is a type of food-poisoning which occurs as a result of eating fish that contains large amounts of histamine. The histamine is produced by bacterial degradation of histadine when the fish – particularly tuna, bonito and mackerel, and also sardines, pilchards and herrings – are stored for prolonged periods at elevated temperatures. The symptoms commonly found are rash, diarrhoea, flushing and headache.

Scorpions

Their venom affects the nervous system, causing pain, salivation, erection of hair, dilated pupils, increased blood pressure, and muscular spasm.

'Scottie Cramp'

A condition apparently confined to the Scottish terrier, and occurring usually for the first time at 4 to 8 months of age. There is cramp following exercise. In mild cases the animal may be seen to be in difficulties when negotiating steps; in severe cases 100 metres' brisk trot will cause the animal to double up and collapse, and in a few instances excitement without exertion will give rise to cramp. Mild attacks often become worse, reaching a maximum severity at 12 or 15 months of age. At around 2 years of age the dog may have outgrown 'Scottie cramp'. The cause is unknown. Intravenous injections of calcium borogluconate, or parathyroid extract administration, have been recommended. The condition could be eliminated by breeders.

Scottish Fold

A breed of droop-eared cat. Although no major problems should be seen, owners are advised to check regularly for ear mites and infection. Some individuals may have a thickening and shortening of the tail that may be accompanied by thickening of the limbs and overgrowth of cartilage at the joints.

Scottish Terrier

A small wiry dog, black, white or brindled. Von Willebrand's disease may be inherited and the breed is prone to craniomandibular osteopathy, deafness and Perthe's disease. Intervertebral disc disease may be found in the neck region; it may possibly be due to the weight of the head in relation to the body in some individuals

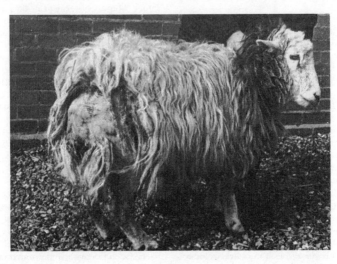

Scrapie.

Scours, Scouring
(see DIARRHOEA)

Scrapie

Scrapie is a disease of sheep mainly confined to the district of the English and Scottish Borders, to Spain, France, and Germany. Sheep imported into Australia, New Zealand, Canada, and the USA have brought the disease with them. Australia and New Zealand are believed to have quickly eradicated the disease. Scrapie is a NOTIFIABLE DISEASE in the UK, which operates a compulsory slaughter policy for infected sheep.

Scrapie, BSE and other 'prion' diseases
It is possible that scrapie has a relationship with the human diseases kuru, Creutzfeldt-Jakob disease and Gerstmann-Straussler-Scheinker syndrome. Material from scrapie-infected sheep, rendered and used in dairy cattle concentrates, is believed to be the origin of BSE in cattle. (See BOVINE SPONGIFORM ENCEPHALOPATHY.)

Diagnosis One method is to detect scrapie-associated fibrillar protein (PrP) by means of a rabbit-anti-sheep PrP polyclonal antibody by Western blot analysis; but consistent results have not, it seems, been obtained.

Experimentally, scrapie has been transmitted to goats, mice, rats, and hamsters.

Cause An infective agent, possibly a prion. Research at the joint AFRC and MRC neuropathogenesis unit, Edinburgh, found that crude extracts of scrapie-infected brain contained accumulations of material known as scrapie-associated fibrils (SAF), which were also found in scrapie-like diseases.

Infection is spread from ewe to lamb and, possibly, by contact with fetal fluids. Signs take about 2 years to appear.

A long-term DEFRA research project is investigating the causes, disease process and epidemiology of scrapie, and the genetic factors making some sheep more susceptible than others. The aim is eradication of the disease from the UK. (See NATIONAL SCRAPIE PLAN.)

Signs The most striking and easily seen symptom of scrapie is the torn, ruffled, and untidy appearance of the fleece, and when very severe, the bruised or scratched condition of the skin. In many cases, especially those occurring during the late spring, the fleece may be almost entirely rubbed off against fences, posts and trees or may be greatly removed by the mouth.

In addition, the condition of the sheep is noteworthy; whereas the remainder of the flock may be in fair bodily condition, the scrapie sheep are thin, gaunt, and apt to become weak on their legs, lagging behind when going uphill, and losing their foothold when descending. Muscular tremors are often seen, and later there is evidence of intense itching.

Occasionally, when startled – as, for instance, when being moved by dogs, or when a gun is fired near the unwary scrapie sheep – convulsive seizures are seen, usually lasting from 3 to 5 minutes, and leaving the animal temporarily dazed.

Screw-Worm Flies

These include *Chrysomyia bezziana* in Australia, *Cochliomyia hominivorax, C. Americana.*

The screw-worm (*C. hominivorax*), a significant parasite of both humans and animals, had not been recorded outside the New World until its accidental introduction into Libya, probably in 1988–9. Hundreds of cases of wound myiasis including many fatalities were recorded in various species of domestic animals during 1989 and 1990.

An international campaign to eradicate the American screw-worm fly from North Africa appears to be succeeding, according to a bulletin from the organisers.

The campaign, begun in December 1990, involved the release of sterile male flies imported from Mexico. The flies were dispersed by air at densities of 500 to 1200 per km^2 over an area of 40,000 km^2. More than 745 million flies have been used and 40 million a week were dispersed during the campaign. (See FLIES; MYIASIS; STRIKE.)

Scrotal

Relating to the scrotum.

Scrub Typhus (Japanese River Fever)

A disease caused by *Rickettsia tsutsugamushi*, and transmitted by mites.

Scur

A loose, horny growth, not attached to the skull, at the site normally occupied by a horn in a horned breed of cattle.

A bull calf with a scur, or with a bony protuberance beneath the skin at the horn site, is not a pure polled animal. Without these, a bull can be expected to breed true as regards the poll character; this can be checked by a progeny test of the bull mated to horned cows – the result should be polled heifer calves or bull calves with scurs or bony protuberances, but no calves with horns.

Sea Lice

Farmed Atlantic salmon, and sea trout, are subject to infestation by sea lice (*Lepeophthirus salmonis* and *Caligus elongatus*) with serious economic consequences. Treatment with parasiticides including hydrogen peroxide and synthetic pyrethroids such as cypermethrin is effective, but must be repeated at intervals depending on circumstances.

Seal

A common marine mammal found around the coasts of Britain and many parts of the world, favouring colder climates. True, or earless, seals are members of the family *Phocidae*. They are susceptible to infection by a morbillivirus similar to that causing canine distemper. In polluted areas, they are liable to suffer mercury poisoning.

Sealyham Terrier

A short-legged breed with a wiry, often white, coat. Retinal dysplasia may be inherited and the breed is prone to deafness and lens luxation.

Season

(see OESTRUS)

Seat-Worm

(see OXYURIS)

Seaweed

A source of AGAR; a food grazed by sheep on the seashore, and sometimes fed to horses and cattle. A source of iodine and other trace elements and (in the case of brown seaweeds) of vitamins A, B_1, B_2, C, and D. Animals do not take readily to seaweed as a rule, nor are they able to digest it well at first, but after a few days it usually proves an acceptable supplement to the ration.

The ruminal microflora of sheep feeding almost entirely on seaweed were devoid of cellulolytic bacteria and anaerobic bacteria which are so numerous in sheep-grazing pasture.

Sebaceous Glands

Sebaceous glands are found in the skin (see diagram under SKIN), and secrete the oily sebum which prevents excessive dryness of hair and skin. The glands are liable to become invaded during some parasitic diseases; sometimes a blocked duct leads to a retention cyst.

Seborrhoea is an excessively oily skin due to over-production by the sebaceous glands.

Secretin

A hormone secreted by the mucous membrane near the beginning of the small intestine when food comes into contact with the latter. On reaching the pancreas via the bloodstream, the hormone stimulates the flow of pancreatic juice.

Secretory IgA

It has been shown that in some infections, especially those of the respiratory and digestive tracts, immunity is conferred by antibody found in the local secretions – and not by the antibody circulating in the bloodstream. For example, the IgA found in secretions is quite different from that found in serum. Secretory IgA is relatively resistant to breakdown by digestive enzymes and has an affinity for mucus. (See IMMUNE RESPONSE, IgA.)

-Sectomy

A word-ending meaning 'surgical removal of'.

Seed Corn, dressed

A number of substances with which seed corn may be dressed may be toxic to animals. For example, corn with a mercury dressing has been fed to pigs with fatal results.

Dieldrin seed dressings lead to poisoning in wild birds and, indirectly, have killed dogs, cats, and foxes which have eaten poisoned birds. (See also under GAME BIRDS.)

Seedy Toe

A condition affecting the hoof of the horse, in which there is a separation of the wall from the laminar matrix below, and the formation in the space so produced of a dry, crumbly, friable variety of horn, which bears some resemblance to pumice-stone. It may occur at any part of the wall of the foot. The cause is uncertain.

Signs In most cases the condition is generally first noticed by the farrier when paring down the wall prior to fitting a new shoe. Lameness is only seen when the extent of the separation is large, or when foreign matter becomes forced up into the space, and causes pressure upon the sensitive matrix.

When struck with a hammer the affected part of the foot gives out a hollow resonating note, and the margins of the separated area can usually be fairly well determined by this means.

Treatment All the soft friable horn should be cleared away and an antibiotic applied within. A suitable shoe should be fitted to cover the base of the cavity. (See HOOF REPAIR.)

Selenium (SE)

A TRACE ELEMENT essential in minute quantities for nutrition, but toxic if fed in excess. In some parts of Britain home-grown animal feeds may not contain enough selenium, and unless concentrates are fed as well, nutritional muscular dystrophy may result. The organic form conjugated to the amino acid methionine is more easily utilised by animals than inorganic salts. In other areas the soil may contain an excess of selenium. The normal level in animal feeds should be around 0.2 ppm; the maximum level of selenium allowed in pig diets without a veterinary prescription is 0.5 mg/kg, this level being specified under the Feeding-Stuffs Regulations 1982.

Supplements of selenium can be given not only in the feed, but also in drinking water, by subcutaneous injection, by BOLUS, and (for lambs) by an oral dose.

Sodium selenate is used by horticulturists as an insecticide, and accordingly there is a possibility of toxic effect occurring in animals. Sterility results, and also loss of hair. These symptoms are also observed in parts of the USA and Eire where the soil contains an excess of selenium. In the acute form of poisoning, animals may be found wandering aimlessly or in circles. Paralysis precedes death.

A horse weighing approximately 450 kg received 25 mg selenium as sodium selenate daily for 5 consecutive days. The horse became lethargic, walked stiffly and was unwilling to undertake pace work. The main signs were loss of hair from the mane and tail, disintegration of the skin of the lips, anus, prepuce and scrotum, and separation of the hooves from the coronary corium. There were strong correlations between the selenium concentrations in blood, hair and hoof parings.

Externally, selenium sulphide is used in wet shampoos for dogs and cats infested with fleas, harvest mites, or cheyletiella mites. (See also VITAMIN E; LATHYRISM; MUSCLES, DISEASES OF; IONOPHORES.)

Retention of placentas in a dairy herd in the north of England was associated with a selenium deficiency.

Sella Turcica

Sella turcica is the name applied to the deep hollow on the upper surface of the sphenoid bone in which the pituitary gland rests.

Semen (Seminal Fluid)

Semen (seminal fluid) consists of the secretions of the accessory sex glands, in which is found the mature spermatozoa (or sperms) from the epididymis. A single ejaculation by a bull may produce semen containing millions of sperms.

The secretions of the accessory sex glands act as a vehicle for the sperms, probably as a nutrient, and neutralise any acidity in the female genital passages.

The accessory glands are the prostate; the ampullae of the vasa deferens (absent in the boar); the seminal vesicles; and (except in the dog) the bulbo-urethral (Cowper's) glands situated on either side of the urethra. (See also under SPERMATOZOA; ARTIFICIAL INSEMINATION.)

Imports of semen in Britain are subject to DEFRA regulations.

Seminal Vesicles
(see under TESTICLE; ACTINOBACILLOSIS).

Sendai Virus

This causes respiratory disease in the mouse but is most noteworthy for its use in experimental cell fusion work.

Senkobo

Cutaneous streptothricosis, caused by *Dermatophilius congolensis*, occurring in tropical Africa in cattle, sheep, goats, and horses. The hair stands erect and matted on small patches along the back. Moist, raw areas are left, then crusts form, and eventually a 'crocodile-skin' effect is produced. The disease occurs in association with tick infestation, and can therefore be controlled by means of an ectoparasiticide. (See DERMATOPHILUS.)

Senna

A standardised preparation of this household laxative has been recommended in treating or preventing constipation in pigs – especially in pregnant sows. A sublaxative dose of 3 g is recommended during the farrowing period.

Sensitisation
(see ALLERGY)

Sepsis
(see SUPPURATION; ANTISEPTICS)

Septicaemia

A condition in which toxic bacteria invade the bloodstream. It is very serious because the organisms and the toxins they produce become widely distributed throughout the tissues, and practically every organ is affected by them. In most cases, septicaemia terminates in death. Examples are ANTHRAX; HAEMORRHAGIC SEPTICAEMIA.

Signs In many cases, especially when the animal is in a weakened state, sudden death, preceded by a very high temperature, may be the only sign of the presence of septicaemia.

Treatment Antibiotics and/or sulfonamides, and antisera (where appropriate) are given.

Septum
A thin wall dividing 2 cavities or masses of tissue.

Sequestrum
A fragment of bone which, in the process of necrosis, has been cast off from the living bone and has died, but still remains in the tissues.

Sequelae
Symptoms or effects which may follow disease or injury. Thus pneumonia may follow a simple influenza, and chorea may follow distemper.

Seroconversion
The appearance in the blood serum of antibodies following vaccination (or natural exposure to some infective agent).

Serous Membranes
Serous membranes are smooth, glistening, transparent membranes that line certain of the large cavities of the body and cover the organs that are contained in them. The chief serous membranes are: (1) the peritoneum, lining the cavity of the abdomen; (2) the pleurae, one of which lines each side of the chest and surrounds the corresponding lung; (3) the pericardium, in which the heart lies; (4) the tunica vaginalis, one on each side, enclosing a testicle; and (5) the mesentery supporting the small intestine.

Serpulina
A group of spirochaetes which includes *Serpulina hyodysenteriae*, the cause of swine dysentery. (See SWINE DYSENTERY; TREPONEMA.)

Sertoli-Cell Tumour
This may be associated in the dog with feminisation, urethral bleeding, and urinary obstruction. (See also SPERMATIC CORD, TORSION OF.)

Sertoli Cells
Cells in the testicular tubules to which spermatids become attached. Their function is believed to be the nourishment of spermatids. (See diagram under SPERMATOZOA.)

Serum
Serum is the fluid which separates from blood when clotting takes place. It is, in effect, defibrinated plasma without the red cells,

platelets or white cells. (For a description of plasma, see BLOOD.) (See also ANTISERUM.)

Serum Gonadotrophin
(see HORMONES)

Serum Sickness
In human medicine this term is applied to the fever, glandular enlargements, oedema, and pain in the joints, which may occur 8 to 12 days after the injection of a 'foreign' serum. Immediate reaction, denoting sensitisation by a previous injection of the same kind of serum, is regarded as anaphylactic shock. (See HYPERSENSITIVITY.)

Serum Therapy
(see ANTISERUM)

Service Period
This is usually taken to mean the interval between giving birth and subsequent service leading to conception. In cattle, an 85-day service period would appear to be the optimum number of days between calving and successful service. If the trend of heat periods after calving is detected at about 6 weeks, and checked again around 9 weeks, the herdsman can, with a fair degree of accuracy, be on the look-out for bulling at or about the 12th week (or 84 to 85 days). In practice, most farmers will serve at 9 weeks to try to maintain a 365-day calving interval. Very early service may produce prolonged infertility.

Setae
Stiff hairs. (See CATERPILLARS; SPIDERS.)

Sewage Sludge
Sewage sludge is often contaminated by heavy metals (cadmium, copper, lead) and should not be used for manuring pasture unless these have been removed. The heavy metals are present as harmless sulphide complexes when first applied to the soil: however, passage through earthworms breaks down the complexes, which can then be absorbed by animals. The process may take several years. Horses on pasture were fatally poisoned by cadmium, lead and copper 5 years after sewage sludge was applied. More rarely, the eggs of *Taenia sagniata* which pass through the filters in some sewage may be present on pasture and lead to cysticercosis in cattle. (See also SALMONELLOSIS; SLURRY; COPPER POISONING in sheep.)

Sex Differentiation
Sex differentiation in the fetus is briefly described under EMBRYOLOGY. (See also under GENETICS; CYTOGENETICS; FREEMARTIN.)

Sex-Hormones
(see HORMONES)

Sex-Inversion
Animals which at birth, and for a variable period afterwards, are of normal sexual structure and function, but which later in life acquire properties of the opposite sex, are said to undergo sex-inversion. This has been seen in Ayrshire cows permanently kept indoors. (See also FEMINISATION.)

Sex Pilus
(see PLASMIDS)

Sex, Predetermined, of Calves
(see PREDETERMINED SEX OF CALVES)

Sexual Cycle
(see OESTRUS)

Shar-Pei
A medium-sized breed of dog originally from China which is characterised by very loose, infolded skin. In the folds, dermatitis may develop if the care of the dog is less than good.

Shavings
(see under BEDDING)

Shearing
In Britain, the usual time for shearing is May in the southern counties, early June onupland semi-arable farms, and during July in mountain flocks.

The newly shorn sheep is very sensitive to cold. This is particularly so with machine shearing which leaves a fleece of about 6 mm depth compared with about 12 mm after hand shearing. In Australia, late-winter and early-spring shearing of ewes has led to a high mortality, so that the practice is being abandoned or the usual shears replaced by 'snow combs' which leave a longer fleece. In Britain, losses of weight or poor gains in lambs shorn during the summer can largely be attributed to an effect of cold.

Chemical 'shearing' Certain drugs, for example cyclophosphamide and mimozone, cause the wool to loosen so that it can easily be plucked. It has been suggested that this could be an economical way of defleecing sheep. However, the sheep is left naked and unprotected against cold. It does not seem that the system has gained wide usage.

Sheep, Abortion and Infertility in
(see ABORTION)

Sheep Breeding and Management
The use of hybrids, referred to under SHEEP, BREEDS OF (British), is a relatively new trend. Another is the housing of ewes for part of the winter before lambing. The number of sheep per flock has increased and a full-time shepherd will be looking after more than 10,000 breeding ewes.

Economic factors have dictated many changes in traditional sheep management. The sheep market has altered greatly; the demand is mainly for lamb, not mutton. However, sheep are still sold through markets on a liveweight basis and are classed as light (25.5 kg), standard (32.1 to 39 kg), medium (39.1 to 45.5 kg) and heavy (45.6 to 52 kg). Wool is now of relatively low value, because of reduced demand.

Efficient sheep production depends on raising the productivity of grassland by improving the quality and quantity of the grazing and improving the growth characteristics of the sheep. Worming regimes must be established to deal with the infestations that affect all grassland used for growing young sheep. Feed available to the lactating ewe must be of sufficient quality to allow a good supply of milk for twin or triplet lambs, and limit initial grass uptake.

Direct and indirect feed costs (including fertilisers, fuel and labour), can account for 60 per cent of the cost of sheep production. This emphasises the importance of the efficiency of feed conversion. In lowland flocks, most food is consumed by the ewes, so the number of lambs weaned per ewe per year is of critical importance. Ideally, the aim is for a relatively small ewe, with good milking potential, which can be crossed with a larger, meat-producing, breed to produce several offspring that grow fast and economically.

While artificial rearing systems for lambs are used, they are not favoured by most breeders except for orphan lambs or those from large litters. Most farmers aim to produce 2 viable lambs that can be naturally reared.

Housing of sheep (In-wintering) Sheep are frequently housed for part of the year, usually before and after lambing. The duration of housing depends on the area and other management considerations. In Scotland, in-wintering of ewes lambing between December and April revives a practice traditional in hill areas until a change was made to wintering them on lowland pastures. That policy proved too costly and led to the flocks being kept on the farms and provided with shelter. Winter housing is also now common on lowland farms. The ewes are kept in groups of 50 to 70, lambing at the same time.

Housing permits greater attention to feeding and care at lambing, and leads to less culling as the sheep are not subjected to the stress of exposure to severe weather and finding their own food. However, the risk of disease and mismothering is higher.

Portable feeding troughs and racks in sheep houses can be used as partitions and leave an unobstructed floor so that pen sizes can be altered according to requirements. The 2 main types of feeder are a hay rack, with sloping sides so that seeds do not drop into the sheep's eyes, with a concentrate trough below (preferred for upland sheep); and a box type with a barrier in front which prevents the ewes from wasting the forage. Troughs should allow a length per ewe of 23 to 25 cm (9 to 10 in) for hill breeds and 30 to 35 cm (12 to 14 in) for lowland breeds. A supply of fresh (i.e. running) water must be provided; sheep will not drink water that is even slightly fouled, or warm. A raised trough fed from a slow running tap, with drainage to the outside, is suitable. About 30 cm (12 in) of trough per sheep should suffice for 40 sheep.

Adequate ventilation is essential. Yorkshire boarding to walls is suitable. If slatted flooring is used, care must be taken that updrafts do not chill sheep and, especially, lambs. The slats must be laid parallel to the door openings.

Lamb survival Lambs have the highest post-natal mortality of all the main farm species. This is partly because they are very susceptible to hypothermia caused by exposure, or lack of food. Problems arise when the environment is colder than the critical temperature of the lamb in the first few hours after birth. This is 32°C (89.5°F) for heavy lambs and 37°C (98.5°F) for light lambs. As most lambs are born at ambient temperatures well below this, they have to increase their metabolic rate to maintain body temperature. Wind chill factor can reduce the effective temperature considerably. A wind speed of 20 km/h (12 mph) can have a cooling effect of up to 20°C (68°F) or more if there is rain. Even when a lamb survives such conditions, it will have suffered a major drain on its bodily reserves, mainly in the form of fat. In bad conditions these may be used up in between 5 and 17 hours.

While a lamb will normally begin to replenish its store of energy within an hour of birth by sucking, work in Australia has shown that the urge to do so is reduced if its body temperature falls below 37°C. In some breeds of sheep, such temperatures occur in weather not unusually

severe for March and April in Scotland. So cold not only increases the demand for energy, but may prevent that demand from being met.

Starvation exaggerates the effect of cold by reducing heat-production capability, so increasing the risk of death from hypothermia.

It may be possible to breed for greater ability to survive under harsh conditions. Experiments suggest that there are significant differences between breeds in their tolerance of body cooling; and within breeds, some individual sheep have a cold-resistance several times greater than that of other individuals. Preliminary trials have indicated that this character is moderately well inherited.

Lambs require between 180 and 210 ml of colostrum per kg bodyweight during the first 18 hours after birth, to provide sufficient fuel for heat production; and immunoglobulins for protection against infections.

Ewes which are well fed during late pregnancy produce more colostrum than their lambs need; those with singletons have enough for a 2nd lamb. By contrast, most underfed ewes do not produce enough colostrum.

Colostrum can be readily obtained by hand milking and stored for subsequent use. Yields are markedly increased when milking is preceded by an oxytocin injection.

Life-saving techniques on the farm. The following recommendations have been made by the Moredun Institute, Edinburgh. Two danger periods should be recognised: (1) from birth to 5 hours afterwards; and (2) 10 hours to 3 days after birth.

During the 1st period, moderate hypothermia (a body temperature of 37° to 39°C; 98.5° to 102°F) usually responds to drying the lamb, feeding it colostrum by stomach tube, and moving it to shelter along with the ewe. Serious hypothermia (below 37°C; 98.5°F) requires in addition that the lamb be warmed in air at 37°C (98.5°F) to 40°C (104°F) until its body temperature has reached 37°C (98.5°F). When removed from the Moredun-type bale-warmer (heated by a domestic fan-heater), the lamb is then given colostrum and, if strong enough to suck vigorously, can be reunited with the ewe. If not strong enough, the lamb must be housed for a day or two in its own cardboard box in an intensive care unit. There colostrum is given 3 times daily, and warmth provided by an overhead infra-red lamp.

During the 2nd danger period, when serious hypothermia is then usually due to depressed heat production as a result of starvation, and often complicated by low glucose levels in the blood, treatment consists of drying the lamb, the injection of glucose, and warming – in that order.

Further details of bale warmers, lamb warming boxes, the Moredun lamb thermometer (which indicates by flashing, coloured lights whether a lamb has hypothermia, and if so how badly), and techniques can be obtained from the Moredun Research Institute,Pentlands scientific Park, Bush Loan, Penicuik, Midlothian EH26 QPZ .

Worm control Most sheep at pasture are infected with roundworms. These, if numerous, can cause outbreaks of scouring and obvious unthriftiness. Subclinical infestations of the stomach or intestine can reduce the weight gain of growing lambs by 20 to 50 per cent. (See WORMS, FARM TREATMENT AGAINST.)

Winter feeding Research has indicated the wisdom of hand feeding with starchy concen-

trates (rather than high protein or high roughage rations) to obviate the hill ewe burning up her own tissues in order to keep warm and alive during very cold weather. (See under ABORTION, FEED BLOCKS.)

For other aspects of sheep husbandry, and related health and disease problems, see ABORTION; BARLEY POISONING; BRACKEN POISONING; 'BROKEN MOUTH'; CASTRATION; CLOTHING OF ANIMALS; COBALT; COLOSTRUM; CONTROLLED BREEDING; COPPER; COPPER POISONING; DIET AND DIETETICS; DIPS AND DIPPING; DOCKING, DRENCHING; EXPOSURE; FEED BLOCKS; FLEECE, FLUSHING OF EWES; GENETICS; HOUSING OF ANIMALS; INFECTION; INFERTILITY; ISOLATION; LIGHTNING STRING; LUMPY WOOL; NOTIFIABLE DISEASES; OESTRUS; PARASITES; PARTURITION, DRUG- INDUCED; PASTURE, CONTAMINATION OF; PASTURE MANAGEMENT; POISONING; SEAWEED; SHEARING; SHEEP, DISEASES OF; SHEEP-DOGS; SOIL-CONTAMINATED HERBAGE; STELL;

NAMES OF SHEEP GIVEN ACCORDING TO AGE, SEX, ETC.

Periods	Male		Female	Remarks
	Uncastrated	Castrated		
Birth to weaning	Tup lamb Ram lamb Pur lamb Heeder	Hogg lamb	Ewe lamb Gimmer lamb	A sheep until weaning is a lamb
Weaning to shearing	Hogg (also used for the female) Hogget (also used for the female) Haggerel or hoggerel Tup teg Ram hogg Tup hogg	Wether hogg Wedder hogg He teg	Gimmer hogg Ewe hogg Sheeder ewe Ewe teg	Hogget wool is wool of the first shearing
First to second shearing	Shearing, or shearling, or shear hogg Diamond ram Dinmont ram tup One-shear tup	Shearing wether Shear hogg Wether hogg Wedder hogg Two-toothed wether	Shearing ewe Shearling gimmer Theave Double-toothed ewe Double-toothed gimmer Gimmer	'Ewe', if in-lamb or with lamb; if not a 'barren gimmer'; if not put to a ram is a 'yield gimmer' (Scotland)
Second to third shearing	Two-shear ram Two-shear tup	Four-toothed wether Two-shear	Two-shear ewe	A ewe which has ceased to give milk is a 'yeld ewe'; taken from the breeding flock she is a 'draft ewe' or a 'draft gimmer'
Third to fourth shearing	Three-shear ram Three-shear tup	Six-toothed wether Three-shear wether	Three-shear ewe Winter ewe (Scotland)	
Afterwards	Aged tup or ram	Full-mouthed, full-marked or aged wether or wedder	Ewe Ewe	After fourth shearing 'aged' or 'three-winter'

STOCKING RATES; STRESS; TRACE ELEMENTS; TROPICS; VAGINA (for rupture of); VITAMINS; WATER; WEANING; WOOL BALLS; WORMS, FARM TREATMENT AGAINST.

Clipping (see SHEARING; CLOTHING FOR ANIMALS; WOOL SLIP)

Sheep, Breeds of

Introduction Sheep are maintained, generally speaking, with the object of producing both wool and meat. In some countries' ewe's milk is valued for cheese-making. In the UK the importance of the fleece tends to be disregarded.

Hardiness, prolificacy, milking capacity of the females, and activity are all important. What will constitute the most profitable type must be carefully considered in relation to local conditions.

British breeds of sheep British breeds – some 40 are registered – offer a wide choice of types, adapted to almost every conceivable set of conditions under which sheep are maintained in the country, from the highest mountain grazings in Scotland and Wales to the richest lowland pastures, or the dry arable farms of the Wolds. However, crossbreeds are increasingly popular.

Cambridge This breed was developed at the University of Cambridge by Professor John Owen in collaboration with Alun Davies. The breed is now regarded as one of the most prolific in the world with litter sizes of 1.7, 2.5 and 2.9 for 1-, 2- and 3-year-old females respectively. Both sexes are polled, ewes weighing 70 kg (154 lb) and rams 90 kg (98 lb). (See also TEXEL; COOPWORTH.)

The British breeds are commonly classified as Longwools, Downs, other Shortwools, and Mountain breeds.

Longwool breeds include Leicester, Border Leicester, Lincoln, Wensleydale, Kent or Romney Marsh, Devon Longwool, South Devon, and Roscommon.

Downs breeds include Southdown, Suffolk, Hampshire, Dorset Down, Shropshire, and Oxford.

Other Shortwool breeds include Dorset Horn, Wiltshire Horn, Ryeland, Devon Closewool, and Kerry Hill.

Mountain breeds include Scottish Blackface, Cheviot, Swaledale, Herdwick, Lonk, Welsh Mountain, Exmoor, and Dartmoor.

UK sheep population A rapid rise in sheep numbers followed the imposition of dairy milk quotas, plus the granting of various subsidy payments. At December 1994, MAFF recorded 29.5 million of which 20.1 million represented ewes in the breeding flock. The summer census annually lists the population at 35 to 40 million. However, the virtual collapse of the sheep market in the later 1990s led to a drop in numbers. A further fall followed the foot-and-mourh diseases outbreaks of 2001, since when restocking has revived numbers.

Sheep Dipping
(see DIPS AND DIPPING)

Sheep, Diseases of
(see under ABORTION; ACTINOBACILLOSIS; ANTHRAX; ARTHRITIS; BALANITIS; BLACK DISEASE; BLACK-QUARTER; BLOUWILDEBEESOOG; BLUE TONGUE; BORDER DISEASE; BRAXY; 'CAPPIE'; CASEOUS LYMPHADENITIS; ENTEQUE SECO; EYE DISEASES OF; FOOT-AND-MOUTH DISEASE; FOOT ROT; GAS GANGRENE; HYPOMAGNESAEMIA; JAAGSIEKTE; JOHNE'S DISEASE; JOINT-ILL; LAMB DYSENTERY; LIVER-FLUKE; LOUPING-ILL; MILK FEVER; MOREL'S DISEASE; OVINE EPIDIDIMYTIS; OVINE INTERDIGITAL DERMATITIS; NEMATODIRUS; PARASITES; 'PINING'; PNEUMONIA IN SHEEP; PREGNANCY TOXAEMIA; PULPY KIDNEY; 'REDFOOT'; 'RINGWOMB'; SCALD; SCRAPIE; SHEEP SCAB; SWAYBACK; TICKS; TICK-BORNE FEVER OF SHEEP; TOXOPLASMOSIS; UDDER, DISEASES OF; WATERY MOUTH; WESSELSBRON DISEASE; also ARIZONA INFECTION; ENZOOTIC OVINE ABORTION; HAEMORRHAGIC SEPTICAEMIA; MAEDI/VISNA; 'MILKSPOT LIVER'; PULMONARY ADENOMATOSIS; RIFT VALLEY FEVER; ULCERATIVE DERMATOSIS and under RAM.)

Sheep Health Scheme
A preventive medicine and productivity monitoring scheme for maintaining herd health; it is operated by Scottish agricultural colleges. A Premium Health scheme is operated for flocks seeking accreditation as free from chlamydial abortion. A maedi/visna accreditation scheme is also available; it involves certification by a veterinary surgeon that movement records have been checked, flock security rules obeyed and blood samples taken.

Sheep Ked (Melophagus Ovinus)
Sheep ked (Melophagus Ovinus) is a wingless blood-sucking parasite. (See KED.)

S

Sheep, Legislation Affecting

Agriculture (Miscellaneous Provisions) Act 1968
Animal and Animal Products (Import & Export) Regulations 1998
Animal Health Act 1981
Anthrax Order 1991
Artificial Breeding of Sheep & Goats Regulations 1993
Diseases of Animals (Approved Disinfectants) (Amendment) Order 1997
Foot and Mouth Order 1983
Fresh Meat (Hygiene & Inspection) Regulations 1995
Market Sales and Lairage Order 1925
Products of Animal Origin (Import & Export) Regulations 1992
Protection of Animals Act 1911
Protection of Animals (Anaesthetics) Act 1954 (amended 1982)
Sheep and Goats Spongiform Encephalopathy Order 1998
Sheep and Goats Spongiform Encephalopathy Regulations 1998
Sheep Scab Order 1997
Specified Diseases (Notification & Slaughter) Order 1991 (amended 1992)
Veterinary Surgeons Act 1966
Welfare of Animals at Markets Order 1990 (amended 1993)
Welfare of Animals (Transport) Order 1997
Welfare of Livestock (Prohibited Operations) Regulations 1982, 1987
Welfare of Livestock Regulations 1994
Zoonoses Order 1989

Sheep, Names Given According to Age, Sex, etc.

There are probably more names for any given class of sheep than is the case among any of the other domesticated animals, and it is almost impossible to give a list that will include all the various designations that are used, but the table gives a list of commoner terms.

Sheep Pox

(see POX)

Sheep Scab

The popular name for psoroptic mange. Sheep scab was formerly a notifiable disease in the UK, from where it was eradicated in 1952. It reappeared in 1973 and, following the abolition of compulsory dipping, has again become a serious problem. In the late 1990s, as many as 25 per cent of sheep pelts showed evidence of damage associated with scab. Although sheep scab is no longer a notifiable disease, control is

exercised through local authorities. It is an offence under the Protection of Animals Acts and the Welfare of Animals (Northern Ireland) Act 1972 to expose an infected sheep for sale; the charge would be one of causing unecessary suffering.(see MANGE – Mange in sheep).

Sheepdogs

Sheepdogs are popularly regarded as exceptionally healthy, but a survey in Scotland showed that at least 11 per cent were suffering from 'BLACK TONGUE' as a result of an inadequate diet. On average, this consisted basically of 225 g (8 oz) oatmeal, 225 g (8 oz) maize, and (by no means always) 225 ml (8 oz) of milk; the first 2 ingredients being made into a brose or mash by pouring on boiling water. The occasional rabbit, or piece of boiled mutton from a dead sheep, or – at lambing time – the afterbirths, were not sufficient to prevent 'black tongue'.

Sheepdogs may walk or run 90 miles per day at lambing time and must have meat if stamina and health are to be maintained. Even fishmeal is of service – also dried blood – if meat or fish are unobtainable. (See also under GID; RICKETS.)

Sheepdogs may become infected with brucellosis as a result of eating infected cattle afterbirths; through eating dead sheep they may become infested with the tapeworm causing HYDATID disease. Regular worming is essential. (See also ORF; ANTHRAX; BOTULISM.)

Sheep, Winter Coats for

(see CLOTHING OF ANIMALS)

Shelters, Need for

(see under EXPOSURE, TROPICS; also STELL)

Shepherds

Occupational hazards include the following diseases: CAMPYLOBACTER   INFECTIONS; CHLAMYDIA; HYDATID DISEASE; LISTERIOSIS; LOUPING-ILL; ORF; PASTEURELLOSIS; Q FEVER; SALMONELLOSIS; TOXOPLASMOSIS. (See also ZOONOSES.)

Shepherdesses, if pregnant, are at risk when helping with lambing. (See CHLAMYDIA.)

Shetland Sheepdog

A small breed resembling a toy rough collie. Progressive retinal atrophy and distichiasis are inherited dominat traits and collie eye anomaly and patellas luxation are recessive traits. Haemophlia and deafness may also be found.

Shigellosis

Infection by one of the Gram-negative *Shigella* bacteria. (See Sleepy foal under FOALS, DISEASES OF – Septicaemia.)

Shih Tzu

A small dog with short muzzle and long flowing hair; it originates from Tibet. The breed is prone to cleft palate and interverbral disc disease.

'Shipping Fever'

A disease of cattle caused by a virus and/or *Pasteurella multocida* or *P. haemolytica*. 'Shipping fever' is very common in American feedlots, among cattle 6 months to 2 years old, and often follows the stress of transport, castration, de-horning, winter weather, change of food, etc. In the USA the term 'bovine respiratory disease complex' is a synonym. (See PASTEURELLA.)

Signs include fever, loss of appetite, weakness, followed by nasal discharge, a discharge from the eyes, distressed breathing, coughing, and signs indicating bronchopneumonia. Mortality is usually 1 to 2 per cent, but may exceed this if cases are neglected .

Treatment And Prevention Antibiotics and sulfa drugs are used. Immunisation has been tried using myxovirus parainfluenza-3 and *P. septica*, for example.

'Shivering'

A nervous disease of horses. It runs a slowly progressive course, and constitutes an unsoundness.

Cause This is unknown, though it seems that there may be a hereditary predisposition to it.

Signs In a well-marked case, the muscles of the hindquarters are seen to quiver or tremble. At the same time, the tail is usually elevated and also shows the quivering movements. In advanced cases it may be difficult or impossible to pick up either of the hind-feet, and shoeing is only accomplished with difficulty. When the hind-limb is raised from the ground during backing, in many cases it also quivers, or 'shivers', and in some instances one or both of the fore-limbs, or the muscles of the fore-quarter, exhibit the same feature.

Shivering in the dog may occur, especially in fox terriers, for no apparent reason and may be unconnected with either cold or fear. At the prospect of a walk the dog may suddenly cease trembling.

Shock

Shock is, clinically, an abrupt fall in blood pressure (acute hypotension).

Signs include weakness, pale and cold mucous membranes, subnormal temperature but no shivering; a weak and rapid pulse; shallow breathing at an increased rate; cold extremities.

Cause Shock may follow severe trauma, haemorrhage, surgical operations, a sudden decrease in the heart's pumping capacity, burns and scalds, toxaemia. (See also ELECTRIC SHOCK; ANAPHYLACTIC SHOCK.) Pain, fright, and any airway obstruction may exacerbate the condition.

Treatment Although corticosteroids are often used, it has been stated that there is little or no evidence that they are effective. A blood transfusion, adrenalin, plasma substitutes based on gelatin and dextrans, and lactated Ringer's solution given intravenously, may each have a place in treatment, as appropriate.

The patient must be rested and kept warm.

Shoeing of Cattle

This may be undertaken to reduce weight-bearing on an injured claw, especially where there is a fracture of a phalanx. Draught cattle may also be shoed.

Shotgun Injuries

(see GUNSHOT INJURIES)

Shoulder

Shoulder is the joint formed between the scapula and the upper end of the humerus. (See DISLOCATION.)

Shoulder-Blade

(see SCAPULA)

Shovel Beak

A disease occurring in intensively reared chicks fed dry mash. It affects usually birds of 2 to 8 weeks old. The upper or lower beak (or both) may be deformed, with ulceration or necrosis. Infection with *Fusiformis necrophorus*, *Staphylococcus aureus*, or *Clostridium welchi* may follow.

Shying

(see 'VICES')

SI Units

The *Système International d'Unités* was adopted by the *Conférence Générale des Poids et Mesures* in 1960. Based on 7 units – metre, kilogram, second, ampere, degree kelvin, candela, and mole – it admits only 1 unit for any 1 physical quantity. Derived units in any science or technology can be made up from the 7 basic units by division or multiplication without numerical factors being involved. The SI unit joules replaces calories. The 7 basic SI units and their symbols are as follows:

(length)	metre	m
(mass)	kilogram	kg
(time)	second	s
(electric current)	ampere	A
(thermodynamic temperature)	degree kelvin	°K
(luminous intensity)	candela	cd
(amount of substance)	mole	mol

(See under METABOLISABLE ENERGY.)

Sialocoeles

Cyst-like swellings, usually lined by granulation tissue rather than epithelium, containing saliva.

Sialogogues

Sialogogues are substances which produce a copious flow of saliva, e.g. pilocarpine and arecoline.

Sickness

(see VOMITING)

Sidebones

Ossification of the LATERAL CARTILAGES of the horse's foot. When this occurs in a young animal, it is looked upon as an unsoundness. In old horses, all cartilages, not only in the foot, tend to become ossified as an almost natural course of events, and sidebones are accordingly not looked upon as so serious.

Causes Heredity is considered as a predisposing cause, but in many instances no such relationship can be shown. It has been suggested that a vitamin D deficiency in foalhood may be partly responsible.

Signs Ordinarily, the upper part of each cartilage can be felt at the coronet as a flexible ridge or edge, lying immediately below the skin, but when the cartilage has ossified, this ridge is no longer flexible, and is more or less thickened as well. In some instances the ossified cartilage can be easily seen when the feet are viewed from the front. The condition is more common by far in the fore-limbs, and may occur on the outside or inside, or in both places, on one or both of the fore-feet.

When sidebones have formed, there is no lameness, pain, heat, or other signs of inflammation, but when forming, there may be pain over the quarters involved, and lameness –

characterised by the taking of a shorter step by the affected foot, and the tendency to do this may result in a peculiar short and long step.

Treatment As a rule, in horses with wide open feet and well-developed frogs, no treatment is required. The sidebone does not interfere with slow work of a regular nature. (See also RING-BONES.)

Side-Effects

The side-effects of a drug are those produced in addition to that for which purpose the drug is given. Examples: deafness in humans following the administration of streptomycin; moniliasis after the use of chlortetracycline; aplastic anaemia after the use of chloramphenicol. (See also IATROGENIC DISEASE.)

Silage (Ensilage)

Silage (ensilage) is a succulent food. It has been classified as follows: Grade I containing 15 per cent and over crude protein, and made from young grasses, none in flower, clover, lucerne, or sainfoin in bud stage; Grade II containing 12 to 14.9 per cent crude protein, and made from grasses in their flowering stage, late autumn grass, clover passed full flower, marrow stem kale, pea pods, cereal-legume crops cut when cereal is 'milky'; and Grade III containing less than 12 per cent crude protein, and made from seeding grasses, stemmy clover, maize, pea haulm and pods, sugar-beet tops, potatoes.

Grade I makes a substitute for cake, whereas Grade III is good enough only as a substitute for roots, straw, or low-grade hay.

Ensilage involves fermentation. Lactic, acetic and butyric acids are produced: in good silage, lactic acid predominates. Silage with a high butyric-acid content must be fed with caution, and may be recognised by its to unpleasant smell and lighter colour – yellowish-green instead of dark brown.

The Dorset wedge system of silage-making has enabled better quality to be achieved.

ADAS comments: 'Most farmers still make silage at the wrong time.' This criticism refers to not cutting at the optimum stage of growth but tending to delay until there is more to cut. Wilting, judicious choice of harvester, type of silo, sealing, consolidation, and use of additives are all being applied by the more progressive farmers.

As with hay, there are extremes of quality in silage. At the Rowett Research Institute cows have maintained a yield of up to 23 litres (5 gallons) daily for 2 months while receiving no other feed. With the average quality silage it would, however, be unrealistic to expect to be able to dispense with supplements.

Acetonaemia is often seen in cattle receiving large quantities of silage of low quality. Hay should be made available as well; also 55 g (2 oz) per head of bone flour with salt added.

When self-feeding of silage is practised, care must be taken that conditions underfoot do not become dirty and slushy to an extent where softening of the horn of the hoof occurs and foot troubles develop.

Silage must be free of ragwort. (See under RAGWORT POISONING; also RETICULITIS, TRAUMATIC.)

Listeria in silage
LISTERIOSIS in ruminants has often been associated with silage feeding. In a survey carried out in Scotland, *Listeria monocytogenes* was isolated from 2.5 and 5.9 per cent of samples of clamp silage obtained in two successive years.

Silage Effluent
Silage effluent has been described as one of the strongest of all agricultural wastes and pollutants. Some 16,000 litres (3500 gallons) of clean water are needed to dilute 4.5 litres (1 gallon) of silage effluent to bring it to the recommended level for treated ('safe') effluents.

In a wet season a 400,000-kg (400-ton) silage clamp with grass at 1 to 15 per cent dry matter at ensiling may produce 182,000 litres (40,000 gallons) of effluent, most of which discharges in the first month. It takes only a little of this effluent to kill fish and other forms of aquatic life if it reaches a stream.

'Silent Heat'
(see under OESTRUS DETECTION; INFERTILITY)

Silica Contamination
Silica contamination can be a problem with sugar-beet tops and other arable residues. Crops windrowed and then picked up may contain up to 30 per cent silica. Direct loading might keep the figure down to 10 per cent. (See also SOIL-CONTAMINATED HERBAGE, SAND, COLIC.) Silica is silicon dioxide, present in sand.

Silicon
A non-metallic element. In the form of silicic acid or its derivatives, silicon is essential for growth, and is found mainly in connective tissue. It has been suggested that lack of sufficient silicon may be a factor in the cause of atherosclerosis in man. (See also SILICA CONTAMINATION.)

Silicone implant repair
A year-old Arabian filly had a depression over its right frontal sinus as the result of an injury sustained 6 months earlier when it ran into a steel pipe and the frontal bone had been broken. A heat-vulcanised silicone implant was used to repair the deformity and the normal facial contour was restored by suturing the sculpted implant to the periosteum over the defect.

Silicone Solution
An anticoagulation solution used in connection with blood transfusion apparatus and syringes to prevent clotting.

Simian Haemorrhagic Fever
(see MONKEYS, DISEASES OF; EBOLA VIRUS)

Simmental
A dual-purpose breed of Swiss cattle, now to be found throughout Europe and in the USA. In Germany the Simmental has been developed with emphasis on beef production.

Simulium
(see under FLIES). In the UK, the gnat *S. ornatum*, which breeds in running water and is difficult to control, sometimes causes eye lesions in cattle.

Sinus
Sinus is a term applied to narrow hollow cavities (especially in bones) occurring naturally in the body, or produced as the consequence of disease. (See SINUSES OF THE SKULL; also FISTULA.)

In pathology, sinus refers to a blind infected tract, leading from a site of suppuration to the surface of the skin or of a mucous membrane.

Sinuses, Diseases of the
The sinuses of the head are lined with a membrane which is continuous with that of the nasal cavities, and which acts as a periosteal covering for the bone.

Causes Sinusitis may arise as a result of a spread of inflammation from that affecting the nasal mucous membrane. It may follow strangles in the horse; occasionally the cause is a diseased tooth, the root of which has suppurated and the pus burrowed through the thin plate of bone that separates the tooth socket from the sinus cavity. In other cases, the cause is a penetrating injury from the outside, such as is occasioned by a blow on the forehead which fractures the external plate of bone and allows the ingress of infection. Animals living near the seashore or in sandy and windy localities are sometimes afflicted with collections of fine sand in the sinuses. In sheep, and sometimes in the horse, sheep-nostril fly larvae of the Oestrus family may be found in the sinuses, and are generally associated with pus formation. In dogs especially, but also in other animals, tumour formation is often accompanied by the presence of pus in the sinuses, and the condition may be complicated by a FUNGAL infection. In the dog, a foreign body such as a grass seed may give rise to the discharge from one nostril which is characteristic. Either cancer, or a fungal infection which may follow, can lead to distortion of the dog's or cat's face. (See also MITES linguatula serrate LEECHES.)

Signs The most prominent sign of the presence of any amount of pus in the sinuses is the usually slight, but continual, dribbling of discharge from one or both nostrils. This discharge is usually more marked when the animal lowers its head.

Treatment This consists of opening, under anaesthesia, the diseased sinus by trephining the bone over the surface, and irrigation and evacuation of the cavity. When a tooth has been the primary cause of the condition it is extracted, and its cavity temporarily plugged with gauze until healthy tissue fills up the space between the tooth socket and the sinus. Parasitic inhabitants are removed, either by the injection of fluids that will kill them, or by picking each out separately with forceps. Chloroforming the animal will often kill such parasites.

Sinuses of the Skull,

The sinuses of the skull, also called the paranasal sinuses, are directly or indirectly connected with the nose. There are 4 pairs: (1) maxillary; (2) frontal; (3) spheno-palatine, or sphenoid; and (4) ethmoidal.

Sinusitis

Inflammation of the sinuses.

Sinusitis, Infectious

A disease of turkeys, poultry and pheasants caused by *Mycoplasma gallisepticum*. The obvious sign is a swelling of the sinuses below the eyes, but the disease will also be present in the lower respiratory tract. While local treatment (e.g. draining the sinuses) is helpful, generally administration of antibiotics is necessary. The disease is egg-transmitted and may spread from egg to egg in the hatcher. Infected birds always remain carriers. Eradication has been carried

out in the commercial breeding stock of major suppliers.

Swollen sinuses may also be seen in certain paramyxovirus infections, from which infectious sinusitis must be differentiated.

Sire Identification
(see DNA – 'Fingerprinting')

Sitfasts
(see SADDLE-SORES)

Skim Milk

This is a valuable food, retaining, as it does, the solids-not-fat after most of the fat has been removed. These solids include the valuable milk-protein, the sugar lactose, valuable minerals, and vitamins of the B group. It is poor in the fat-soluble vitamins A and D, and also in vitamin E; and if given along with cod-liver oil to beef stores, may lead to cod-liver oil poisoning or MUSCULAR DYSTROPHY.

Skim milk is a useful food for pigs, but is not suitable on its own. It can be fed ad lib to suckling pigs; weaners may receive 3 litres (5 pints) per day; fatteners from 14 weeks to slaughter, about 3.5 litres (6 pints).

Skim milk is, if from infected cattle, a source of tuberculosis in pigs, and pasteurisation may be desirable in many countries.

For sows and piglets, skim milk should be fresh or completely sour; 0.1 per cent formalin is sometimes added to skim milk for fattening pigs.

Skin

Skin, the protective covering of the body, is continuous at the natural openings with the mucous membranes. It consists of 2 main layers, which differ in structure and origin.

The epidermis This is a cellular layer of non-vascular, stratified epithelium of varying thickness, covering the outer surface of the body, which presents the openings of the cutaneous glands and of the hair follicles. In animals it is divisible into 2 layers, the outer, hard, dry stratum corneum, and the deeper, softer, moist stratum germinativum. The cells of the latter are pigmented, and by their growth compensate for the loss by exfoliation or shedding of the surface cells from the stratum corneum, which forms the scurfy deposit upon an ungroomed horse. This inner layer consists of the part of the skin which is living, and is formed by several layers of cells set upon the corium and nourished by it. The cells continually multiply, and are slowly pushed upwards to

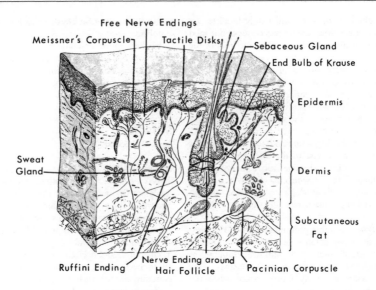

The nerve supply to the skin. (In Muller, Christensen and Evans, *Anatomy of the Dog*, courtesy of W. B. Saunders Co.)

replace the constant wear and tear which occurs on the cells at the surface. There are no blood vessels in the epidermis, but there is a ramification of the surface sensory nerves which supply the skin with its delicate sense of perception. A blister is a collection of fluid separating the stratum corneum from the stratum germinativum.

The dermis (corium) consists of a network of fibrous tissue and elastic fibres. It is very vascular, contains the hair follicles, the sudoriferous (or sweat) glands, and the sebaceous glands, as well as a certain amount of involuntary muscle. The most superficial part is known as the corpus papillare, on account of the presence of numbers of tiny papillae, which are received into corresponding depressions in the epidermis. These papillae contain loops of blood vessels, which nourish the epidermal cells, and numerous sensory nerves, which act as tactile organs, affording sensations of touch, pain, temperature, etc.

The sweat glands are situated partly in the deeper parts of the corium, known as the tunica propria, and partly below it in the layer of subcutaneous fibro-fatty tissue. In this deepest layer, which forms the bulk of the skin, or lying in the deeper part of the corium, there are certain tactile bodies, known as Pacinian corpuscles. The fibrous tissue of the skin consists of interlacing bundles of white fibrous tissue which form a dense felt-work. Here and there

elastic fibres are mixed with them, and these serve to give the skin its pliability, and at the same time keep it in place and stretched reasonably tightly.

Hair Practically the whole of the body of each domesticated animal is covered by hair, except in the pig. Portions of the skin which appear to be bare are found on close inspection to be covered with very fine hair of delicate texture. The hairs are constantly being shed and replaced by others, while at certain periods of the year in the horse, and to a lesser extent in the other animals, they are cast off in great numbers, and constitute the 'shedding' or 'casting of the coat'. This normally occurs twice a year – once in the autumn, when it is more marked, and again in the spring with the first warm weather of the year.

Hairs are of several kinds: in the first place there are the ordinary hairs which, on account of the small amount of pigment that each carries, give the coat its characteristic colour; and there are different kinds of special hairs. Among these ordinary hairs scattered over almost the whole body are: tactile hairs of the lips, nostrils, and eyes; cilia, or eyelashes, growing from the free rim of the eyelids; tragi, in the external ear; and vibrissae, round the nostrils. In addition to the ordinary and tactile hairs, certain regions carry specially long and coarse hairs, such as the mane (juba), the forelock or foretop (cirrus capitis), the tail, where the hairs (cirrus caudae) are very large and long, and the 'feather' of the fetlocks and cannons (cirrus pedis), which gave the name of this region (fetlock = feet-lock – a lock of hair on the foot).

Each hair has a shaft, the part above the surface, and a root, embedded in the hair follicle. Below this is a little fibrous papilla possessing blood vessels, which is capped by the expanded end of the hair root, and known as the hair bulb. The follicles are set somewhat obliquely in the corium and at varying depths; the long tactile hairs reaching down to the underlying muscle. Most of the follicles have little bands of plain muscle attached to one side, known as the arrectores pilorum; these serve to erect the hairs during anger, fear, or extreme cold, and also to express from the sebaceous gland a small portion of sebaceous secretion.

Glands of the skin are of 2 kinds: sweat and sebaceous. The former are scattered over the body in nearly all animals, being most numerous in the horse, and least in the dog (which is essentially a non-sweating animal), where the largest are found only on the pads of the feet. Each sweat or sudoriferous gland consists of a long tube, usually greatly coiled in its inner part, which has a duct leading up to the surface of the skin. (See PERSPIRATION.)

The sebaceous glands, except in certain places, open into the follicles of the hairs a little way below the surface. Each consists of a little bunch of small sacs, within which fatty or oily material is produced. This secretion is forced from the sacs by the contractions of the arrectores pilorum muscles, and during exercise it also escapes on to the shafts of the hairs. Its function is to keep these pliable and lubricated and prevent them from becoming brittle through drying. A copious secretion from the sebaceous glands results in a sleek shining coat, such as is associated with a well-fed and well-groomed horse.

Appendages of the skin In addition to hair, the skin possesses certain appendages, which in reality are modified hair only. Thus, horns, hoofs, claws, nails, ergots, chestnuts, and other horny structures are closely packed epidermal cells which have undergone keratinisation or cornification. Spurs of poultry are horny epidermal sheaths covering a centre of bony outgrowth from the metatarsal in the case of poultry. Feathers are highly specialised scales. The down feathers of the chicken are simple, and consist of a brush of hair-like 'barbs' springing from a basal quill or 'calamus'. From the whole length of each barb a series of smaller 'barbules' comes off not unlike the branches of a shrub. The adult or 'contour feathers' are formed at the bottom of the same follicles that lodged the down feathers, which by the growth of the adult feather become pushed out of place. At first they are nothing more than enlarged down feathers, but soon one of the barbs grows enormously, and forms a main shaft or 'rachis' to which the other barbs are attached on either side. From the sides of the barbs grow the barbules, just as in the down feathers; and these, in the case of the large wing feathers ('remiges') and the tail feathers ('retrices'), are connected by minute hooks so that the feather 'vane' has a more resistant surface for flight than in the case of the breast feathers, for instance. Moulting in birds occurs periodically, when the bird casts off the old feathers and gets a complete new set.

Functions of the skin The main use of the skin is a protective one. It covers the underlying muscles, protects them from injury, and by virtue of its padding of fat prevents them from extremes of temperature. The hair, fur, wool, or feathers assist this heat-regulating mechanism still further, and usually the growth of the coat is determined by the temperature of the surroundings. For example, when horses are kept out of doors during winter they grow long thick coats, while when kept in warm stables and covered with rugs they assume a close sleek coat: and the same applies to other animals.

Heat regulation is one of the most important functions of the skin. When cold air, water, or other cooling substances come into contact with a large area of the skin, the numerous blood vessels of the skin immediately contract, reducing the amount of blood circulating in them, and therefore reducing the amount which will be exposed to the cooling action from outside. On the other hand, when the surrounding medium is at a higher temperature than the normal – i.e. when it is approaching body heat, or rises above it – the blood vessels of the skin dilate, more blood is brought to the surface, and this stimulates sweating, or excretion; when the perspiration evaporates, especially when the surrounding atmosphere is dry, considerable cooling of the skin surface occurs. (See TEMPERATURE; TROPICS; HYPOTHALAMUS.)

Skin, Diseases of

The majority of the commoner diseases of the skin in animals are due either to parasitic invasion, or to conditions of an allergic origin, e.g. eczema. These are treated under separate headings – e.g. mange, of all varieties, is dealt with under MITES; ECZEMA; URTICARIA; RING-WORM; ACNE; see also TUMOURS; IMPETIGO; POX; BRIDLE INJURIES; SPOROTRICHOSIS; SWINE ERYSIPELAS; LIGHT SENSITISATION; DER-MATOPHILUS; GRANULOMA; ABSCESS; HYPERK-ERATOSIS; LUPUS; AUTO-IMMUNE DISEASE; CUTANEOUS ASTHENIA.

Cats may suffer from cancer of the sweat glands.

Skin Disorders in Cattle
These include squamous-cell carcinoma (which may also affect the eye), iodism, persistent BVD infection, vitamin E deficiency, vitamin A deficiency, papillomatosis, lice infestation, ringworm and the effect of a snake-bite.

Skin Grafting Transplantation
The pedicle technique, in which the transplant is attached at one end to adjacent skin, has been applied in cats and dogs. A broad flap of skin is formed by incision to cover the denuded area, with a narrow strip to form the pedicle or bridge to carry the blood supply to the broad flap or graft. The edges of the pedicle are sutured; the flap is sutured to adjacent skin.

In horses, skin grafting has also been carried out using free, whole-thickness grafts of skin taken from other sites in the same animal. Such grafts will give rise to normal hair growth.

In a cat a badly damaged tail was used as a source of skin for a graft before tail amputation – extensive skin loss having resulted from a fan-belt accident.

Skin, Poisoning Through
(see under POISONING; HYPERKERATOSIS)

'Skin Tuberculosis'
This is characterised by the appearance of swellings, varying in size from that of a pea to that of a tangerine, on the limbs and occasion-ally on the trunk of cattle. Lesions are often mul-tiple and in the form of a chain, often along the lines of the lymphatic vessels. They are unsightly but appear to cause the cow no discomfort and their economic importance lies only in the fact that they apparently sensitise the animal to mam-malian and/or avian tuberculin, thus complicat-ing the interpretation of the tuberculin test. This, indeed, may give rise to anxiety on the part of the owners of attested herds. A re-test after an inter-val of 30 to 60 days will, however, in the absence of tuberculosis, usually give a reaction justifying retention of the animal within the herd.

Microscopically, the lesions of 'skin tubercu-losis' closely resemble those of tuberculosis, and

acid-fast bacilli resembling *Mycobacterium tuberculosis* are present in them.

Skull
The bony structure of the head. Excavated in it there are large irregular spaces known as sinuses. (See SINUSES OF SKULL.)

General arrangement of the skull The skull is divided into 2 parts: (1) the cranium; and (2) the face. The former consists of the posterior part, which encloses the brain.

Most of the bones of the skull are flat bones developed from a structure which is partly car-tilage and partly fibrous membrane. Centres of ossification appear in these during early life, and soon after birth the greater part of each bone has assumed its eventual outline, but is separated from its neighbours by an intimately dovetailed joint. These joints, none of which is movable, allow growth until the animal is adult, when bony fusion usually occurs, and the joints become obliterated. Many of these joints – 'sutures', as they are called – can be felt in the skull of a newly born animal, particularly over the dome of the head in a foal or puppy, and for a time constitute especially vulnerable parts of the skull.

The bones of the cranium – those which enclose the brain and its membranes – are 10 in number: 4 single and 3 paired. They are occip-ital, sphenoid, ethmoid, interparietal (single), and parietals, frontals, and temporals (paired). The occipital lies at the posterior lower aspect of the skull, and forms the hinder wall of the brain cavity. Through it passes the spinal cord, which emerges by the foramen magnum, and to a roughened prominence above this foramen is attached the very powerful 'ligamentum nuchae', which supports the head. On either side of the foramen are the occipital condyles which articulate with the atlas – the first of the cervical vertebrae. The lower part of the occipital – the basilar *part* – runs forward along the base of the brain to meet the body of the

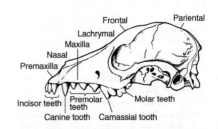

The dog's skull, and teeth of the upper jaw.

sphenoid bone. The inner surface is adapted to the cerebellum – the most posterior upper part of the brain, while above the basilar portion lies the medulla which is continued backwards into the spinal cord. It has the form of a body with 2 pairs of wings and 1 pair of projections. It is supposed to resemble a bird with 2 pairs of wings in flight trailing its legs behind it. The body is continuous with the basilar part of the occipital, and helps to form the base of the brain.

Skunks

Skunks and foxes are now the 2 most important wildlife hosts of the rabies virus in the USA.

Slag

(see BASIC SLAG)

Slatted Floors

These were tried in England in the 19th century and described in the *RASE Journal* of 1860, and had been used for many years in Norway, before being re-introduced in Britain as a means of saving money on straw. The current practice is sometimes to sprinkle sawdust on the slats (of wood or concrete), but to use no straw. The use of slatted floors can hardly be regarded as anything but a retrograde step from the animal husbandry point of view, however attractive commercially. The animals obviously cannot rest as comfortably as on straw, and if strict precautions are not taken (as in Norway) they may be subjected to severe draughts with resultant ill-health and poor food conversion ratios. Teat and leg injuries, and injuries or abnormalities of the feet, may also develop in animals on slats. (See also EPIPHYSITIS.)

The space between the slats is critical, and there must be no sharp edges on the concrete. (See LAMENESS.)

A slatted dunging area and a bedded area are satisfactory. (See also under SOW STALLS and SLURRY.)

Slaughter

(see under EUTHANASIA; STUNNING). Specified intervals between cessation of treatment of food animals with certain drugs are required before slaughter. (See IVERMECTIN.)

Sleep (Horses)

The rest obtained by horses sleeping in an erect position is, actually, not sufficient for their needs. They require complete relaxation of their muscles, and this can only be furnished in the recumbent position. When from fear, ankylosis of vertebrae, or other cause a horse does not lie down, it should be placed in slings, or given some form of support, such as a rope between the heel posts upon which the hindquarters may bear, so that it may obtain the requisite rest.

On board ship, and for surgical or other reasons, horses may be kept standing without harm for considerable periods, but they should be exercised for a short while 2 or 3 times daily, in order that the muscles may be prevented from becoming stiff. Horses are liable to fall while standing asleep, and may, in rare cases, actually come to the ground through the relaxation of their extensor muscles; what happens more frequently is that they knuckle over on to their fetlocks, recovering themselves almost at once, but not before a slight injury has been inflicted to the skin over the joint. The fall always occurs in front, not behind, probably because of the extra weight carried by the fore-legs.

'Sleeper' Syndrome (Haemophilosis)

This takes the form of a septicaemia, is caused by *Haemophilus somnus*, and occurs in cattle in feedlots in the USA. The syndrome is associated with an encephalomyelitis; as well as brain and spinal cord, many other tissues may be involved. It has also been seen in the UK.

Sleeping Sickness

Human trypanosomiasis transmitted by tsetse flies and caused by *Trypanosoma gambiense* and *T. rhodesiensis*. (See TRYPANOSOMES; TROPICS; FLIES.) Sleeping sickness caused by *T. rhodesiensis* can also be transmitted from person to person.

'Sleepy Foal Disease'

Infection with one of the Gram-negative bacteria (see under FOALS, DISEASES OF).

Slings

A device whereby a large animal may be kept in the standing position for long periods without becoming completely exhausted. The apparatus consists essentially of a broad strong sheet which passes under the animal's chest and abdomen, supported by a block-and-tackle or other means to a beam overhead. Connected with this there are 2 strong straps, one passing round the front of the chest, and the other passing round the buttocks. These latter serve to hold the sling in position, and prevent the animals from struggling free. The whole is adjustable so that it may fit animals of different sizes. The sling is often made with a metal or

S

wooden bar along each end of the sheet; these bars serve to distribute the weight of the animal along the whole width of the sheet, and afford a rigid means of attachment to the cross-beam of the slings, to which the chain or rope of the block-and-tackle is attached.

In addition to the above use, slings are one of the means of lifting a horse that has either fallen or lain down in a stable and is unable to rise. The horse is placed so that the slings may be pulled under it, or is rolled on to them, and after the chest and breeching straps are arranged, the horse is lifted by the block-and-tackle high enough to be able to use its feet. It sometimes happens that if the horse has lain for a considerable time it refuses to support its weight on its feet, but hangs 'like a herring' in the slings. In such cases it may be necessary to startle the horse, when it will generally make a lunge and 'find its feet'.

Slings are employed in a variety of conditions, e.g. fractures.

When slings are applied to an animal, they should not be fixed up so tightly that the animal is unable to walk a step or so in each direction. They are only required as a means of support for the animal when it so desires, and not as a suspensory apparatus which is always in use. The animal soon learns to lean on the slings and rest its feet. The hand should be able to be passed under the sling webbing when the animal is standing immediately under the centre of the block-and-tackle, and neither the chest strap nor the breeching should be buckled up tightly. It is generally necessary to secure the head of the animal by a halter to restrict its movements, and to supply a suitable manger or other receptacle from which it may feed easily.

(See also 'DOWNER COW' SYNDROME for a means of lifting a cow.)

Slink Calves

Immature or unborn calves improperly used for human food. The flesh of slink calves is often called slink veal.

'Slipped'

A colloquial expression meaning aborted; also dislocated (see below).

'Slipped Shoulder'

(see DISLOCATION and SUPRASCAPULAR PARALYSIS).

Slipped Stifle

Slipped stifle is the popular term for dislocation of the patella. It may be partial, when the patella slides in and out of the trochlear depression on the femur with each step; or it may be complete, when the patella becomes fixed above the outer lip of the pulley-like trochlear surface, causing all the joints of the affected leg to become straightened, and the limb to be held pointing behind. Dislocation of the patella is a common condition in the dog.

'Slipped Tendon'

A condition seen in chickens, turkey poults, and ducklings, in which there is displacement of tendons and an inability of the leg to support the bird's weight. It is due to a manganese deficiency, and may arise from feeding lime to excess. The incidence is higher in bronze and black turkeys and in dark-coloured chicken breeds, as extra manganese is necessary to synthesise the pigment melanin.

Slope Culture

A method of growing micro-organisms on solid media (e.g. agar) in tubes which are usually arranged in racks at the correct angle for the agar to solidify on cooling.

Slough

Slough means a dead part separated by natural processes from the rest of the living body. The slough may be only a small part, such as a piece of skin that has been burnt by heat or chemicals, or it may be a whole foot. (See GANGRENE.)

Slow-Milking Cows

(see under MILKING MACHINES)

Slow Reacting Substances (SRS)

Also called leukotrienes, they are substances released in an anaphylactic reaction which induce prolonged smooth-muscle contraction. The effect is seen in asthma.

Slugs

The common field slug *Agriolimax meticulatus* is of veterinary interest as intermediate host of the sheep lungworm *Cystocaulus ocreatus*. (For the danger of slug poisons, see METALDEHYDE.)

Slurry

Slurry is the liquid mixture of urine and faeces, together very often with washing-down water and rain-water, which has to be disposed of from pig, beef and dairy units. Deaths of pigs have been reported following agitation of slurry during the emptying of tanks or pits under the piggery slats. It is recommended that slurry should never be allowed to come within 45 cm (18 in) of the slats, and that especially in hot weather emptying should be carried out at least every 3 or 4 weeks. Methane, hydrogen sulphide, ammonia, and carbon dioxide may all be given off as the result of bacterial action on slurry, giving rise to a mixture both lethal and explosive.

Cows, too, have been overcome by slurry gas.

For methods of slurry disposal, see DAIRY HERD MANAGEMENT. (See also under SALMONELLOSIS; PASTURE CONTAMINATION OF; 'MILKSPOT LIVER'; SILAGE.)

Smear Preparations
A film of blood, pus, etc., smeared on to a slide, fixed – and if necessary stained – for microscopical examination.

Smedi
An acronym for stillbirth, mummification, embryonic death, infertility in pigs – a syndrome caused by infection with subgroups of enteroviruses A, B, or C.

Smegma
Sebum with a distinctive odour found in the region of the clitoris and penis. For a test using smegma, see EQUINE CONTAGIOUS METRITIS.

Smell
Smell is detected by the dissolving of minute particles of oderiferous substances, gaseous or solid, in the mucus lining the nose. This triggers a response in the hair-like processes attached to the nerve cells which is transmitted to the brain by the olfactory nerve. The sense of smell is much more highly developed in dogs and cats than in humans. They have a formation at the roof of the nasal passage (the subethmoidal shelf) that extends the range and accuracy of smell detection. The act of 'sniffing', familiar in the case of the dog especially, simply ensures that the particles are rapidly and forcibly drawn upwards into the nose. Smells may be air-borne or ground smells, those left on solid objects by an animal, person or object. The response to a smell can differ in different animals: thus the smell of fish, blood, and offal has a remarkably stimulating effect upon the carnivorous animals, while grass, grain, and vegetable substances stimulate the sense organs of herbivorous creatures particularly. The odour of flesh, blood, etc., is repulsive to the herbivora, and may cause great nervousness and fright. Most of the wild grass-eating animals have remarkably well-developed powers of smell, and are able to locate their enemies at great distances – over 1 kilometre – but they also detect ground smells which are important in marking out territory. It is through the sense of smell

that the male is attracted to the female during the season or oestrus of the latter; the odour at this period is most persistent, and can be appreciated at great distances. Females recognise their offspring by their sense of smell, and dams whose young have died can often be deceived and persuaded into accepting other young animals by clothing these in the skins of the dead ones. This fact is made use of in the case of ewes which have lost their lambs. (See JACOBSON'S ORGAN; PHEROMONE.)

Smells as Evidence of Disease
In certain cases the presence of a smell connected with an animal is almost a diagnostic feature of disease. Thus in decay of the teeth or decomposition of bone there is a characteristic smell which, when once it is appreciated, can never be forgotten, although it is difficult to describe. The breath, urine, and the milk of a cow suffering from acetonaemia have a characteristic sweetish sickly smell. Poisoning by certain drugs, e.g. carbolic acid, can be diagnosed to some extent by the smell of the drug that is left in the mouth or on the skin. The urine of the horse has the smell of violets after the administration of turpentine in large quantities.

It has been suggested that dogs might be trained to recognise certain smells associated with human diseases, and so aid diagnosis at an early stage.

Smog
This is the popular name for fog containing a dangerously high proportion of sulphur dioxide and other harmful gases derived from coal fires and factory chimneys. (See also OZONE for a further description of smog.)

Smooth Collie
This breed, originally a shepherding dog, can inherit, like other collies, collie eye anomaly. Central progressive retinal atrophy is a dominant trait.

Snails
One or two species are of veterinary interest in connection with LIVER-FLUKES and tapeworms.

The giant African snail (*Achatina fulica*) is commonly kept in UK schools to show to biology class pupils; however, it is a potential human health risk. Third-stage larvae of *Angiostrongylus cantonensis*, passed out in rats' faeces, are infective for mammals, and in the Far East have caused meningitis in people; though the majority of cases have occurred through eating uncooked snails. Snails are farmed for food in Britain, as well as in France and elsewhere.

Snakes

Limbless reptiles, widely distributed and differing greatly in size. Many are poisonous. Broadly speaking, those which have 2 rows of small, solid, equal-sized teeth on either side of the upper jaw are non-venomous; while those with 1 row of small teeth on either side of the upper jaw, and 2 or more large, curved, hollow or grooved fangs on the outside of the smaller teeth, should be considered venomous.

Signs Two kinds of symptoms are produced, depending upon the kind of venomous snake involved. In those of the cobra type there is a period of excitement immediately after the bite, lasting only for a few minutes and followed by a period of normality. Then nervous excitement appears, convulsive seizures follow, and death takes place from asphyxia. If death does not occur at once, dullness and depression are seen and death or recovery takes place some hours later. There is usually little pain at the site of injury, and practically no local reaction in rapidly fatal cases.

The symptoms of bite by the adder (*Vipera berus*) – the only poisonous snake found in Britain – are similar, except that there is local pain and considerable swelling. The skin becomes a livid colour, tumefied, and if in a limb there may be severe lameness. The dog often appears to be frightened.

With most snakes, the venom is, of course, introduced by their fangs, which have either a groove on the surface, as in cobras, or a canal down its centre, as in adders.

The African Ring-hals, however, squirts its venom with uncanny accuracy for a distance of about 2 m (6 ft) into the eyes of its victim; the snake rising and opening its mouth wide, its head thrown back.

The rattlesnake venom contains compounds possessing zinc, plus an enzyme which causes destruction of muscle tissue.

In Australia, snake bite was diagnosed at the University of Melbourne in 41 cats over a 6-year period – the tiger snake having been positively identified in 7 of these cases. Symptoms included weakness, dilated pupils and absence of normal reaction to light by the pupils, with vomiting and laboured breathing in some instances. Paralysis and a subnormal temperature suggest a fatal outcome. A high rate of recovery followed the use of 3000 units of tiger snake antivenin.

Animals susceptible Dogs are the animals most frequently killed by snake-bites, both at home and abroad, and sporting dogs suffer more than others. Sheep, cattle, and horses come next in frequency, whilst cats and pigs are only very rarely killed. The reasons for this appear to be that hunting dogs most often disturb snakes, and that grazing herbivorous animals, moving only slowly over a tract of country, disturb snakes less; while the cat is not often attacked because of its greater caution when hunting, and because of its superior agility. Pigs apparently are least often killed because of the protection they possess in a hard tough skin, with a padding of fat immediately below it.

Sneezing

Sneezing is a sudden expulsion of air through the nostrils, designed to expel irritating materials from the upper air passages; the vocal cords being kept shut till the pressure in the lungs is high, and then suddenly released, so that the contained air is driven through the throat into the nose. Entrance to the mouth is prevented by the soft palate closing the exit from the mouth.

Sneezing is induced by the presence in the nose of particles of irritating substances, such as pungent odours, smoke, dust, spores of certain species of fungi, pollen from some grasses, etc. It is also the forerunner of chills, colds, influenza, etc., when it is usually accompanied by a running at the nostrils, and it is a sign of the presence of certain parasites, such as *Oestrus* larvae in sheep and horses, and rarely *Linguatula* in dogs. In pigs, sneezing is an important sign of atrophic rhinitis and Aujeszky's disease.

S-N-F
(see SOLIDS-NOT-FAT)

Snood
The long fleshy appendage extending from the front of a turkey's head over its upper beak.

'Snow Blindness' in Sheep
(see under EYE, DISEASES OF – Keratitis)

Soapwort Poisoning
Soapwort poisoning may occur when the soapwort plant (*Saponaria officinalis*) grows abundantly in pasture. The plant contains the glycoside saponin, which causes frothiness when stirred in water. When saponin is introduced into the body it causes dissolution of the red blood cells, stupefaction, paralysis, vomiting, and purging with the passage of large amounts of frothy faeces, which are mixed with blood.

Soay

A breed of small brown sheep, named after the isle of Soay in the Outer Hebrides, where they have existed since before the Roman occupation of Britain. Their fleeces, which weigh 1 or 2 kg each, are much favoured by hand spinners. The ewes produce only single lambs but mother them very well. The breed has found favour in Cornwall, where they do not graze clover in a grass/clover mixture, so that the hillsides are never overgrazed.

Social Behaviour

(see BUNT ORDER)

Sodium (Na)

A metal, the salts of which are white, crystalline, and very soluble in water. Common salt, or sodium chloride, is contained in the fluids of the body under natural circumstances, and therefore the salts of sodium, when used as drugs, act not through their metallic base but according to the acid radicle with which the sodium is combined. Generally speaking, the salts of sodium act in a manner very like corresponding salts of POTASSIUM but are better tolerated.

Sodium carbonate (washing soda) is an irritant internally, and is therefore never given by the mouth except, in an emergency, as an emetic for the dog. A solution of sodium chloride 0.9 per cent is called 'normal saline', as it is isotonic with body fluids.

Sodium Arsanilate

Sodium arsanilate is an organic preparation of arsenic used for the treatment of coccidiosis in poultry. It has been used by intramuscular and intravenous injection for treatment of certain diseases caused by the presence of trypanosomes in the blood.

Sodium Deficiency

This may occur in dairy cattle in the UK in July. (See also SALT – Salt licks; METABOLIC PROFILE TESTS, 'LICKING SYNDROME'.)

Sodium Metabolism

Sodium is important in maintaining osmotic pressure in the body fluid outside cells, and so controlling body fluid volume. (See also KIDNEYS – Function, and ALDOSTERONE.)

Sodium Monofluoroacetate

A rodenticide also known as '1080'. If ingested by dogs, symptoms of poisoning include yelping, sometimes vomiting, and convulsions. This compound was sometimes used in wild-life rabies control operations against foxes, etc.

Sodium Nitrite

(see under NITRITE POISONING)

Sodium Propionate

(see under PROPIONATE)

Soft Palate

For a condition of this causing distressed breathing in the racehorse, see under PALATE; likewise for prolonged soft palate in the dog.

Soil-Contaminated Herbage

Experiments in Australia and New Zealand with intensively grazed sheep were undertaken to investigate tooth wear in ewes and wethers at various stocking densities. It was found that 'tooth wear was low when soil content of faeces was low and they rose to a peak simultaneously'. Moreover, in the majority of cases, soil content of the faeces was highest where stocking rates were high; when stocked at 9 adult sheep to 4000 sq m (1 acre), the daily intake of soil per head could be as much as 370 g (13 oz) in the rainy season.

In Britain, it has been suggested, July thunderstorms over first-year leys may – by a combination of splashing by rain and poaching by feet – produce a herbage that is seriously contaminated with soil. This could well irritate the sensitive lining of the gut in young lambs, with consequent scouring; this is often seen among lambs believed to be reasonably free from parasitic worms. (See also SAND, COLIC; SILICA CONTAMINATION.)

Solids-not-Fat (S-N-F)

These include the protein casein, milk-sugar, and minerals.

Deficiencies of solids-not-fat lead to difficulties in processing the milk, and render it unsuitable for manufacture into high-class products. Milk produced by a cow affected with mastitis, or by one approaching the end of a lactation, is particularly undesirable.

Maintaining the S-N-F percentage at a satisfactory level is a more difficult problem for the milk producer than rectifying variations in the butterfat percentage. The causes of S-N-F deficiency are not always apparent, and attempts at remedying them may have no rapid effect.

Factors involved include breed of cow, her inherited capacity, age, stage of lactation, the season of the year, feeding, management, and attacks of mastitis.

The diet should contain adequate fibre as well as protein. There is some evidence suggesting that an all-silage diet may lower S-N-F, unless the silage is of the highest quality.

Hay, as well, is desirable. (See RATIONS FOR LIVESTOCK – Winter rationing.)

The percentage of solids-not-fat is relatively high in October and November, after which time it begins to decline and falls to a minimum in February and March. It then starts an upward trend, reaches a high level in May, and may drop again in July and August.

Milk from cows of the Jersey and Guernsey breeds is relatively high in solids-not-fat. British Friesians, as a rule, give milk low in S-N-F. Inherited capacity is important.

The percentage of solids-not-fat in milk varies according to the stage in the lactation. It is high at the beginning, but falls rapidly to a low level within 6 to 8 weeks after calving. Thereafter, it rises gradually if the cow is pregnant, while it tends to decline further if she is not again in calf. Towards the end of the lactation, when the cow is drying off, it may fall very low.

Somatic

Somatic means all the cells belonging to the body except the germ cells in the gonads.

Somatic Nerves

Sensory or motor nerves of the somatic division of the central nervous system; they deal with awareness of sensation and with voluntary control of muscles. (See CENTRAL NERVOUS SYSTEM.)

Somatostatin

A peptide hormone, produced by the hypothalamus at the base of the brain, which acts as a brake on growth by regulating release of growth hormone directly responsible for tissue growth. Animals immunised against somatostatin are not subject to this 'braking' effect, and it has been suggested that this technique might be more effective than conventional growth promoters used in meat production.

Somatotrophin

A growth hormone, produced by the pituitary gland, which stimulates growth of all body tissues, and influences mammary-gland development. Like insulin, somatotrophin helps to maintain correct glucose levels in the blood.

In the 1930s the National Institute for Research in Dairying found that the hormone could increase the milk of dairy cows. In 1983 research was being directed towards production of growth hormone by genetic engineering techniques, with the aim of producing a commercial product which could increase milk yields. This research was successful and trials showed that in cows, fodder was metabolised

more efficiently, producing higher milk yields for a given quantity of feed. However, the argument that this increased efficiency was beneficial did not prevail against UK and EU welfare concerns about its use. Although used in the USA and elsewhere, there is a moratorium on the use of somatotrophin in the EU. (See SOMATOSTATIN; PITUITARY GLAND.)

Sorbitol

A sugar alcohol found in fruits and berries, it is one of the intermediate products in the conversion of glucose to fructose. In severe diabetes mellitus, it is deposited in the lens of the eye.

Sorbitol Dehydrogenase (SDA)

A liver enzyme; raised levels indicate liver damage, particularly in horses. Also called L-iditoldehydrogenase.

Sore Throat

Sore throat is a popular term for laryngitis or pharyngitis, which is often present during catarrh, strangles, influenza, etc. (See THROAT – Throat diseases.) A person with an infected throat may pass the infection to the udders of cows being milked, setting up mastitis.

Sores

(see ULCERS)

Sorghum

Widely grown fodder and grain plant. Poisoning in horses has been recorded in horses grazing pasture containing *Sorghum* species. Hindquarter weakness and paralysis of the bladder may result.

Sorrel Poisoning

(see DOCKS, POISONING BY; SOURSOB)

'Sound'

A blunt metal rod, either curved or straight, which is used for passing along a natural channel or duct of the body. They are generally used to discover whether there are any hard or solid foreign bodies present.

Sounds

Sounds are made both normally and abnormally by some of the organs of the body. For example, during the normal heartbeat there can be distinguished 2 definite sounds. The first of these, known as the 'first heart sound', is a long booming noise, similar to the syllable *lŭb*, which is heard when the ventricles are contracting and the atrio-ventricular valves are closing, and which is produced by these processes. The 'second heart sound' is a short, sharp, sudden sound, similar to the syllable *dûp*, and is heard at the end of the contracting period of the ventricles, when the semilunar valves at the bases of the pulmonary artery and the aorta are closing.

Respiratory sounds are also present normally. The sound made by the air entering the alveoli is generally called the respiratory, or vesicular, murmur. It is a soft, low, quiet blowing sound, which can be imitated by the gentle blowing of air from a pair of bellows. In addition to the friction of the air in the alveoli there is also a sound produced by the air in its course down the trachea and along the greater bronchi.

During disease there are unusual sounds produced, especially by the organs in the chest: for these see RALES; HEART DISEASES; LUNGS, DISEASES OF; etc.

Soursob

The Australian name for *Oxalis cernua*, a member of the sorrel family, found in Australia, South Africa, the continent of Europe, and now the West of England. It has caused fatal poisoning in sheep.

Sow

A female pig that has had one or more litters.

Sow Stalls

Sow stalls have been widely used for dry and pregnant sows, and ensure that each animal obtains her fair share of food. However, in partly slatted stalls, high culling rates have sometimes resulted from defective slats causing foot and leg injuries, leading in some instances to partial or complete paralysis of the hind-quarters. Also the sow is cramped, and cannot move out of draughts; so the use of these stalls can lead to stress. They became illegal in the UK on January 1, 1999 by a unilateral decision of the British government. Leading retailers agreed to obtain pig meat only from sources where stalls are not used. As a result, Denmark and the Netherlands are bringing in legislation to ban sow stalls. (See THIN SOW SYNDROME.)

Sows' Milk

The production of colostrum lasts for about 5 days, during which time the milk composition changes rapidly to 'normal'. In fact there is no such thing as 'normal' milk because its composition changes continually throughout lactation. The protein and mineral contents rise steadily, while lactose and fat contents fall.

Sows' milk is very rich in fat, reaching a peak at about the 3rd week of lactation; levels may reach as much as 17 per cent. This high fat level

may be significant in the frequent occurrence of piglet scours at about 3 weeks of age.

Although inadequate in iron, sows' milk appears otherwise to be an ideal feed for young pigs, allowing an efficiency of feed conversion on a dry matter basis of some 300 g (0.8 lb) feed per 450 g (1 lb) of gain. However, the sow is unable to produce sufficient milk to allow the piglet weight-gain expected. Thus, an average yield is about 45 kg (100 lb) milk per piglet suckled, or 9 kg (20 lb) dry matter in 8 weeks which, at an efficiency of conversion of 0.8, is sufficient to allow a weight gain of 11.3 kg (25 lb). With an average birth-weight of 1.4 kg (3 lb) this would allow the production of 13 kg (28 lb) weaners at 8 weeks. So to produce an 18 kg (40 lb) pig at this age it must have consumed some 11 kg (24 lb) creep-feed at an efficiency of feed conversion of about 2:1.

The major requirement of a creep-feed is energy as the sow's milk should provide adequate protein. An early-weaning diet, on the other hand, requires to have a high protein content, which will vary with the age of pig to which it is given.

Sows' Milk, Absence of,

The absence of milk following farrowing may be due to prior feeding with excessive quantities of fodder beet, or to inflammation of the uterus (metritis). Another cause is an endocrine failure. Post-parturient fever is an important cause. Wet, cold floors and cold, draughty premises appear to predispose sows to mastitis and agalactia.

In herds where agalactia is common, administration of prostaglandin (PG) $F_{2\alpha}$ to induce parturition reduces the number of cases of lactation failure.

In parts of Africa, heavy losses of piglets have resulted from this failure of the sows' milk supply, and the cause was traced to the fungus ergot, parasitic on bulrush millet ('MUNGA'). (See PREDNISOLONE; POST-PARTURIENT FEVER; ERGOT OF MUNGA.)

Soya Beans

Soya beans are rich in protein and fat. Soya flour contains about 40 protein and 20 fat, and is a good source of thiamine, riboflavin, vitamin A, and lysine.

Spanish Fly

(see CANTHARIDES)

Sparganosis

Infestation with *Spirometra* larvae of muscles and subcutaneous tissue. The adult worms infest dogs, cats, and wild carnivores in Australia, the Far East, and North and South America.

Sparganosis is a ZOONOSIS, as people can become infested through eating pork or drinking water containing the larvae at one stage in their development.

Spasm

An involuntary and, in severe cases, a painful contraction of a muscle, or of a hollow organ with a muscular wall. Further information is given under ASTHMA; COLIC; CHOREA; CONVULSIONS; CRAMP; EPILEPSY; MUSCLES, DISEASES OF; SPINE AND SPINAL CORD, DISEASES OF; STRYCHNINE; TETANUS; TETANY; RABIES; HYPOMAGNESAEMIA.

Spastic

Spastic is a term applied to any condition showing a tendency to spasm, such as 'spastic gait'.

In British Friesian cattle, an inherited spastic form of lameness may appear when the calf is 6 or 8 weeks old, but sometimes not until it is 6 months old. Before long, the toe may not touch the ground as the calf walks, and the affected hind-leg is held backwards. Later, the leg becomes shortened and useless. If, however, the case is treated early enough, a simple operation will correct the deformity and prevent these unfortunate sequels. But of course, that calf, grown to maturity, can transmit the deformity to a proportion of its offspring. The condition has also been seen in Shorthorns and Aberdeen Angus crosses. (See TENOTOMY.)

Spavin

General name for diseases of the hock-joint (see BONE SPAVIN; BOG SPAVIN).

Spaying

Surgical removal of the ovaries, and usually of the uterus also, carried out mainly in cats and bitches. (See OVARIO-HYSTERECTOMY for reasons for the operation.)

Also, mares to be used in cavalry regiments, or polo pony mares, as well as certain thoroughbred racing mares, where the occurrence of oestrus and its associated phenomena would interfere with the proper performance of work, and mares which are suffering from some definitely hereditary disease, are subjected to the operation.

In 'nymphomania', ovariotomy, when performed before the symptoms have been in existence for long, usually results in a complete cessation of the kicking, squealing, and fractiousness which generally render the mare unfit for work.

In the past it was common practice to spay both cows and sows – the former giving a continuous milk supply for 18 months or even much longer.

Cats are spayed to prevent the birth of unwanted kittens, adding to the problems of stray and feral cats. The operation is almost invariably satisfactory, and involves few if any disadvantages.

Bitches are spayed to a less extent than cats. The operation may be requested by the owner on account of domestic difficulties or convenience, or it may be advised as a means of preventing pyometra. Bitch puppies can be spayed as early as 8 to 10 weeks of age; kittens also, though probably most are spayed between 3 and 4 months of age.

Ovario-hysterectomy is performed usually through a flank incision.

Spectacles,

Spectacles, so-called, of plastic material are sometimes used to prevent poultry from resorting to cannibalism, etc. 'Spectacles' for horses used in mines are really eye-shields. (See also LENSES, CONTACT.)

Sphinx

A breed of cat originating from Canada, also kown as the Canadian hairless cat. Although it looks hairless, it has a short, soft, downy coat. This provides insufficient insulation and the breed needs a warm environment and protection from sunburn. The breed has a high pain threshold and should not be given the opportunity to engage in fights.

Speculum

Speculum is an instrument designed to aid the examination of the various openings of the body surface. Many are provided with small electric lamps which illuminate the cavity under examination.

Speeds Of Animals

RACING CAMEL In Australia the record is ¼ mile in 27 seconds.

CHEETAHS 100 km/h (62 mph).

GREYHOUNDS The record is 66 km/h (41 mph).

OSTRICHES can achieve a speed of 72 km/h (45 mph) over short distances.

PIGEONS can fly at 74 km/h (46 mph).

PORPOISES can swim at 64 km/h (40 mph).

PRONGHORN ANTELOPE 56 km/h (35 mph) for 6 km (4 miles); 88.5 km/h (55 mph) for 0.8 km (H mile).

RACEHORSES have reached 69 km/h (43 mph).

KILLER WHALE 30 knots.

(with acknowledgements to *Guinness World Records*)

Speedy-Cut

Speedy-cut is the name given to the injury that results from a horse striking the inside of the carpus or metacarpus with some part of the inside of the shoe of the opposite foot. (See BRUSHING AND CUTTING.)

Spermatic

Adjective used to describe blood vessels, nerves, and other structures that are associated with the testicle.

Spermatic Cord

(see INGUINAL CANAL and the illustration under PENIS)

Spermatic Cord, Torsion of

This has been reported, as a rare condition, in the dog. In a review of 13 cases, the testicle involved was intra-abdominal in 11 dogs, and inguinal and scrotal in others. In most cases the torsion appeared to result from enlargement of the testis due to tumours. Two of the dogs died – one of uraemia due to retention of urine, the other from shock – and a 3rd after surgery. However, 10 dogs recovered completely after castration.

Spermatid

A developing stage of the maturing spermatozoa.

Spermatozoa (Sperms)

Spermatozoa (sperms) are the motile male sex cells which, having matured in the epididymis, are ejaculated at orgasm and are normally capa-

ble of fertilising the ovum or egg. The sperms are derived from non-motile cells in the seminiferous tubules of the testicle. The first-stage cells, Spermatogonia, divide to form the primary spermatocytes. When these latter in turn divide, the chromosomes become paired, one from each pair being found in the resulting secondary spermatocytes, which accordingly have half the number of chromosomes found in all the somatic cells. The spermatid is a further stage of development which includes acquisition of the flagellum or tail which provides the sperm with its motility. For their journey to the Fallopian tubes, it appears that the sperms are not wholly dependent upon their own motive powers; the muscles of the female genital organs apparently assist onward movements of the semen.

Each spermatozoon has 3 main parts: the head, containing the cell's nucleus; a middle portion; and the tail. (See also SEMEN; REPRODUCTION; and ARTIFICIAL INSEMINATION.)

In the bull, it takes about 50 days from the time a sperm begins to be formed in the testicle to the time it appears in semen.

All normal semen contains some genetically deleterious diploid spermatozoa, distinguishable by their large size.

Fever may result in increased numbers of abnormal spermatozoa. For example, in Australia many abnormalities have been found in the middle portions of sperms from bulls suffering from bovine ephemeral fever.

Spermiophages

Spermiophages are macrophages which engulf sperms, thereby causing infertility. They have been found in both human and canine semen.

SPF

Specific pathogen-free. In Britain as in the USA, SPF pigs are available for repopulating farms where disease has become a problem. SPF piglets are removed from the uterus by surgery in a sterile manner, reared in elaborate isolation premises, and immunised and prepared for a normal farm environment. (See also 'DISEASEFREE' ANIMALS.)

Sphenoid

Sphenoid is a bone lying along the base of the skull in front of the occipital bone, and immediately above and slightly behind the throat.

Sphincter

A circular muscle which surrounds the opening from an organ, and by maintaining constantly a

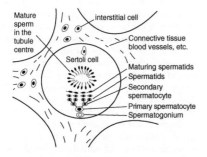

Sperm formation in the testis. (From D. F. Horrobin, *Medical Physiology and Biochemistry*, courtesy of the author and Edward Arnold.)

state of moderate contraction prevents the escape of the contents of the organ. The muscle fibres forming the sphincter relax when the contents of the organ are due to be discharged to the outside past the sphincter. Sphincters close the outlet from the stomach, bladder, and rectum, and regulate the escape of the contents from these organs. Under certain conditions the nervous mechanism which keeps these sphincters shut is liable to become upset, so that faeces and urine, for instance, can escape freely. This incontinence is one of the important symptoms seen in fracture of the spinal column, and in some forms of paralysis.

Sphygmograph

Sphygmograph is an instrument used for recording the pulse.

Spica Bandage

(see BANDAGES)

'Spider Syndrome'

A name given by Minnesota sheep breeders to a crippling congenital disease seen mostly in black-faced lambs. The forelimbs may be bent, spines 'twisted', rump angled steeply from *tuber sacrale* to *T. ischii*.

Spiders

In the USA and South America, dogs are often bitten by the black widow spider (*Latrodectus mactans*), which tends to lurk among piles of logs or in dark outhouses. The bite is extremely painful, and may be followed by vomiting, laboured breathing, weakness, and paralysis. Death follows within hours or days, unless the antivenin is administered.

In the USA bites by the spiders of the suborder Labido are fairly common in horses and dogs, the bites being mostly on the head. Cats are mostly bitten on the face or forepaws. Two puncture marks provide a clue aiding diagnosis. Within minutes or hours, signs of neurotoxicity appear and may last for several days. Myalgia, abdominal rigidity, vomiting, panting, disturbance of vision, and shock occur.

Another spider, the brown recluse (*Loxoceles reclusa*), causes an erythematous lesion, from which a central blister emerges; the skin there turns purple or black. Convulsions followed by death are not uncommon – the preliminary signs being those caused by the Labido spider.

Several of the larger 'bird-eating' spiders have setae, which they brush off their abdomens with their hind-legs. These setae (described under CATERPILLARS) can give rise to dermatitis, pharyngitis, and eye inflammation.

Such spiders are becoming popular as pets, and veterinary advice is increasingly sought on their care.

The Sydney funnel-web spider (*Atrax robustus*) is poisonous to a degree which varies with its sex. The male is much more poisonous than the female. Seventy-five per cent of mice, and 95 per cent of guinea pigs, died after being bitten by male spiders, but only 20 per cent or so after bites by females.

Spina Bifida

A congenital abnormality of the vertebral column, involving a defect in closure of the arch formed by the dorsal laminae of one or more vertebrae. The worst lesions prove lethal. Symptoms of less serious lesions include paresis or paralysis, and incontinence. The condition has been found in dogs.

Spinal Anaesthesia

(see under EPIDURAL)

Spinal Column,

The spinal column, the chain of bones reaching from the base of the skull along the neck and back to the tip of the tail, is composed of the vertebrae, and forms the central axis of the skeleton. Through the spinal canal, formed by the arches of adjacent vertebrae, runs the spinal cord, which gives off the spinal nerves running to various parts of the body. (See BONES; NERVES; SPINAL CORD.)

Spinal Cord

The spinal cord is the posterior part of the central nervous system and is situated within the spinal canal of the SPINAL COLUMN. It forms the direct continuation of the medulla of the brain, being usually arbitrarily held to commence at the foramen magnum, the large opening in the occipital bone at the back of the skull. Posteriorly, it ends about the middle of the sacrum, although in this region the cord has lost its original form, and consists of a bundle of nerves, the actual termination being at about the level of the joint between 5th and 6th lumbar vertebrae, the continuation of bundles behind this being known as the cauda equina, owing to its supposed likeness to a horse's tail. The spinal cord is thus considerably shorter than the spinal column which houses it. During its course in the horse it gives off 42 pairs of spinal nerves, each of which takes origin by means of a dorsal and ventral root, which join each other, before emerging from the spinal canal. These spinal nerves, according to their position, are known as cervical (8), thoracic

(18), lumbar (6), sacral (5), and coccygeal (5). The cord itself is divided into cervical, thoracic, lumbar, and sacral parts. Like the brain, the cord is surrounded by 3 membranes, the dura mater, arachnoid, and pia mater, from without inwards. In the spaces of the arachnoid is a quantity of cerebro-spinal fluid, and between the outside of the dura and the inside of the bony canal is a padding of fat and blood vessels, which together prevent injury to the spinal cord itself during the movements of the spinal column.

On cross-section the spinal cord is found to be composed partly of grey, but mainly of white, matter. It differs from the arrangement in the brain in that while in the brain the grey matter is on the outside of the white mass, in the cord the white matter is superficial. The arrangement of grey matter, as seen in section transversely across the cord, resembles the capital letter H 'horn', and the masses at each side are joined by a wide bridge of grey matter known as the 'grey commissure'. In the middle of this commissure lies the 'central canal' of the cord, which communicates with the ventricles of the brain.

Microscopic structure The grey matter consists greatly of 'neuroglia' cells, the supporting scaffolding fibrous-tissue cells of nerve regions, and in the meshes formed by these cells lie the large multipolar motor nerve cells, and the fibres which spring from them and unite one cell to another, or pass out of the cord to form the fibres of the nerve trunks. The white matter is composed almost entirely of bundles of nerve fibres, most of which possess a myelinated sheath, the white colour being due to the appearance of these sheaths in the mass. (See NERVES.) There is also in the white matter a certain amount of supporting tissue. Blood vessels are found in both white and grey matter.

Functions The spinal cord conveys nerve impulses to and from the brain, but it also deals with spinal reflex actions. For example, sensation of pain in a dog's paw will cause the animal to snatch the paw away from the source of pain, e.g. a hot cinder. Such protective action is a spinal reflex, involving sensory and motor nerves, taken without reference to the brain. (See also CENTRAL NERVOUS SYSTEM and BRAIN.)

Spine and Spinal Cord, Diseases and Injuries of

These will be considered together, because the chief danger of injury to or disease in the spine is that the spinal cord and its nerves may be simultaneously injured or diseased.

Fracture of the spinal column is probably the commonest severe injury that affects this part. It may be encountered in any animal, but is probably commonest in the horse and dog. It usually occurs as a result of external violence, such as falls, falling timber, running into stationary objects and other run-away accidents, in the larger animals; in the smaller animals it is often occasioned by run-over accidents, kicks or blows from large animals, falls from great heights, etc. It may occur from powerful muscular contractions when a horse is cast, or falls in a loose-box, and cannot easily regain its feet; while suddenly pulling up during a gallop in a hilly field occasionally causes it in saddle-horses. Paralysis of the hindquarters, with loss of sensation, and often local sweating behind the injury, are symptoms of fracture, in addition to severe shock, occasioned by the laceration of the cord. (See also FRACTURES; PARAPLEGIA; PARALYSIS.)

Concussion of the cord, occasioned by factors similar to but milder than those which cause fracture, is also common. Generally speaking, if the onset of the symptoms of paralysis occurs a day or two after the accident, instead of at the time, concussion, with or without haemorrhage, should be suspected, and hope of recovery can usually be entertained so long as there is not much systemic disturbance. (See also HORSES, BACK TROUBLES IN.)

Intervertebral disc protrusion Each intervertebral disc, which has a soft, pulpy centre and a fibrous or gristly outer ring, acts as a shock-absorber between the vertebrae, and supports the spinal cord between them. The nature of the usual disc injury is one of partial or complete rupture, with compression of the spinal cord to a lesser or greater extent. The injury is most common in Pekingese, dachshunds, Sealyhams, and spaniels. It also occurs in cats.

The cause would appear to be a gradual wear of the disc with age, and perhaps the extra strain on the spine which may be imposed upon the short-legged breeds. In some cases there is no history of violence; in others, a sudden muscular effort, e.g. in jumping to catch a ball, is the cause.

Symptoms consist of pain and weakness or paralysis of the hindquarters, and may appear shortly after the dog has been observed to jump, slip, or fall; or they may appear in cases where the owner has not observed any violent

S

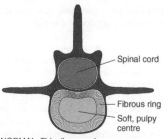

NORMAL: This diagram shows a cross-section through the vertebral column, with the spinal cord above and the disc below.

Labels: Spinal cord, Fibrous ring, Soft, pulpy centre

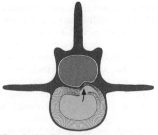

PARTIAL RUPTURE of the intervertebral disc, with pressure being exerted upon the spinal cord.

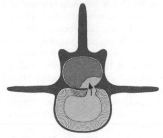

COMPLETE RUPTURE of a disc, with severe compression of the spinal cord.

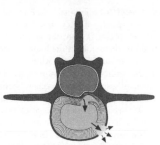

"FENESTRATION" OPERATION sometimes performed to relieve pressure on the spinal cord by making a counter opening.

Intervertebral disc lesions.

movement whatsoever: for example, a dog apparently normal at night may be found paralysed in the morning.

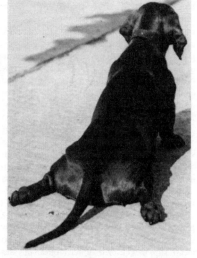

Paralysis due to a ruptured intervertebral disc.

The muscles which control the passage of urine and faeces may become paralysed.

In uncomplicated cases, natural recovery may take place within a fortnight. Where paralysis persists, the outlook becomes progressively less hopeful, though a complete recovery after 12 months is not unknown. It is essential that veterinary attention is given as soon as possible.

A 'fenestration' operation is occasionally performed to reduce pain by relieving pressure upon the spinal cord, but it is not of much use for paralysis. Other measures are for the treatment of paralysis generally.

Cervical spondulopathy (or 'wobbler' syndrome) in the dog is most commonly seen in the Great Dane but also occurs in other breeds, especially the Dobermann. It is usually first seen between 8 and 12 months, and the clinical signs include hind-limb incoordination, abduction of the limbs, a prancing gait, and dragging of the feet causing wearing of the toe nails. Diagnosis of cervical spondylopathy is confirmed by radiography. Lesions include stenosis of the vertebral canal, exostosis of the articular facets, and subluxation.

Hemivertebra 'Wedge-shaped' vertebra; in many cases this condition in dogs gives rise to no obvious symptoms, but in others the condition is characterised clinically by progressive hind-leg weakness, spinal pain, abnormalities of the nervous system and evidence of muscle atrophy or other abnormalities of conformation. Confirmation of the clinical diagnosis is by radiography. Breed incidences are reported. The occurrence of the disorder in certain families of dogs suggests also that it may be hereditary.

Ankylosis of the vertebrae is not rare in horses. It originates from diffuse inflammation of the spinal column, frequently due to rheumatic causes, and one after another of the vertebrae becomes fused to its neighbour in front or behind. In severe cases practically the whole of the thoracic and lumbar regions of the horse may fuse into a rigid bar. Such horses usually can perform straightforward work for some time, but are unable to carry any weight, to back heavy loads, or to lie down or rise with ease. They may develop into 'shiverers', but so long as the spinal cord is not compressed, they may live for years.

Pachymeningitis, or inflammation of the membranes of the cord, sometimes occurs in old dogs. It is called 'ossifying pachymeningitis' in these animals, because of the tendency for bone to be deposited in the dura mater.

Abscess in the cord, or in one of the vertebrae, may be discovered only at a knackery or at autopsy; or it may lead to symptoms of paresis/paralysis. (See also ABSCESS; SPINA BIFIDA.)

Spirillum
A bacterium with a wavy shape. (See RAT-BITE FEVER.)

Spirit
(see ALCOHOL POISONING; and SURGICAL SPIRIT)

Spirocerca
Worms which are found in nodules on the oesophagus. In the dog they may sometimes give rise to cancer (sarcoma) of the oesophagus; and also to fatal haemorrhage. (See ROUNDWORMS.)

Spirochaete
Spirochaete is one of the names applied to bacteria possessing a more or less spiral or wavy outline. Another term applied to this group is 'spirillum'. There are 3 genera which are important causal agents of disease: *Borrelia*, *Treponema*, and *Leptospira*. The 1st has large wavy spirals and is flexible, the 2nd has regular rigid spirals, while the last has small spirals and one hook-like end.

Many spirochaetes produce disease in man and animals, the best known among which is *T. pallida*, the cause of syphilis in man. *T. cuniculi* in rabbits causes 'rabbit syphilis', in Britain, on the continent of Europe and in America. *B. galinarum* is responsible for a form of spirochaetosis affecting fowls in the tropics and subtropics, and is transmitted by the fowl tick. *L. canicola* causes nephritis in dogs and canicola fever in man; *L. icterohaemorrhagiae* causes Weil's disease in man and jaundice in dogs. Leptospirosis also occurs in cattle and pigs, and there are many serotypes. (See LEPTOSPIROSIS and, for infection with *Treponema* in pigs, SWINE DYSENTERY.)

Spirochaetosis of Fowls
Spirochaetosis of fowls is met with in Africa, Asia, the West Indies, South America, Australia, and Europe. It occurs in fowls, ducks, geese, and turkeys. Canaries and other birds are susceptible to artificial infection.

Transmission The disease is transmitted from diseased to healthy fowls by the fowl tick *Argas persieus*, one of the most important parasites of poultry. The ticks are very active at night, and may travel long distances to reach a host. They remain hidden during the day in crevices and underneath the bark of trees. Myriads of these ticks may attack fowls on the roost, a large quantity of blood being sucked – the affected birds becoming weak and unthrifty and having ragged plumage.

If, however, the ticks have fed on a bird affected with spirochaetosis, they become carriers of this disease and may transmit the infection through the egg to the next generation of ticks.

Signs Affected fowls show diarrhoea, loss of appetite, loss of power of the head, and may die in convulsions. A more chronic course is also described, birds becoming paralysed and emaciated, and dying in about a fortnight.

Treatment Antibiotics are effective.

Preventive Treatment This consists of ridding the premises of ticks.

Spirochaetosis of Pigs
(see under PORCINE ULCERATIVE SPIROCHAETOSIS and SWINE DYSENTERY).

Spirometra

A tapeworm which infects cats, dogs, and occasionally people.

Splanchnic

Splanchnic means relating to the viscera (internal organs) of the body – as distinguished from its framework.

Splayleg, Congenital

Congenital splayleg of piglets may involve either the fore-legs or all 4 legs. Recovery from this defect can be expected if the piglet can manage to keep out of the sow's way. (See VITAMIN E.)

Spleen

A soft, highly vascular, plum-coloured organ, possessing a smooth surface formed by a dense fibrous capsule over which the peritoneum is closely applied.

Structure Beneath the outermost covering of peritoneum lies the dense fibrous-tissue coat, from the inner surface of which numerous strands or 'trabeculae' run into the organ. The fibrous coat and the trabeculae possess elastic fibres and a fair number of plain muscular fibres. The trabeculae branch and rebranch throughout the substance of the organ, and in the meshes so-formed lies the spleen-pulp. This consists of delicate connective-tissue fibres passing between the trabeculae, and numbers of leucocytes and red blood corpuscles. Blood vessels run through the trabeculae and end in areas where the blood cells appear to be highly concentrated; these concentrations are known as Malpighian corpuscles or bodies. The blood escapes into the pulp of the spleen instead of travelling through capillaries everywhere as in other organs.

Functions The spleen destroys old red blood cells, acts as a blood store, and appears to play some part in the formation of lymphocytes.

An animal is able to survive after removal of the spleen. There is a compensatory increase in the lymph nodes all over the body, and, after a period of adjustment, life continues normally.

The spleen is apparently concerned also with bodily defence, and resistance to liver-fluke infestation is reduced after removal of a sheep's spleen. (See RETICULO-ENDOTHELIAL SYSTEM.)

Spleen, Diseases of

It is often only at post-mortem examination that spleen diseases are revealed in the large animals. In anthrax it becomes greatly enlarged, and also in babesiosis. In the dog, splenectomy is occasionally performed in cases of tumour formation or injury. Rupture of the spleen, with resultant internal haemorrhage, occurs in small animals which have fallen from a height or have been involved in a road accident.

Splenectomy

Surgical removal of the spleen.

Splinting Materials

For the immobilisation of limbs to achieve external fixation of fractured bone, or to provide additional support for internal fixation, plaster of Paris and resin-impregnated materials are used.

For large-animal use, plaster of Paris has several disadvantages: it does not achieve its maximum strength for up to 24 hours after application, and is liable to break. The cast is often heavy and cumbersome, and will soften in contact with moisture.

A number of proprietary splinting materials are available, which offer advantages of strength, lightness and transparency to X-rays. They include: Baycast (Bayer), a polyester cotton bandage impregnated with a water-activated prepolymer resin; Scotchcast, which consists of polyurethane resin on a fibreglass bandage; Hexcelite, a thermoplastic material, stated to be easily applied and very strong.

Splints in Horses

The splint-bones are the rudientary 3rd and 4th metacarpals; 'splints' is the common name given to exostoses (bony outgrowths) on the splint-bones producd by inflammation.The inflammation itself may be caused by a knock or a minute fracture. They are more common in young horses and slight or severe lameness may be seen. Splint formation usually starts in the periosteum or ligament. The amount of new bone formed depends on the extent and duration of the inflammation.

The lameness disappears as the inflammation subsides. The causes include an inherited defect.

Signs Usually, lameness appears before any bony enlargement can be seen or felt, although pressure over the region of splints causes pain. This lameness usually increases with exercise. The horse may walk sound, but trots lame to a surprising extent, considering the apparently 'sound' walk. Later on, a soft putty-like swelling can be felt, and this becomes harder with time, until it can be finally recognised as bone. In knee-splint the leg is carried to the outside, and appears stiff. As a rule splints are not serious, since with rest and treatment the bony fusion becomes complete, and the horse goes sound. When they are placed high up, however, there is a danger that the new bone formation may involve the knee-joint, and when they are situated far back, so as to interfere with the tendons, they may produce permanent lameness and injury to the tendon. In a horse under 6 years old they should be looked upon as liable to cause future trouble, but in a horse over 6 years old they can be disregarded unless lameness is present.

Treatment Most mild cases require nothing further in the way of treatment than a rest from work, and later a run at grass for a fortnight or so. Topical applications of anti-inflammatory preparations or hot fomentations may help to relieve pain during the acute stage.

Spondylitis
Inflammation of a vertebra, due to trauma or an infection.

Spondylosis A degenerative condition of the spine which can lead to ANKYLOSIS.

Spondylopathy
Disease of the vertebrae such as may cause compression of the spinal cord, disc degeneration, and narrowing of the intervertebral space.

Sponges
In modern stables it is recognised that if a contagious disease breaks out, the sponge used for a number of horses is an important factor in the spread of the disease, and consequently a piece of flannel or other material which can be boiled is generally used instead for 'quartering' (see GROOMING). A sponge used at the end of a hosepipe for udder-washing of cattle led to an outbreak of mastitis due to *Pseudomonas aeruginosa*.

Spongiform Encephalopathy (Human)
The human spongiform encephalopathies – Creutzfeldt-Jakob disease (CJD), Gerstmann-Straussler-Scheinker syndrome (GSS) and kuru – are pathologically very similar to scrapie in sheep and to bovine spongiform encephalopathy (BSE). Like them, they are transmissible, although there is very little evidence of person to person transmission, except in a very few iatrogenic cases, such as the grafting of corneal or dura mater tissues from donors subsequently shown to have had CJD, and the use of human growth hormone prepared from the pituitary glands of patients dying with CJD. Kuru was transmitted by cannibalism in Papua New Guinea.

(See also BOVINE SPONGIFORM ENCEPHALOPATHY; FELINE SPONGIFORM ENCEPHALOPATHY.)

Sporadic Disease
A sporadic disease is a disease occurring in single cases here and there, as distinct from disease occurring as an enzootic, throughout a district, or epizootic, through a country or large tract of land.

Spores
Reproductive cells of protozoa, bacteria, and fungi, etc., usually able to withstand an adverse environment.

Sporidesmin
A poisonous substance, isolated from the fungus *Pithomyces chartarum*, which causes facial eczema and liver damage in sheep and cattle in New Zealand and Australia.

Sporotrichosis
A fungal disease of horses, cattle, dogs, cats, and man, caused by *Sporothrix schenckii*. This gives rise to nodules under the skin, and thickening of the lymphatics with ulceration. In the dog, liver, lungs and bone may show lesions. Of 19 people reported to have acquired this infection from cats, 14 had no history of traumatic injury at the site; 12 were veterinarians or assistants/nurses. All had a localised cutaneous lymph-node infection, lesions resolving in 1 to 10 months after potassium iodide treatment. One patient had a deep ulcer on a finger. Although rare, infection through inhalation has been recorded in people.

Sporozoa
This is a group of Protozoa which are all parasitic and produce spores at some stage of their life-cycle. It is divided into a number of orders, of which only 2 are important. These are the Haemosporidia which are parasites of the red blood cells, and the Coccidia which are parasites of epithelia.

Spotted Fever
(see ROCKY MOUNTAIN FEVER)

Spotted Horse
(see under APPALOOSA)

Sprained Tendons
Sprained tendons is an extremely common condition in both the heavy and the light draught

S

horse. The flexors, superficial and deep, are mostly affected.

Causes The superficial flexor tendon is sprained during maximum weight-bearing by the limb, and the deep flexor becomes sprained at the period of thrust.

Signs There are the usual signs of inflammation – heat, pain, swelling. A horse with a badly sprained deep flexor may walk almost sound, but goes pronouncedly lame when made to trot. A localised sprain of the check ligament and its insertion into the deep flexor tendon often produces acute lameness, but the condition is not as serious as a sprain of the tendons lower down. From an owner's point of view, however, differential diagnosis between the various forms and situations of sprain is not important.

Treatment A firm elastic support bandage, and adequate rest. A poultice, spread on cotton-wool and applied hot, before bandaging, is a traditional remedy.

Generally a horse with a badly sprained tendon is not fit for work for a month to 6 weeks, although it may be apparently sound before this time.

Chronic sprained tendons are often incurable, but good results have sometimes been obtained with DIATHERMY.

Sprains

Sprains involve the wrenching of a joint, often with the simultaneous tearing of a ligament. The term is also applied to an inflammation of a tendon, generally the result of an excessive stretching of its fibres. (See SPRAINED TENDONS; SYNOVITIS.)

Spray 'Drift'

By this is meant droplets of spray liquid carried by the wind to fields adjacent to that which is being intentionally sprayed with some farm chemical for purposes of weed control, pest control, haulm destruction. It is a potential cause of poisoning in grazing animals. (See SPRAYS USED ON CROPS.)

Spray Race

A race which can be used for spraying sheep or cattle. Nozzles are arranged at intervals and fed with suitable parasiticide liquid by means of a pump. The system has not been found as satisfactory as dipping for sheep scab.

Sprays used on Crops

Sprays used on crops include weedkillers such as DNOC, insecticides such as parathion, and potato-haulm destroyer such as arsenites. Such substances constitute a hazard to livestock which gain entry into fields. (See POISONING; INSECTICIDES; WEEDKILLERS).

'Spreading Factor'
(see HYALURONIDASE)

Spring Viraemia of Carp

A serious viral disease to which farmed or ornamental fish are particularly susceptible. It is transmitted by lice which parasitise carp. Clinical signs vary, but affected fish swim erratic-ally, may be swollen, and have small red spots on the skin. It is a NOTIFIABLE DISEASE.

Spur Veins

The veins liable to damage by the horseman's spurs.

Spurges, Poisoning by

The various species of spurges (*Euphorbia* spp.) are, apparently, mostly poisonous, though not to the same extent. Animals are not likely to eat them because of the acrid milky sap. Species which have been blamed for causing poisoning are as follows: caper spurge, *E. lathyris*; Irish spurge, *E. hibernica*; petty spurge, *E. peplus*; and the sun spurge, *E. helioscopia*. Of these, the first seems to be the most dangerous.

Signs Inflammation and swelling of the mucous membranes of the mouth and tongue, pains in the abdomen, coldness of the extremities of the body, dizziness, fainting, leading to unconsciousness and death in 2 or 3 days. In one of the South African spurges, *E. genistoides*, the typical symptom, in addition to these mentioned here, is an acute inflammation of the urethra, accompanied by frequent and painful attempts at urination. Symptoms of acute enteritis may also be seen.

Treatment Veterinary advice should be sought at once and, since the milk of affected cows may cause illness to people drinking it, it should not be used for either human or animal consumption.

SRM (Specified Risk Material) In the case of bovines, for animals aged 12 months or more this is the skull including brain, eyes, tonsils and spinal cord. For bovines over 6 months, the spleen, thymus and intestines are also included. SRM must be stained to prevent its consumption and destroyed by incineration or rendering. For sheep and goats older than 12 months, SRM includes the skull, including

brain, eyes, tonsils and spinal cord; the spleen of any age of sheep or goat is included. The tongue is exempt, provided it is removed immediately after slaughter.

St Bernard

A very large dog with a massive head and drooping ears, traditionally used for mountain rescue work in the Swiss Alps; the rough-coated variety is commoner. The breed is prone to 'diamond eye' – a combination of entropion and ectropion. Wobbler syndrome (cervical spondylolithesis) is inherited as a recessive trait and haemophiolia B is a sex-linked recessive trait. Other inheritable conditons include ununited anconeal process and a progressive posterior paralysis (Stockards disease).

'Stable Cough'

(see EQUINE INFLUENZA)

Stable Fly

Stable fly is a serious pest to horses and other animals, and transmits diseases such as surra and anthrax in the tropics. (See FLIES – Fly control measures; SUMMER SORES.)

Stable Vices And Tricks

(see 'VICES' AND VICIOUSNESS)

Stables for Racehorses

A survey of 96 racehorse stables in the south-west of England showed that a 'typical' race-horse is kept in a loose-box with a floor area of 12 m² and is bedded on straw; it shares its airspace of 39 m³ with 7 other horses. In calm conditions, with the top door of the stable open, natural convection would provide 6.6 air changes/hour, but with the door closed, only 2.2 changes. The top door should rarely, if ever, be closed. It has been suggested that present-day stables are based on designs which are worse than the best available in the 19th century. (See also BEDDING.)

Staffordshire Bull Terrier

A medium-sized muscular breed with a smooth coat, often mainly white. Cataract may be inherited and the breed is prone to cleft palate. The American pit bull terrier was derived from the Staffordshire, which it resembles; it is advisable to keep a pedigree record to avoid confusion and impounding under the Dangerous Dogs Act.

Stag

In deer, it is a male of some species; the female of those species is always called a hind and the young, calves. It is also the British term for a male turkey.

Staggers

Erratic gait caused by incoordination of the limbs, as in 'rye-grass staggers'. It may be seen in hypomagnesaemia.

'Staggers Weed'

A poisonous South African plant. (See 'PUSHING DISEASE'.)

Staining

For differentiation of bacteria, see ACID-FAST ORGANISMS; GRAM-NEGATIVE.

Stallion

An adult male horse, uncastrated, over 4 years old.

Standard International Units

(see SI UNITS)

Staphylococcus

(see BACTERIA)

Staples for Wound Closure

These have long been used in human surgery in place of stitches and are also used as wound closures in some types of surgery for animals.

Starch

(see CARBOHYDRATE; DIET AND DIETETICS; DIGESTION)

Starch Equivalent

This term is no longer used, and the starch equivalent in the UK was replaced in 1975 by units of METABOLISABLE ENERGY as part of the introduction of metric and SI UNITS.

Starch Gel Electrophoresis

This is one of the commonest techniques for studying the genetic variation in serum proteins. (See ELECTROPHORESIS.)

Stargazer

The term applied to a newly hatched chick or poult where the head is permanently held back with the beak pointing directly upwards. Affected birds may twist their heads continuously. The cause is a deficiency of thiamine.

Staring Coat

Dry, dull, scurvy hair or fur. A common sign of poor condition of whatever cause. In the dog, one cause is lack of suitable fat in the diet. As a first-aid measure, offer bread and butter or dripping (but not margarine) for a few days as an 'extra'. It is seen in, e.g., cattle, often as the result of parasitic gastroenteritis. (See also under WORMS.)

Stasis

Stasis is a term applied to stoppage of the flow of blood in the vessels or of the food materials in the intestinal canal.

'Steaming up'

A term used by dairy farmers to describe the practice of feeding a concentrates ration 4 to 5 weeks before calving in order to provide for growth of the fetus and provide reserves against the onset of lactation. Nowadays, it is generally considered that 'steaming up' is not to be encouraged as it tends to lead to poor dry matter intakes after calving, and fatty liver and acetonaemia. Usually, the aim is to provide small quantities (3 to 5 kg; 6½ to 11 lb dry matter) of the production ration in a complete diet for about 2 weeks prior to calving. Concentrate should not usually be fed at more than 2 to 3 kg (4½ to 6½lb) daily in two feeds for a similar period. For detailed advice on 'steaming up', see under ACETONAEMIA – Prevention.

Excessive 'steaming up' is regarded as one cause of LAMINITIS and lameness.

Steatitis

A yellow discoloration of fat occurring in cats, mink, and pigs fed mainly on fish scraps or tinned fish. Listlessness, tenderness over the back and abdomen, and a reluctance to move are observed. In cats, steatitis may follow prolonged and continuous feeding not only with red tuna or pilchards, but also with white fish such as coley. The symptoms include stiffness and pain. Steatitis in horses has also been reported. Pathological changes in the fat taken from the abdominal wall was found in 44 of 173 horses and ponies examined post-mortem at the Institute of Veterinary Pathology, Utrecht, over a 2-year period. Steatitis was found in fetuses from normal mares, and in adult horses. Subclinical steatitis was the most common type, but a few deaths were attributed to this cause. Lesions varied from the presence of macrophages in the fat, to some fibrosis in addition, and to necrosis.

Treatment includes a change of diet and a vitamin E supplement.

Steatorrhea

Fatty faeces.

Stell

A circular stone or corrugated metal shelter for sheep or cattle, built on moorland or hill, and affording good protection against snow drifts. Stells were in use in the early 19th century, if not earlier. (See diagram, page 665.)

Stenosis

Stenosis is any unnatural narrowing of a passage or orifice of the body. It is specially reserved for application to the heart valves, and to the opening through the larynx – the glottis – but is applied to any of the large arteries, as well as to the parotid ducts. (See HEART DISEASES; LARYNX; PAROTID GLAND; PYLORIC STENOSIS.)

Stenson's Duct

Stenson's duct is the duct which carries saliva from the parotid gland into the mouth. (See PAROTID GLAND.)

Stent

A device used to support or to keep in place a skin graft or other surgical suture. Stents woven in the form of a tubular mesh from surgical-grade stainless steel, and self-expanding when released from a small-diameter delivery catheter, were developed for endovascular use, but are also used to relieve urethral stricture in human patients.

Stephanofilariasis

A chronic skin disease occurring in cattle in parts of the USA, and caused by the nematode worm *Stephanofilaria stilesi*. The intermediate host is the horn fly.

Sterilisation

(see CASTRATION; also SPAYING for sterilisation in the sexual sense).

With reference to sterilisation in its other sense, see DISINFECTION; ANTISEPTICS; ASEPSIS; WOUNDS. For most general purposes the best sterilising agent is boiling water. Boiling should be continuous and should last for 30 minutes in order to kill vegetative bacteria, viruses, and most other types of micro-organisms. Surgical instruments and dressings are usually sterilised in an autoclave which reaches temperatures in excess of 100°C.

Sternum

The breastbone. This forms the floor of the chest (in quadrupeds), provides attachment for the pectoral muscles, and for the costal cartilages of the sternal (true) ribs. (The asternal (false) ribs are not directly connected to the sternum.) The sternum comprises sternebrae

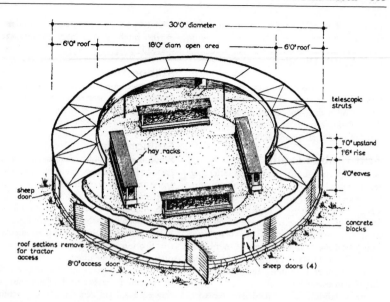

Of metal construction, on a base of concrete blocks, this modified stell at the Rowett Research Institute, Aberdeenshire, was designed by Dr E. Cresswell. Sheep doors and a doorway for tractor access are shown.

– segments which fuse together with advancing age. The horse and dog each have 8 of these; the cow 7; pig and sheep, 6.

Steroids

Chemical substances closely related to the sterols, e.g. the sex hormones, hormones of the adrenal cortex, bile acids. (See also CORTICOSTEROIDS; DIABETES.)

Prescribing steroid hormone products (where allowed)

Steroid hormone growth promoters are substances with an androgenic, oestrogenic or gestagenic action. In general they must not be administered to farm animals. 'Farm animals' includes cattle, sheep, pigs, goats, horses, poultry, the wild animals of these species and any ruminants raised on a holding.

The prohibition does not apply to:

(a) the administration for therapeutic treatment by a veterinarian in the form of an injection of oestradiol-17-beta, progesterone or testosterone or derivatives of these substances which readily yield the parent compound on hydrolysis after absorption at the site of application;

(b) the administration of a steroid hormone product for the termination of unwanted gestation or the improvement of fertility;

(c) the administration of a steroid hormone product by, or under the direct responsibility of, a veterinarian for the synchronisation of oestrus or the preparation of donors or recipients for the implantation of embryos.

For the purposes of the controlling regulation, the term 'injection' does not include implantation and the term 'therapeutic treatment' has a very restricted meaning – i.e. the treatment of a fertility problem diagnosed by a veterinarian in an animal not intended for fattening.

A small range of products is licensed in the UK for the purposes listed above. **The regulations are subject to change; the current status of hormonal products should be checked.**

Sterols

Solid alcohols, waxy substances derived from animal (and plant) tissues, e.g. cholesterol, ergosterol.

Stertor

Noisy breathing resembling snoring.

Stick Insects

Slow-moving green or brown insects that resemble twigs, often kept as 'pets'. They are vegetarian and must have fresh food that is not allowed to wilt. Hygiene is important in their care.

Stiff Lamb Disease
This is a mild disease occurring in East Anglia due to infection with *Erysipelothrix rhusiopathiae*, the cause of swine erysipelas. The same name is also applied to muscular dystrophy, a condition similar to that occurring in cattle as a result of vitamin E deficiency.

'Stiff-Limbed Lambs'
This is a hereditary condition affecting newly born lambs, to which the name *Myodystrophia fetalis deformans* has been given. It is commoner among Welsh Mountain sheep than among other breeds. The condition is an arrest of the development of muscular tissue during fetal life, and a replacement by fibrous tissue. This contracts and pulls the limb into an unnatural, stiff attitude, and gives rise to difficulty in parturition.

The condition is a Mendelian recessive lethal. It has been reported from Britain and America as affecting cattle, but it is not at all common in them.

Stiff Sickness
(see STYFZIEKTE)

Stifle
The joint corresponding to the human knee. (See BONES and JOINTS.) In horses, stifle lameness is often the result of OSTEOCHONDROSIS dissecans or of subchondral bone cysts.

In 42 cases of stifle lameness in cattle, the diagnoses included subchondral bone cysts (18 cases), joint instability (15), degenerative joint disease (12), cranial cruciate ligament injury (9), sepsis (9), collateral ligament injury (3), femorotibial luxation (2) and intra-articular fracture (2). The prognosis for animals with bone cysts was good, irrespective of treatment (75 per cent recovered), while it was much poorer for animals with sepsis (22 per cent) or joint instability (27 per cent).

Stilbenes
Substances consisting wholly or partly of stilboestrol, hexoestrol, dienoestrol, or benzestrol. (See HORMONES IN MEAT PRODUCTION.)

In accordance with an EU directive, the sale of veterinary medicines, veterinary products or animal feeds containing these stilbenes was banned in 1982 in the UK for use in food animals.

An exemption allows the limited use of stilbenes in companion animals for treating enlarged prostate glands, adenoma, misalliance in the bitch, and urinary incontinence in spayed bitches.

Stilboestrol
An oestrogen formerly used both therapeutically and as a growth promoter in food animals. (See HORMONES; HORMONE THERAPY; HORMONES IN MEAT PRODUCTION; STILBENES.)

Stillborn Pigs
Breeding stock should, of course, have access to pasture, but if for any reason this golden rule is going to be broken, then rations should be supplemented in summer as well as in winter, with vitamin A. In a group of 20 gilts which were suddenly switched from succulent feeding to dry, fibrous grazing late in pregnancy, severe constipation resulted, and there were dead piglets in 19 of the litters.

A survey carried out by the Veterinary Investigation Service in England and Wales showed a 4.8 per cent incidence of stillbirths out of a total of 4394 piglets born in 371 litters. The incidence varied widely from herd to herd, as would be expected – ranging from 0.4 to 12.9 per cent. Constipation appears to be a cause of stillbirths, and SENNA may be used.

There are several infections which give rise to abortion and stillbirths. (See AUJESZKY'S DISEASE; ABORTION; MUMMIFICATION; INFERTILITY; CARBON MONOXIDE.)

Stimulants
Heart 'stimulants' include caffeine, digitalis, etc. (See also RESPIRATORY STIMULANTS.)

Stings
(see BITES AND STINGS)

Stirk
A young female bovine of 6 to 12 months old, sometimes a male of the same age, in Scotland.

Stitching
(see SUTURE; WOUNDS)

Stockard's Disease
An inheritable posterior paralysis found in individuals of cetain breeds of dog.

Stocking Rates
During the peak of grass growth from early April to mid-June, 8 to 10 ewes and their lambs can be carried per acre (4000 m²). But this is a maximum figure for this period only. For cattle, continuous grazing, the figure is perhaps 1 to 3 acres (12,100 m²).

In Britain, 'most grass is greatly under-stocked during the grazing season, chiefly due to the lack of capacity to carry more stock over winter.

'Good farmers, using intensive grass-farming methods, require 1½ acres (6000 m²) or more per cow, even when winter feeding is supplemented considerably with concentrates.

'Estimates in New Zealand have suggested that dairy cows at 1.2 per acre may consume as little as 30 per cent of the available herbage.' (Director, Grassland Research Institute, Hurley.)

The most skilful dairy farmers were soon achieving 0.9 to 1.0 acre per cow without purchasing more than 10 to 15 per cent of their winter feed requirements other than production concentrates.

Stockmen/Women

For health hazards see under COWHERDS; SHEPHERDS; MEAT-HANDLERS; ZOONOSES.

Stomach

Functions of the stomach (see RUMEN;
RUMINAL DIGESTION; RETICULUM; OMASUM; ABOMASUM.) Broadly speaking, the function of the stomach is to store, warm, soften, and prepare food materials, and then to pass them on in regulated amounts into the intestine, where the more important digestive processes and absorption occur.

Stomach, Diseases of

In all animals bacterial diseases, such as SALMO-NELLOSIS, may be involved in diseases of the stomach; likewise parasitic worms.

Horse In view of the comparatively simple arrangement of the stomach, and the natural fastidiousness of the horse in the matter of food, stomach disease is not so common as in some other animals.

Gastritis is usually brought about by the ingestion of irritant, poisonous, or otherwise harmful substances, or by the presence of bots, or spread of disease from other parts of the body. (See also SALMONELLOSIS; ROUNDWORMS.)

Signs Attacks of violent abdominal pain, occurring shortly after feeding or even before feeding is completed, indicate that the stomach is affected. Dullness and depression are noticed; patchy sweating may break out; food is refused; the temperature rises slightly in mild cases, and to as high as 41°C (106°F) in severe instances.

Usually within 2 to 3 hours after taking food the acute pain ceases, but the horse remains dull, and gives the impression that it is affected with a dull ache rather than with acute pain. Vomiting does not usually occur unless the stomach is ruptured or the oesophagus is dilated.

Impaction of the Stomach is a condition in which engorgement of the stomach with food takes place. It may be due to lack of vitality (atony) in the muscular walls, to impaired gastric secretion.

Signs Signs of impaction may occur, suddenly or gradually. There is depression, uneasiness, and perhaps colic, in those cases where a horse over-eats. (See COLIC.)

Sometimes a horse obtains relief by vomiting through the nostrils a quantity of the impacted material, which reduces the amount in the stomach so that the remainder can be dealt with in the usual way.

Prevention It is easier to prevent impaction of the stomach than it is to cure it.

Whole beans, peas, wheat, or barley should not be used for horses. Horses should always be allowed as much water as they desire to drink, and should be watered before feeding in all

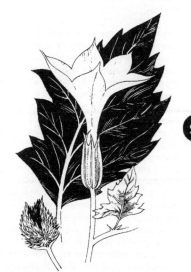

Thorn apple (*Datura stramonium*), which is also known as the Jamestown or jimson weed. The flower may be white or purple. On the left is a fruit capsule. Well-developed plants may be 1.6 m (5 ft) high. (See entry for Stramonium, page 670.)

S

cases. Diseased or rough and irregular teeth should be treated.

Tympany of the stomach When vegetable food ferments from any cause, gas is produced. Certain foods, especially when unsound, undergo fermentation in the stomach instead of digestion, and the gas so formed is liable to collect in that organ often under pressure producing great distension. Foods which ferment easily are succulent green crops, clovers, lucerne, and potatoes eaten in quantity.

Signs There is no remission of pain, such as is usually seen when the intestines are tympanitic. Horses may roll, plunge, and paw the ground during the earlier part of the attack. Respirations increase in rate, and become laboured. The abdomen becomes tense and often swollen, and in many instances horses assume a crouching attitude with their hindquarters, not unlike the way in which a dog sits. When the tympany is severe, unless relief is afforded by the passage of the stomach-tube, rupture of the stomach may occur, and death follow. (See COLIC.)

Rupture of the stomach may also occur when a horse falls violently to the ground soon after a big feed, i.e. when the stomach is full.

Signs The distress characteristics of engorgement and tympany suddenly cease when the stomach ruptures, and for a short time the horse appears so much better that the owner imagines recovery will result. After a short time, however, the more serious symptoms of peritonitis and shock occur. Profuse perspiration usually breaks out; the pulse changes to what is called a 'running down pulse', i.e. there are a few strong beats which gradually become weaker until they are almost imperceptible, and then a succession of strong beats return; this is repeated rhythmically. Ears and feet become cold and clammy to the touch; respiration is blowing; and the expression on the face of the horse is one of anxiety. Vomiting is said to characterise rupture of the stomach, but it is probable that in most cases the vomiting occurs before the rupture takes place; the food material escapes into the abdominal cavity after rupture has occurred rather than up into the pharynx and nostrils. (See also COLIC.)

Treatment is usually regarded as useless; euthanasia is advisable.

Cattle Acute indigestion with acidosis, and sometimes impaction of the rumen, may follow overeating of grain or green foods. (See ACIDOSIS.)

Tympany of the rumen (bloat) consists of a collection of gas in the rumen. (See under BLOAT for symptoms, prevention and treatment.)

Inflammation of the rumen (see also RUMEN ULCERATION) may be due to ingestion of irritant poisons, of either chemical or vegetable origin, to penetrating foreign bodies, or to the spread of inflammatory conditions from other parts in specific diseases.

Foreign bodies in the reticulum are of great importance in both young and adult cattle, because of the close proximity of this organ to the pericardium and heart. In the reticulum 2 things may happen: they may fall to the lowermost part of the sac and remain there for an indefinite period, or they may slowly penetrate its wall and wander forwards through the diaphragm. Their subsequent course is described under HEART DISEASES – Traumatic pericarditis of cattle. (See also HAIR-BALLS)

Inflammation of the abomasum, abomastitis, or gastritis, is caused by a lack of long-fibre roughage and the too-rapid introduction of concentrate diets after calving; it may also be caused by parasitic roundworms. (For the causes, symptoms, and treatment of parasitic gastritis in cattle and sheep, see PARASITIC GASTROENTERITIS.)

Displacement of the abomasum may be associated with stenosis of the sigmoid curve of the duodenum in cattle. The abomasum is then found to be distended with fluid and gas, and displayed to the right.

Signs include a distended abdomen, loss of appetite, loss of weight, and depression of milk yield, and may sometimes be successfully treated by casting the cow and, with her lying on her back, rotating or rocking her through an angle of 45° from the vertical each way. Surgical treatment may be necessary. (See TYMPANITIC RESONANCE.)

Ulceration is a condition by no means rare in cattle. It is sometimes associated with displacement of the abomasum, and may give rise to symptoms a few days after calving. Death follows perforation. Symptoms are similar to those given above. Ulceration is not uncommon in calves after weaning, giving rise to capricious appetite and sometimes evidence of abdominal pain. *Fusiformis necrophorus*, *Actinomyces pyogenes*, and *Pasteurelle* organisms in other parts of the body may be associated.

Sheep The diseases of the stomachs of the sheep resemble in general those of the same organs in cattle.

Braxy is characterised by a patch of acute inflammation in the wall of the abomasum, usually about the size of the palm of the hand, where the mucous membrane is to a large extent destroyed.

Another form of gastritis is due to parasitic worms in the young lambs. (See WORMS.)

Pigs

Gastritis Irritating or poisonous substances, specific disease, or parasites are among the causes. Salt poisoning is a cause of gastritis, as are also poisonings by arsenic, copper, saltpetre, sheep dips, etc. During the course of swine fever, swine erysipelas, foot-and-mouth disease, and even tuberculosis, the wall of the stomach may become involved, and inflammation may result. (See under GASTRIC ULCERS.) Parasites may also cause this condition. (See WORMS, TREATMENT AGAINST; MUCORMYCOSIS.)

Signs Vomiting is the first and most important symptom of stomach disturbance. Thirst, depression, and sometimes skin discoloration are other symptoms. Convulsions and twitching of the limbs may be seen in young pigs.

Treatment All solid foods must be withheld, and soft light foods given instead. Whole milk is one of the best. Where the condition is believed to be due to poisonous substances, the appropriate antidotes must be given. (See ANTIDOTES.)

Dogs Gastritis may be bacterial in origin, caused by parasitic worms, irritating substances which include poisons, or be associated with foreign bodies. It is probably less common than enteritis or nephritis, both of which may give rise to vomiting.

Causes Gastritis/gastroenteritis may be a complication of distemper, canine virus hepatitis, or may arise during salmonellosis and other bacterial disease; or follow the eating of infected or decomposing food.

Ulceration of the stomach in dog and cat may be associated with gastritis – sometimes with tuberculosis, malignant growths, and actinobacillosis. Ulcers similar to peptic ulcers in human beings, and leading to perforation, occur occasionally.

Signs As a rule, a severe attack of vomiting immediately after a feed, and refusal to touch food subsequently. Thirst is nearly always excessive, and if gratified, vomiting usually follows.

If capillary haemorrhage occurs into the stomach, perhaps as the result of retching, the blood which slowly oozes from its walls collects in the cavity of the stomach, undergoes partial digestion, and becomes changed into a brownish granular material, strongly resembling moist coffee grounds. This always has a most foul and objectionable odour. The dog itself becomes extremely miserable, dragging itself slowly from place to place, and showing preference for cold places where it may lie stretched out with its hind-legs straight behind it, so that the lower wall of the abdomen is in close contact with the cold surface, e.g. a stone step, or linoleum in a passage. Constipation usually occurs unless the intestines become involved, when diarrhoea is noticed. Pressure on the abdomen causes pain, and sometimes a dog lifted by the hand under the abdomen cries out. The temperature is raised at first.

Treatment Hot packs applied to the abdomen soothe pain. Dogs affected with gastritis should be under the charge of a veterinary surgeon, who will vary the treatment according to the circumstances.

At first food is better withheld. (See PYLORIC STENOSIS; GLUCOSE; NORMAL SALINE; PROTEIN, HYDROLISED.)

Foreign bodies in the stomach may include pieces of carpet or other fabric, the rubber from a golf ball, the covers of tennis balls, bones, pieces of wood, etc. A depraved appetite may be due to hunger, a mineral or vitamin deficiency, rabies, or to bad habits – such as picking up and swallowing pebbles (often misguidedly thrown by the owner).

Signs Ineffectual attempts to vomit, accompanied by painful retching, an arched back, salivation from the mouth, and signs of discomfort. Sharp-pointed bodies may cause perforation of the stomach walls, peritonitis, and death. (See PERITONITIS.)

In small toy dogs it is quite usual for symptoms of acute nervous excitement to be shown.

With chronic gastritis due to swallowed pebbles, symptoms are those of occasional vomiting, discomfort, and even a rattling sound as the dog walks.

First-aid An emetic, e.g. a crystal of washing soda and water.

Treatment Apomorphine given by hypodermic injection will rid the stomach of the greater part of fibrous or soft ingesta, but where sharp-pointed foreign bodies have been swallowed, obviously it is unsafe to give emetics. To remove these and large rounded objects which cannot be easily vomited, surgery will be necessary.

Torsion of the stomach Except in the giant breeds of dogs, torsion or twisting of the stomach is rare. The abdomen becomes painful to the touch, swelling may be apparent, and vomiting likely to occur. The dog is soon in a very distressed condition, and needs emergency treatment or death will result.

Pyloric stenosis and pylorospasm (see under these headings for disease affecting the pylorus of the stomach)

Stomach-Tube

A flexible, often rubber, tube used for introducing into the stomach (either through the mouth or more often through the inferior meatus of the nostril on one side), with a view to relieving tympany, or introducing medicines in the treatment of disease. It is about 3 m long for horses and cattle, and about 10 to 15 mm in diameter (proportionately smaller for other species).

A tube which possesses 2 channels is sometimes used to attempt to remove from the stomach portions of poisonous plants which may have been eaten. Water is pumped down through one channel, and when the stomach is full it runs from the other carrying with it small pieces of the harmful material. It is not possible to empty completely the stomach by the double stomach-tube, but considerable amounts of the harmful material may be removed.

The stomach-tube is extremely useful in those cases of colic which depend upon disturbances in the stomach, and if warm water is introduced by it in impaction of the large colon, peristalsis can often be stimulated. (But see DEHYDRATION.)

Its use demands care and a knowledge of the structure of the nasal passage, pharynx, gullet, and stomach.

Stomatitis

Inflammation of the mouth and gums (gingivitis), tongue (glossitis) or lips (cheilitis). (See BOVINE PAPULAR STOMATITIS; FOOT-AND-MOUTH DISEASE; VESICULAR STOMATITIS; SWINE VESICULAR DISEASE; MOUTH, DISEASES OF; FELINE STOMATITIS.)

-Stomy

A suffix signifying formation of an opening in an organ by operation, e.g. gastrostomy and colostomy.

Stones

(see CALCULI and FOREIGN BODY)

Storing Feeds

(for safe storage periods see under DIET AND DIETETICS).

Stot

A steer.

Strabismus

A condition in which each eye appears to be looking in a different direction. Also called squint.

Straights

Single feeding-stuffs of animal or vegetable origin, which may or may not have undergone some form of processing before purchase, e.g. flaked maize, soya bean meal, fish meal, barley.

Strain

The over-stretching of muscle fibres. Often a few of these are ruptured. A painful condition requiring rest. The same is true of overstressed tendons. (Compare a SPRAIN which involves ligaments of a joint.)

Stramonium

Stramonium is the leaf of *Datura stramonium*, which is popularly known as the thorn apple or the Jamestown or jimson weed. It contains the alkaloid daturine, which is almost identical in its actions with atropine.

The plant has caused fatal poisoning in pigs in Britain. However, the fatalities which have been reported appear to be the result of ingestion of large quantities of the plant in the absence of other food.

Strangles

Strangles is an acute contagious fever of horses, donkeys, and mules.

Cause *Streptococcus equi.* Strangles is commonest and most serious in horses under 6 years of age. Mature horses living in a stable where an outbreak has occurred are frequently unaffected.

Signs Typical attacks begin with dullness, lack of appetite, rise in temperature to between 39.5° and 40.5°C (103° and 105°F) and congestion of the visible mucous membranes, especially of the nose and eyes. Nasal discharge is at first thin and watery, but soon becomes thicker, and profuse. There is often a cough. One or both of the submaxillary nodes, or perhaps one of the pharyngeal nodes, becomes enlarged, hot, tense, and painful to the touch; until a soft spot, usually over a most prominent part of the swelling can be detected. This indicates the 'pointing' of the abscess. Following its resolution the horse improves greatly; temperature falls, appetite returns, and the animal becomes much brighter.

Complication: occasionally a suppurative pneumonia occurs. There may also be abscess formation in the liver or other abdominal organs.

Treatment The owner should call in a veterinary surgeon. Immediate isolation of the affected horse is necessary. (The box or stall where it stood must be disinfected as carefully and thoroughly as possible, and should be left vacant for 3 to 4 weeks afterwards.) The sick horse should be clothed and made comfortable. Soft foods, such as mashes, are indicated, as swallowing may be painful. (See NURSING OF SICK ANIMALS.) Antibiotics and/or sulfa drugs are used.

Prevention An efficient vaccine can be produced only if encapsulated *S. equi* is used (i.e. from very young cultures) and the capsule not destroyed by formalin and excessive heat. In older cultures, the capsule is lost and the organism no longer invasive.

Human Infection by *S. equi* has been recorded.

Strangulated Hernia

The term is applied to a loop of intestine becoming trapped in a hernia, so that the blood supply to that section of it is cut off. (See HERNIA; 'GUT-TIE'; VOLVULUS; INTESTINES, DISEASES OF.)

Strangury

Difficulty and pain in passing more than a few drops of urine at a time. It is a sign of an inflammatory condition situated in the kidneys, bladder, or urethra.

Straw
(see under BEDDING; DAIRY HERD MANAGEMENT; DEEP LITTER)

Straw feeding of cattle Straw is commonly included in diets, particularly when treated with sodium or ammonium hydroxide. It has been used in a strict maintenance diet of 2 kg (4 lb) each of barley and a low protein-mineral-vitamin concentrate with some 4.5 to 5.5 kg (10 to 12 lb) barley straw.

Experimentally, up to 30 per cent of ground straw has been incorporated into beef rations, along with 10 to 20 per cent molasses, 45 per cent cereals, and 5 per cent total minerals, vitamins and urea to provide a complete ration. Fed *ad lib*, this is claimed to have consistently given daily liveweight gains in excess of 1.3 kg (2.8 lb) with Friesian steers in commercial trials.

The main snag with feeding ground straw is its tendency to produce frothy bloat (with loss of appetite and loss of weight in subclinical cases). This has been overcome, it is claimed, by inclusion in feeds of an anti-bloat preparation (Poloxalene).

(See also NITRITE POISONING.)

Straw is a very useful bedding material for livestock.

'Strawberry Foot-Rot'

The colloquial name applied to a condition caused by the fungus *Dermatophilus pedis* or *D. congolensis*.

'Stray Voltage'
(see under ELECTRIC SHOCK)

Streams

As a source of drinking water for cattle these should always be suspect, since they often carry infection from one farm to another, e.g. COCCIDIOSIS; JOHNE'S DISEASE; SALMONELLOSIS.

'Street' Virus

This term refers to the naturally occurring rabies virus, such as may be isolated from a rabid dog.

Streptococcal Meningitis
(see under PORCINE STREPTOCOCCAL MENINGITIS)

Streptococcus

A micro-organism which under the microscope has much the appearance of string beads. It is responsible for strangles, mastitis, acute abscess formation, etc. (See BACTERIA.)

Streptococcus Suis

Streptococcus suis infection is a cause of meningitis and lymphadenitis in pigs.

Streptodornase, Streptokinase

Enzymes used to dissolve pus, fibrin, and blood clot in infected wounds. They have also been used in the treatment of mastitis.

Streptomycin

An aminoglycoside antibiotic obtained from *Streptomyces graces*. Active almost entirely against Gram-negative organisms, streptomycin has given good results against infection with *Corynebacterium (Actinomyces) pyogenes*, *Staphylococcus pyogenes*, *C. renale*, *E. coli*, and *Pasteurella septica*.

It has been used in cases of calf pneumonia and calf scours, some types of bovine mastitis, and complications of viral diseases in the dog, and in septic conditions in the cat. (In medical practice, streptomycin is regarded as one of the most toxic of the antibiotics in common use. It may cause deafness and vestibular disturbance in dogs and cats.) Resistance to this antibiotic develops readily and is usually multiple. For these reasons, other anti-biotics are to be preferred when suitable.

Streptothricosis

Infection with streptothrix organisms. In Britain, the name is applied to the disease in cattle equivalent to lumpy wool or wool rot, caused by *Dermatophilus dermatonomus*. A scurfy, scaly condition of the skin is produced, and scabs come away with a bunch of hairs attached if plucked. Anything which lowers the resistance of a hitherto healthy animal facilitates infection; and prolonged wetting, insect bites, thistle pricks, and other tiny breaks in the skin may all predispose to infection.

In the tropics, the name is applied to infection with *D. congolensis*.

The onset of the rains brings an increase in the incidence and severity of the disease, which is of great economic importance in Central and West Africa. Flies, ticks, and thorn bushes appear to play some part in the production and spread of the disease. Zebu cattle, as exotic cattle, appear highly susceptible; while N'dama and Muturu humpless cattle are resistant. It seems that infection does not give rise to later immunity.

Treatment with antibiotics or sulfonamides offers most chance of success, but is impracticable in many areas. (See DERMATOPHILUS.)

Streptothrix

Dermatophilus congolensis (see STREPTOTHRICOSIS and SENKOBO)

Stress

In human medicine it is now recognised that mental stress, anxiety and frustration can exert a profound effect for the worse upon bodily health. Similar effects may be found in animals. Stress can adversely affect production in food animals and behaviour in companion animals.

On a farm in New Zealand where theoretical considerations were all against high milk yields, the yields were, in fact, extremely high. After a detailed investigation it was concluded that the reason could only be sympathetic handling at milking time by the farmers – father, son, and daughter – who were strikingly 'in harmony' with their cattle.

By contrast, on another New Zealand farm where everything – staff, milking machines, and herd management – remained the same, the strangeness of a new milking shed was apparently the sole cause of a 15 per cent reduction in milk yield. (See also CALF HOUSING.)

Stress is recognised as a predisposing cause of diseases in pigs, following the mixing of litters, castration, etc.; and in all species following parturition.

Subjection of animals to noise in intensive livestock production, or in the course of transport, can be a source of stress. Reduction of noise could have considerable economic benefits. (See TRANSPORT STRESS.)

Sheep Problems can arise in paddock grazing. The grassland breeds need a greater space, if stress is to be avoided. They are the hedge-breakers and fence-testers. They 'work away' at weak places with a will to escape.

Where a very large number of sheep are dealt with in one unit, it has been shown that it is especially desirable to reduce the flock to units of 80 ewes during the intensive management period at grass. Stress can result in a subclinical infection turning into overt illness. (See also BUNT ORDER; INTENSIVE LIVESTOCK PRODUCTION; INFECTION.)

Dogs Stress may result from being left tied up for long periods, or alone in an otherwise empty house; sometimes from ill-treatment by one member of a family. Dog fights are another cause, or merely the presence of a large dog in the vicinity, known to be a fighter. Being lost or abandoned, placed in boarding

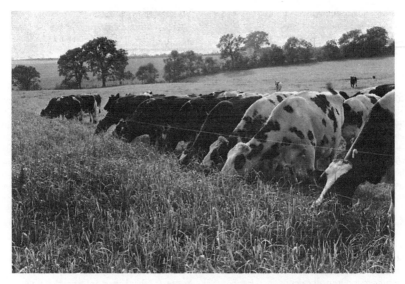

Controlled grazing, showing use of an electric fence. (*Farmers Weekly*.)

kennels, change of ownership, etc., can all cause stress. Diarrhoea, sometimes vomiting, and 'compulsive' polydipsia may result.

Cats The presence of a particularly aggressive tom (perhaps newly arrived in the district); the addition of another cat or dog to the household, or a mother paying less attention to the cat after the birth of a baby; or too many cats in the same house or confinement in a boarding cattery – these are all potential causes of stress.

During times of stress, a cat may develop a transient hyperglycaemia. This could lead to a mistaken diagnosis of diabetes.

Stricture
An abnormal narrowing of one of the natural passages of the body, such as the oesophagus, bowel, or urethra.

Strike
Blowfly myiasis, the condition resulting from infestation of the living skin of sheep by the larvae of blowflies which, in certain circumstances, lay their eggs in the wool. The flies are, apparently, attracted by putrefactive odours, and strike accordingly most often occurs in the region of the hindquarters in sheep which have been scouring. Some cases of strike begin, however, in the clean wool covering the shoulders and loins; and other parts may be affected.

Where there is sufficient moisture the eggs hatch in about 12 hours and the resulting larvae attack the skin with their mouths and secretions, causing raw areas. The consequent moisture favours the larvae, and their excreta attracts further blowflies which give rise to further generations of larvae.

Signs A characteristic twitching of the tail is seen when the hindquarters are affected. Tufts of white wool, discoloured wool, and the odour are indications of strike in other parts of the body. Death may occur within a week, and the mortality may be high among hill sheep especially, as the trouble may in them go undetected.

Treatment consists in the use of a dressing which will kill the larvae and facilitate healing of the wounds.

Prevention (see DIPS; INSECTICIDES)

String as a Foreign Body
It might reasonably be thought that string would be the least dangerous of foreign bodies, but such is not the case. Gravy-soaked string may inadvertently be included in a dog's or cat's meal of chicken scraps or leftovers from a joint of beef. Occasionally string will form a loop around the base of the tongue, but more often it will pass into the stomach, causing local inflammation and sometimes obstruction. In

the intestine, swallowed string is apt to lead to an accordion-pleated appearance of the bowel wall, which may perforate. One dachshund had no fewer than 15 such perforations, each of which had to be sutured during the course of a life-saving operation.

Stringhalt

Stringhalt is the sudden snatching up of one or both hind-legs of the horse when walking or, less often, when trotting.

All classes and ages of horses may be affected, although it is perhaps commonest in older horses. It often appears about the time when maturity is reached, i.e. 5 to 6 years or a little sooner.

Causes The cause of stringhalt is unknown.

An Australian form of stringhalt is seasonal in incidence, and possibly associated with plant poisoning. Several horses in a locality may be affected. Recovery occurs after weeks or months, but not in all cases.

Neither pain nor lameness is associated with stringhalt, but the condition constitutes an unsoundness, and is incurable.

Strip-Cup

(see MASTITIS)

Strip-Grazing

Strip-Grazing of cattle behind an electric fence tends to give greater production per acre, but it carries with it a risk of worm infestation under lush condition unless a back-fence is brought up at 5-day periods, and 'resting pastures' avoided. The use of an electric fence for strip-grazing on 'early-bite' is valuable. It induces the cattle to eat the whole plant instead of nibbling off the most succulent leaf-tips which predisposes to bloat. (See illustration, page 673.)

Stroma

Tissue which forms the structure of an organ but does not play a part in its function. For example, the stroma of a secretory gland does not itself secrete.

Strongyles

Roundworms (red worms) of the family Strongylidae. They are parasitic in many farm animals and can cause anaemia, unthriftiness, debility, intermittent colic. (See FOALS, DISEASES OF; and under ROUNDWORMS.)

Strontium

(see under RADIOACTIVE STRONTIUM)

Struvite

A magnesium-aluminium-phosphate compound found in urinary calculi (see FELINE UROLOGICAL SYNDROME).

Strychnine

Strychnine is one of the 2 chief alkaloids of the seed of *Strychnos nux-vomica*, an East Indian tree – the other being brucine, which is less powerful and not used medicinally, although its actions are similar to those of strychnine. Strychnine itself is a white crystalline substance, possessing an intensely bitter taste. Strychnine (or nux vomica) was at one time much used as a tonic, especially during convalescence from debilitating illnesses, in pneumonia, and in atony of the bowels.

It is now used only for the killing of moles, under strict control.

Strychnine Poisoning

Signs In the larger animals the symptoms consist of convulsive seizures, characterised by a pronounced spasmodic contraction of the muscles of the limbs and trunk, and by a drawing back of the head and hollowing of the back (opisthotonus). In the horse, the eyeballs roll and the eyelids are seen quivering and often becoming drawn back, exposing the white of the eye. In the smaller animals the same symptoms are seen, but the seizures are of a more violent nature, and the periods of relaxation are shorter.

First-aid If a large dose has been taken, an emetic should be given at once to the smaller animals, preferably apomorphine given hypodermically; the larger animals should have their stomachs emptied as far as possible by the use of the stomach-tube. Tannic acid or strong tea is indicated for immediate first-aid.

Treatment Expert advice should be sought without loss of time. The patient should be anaesthetised.

Stud Tail

An over-production of sebum by the modified sebaceous glands on the dorsal aspect of a cat's tail. The fur tends to become matted, and bare patches may occur. The precise cause is unknown, but it has been suggested that close confinement, and a consequent failure of the cat to groom itself, leads to 'stud tail'. Prolonged treatment may be necessary, on the line of that for acne.

Stunning, Electric, of Cattle

This is practised in Sweden and the Netherlands by means of the Elther apparatus (prior to Jewish ritualistic slaughter or otherwise). It is used also for calves, sheep, and goats.

Stunning, Electric, of Pigs

This has been practised extensively since the 1930s, and involves the use of brine-soaked electrodes, applied on each side of the pig's face, by means of which the electric current is passed. A voltage of not less than 75 is recommended and a current of not less than 250 milliamperes, assuming 50 cycles-per-second alternating current. An electroplectic fit is caused, with anaesthesia lasting for about 60 seconds, when conditions are satisfactory. After 60 seconds, there may be a half-minute period of paralysis during which sensation is present. Therefore, the pigs must be stuck during the first 60 seconds. If care is not taken and the apparatus be faulty or unsuitable, paralysis only, and not anaesthesia, may result; the pig being conscious when stuck.

High-voltage stunning The trend towards the use of 180 to 600 volts has been impeded by the commonly held belief that it might adversely affect 'bleed out'. However, the ARC's Meat Research Institute has shown that this need not be so.

Stunted Chick Disease

This syndrome in chickens was first recognised by Kouwenhoven and others in 1978, and has since been found to occur worldwide. The cause is believed to be a virus, possibly exacerbated by *Campylobacter* spp. and spirochaetes.

Sturdy

A neurological disease in sheep caused by *Coenurus cerebalis*, it is also known as GID.

Stye

(see EYE)

Styfziekte

Styfziekte is a name meaning 'stiff sickness', which is used to describe either the symptoms associated with chronic aphosphorosis, which is the forerunner of lamziekte in South Africa, or those associated with a mineral deficiency in certain parts of northern Nigeria.

Subclinical

A disease is said to be subclinical when the symptoms are so slight as to escape the notice of the animal-owner. Examples: subclinical mastitis, which by lowering the milk yield of a herd of cows may be of considerable economic importance; similarly, a subclinical infestation with parasitic worms. (See also STRESS.)

Subcutaneous

Subcutaneous means anything pertaining to the loose connective tissue lying under the skin, such as a subcutaneous injection, where the injected fluid is introduced below the skin. (See under INJECTIONS.)

Subluxation

A partial dislocation. Atlantoaxial subluxation is a cause of neck pain and muscle dysfunction in some toy breeds of dogs.

Treatment In 13 cases the atlas and axis were stabilised with a wire suture; in 10 cases lag screws were used for fixation of the ventral articular facets. Nine of them recovered within 2 months.

Sucking (Intersucking)

This habit or 'vice' occurs among dairy calves. If allowed to go unchecked, the practice may become habitual, involving a risk to the health of the calves, and, if persisting into adulthood, the welfare of the herd in general may be affected. In a herd of 50 Friesian cows the habit grew so pronounced that the herd became uneconomic and had to be dispersed. Cattle of all ages were involved and milk loss was considerable. Purchased calves acquired the same habits after a short while. Intersucking is a problem in only a small proportion of herds, usually those of above average size, where the calves are bucket fed, or where they are grouped at or shortly after birth.

The most effective remedy is to separate the calves after feeding, but if this is not practicable, mechanical devices or the provision of dry food are good alternatives. It seems that a useful preventive measure is to delay grouping calves until they are more than 4 weeks of age.

Suckling

(see CALF REARING)

Sudden Death

(see under DEATH)

Sudorifics

Sudorifics are drugs and other agents which produce a copious flow of perspiration. (See DIAPHORETICS.)

Suffocation

(see ASPHYXIA and CHOKING)

Sugar

Sugar is a substance containing the elements carbon, hydrogen, and oxygen, and belonging therefore to the chemical group of carbohydrates. This group includes three main subdivisions as follows:

(1) Monosaccharides, or glucoses ($C_6H_{12}O_6$):
   e.g. Dextrose or grape-sugar,
      Levulose.

(2) Disaccharides, or sucroses ($C_{12}H_{22}O_{11}$):
   e.g. Cane-sugar,
      Lactose or milk-sugar,
      Maltose or malt-sugar.

(3) Polysaccharides, or amyloses ($C_6H_{10}O_5$)n:
   e.g. Starch,
      Glycogen (animal starch),
      Dextrin and other gums.

Glucose is the form of sugar present in the blood, and reserves are stored in the liver in the form of glycogen.

Starch is mentioned under a separate heading, and its use as a food-stuff is described under DIET AND DIETETICS.

Sulfaquinoxaline

Mixed in food or drinking water, for the control of coccidiosis in poultry.

Sulfasalazine

(see EYE, DISEASES OF – 'Dry eye')

Sulfonamides

A group of drugs which are, to susceptible organisms (e.g. streptococci), bacteriostatic (rather than bactericidal); that is to say, they prevent the multiplication of bacteria rather than killing them. Sulfonamide drugs are all synthetic and closely related to p-aminobenzoic acid, which is believed to be essential to bacteria, and which is absorbed by them; and it is believed that the sulfonamides are absorbed by the bacteria similarly, with the result mentioned above. Individual sulfa drugs do not have specific action against specific bacteria; their differences lie in the differing concentration or level which can safely be obtained in the animal's bloodstream, and their excretion route.

Uses Sulfonamide drugs are extensively employed in veterinary medicine for dressing wounds, for the prevention of post-operative sepsis, and in the treatment of pneumonia, metritis, enteritis, 'joint-ill', foul-in-the-foot of cattle, and arthritis in young pigs, etc. They must be used in full dosage, or resistant strains of bacteria may be set up.

Residues Traces of sulfonamide are occasionally found in pig kidneys. Where sulfa drugs are prescribed for farm use, management procedures should be examined to avoid risk of residues. Likely causes of residue problems include: sows having access to medicated creep in farrowing pens; barrows used to carry medicated feed being used for carrying feed for finishing pigs without being cleaned; failure to clean pens used for medicated pigs before restocking.

Toxicity Sulfonamides may have an adverse effect upon the host's cells as well as upon the invading organisms. For this reason (and to avoid giving rise to resistant strains), sulfonamides should be used only under veterinary advice and not indiscriminately. Fortunately, however, domestic mammals, with the exception of the goat, show few signs of intolerance. Sulfanilamide is, however, highly toxic to birds.

Names of individual compounds The list of these is being continually extended, but mention may be made here of:

Sulfadiazine. Has been used in the treatment of calf pneumonia, etc.

Sulfadimidine. Of value in foul-in-the-foot in cattle, pneumonia, enteritis. Is readily accepted in the food by all animals.

Sulfaguanidine. Used in the treatment of white scour of calves, necrotic enteritis in pigs, and enteritis in other animals. Readily taken in the food.

Sulfamerazine. Has been used in the treatment of calf pneumonia, etc.

Sulfamethoxipyridazine. Used to treat coccidiosis in sheep.

Sulfanilamide. Of value as a dry dusting powder for wounds, teat sores, etc. May be combined with 1 per cent neutral proflavine sulphate.

Sulfaquinoxaline. Used in the control and treatment of coccidiosis in chickens and turkeys.

Sulfathiazole. Has been used in the treatment of calf pneumonia.

Sulpha (Sulfa) Drugs

(see SULFONAMIDES) The International Nonproprietary Name (sulfa-) has superseded the original UK form (sulpha-).

Sulphur

Sulphur is a non-metallic element which is procurable in several different allotropic forms, e.g. 'flowers of sulphur'. As a parasiticide, sulphur has been largely replaced by more effective substances, although proprietary organic preparations of sulphur are still used in the treatment of mange.

Internally, sulphur was at one time a popular laxative and mild tonic, and no doubt still enjoys a vogue among some animal-owners.

Poisoning Overdosage must be avoided: 85 g (3 oz) of flowers of sulphur has killed cattle. Dosing by guesswork on the part of a shepherd killed 140 ewes in a single flock.

Accidental poisoning by sulphur occurred in 14 horses, 2 of which died.

Sulphur Dioxide

A poisonous gas which is a constituent of diesel engine exhaust fumes. (See SMOG.)

Summer Mastitis

Summer mastitis is caused by *Actinomyces pyogenes* and *Peptococcus indicus*. Both the headfly and *P. indicus* are implicated in the aetiology of this disease. (See MASTITIS; FLIES.)

Summer Sores

Summer sores in horses are caused by infective *Habronema* larvae deposited in wounds by stable- or house-flies. They are very itchy. Eyelids may be affected. The infestation results in the formation of fibrous nodules which may later ulcerate. Summer sores are uncommon in Britain.

Sunburn

(see LIGHT SENSITISATION; EYE, DISEASES OF; CANCER). This is a hazard for a number of animal species. White pigs must be protected from sunburn by providing shade. Small animals, particularly those with short coats, can be affected: Mexican hairless dog, shar-pei, sphinx cat etc. A type of sunburn can occur in some fish in clear water where no shade is available.

Sunlight

(see under RICKETS; INFERTILITY; LIGHT SENSITISATION; TROPICS)

Sunstroke

(see HEAT-STROKE)

Superfetation

The presence in the uterus of fetuses of different ages, due to successive services.

For example, a cow is got in calf at one service, comes on heat again, and settles to a further service – in due course producing a calf as the result of the first mating, but more often than not having little or no milk. She later calves again, as the result of the second mating, and this time lactation begins. Calves born in this way are not, of course, twins. Although contemporaries within the dam, they are of different ages, and can have different sires.

An elderly cow, which had always had single calves, was 'put to AI again and subsequently on 3 occasions at normal intervals, after which she appeared to hold'.

Presuming that she had held to the last service, her owners were very surprised to find her one morning, 2 months before she was expected to calve, licking a full-term heifer calf which was 'quite obviously hers'. The milk yield was poor, and so the cow was left at grass to suckle her calf. Two months later she 'suddenly bagged up well and calved a live, full-term bull calf in circumstances that left no doubt it was hers also'.

Subsequent blood tests, carried out in Copenhagen, showed that the first calf was not by the AI centre's bull as stated. The second was.

The remarkable features of this example of 'double pregnancy' are that artificial insemination did not disturb a 2-month embryo; and the stress and exertion of calving did not affect a 7-month fetus, either.

Superinvolution

Superinvolution is the contraction of the uterus after parturition when the shrinkage proceeds beyond the normal, and the organ is less in size than before conception. It may proceed to such an extent that the dam is subsequently unable to breed, or it may result in a reduction in size of the organ, which is not very important.

Superovulation

The production of extra (mammal's) eggs. It can be induced by means of hormones. (See TWINNING.)

Superpurgation

Superpurgation is excessive purgation which continues for some considerable time, and may end fatally. It is most serious in the horse, where it may follow the administration of aloes. It may also arise through the ingestion of food-stuffs which are unwholesome, such as sprouted potatoes and decomposed mouldy oats; and it may result from horses breaking out from a stable and getting into a field of clover or lucerne. (See PURGATIVES; LAXATIVES; COLIC.)

Supplementary Feeding

(see FLUSHING OF EWES; FEED BLOCKS; UREA; SUPPLEMENTS; CREEP-FEEDING)

Supplementary Veterinary Register

(see under VETERINARY SURGEONS ACT 1966)

Supplements

Products for use at less than 5 per cent of the total ration in which they are included, and designed to supply planned proportions of vitamins, trace minerals, one or more non-nutrient additives and other special ingredients.

Suppository

A suppository is a small conical mass made of glycerine or a similar substance, and containing drugs intended for introduction into the rectum.

Suppuration

The formation or discharge of pus (see under ABSCESS; CELLULITIS; FISTULA; INFLAMMATION; PHAGOCYTOSIS; WOUNDS).

Suprarenal Bodies

(see ADRENAL GLANDS)

Suprascapular Paralysis

Suprascapular paralysis occurs as a result of injury to the suprascapular nerve. The term 'slipped shoulder' is applied to the symptoms which are shown in a typical case. The supraspinous and infraspinous muscles act as ligaments of the shoulder-joint, and when they are paralysed the shoulder slips outward each time the foot is placed upon the ground and when weight is put upon it. After the paralysis has been in existence for some few days, 2 distinct hollows appear over the shoulder, due to atrophy of the muscles, and the spine of the scapula stands out prominently between these hollows. When viewed from in front the animal appears to have lost the symmetry of the 2 shoulder regions. In typical cases there is difficulty in bringing the limb forward, and often the leg appears to swing outwards with a circular movement. When a horse stands quietly, the affected limb is usually brought well under the body, and may even take up a position across the middle line of the body. The paralysis may disappear in 6 weeks; but in more severe cases, 18 months may elapse before the horse is fit for work.

First-aid Fomentations, or application of a liniment may be helpful until the acute symptoms subside; thereafter a run at grass generally results in improvement.

In the dog there may be permanent paralysis, sometimes requiring amputation of the leg or other surgery.

Suramin

A drug used against trypanosomes.

Surfactants

Substances that reduce the surface tension of a liquid; soap and detergents are examples. Surfactants are used in frothy bloat to allow the release of gas from the bubbles which are formed.

Surgical Spirit

A preparation of alcohol used, for example, as a skin cleanser before giving an injection. It consists of industrial methylated spirit with the addition of castor oil (2.5 per cent), methyl salicylate (0.5 per cent) and diethyl phthalate (2 per cent).

Surra

Surra is a disease of most economic importance in camels and horses, but it can affect all the domestic animals. The disease occurs in Africa (north of the tsetse fly belt), Asia, Central and South America. In the latter, *Trypanosoma equinum* is responsible; elsewhere it is caused by *T. evansi.*

The infection is spread by blood-sucking flies, such as tabanids and stable flies. Vampire bats are believed to transmit the infection also. Animals which eat the meat from carcases infected with trypanosomes may themselves become infected in the case of surra.

In the Sudan, surra affects mainly camels, which die within weeks or a few months, after showing symptoms of fever, anaemia, progressive emaciation, oedema, and paralysis. In Asia, surra in camels is often a chronic disease which may persist for years.

In horses, symptoms are similar, but the dropsical swellings (oedema) are especially noteworthy, affecting several parts of the body (as they do also in the dog). Mortality is high, and occurs in horses after a matter of weeks or months. Loss of power in the hind limbs, and exaggerated heart sounds may precede death.

In Central America the names 'murrina' and 'derrengadera' have been used for vampire-bat and fly-transmitted infection with *T. equinum.*

Treatment involves use of drugs such as antrycide, diminazine and suramin which have specific action on trypanosomes. Fly control is also important in reducing the incidence of the disease.

Suspected Adverse Reaction Surveillance Scheme (SARSS)

In the UK, the Veterinary Medicines Directorate monitors reports of unusual unexpected adverse reactions to veterinary medicines and lack of efficacy. The manufacturers are kept informed of such reports so that they can take appropriate action.

Suture

Suture is the name given either to the close union between 2 adjacent flat bones of the skull at their edges, or to a series of stitches by which a wound is closed. (See WOUNDS.)

Swabs

Swabs are used for sampling mucus, etc., for diagnostic purposes; the material subsequently being cultured so that pathogenic organisms, if present, may be identified. For swabbing as a guide to infertility in the thoroughbred mare, see under EQUINE GENITAL INFECTIONS.

Swallowing

As soon as food ready for swallowing enters the pharynx, it touches areas of mucous membrane supplied with nerves which automatically inhibit breathing, in order to prevent food going the wrong way; close the larynx, which is pulled forwards and upwards, while the base of the tongue folds the epiglottis over the opening of the larynx. The pharynx is shortened and its muscles force the food into the oesophagus, where peristalsis takes the food to the stomach.

Swallowing is one-third voluntary and two-thirds reflex. The voluntary part is placing the food on the upper surface of the tongue which is raised, tip first, against the hard palate towards the rear. At the same time the soft palate is raised, closing the gateway to the nose. The base of the tongue forces food into the pharynx. The next 2 stages of swallowing are involuntary, reflex actions. (For difficulty in swallowing, see DYSPHAGIA.)

Swamp Cancer

A condition affecting horses in Australia. The lesion is, in fact, a fungal granuloma caused by *Hyphomyces destruens*.

Swamp Fever

(see EQUINE INFECTIOUS ANAEMIA)

Swayback

Swayback is a copper deficiency disease seen in the last 3rd of pregnancy in the ewe or in newborn and young lambs. It is characterised by progressive cerebral demyelination, which results in paralysis and often death. It occurs in many parts of the UK.

Signs A staggering gait or inability to walk. Severely affected cases all die. Newborn lambs cannot rise and suckle.

Treatment None.

Prevention Allow the pregnant ewes access to copper licks or give injections of a suitable copper preparation.

Sweat (Perspiration)

The excretion produced by the sudiparous glands of the skin; it exerts a cooling effect by evaporation. In the horse, there are parts of the skin which sweat more readily than others, e.g. the bases of the ears, under the fore-arm, and around the dock, and generally speaking, fore-parts of the trunk sweat more quickly than do the hinder parts. Mules and donkeys do not sweat readily, and when they do it is generally confined to the bases of the ears. In cattle, sweating occurs chiefly at the neck and over the chest. In Brahman cattle the hump is an important sweating site. Panting (and loss of water vapour from the lungs) is the chief means of heat loss in sheep, but they do sweat. The dog, cat, and pig are, for all practical purposes, non-sweating animals, though sweating may occur from the pads of the feet of dogs and cats; dogs rely mainly on panting. (See also ANHIDROSIS; HYPERTHERMIA; HYPOTHALAMUS; TROPICS.)

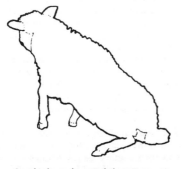
Swayback – a characteristic posture.

Sweat Glands

(see SKIN). Like all other tissue, the sweat glands can become the site of cancer. For example, 10 cases were diagnosed in cats at the New York State College of Veterinary Medicine during a 2-year period. Head, neck, pinna of the ear and base of the tail were affected in cats aged 6 to 17 years.

Sweating Sickness

This is a tick-borne disease of cattle in southern Africa, affecting mainly calves. (Sheep can also become naturally infected.)

Signs Fever, eczema. (See also TICKS.)

Swedish Red and White Cattle

This is the main breed of Sweden. The herdbook dates from 1928, when the Swedish Ayrshire and the Swedish Red-White breeds – similar in origin and characteristics – were amalgamated. Each was the result of breeding from old Swedish stock to which had been introduced some Dairy Shorthorn and Ayrshire blood.

It is a long-lived breed, with an overall milk yield average in excess of 4300 litres (950 gallons) at 4.1 per cent butter fat.

There is very little white in the coat-colour; and some animals are entirely red.

'Sweet Itch'

A seasonal inflammation of the skin of horses, caused by hypersensitivity to the bites of *Culicoides* midges. Lotions containing benzoyl benzoate or pyrethrins are used to control the midges; calamine and antihistamine cream helps relieve the symptoms

Fly repellents are effective for such short periods as to be worthless for control, probably best achieved by stabling in the early evening; a Vapona strip being hung in the stable to kill any midges entering.

Sweet Vernal Grass (Anthoxanthum Odoratum)

Hay containing this has caused poisoning owing to its DICOUMAROL content. The dicoumarol content of the grass varies, but may increase in hay which has become overheated or mouldy.

Swill

The feeding of unboiled swill – a practice which is illegal in the UK – is a frequent source of swine fever, swine vesicular disease, and foot-and-mouth disease infections. Scouring and deaths occurred among swill-fed pigs on premises where it was the practice to use daily only 2275 litres (500 gallons) out of a total of 9095 litres (2000 gallons) of steam-sterilised swill, the remainder being stored. There was no further trouble after the tank was emptied and the swill fed as soon as possible after processing.

'Swimmers'

The colloquial name for puppies showing the juvenile femoral rotation syndrome. They are unable to rise on to their hind-legs at the usual age, due to the head and neck of the femur being wrongly positioned on the shaft. Sometimes the name 'flat pup' syndrome is applied.

Swine Dysentery

An important disease, characterised by haemorrhagic enteritis, and dependent for its cause upon synergism between the spirochaete *Serpulina hyodysenteriae* and *Bacteroides vulgatus* and other bacteria.

About 1 in 3 pigs in a herd become ill, and the mortality rate is 10 to 60 per cent. Chronic scouring, without dysentery, may persist. The faeces are greyish.

Prevention and *Treatment* Antibacterials such as tiamulin or dimetridazole may be added to drinking water or the feed of susceptible animals, or tiamulin given by injection.

Swine dysentery and chickens

Retarded growth rate and delayed onset of egg production in pullets have, as one of the causes, infection with *S. hyodysenteriae*. Pullets reared on deep litter with indirect contact with pigs have become infected.

Swine Erysipelas

Swine erysipelas is an infectious disease of pigs and characterised by high fever, reddish or purplish spots on the skin, and haemorrhages on to the surfaces of certain of the internal organs in acute cases; and by general debility, lameness, and difficulty in breathing in chronic cases. In these latter there are usually found characteristic cauliflower-like masses on the valves of the heart.

The disease may occur in man; also in chickens, turkeys, ducks, pheasants and grouse. According to American research, dogs are susceptible to one strain of the organism, which gives rise to bacterial endocarditis.

Incidence In Europe it is usually prevalent both in the acute form and in the chronic, and at times it assumes the nature of an epizootic, sweeping throughout large territories, and leaving a high percentage of death in its wake. In the UK the chronic form is usually met with in small outbreaks in different parts of the country, but from time to time in certain areas, especially in East Anglia, and during hot dry summer weather, it breaks out in a more menacing form, and large numbers of pigs become affected with the acute form, and considerable numbers die.

Cause *Erysipelothrix rhusiopathiae*, which may also infect sheep at shearing or dipping time through small wounds or abrasions.

Signs There are 3 recognised forms of swine erysipelas: the subacute, the acute, and the chronic. Mild or subacute attacks come on suddenly; there is high fever, loss of appetite, dullness, a tendency to lie buried in the litter, and when moved, to do so reluctantly: the skin over the chest, neck, back, and over the thighs becomes flushed at first, and soon changes to a red or purple colour. The outlines of the areas affected are often square, or they may be the shape of the playing-card diamond, from which the disease gets one of its names – 'diamond disease'. The areas are usually raised above the level of the surrounding skin, are painful to the touch at first, but not so later, and, appearing about the 2nd or 3rd day of the attack, last for 4 days, and then disappear. Recovery may be followed by the chronic form. In some cases, pigs may show painful swellings of the knees and hocks, but this is not invariable. Young pigs between 3 and 5 or 6 months old are most commonly attacked; it is rare before 3 months, but may occur in older animals.

Acute type, or septicaemic type, often results in sudden death.

Chronic type is the most insidious, and pigs affected with it are probably responsible for causing most of the outbreaks of the previous types, since, being bad thrivers, they are often disposed of through the open market and bought by owners of clean herds. They feed, but do not always finish their food; they have a normal temperature, but are easily distressed when made to take exercise. Breathing becomes shallow, and a cough generally develops. The pulse becomes thready, and if the heart is listened to, a flowing murmur can be heard over the left side of the chest. This is due to the vegetative (or verrucose) endocarditis, which is almost the characteristic feature of post-mortem examination of pigs dead from chronic swine erysipelas. The chronic form may last for several weeks, or even for 2 or 3 months, especially in strong robust young breeding

gilts, but towards the end emaciation and prostration become very obvious.

Infertility, involving abortion, stillbirths, and mummified fetuses, commonly results from erysipelas.

Treatment Antibiotics have been used.

Prevention Avoid any pigs in the open market which appear to be thin and not thriving, especially sows and boars, or older pigs. Any showing wrinkling of the skin of the ears, or patches or flushing on the skin, those which have swollen joints, or those which have diarrhoea, should not be bought. Pigs showing extreme breathlessness upon mild exertion should be likewise avoided.

Vaccinate piglets from non-immune sows at 7 days old, repeated at 4 weeks; pregnant sows and gilts should be vaccinated at 6 and 3 weeks before farrowing and a booster given 3 weeks before subsequent farrowings.

Arthritis and heart disease may be a result of pigs becoming hypersensitised to the bacteria, and not the result of attack by the bacteria themselves. This must be borne in mind when prescribing the vaccine.

Public health Stockmen exposed to infection must be careful to wash their hands.

Swine Fever (Classical Swine Fever)
Also called hog cholera or pig typhoid, this is a highly infectious and contagious disease of pigs. It is a NOTIFIABLE DISEASE in Britain and the EU.

Cause The cause of swine fever is a pestivirus (a member of the Togavirus family). Secondary bacterial invaders include *Salmonella suipestifer* and *Pasteurella suiseptica*. None of these secondary organisms is, however, necessary for the production of swine fever.

It inevitably happens that pigs harbouring the virus of swine fever, but not yet showing symptoms of the disease, are slaughtered for human food. Under such circumstances, the virus can survive in the skin and muscle for 17 days. In frozen pork the survival time has been quoted as over 4 years; in bacon, 27 days. No wonder that unboiled swill is responsible for so many outbreaks.

At public markets, the urine of infected pigs often drains into adjoining pens and alleyways. The urine may, too, get splashed on to clothing, boots, etc., and droplets of it find their way into lorries and on to farms. In one instance about 30 outbreaks, spread over 10 counties, arose from the sale of a single infected pen at a large market.

It seems probable that the virus may be carried by rats and mice for short distances at least. Horse-flies can carry the virus, which – according to an American report – can be harboured by larvae of the pig lungworm. These larvae are, in turn, harboured by earthworms.

The use of antibiotics contained in feeding-stuffs has had the effect of masking the classical symptoms of swine fever, and is sometimes said to have extended the incubation period.

Signs In young pigs the disease is often acute or peracute, while in older pigs it tends to assume a chronic form, although they also may be affected with the severe rapidly fatal form.

Acute type: After an incubation period of 5 to 10 days, signs of the disease include thirst, sometimes vomiting, shivering, loss of appetite. There is a tendency to lie with backs arched and tails uncurled. If forced to move, pigs are seen to be unsteady on their legs. If their temperature is taken, it is found to be high. Initial constipation is usually followed by diarrhoea, with a foul odour. There is often a discharge from the eyelids. The skin becomes reddened or purplish. Some pigs may cough or show laboured breathing. Convulsions may precede death. The mortality rate can be as high as 90 per cent.

Pneumonia is a common post-mortem finding and 'button ulcers' may be present in the intestines.

Chronic Type The pigs are dull and unthrifty, lose weight, have a variable appetite; coughing and/or diarrhoea may be other signs. The temperature may be only slightly raised or as high as 41°C (106°F). A partial recovery may be followed by relapse and death.

Subclinical Swine fever may exist in a herd in a subclinical form; pregnant sows showing no obvious signs (though fever may be present), and the disease remaining unsuspected until the finding of a few dead piglets, or of others showing muscular tremors.

Death of the fetus may occur (see MUMMIFI-CATION) or weak or deformed piglets may be born. If infected late in pregnancy, piglets may die without signs of swine fever. Meanwhile, being viraemic, they may have infected others. Infection of a pregnant sow can be followed by the presence of virus in her piglets, either stillborn or living. The sow is not a carrier in the usually accepted sense, since after the birth of her piglets the virus – having crossed the placental barrier – no longer remains within her

body. A period of 56 days may elapse between the last deaths on a farm and a recrudescence of the disease.

Diagnosis The fluorescent antibody test.

Prevention Swill must be boiled for at least an hour, and it must be prepared only in regis-tered premises for pieces of infected pig meat may otherwise give rise to an outbreak of the disease. NB: Swill feeding is illegal in the UK since the 2001 outbreaks of foot-and-mouth disease. Pigs introduced into a herd should be from premises shown to be free from the disease. Visits by pig-dealers should be discouraged.

Control A swine fever eradication pro-gramme, with compulsory slaughter, and compensation, was introduced in 1963. The disease was eradicated in 1966, but re-appeared briefly in Yorkshire in 1971; and a single outbreak occurred in 1986. In 2000, a serious outbreak occurred in East Anglia, resulting in the imposition of movement restrictions on animals from affected areas and the slaughter of thousands of pigs. Sixteen areas were affected, the first case being confirmed on August 8; the final restricted area was cleared on December 30. The outbreak might have originated from a pork pie, made from imported pork, discarded where free-range pigs could have consumed it.

Swine Fever, African

This disease, formerly indigenous in the African continent, appeared in Spain and Portugal during 1960.

During 1978 there was an outbreak in Malta; eradication was effected by slaughter of the entire pig population and restocking in a quarantine station on the island of Comino. An outbreak in Sardinia, also in 1978, spread into the wild boar population, in which it remains endemic. The risk of introduction to other countries is a serious one; there were 5 outbreaks in Belgium in 1985. The disease may be caried by airline meals or by passengers.

The disease is also known as wart-hog disease, as these animals besides bush-pigs are affected. In some parts of Africa, pig-raising has had to be abandoned on account of the disease, which is highly contagious, nearly always fatal, and gives rise to carriers – those few that survive often transmitting the infection to other pigs for a year or more.

Cause A pestivirus, resistant to heat, drying, and putrefaction, and which can survive in smoked or partly cooked sausage and other pork products. The virus attacks blood-vessel cells and the disease is accordingly characterised by haemorrhages.

Signs After an incubation period of 5 to 15 days, there is fever, the pig running a temperature of 40.5°C (105°F) or so. This is followed by blotching of the skin, depression, anorexia, diarrhoea and weakness of the hind-quarters with a disinclination to rise. Death may occur within a day or two. Clinically, the disease is indistinguishable from acute classical swine fever.

Control African swine fever is a NOTIFIABLE DISEASE; control is by slaughter.

At the beginning of 1978 there were approximately 80,000 pigs in the islands of Malta and Gozo, supplying the inhabitants with all their requirements of fresh pork and bacon. By the end of January 1979 there were no pigs at all.

It was the first time that any country had slaughtered all the surviving members of a species in order to eliminate a disease – in this instance, African swine fever. The decision to slaughter all survivors was taken when the pig population had fallen to 13,975. Swill feeding and the movement of weaners to fattening premises helped to spread the disease.

Swine Influenza

A common problem which can rapidly spread through a pig unit; affected animals usually recover within a week, but other respiratory problems may be precipitated. An H1N1 virus was causing the disease in Europe in 1986, and was isolated from an outbreak involving a 400-sow unit in the UK. Morbidity was nearly 100 per cent, but all recovered. H3N2 virus is also present in the UK..

In many outbreaks, several deaths are to be expected. (See also INFLUENZA and ENZOOTIC PNEUMONIA.)

Cause An orthomyxovirus; important secondary invaders include *Haemophilus influenzae suis*, *Pasteurella suiseptica*, *Brucella bronchiseptica*, and streptococci.

Signs Coughing, fever, anorexia, laboured breathing. (See also INFLUENZA.)

Swine Plague

Swine plague is the term applied to what in Britain is considered to be the pneumonic form of swine fever, but what in America and the continent of Europe has been regarded as a separate disease. (See SWINE FEVER.)

Swine Pox

A virus disease identified by lesions on the abdomen, in adults, and on the face in piglets,

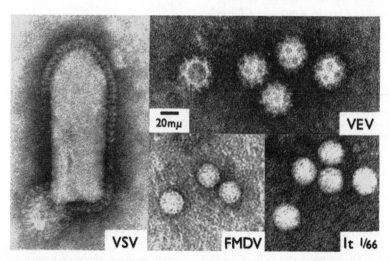

The virus causing swine vesicular disease is shown bottom right, labelled It 1/66. Extreme left is the bullet-shaped virus of vesicular stomatis (VSV), and top right is the virus of vesicular exanthema (VEV). Centre bottom picture shows foot-and-mouth disease virus. All these viruses affect pigs and have to be differentiated. (The scale shown 20mm = 0.00002 mm. Photographs by electron microscope, with acknowledgements to C. J. Smale and the Animal Virus Research Institute, Pirbright.)

in which the disease is more serious; they also have conjunctivitis and some may die. The cause is infection with swine poxvirus and/or vaccinia virus (see POX).

Swine Vesicular Disease (SVD)

A NOTIFIABLE DISEASE. An enterovirus disease whose signs resemble those of foot-and-mouth disease. It first appeared in the UK in 1972. In the Staffordshire outbreak of that year it was at first mistaken for foot-and-mouth disease, from which it cannot be differentiated on clinical grounds alone. However, it was shown at the Animal Virus Research Institute, Pirbright, that the virus was not that of foot-and-mouth disease but related to an enterovirus which had caused outbreaks in Italy and Hong Kong.

All cases in the UK were linked either to swill feeding of pigs or to the movement of pigs from infected to clean premises. The disease appears to be spread rapidly through contact, with an incubation period of perhaps 4 to 8 days. Airborne infection appears less likely than with foot-and-mouth disease.

A similar disease has been reported in Austria among pigs imported from Poland, and also in France.

SVD virus is very closely related to Coxsackie B5 virus, which causes not only influenza-like symptoms in man but also sometimes heart disease and meningitis. It is thought possible that SVD arose as a result of pigs becoming infected by people ill because of Coxsackie B5 virus, which locally then became adapted to pigs or underwent mutation.

SVD has been transmitted to laboratory workers, so precautions must be taken.

Control Experience has shown that the incidence of the disease has been quickly reduced by the imposition of Controlled Area measures, and this fact led to the Movement and Sale of Pigs Order 1975, and subsequent legislation, designed to slow down the movement of pigs so that infection can show up and be dealt with before it spreads further.

Licences are required for all movement of pigs; entry of pigs on to a farm precludes movement of animals off that farm for 21 days, except for those going direct to slaughter. Swill-fed pigs can move only to a slaughterhouse. All pigs consigned to a slaughter market or to a slaughterhouse must be marked with a red cross of specified dimensions.

Sporadic outbreaks have occurred since the original outbreak. The infection can be subclinical.

Mode of Infection Although the SVD virus belongs to the enterovirus group, it has been difficult to obtain evidence for infection by mouth. Many experiments, in which precautions were taken to prevent entry of virus by other routes, have failed to produce the disease. In contrast, infection by rubbing or scarification of the skin regularly produces infection, and it seems that the most likely route of infection in the field is through damaged skin.

Swinge Coat

An abnormality in which the hair is short, sparse and curly.

Swollen Head Syndrome of Chickens (SHS)

Signs An oedematous swelling beginning round the eyes and progressing to the inter-mandibular tissue. There is coughing and a nasal discharge. Opisthotonus may be seen. If picked up the birds become incoordinated, roll over, and have difficulty in regaining a normal posture; diarrhoea may be seen. The disease lasts about 2 weeks.

Cause A paramyxovirus.

Symbiosis

Symbiosis means an obligatory association between 2 different species for their mutual benefit.

Sympathetic Nervous System

(see CENTRAL NERVOUS SYSTEM; AUTONOMIC NERVOUS SYSTEM)

Symphysis

A joint, in which bones are united by a flattened disc of fibro-cartilage.

Syn-

Syn- is a prefix signifying union.

Synapse

(see NERVES)

Synchronisation Of Oestrus

(see CONTROLLED BREEDING)

Syncope (Fainting)

Syncope (fainting) is generally due to cerebral anaemia occurring through weakened pulsation of the heart, sudden shock, or severe injury.

It is common in dogs and cats, especially when old; cases have however been seen in all animals.

Syncytial Viruses

(see RESPIRATORY SYNCYTIAL VIRUS)

Syncytium

Tissue composed of a mass of nucleated protoplasm without cell boundaries, such as the outer layer of the trophoblast of a placenta; or a mass of cells united by protoplasmic bridges.

Syndrome

A group of symptoms.

Synechia

Adhesions in the eye, e.g. involving the tissues of the iris to the cornea or lens (see EYE, DISEASES OF – Iritis).

Synergism

Synergism is the opposite of antagonism. Synergism between drugs, e.g. trimethoprim and sulfadiazine, may be of practical value, for with the two it may be possible to obtain the required effect with a dosage of one which, if used alone, would be insufficient, but which cannot be increased because larger amounts would cause side-effects. Another advantage of using two drugs is the possibility that this would tend to prevent the multiplication of strains resistant to one of the compounds.

The word 'synergism' is also used to describe an interaction between a virus and bacteria in their combined invasion of, for example, the lungs; implying that the result of the 'combined forces', as it were, is greater than the sum of the effects produced by the agents individually. Synergism occurs in calf pneumonia between *Mycoplasma bovis* and *Pasteurella haemolytica*. (For another example, see SWINE DYSENTERY.)

Synostosis

Synostosis is the term applied to a union by bony material of adjacent bones usually separate. It may occur in the spinal column in old animals. (See also HORSES, BACK TROUBLES IN.)

Synotia

The (virtual) absence of head in a stillborn animal.

Synovial Membrane

Synovial membrane forms the lining covering the surfaces of the opposed articular cartilages, which enter into the formation of a joint. (See JOINTS.)

Synovitis

Inflammation of the membrane lining a joint. It is usually accompanied by effusion of fluid within the synovial sac of the joint. It is found in various injuries and inflammation of joints.

Synovitis, Infectious

This is a disease of chicks, of about 2 to 10 weeks old, and of turkeys; first diagnosed in Britain in 1959.

Cause *Mycoplasma synoviae.*

Signs Reluctance to move, lameness, swelling of joints, anorexia.

The confined conditions under which broilers are raised appear to render them particularly susceptible to this disease. Mortality is low, but a third of the survivors may be downgraded, so that severe financial loss may be caused. Control depends upon hygiene, and being careful about the breeding stock.

Syringe, Hypodermic

A pump-like device used to introduce solutions to, or withdraw them from, the body. (see INFECTIONS, DETERGENT RESIDUE; also PROJECTILE SYRINGE)

Systole

Systole means the contraction of the heart as opposed to the resting phase, which is called 'diastole', and which alternates with the former contracting period. In the cardiac cycle systole takes about one-third, and diastole about two-thirds, of the whole period of the heartbeat. (See HEART DISEASES.)

T

T-Cells
LYMPHOCYTES from the thymus gland concerned with cell-mediated immunity. (See IMMUNE RESPONSE.)

T₂ Toxin
This fungal toxin may poison cattle or poultry eating stored corn containing the fungus *Fusarium tricinctum*. In cattle, the toxin may cause multiple haemorrhages and sometimes death; in poultry, there may be mouth lesions.

Tachycardia
Tachycardia is a disturbance of the heart's action which produces great acceleration of the pulse.

Tachypnoea
An increase in the rate of breathing due to some pathological condition. (See BREATHLESSNESS; PARAQUAT POISONING.)

Taenia
(see TAPEWORMS)

Tail, Amputation of
Amputation of the tail (docking) is, or has been, undertaken for a variety of reasons. In the UK the Royal College of Veterinary Surgeons has ruled that docking a puppy's tail is an unethical procedure except when it is done for prophylactic or therapeutic reasons. Docking by lay persons is illegal. In cattle, amputation of the tail is illegal except following injury and must, except in an emergency, be undertaken by a veterinary surgeon. Pigs' tails are often docked to prevent tail-biting. Lambs tails are docked to prevent faecal soiling and fly strike (see under DOCKING; LAW; WELFARE CODES).

Tail-Biting
In pigs this 'vice' can be of great economic importance. There are various reasons why it occurs: boredom, absence of bedding, and overcrowding (floor space of less than 1.5 m² (5 square feet) per pig), are regarded as conducive to tail-biting. High temperature and humidity are possible causes. Bitten tails require amputation or dressing if pyaemia is to be prevented.

Tail sores in pigs
These may follow tail-biting by 1 or 2 pigs out of a large batch, and if untreated can lead to pyaemia.

In 6 months, out of 135 pig carcases condemned in an Oslo abattoir, 56 were affected with pyaemia – and of these, 43 had tail sores.

Talfan Disease (Teschen Disease; Porcine Viral Encephalomyelitis)
This disease of pigs was first recognised in the Czech Republic and occurs throughout Europe. In the UK, it was made a NOTIFIABLE DISEASE in 1974. Its cause is an enterovirus. Experimentally, the incubation period is stated to be 12 days. Piglets 3 weeks old and upwards are affected; adult pigs may be infected but show no clinical signs. By no means all piglets in a litter or on a farm become ill, and the mortality is usually low. The main symptom is weakness or paralysis of the hind-legs. There is little or no fever or loss of appetite. Recovery occurs in a proportion of animals which are hand-fed. The disease is present in Britain to a small extent, and apparently may be associated with abortion.

Tampan
A soft tick of the family Argasidae. (See TICKS.)

Tamponade, Cardiac
A rapid accumulation of blood or other fluid in the pericardial sac, compressing the heart and sometimes suddenly arresting its function.

Tannin (Tannic Acid)
Tannin (tannic acid) is a non-crystallisable white or pale-yellowish powder, which is soluble in water and glycerine. It is prepared from oak-galls, and is found in strong tea or coffee. When brought into contact with a mucous surface, tannin causes constriction of the blood vessels. When brought into contact with many poisonous alkaloids it renders them temporarily inert by forming the insoluble tannate, and so is a valuable antidote.

Uses Tannic acid has been used in diarrhoea and dysentery in young animals, usually as catechu or kino – 2 vegetable drugs which contain a large amount of tannin. It is often administered, in the form of strong tea, as the first step in the antidotal treatment of poisoning by ALKALOIDS.

Tannic-acid jelly is a valuable burn dressing. It lessens the absorption of breakdown products from the burned area and hence diminishes the

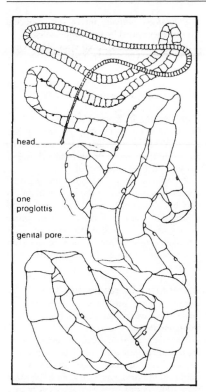

head

one
proglottis

genital pore

A typical tapeworm. Each segment is called a
proglottis. (From H. T. B. Hall, *Diseases and
Parasites of Livestock in the Tropics*, Longman.)

secondary effects of a serious burn. It is not
suitable for extensive areas owing to the danger
of liver damage if large quantities are absorbed.

Tapetum
(see EYE)

Tapeworms
An intestinal parasite commonly found in
vertebrates. Their life-cycle requires 2 hosts,
sometimes 3. The presence of the adult worm
may give rise to few if any symptoms or, on the
other hand, to anaemia, indigestion, and
nervous symptoms – or even to blockage of
the intestine. The cystic stage of tapeworms
may involve the brain. Tapeworms are of
considerable public-health importance.

A typical tapeworm has a head or scolex,
provided with suckers and, in some species,
with hooks also.

Behind the scolex follows a neck, and behind
that are the segments, each being called a proglottis. The segments nearest to the head are the
smallest, and are immature. Next follow mature

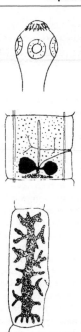

Taenia. Head, mature and gravid segments.

segments, and lastly the gravid segments containing eggs. These older segments fall off and are
passed out of the host's body in the faeces.

Taenia. This is the common genus of worms
found in dogs and cats, and includes:

T. pisiformis (*T. serrata*) is one of the commonest. Its cystic stage, *Cysticercus pisiformis*, is
found in rabbits and hares.

T. hydatigena (*T. marginata*) is the largest
form, with mature segments wider than long.
It may reach a length of over 5 metres (16 feet).
Its cystic stage, *C. tenuicollis*, occurs in the
viscera of various animals, especially sheep,
cattle and pigs. *T. ovis* is frequently mistaken
for the last form, from which it can be
distinguished only by microscopical examination. Its cysticercus, *C. ovis*, is found in the
muscles and organs of sheep and goats. It is a
small form, easily overlooked.

T. multiceps (*T. coernurus*) is a more delicate
form than the others, semi-translucent. The
intermediate stage is a coenurus, found in the
nervous system of sheep and other ruminants
and man.

T. serialis is a more robust form, its coenurus
being found in rabbits and hares. Only 1
species is common in the cat, *T. taeniaeformis*
(*T. crassicollis*). The cystic stage *C. fasciolaris* is
found in the liver of rats and mice.

T

T. saginata is a tapeworm of man which produces cysticercosis infection in the muscles of cattle; this is *C. bovis*, known as measly beef. *T. solum* is another tapeworm of man, the intermediate stage of which (metacestode) is found in the skeletal and heart muscles of pigs, producing measly pork.

Diphyllobothrium. D. latum is the broad tapeworm of man, the dog, and the cat. It is rare in Britain, but has a wide distribution. Several species are found, but this is the commonest. The life-history is interesting. The ciliated larva liberated from the egg is swallowed by a crustacean, *Cyclops strenuus* or *Diaptonius* spp., in which it becomes an elongated form with a terminal sphere containing three pairs of hooklets, called a 'procercoid larva'. The crustaceans are swallowed by a fish, when the larva, migrating to the muscles, becomes an elongated infective larva called a 'plerocercoid'. The fish is eaten by a suitable host, and the adults develop. In man, the tapeworm may attain a length of 18 metres (60 feet), and it may cause a grave form of anaemia (bothriocephalus anaemia) associated with gastric and nervous symptoms.

D. mansoni is also widely distributed and has a similar life-history, but the infective stage is found in many hosts, including man, pig, and carnivores. It is common in frogs in Japan. The adult worm is found in carnivores.

Treatment of dogs infested with tapeworms is very important, because some of the species in their intermediate stages are dangerous to food animals. Farm dogs should never be allowed to harbour tapeworms. Routine use of anthelmintics is essential: a wide range is available, many based on praziquantel or dichlorophen. All material passed should be destroyed.

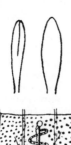

Diphyllobothrium. Head and segment.

Dipylidium caninum infests cats also; and may be transmitted by swallowing a flea.

In pigs, cattle, and sheep cysts of the tapeworm *Taenia hydatigena* (which infests the dog and may occasionally attain a length of 5 metres (16 ft)) may be so numerous in the liver that the latter ruptures, causing death.

Tapeworms in horses Three species occur in horses, all belonging to the genus *Anoplocephala. A. perfoliata* and *A. mammillana* are not uncommon in Britain, while *A. magna* is also sometimes encountered.

A. perfoliata, a stoutish worm with large head and no hooks, is a cause not only of unthriftiness but occasionally also of ileal and caecal obstruction, and/or intussusception, where numerous *A. perfoliata* are present. The infection may therefore be more serious than is generally supposed. The intermediate host is a mite.

Tapeworms in ruminants All the tapeworms of ruminants have 4 suckers and no hooks. In *Moniezia* the intermediate host is a free-living mite.

The segments of *Moniezia* worms are much broader than they are long. The worms may attain a length of several metres/yards, with a minute head little larger than a pin-head. More than 1000 worms have been recorded from a single host. Numerous species have been recorded. *H. giardi* is found in Europe, Australia, and Africa and is from 1 to 2 metres (3 to 6 ft) long.

A closely related form, *Thysanosoma actinoides*, is found in North America. It is about 30 cm (1 ft) long, and is found in the liver. The sheep show general symptoms of malnutrition.

Bovine cystercercosis in Denmark Studies were conducted on 14 farms with a history of this disease. On 6 of the farms the source of infection was sludge from septic tanks applied to pasture or crops. In 2 herds the cattle grazed pasture near a sewage plant; while on 3 farms people defecating on pasture was a possible source.

Tapeworms in poultry A number of tapeworms have been found in poultry, of which the commonest are *Davainea proglottina*, which has a larval stage in slugs and snails and is widely distributed, and several species of *Raillietina*, with the larvae in house-flies, dung beetles and ants. The following are also common in many countries: *Amoebotoenia*, with larvae in earthworms; and *Hymenolepis* of various species, some of which may be very numerous in individual birds.

'Measles' in beef

'Measles' in beef due to the presence of the cyst stage (*Cysticercus bovis*) of the tapeworm *Taenia saginata*, which is a parasite of man. Cattle swallow the eggs of the adult tapeworm, and these hatch in the intestines, liberating young embryos, which burrow until they settle in muscle fibre or connective tissues. Here they appear as small oval cysts, containing fluid, and each possessing the head of a potential tapeworm.

'Measles' in pork

'Measles' in pork is due to the presence of the cyst stage (*Cysticercus cellulosae*) of the tapeworm of man, *Taenia solium*. It is extremely common among pigs in eastern lands, which have access to garbage and human faeces, from whence they pick up the eggs passed through the human intestines. The eggs undergo a development similar to those of the beef-measles tapeworm. Man may also himself harbour the cystic stage.

Cysticercosis in man

Cysticercosis in man Very high sporadic infection rates have been found in Africa with *Taenia saginata* and *T. solium*, the 2 tapeworms of major importance in man. Where *T. solium* is present, serious human infections with the cysticercus stage may be observed, as well as mild infections with the adult tapeworm. When it occurs in beef cattle, the cysticercus of *T. saginata* is a major economic problem and a serious obstacle to the export of meat.

A single human carrier of *T. saginata* led to an outbreak of cysticercosis among cattle on a large farm in the USA.

Coenuriasis (gid or sturdy) in sheep

This disease is caused by the pressure of cysts of the tapeworm *Taenia multiceps* on cells of the brain (or spinal cord).

Sheep become infested by swallowing the unhatched eggs, excreted in a dog's faeces, while grazing. In the digestive tract the eggs hatch, and pass via the bloodstream to various parts of the body; only those reaching the central nervous system develop. Here they form small cysts, each containing 1 tapeworm head: this larval stage is known as *Coenurus cerebralis*. Over a period of months, each cyst increases in size, and more heads are budded from the lining membrane of the translucent cyst wall. Eventually a single coenurus may contain 50 or 100 or more tapeworm heads (scolices) projecting inwards.

The life-cycle is completed if a dog eats the head of an infested sheep.

Signs These include impairment of vision, a staggering or high-stepping gait, circling, and standing with head lowered, raised, or pressed against an object. Backward somersaults have been recorded. Recumbency and opisthotonus may occur. A softening of the bone of the skull, due to internal pressure of the cysts, is found in a proportion of cases.

Diagnosis Where there is no softening of the skull, a guide to the location of the cyst may be given by interpretation of the neurological signs as indicated by the sheep's behaviour. An intra-dermal test has been used: 0.1 ml of cyst fluid is injected into a shaved area of skin. Thickening of the skin within 24 hours indicates the presence of a cyst in the animal.

Treatment Physical removal of the cyst may be attempted. The sheep is anaesthetised and, in the absence of any skull softening, a trephine used to remove a disc of bone 1.5 cm (0.6 in) in diameter. Draining the fluid from the cyst before its removal obviates the need to enlarge the hole. The cyst is then removed completely. (If this is not done, the remaining cyst wall is apparently capable of replacing the fluid.)

Hydatid disease

Hydatid disease is caused by the cystic larval stage of the tapeworm *Echinococcus granulosus*, of which the dog and fox are the usual hosts. Eggs released from tapeworm segments passed in the faeces by these animals are later swallowed by grazing cattle, sheep and horses, which may become infested also through drinking water contaminated by wind-blown eggs.

People become infested through swallowing eggs attached to inadequately washed vegetables, and possibly eggs may be inhaled in dust or carried by flies to uncovered food. The handling of infested dogs is an important source. In Beirut, the risk is put at 21 times greater for dog-owners than others, by the World Health Organisation, which states also that in California nomadic sheep-rearers are 1000 times more likely to have hydatid disease than other inhabitants of the state. (WHO Technical Report 637).

There have been successful campaigns to control human hydatid disease in both Cyprus and Iceland, by compulsory treatment and/or banning of dogs.

Swallowed eggs hatch in the intestines and are carried via the portal vein to the liver. Some remain there, developing into hydatid cysts; others may form cysts in the lungs or occasionally elsewhere, e.g. spleen, kidney, bone-marrow cavity, or brain. Inside the cysts, brood capsules, containing the infective stage of the tapeworm, develop, and after 5 or 6 months can infest dog or fox.

In Wales, where the incidence of hydatid disease is relatively high, farm dogs and foxhounds are important in its spread.

Only some 7 people are known to die from this disease in England and Wales each year – a figure which would probably be higher were diagnosis less difficult. Condemnation of sheep and cattle offal from this cause runs into hundreds of thousands of pounds annually. Routine worming of dogs is essential for control.

E. granulosus is far from being a typical tapeworm, as it has only 3 or 4 segments and a total length of a mere 3 to 9 mm (0.12 to 0.35 in), so that the dog-owner will not notice the voided segments.

A problem of diagnosis also arises, in that this worm's eggs are indistinguishable from those of *Taenia* tapeworms. Examination of a dog's faeces following dosing with arecoline would reveal the intact tapeworm. However, this drug has now been replaced by more modern drugs which destroy the tapeworm but leave it unrecognisable.

Dichlorophen, praziquantel, nitroscanate, and benzimidazoles are used for treatment.

Equine hydatidosis in Britain is caused by a strain of *Echinococcus granulosus* which has become specifically adapted to the horse as its intermediate host, and is often referred to now as *E. granulosus equinus*. This apparently is of low pathenogenicity for man.

In a survey covering 1388 horses and ponies examined at 2 abattoirs in the north of England, 8.7 per cent were infected. Prevalence of infection was closely related to age, rising from zero in animals up to 2 years old to over 20 per cent of those over 8 years old.

Sixty-six per cent of the infected animals had viable cysts.

Treatment of human patients Hydatid disease is one of the rare parasitic conditions that can be treated by surgery. However, the result is often incomplete, with frequent local recurrences or accidents of secondary dissemination. Repeated interventions are often mutilating and do not guarantee a definite cure. Mebendazole is reported to have been used successfully in patients.

Tapping
(see ASPIRATION)

Tar
Recently applied tar, in the form of asphalt on roads and pavements, often causes irritation between a dog's toes, causing the animal to lick or bite the part. The tar must be removed with a bland fat or oil. Crude tar should never be used on an animal's skin. (See also PITCH POISONING.)

Tarantulas
These include the Chilean rose spider (*Grammostola spatulatus*). If found lying on its back, this creature should not be assumed to be dead, but merely moulting. In the UK, tarantulas are being kept as pets; in Australia wild tarantulas ('red-back' spiders) bite a few hundred people each year. An antivenin is available. (See also PET ANIMALS ACT 1971; PETS.)

Tarsorraphy
An operation for producing union of upper and lower eyelids. It is performed as a permanent measure after enucleation of an eyeball; and sometimes as a temporary expedient to give protection to an ulcerated or perforated cornea (but see LENSES, CONTACT).

Tarsus
The hock. (See under BONES.)

Tartar
Tartar is the concretion that often forms upon the crowns and upon the necks of the teeth, as well as upon exposed portions of the roots. The material is of a brownish, yellowish, or greyish colour, and consists chiefly of phosphate of lime which has been deposited from the saliva, with which are mixed numerous food particles and bacteria of a harmful nature. Tartar is most often seen in the mouths of dogs and cats, although the herbivorous animals may also be affected.

It is important that accumulated tartar be removed from time to time, for if it is allowed to collect for an indefinite period the gums shrink before the advancing deposit, the root becomes exposed and ultimately affected, and the tooth loosens and falls out. In addition to this, there are generally signs of systemic disturbance, such as a bad smell from the breath, indigestion from inability to feed properly, and in bad cases, great irritability and loss of condition. (See TEETH, DISEASES OF.)

Tasmanian Grey
An Australian breed of beef cattle, similar to the Murray Grey but developed from Aberdeen Angus and White Shorthorns.

Taste
This special sense is dependent upon the taste buds, located in the crevices of the papillae. The taste buds have minute projections – the endings of nerve fibres. It is necessary for the purpose of taste that the substance should be dissolved in a fluid, and it seems that this is one of the functions of the saliva. The sense of taste is closely associated with the sense of smell. (See TONGUE; SMELL; JACOBSON'S ORGAN.)

Tattooing
Identifying marks or numbers may be applied to animals by tattooing. On black skins, tattooing is not an effective method, and the use of nose prints has been tried for cattle. The tattooing of dogs is widely practised in France (where it is compulsory for the Kennel Club's register of pedigree dogs), and in Canada and the USA.

Tattooing, usually in the ear, is used to identify cattle, pigs, sheep and goats. It is not entirely free from the risk of introducing infection, e.g. blackquarter, tetanus. FREEZE-BRANDING and MICROCHIPPING are alternative methods. (See also DANGEROUS DOGS ACT 1991.)

Taurine
An amino acid essential to maintain the health of cats, and which must be provided in the food. In the USA, feeding of cats on canned dog foods is reported to have led to a taurine deficiency, resulting in degeneration of the cat's retina.

However, a level of taurine in the cat's diet sufficient to prevent degeneration of the retina may be insufficient to prevent the heart disease, dilated cardiomyopathy (DCM). Most modern proprietary cat diets contain adequate amounts of taurine.

Taxis
Taxis is the method of pushing back into the abdominal cavity a loop of bowel which has passed through the wall as the result of a rupture or hernia.

Tear-Staining
Tear-staining of the face in the dog may be due to atopic disease or to blockage of a lacrimal duct.

Tears
(see EYE; for 'soapy' tears, see ALGAE POISONING; see also NAPHTHALENE POISONING)

'Teart' Pastures, Soils
(see under MOLYBDENUM)

Teaser
(see under VASECTOMISED)

Teat Canal
One of the most important defences against bovine mastitis, as almost all infection enters the cow's udder by this route. The constant production and shedding of cells lining the canal helps to remove pathogenic bacteria. (See also MASTITIS IN THE COW; ORIFICES, IMMUNITY AT.)

Teat Dipping
First practised by a veterinary surgeon in 1916, this has proved a useful measure for the control of mastitis in cattle. Teats are dipped usually after milking, to help prevent streptococcal and staphylococcal infection. However, pre-milking teat dipping has been advocated as a means of reducing coliform mastitis. Results in the UK are reported as variable.

The liquid chiefly used for the purpose is an iodophor, but good results can be obtained with hypochlorite teat dips containing 1 per cent available chlorine. (See under MASTITIS IN COWS.)

Teat Necrosis
This is seen in piglets under intensive conditions of rearing, and is sometimes accompanied by skin necrosis affecting the limbs. Inadequate bedding and abrasive concrete may be contributory factors.

Teats, Cow's
(see under MAMMARY GLAND; also VIRAL INFECTIONS OF COWS' TEATS; MASTITIS)

Teats, Diseases of
(see BOVINE HERPES MAMMILLITIS; TEAT NECROSIS, VIRAL INFECTIONS OF COWS' TEATS)

Teeth
Teeth are developed in connection with the mucous membrane of the mouth, being actually calcified papillae. They are implanted in sockets or 'alveoli' in the upper and lower jaws, being only separated from actual contact with the bone by a layer of 'alveolar periosteum'.

The incisors are implanted in the incisive bones of the upper jaw, and in the anterior part of the mandible; they are situated in the front of the mouth, and used for grasping and cutting. They are absent from the upper jaw of cattle, sheep, and goats, as well as other ruminating animals.

The canines are situated behind the incisors, and are used mainly for fighting purposes, being most developed in carnivores and omnivores. They are useless to the domesticated herbivorous animals, and in them are usually of small size. They are not present in the upper jaws of ruminants, and in the lower jaws have the shape and function of incisors.

The molars are the remaining teeth, situated further back in the mouth. They are used mainly for chewing, and are specially adapted for this purpose by having broad strong irregular tables or grinding surfaces. The term 'cheek teeth' is often applied to these teeth, since, strictly speaking, they are composed of 'pre-molars', which are represented in the milk dentition, and 'molars', which are not so represented. (See DENTITION.)

Each tooth has a portion covered with enamel, the 'crown'; a portion covered with cement, the 'root'; and a line of union between these 2 parts known as the 'neck'. A constriction occurs at the neck in the temporary incisors of the horse, in the incisors of the ruminants, and in incisors and molars of the dog and cat; in the remaining teeth there is no such constriction.

Structure Teeth consist of 4 tissues. In the middle of the tooth is the 'pulp', occupying the 'pulp cavity'. It is soft and gelatinous, well supplied with blood vessels and nerves, and is large in the young tooth. It nourishes the remaining tissues, and forms dentine for as long as the pulp cavity is open. In later life it is small

Tooth structure. (From de Coursey, *The Human Organism*, McGraw-Hill.)

or absent, the pulp cavity having filled with dentine formed from the pulp. The 'dentine' forms the greater part of the tooth. It is hard, yellowish, or yellowish-white in colour, and is surrounded in the crown by enamel, and in the root by cement. The 'enamel' consists of a comparatively thin layer of a brilliant white colour and extremely dense and brittle, which forms a cap to the dentine, or is arranged in layers through it. The 'cement' is always the outermost layer of a tooth, being formed on the outside of the dentine in the root, and filling up the irregular spaces and hollows of the crown. The implanted part of a tooth is fixed into the socket by a layer of vascular fibrous tissue, which serves as the periosteum both of the tooth root and of the lining of the alveolus. It is known as the 'alveolar periosteum'.

Enamel is the hardest tissue in the body, and consists mainly of phosphate of lime. It is composed of prisms placed side by side, with one end resting on the dentine and the other end towards the free surface in a simple tooth, such as the canine of a dog. Cement is practically of the same structure as bone, without possessing Haversian canals.

Arrangement and form For times of cutting of the various teeth, see DENTITION.

Teeth, Diseases of

Most diseases or disorders affecting the teeth are associated with pain or discomfort, which results in absence of appetite, capriciousness in feeding, or other disturbances.

Irregularities In certain cases, the incisor or molar teeth develop out of their normal positions in the jaw, with the result that perfect apposition between the upper and lower teeth is not possible, and the rate of toothwear is not uniform. In other instances, extra or 'supernumerary' teeth are formed; in the incisor region these are usually placed behind the arch of normal teeth, while extra molars may be found as projections from the gums on the inside or the outside of the line of normal teeth.

When the temporary teeth are shed, it sometimes happens that the permanent teeth erupt irregularly to one side or behind the temporaries, and are distorted accordingly. This frequently happens in puppies, and to a lesser extent in the herbivora. In the former, trouble is likely to be experienced between 3½ and 5 or 6 months, and in young horses at 2½ and 3½ years of age. In such cases it is necessary to extract any temporaries which persist, so that the permanent teeth can arrive in their proper places in the mouth.

In dogs frequently, in sheep sometimes, and in other animals less commonly, there may be a discrepancy in length between the upper and lower jaws. When the upper jaw is too long, the condition is known as an 'overshot jaw', and when the lower jaw projects too far forward, it is popularly spoken of as an 'undershot jaw'. In bulldogs, pugs, and other breeds of dogs with very short upper jaws the undershot condition is practically normal, while in certain breeds with extremely long upper jaws, such as the greyhound and show collie, overshot jaws are very common.

Abnormal wear, which is due to malformations of the jaws, to excessive softness of the teeth, or to the direction of the teeth, is another mechanical cause of tooth disorder. (See SOIL-CONTAMINATED HERBAGE with reference to sheep.)

Abnormal wear varies in different cases, and is productive of some well-known conditions, as follows: (1) shear mouth, in which the molar teeth of the upper and lower jaws wear so that in time they appear like the blades of a pair of sheep-shears, the upper row being worn away on its inner border, and the lower one along its outer border; (2) step mouth, where the cheek teeth, instead of being all at the same level, are arranged with some higher than others, somewhat like steps – a high tooth in the lower jaw being opposite a short one in the corresponding upper jaw; (3) overhanging upper jaw, which is where the first upper cheek tooth on either side is placed too far forward in the mouth, and does not come into accurate apposition with the tooth immediately below it, causing the formation of a hook – at the same time the last lower cheek tooth is situated too far back and also forms a hook; and (4) curved tables, where the line of cheek teeth in the upper jaw shows a convexity in its centre, and a corresponding concavity exists in the lower row.

Signs In most of these instances the animal affected (almost always a member of the horse tribe), instead of chewing its food and swallowing it in the usual way, rolls it round and round in the mouth until it collects into a sodden mass, often about the size of a couple of fingers, and puts it out of the mouth instead of swallowing it. (See QUIDDING.) Pain may be shown when the hand is passed along the outside of the cheek, especially when pressure is put upon the line of teeth.

Treatment Rasping the teeth by means of a special tooth-rasp will reduce smaller irregularities, and bring the teeth back into their proper function.

Caries is **not** synonymous with tooth decay, although the term – borrowed from human dentistry – is often used in veterinary practice to include all tooth decay.

Caries is the destruction of the tooth enamel and invasion of the dentine by bacteria, resulting in the formation of a cavity. True caries has been confirmed in dogs but is comparatively rare in farm animals.

Neck lesions in cats' teeth A painful condition affecting middle-aged to elderly cats, characterised by cavitation of the necks of teeth. This makes extraction difficult because of the risk of breakage of crowns.

Inflammations of the periosteum lining the root cavity of a tooth are common. They may be due to small particles of food getting forced down into the socket of the tooth, to fractures or fissures of the teeth, to caries, tumour formation, depositions of tartar, and to certain specific diseases, such as actinomycosis, etc.

Signs These vary from a slight redness of the gum around the root of the tooth, which is painful when pressed by the finger, to a large suppurating tract running alongside the root of the tooth down into its socket, and perhaps through the skin to the outside or into one or other of the sinuses. Abscess formation in the tooth socket may take place, and the abscess may burst into the mouth, to the outside through the skin, or up into a sinus. In many cases there is a distinct bulge of the surface above the diseased tooth, which may give to the face a one-sided appearance.

Treatment The affected tooth or teeth must be extracted, and the areas of suppuration cleansed and curetted if necessary. The cavity usually has to be packed with antiseptic gauze afterwards for a few days until it begins to fill by healthy granulation tissue.

Periodontal disease is a name for chronic infection of the periodontal membrane. It is one form of inflammation of the periosteum, or alveolar periostitis. It causes loosening and shedding of the teeth, pain, failure to masticate, and loss of weight.

Odontomata are tumours formed in connection with the root of one tooth, or they may be found in the jaw, sinuses, or even involving part of the nasal passage, and be composite or compound, when multitudes of small rudimentary teeth are present. They cause swelling and bulging of the surface of the face, and can only be treated surgically.

Porphyria gives rise to a pink or brown discoloration of teeth. (See under BONE, DISEASES OF.)

Toothache is most spectacular in the dog, which rubs its mouth along the ground, paws at its nose or mouth, works its jaws, salivates, and may whine or moan.

A veterinary surgeon will offer a diagnosis and initiate the necessary treatment.

'Broken mouth' is important in hill sheep. (See under main dictionary heading.)

Fractures of the canine teeth in dogs are not uncommon. If the pulp is exposed, subsequent infection can lead to a painful abscess. Extraction of the remainder of the tooth obviates this but, for show dogs or guard dogs, is undesirable. Metal crowns have been applied to dogs' teeth, but are liable to be dislodged.

Tooth transplantation has been used in veterinary practice but the results are seldom lasting, due to root resorption and bone replacement. Fracture of the transplanted tooth is likely after a couple of years or so.

Teeth, Ewes', 'Trimming'

It has been estimated that between 60 and 70 per cent of culling of ewes is on account of their teeth. A small percentage will involve loss of molars or incisor wear, but the vast majority will be incisor loss.

Ewes have been treated for 'bite correction' by means of an electric grinder, a practice that originated in Australia. The procedure has been strongly condemned on welfare grounds.

(See also 'BROKEN MOUTH'.)

Teeth Scaling

The use of ultrasonic dental scalers is widely accepted in veterinary dentistry. During the scaling, an aerosol of water droplets is formed, with a variable amount of periodontal debris spattered from the patient's mouth. In the debris there are likely to be viruses and/or bacteria – a danger for operator, assistant, or subsequent patient unless precautions are taken. An aerosol of mouth flora can remain airborne for up to 30 minutes following scaling.

It is recommended that: (1) the working area should be well ventilated – preferably with forced air extraction; (2) masks should be worn at all times by anyone in the working area; and (3) a 0.2 per cent chlorhexidine solution should be used as the coolant supplied to the scaling equipment.

Telogen

The resting phase in the cycle of hair growth.

TEM

Triethylenemelemine, a gametocide which, in America, has been used in field trials for the control of birds. The chemical is mixed with corn, and has the effect of making the male bird infertile. The birds continue to defend their territories and nest, but do not produce any young.

Temperament, Change in

This may follow a brain tumour or infection, as occurs in BOVINE SPONGIFORM ENCEPHALOPATHY and RABIES, for example. A horse may become bad-tempered as the result of EQUINE VERMINOUS ARTERITIS. Poisoning may cause frenzy or aggressiveness, e.g. BENZOIC ACID poisoning in the cat. (See also BRAIN DISEASES; STRESS; FUCOSIDOSIS.)

Temperature, Air

(see under HOUSING OF ANIMALS; HEAT EXHAUSTION; TROPICS)

Temperature, Body

Body temperature is controlled by the heat-regulating centre in the brain – the hypothalamus, which also influences blood circulation, secretion of urine, and appetite – all 3 of which have a bearing on body temperature.

Heat is produced by the muscles and by the digestive organs, and during very cold weather or exercise, heat from the former increases, while that from the liver and other digestive organs decreases. The animal may also absorb heat from the sun's rays.

Heat is lost by evaporation of water, and by sensible heat loss (see under HEAT LOSS). Water loss is achieved via the lungs and the skin, e.g. by panting and sweating. (The dog is, for all practical purposes, a non-sweating animal apart from the pads of its feet, and has to rely mainly on panting.)

Diurnal variations in body temperature are normal; in the early hours of the morning it is usually at its lowest, and at its highest in the late afternoon.

For ordinary practical purposes the usual average temperatures of animals are given as follows:

Horses	38.0°C (100.5°F)
Cattle	38.9°C (102.0°F)
Sheep, goats	40.0°C (104.0°F)
Pigs	39.7°C (103.5°F)
Dogs	38.3°C (101.0°F)
Cats	38.6°C (102.0°F)
Rabbits	38.2°C (100.8°F)
Fowls	41.6°C (106.9°F)
Small birds	42.5°C (108.6°F)
Elephants	36.4°C (97.6°F)
Camels	37.5°C (99.5°F)

Temperature-taking The most satisfactory place is within the rectum. In females the thermometer may also be inserted into the external part of the genital canal; as a rule, the vaginal temperature is about half a degree higher than the rectal temperature, so that when a series of temperatures is to be taken, one site or the other should be selected.

With dogs and cats, one person should hold the animal, preferably on a table, while another inserts and holds the thermometer. In each animal, after the bulb of the thermometer has been lubricated with a little soap or Vaseline, etc., the tail is raised vertically by the left hand, and the thermometer is inserted through the anal ring and into the rectum, by a screwing movement if any resistance is encountered. It is held in position for 30 seconds, or 1 minute, according to the make of the thermometer, and then withdrawn. With a piece of cotton-wool any adherent faeces are wiped away, and the temperature is read off. Subsequently, the thermometer should be washed in cold water, and a cold solution of disinfectant used to disinfect it.

For purposes of temperature stress research, American scientists use a special ear thermometer in cattle. As in similar medical research, this tympanic thermometer is more reliable than the rectal thermometer, and can sense changes as small as 0.05°C (⅒°F).

Temperature in disease A high temperature is one of the classic symptoms of fever, and in greater or less measure accompanies practically all acute cases of disease. A comparatively steady rise in temperature is as a rule succeeded by a correspondingly steady fall, and is to be looked upon as a more favourable sign of the natural course of a disease than when the temperature rises and falls with greater suddenness. The reduction of temperature in simple fevers is in almost all cases much slower than the rise. A wavering temperature, which shows little tendency to come down to normal, generally indicates that there is some active focus of disease, such as an abscess, which the body cannot overcome. Sudden rise in temperature in an animal which has shown a steady fall previously is an indication of a relapse or recurrence of the disease. (See also FEVER; HYPERTHERMIA; HEAT-STROKE; TROPICS.)

Fall of temperature may be occasioned by great loss of blood, starvation, collapse, or coma; it is characteristic of certain forms of kidney disease. Certain chronic diseases in which emaciation is marked are also associated with a subnormal temperature. (See also HYPOTHERMIA.)

Temperature, near calving time A healthy cow – even though showing the familiar signs – is unlikely to calve during the next 12 hours if her temperature is 39°C (102°F). This is a useful guide to herdsmen. (See also under FEVER; HOUSING OF ANIMALS, etc.)

Temperature Control in Animal Housing
(see CONTROLLED-ENVIRONMENT HOUSING)

Temperature-Sensitive (TS) Viruses
(see VACCINE)

Tenderness
Tenderness is pain that is felt only when a diseased or injured part is handled.

Tendon
Tendon is the dense, fibrous, slightly elastic cord that attaches the end of a muscle to the bone or other structure upon which the muscle acts when it contracts. Tendons are composed of bundles of fibrous tissue, white in colour, and arranged in a very dense manner, so as to be capable of withstanding great strains. Some are rounded; some are flattened into ribbons; others are arranged in the form of sheets; while those of a 4th variety are very short, the muscle fibres being attached almost directly on to the bone or cartilage which they actuate. Most tendons are surrounded by sheaths lined with membrane similar to that found in joint cavities, i.e. synovial membrane. In this sheath the tendon glides smoothly over surrounding parts. The fibres of a tendon pass into the fibres of the periosteum covering a bone, and blend with them. One of the largest tendons in the animal body is the Achilles tendon, which runs

from the large muscles at the back of the stifle down to the point of the hock; it is often called the 'hamstring', and is the structure that is injured in the condition known as 'hamstrung'.

Tendons, Diseases and Injuries of

(see also under MUSCLES; SPRAINED TENDONS) In most cases the injuries to which tendons are liable are in the nature of minute lesions in which fibres have been torn across through over-extension of the tendon as a whole. Accompanying these there are often slight haemorrhages or extravasations of blood into the substance of the tendon, and the tendon itself is thickened at the injured part or, when severe, practically over the whole of its length. At the same time, a certain amount of damage has usually been sustained by the tendon sheath, or by its lining, and an unusually large amount of the lubricating synovial fluid is thrown out, which fills the tendon sheath to the point of dilatation, causing it to stand out on the surface of the limb.

When recovery occurs, the swelling subsides, fluid is absorbed, and the broken ends of the fibres become attached by strands of fibrous tissue to other intact fibres nearby. Pain disappears, and the animal becomes sound. Sometimes, however, permanent thickening results. (See also KNUCKLING.)

Certain of the tendons of the horse's limb are liable to become ruptured when subjected to great or sudden strains. Suture of the ruptured ends of the tendon has given good results when performed early, and when a sufficient amount of support can be provided by splints or other means. (See CARBON FIBRE.)

Severing of tendons in dogs' legs has been successfully treated. (See also TENOSYNOVITIS.)

Tenesmus

Straining to pass urine or faeces with little or no result.

Tenosynovitis

Tenosynovitis is inflamation of the tendon and its sheath. It affects the legs of broiler chickens and is usually caused by a virus. Tendons may enlarge and cease to function. (See also SYNOVITIS.)

Tenotomy

The surgical severing of a tendon.

TEPP

Tetra-ethyl pyrophosphate, used in agriculture as a pesticide, is a potential danger to livestock.

A Texas rancher diluted 1 volume of TEPP with water to make 120 volumes, and sprayed 20 head of cattle. All were dead within three-quarters of an hour. Symptoms of poisoning in a puppy comprised drowsiness, muscular incoordination, and vomiting. The antidote is atropine sulphate.

Teratogenic

Teratogenic agents, called teratogens, are those known to cause congenital defects when the pregnant mother is exposed to them. The most notorious is thalidomide but there are many others, not all of them drugs: alkaloids found in some plants, e.g. hemlock, viruses and radiation can all be teratogenic.

Teratoma

Teratoma is a developmental irregularity in which the embryo, instead of growing normally in the uterus, develops structural defects or, in extreme cases, develops into a seriously deformed fetus. The latter are comparatively common in cattle, and give rise to difficulty at parturition. 'Teratology' is the study of congenital deformities. (See also under TUMOURS.)

Termites

Whitish, ant-like insects of the tropics. Some species feed on wood, damaging buildings.

Control Heptachlor and chlordane.

Terrapin

A small aquatic turtle, of which the diamond-backed terrapin (*Malaclemys terrapin*) is typical. Males are smaller than females, reaching about 14 cm (5½ in) to the female's 32 cm (9 in). They are popular domestic aquarium pets; however, they should be handled with care as cases of salmonella poisoning in members of households in which they are kept have occurred.

Tervueren

A breed of dog originally from Flanders. Epilepsy has been recorded in some individual dogs.

Teschen Disease (Porcine Viral Encephalomyelitis)

(see TALFAN DISEASE)

Testicle (Testis)

Testicle (testis) is the essential male generative gland or gonad, which, along with the epididymis and its associated structures, lies in the scrotum in each of the domesticated animals.

Normally, in the fetus or soon after birth,

the testicle, guided by the fibrous cord known as the gubernaculum, moves down from a position close to the kidney to a 'cooler climate' in the scrotum. Into this it is pulled by the gubernaculum, which either fails to lengthen or actually shortens.

In some animals, e.g. foals, one or both testicles may go up again through the inguinal canal. This occurs occasionally in pigs, in which a returning testicle has been known to become a mere vestige by the age of 6 months.

In certain of the wild animals, such as the rat, and in many tropical animals, e.g. the elephant, the testes are found in the abdominal cavity, either permanently or temporarily between periods of sexual activity. In the foal the testes appear in the scrotum usually very soon after birth, but they are subsequently drawn up into the abdomen, and do not reappear until between 5 or 6 months and 10 to 12 months. In a certain proportion of cases the testes are retained in the abdomen until 2 years of age, and then descend into the scrotum; in a number of cases they do not descend at all. The name 'rig', or 'cryptorchid', is applied to such animals, and the condition is known as 'cryptorchidism'. (See CRYPTORCHID.)

The testes consist of a dense fibrous coat, the 'tunica albuginea'. Blood vessels run throughout the fibrous tissue, and nourish microscopic tubules, lined by layers of specialised cells which form the spermatozoa. The tubules, known as 'seminiferous tubules', are connected with each other near the centre of the testes, and communicate with the coiled tubes of the epididymis, from which springs the vas deferens connecting with the urethra at the opposite end. In the epididymis the sperms mature. The 'spermatic cord', which consists of the vas deferens, spermatic artery, veins, and nerves, enclosed in the layer of serous membrane (tunica vaginalis), passes upwards through the inguinal canal and enters the abdomen, whence it runs back to the region of the neck of the urinary bladder, opening finally into the urethra. Along the course of the urethra are the openings of the ducts from the secondary sexual glands – seminal vesicles, prostate, and bulbo-urethral glands – which pour out a secretion which mixes with, nourishes, and protects the masses of spermatozoa coming from the testes.

Externally, the testicle is covered by a layer of serous membrane, lying immediately outside the tunica albuginea, and known as the tunica vaginalis propria, which also covers the epididymis. On the outside of this tunic is the tunica vaginalis communis, or the parietal layer.

Outside this is a fairly thick layer of scrotal fascia, in which is deposited the 'cod-fat' of the bullock and wedder. A strong reddish, fibroelastic tunica dartos forms the next outermost layer, and provides the septum between the right and left pouches of the scrotum. Finally, on the outside, there is the practically hairless, thin, elastic, oily-feeling skin of the scrotum.

Functions The essential function of the testis is to produce sperms. (See SPERMATOZOA.) Between 60 and 80 million sperms are discharged at each copulatory act by the stallion at the beginning of the breeding season. Since a stallion may serve more than 100 mares during the season, many of them upon 2 separate occasions, it will readily be understood that the testes are extremely active organs, and make a considerable demand upon the vitality of the body generally. The necessity for a recuperative period in breeding males will also be obvious.

The other function of the testis is that associated with elaboration of the male sex-hormones, resulting in the production of the secondary sexual characteristics, such as the arched neck and great body size of the stallion, the broad forehead, massive development of horns, and deep voice of the bull, the horns of the ram, and the tusks of the boar, etc., as well as the instinctive desire for sexual intercourse. The chief hormone is testosterone.

(See also REPRODUCTION; ENDOCRINE GLANDS; ARTIFICIAL INSEMINATION.)

Testicle, Diseases of

During service, an irritable mare may kick a stallion and rupture one of the testes, or seriously injure it. Damage may also be occasioned to these organs by the bites of dogs when fighting, by gores from cattle, or by injuries from the tusks of boars, gunshots, etc. However, infection is probably most common.

Orchitis, or inflammation of the testis, may be the result of infection (e.g. by *Actinobacillus seminis, Brucella abortus, B. suis, Corynebacterium pseudotuberculosis*, tuberculosis) or of trauma which – if the skin is broken – may itself lead to infection. A viral infection of bulls – infectious orchitis – was reported in the former Czechoslovakia. Necrotic orchitis in the bull has been caused in Britain by actinobacillosis. The testis, being enclosed in a fibrous, comparatively non-elastic capsule, is not able to swell to a great extent, although the loose tissues of the scrotum often do. The scrotum becomes reddened in animals which have unpigmented skin in the inguinal region, and the whole area is very painful to the touch.

Treatment Antibiotics or other therapy may be needed to deal with an infection.

Epididimytis (see under main dictionary heading, and under RAM)

Hydrocele is a local oedema affecting usually one tunica vaginalis, and distending that side of the scrotum with fluid. It is most frequently encountered in the dog, although it may affect other animals.

Hypoplasia (see under INFERTILITY)

Tumours affecting the testicle and/or scrotum include CARCINOMA, SARCOMA, FIBROMA, PAPIL-LOMA, SEMINOMA, and SERTOLI-CELL TUMOUR.

Torsion (see under SPERMATIC CORD, TORSION OF)

Testosterone

The hormone, secreted by the testicle, which controls development of the secondary sex organs, sex characteristics and libido. (See ENDOCRINE GLANDS; HORMONES.)

Tests

(see LABORATORY TESTS)

Tetanus (Lockjaw)

Tetanus (lockjaw) is a specific disease of the domesticated animals and man, caused by *Clostridium tetani*, which obtains access to the tissues through a wound. Horses are most commonly affected. The organism is present in most cultivated soils, especially such as receive heavy dressings of farmyard manure.

In certain districts, tetanus is so common that it is usual to take precautions by inoculating horses with antitoxin whenever they receive even comparatively slight wounds, and always before castration or major operations. Lambs are lost each year after docking and castration, or before the umbilicus (navel) has closed after birth, from tetanus.

Cl. tetani is an anaerobe, i.e. it thrives only in an absence of oxygen. Its serious effects are produced by a toxin, which is absorbed into the general circulation and exerts its effects upon the nervous system of the brain and spinal cord. This toxin is one of the most powerful known.

Deeply punctured wounds, from which oxygen is excluded, are much more serious than even large superficial wounds, the surfaces of which are exposed to the action of sunlight and fresh air. Picked-up nail wounds, cracked heels, injuries from the prongs of stable-forks, etc., are examples of wounds which often become contaminated with *Cl. tetani*. Tetanus may occur in an animal which has had a slight wound which appeared to heal without any complication. It may follow tattooing. Cases are met with where no wound can be found on the surface of the body, nor is there any history of an accident; such cases are probably the sequel to injuries inflicted by worms in the intestinal wall, or to slight scratches from unusually hard or rough herbage.

Intramuscular injections are a potential route of infection when sterile precautions are neglected.

Signs

Horses become stiff and disinclined to move. There is difficulty in turning the head round to the side, and the fore-legs are splayed outwards as though to enable the unfortunate animal better to retain its balance.

The ears may be turned in towards each other.

If the head is lifted sharply up, by placing the hand under the chin, the haw or 3rd eyelid (nictitating membrane) is seen to flicker across the eye to an extent much greater than usual.

Fixity of the jaws, or trismus, which has been responsible for the popular name given to tetanus (i.e. lockjaw), is not always in evidence in the early stages of an attack.

The tail may be held out quivering, and OPISTHOTONOS may be evident.

During the course of an attack, faeces and urine are usually withheld, and digestive disturbances may occur, sometimes resulting in fatal collections of gas in the large intestines.

(See HYPERAESTHESIA – another sign.)

Cattle Early signs include a raising of the tail-head and, in some cases, bloat. The gait becomes stiff and the animal may have difficulty in feeding because it cannot easily lower its head because of stiffness in the neck. Trismus (lockjaw) is a late sign. Tetanus in cattle is not, however, at all common; occasionally outbreaks occur, possibly due to rough, abrasive feed which allows entry of the infection through the gut.

Sheep The signs are similar to those in cattle. As the disease progresses, standing is difficult; the affected animals lie on their sides, rapidly become tympanitic, and die after a very short

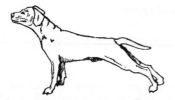

Diagram of attitude assumed by a dog affected with tetanus. The hind-limbs are kept well out behind the body, the tail is held rigidly or quivering, and the muscles of the face are drawn into a sardonic grin – the 'risus sardonicus' of ancient authors.

illness. In lambs after castration or docking, the disease is very rapid in its effects, and several are affected at the same time.

Pigs Tetanus is not common.

Dogs The owner may notice something peculiar about the eyes and mouth, and either stiffness or recent lameness. Later, the limbs are usually stretched out as far from each other as possible, in a sawhorse position. Squinting and grinning are common, but closure of the jaws is not always in evidence. When it is present it is complete, and death practically always follows. Hyperaesthesia is also very marked. The ears may be bent inwards (as in the horse).

Treatment Farm animals should be placed in a darkened loose-box, away from noise, and with food and water placed at a new level which they can reach despite their stiffness.

If nursed at home, a dog should be in a room where there are no bright lights, noise, television, or family activity.

Tetanus antiserum, penicillin, and muscle relaxants (such as acepromazine, which can obviate exhaustion and save life) are all needed. Treatment must also include glucose saline injections, e.g. in a dog which cannot drink or eat; and large animals similarly. (See DEHYDRATION, NORMAL SALINE.)

Prevention Vaccination is effective, and on land where tetanus is rife, the most susceptible animals should be immunised.

Lambs are given antitoxin on the day of docking or castration. Vaccine can be injected at a different site on the same occasion.

Horses The usual practice is to give 2 injections at an interval of 4 to 6 weeks, with a booster dose 6 or 12 months later. Further booster doses may be required. It is practicable

to vaccinate pregnant mares so that later their newborn foals will be protected against tetanus infection via the navel. (See also under IMMUNITY.)

Prognosis In the absence of first-class nursing and intensive care, not many animals (other than cattle) recover from tetanus.

If an animal regains the ability to drink, that can be regarded as a favourable sign.

Tetany

Tetany is a condition in which localised spasmodic contraction of muscles takes place. There may be twitching or convulsions. Tetany occurs when the level of blood calcium falls below normal. (See also under PARATHYROID; HYPOMAGNESAEMIA; TRANSIT; MILK FEVER; RABIES.)

Tethering

The Cruel Tethering Act 1988 makes it illegal to tether a horse, ass or mule in such a way as to cause suffering. The animal must have enough to eat and be supplied with fresh water regularly. The tether must not be able to cause injury, e.g. by being too tight or too short.

Tetracyclines

Tetracyclines are bacteriostatic antibiotics with a wide range of activity which includes Gram-positive and Gram-negative bacteria, certain protozoa, rickettsia, and mycoplasma. Tetracyclines are absorbed from the gut, but oral administration may upset the gut flora. They are irritant when injected.

Tetracyclines cause fluorescence in bone and teeth. In late pregnancy or in young growing animals, high dosage can result in teeth discoloration and can interfere with the formation of enamel.

Horses treated with tetracyclines while suffering from stress may become affected with diarrhoea and die. (See DIARRHOEA in horses.)

In cats, tetracyclines occasionally cause severe loss of hair.

Tetraiodophenolphthalein

Tetraiodophenolphthalein is used in radiography of the gall-bladder and bile-ducts for diagnostic purposes.

Texas Fever

Texas fever is a tick-borne disease. (See BABESIA – Babesiosis.)

Signs Stained urine (red-water), high temperature, no appetite, and constipation followed by diarrhoea. Cerebral symptoms may be evident. The animal dies within 3 to 10 days. On post-mortem examination the blood is bright red and abnormally fluid, while the tissues are paler. The spleen is enlarged from 2 to 4 times its normal size and is reddish-brown ('anthrax spleen'). The liver is swollen and pale and the gall-bladder is distended with thick, viscid, dark-coloured bile. The muscles are normal.

The chronic form is similar but milder, and occurs in late autumn. Recovery is frequent, but convalescence is long (although it is stated to be very short in Argentine cattle).

Treatment is fairly effective. Imidocarb is one of several proprietary preparations that have replaced the trypan blue formerly used.

Transmission is by the following ticks:
Boophilus (Margaropus) annulatus (North America)
B. microplus (South America)
B. australis (many countries)
B. argentinus (South America)
B. calcaratus (Asia)
B. decoloratus (South Africa)
Rhipicephalus appendiculatus (South Africa)
R. evertsi (South Africa)
R. bursa (North Africa)
Haemaphysalis punctata (Europe)

Texel

A Dutch breed of sheep, and the most common breed in Europe. Noted for its milk production, it has good growth rate and meat potential.

TGE

(see TRANSMISSIBLE GASTROENTERITIS OF PIGS)

Thalamus

A part of the brain consisting of 2 large ovoid structures at the base of the cerebrum (see under BRAIN).

Thallium

Thallium sulphate is used in poison baits to destroy rats, ants, and other pests, and accidental poisoning in domestic animals may occur. Thallium poisoning in dogs gives rise to gastroenteritis, profuse vomiting, and severe pain. If death does not immediately follow, there may be a brick-red discoloration of lips, skin of groin or axilla. Hair begins to fall out. In human medicine, thallium poisoning has been successfully treated with prussian-blue.

Theave

A sheep between 1st and 2nd shearing (see under SHEEP).

Theileriosis

Infection with tick-borne parasites of the *Theileridae*.

The parasites vary in shape, some being spherical, others ovoid, pear-shaped, or elongated rod-like. Division by binary fission within the blood corpuscle may occur. Sexual multiplication occurs within the tick which transmits the parasite when it bites a new host.

There are several species in cattle and in sheep, including:

T. parva (EAST COAST FEVER in tropical Africa).
T. mutans (Benign bovine theileriosis).
T. lawrencei, causing CORRIDOR DISEASE.
T annulata, causing MEDITERRANEAN FEVER.
(See also TZANEEN DISEASE.)

Theine

Theine is the alkaloid which gives its stimulant properties to tea. It is the equivalent of CAFFEINE.

Thelazia

(see EYEWORMS)

Theobromine

Theobromine is the alkaloid upon which the stimulant action of cocoa and chocolate depends. Horses fed a supplement of vitamins and minerals incorporated in a material containing ground cocoa shells have tested positive for this alkaloid.

Thermography

The mapping of temperature over surfaces. Infra-red thermography, using a camera, has been tested in the diagnosis of orthopaedic lesions in horses.

Thermolabile

Subject to the loss of characteristic properties when heated.

Thiabendazole

(see ANTHELMINTICS)

Thiamin (Thiamine)

Thiamine hydrochloride, or vitamin B_1. A secondary deficiency occurs in bracken poisoning and horse-tails poisoning in horses, and in pigs due to the enzyme, thiaminase. Thiaminase-producing bacteria have been isolated from sheep dying from polioencephalomalacia (cerebrocortical necrosis). (See also 'CHASTEK PARALYSIS'.)

Thiaminase is present to a varying degree in raw fish. Accordingly, fish should be cooked before it is fed to cats, etc.

Signs of this deficiency include loss of appetite, a staggering gait, and muscular spasms.

Thin Sow Syndrome

Groups of sows or gilts lose weight, usually in the middle or later stages of pregnancy, and remain emaciated for perhaps 6 months or more. Prolonged under-feeding may eventually result in some sows being unable to cope with adverse conditions encountered at times of stress, e.g. weaning. It has also been suggested that infestation with the stomach worm *Hyostrongylus* or with the nodular worm *Oesophagostomum* may be a cause. The use of sow stalls, in which animals cannot move away to escape draughts, is another possible cause.

Thiopental

A widely used anaesthetic for horses, dogs and cats. It is administered intravenously, as an aqueous solution of the sodium salt; other routes cause necrosis of the tissues.

Thiouracil

An antithyroid agent which lowers the rate of metabolism. It has been used as a growth promoter; such use is banned in the EU.

Thiourea

This is naphythyl antu, a rat poison which causes oedema of the lungs. It is dangerous to domestic animals and birds.

Thirst

(see WATER; DIABETES; SALT POISONING; COMPULSIVE POLYDIPSIA)

Thogoto Virus

Thogoto virus is a cause of abortion in ewes in Africa. It was first isolated from a tick, *Rhipicephalus appendiculatus*, near Thogoto in Kenya. In one flock of some 600 Dorper ewes, more than 200 aborted over a 2-month period.

Thoracic Duct

The thoracic duct is the large lymph vessel which collects the contents of the lymphatics proceeding from the abdomen, hind-limbs, part of the thorax, etc., and which discharges its contents into the left innominate vein. (See aspiration under PARACENTESIS.)

Thoracocentesis

Draining off from the thorax of the fluid found in certain diseases of the chest. (See aspiration under PARACENTESIS.)

Thoracotomy

A surgical operation involving opening of the chest cavity.

Thorax

(see CHEST)

Thorn Apple

(see STRAMONIUM)

Thorough-Pin

Thorough-pin is a distension of the sheath of the deep flexor tendon where it passes over the arch of the tarsus (hock). It is characterised by swellings, one on either side of the hock, about the level of the 'point of the hock' (summit of the tuber calcis), and lying in front of the strong Achilles tendon.

Thread-Worm

Thread-worm is a popular term for *oxyuris* worms. (See ROUNDWORMS.)

Threonine

One of the essential amino acids.

Throat

(see PHARYNX; also under LARYNX; NOSE AND NASAL PASSAGES; MOUTH)

Throat diseases Most of these will be found under separate headings such as choking; larynx, diseases of; tonsillitis. For 'sore throat', see PHARYNGITIS.

Thrombasthenia

This is a rare, congenital disorder of the blood, occurring in man and dogs, in both sexes (compare HAEMOPHILIA). It arises from a defect of the platelets, and gives rise to prolonged bleeding resulting in anaemia. It has been described in foxhounds, otterhounds, etc.

Thrombocytopenia

A condition of the blood in which the number of platelets is below normal. Causes include viral infections, poisoning, auto-immune disease. The signs may include petechial haemorrhages and fever.

Thrombosis

The blocking of a blood vessel by a blood clot. It may follow atheroma, or some injury to the vessel. In cats, thrombosis of the femoral arteries is by no means rare, and causes paralysis of the hind-legs and often pain. There is complete absence of pulse in the arteries. In dogs, thrombosis of the iliac and femoral arteries occurs occasionally. Euthanasia is nearly always necessary. (See also PARAPLEGIA.)

Aortic-iliac thrombosis is seen in the horse; the worm *Strongylus vulgaris* may be a cause.

Thrombosis of a blood vessel in the brain is a cause of apoplexy (in human medicine a stroke). (For thrombosis of the vena cava in cattle, see under VENA CAVA.) (See also under ANTICOAGULANTS.)

Thrombus

A blood clot in a blood vessel or the heart.

Thymus Gland

Situated in the anterior part of the chest cavity, this gland attains its largest size during early life and thereafter gradually dwindles. The thymus has a role in immunity, as it removes young T-cells that happen to reccognise the body's own components as foreign. Failure of this function can result in auto-immune disease. (See T-CELLS, which are thymus derived; also LEUKAEMIA.)

Thyroid Cartilage

The thyroid cartilage is the largest cartilage of the larynx, and forms a well-marked prominence at the upper end of the trachea. It gives attachment to one end of each of the vocal folds, which are concerned in the production of voice. (See LARYNX.)

Thyroid Gland

This is a very highly vascular ENDOCRINE GLAND, situated near the thyroid cartilage of the larynx. The gland usually consists of 2 lobes, one on either side of the larynx, joined by an isthmus in some species and individuals.

Located within or near the thyroid gland are the PARATHYROID GLANDS.

Minute structure Each lobe is enveloped in a thin capsule of fibrous tissue, strands from which pass into the organ, dividing it into lobules.

Function The most important hormone secreted by the thyroid gland is an iodine-containing compound called thyroxin. This increases the rate of metabolism, and is released when an animal is exposed to cold, for example. In hot weather, thyroid activity is reduced. Thyroxin is essential for growth and reproduction, and influences lactation.

Secretion of the hormone is controlled wholly or in part by a hormone from the anterior lobe of the pituitary gland. (See also PARATHYROID GLANDS.)

Thyroid Gland, Diseases of

Enlargement of the thyroid gland is known as GOITRE. Goitre may occur when there is either too little or too much of the thyroid hormone, thyroxin, produced.

Dwarfism in young animals (cretinism) can result from failure of the gland to produce sufficient thyroxin.

Hypothyroidism An insufficiency of thyroxin is known as hypothyroidism, and may be associated with insufficiency of iodine in the diet (see GOITRE). The rate of metabolism is slowed, while there is an increase in body weight, loss of hair, and lethargy.

One form of hypothyroidism, MYXOEDEMA, affects the skin, causing its deterioration.

Treatment includes the use of thyroid extract; and iodides if appropriate.

Hyperthyroidism, or excess thyroxin in the blood, is characterised by loss of weight, sometimes an increase in appetite, polyuria, thirst, increased rate of metabolism and heartbeat. Enlargement of the gland may be detected on palpation. The animal may become restless or irritable. Protrusion of the eyeballs (exophthalmic goitre) may occur.

Hyperthyroidism is seen in elderly cats. They are mostly thin, and it is this loss of weight which causes the owner to seek veterinary advice in many instances. In addition to the symptoms mentioned above, diarrhoea may occur.

Treatment is surgical: removal of one gland, or ligation of the anterior arteries; alternatively, the use of drugs such as sodium fluoride or methylthiouracil.

Tumours of the gland include ADENOMA; sarcoma and carcinoma (see under CANCER); and EPITHELIOMA.

Thyroxine

The active principle of the THYROID GLAND. It is used in pharmaceutical preparations to correct hypothyroidism, a common endocrine deficiency in dogs.

Tiamulin

A macrolide antibiotic active against *Treponema hyodysenteriae* (swine dysentery), various Gram-positive organisms, and *Mycoplasma hyosinoviae* (a cause of arthritis in pigs). It must not be used at the same time as MONENSIN or SALINOMYCIN.

Tibia

The tibia is the larger of the 2 bones which lie between the stifle and the hock. In animals which possess fewer than 5 digits in their hind-limbs, the tibia has become modified so that it sustains the greater part of the weight borne by the limb – the fibula, its complementary bone, having become reduced in size and importance. The tibia lies just below the skin on the inside of the limb, in such a position that it is liable to be injured by kicks, blows, etc., and in this connection is of more importance than those bones that are surrounded by massive muscles which afford some protection. It is not uncommon for the tibia to become fractured, but the parts remain held together by the very dense periosteum that covers the bone. In the smaller animals, the setting of the fractured bone is a routine. (See BONES; FRACTURES.)

Tibial dyschondroplasia A crippling deformity occurring in certain strains of chickens, ducks, and turkeys selected for high growth rates. It is due to a cartilage abnormality.

Tick-Bite Fever of Man in Africa

Cause A RICKETTSIA. Local reactions, swelling of lymph nodes, occur in some individuals. So far as is known, tick-bite fever is not fatal.

The bont tick, bont-legged blue tick, yellow dog tick, and the brown tick – all common in East Africa – transmit this disease. It can be transmitted to the guinea-pig by inoculation of blood.

Tick-Borne Encephalitis (TBE)

A meningioencephalitis following infection by a flavivirus transmitted by the sheep/cattle tick *Ixodes ricinus*. The ticks become infected by field mice, voles, shrews, and occasionally moles. It occurs throughout continental Europe, being especially prevalent in mountainous regions with coniferous forests. It is more common in humans than in animals, but the infection in dogs has been confused with rabies.

The human illness resembles influenza in its symptoms, with a high fever. This may be followed by meningitis. Mortality is about 1 per cent.

In differential diagnosis, the flavivirus causing TBE has to be distinguished from louping-ill virus.

Tick-Borne Fever of Cattle

Tick-borne fever of cattle is caused by *Cytoectes (Erlichia) phagocytophila*, transmitted by the common sheep tick, *Ixodes ricinus*. Symptoms of this infection are high but transient fever, and a considerable reduction in milk yield. Abortion may also occur. Oxytetracycline is used in treatment. (Red-water, caused by *Babesia divergens*, often occurs simultaneously.)

Tick-Borne Fever of Sheep

Tick-borne fever of sheep is a disease caused by *Cytoectes phagocytophilia* transmitted by the tick *Ixodes ricinus*.

Tick-borne fever is a mild febrile disease of sheep in which the essential symptom is a rise in temperature occurring after an incubation period of 4 to 8 days, and lasting about 10 days, when it subsides. During this period (which may be prolonged) there is dullness and listlessness, and a considerable loss of weight may occur. Death occurs in only a small percentage of cases; most sheep recover unless some other complicating condition such as louping-ill supervenes. Abortion is an important result of infection in many instances, and may affect 50 per cent of breeding stock introduced from tick-free areas.

Rickettsiae can be demonstrated in the polymorphonuclear white cells of the blood.

The importance of tick-borne fever is that it is capable of rendering the vasculo-meningeal barrier of the central nervous system vulnerable to the virus of louping-ill. Without its presence, though the louping-ill virus may be introduced into the bloodstream (by the bite of a tick), it cannot pass this barrier to attack the nerve cells and so produce the typical nervous symptoms. It has been shown that both infective agents – that of tick-borne fever and of louping-ill – frequently exist together in ticks found on animals on farms where louping-ill is common, and it is probable that under natural conditions the great majority of adult sheep on such farms have been infected with tick-borne fever infection and have recovered.

Tick-borne fever increases the susceptibility of lambs to tick pyaemia, often caused by infection with *Staphylococcus aureus* following tick bites. Abscesses occur in the joints and elsewhere, causing lameness, unthriftiness, and death.

Tick Paralysis

Tick paralysis affects man, cattle, sheep, horses, pigs, dogs, cats, and poultry.

It occurs in Africa, Australia, and Canada, and is caused by the presence on the animal of various species of *Ixodes* (especially the dog tick) in South Africa and Australia, and *Dermacentor* in America. In East Africa, the bont-legged tick (*Hyalomma spp.*) and possibly the Red tick (*Rhipicephalus evertsi*) cause paralysis.

The paralysis is caused by toxin(s) present in the saliva of ticks.

In human beings, 3 or 4 days after the ticks attach themselves, paralysis of the legs occurs, then paralysis of the arms takes place, later the chest and neck become involved, and ultimately the heart and respiratory centres are attacked. In the sheep, the parts are affected in the same general sequence.

This form of paralysis is peculiar in that symptoms disappear within 2 to 6 days after the ticks are removed, and recovery takes place subsequently. Individual lambs, for example, can be reinfected and recover more than once, if the ticks are removed by hand. They are usually not easily seen unless a deliberate search is made in the wool over the vertebral column from the base of the skull back to the tail.

In the dog, they may cause QUADRIPLEGIA.

Tick Pyaemia
(see TICKS; TICK-BORNE FEVER OF SHEEP)

Ticks
These are among the most serious parasites of domestic animals. In the tropics they transmit bacterial, protozoal and viral diseases; in the UK, tick-borne fever, red-water fever and louping-ill. Tick pyaemia is caused in sheep by the transfer of staphylococcal infection. Lyme disease is considered to be partly tick spread.

Some cause illness by means of a toxin, while all feed on the host's blood – which can result in a serious anaemia. Large numbers of ticks also worry the host, and cause unthriftiness. Suppurating wounds may also result. In the British Isles, *Ixodes ricinus* is the main tick found, although *Haemophysalis punctatis* is present in some southern coastal areas.

Life-cycles On this basis, ticks can be divided into 3 groups:

1-host ticks, such as *Boophilus*, which spend all 3 stages of their life-cycle on the same animal. Larvae having attached themselves to the host, they feed on it, moult, feed again on it as nymphs, moult, and the adult ticks also feed on it – the females subsequently dropping to the ground to lay their eggs.

2-host ticks: these, such as some *Hyalomma* species, feed as both larvae and nymphs on the same host, but then moult on the ground; emerging adults find and feed on a 2nd host.

3-host ticks: larva, nymph, and adult each feeds on a different host, with moulting taking place on the ground between each stage in the life-cycle. *Ixodes* and *Dermacentor* species are included in this group.

Family Ixodidae (hard ticks) In this family the dorsum of the body is more or less protected by a hard shield of chitin, and in some species the male has ventral plates also.

The principal species attacking the domestic animals are dealt with below. (See also DOG TICKS for those occurring in Britain.)

Ixodes. There are over 50 species in this genus, including the following:

(a) *I. ricinus* attacks all the domesticated animals and is found in most parts of the world. It is known locally as the castor-bean tick, or European sheep tick. A 3-host tick, it leaves its host before each moult, and then seeks a new host. In this way 3 animals are attacked by the same tick: one as a larva, one as a nymph, and one as an adult. The animals attacked need not be of the same species. This tick transmits tick-borne fever in sheep, louping-ill, and causes tick paralysis in sheep and cattle. It can also transmit Babesia, the cause of red-water.

(b) *I. hexagonus* attacks especially the dog, but is found on other hosts, notably sheep. It

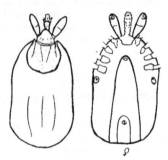

Ixodes. (Dorsal and ventral views of a small female. × 8.) In this and subsequent drawings of ticks only the fore parts of the legs are shown in diagrams of the ventral surface.

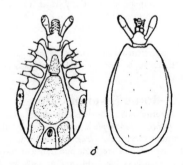

Ixodes. (Ventral and dorsal views of male. × 12.)

occurs in Europe, North Africa, and America; it is common on hunting dogs in France. In addition it is a transmitter of babesiosis.

(c) *I. canisuga* is the common species found on the dog in Britain. It occurs also in Western Europe and North America. Like the last species, only females are found on the host. It is known popularly as the British dog tick.

(d) *I. pilosus* attacks all the domestic mammals in South Africa. It is a reddish-brown tick, with the body larger behind than in front. It is known locally as the russet tick, and is a causal agent of tick paralysis.

(e) *I. rubicundus*, another South African tick, which is found only on sheep, also causes tick paralysis.

(f) *I. holocyclus*, in Australia and India, is found on ruminants, dogs, and pigs. It is the cause of Australian tick paralysis, symptoms of which may appear within an hour of attachment. It transmits Q fever.

Haemaphysalis. The following species are important:

(a) *H. punctata* (*H. cinnabarina* var. *punctata*) is a common tick in Europe, North America, and North Africa on all the domestic animals. The life-history is identical with that of *H. leachii*. It transmits *Babesia bovis* in Britain.

(b) *H. leachii* is a 3-host African species which has been found in Western Asia and Australia. It attacks carnivores, but is sometimes found on ruminants. In East Africa it is called the yellow dog tick; it is also known as the South African dog tick. It transmits canine babesiosis, Q fever, and tick-bite fever.

Dermacentor. The following species are important:

(a) *D. reticulatus* is common in Europe, but also occurs in North Asia. It attacks ruminants, and also the dog and the horse. It is occasionally found in Western England. It transmits equine and canine babesiosis.

(b) *D. variabilis* (*D. electus*) is found on dogs in North America. It also occurs on cattle and horses. It is known as the American dog tick.

(c) *D. occidentalis* occurs in western North America on various domestic mammals. It is considered by some authorities to be *D. reticulatus*.

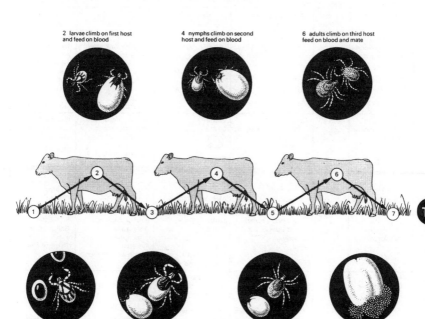

2 larvae climb on first host and feed on blood

4 nymphs climb on second host and feed on blood

6 adults climb on third host feed on blood and mate

1 eggs hatch, larvae emerge

3 engorged larvae fall to ground and moult, nymphs emerge

5 engorged nymphs fall to ground and moult, adults emerge

7 engorged female falls to ground and lays eggs

Life-cycle of a 3-host tick, *Ixodes ricinus*. (Reproduced with permission from H. T. B. Hall, *Diseases and Parasites of Livestock in the Tropics*, Longman.)

(d) *D. venestus* is found in the Rocky Mountain District of North America and is called the Pacific Coast tick. Adults are found on various mammals, including man. It is the transmitter of Rocky Mountain spotted fever in man, and of canine babesiosis. It is the cause of American tick paralysis. It is a 3-host tick.

Rhipicephalus. The following species are important:

(a) *R. sanguineus* is found in all parts of the world on dogs and ruminants. It is brown in colour. It is known as the European brown tick and also as the European dog tick – a name shared with *Ixodes hexagonus*.

(b) *R. appendiculatus* is found in Africa, where it attacks cattle, sheep, goats. It is called the brown tick, and is a 3-host tick. This species transmits East Coast fever, corridor disease, mild gall sickness, red-water, Nairobi sheep disease.

(c) *R. bursa* is found in North Africa and Southern Europe on all animals. It is a 2-host tick. It transmits ovine babesiosis in Europe.

(d) *R. capensis* is found in South Africa on cattle, horses and dogs. It is called the Cape brown tick. The life-cycle is similar to the 2nd species. It can transmit *Theileria parva*.

(e) *R. simus* is found in Africa on dogs and herbivores. It is called the dark pitted tick. Its life-cycle is similar to the 2nd species. It can transmit *Theileria parva*, *Anaplasma marginale*, *T. mutans*.

(f) *R. evertsi* in Africa may be found on all the domestic mammals except pigs. It has orange-red legs with round convex distinct eyes. The scutum is black and densely pitted. The underside of the male is red; the females are brown or reddish brown. It is called the red tick or the red-legged tick. This 2-host species transmits *Nuttallia equi* and *T. parva*, causing East Coast fever, babesiosis, spirochaetosis.

Boophilus

(a) *B. decoloratus* is found on cattle and other animals in Africa. It is a 1-host tick, called the blue tick. This tick, which may be a variety of *B. annulatus*, transmits *Babesia bigemina*, *Anaplasma marginale*, and *Spirochaeta theileri*.

COMMON TICKS IN EAST AFRICA

Tick species	Number of hosts	Preferred site of attachment	Animal affected	Parasite	Disease transmitted
Brown-ear tick (*Rhipicephalus appendiculatus*)	3	Ears, base of horns, around eyes, tail brush, and heels	Cattle	*Theileria parva*	East Coast fever
			Cattle	*Theileria lawrencei*	Corridor disease
			Cattle	*Theileria mutans*	Mild gall-sickness
			Cattle	*Babesia bigemina*	Red-water
			Sheep and goats	Virus	Nairobi sheep disease
			Sheep, cattle, and goats		Louping-ill
			Man	*Rickettsia*	Tick-bite fever
Red-legged tick (*Rhipicephalus evertsi*)	2	Larvae and nymphae in ears Adults perineal region	Cattle	*Babesia bigemina*	Red-water
			Cattle	*Theileria parva*	East Coast fever
			Cattle	*Theileria mutans*	Mild gall-sickness
			Horses	*Babesia nuttali* } *Babesia caballi*	Biliary fever
			Cattle, horses sheep, and goats	*Spirochaeta theileri*	Spirochaetosis
			Lambs	?Tick toxin	?Paralysis
Yellow dog tick (*Haemaphysalis leach*)	3	Whole body	Dogs	*Babesia canis*	Biliary fever
			Man and animals	Virus	Q fever
			Man	*Rickettsia*	Tick-bite fever
Blue tick (*Boophilus decoloratus*)	1	Face, neck, dewlap, and sides of the body	Cattle	*Babesia bigemina*	Red-water
			Cattle	*Anaplasma marginale*	Gall-sickness
			Man	*Rickettsia*	Tick-bite fever
			Horses, cattle, Goats and sheep	*Spirochaeta theileri*	
Bont tick (*Amblyomma* spp.)	3	Larvae and nymphae on head and ears Nymphae and adults on perineum, udder, scrotum, and tail	Cattle/Sheep/ Goats	*Rickettsia ruminantium*	Heartwater
			Sheep	Virus	Nairobi sheep disease
			Man and animals	Virus	Q fever
			Man	*Rickettsia*	Tick-bite fever
Bont-legged tick (*Hyalomma* spp.)	2 or 3	Adults on perineum, udder, scrotum, and tail brush	Cattle, sheep, goats, and pigs	Tick toxin	Sweating sickness
			Man and animals	Virus	Q fever
			Man	Tick toxin	Tick paralysis
			Man	*Rickettsia*	Tick-bite fever

(b) *B. australis* is found in Australia, India, Africa, and tropical America. It is called the Australian blue tick. It also is probably a variety.

(c) *B. annulatus* is the Texas fever tick, and is found in southern North America.

The tick remains on the host for 3 to 9 weeks. It transmits *B. bigemina.*

Hyalomma. This genus has an oval body with longish pedipalps and distinct eyes.

(a) *H. aegyptium* is found on all the domestic animals in Africa, Southern Europe, and Asia. It has a brown scutum. Only adults are found on the domestic animals, the younger stages being found on small mammals. It is called the striped-leg tick, or the bont-leg tick. The tick produces ulcerating sores in cattle, and is frequently the cause of lameness in sheep and goats owing to its attachment between the claws. It is believed to transmit both species of *Theileria,* and equine and bovine babesiosis.

(b) *H. truncatum,* the African bont-legged tick, is usually a 2-host, occasionally a 3-host parasite. Cattle and goats are the main hosts. It transmits sweating sickness and Q fever. A toxin is thought to be produced by this species capable of causing necrosis of skin and mucous membrane at the site of bites, as well as some degree of paralysis. The necrosis may be extensive. In one case, in a terrier bitch, it extended from vulva to umbilicus, with exposure of the urethra and much sloughing.

Amblyomma. In this genus the body is broadly oval.

(a) *A. hebraeum* is an African tick attacking all the domestic mammals. It has a conspicuously marked scutum, yellowish with a red and blue tinge, and brown or black markings. The eyes are flat and flush with the body. It is called the bont tick. This species causes ulcerating sores at the points for attachment, and is a frequent cause of sore teats. It conveys heart-water to ruminants.

(b) *A. variegatum* is an African species attacking herbivores. It has distinct convex eyes. The scutum is reddish yellow bordered with green with black markings. It is called the variegated tick. Its life-history is as above. It also transmits heart-water, Nairobi sheep disease, and Q fever.

(c) *A. lepidum,* an African 3-host bont tick, apparently transmits no diseases but gives rise to unpleasant sores.

(d) *A. gemma,* an African 3-host bont tick which infests cattle, camels, and other domestic animals. It can transmit both heart-water and Nairobi sheep disease.

(e) *A. cayannense* in South and Central America attacks all the domestic mammals. It is a most vicious biter, and transmits equine nuttalliosis.

(f) *A. americanum* is similar to the last species, but the scutum has a silvery white spot, giving it its popular name of the lone star tick.

An American species of *Amblyomma* transmits *Anaplasma argentinum.*

Family Argasidae (soft ticks) This family is distinguished from the hard ticks by the absence of a scutum and by the fact that the males and females are almost indistinguishable. Looked at from above, the capitulum is invisible in the adult, whereas in the Ixodidae the head is always visible.

Only 2 genera exist in this family, *Argas* and *Ornithodorus.* The adults do not permanently attach themselves to 1 host, like the hard ticks, but resemble the bed-bug in habits. The female also generally lays more than one batch of eggs.

Some ticks in this family are carriers of spirochaetal diseases to man and birds.

Argas.

(a) *A. persicus* (*A. miniatus*) is the well-known fowl tick, or blue bug, or tampan. It is practically cosmopolitan in its distribution.

It is essentially a bird tick, but will bite man and other mammals (horses and cattle) on occasion. It particularly attacks chickens. A large number on a fowl will suck so much blood that the bird will die from anaemia. It is the carrier of fowl spirochaetosis, and fowl piroplasmosis.

The tick normally feeds at night, spending the day in crevices, and accordingly is seldom seen – as is the case with bed-bugs, which also attack chickens. It is easily distinguished from this pest by the presence of 8 legs – the bed-bug being an insect, and in consequence having

T

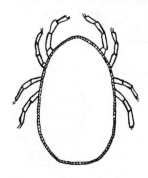

Argas. × 4.

only 6 legs. The larval tick (seed tick) remains several days on the host, and is more frequently seen. The adults can live for 2 years without food.

(b) *A. reflexus*, a closely related species, is found mainly on pigeons, but also attacks poultry and man. It is found in Europe, Africa, and America.

Ornithodorus.

(a) *O. savignyi*, the sand tampan, is a soft tick of great economic importance in Africa, Asia, and the Near East. The tick lives below the surface of the sand, emerging to feed on the blood of cattle, other domesticated stock, wild animals, and man. The tick's saliva contains a potent toxin and this, together with massive blood loss, readily kills young or debilitated animals. Amitraz, cypermethrin and ivermectin are among effective controlling agents.

(b) *O. megninii* is the spinose ear tick of America and South Africa. The larvae creep into the ear of some mammalian host, and in a few days moult. The nymphs, which are covered with minute spines, may live for 1 to 7 months in the ear, increasing in size from 3 to 17 mm (⅛ to ⅔ in). They finally drop to the ground, moult, mate, lay their eggs, and die. The adult is not parasitic. The eggs hatch in about 10 days. As many as 80 ticks have been found in a single ear. The irritation is considerable and heavy losses may result. A modern treatment is IVERMECTIN.

(c) *O. coriaceus* (pajaroello) is a venomous species (found in North America) which causes a very painful bite.

Transmission of disease When an infected tick feeds upon a calf, it transmits the parasites – or causal organisms – of the tick-borne disease in question. The calf soon becomes ill, and either dies or recovers. As a rule, recovery is associated with immunity. However, relapses may occur in animals thought to be immune to red-water, for example.

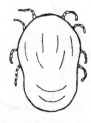

Ornithodorus. × 3.

With the exception of ticks of the *Boophilus* species, larvae hatching from a tick's eggs will not immediately be infective because these larvae have not yet fed on any host; but as soon as they start feeding they may ingest the causal organisms of a tick-borne disease. When they moult and become nymphs, they may then be capable of transmitting disease. Similarly, when the nymph, on moulting, becomes an adult tick, it will be infective if there were already parasites in its blood.

Not all tick vectors will transmit all causal organisms; and, of course, not all species of host are susceptible to the same causal organisms.

An infective 3-host tick feeding on a nonsusceptible host 'cleans' itself of infection and will not transmit disease in the next stage of its life-cycle. This fact provides a useful control measure.

The specific parasites transmitted by the ticks are not passed on mechanically, but must undergo a special development in the tick. This is easily understood when it is realised that any one stage in the life-history of a hard tick bites only one animal. Accordingly, a tick infected in one stage must be capable of producing the disease in some succeeding stage, which depends on the tick.

Control of ticks In many tropical countries, energetic measures for the regular and frequent dipping of cattle and sheep are necessary. In order to achieve adequate control of the tick-borne diseases, it is important that hand-dressing of certain parts of the body should be carried out in addition to the dipping or spraying. This applies to inside the ears, around the base of the horns, around the eyes, anus, etc.

The acaricides, or tick-killing chemicals, have comprised: (1) arsenical compounds; (2) chlorinated hydrocarbon compounds; (3) the organo-phosphorus compounds; and (4) avermectin compounds.

Dipwashes containing arsenic are unsuitable for spraying because of the danger of pasture contamination. Although cheap, stable, and soluble, arsenic compounds are very poisonous: another disadvantage is that some species of ticks acquire a resistance to arsenic preparations. Accordingly, a change to chlorinated hydrocarbons followed. Of these, BHC and toxaphene have been widely used. Unfortunately, ticks can become resistant to these too. (See also BHC.)

Organophosphorus compounds tend to be expensive, and are used mostly against ticks resistant to other acaricides.

Coumaphos; cypermethrin, a synthetic pyrethroid; diazinon, an organophosphorus compound – these are among a range of substances formulated for application against ticks

For tick control in temperate regions, see also DIPS AND DIPPING and DOG TICKS.

Systemic Acaricides are a useful alternative to spraying or dipping. 'Pour-on' or 'spot-on' formulations of acaricides such as amitraz and ivermectin are applied along the dorsal ridge (pour-on) or to the base of the head, between the shoulder blades (spot-on). The drug is absorbed through the skin and carried by the blood circulation to all parts of the body.

Ticks in Buildings

Ticks in buildings, such as quarantine premises, kennels in the tropics, private houses, etc., can be eradicated by placing a block of dry ice on the floor and closing all doors and windows. Adults, nymphs, and larval ticks will be found, after a time, clustering around this source of CO_2 and can then be easily collected and destroyed.

Timber

(see WOOD PRESERVATIVES; BEDDING – Pigs, and Dogs and cats)

Tincture

Tincture is an alcoholic solution, e.g. tincture of iodine.

Tinea

(see RINGWORM)

Tissue Culture Vaccines

(see VACCINES)

Tissues of the Body

Tissues of the body include 5 groups:

(1) Epithelial tissues, including the cells covering the skin, those lining the alimentary canal, those forming the glands, etc. (See EPITHELIUM.)

(2) Connective tissues, including FIBROUS TISSUE, FAT (adipose tissue), BONE, and CARTILAGE. (See main dictionary headings.)

(3) Muscular tissues (see MUSCLES).

(4) Nervous tissues (see NERVES).

(5) Fluid tissues (see BLOOD; LYMPH).

Titre

The extent to which an antibody-containing biological substance can be diluted before losing its power of reacting with a specific antigen. 'High titres' indicate, in practical terms, that a patient's blood serum contains high levels of antibody, e.g. to the rabies virus.

TLC

'Tender loving care' – the indefinable quality that good nursing brings to recovery. Also, thin layer chromatography.

Toadfish (Puffer Fish)

Members of the Tetraodontidae which contain a poison, tetrodotoxin; if eaten, can cause paralysis.

Toads

Toads have a defensive venom which is secreted by skin-glands and by the parotid salivary gland. The principal toxic substance is BUFOTALIN. Symptoms of poisoning in the dog are profuse vomiting followed by the emission of ropy saliva and by loss of consciousness, which may persist for a couple of hours. Adrenalin has been used in treatment.

The Central American toad, *Eufo marinas*, is very large, and has a powerful venom which can cause prostration, convulsions, and death within 15 minutes.

Toadstools

Toadstools can cause severe poisoning if eaten. In one recorded instance, a cairn terrier died after eating *Nolanea sericeum* toadstools growing on a lawn. Death occurred within 3 hours.

Signs of poisoning by this fungus are severe vomiting and abdominal pain.

Tobacco

(see NICOTINE) Stalks of tobacco plants fed to pigs have resulted in piglets born with limb deformities.

Tocopherol

Vitamin E.

Toes, Curly

Also called curly toe disease and curled toe paralysis, it is a condition arising in chicks from a deficiency of riboflavin. The toes curl underneath the feet. (See VITAMINS.)

Toes, Twisted

Also called crooked toes, it is a condition seen in chicks – one or more toes twisting inwards or outwards. There is, at least, a hereditary disposition to this abnormality, but it may occur in temporary and reversible form where infra-red brooders are in use.

Togaviruses

Formerly known as arboviruses, this group includes ALPHAVIRUSES, BUNYAVIRIDAE,

ORBIVIRUSES, and PESTIVIRUSES. (See table under VIRUSES.)

Tom
A male cat. In North America, male turkeys are also called toms.

Tomography
Body section radiography. (See X-RAYS – Computed tomography.)

-Tomy
-Tomy is a suffix indicating an operation by cutting.

Tongue
(see also MOUTH) is a muscular and fibrous organ, richly supplied with blood vessels and nerves, and covered with a highly specialised mucous membrane. Its shape varies in the different animals, but in all it consists of a free part or 'tip'; a middle part, the 'body'; and a hinder part, the 'root'. In the horse the tongue is long and spatulate, with a blunt tip, freely movable, and there is a definite narrowing just behind the tip. In the ox the tip is short, and pointed or conical; mobility and pliability are not so great, and on the upper surface is a hump-like eminence or 'dorsum', divided from the tip by a distinct, deep, transverse groove. The dorsum is of the greatest use in swallowing, and in bringing the small balls of cud from the back of the mouth forward for chewing by the cheek teeth.

Tongue, Diseases of
(see under MOUTH, DISEASES OF; SALIVATION; RANULA; 'CURLED TONGUE' in turkey poults)

Condition of the tongue The tongue of any animal in health should be of a pink glistening appearance, soft and moist to the touch in the horse, sheep, pig and dog; rough in the cow and cat. (There are a few breeds of dogs, such as the chow, in which the tongue is normally black or bluish.) When handled the tongue should possess a considerable power of retraction; a weak flabby tongue usually indicates general muscular weakness. When at rest the tongue should touch the inner edges of all the lower teeth. When it becomes greatly swollen it presses against the teeth and these leave indentations around its margin. In cattle there is a raised part or 'dorsum' behind the free tip, which is instrumental in forming the food into boluses for swallowing.

Inflammation of the tongue (glossitis) is usually accompanied by SALIVATION, and

may result from injuries, irritant or corrosive poisons, infections, and vitamin deficiencies.

Glossitis may be accompanied by the formation of vesicles which burst, leaving ulcerated areas. (See FOOT-AND-MOUTH DISEASE; SWINE VESICULAR DISEASE.) Ulcers are also a symptom of cattle plague (see RINDERPEST), MUCOSAL DISEASE, and ORF in sheep. FELINE CALICIVIRUS may cause tongue ulcers in the cat.

Raised irregular swellings or abscesses on the tongues of cattle suggest ACTINOBACILLOSIS.

Ulcers along the free edges of the tongue may be produced by diseased teeth.

In the disease called calf diphtheria (necrosis of the pharynx), the tongue may be the seat of raised areas of false membrane which will also be seen in other parts of the mouth.

The tongue may be injured or wounded from too severe a bit in the horse, or from carelessness in breaking in a young colt. In such cases there is usually a distinct mark across the tongue's upper surface, behind which the organ appears normal, and in front of which it is reddened and swollen.

Foreign bodies, such as fish-hooks, needles, wire, splinters of bone, etc., may become fixed in the tongue, and lead to protrusion of the organ, difficulty in swallowing, salivation, and a disinclination on the part of the animal to allow the mouth to be handled or examined.

In canine LEPTOSPIROSIS/kidney failure there are often areas of necrosis around the tip (which may slough off), and a foul odour.

A brown discoloration may be present in the above condition. (See also 'BROWN MOUTH'.) A soapy-white appearance of the tongue, again accompanied by an unpleasant odour, often indicates some digestive disorder.

Curled tongue is an inherited defect in turkeys which has largely disappeared from the main hybrids. It may, however, still surface in the more traditional types – for example, broad-breasted bronze or Norfolk black. (See also 'BLACK TONGUE'; BLUETONGUE (a specific disease of sheep and cattle); MYOTONIA; ASPHYXIA.)

'Tongue Worm'
'Tongue worm' is the colloquial name for *Linguatula serrata*, a parasite of the nose of the dog and other animals. (See MITES.)

Tonic
Tonic means, in one sense, a continuous muscular spasm, as compared with CLONIC. (See also TONICS.)

Tonics
A name applied to a variety of medicines or other substances believed to help improve health. In

human medicine, the term is often applied to bitter herbal extracts that may stimulate the appetite.

Turning out to grass is itself a tonic to animals that have been confined indoors. (See also under PROTEIN, HYDROLISED; VITAMINS.)

Tonsillitis

Inflammation of the tonsils, a symptom of e.g. canine viral hepatitis. The dog may retch or cough, and be slightly feverish.

Tonsils

Tonsils are collections of lymphoid tissue, situated between the anterior and posterior pillars of the soft palate at the back of the throat. In the horse there is not a compact tonsil, as in man, the dog, etc., but a diffuse collection of lymphoid tissue, mucous glands, etc., causing elevations on the surface, in which are seen the numerous depressions or crypts which characterise the tonsil and differentiate it from other lymphoid tissue. In the sheep the tonsil is bean-shaped and does not project into the throat, as in most other animals. In health, the dog's tonsils are not conspicuous, being situated in a depression; but when inflamed they appear as 2 bright red lumps.

Toothache

(see TEETH, DISEASES OF)

Topical Applications

Topical applications of a drug are those made locally to the outside of the body.

Topping of Pastures

Mowing the top growth on an overgrown pasture. This practice is beneficial from a veterinary point of view in that it is unfavourable to the survival of parasitic worm larvae.

Torsion (Twisting)

Torsion (twisting) occasionally involves the intestine (see VOLVULUS); the pedicle of the spleen; the stomach; uterus; and spermatic cords.

Torticollis

A lateral deviation of the neck.

Tortoises

In Britain an amendment to the Endangered Species Act, in 1982, required that every buyer of tortoises must sign an undertaking to provide them with appropriate care, attention, and living quarters necessary for their survival. Failure to comply can result in a fine of up to £400 for an offending supplier, pet trader, or private individual. This little piece of legislation may help to mitigate the extremely high mortality of tortoises imported into the UK, often due to their being crammed into unsuitable containers for their journey here and badly looked after subsequently.

It has been suggested that outbreaks of viral disease are present among tortoises (*Testudo* species) in the Mediterranean region.

Imported tortoises should be carefully examined for the presence of exotic ticks.

Tortoises and turtles have been known to infect dogs, cats, and people with salmonellosis. (See also AMERICAN BOX TORTOISES; PETS.)

For euthanasia, an injection into the abdomen of pentobarbitone sodium is recommended.

Tortoiseshell Cats, Male

Although nearly all tortoiseshell cats are female, males do occasionally occur. It appears that the most common chromosome complements are 39XXY, 38XY/38XX, 38XY/39XXY and 38XY/38XY. A 38XY is needed for the cat to be fertile.

Touch

This sense depends upon receptors at the end of nerves, or upon the nerve endings themselves:

Touch sense proper, by which touches or strokes are perceived, such as the lightest sensation caused by a fly settling on the skin. The size and shapes of bodies in contact with the skin which are not seen is also appreciated by this sense.

Pressure sense, by which the weight of heavy objects and their hardness can be determined.

Heat sense, by which the heat of the surrounding atmosphere, or of bodies in contact with the skin, is appreciated as being above that of body temperature. (Receptors for warmth in the human body number about 16,000 as compared with 150,000 for detecting cold.)

Cold sense.

Pain sense.

Muscle sense, by which the weight of an object can be tested, and the amount of energy necessary for an effort can be gauged.

Sense of position, by which, without using the powers of vision, the attitude and position of any part of the body is known.

The distribution of the sense organs which are concerned with the reception of these sensations is very widespread. There is no part of the surface of the body, except the horns, hoofs and claws, which can be cut without giving evidence of pain, and there is no part, including horny structures, which is insensible to touch.

T

Pain is detected, it seems, by free nerve endings in the layers of the skin, connective tissue, and cornea. The sense of touch is apparently dependent upon Meissner's corpuscles, situated under the epidermis; upon Merkel's discs in tongue, lips, muzzle. Tactile hairs on muzzle, etc., function through free nerve endings surrounding the hair follicle. Pacinian corpuscles in connective tissue, penis, clitoris, etc., react to pressure and contact. Receptors for heat and cold are named Ruffini's corpuscles and Krause endbulbs, respectively. (See also SKIN; HYPERAESTHESIA; PARALYSIS.)

Tourniquet

A tourniquet is an appliance for the temporary stoppage of the circulation in a limb or appendage of the body, for use only in very severe haemorrhage. Application of a tourniquet is a risky procedure, best not undertaken by the animal-owner unless raising the limb and application of a pressure pad has failed to control the haemorrhage, which appears to be endangering the animal's life. It is to be avoided on cats.

In emergencies, a handkerchief may be tied round the part, the knot being arranged above the principal artery, and a rigid object, piece of wood, pencil, etc., used to twist the loose part up tightly.

A tourniquet must not be left in position around a limb for longer than 20 minutes, or gangrene of the lower part will result. Occasionally, a circular bruise may occur under a tourniquet, especially in the limbs of horses; this, after healing, leaving a ring of white hair marking the place where the tourniquet was applied. Such a circular mark is due to a destruction of the pigmentary apparatus of the hair follicles. (See also BLEEDING.)

Toxaemia

The presence of toxins in the bloodstream.

Toxaphene

A chlorinated hydrocarbon insecticide which remains active for a long time on the hair of cattle, and of value against ticks also.

Toxascaris

(see under TOXOCARA)

'Toxic Fat Syndrome'

'Toxic fat syndrome' of broiler chickens, mainly between 3 and 10 weeks old, has occurred in the USA and Britain. It is associated with oedema of the pericardium and abdomen, a waddling gait, squawking, laboured breathing, and

sudden death. Mortality may reach 95 per cent. It has been seen in chicks only a few days old.

This condition has to be differentiated from round heart disease, which usually occurs sporadically among older birds and is not associated with the feeding of fat-supplemented rations.

Toxicology
The study of POISONS.

Toxins

Toxins are POISONS produced in animal tissues, by some bacteria, ticks, and fungi. Waste products, not removed from the body during liver or kidney failure, are also sometimes referred to as toxins. (See TETANUS; BOTULISM; TICKS; MYCOTOXICOSIS; VENOM; TOXOID; MOULDY FOOD.)

Toxocara

A genus of roundworm which includes *Toxocara canis*, a parasite of dog and fox, *T. cati*, and *T. vitulorum* of cattle (the last-named not present in the UK). Infection with these worms is known as toxocariasis. This is important not only from the veterinary aspect but also as regards public health, since toxocara worm larvae cause visceral larva migrans in man.

In dogs, *T. canis* is primarily a parasite of the young puppy, which commonly becomes infected before birth by larvae crossing the bitch's placenta. Post-natal infection may occur through the milk. During the first few weeks of the puppy's life, the life-cycle of toxocara is completed, adult worms being found in the intestine. (In severe infestations, complete impaction of the bowel has been known to occur in puppies as young as 7 weeks.)

Larvae acquired prenatally from the bitch arrive in the puppy's intestine within 3 days of birth, and mature at about the 9th day. Egg production begins when the puppy is about 2 months old. The number of worm eggs excreted by the puppy may be as many as 15,000 per g of faeces.

As the puppy becomes older, the degree of infestation diminishes. It seems that larvae from ingested eggs migrate within the tissues but are unable to complete the life-cycle. Some of these larvae must remain viable, or prenatal infection could not occur in succeeding generations. Mature male dogs are more likely to carry patent infection than adult bitches, but the lactating bitch apparently experiences a hormonal suppression of immunity, resulting in a brief patent infection of *T. canis* from larvae present in the body. One survey found that of 740 unwanted Glasgow dogs examined after euthanasia, just under 21 per cent carried *T. canis*.

Control This is dependent upon what action dog-owners take or fail to take. Several anthelmintics are effective against the adult worm, including piperazine. Pups should be treated at 2 weeks old, before eggs are passed in the faeces, and at 3, 6, and 8 weeks.

Nursing bitches should be dosed when the puppies are 2, 4, 6 and 8 weeks old. Febendazole is a suitable medication; it prevents migration of larvae into the milk. Adult dogs should be wormed every 2 to 3 months.

In kittens, damage, sometimes severe, may affect the glomeruli of the kidneys as a result of larvae of *T. cati*.

Public health Toxocara eggs are sticky and readily adhere to children's hands, blankets, dog baskets, etc. Fortunately the eggs are not immediately infective when excreted in canine faeces, but require a period of weeks to become so. Two larval moults occur before hatching of the egg, so the infective stage is the 3rd stage larva.

The danger of transmission lies in the fact that the eggs are very resistant and can survive for long periods in the soil. Garden soil, and that of parks, playing fields, and grass verges, is an important source of eggs and larvae. About 7 per cent of soil samples from public parks

have been found to contain viable toxocara eggs, although in one survey the figure was as high as 24 per cent.

Children can easily become infected through not washing their hands after contamination by such eggs – many of which will have undergone development, rendering them infective. The World Health Organisation (WHO) has stated: 'Many patients with proven toxocariasis have not owned or had close contact with a dog or cat,' but have become infected from eggs in soil. Moreover, 'even though toxocara eggs are unlikely to mature on an animal's coat, infective eggs from the soil may adhere to the hair so that contact with it can lead to infection'.

Prevalence in man Human toxocariasis is encountered throughout the world. Surveys have demonstrated that about 2 per cent of people over 10 years old in London, and over 30 per cent in various African cities, showed a positive reaction to a toxocara skin test.

A medical/veterinary team compared the results of blood tests made on 102 dog-breeder volunteers, at the 1977 Windsor championship dog show, with samples from 922 non-dog-breeders. Antibodies to *T. canis* were found in over 15 per cent of the dog-breeders' samples, as compared with only 2.6 per cent of the controls.

Visceral larva migrans affects, states WHO, mainly children between 18 months and 3 years of age. Tumours – eosinophilic granulomata – are

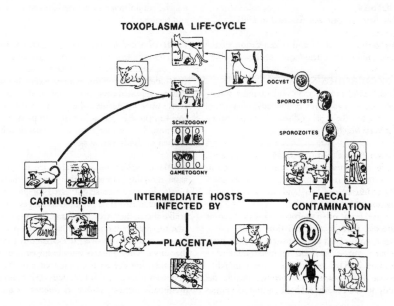

TOXOPLASMA LIFE-CYCLE

formed in organs such as the liver, lungs, eye, and occasionally the brain. In some patients blindness is caused; in others the symptoms may resemble those of asthma or epilepsy. Debility and occasionally partial paralysis may occur. Eosinophilia is usually present.

About 50 cases of ocular toxocariasis are reported each year in England and Wales.

A young woman, who had kept dogs and rabbits for many years, presented with blurred vision in one eye. This condition was treated with corticosteroids. She developed a transient swelling and stiffness of the right elbow and the left ankle and wrist. In the subsequent 18 months she suffered repeated episodes of choroiditis in the left eye and arthralgia. A toxocaral fluorescent antibody test was positive and after treatment with diethylcarbamazine citrate her symptoms subsided.

Diagnosis An immunofluorescent test or the ELISA test may be used in human medicine. Diagnosis of toxocara affecting the eye may be difficult. In one case, fragments of a larva were not found until the 186th section of an eye had been made.

Toxoid

A toxin which has been rendered non-toxic by physical or chemical means, while retaining its antigenic properties. An example is TETANUS toxoid for immunisation.

Toxoplasma Eye Infection in Horses

The first UK case was reported in 1991.

Signs Inflammation and degeneration of the retina and of the sclera (white of the eyeball).

Toxoplasmosis

This is a disease of man and of most warm-blooded animals. It is a major cause of abortion in ewes but the signs of disease in other species can vary widely.

Cause A coccidian (see COCCIDIOSIS) parasite, *Toxoplasma gondii*, closely related to the genus Isospora. The reproductive cells (gametes) form in the intestine of cats (and probably of other members of the cat family).

Cats (and other carnivores) can become infected through the ingestion of the cystozoites within cysts in the muscles of their prey; or they can – like other animals and man – become infected by oocysts present in feline faeces. (The oocysts can survive outside the body for 17 months.) The ingestion of oocysts is probably the major source of human urban toxoplasmosis in the UK.

T. gondii has been isolated from the milk of bitches, cows, ewes, and sows, and it has been shown that the young of these may be born already infected. The parasite can live in ticks and lice, so that the spread of toxoplasmosis by these is not unlikely. The parasite has been recovered from the semen of rams.

For diagnosis, laboratory techniques are essential, e.g. using Sabin-Feldman dye, latex agglutination tests.

Sheep After ingestion of feed or water contaminated with toxoplasma oocysts, susceptible (seronegative) sheep become, and remain, infected for life. Infection of the ovine placenta and conceptus occurs only when the initial infection establishes in susceptible pregnant sheep, following ingestion of oocysts. The oocysts encyst in the digestive tract and the released sporozoites penetrate the cells lining the gut so that tachyzoites eventually reach and infect the placenta and fetus.

Infection in very early pregnancy causes fetal resorption and the ewes subsequently appear to be barren, while infection between about 50 and 120 days' gestation presents the clinical picture typical of the disease, with the premature birth of stillborn and weakly lambs, outwardly of quite normal appearance, often accompanied by a mummified fetus.

Treatment Decoquinate (Deccox; Merial) may be administered in the feed for prophylaxis and treatment.

Control A live vaccine containing tachyzoites of *T. gondii* (Toxovax; Intervet) is available. It may be used in ewe lambs over 5 months old and older ewes not less than 6 weeks before mating; repeat dosing may be needed after 2 years. *Warning*: Accidental exposure to the vaccine can cause infection in man – in particular, abortion. The vaccine must not be handled by women of child-bearing age.

Goats Toxoplasmosis causes abortion and perinatal mortality similar to that seen in sheep. Goats also appear to stay infected for life, but experiments carried out in the USA suggest that, unlike sheep, they may, in subsequent pregnancies, pass infection on to their kids in utero and may even abort with overt toxoplasmosis more than once. Infection can spread also via semen and milk, but the relative importance of these 2 routes within a herd is uncertain, as is the risk to humans ingesting milk from infected goats.

Signs Toxoplasmosis may be subclinical – no symptoms being shown, but a degree of immunity being acquired; or the infection may give rise to very varied symptoms which, in different cases, have included coughing, distressed breathing, mastitis, abortion, fetal degeneration, stillbirths, diarrhoea, and encephalitis.

An Australian report noted that 7 out of 48 penned ewes aborted because of infection with *T. gondii*. They had been eating grain contaminated by faeces from cats which lived in the feed shed.

In a Canadian farm outbreak only 12 out of 50 chicken, reared indoors, survived 3 months after being turned out into the farmyard for the summer. Antibodies to toxoplasma were found in the chickens, in 23 out of 24 of the cows, in all the farm cats, a mare, the farmer, his wife and daughter, but not their son. The source of infection in this outbreak was considered to be wild birds, many of which had been found dead around the farmyard.

Cats The infection is often subclinical. Acute feline toxoplasmosis may prove fatal, a few days after symptoms such as a high fever, lethargy, loss of appetite, and dyspnoea. Chronic toxoplasmosis is often a relapsing disease, with loss of appetite, anaemia, nervous symptoms, abortion or sterility. Heart disease and liver disease may be found. The fever does not respond to antibiotics. Dyspnoea may be seen in the terminal stages.

Public health Probably all practising veterinary surgeons, and many cat-owners, have had antibodies to toxoplasma in their blood serum; yet of these people only a small percentage were ever ill as a result of the infection (though a proportion may have suffered malaise).

The World Health Organisation (WHO) has stated that the only real danger to human health appears to be: (1) acute, generalised toxoplasmosis, especially in patients undergoing immunosuppressive therapy; and (2) congenital infection which can lead to miscarriage, stillbirth, or abnormality in the baby.

In the USA 3000 of the 3 million babies born each year are reckoned to have congenital toxoplasmosis, but many of the babies are well or only mildly affected.

Medical opinion is that pregnant women should be advised against eating or handling raw or undercooked meat, and should not themselves empty cat litter trays.

There is danger for the baby only if the mother becomes infected during pregnancy; if infected previously, there is no such danger.

The immunosuppression occurring in AIDS has resulted in some deaths from toxoplasmosis.

In a family outbreak of toxoplasmosis, attributed to the eating of lamb served rare, the husband suffered fatigue, malaise, muscle pains, headache and fever. After 11 days in hospital he was discharged, the cause of his illness undetermined. Some weeks later toxoplasmosis was diagnosed, following an immunofluorescent test. A complement fixation test and a Sabin-Feldman dye test were also positive. Three months later an eye lesion affecting the retina was discovered. Treatment involved the use of prednisone, sulfadiazine, and pyrimethamine, but while the lesion decreased in size, vision was not restored to normal. The wife's illness left her tired and lethargic for nearly 10 weeks, with weakness, fever and a rash. Neck swelling, with lymph node enlargement, was a feature of illness in 2 boys. The family had no pet animals.

(See also CANARY.)

Trabecula
A band of fibrous tissue.

Trace Elements
Trace elements are those of which minute quantities are essential for the maintenance of health in animals (or plants). They include iron, manganese, iodine, cobalt, copper, magnesium, zinc, selenium. (See under HYPOMAGNESAEMIA; PIGLET ANAEMIA; 'PINING'; IODINE; HYPOCUPRAEMIA; perosis (see under 'SLIPPED TENDON'); ZINC; SALT – Salt licks.) Calcium and phosphorus are also needed, but in much larger quantities than is the case with trace elements. (See also VITAMINS – Vitamin E.)

Trachea
Trachea is another name for the windpipe. (See NOSE AND NASAL PASSAGES.)

Foreign bodies have included a spanner in a dog's trachea; a chip of stone in a cat; a snail; and – not strictly 'foreign' – a cat's own tooth. An incision into the trachea, to admit an endoscope from the outside, was necessary in this last case.

Trachea, Diseases of
These include hypoplasia, with a narrow lumen – a congenital defect in several breeds of dogs.

Signs A chronic moist cough, wheezing, dyspnoea, aversion to exercise.

Tracheal Worms
In the dog, infestation with the worm *Filaroides osleri* gives rise to a persistent cough, and

sometimes to retching. The cough may be like that in kennel cough, and hoarse. This disease occurs in Britain. Diagnosis depends on use of an endoscope (which can reveal the characteristic pink nodules), or of X-rays. Treatment can be successful, using an appropriate anthelmintic, e.g. oxfendazole.

Another tracheal worm, which seldom gives rise to symptoms, is *Capillaria aerophilia*. (See also under COUGH.)

Tracheitis

Inflammation of the TRACHEA. The trachea may be severely damaged as the result of a dog fight, involving bites of the neck.

Tracheostomy

Tracheostomy refers to an artificial opening into the trachea, and is usually taken to include the insertion of a tracheostomy tube to overcome nerve dysfunction. Tracheotomy is the surgical procedure of creating a tracheostomy, although some authors use these words interchangeably.

Severe upper respiratory obstruction presents as an anxious, sweating horse with possibly stridulous breathing noises at rest, flared nostrils, extended neck, increased costo-abdominal respiratory effort, cyanosis and functioning accessory muscles of respiration. Particularly if the last 2 signs are present, a temporary tracheostomy is imperative.

Permanent tracheostomy A tracheostomy tube is used to bypass a permanent upper-airway obstruction. A permanent tracheostomy is most commonly used in performance animals to bypass performance-limiting, less severe respiratory obstruction, e.g. cases of laryngeal paralysis non-responsive to conventional surgery. The term 'permanent tracheostomy' is not absolute because for ease of management many owners request the removal of 'permanent' tracheostomy tubes at the end of each working season, with replacement at the beginning of the following season.

In one survey, of 34 cases of permanent tracheostomy involving 11 dogs and 23 cats, the pet-owners assessed the results as good in 16, and fair in 6, cases. The most common post-operative problem was occlusion of the trachea by a fold of skin.

A surgical accident Abscesses due to *Streptococcus equi* caused upper-airway obstruction in a 2-month-old Standardbred foal. Unfortunately, while attempting surgical relief, 4 mid-cervical tracheal rings were completely severed. This led to dyspnoea and a loud respiratory noise even with mild exercise; an endoscopic examination showed that the lumen of the trachea was now key-shaped for a distance of 6 cm.

When 6 months old, the foal was referred to the Ohio State University veterinary hospital, where it was found that the severed ends of the 4 tracheal rings had not healed but were connected solely by fibrous tissue.

In order to effect repair, a prosthesis was made by cutting in half longitudinally a 60 ml plastic syringe, and then cutting segments 2 to 5 cm in length, with 2 mm holes drilled to take sutures.

Two ¾-thickness incisions were made transversely at 1 cm intervals in each ring on both sides of the defect, and sutures placed, avoiding penetration of the tracheal mucosa.

Nine days after surgery, endoscopy showed the tracheal lumen to be nearly normal and the mucous membrane free from inflammation. Ten months later the surgical site was normal. As a 2-year-old, the colt was raced successfully.

Tracheotomy

Tracheotomy is indicated when some foreign body has gained entrance into the trachea or larynx and hinders the flow of air; it relieves breathing when an abscess develops at the back of the throat in strangles in horses, and threatens to occlude the passages; it is also undertaken in oedema of the glottis, in roaring, and in other conditions.

An incision is made into the trachea, through the skin and muscles, usually in the middle line (in cattle sometimes at the side), and a tracheotomy tube is inserted and fixed in place.

The air in the stable must be kept as clean and free from dust as possible, and during foddering or bedding operations a plug should be put into the tube to prevent pieces of chaff, hay seeds, etc., from getting drawn in by the inspired air.

Trachoma

(see EYE, DISEASES OF)

Track Leg

A condition seen in the racing greyhound. There is a swelling of the triceps muscle or the semitendinosus muscle – due to sprain. Prolonged rest is necessary.

Training

(see MUSCLES; EXERCISE)

Tranquillisers

This term usually implies drugs which reduce anxiety without inducing sleep or drowsiness.

They include benzodiazepines such as diazepam and azapirones such as buspirone. They are used in veterinary practice to calm or restrain vicious or nervous animals; to obviate travel sickness; and to facilitate the induction of anaesthesia. Their use is not permitted at Kennel Club shows.

(For horses, see DETOMIDINE.)

Tranquillisers have been administered to cattle, zoo and wild animals, by firing a hypodermic syringe from a cross-bow, gun, or blow-pipe. (See DART GUNS; also PIGS, SEDATION OF; ROMPUN.)

Natural tranquillisers At the Institute of Animal Physiology, during investigation of the hormones contained in extracts of ovarian tissue, several steroids have been found which exert a strong sedative effect on the central nervous system. Variations in secretion rates of these steroids during the reproductive cycle may be partly responsible for cyclic variations in behaviour, states the AFRC. Slight tranquillity could occur when the blood concentration of the steroids is relatively high; restlessness or even aggressiveness might result from a low concentration.

Transferable Resistance
(see under ANTIBIOTIC RESISTANCE; PLASMIDS)

Transferrin
A beta-globulin present in blood plasma and acting as a carrier of iron. (See also IRON.)

Transfusion of Blood
(see under BLOOD TRANSFUSIONS)

Transgenic Animals
Those bred by genetic engineering methods involving the isolation of genes from one animal, modification of them in the laboratory, and introduction of them into animals of the same or different species. (See also RETROVIRUS.)

Transit Tetany
Transit tetany is the result mainly of HYPOCAL-CAEMIA, which is precipitated by the stress of long travel. It is seen in ruminants and, more rarely, in horses.

In lactating mares (also known as lactation tetany), it may occur about 10 days after foaling or a day or two after weaning. It can also occur, it has been said, in fillies and colts.

In ruminants, prolonged travel may induce hypocalcaemia or hypophosphataemia in cattle, with hypocalcaemia, hypomagnesaemia and hypoglycaemia in ewes.

Signs These vary according to the extent to which the blood calcium level is reduced. A slight reduction causes the mare to be excitable, but a further fall produces muscular incoordination and staggering, and the animal appears obviously distressed. Sweating may occur; rapid and noisy breathing and, in the mare, flared nostrils are other signs. A stiff gait, raised tail, and spasms similar to those of tetanus occur.

Another similarity is that eating and drinking may become impossible. Recumbency, coma, and death follow within a couple of days. While mild cases recover, the mortality is high in untreated animals showing the more severe signs.

Treatment The animal should be kept quiet and the appropriate dose of a mineral replacement solution, e.g. calcium borogluconate 20 per cent, given subcutaneously or by slow intravenous injection.

Translocation
In CYTOGENETICS, this means transfer of a broken-off fragment of one chromosome to another. A cause of some congenital diseases.

Transmissible Gastroenteritis of Pigs (TGE)
Transmissible gastroenteritis of pigs (TGE) is a rapidly fatal disease in young piglets. The cause is a coronavirus; mortality decreases with age of the piglet. For example, mortality may be 90 per cent in the first week of life, 50 per cent in the second, 25 per cent in the third, and zero in older pigs.

Foul-smelling watery diarrhoea, vomiting and loss of appetite are the main signs in piglets. Adult pigs are usually little affected, although fattening pigs require extra water during an outbreak.

TGE is typically but not exclusively a disease of the winter months. Epidemics occurred in winter every 5 to 7 years between 1956 and 1983. Apart from 2 incidents in 1996, the UK was free from TGE until a single incident in 1999. The absence of disease from Britain and continental Europe since the mid-1980s has been attributed to the emergence in 1986 of porcine respiratory coronavirus. This is an apparent mutant of TGE virus and is believed to have effectively immunised the pig population against TGE. The reservoir of virus may be as a subclinical infection in large herds.

There is no specific treatment, but losses may be reduced by extra care and management: warmth and extra fluids; good-quality milk replacer/creep pellets; early weaning into warm accommodation; cross-suckling affected piglets onto recovered sows; using antibiotics to control secondary infection.

Control TGE is spread by direct or indirect contact with infected faeces; strict attention to disinfection and hygiene is essential. Sows due to farrow, and sucking piglets under 7 days old should be isolated. Exposure of uninfected pigs to recently infected stock may help to develop herd immunity.

Transmissible Mink Encephalopathy

A spongiform encephalopathy which has been reported in mink in the USA. The affected mink were fed bovine offal.

Transplants

(see EMBRYO TRANSFER and SKIN GRAFTING TRANSPLANTATION)

Transponder

An electronic device which stores information that can be read by a suitable scanner. In miniaturised form, transponders are the basis of identity MICROCHIPS.

Transport Stress

Stress caused by transportation can adversely affect the welfare and health of farm animals and the meat quality of the carcase. A method has been developed for measuring the adverse nature of the noise and vibration components of transport, using operant conditioning. The equipment is a modification of a machine originally developed for testing tractors, and consists of a pen which is tilted up and down in all directions, generating a noise of 80 decibels. It was found that pigs soon learn to press a panel with their snouts in order to obtain a 30-seconds respite from vibration and keep the machine immobile for 70 to 80 per cent of the time. The animals switch the machine off more frequently when the speed of vibration is increased and also when they have eaten a large meal just before the test. During an hour-long session the frequency with which the machine was switched off tended to increase, showing that aversion to the conditions does not diminish with time. Pigs which have experienced the machine will press the switch when exposed to a recording of the noise even when there is no movement. In contrast, naive animals do not learn to operate the switch when exposed to the noise alone. The advantage of this technique is that specifications for improved methods of transport can be based on the animal's own preferences. (AFRC.)

Traumatic Pericarditis

(see HEART DISEASES)

Travel Sickness

Travel sickness is observed in dogs and cats – some individuals being particularly susceptible – and may be relieved by the administration of a suitable tranquilliser prior to the journey. Fitting a chain to a car so as to act as an earth has been recommended, but may be less effective than periodic stops and adequate ventilation. It may also occur in horses on long sea voyages. (See also TRANSIT TETANY.)

Treads

Treads are injuries inflicted at the coronet of the horse's foot, either by the shoe of the opposite foot, or, when horses are worked in pairs, by the adjacent horse. When situated in the posterior half of the foot, the upper free edge of the lateral cartilage may be damaged and a QUITTOR result.

Trefoil

Consumption of the plant is a cause of LIGHT SENSITISATION in Australia.

Trematode

An unsegmented flat worm or fluke. (See LIVER-FLUKES; LUNG-FLUKES; RUMEN-FLUKES; SCHISTOSOMIASIS.)

Trembling in Dogs

(see under SHIVERING)

Tremors

Very fine jerky contractions of a muscle or of some of the fibres of a muscle. They are often seen in nervous animals when frightened, and they are one of the signs of viciousness in a horse when seen on the quarters, especially when the horse is watching out of the corner of its eye. Tremors are, however, encountered in certain nervous disorders, such as shivering in horses and chorea in dogs. (See also 'CRAZY CHICK' DISEASE.) HYPOMAGNESAEMIA in cattle, and RABIES in many species, also give rise to tremors. (For tremors in pigs, see SWINE FEVER.)

Trephining

Trephining is an operation in which a small disc of bone is removed from the cranium to permit the elevation of a depressed portion, or to allow access into the brain cavity. In certain purulent conditions of the air sinuses of the horse's head, trephining may be required to give drainage for the pus.

Treponema

A genus of spiral organisms of the family Treponemaceae, which includes also *Borrelia* and *Leptospira*. (See also SWINE DYSENTERY.)

Triatomid Bugs

Triatomid bugs are the most important vectors of human trypanosomiasis in South and Central America.

Trichiasis

Ingrowing eyelashes (see EYE, DISEASES OF).

Trichinosis

Trichinosis is an infestation of the muscles of the pig, man, dog, etc., with the larvae of *Trichinella spiralis*, a small roundworm. Pigs become infected by eating infected rats, or raw swill or garbage containing pieces of infected pork. Trichinosis constitutes a serious problem among sledge-dogs in the Arctic and may follow the eating of walrus, bear, seal, or fox-meat. A temperature of –15°C for 20 days is needed to kill the larvae.

Infection in man occurs through the eating of raw or undercooked meat. Human symptoms include pain in muscles; myocarditis, meningitis, encephalitis, and rarely death have occurred.

An outbreak of trichinosis in Paris, involving 300 proven cases, followed the eating of horsemeat either raw or served rare. All this meat had come from 2 shops, and originated from a single horse imported from the USA. The main symptoms in this outbreak were fever, muscle pain, swollen face and eyelids, a rash, and digestive system upsets.

The disease has not been seen in the UK for some years, but outbreaks have occurred. (See ROUNDWORMS.)

Trichocephalus (Whip-Worm)

Trichocephalus (whip-worm) is the name of a worm that infests the caeca of various animals. (See ROUNDWORMS.)

Trichodinella and Trichodinia

Trichodinella and trichodinia are skin parasites of fish. Their sharp, rasping teeth damage the skin.

Trichoglyphs

(see WHORLS)

Trichomonas

The flagellates of the genus *Trichomonas* are usually pear-shaped, with 3 to 5 anterior flagella, an undulating membrane and, in some species, 1 free flagellum directed backwards.

Species of this genus very commonly occur in the intestinal canal of many different species of mammals and birds.

Trichomoniasis *Trichomonas fetus* causes abortions, pyometra, and sometimes sterility in cattle. The cow becomes infected by the bull at coitus, or vice versa.

Signs A transient vaginitis, which is often overlooked. If conception has not occurred, a chronic form of endometritis follows. If the cow is pregnant, the fetus dies and is either aborted 1 to 4 months later or retained in the uterus, where it becomes macerated and a pyometra develops.

Control of the disease includes the disposal of infected bulls, withholding all breeding operations on infected cows for at least 3 months, and the serving of non-infected cows and virgin heifers by a 'clean' bull. Freezing bull semen to –79°C, in the presence of 10 per cent glycerol, kills *T. fetus* but allows the spermatozoa to survive. This method of deep-freeze, commonly practised at AI centres, is one way of getting rid of the infection from semen.

Avian trichomoniasis, caused by *T. gallinae,* affects the oesophagus of budgerigars, pigeons, etc, causing necrotic lesions with retching and vomiting. Also known as canker or roup. In pigeons, which feed their young on 'crop milk', squabs are easily infected which led to the belief among pidgeon-fanciers that the disease was inherited. It can be treated with dimetridazole or nifursol.

Trichophyton

(see RINGWORM)

Trichostrongylosis

Parasitic disease caused by infection with *Trychostrongylus* worms. It can affect most

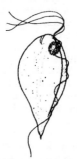

Trichomonas fetus.

mammals, causing poor growth, lack of condition and diarrhoea.

Trichostrongylus
A large group of parasitic worms which infest both people and their domestic animals, and which cause persistent diarrhoea.

Trichothecenes
Trichothecenes are fungal metabolites which contaminate animal feeds and human foods. Examples are deoxynivalenol and nivalenol. The most potent toxin is T_2 TOXIN.

Throat irritation and digestive disorders are caused in people. Baking does not destroy the toxin.

Tricuspid Valve
The tricuspid valve is the valve lying in the heart between the right atrium and the right ventricle, which possesses 3 cusps or flaps. (See HEART.)

Trigeminal Nerve
Trigeminal Nerve is the 5th of the cranial nerves. (See NERVES.)

Trimethoprim
A drug which inhibits the growth of many bacteria and some protozoa through reducing their synthesis of folinic acid (necessary for synthesis of nucleic acids). Effective against many Gram-positive and Gram-negative bacteria. One part of trimethoprim is combined with 5 parts of sulfadiazine, with which it is synergistic, in co-trimazine. Several other preparations of trimethoprim with one or other of the sulfa drugs also exist.

Triorchidism
A condition in which 3 testicles are present. This was found in a cock – all 3 being functional, and structurally independent. A case in which there was duplication of the right testicle was seen in a calf. (In man, triorchidism is not extremely rare, and even 5 testes in a scrotum have been recorded.)

Triplet Calves
In the UK in 1985 a Friesian cow had triplets. After initial breathing difficulties, all 3 survived and were described as 'fine, strong calves'. Quintuplets have been recorded.

Triploid
An animal having one and a half times as many chromosomes in its cells as a normal (i.e. diploid) animal. (See COLCHICINE.)

Triploidy accounts for up to 13 per cent of embryonic loss in animals, and for 20 per cent of all chromosomally-caused spontaneous human abortion (ARC). (See CHROMOSOMES; CYTOGENETICS.)

Trismus
The locking of the jaws, which is characteristic of TETANUS.

Trisomy
The presence in triplicate of a particular chromosome. In the cow, such a condition would be denoted as 61,XXX.

X-trisomy is associated with nymphomania and infertility in cows.

Trixacarus Caviae
The mange mite which is a parasite of guinea-pigs.

Trixylphosphate
A substance used in the manufacture of plastics. Poisoning of cattle has occurred through contamination of molasses with this substance. Symptoms included diarrhoea, coughing, unsteady gait, partial paralysis.

Trocar
A sharp-pointed, rod-like instrument used with a cannula to puncture the wall of a body cavity. It is often used to release gas in cases of bloat in ruminants.

Trochanter
One of the protuberances on the femur which serve as attachment sites for hindquarter muscles.

Trochlear Nerve
The 4th cranial nerve (see NERVES), also known as the pathetic nerve. It controls the superior oblique muscle of the eye.

Trombiculosis
Infestation with *Trombicula autumnalis*, the harvest mite.

Trophic
Relating to nutrition; neurotrophic means the influence that nerves exert upon the tissues to which they are distributed, for health and nourishment.

Trophins
Gland-regulating hormones.

Trophoblast

The outer layer of BLASTOCYSTS which make contact with the wall of the uterus, and through which nutrients and waste products are exchanged between fetal and maternal circulations. (See also SYNCYTIUM.)

Tropics, Livestock Production in the

Livestock farming in the tropics, and even in some subtropical developing countries, is beset with difficulties not experienced to anything like the same degree in developed countries having a temperate climate.

In developing countries there is often the additional problem of limited financial resources. Money may not be available for measures to counter or ameliorate adverse conditions for animals; to provide adequate supplies of safe drinking water, good-quality feeds, vaccines, prophylactic drugs; or to support disease eradication programmes on a large scale. Veterinarians are usually few in number in relation to the large areas in which they are needed (see VETERINARY PROFESSION), and faced with great distances to cover and an absence of local laboratory services.

Heat Animals can survive in temperatures of up to 60°C (140°F). Temperatures above that are lethal. Cattle in Death Valley, California, and in Queensland, Australia, for example, exist at temperatures of 52° to 58°C (125° to 136°F). Such heat, however, is far above the comfort zone – estimated as air temperature at between 21° and 26°C (70° to 79°F); or 13° to 18°C (55° to 64°) for adult cattle.

High temperatures impose stress upon the animal's physiological processes and productive capacity.

Records for more than 12,000 inseminations over a 2-year period in a Florida herd indicated a sharp decline in conception rates of cows when a maximum air temperature the day after artificial insemination exceeded 30°C (86°F) (35°C (95°F) for heifers).

Besides air temperature, radiation, air movement, and humidity all influence the animal's immediate environment. Body temperature is controlled by the heat-regulating mechanism (see HYPOTHALAMUS), and affected not only by environmental heat but also by the heat generated in the tissues (see METABOLISM). The more the animal eats, the more heat its body will produce. Water intake also plays a part in the physiological reactions; as does sweating, but in this respect cattle are less efficient than people. In great environmental heat, the point may be reached where normal body temperature cannot be maintained, and it rises – a state of HYPERTHERMIA. Death may result.

Even at non-lethal levels, tropical heat is a limiting factor so far as fertility and yields of milk, meat and eggs are concerned. Poor feed, and water deprivation, can further depress growth rates, fertility, and yields. Humidity can increase heat stress.

Signs Heat stress may cause the body temperature to rise to 42° to 43°C (110°F) in cattle. The earlier symptom of rapid breathing progresses to panting. The mouth may be kept open, tongue lolling out, and frothy saliva may be in evidence. Appetite is lost. Cattle may remain standing, huddling together.

Preventive Measures If heat stress is to be avoided or minimised, livestock must have shade (from trees or shelters) to protect them from the sun's rays. Cooled drinking water is beneficial to all livestock in tropical heat. Pigs need to be able to wallow – their normal, instinctive method of cooling themselves. Cool water sprays can help dairy cattle to withstand high temperatures. Grazing should take place at night rather than during the day.

Zero-grazing may be practicable in some places, and beneficial too.

Poultry in the tropics grow larger combs and wattles than do similar birds in temperate climates, as a physiological means of body cooling. At very high temperatures they dip combs and wattles into water, for an extra cooling effect. It has been suggested that the design of drinkers in intensive poultry units should be such as to make possible this beneficial practice.

Antibiotics and poultry In developing countries in the tropics, the widespread use of antibiotics – especially the tetracyclines – in modern battery poultry units has been blamed for encouraging the proliferation of drug-resistant bacteria. Where indiscriminate use is coupled with poor sanitation and low personal hygiene, the situation may constitute a danger to public health.

In a study in Nigeria of *E. coli*, 1248 strains isolated from battery hens at the University of Ibadan, and 2196 strains from a commercial poultry farm, were resistant to tetracycline, streptomycin, and also sulfonamides. By contrast, all strains isolated from free-range town and village poultry were sensitive to these drugs.

Altitude In some regions, altitude mitigates the effect of heat. The uplands of Jordan are regarded as suitable for intensive poultry production; and Iran's uplands, with their dry climate, make dairy farming practicable despite very high summer temperatures of 43°C (109°F) upwards, and very cold ones in winter.

When temperature falls during night-time hours, cattle may withstand a higher day-time temperature than they otherwise could.

Very high altitudes, e.g. in the mountains of Peru, can themselves be an obstacle to livestock production. (See ALTITUDE; MOUNTAIN SICKNESS.)

Stock improvement When high-yield stock are imported into tropical regions from countries having a temperate climate, disappointment often follows. At first, yields – whether of beef, milk, pork, or eggs – are better than those of the indigenous stock, as expected; but before long, in many instances, the initial gains are offset by a high mortality rate. The exotic animals may not be able to tolerate the heat, may not produce so well when fed on local feeds of lower quality, and will have no resistance to many local diseases and parasites, especially ticks. (For cattle resistant to heat and ticks, see DROUGHTMASTER; ZEBU; SANTA GERTRUDI; AFRICANDER.)

In many situations it is often preferable to improve indigenous stock first, before introducing new blood from overseas, by selective breeding and better management; ensuring that they are better fed and not deprived of adequate quantities of drinking water. After improvement has been obtained by these means (but not before), cross-breeding with exotic high-performance stock may be begun, preferably on a small-scale trial basis to start with. Use may be made of AI.

Animal power In India it is estimated that work animals provide as much energy as the entire electrical system of the country. The number of work animals is estimated to be 70 million bullocks, 8 million buffaloes, 1 million horses and 1 million camels. Throughout the Far East animal power remains the major factor in agriculture. Small farms, difficult terrain, lack of roads and the structure of the rural economy in many countries mean that situation is unlikely to change in the foreseeable future. (See WATER BUFFALOES.)

Animal feeds In poorer countries the cost of importing cereal grains or high-quality protein feeds may be prohibitive, and local stock will then be dependent on feeds which may restrict their yields – though obviously this is not always the case.

Imported feeds sometimes deteriorate to some extent during long sea voyages and subsequent storage in a hot and often humid climate. There may, for example, be a serious loss of vitamin E, so that a supplement is required if ENCEPHALOMALACIA is to be avoided. (See also VITAMINS.)

Local crops such as groundnuts, cotton seed, sorghum and sunflower seed may be contaminated by AFLATOXINS, so that precautions are needed. Groundnuts may be affected in this way through being left too long in the ground before harvesting, or during subsequent storage.

Minerals In many parts of the tropics, milling and processing facilities are lacking – at any rate in the more remote areas; this fact makes feed supplementation more difficult. Mineral and trace element supplements are necessary for avoidance of deficiencies. In South Africa many years ago, Sir Arnold Theiler showed that the need of cattle for phosphorus drove them to eat the bones of dead animals, and many cattle became infected with botulism in that way and died. (See LAMZIEKTE.) In several parts of the world a deficiency of copper in the herbage has impeded livestock production, and appropriate dressings of the land have brought great benefit. (See TRACE ELEMENTS.)

Some tropical crops Apart from the crops mentioned above, many others – or their by-products – are used. For example, cattle may have the leaves of shade trees, or sugar-cane; pigs may be given dried leaf meal, banana waste, coca pod husks, or sweet potatoes; poultry may receive millet (if any can be spared from human food requirements) or sago.

(See GOSSYPOL – Gossypol poisoning; CASTOR SEED POISONING; COCOA POISONING.)

Tropical diseases In some tropical regions the presence of animal parasites and their vectors makes livestock production difficult, costly, or even impracticable. This is true of the African tsetse-fly belt, extending roughly from latitude 15°N to 30°S. Here control of trypanosomiasis (see TRYPANOSOMES) is dependent on drugs for prevention, drugs for treatment, and use of insecticides against flies. Aerial spraying, bush clearance, and attempts to eradicate reservoirs of infection among wild animals will, if undertaken, obviously add to the cost, which in some territories may be beyond local resources. For many years control of tsetse flies had been successfully achieved by aerial spraying with insecticides, but the ever-rising cost of these, and of aviation fuel, has led to the abandonment of many such government schemes. Fly traps have had to be used instead. The Manitoba trap designed specially for tabanids is reported to be very successful; another widely used trap is the Laveissire. In other territories long-term, government-controlled campaigns have proved successful in maintaining and extending production.

Humpless cattle, such as the N'Dama, in West Africa had long been regarded as historic relics, and their reduced susceptibility to trypanosomiasis as a biological oddity. It has been shown, however, that despite their relatively small size, N'Dama cattle could survive and be productive in endemic trypanosomiasis areas where Zebu cattle died.

Comparative studies on 2 types of large East African zebu (*Bos indicus*) Boran cattle, on a beef ranch in Kenya, indicated that a Boran type bred by the Orma tribe has a superior response to tsetse fly challenge. The Orma Boran when compared with an improved Boran was found to have lower trypanosome infection rates and, when untreated, better control of anaemia as well as decreased mortality.

In areas where trypanosomiasis is endemic in susceptible cattle, sequential use of such drugs as diminazine and suramin has been effective in controlling the disease without causing drug resistance to develop.

Trypanosomes cause disease also in Asia and Central and South America.

Ticks are of great importance in the tropics, transmitting numerous protozoal parasites, viruses, and rickettsias. (See under TICKS.)

Among the major diseases caused by viruses are cattle plague (rinderpest), African swine fever, foot-and-mouth disease, and various types of encephalitis. Bacterial diseases include anthrax, botulism, haemorrhagic septicaemia (pasteurellosis), and salmonellosis. A notable mycoplasmal disease is contagious bovine pleuropneumonia; another is contagious agalactia of sheep and goats.

Vaccine storage/transport One of the problems of veterinary medicine in the tropics is the storage of vaccines at a sufficiently low temperature (below 8°C (46°F)). With the high cost and scarcity of kerosene or liquid propane gas in many rural areas, and the fact that electricity supply is often unreliable or non-existent, there is scope for solar refrigerators. Under a WHO scheme these have been tried in 13 countries. Photo-voltaic panels exposed to

the sun supply electricity direct to an ordinary commercial refrigerator.

Sterilisation In the tropics the sun's rays can be used for sterilisation purposes. Research at the American University of Beirut showed that oral rehydration solution, for treating dehydration, can be sterilised in plastic bags or transparent plastic or glass vessels by exposure to sunlight. In an experiment such a solution, contaminated with fresh sewage, proved to have a zero coliform count after 1 hour. It appears that the sterilising effect is not heat, since the temperature of the solution rises by less than 5°C (41°F) after 2 hours, but is rather solar radiation in the near ultra-violet range.

Another application is the Solomon solar steriliser which uses only solar energy to boil water and sterilise needles and syringes. The prototype consisted of a metal-lined plywood box topped with a truncated pyramid of glass. The steriliser, in use in the Solomon Islands, is easily constructed, has no moving parts, and requires no fuel; but it does need orienting to the sun every half-hour. (World Health Organisation.)

Carcase disposal, following post-mortem examinations, may present problems in undeveloped areas. An Australian veterinarian working at an Indian sheep project found the answer. If unsuitable for boiling as dog food, and yet not likely to spread infection, the carcase is dragged out into the open. He timed events on one occasion. 'At 2.46 p.m., post-mortem examination completed; no vultures to be seen in a clear sky. At 2.50 the first arrived; at 2.53 there were approximately 40 vultures around the carcase; at 2.58 carcase stripped to bones and sinew – vultures leaving.'

Trypanocide
A drug which will kill TRYPANOSOMES within the host's body.

Trypanosomes
Trypanosomes are small single-celled parasites found in the bloodstream in certain diseases that are classed together as the trypanosomiases.

The trypanosome is of an elongated shape with a single flagellum and an undulating membrane. There are 2 nuclei – a large nucleus (macronucleus or trophonucleus) near the centre of the body; and a small kinetoplast (micronucleus) at the posterior end remote from the flagellum. In some forms there is no free flagellum.

Transmission is generally by the bite of an insect (except in the case of dourine). The transmission may be mechanical, i.e. carried directly from an infected animal to an uninfected one by the bite of a blood-sucking fly; or cyclical, when the insect host is not infective for a definite time after ingestion of the parasite. In this case the parasite passes a definite part of its life-cycle in the fly. In many cases transmission may be both mechanical and cyclical. Thus the tsetse fly may have two infective periods, one immediately after biting a sick animal and the second some time later (about 20 days) after the trypanosome has progressed to its infective stage along normal lines.

Life histories of trypanosomes In the blood of the mammalian host, the trypanosomes reproduce by splitting lengthwise (longitudinal fission). A quantity of blood is

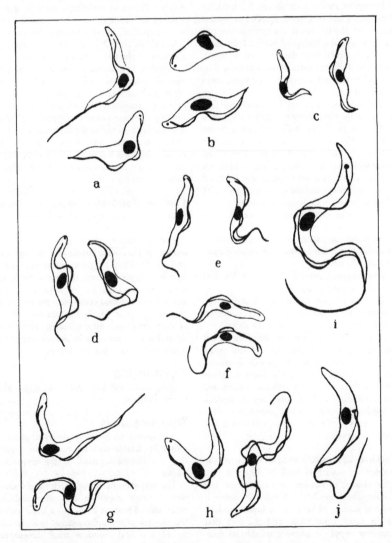

Some typical trypanosomes (drawn to the same scale and magnified 2000 times): (a) *Trypanosoma brucei*; (b) *T. montgomery*; (c) *T. congolense*; (d) *T. vivax*; (e) *T. simiae*; (f) *T. equinum*; (g) *T. equiperdum*; (h) *T. evanis*; (i) and (j) *T. theileri*.

sucked up by the tsetse fly, a species of *Glossina*, and in that host the flagellates undergo a developmental cycle. The location chosen by the parasite for its development varies with the species. Thus some will develop only in the salivary glands, others in the gut, and still others in the proboscis. After some time they assume the infective form, and are ready to be passed with the salivary fluids into the bloodstream of a suitable vertebrate host.

African trypanosomiasis Tsetse-borne trypanosomiasis renders approximately 10 million square km of prime African land unsuitable for cattle production. It has been estimated that if this disease could be controlled, the infested area would increase its cattle holding capacity from 20 million head to 140 million head.

The disease is of greatest importance in cattle, which are hosts of the following trypanosomes: *Trypanosoma congolense*, *T. vivax*, *T. uniforme*, and *T. evansi*.

Usually a chronic disease, acute cases also occur, and the mortality may be high. (See also PREMUNITION; and, for resistant breeds, TROPICS.)

Signs These include intermittent fever, anaemia, anorexia or pica, a progressive loss of condition, and increasing weakness. (See under CHANCRE for the hard swelling which is often the first pointer to trypanosomiasis.) Lymph nodes are enlarged in many cases, the coat harsh, and abortion may occur.

Some cattle recover, but in others apparent recovery is followed later by a relapse and death. In acute cases, death may occur within a fortnight.

Horses Additional signs include oedema of the limbs and abdomen, and corneal opacity. Species of trypanosome infecting horses are *T. brucei*, *T. vivax*, and *T. evansi*. (See also DOURINE, caused by *T. equiperdum*, transmitted at coitus, and occurring also in Asia.)

Dogs The eyes may be affected, as in horses. Canine trypanosomiasis is caused by *T. brucei*, *T. congolense*, and *T. evansi*.

Pigs often suffer from acute and fatal trypanosomiasis caused by either *T. simiae* or *T. evansi*.

Control This is difficult, on account of trypanosomiasis existing in wild animals in the vicinity of cattle herds, and the fact that vaccination has not been practicable.

In well-managed herds in areas where tsetsefly numbers are relatively low, drugs are used for preventive purposes against the trypanosomes; but as the latter develop drug resistance, it is usually necessary to change drugs.

In other areas, reliance is placed on drugs for treatment rather than prophylaxis; these can achieve survival of cattle where untreated animals die.

(See also under TSETSE FLY for another aid to control of the disease, and under TROPICS for breeds resistant to trypanosomiasis, and for drugs in current use.)

Diseases caused by trypanosomes are separately described under NAGANA, DOURINE, SURRA and (for human trypanosomiasis) SLEEPING SICKNESS and CHAGAS DISEASE. The latter also affects domestic animals and is described immediately below.

American trypanosomiasis (Chagas disease) Caused by *Trypanosoma cruzi*, this occurs in South and Central America, and also in the southern states of the USA. WHO estimates that at least 7 million people are infected with *T. cruzi*.

The infection can be carried from both wild and domestic animals to people by blood-sucking triatomid bugs; and the latter also cause people-to-people infections. Blood transfusions, and infection of the human fetus in utero, have also to be borne in mind.

Dogs, cats, and guinea-pigs are among domestic animals which are hosts; pigs and rabbits also have the disease. Rats, mice, foxes, ferrets, and vampire bats are other vectors.

Signs Fever, anaemia, emaciation, ascites, with death from heart failure following myocarditis in children.

Trypsin

Trypsin is a proteolytic enzyme of the pancreatic secretion. It changes proteins into peptones. It is said to be helpful in cases of non-specific diarrhoea in dogs.

Tryptophan

One of the essential AMINO ACIDS. Excessively high levels of tryptophan can result in fog fever (atypical interstitial pneumonia).

Tsetse Fly

Tsetse fly is the insect vector which is of such importance in the transmission of African TRYPANOSOMES. (See also FLIES – Glossina; TROPICS.)

Destruction of tsetse flies in the fly-belts – tracts of bush country in which only cattle which have acquired some degree of immunity to trypanosomiasis can survive – has proved an almost insuperable problem. One method is the sterilisation of tsetse flies by the chemicals tepa or metepa, or by gamma radiation, and the release of sterile males. This can be complementary to the use of insecticides. A difficulty at present is the rearing of tsetse flies in sufficient quantities.

Wide use is also made of fly traps, to which tsetse flies may be attracted by means of PHEROMONES or other chemical compounds such as CO_2, acetone, or octenol.

Tubercle

Tubercle is a term used in 2 quite distinct senses. As a descriptive term in anatomy, a tubercle means a small elevation or roughness upon the surface of a bone, such as the tubercles of the ribs. In a pathological sense a tubercle is a small mass, barely visible to the naked eye, formed in some organ as the starting-point of the disease which has been called after the tubercle, viz. tuberculosis.

Tuberculin Test

The tuberculin test, in its original form, came into use in 1890. It was developed by Koch, who grew his tubercle bacilli on broth. Today, Purified Protein Derivatives (PPD) extracted from bovine and from avian tubercle bacilli are used. These greatly improve the reliability of the test, although false positives still occur. Tuberculin (PPD) is prepared from killed bacteria by adding trichloracetic acid; the precipitated tuberculo-protein is allowed to sediment, collected by centrifugation and adjusted to a standard strength.

Tuberculin has in the past been used by instillation beneath the lower eyelid of one eye (the ophthalmic test); or by subcutaneous injection (the subcutaneous tuberculin test). Today, in the UK, the test used is the double intradermal comparative test. Skin is clipped free from hair over an area the size of a 50p piece in 2 places on the neck.

A fold of the clipped skin is gathered up and measured with special callipers. Using a standard tuberculin syringe, 0.1 ml of tuberculin is injected into the skin (not subcutaneously). Avian tuberculin is used for one injection, bovine for the other – the avian tuberculin being given above the bovine. After 72 hours, the test is read by again measuring the thickness of the skin and the nature of the swelling produced by the injection.

A reaction to the avian tuberculin can mean exposure to *Mycobacterium avium* (especially if

cattle are close to woods – pigeons are often infected), the presence of non-specific mycobacterial infection, of Johne's disease or so-called skin tuberculosis. The swelling caused by the avian tuberculin is compared to that caused by the bovine, using the same callipers. If reaction to the bovine is 4 mm or more than the avian, that is considered a positive reaction; a swelling of 3 mm indicates an inconclusive reaction. Reactors are normally slaughtered at a licensed abattoir and certain organs removed for examination, even if there are no visible lesions. Inconclusive reactors are usually retested 75 days after the first test. If a herd being tested has previously been vaccinated against Johne's disease, the State Veterinary Service will normally carry out the test as this vaccination produces a severe reaction to tuberculin.

Testing other animals Tuberculin testing of deer requires special training, as a swelling of as little as 0.5 mm difference, can be considered significant. Poultry can be tuberculin-tested using only the avian tuberculin injected intradermally into the left wattle. Any resulting swelling of that wattle is regarded as significant. Sheep, goats and pigs can be subjected to the double intradermal comparative test, with the avian tuberculin being given on the left side of the neck and the bovine on the right. As pigs are not clipped, a ring made by indelible marker is drawn round the site of the injection. Primates in zoos or research facilities may be tested; only mammalin tuberculin is used and the test carried out under sedation, using the left eyelid. Any swelling is regarded as significant.

Tuberculosis (TB)

A contagious disease of man, all the domesticated animals, many wild animals in captivity, birds, fishes, and reptiles. It is caused by *Mycobacterium tuberculosis* (bovine, human, or avian strains). It is a NOTIFIABLE DISEASE in cattle and deer.

The disease is usually a chronic one, though the miliary form is acute. It is characterised by the formation of nodules or tubercles in almost any or all of the organs or tissues of the body. (See also 'SKIN TUBERCULOSIS'.)

Occurrence The prevalence of tuberculosis in animals bears a direct ratio to the intensity of the methods of agriculture in an area. Cattle closely confined, and housed to a great extent in buildings, are much more often affected than are those living a free open-air life. The cattle in the prairies of North America, on the tablelands of Central Africa, and in the steppes of Eastern Europe, are almost entirely free from its ravages, while it is unknown in many islands (Iceland, Sicily, etc.).

Bovine tuberculosis eradication campaigns have succeeded in several countries.

Animals affected Among the ordinary domesticated animals, cattle and pigs are more commonly affected than are other species. Dogs are rarely infected but have been known to contract TB. Horses and sheep appear to be more resistant, though cases of progressive avian TB have been recorded in both species. Donkeys and mules are only very seldom attacked.

Methods of infection Cattle are infected in 2 chief ways: (1) by the respiratory system; and (2) by the digestive tract. They are susceptible to infection from humans suffering from bovine tuberculosis, and serious breakdowns in attested herds have been traced to farm workers suffering from the disease. Cattle are also susceptible, to a lesser degree, to infection of the human type. (See also under TUBERCULIN TEST *re* avian tuberculosis.) Badgers have been implicated in the spread of bovine TB and long-running tests are taking place in the UK to establish whether this is the case (*see below*, Tuberculosis in wildlife).

Sometimes tuberculosis may be contracted through a wound (e.g. after dehorning) or by direct introduction into the tissues of a penetrating instrument, and an infection of the udder may easily occur through the teat canal. An aerosol infection commonly results from coughing cows, and infected sputum may contaminate feed or be swallowed, thereby spreading infection to the intestines.

Within the body, infection may spread via the lymphatic system or the bloodstream.

Tuberculosis of the vagina occurs in cows, and the disease may be spread from them to healthy cows through the medium of the bull. Infected dung can be a source of infection.

Nature of the lesions A typical lesion is a tubercle – a small nodular swelling whose centre contains either pus or dry yellowish cheesy material. The peritoneum, liver, lymph nodes, lungs, etc., may be affected. Sometimes the disease remains localised to the area of its first infection and does not spread. In other cases the defensive forces of the body overcome and destroy the focus of infection.

Tuberculosis may affect bones and one or more joints, causing arthritis.

Superficial, as well as deep, lymph nodes may become enlarged.

A subclinical infection may occur, and result in overt illness only when stress, under-feeding, exposure or some other infection lowers the animal's resistance.

Cattle As a rule a considerable period of time elapses between infection and the appearance of the first symptoms.

Tuberculosis of the lungs – the commonest type – gives rise to a hard, dry, short cough in the early stages. Later, coughing becomes more frequent and DYSPNOEA is evident.

Appetite is variable. Sometimes a difficulty in swallowing is noticed. Loss of condition follows, with pale mucous membranes, and a staring coat. There may be diarrhoea.

Superficial lymph nodes may become enlarged. Those at the back of the throat or at the corner of the lower jaw, or the glands of the neck, shoulder, or stifle, may be swollen.

Tuberculosis of the udder – which is all-important from the milk standpoint – begins insidiously. The gland slowly becomes diffusely thickened, and more solid to the touch than normally. After milking, it does not feel quite so elastic as it should, and in some cases distinct hard nodules can be felt.

(Tuberculoid mastitis. Over 700 cases of this, due to rapidly growing acid-fast organisms other than *Mycobacterium tuberculosis*, occur in the UK annually – mainly due to not cleaning the teats before introducing antibiotics.)

Tuberculosis sometimes involves the brain or spinal cord, giving rise to symptoms described under MENINGITIS.

Tuberculosis of the bones and joints is not uncommon.

In the skin there occasionally develop hard tumours, about the size of a hazelnut (see also 'SKIN TUBERCULOSIS'), which, if they are opened, are found to contain cheesy or mortar-like masses in their centres. Later, ulcers may develop with the formation of multiple small abscesses in any or all of the organs. The abscesses are millet-seed sized (hence 'miliary'). This form of tuberculosis is rapidly fatal.

Sheep and goats A distressing painful cough, always present, but most noticeable upon exertion; and a gradual, but quite definite, loss of condition, with progressing weakness, are the main symptoms observed in these animals. Sheep are very rarely affected, but milking goats kept in the vicinity of infected cattle not uncommonly develop tuberculosis. There is nearly always a marked anaemia, pneumonia,

T

sometimes diarrhoea, and occasionally an infection of the udder corresponding to that found in cattle.

Horses Tuberculosis in the horse is not very common, but there are certain symptoms which should always lead one to suspect its presence: a gradual emaciation in spite of good food and without any other established possible cause; a slight fluctuating increase in the temperature, an occasional moist weak cough; a tucked-up appearance of the abdomen, or in some cases (where ascites exists) a heavy pendulous condition, 'pot-bellied'.

Cases in which the abdominal organs are affected sometimes terminate by lung complications – i.e. miliary tuberculosis sets in – the animal becomes feverish, distressed in its breathing, refuses all food, and generally dies within a few days. Tuberculosis may also become localised in the skin, lymph nodes, brain, or udder, but these are not common. It is comparatively often found that sooner or later some part of the skeleton (the bones of the neck being a very usual situation) becomes infected.

Occasionally, tuberculosis in the horse may be caused by the human or avian type of the tubercle bacillus.

Pigs Tubercular poultry, or wild birds such as wood-pigeons, are a not uncommon source of infection. A diagnosis may be established by means of the tuberculin test.

Symptoms are as in the horse. Scouring and emaciation may occur. Anaemia is common. As in horses, the bones are especially vulnerable to attack.

Lesions, which, to the naked eye, appear identical with tuberculosis, may be caused by infection with *Corynebacterium equi*. Even the use of a microscope sometimes fails to differentiate between the 2 infections.

Deer Disease caused by bovine or avian tubercle bacilli can be found. The clinical signs, which may not be noticeable until the disease is advanced, include respiratory signs. Caseous lesions are rarely seen as tuberculous lesions are usually filled with pus.

Dogs and cats Where tuberculosis is common in the human population, these domestic animals are liable to become infected – either as the result of receiving tubercle-containing milk, or as the result of infection from sputum or discharges from a human case. Not only may dogs and cats contract the disease from man, but they may occasionally be sources of infection to healthy human beings, and especially to children.

As in other animals, the symptoms are somewhat vague until the disease is well established. The first signs may be no more than a capricious appetite, slight loss of condition, general weakness, and exhaustion when at exercise. Pulmonary tuberculosis usually begins with a short dry cough. It is less common in these animals than the abdominal form (but see PLEURISY).

Tuberculosis of the abdominal organs is indicated by impaired nutrition and anaemia, attacks of diarrhoea and constipation alternating with each other. There may be vomiting, also ascites. Body temperature is very variable.

Joints and sinuses may be sites of infection in the cat. Occasionally skin tuberculosis is seen in dogs and cats, and may take the form of raised plaques with a tendency to ulcerate.

Treatment The treatment of tuberculosis in the domesticated animals is not attempted, for 4 reasons: (1) because of the nature of the disease; (2) because of the ever-increasing danger to human beings who have to attend affected animals; (3) for economic reasons; and (4) for humanitarian ones. However, in zoological gardens, animals are sometimes treated. (See PAS.)

Prevention Good hygiene, good feeding and good ventilation all help. Animals brought in from areas known to be infected should be quarantined on the premises and a tuberculin test carried out by the veterinarian befoe they are allowed to mix with other stock.

History of control in Britain It was not until 1928 that measures to control bovine tuberculosis were introduced by the government. In that year, the Tuberculosis Order, enacted in 1915, came into force, and the attempt to control the disease by the detection and elimination of 'open' cases began. In 1935 the Attested Herds Scheme carried control measures a stage further.

Area Eradication, which began in 1950, and meant, at first, an extension of the Attested Herds Scheme on a voluntary basis, and then the compulsory slaughter of reactors within the prescribed areas, followed.

In October 1960, the whole of the UK was declared one Attested Area – bovine tuberculosis being virtually eradicated from all herds of cattle.

In 1962, the incidence of bovine tuberculosis in herds in England and Wales was

0.14 per cent. The number of reactors slaughtered was 8846.

During 1968, 5,854,915 cattle were tested in 108,452 herds and as a result 2170 reactors (including 2 'affected' animals) and 202 contacts in 1040 herds were slaughtered.

The Tuberculosis Orders 1964 provide for the notification and slaughter of cattle found to be affected with certain forms of tuberculosis – i.e. tuberculosis of the udder; giving tuberculous milk; tuberculous emaciation; chronic cough accompanied by clinical signs of tuberculosis; or found to be excreting or discharging tuberculous material.

Since 1990, TB outbreaks in cattle have been increasing by 20 per cent a year in certain parts of the UK, including the West Country and Staffordshire. The search is on for a vaccine, which, unlike BCG, does not interfere with the diagnostic skin test. Trials of a promising DNA-based vaccine took, place in 2004.

Tuberculosis in wildlife In many countries, complete eradication of TB has been elusive because of reservoirs of infection in wildlife. In Britain, BADGERS (*Meles meles*) can become infected and die from TB. The form of the disease in badgers is variable but is often respiratory; it can be spread between badgers by aerosol (in the breath) or by the shedding of bacilli in the urine. The State Veterinary Service has carried out a long-term policy of eradicating badger populations in the vicinity of cattle herds. This has not resulted in an overall improvement of the situation as the disease has spread from the original infected area. In 1999, following a report by Professor Krebs, a long-term study to evaluate how TB may be spread between cattle, badgers and other wildlife was begun but was interrupted by the 2001 foot-and-mouth disease outbreak. The aims are to establish definitively what proportion of TB outbreaks in cattle is caused by badgers; and whether culling badgers is an effective way of controlling the disease. The trial is in 3 parts: (a) badgers are culled on and around farms following TB outbreaks; (b) those where all badgers are killed; and (c) those where no badgers are culled. Part (a) of the trial was discontinued in late 2003 as interim results showed an increasde of 27 per cent in TB breakdowns in that area compared with the other two.

DEFRA emphasises that the trial will not endanger the viability of the UK badger population of over 300,000; it is estimated that no more than 12,500 badgers will be culled. More than that number are believed to be killed annually in road accidents.

Tuberculosis has been found in other wild animals including deer, foxes and weasels, as well as pigeons and their predators.

The relationship of tuberculosis in animals and man; bovine tuberculosis

This is not a pedantic way of saying 'tuberculosis in cattle', but indicates that one is referring to disease set up by the bovine strain of tubercle bacillus as opposed to the human strain or the avian strain. Man may become infected by any one of the 3 strains. The bovine strain of the tubercle bacillus is particularly pathogenic for children under 16.

In considering statistics dealing with incidence of bovine tuberculosis in humans, it must be borne in mind that bovine tuberculosis can be spread from one person to another, just as it can be from animal to man.

Human infection with tuberculosis may also arise from eating infected meat, but this risk, is, in civilised countries, not great owing to meat inspection services, and cooking of the meat. The protection of the human population from TB involves the tuberculin test, meat inspection and pasteurisation of milk.

Tuberculosis (Amendment) Order 1973

The Tuberculosis (Amendment) Order 1973, made under the Diseases of Animals Act 1950, requires anyone who suspects a carcase to be affected with tuberculosis to notify a veterinary inspector and to retain the carcase (or parts of it) for examination. The purpose of the Order is to enable the herd of origin to be traced. Isolation of suspected tubercular cattle is also empowered.

Tuberculosis, Avian
(see AVIAN TUBERCULOSIS)

Tularaemia

Tularaemia is a disease of HARES, ground squirrels, rabbits, and rats, caused by the *Pasteurella (Francisella) tularensis*, and spread mechanically either by flies or ticks, or by direct inoculation – for example, into the hands of a person engaged in skinning rabbits. In man, the disease takes the form of a slow fever, lasting several weeks, with much malaise and depression, followed by considerable emaciation. It was first described in the district of Tulare in California, but is found widely spread in North America, also in parts of Europe and Japan. Sheep and pigs are attacked and many die. Streptomycin may prove effective in treatment.

Dogs are susceptible, too.

Tumbu Fly
(see under SCREW-WORM FLIES)

Tumour

Malignant tumours are those which tend to grow and spread rapidly, destroying neighbouring tissues and infiltrating the healthy structures near by. They are liable to ulcerate through the skin when superficial, are non-encapsulated, and may spread to distant parts of the body by the blood- or lymph-stream, giving rise to secondary tumours there. (Further information upon malignant tumours appears under CANCER.)

Benign tumours grow slowly at one place, press neighbouring parts aside, but neither invade nor destroy them, only seldom ulcerate through the skin or mucous membrane, have usually a capsule of fibrous tissue surrounding them, and when once completely removed by surgical excision or other means, do not recur.

While this classification serves in a measure to differentiate typical varieties into 2 classes, it is by no means absolutely satisfactory. There are certain kinds of normally benign tumours which may remain comparatively small and circumscribed for a number of years, and then suddenly become malignant.

Benign or simple tumours include ANGIOMA, CHONDROMA, fibroma GLIOMA, LIPOMA, MYOMA, MYXOMA, NEUROMA, ODONTOMA, and PAPILLOMA. The last-named may be benign in the beginning but become malignant later; also MELANOMA and ADENOMA. (See also CYSTS; WARTS; CANCER.) While normally all tumours tend to increase in size – either slowly or rapidly – some grow to a certain size, remain stationary, then decrease in size, and a few may even disappear completely.

Two of the most common tumours of the dog are mammary carcinoma and anal adenoma (usually benign). (See also EOSINOPHILIC GRANULOMA.)

Tumour Angiogenesis Factor (TAF)

This has been isolated from human and animal tumours. It stimulates mitosis in endothelial cells and rapid formation of new capillaries for tumour nourishment. (Unlike a skin-graft, which sends out capillary shoots to join the capillaries of the recipient tissue, a tumour has to rely entirely on the host, and makes use of TAF for this purpose.)

Tungiasis

Infestation with *Tunga penetrans*, the jigger flea. (See under FLEAS.)

Tup

A ram (see under SHEEP).

Turbinate Bones
(see under NOSE and RHINITIS)

Turkey Coryza

A disease of the upper respiratory tract, with sneezing and nasal discharge, whose probable cause is *Bordetella avium.* It occurs in turkey poults, usually in conditions where ventilation is poor and the birds are stressed.

Turkey Viral Hepatitis

This occurs in Europe, the USA, and Canada; and in 1982 isolation of a picorna-like virus causing hepatitis and disease of the pancreas was isolated from an outbreak in Scotland. The infection, which is highly contagious, is often, if not usually, subclinical, but may take an acute form, and prove fatal.

Turkeys

Diseases include Arizona disease, blackhead, coccidiosis, erysipelas, fowl pest, hexamitiasis, haemorrhagic enteritis, moniliasis, Oregon disease, ornithosis, mycoplasmosis, pullorum disease, reticuloendotheliosis, rupture of the aorta, sinusitis, synovitis (see also GROUNDNUT MEAL MANIOC).

Turkey meningoencephalitis occurs in Israel. Influenza viruses cause disease in North American domestic turkeys.

Turkey rhinotracheitis has been seen in several countries, and appeared in the UK in 1985, causing severe financial losses due to deaths, carcase rejections, and lowered egg production. The first sign is sneezing.

Turnips

Like kale, these contain a goitre-producing factor, and if fed in large amounts to pregnant ewes are liable to cause abortion – unless iodine licks are provided. (See VAGINA, RUPTURE OF.)

Turpentine, Medicinal Oil of

Turpentine is the oleo-resin which exudes from various members of the pine family, especially the *Pinus australis, P. taeda,* and *P. sylvestris.* The oil distilled from this oleo-resin is known as oil of turpentine. The natural turpentine is not used in medicine, as it is highly irritating and when the word 'turpentine' is employed, the oil of turpentine is indicated.

In collections of gas in the abdominal organs, medicinal turpentine has been used (e.g. tympany in horses and cattle). Large doses are liable to irritate the stomach and kidneys.

Turpentine should never be given when an animal is suffering from nephritis, inflammations of the bladder, stomach, or bowels, as its active irritant action only increases the already existing inflammation. (See under SMELL.)

Externally, oil of turpentine is used as a constituent of liniments.

Turtles

(see AMERICAN BOX TORTOISES; TORTOISES)

Threat to public health from pet turtles
Serious infection can be transmitted to owners by turtles, including aquatic turtles (terrapins). Six of 28 lots of embryonated eggs of the red-eared turtle (*Pseudemys scripta elegans*) imported into Canada from Louisiana were found to harbour salmonellae. *Salmonella poona* and *S. arizonae* were isolated from the eggs and the packaging moss, and the turtles hatched from the contaminated eggs continued to shed salmonellae into the tank water for up to 11 months. Of the 37 strains of salmonellae isolated, 30 were resistant to gentamicin, probably because of the widespread use of the antibiotic to try to produce salmonella-free eggs for export. Such high levels of antibiotic-resistant salmonellae in turtle eggs could pose a serious risk to human health.

'Twin Lamb' Disease
A colloquial name for PREGNANCY TOXAEMIA.

Twinning, Artificial
In the interests of increased beef production, techniques have been developed to encourage the production of twin calves. A suitable dose of pregnant mare's serum (PMS), injected subcutaneously at a suitable time, e.g. 4 days before oestrus, will on average give twins; but there will be some triplets and singles. The FOLLICLE-STIMULATING HORMONE contained in the serum causes an extra follicle to mature and shed an extra egg with resultant twinning. Over-dosage, however, leads to undesired quadruplets, etc.; or to numerous eggs which pass quickly down the Fallopian tubes without being fertilised; result – no calf at all. There is a risk of stillbirths and of strain on the dam.

Twins (Calves)
Twins tend to run in families. For example, a cow had 3 pairs of twins, her daughter 4 pairs, and a grand-daughter 2 pairs. That might be called twinning at its best. Of course, there is sometimes trouble. Perhaps the condition of the dam is pulled down; or perhaps the 'cleansing' is retained, becomes infected, and infertility follows.

Predicting twins The presence of twins can sometimes be detected by manual examination, but ultrasound scanning is more reliable and allows earlier detection.

The concentration of oestrone sulphate, a hormone produced by a cow carrying a viable fetus and present in blood plasma or milk, can be used to confirm pregnancy.

The concentration is higher in cows carrying twins, but the difference does not become significant until about the 220th day of gestation. However, even at this late stage, the prediction of twins could be used as a guide to increase the feed allowance of cows carrying more than 1 fetus.

In strains not noted for twins, twinning may occur on farms where there is a herd infertility problem.

Identical twins – always of the same sex – result from the division of the fertilised egg into 2; whereas ordinary twins are produced as the result of the fertilisation of 2 eggs.

These 2 eggs may come from the same ovary, when the 2 fetuses may develop in the same horn of the uterus. Sometimes they result in a FREEMARTIN.

There is apparently, with cattle, a close affinity between identical twins – as there undoubtedly is with human beings. In a Swedish study, 6 pairs of twins were split at birth and reared separately for 15 months. At this age they were all put into a field together. Within a few days each twin had found and paired off with its sister. (See ERYTHROCYTE MOSAICISM; also GENETICS; SUPERFETATION; TWINNING, ARTIFICIAL; TRIPLET CALVES.)

Twins (Foals)
In the mare, the presence of twins in the uterus is a common cause of abortion. About 3 per cent of pregnant mares conceive twin fetuses, but the birth of healthy twins is exceedingly rare – about 0.01 per cent.

Twins, Monozygous
Identical twins, from the same ovum.

Twitch
This consists of a loop of soft rope threaded through a hole near the end of a stout piece of wood. The twitch is applied to the horse's upper lip, where it compresses the sensitive nerves. It used to be thought that the twitch merely diverted the horse's attention away from other parts of the body, but this view is now disputed. It is thought that pain perception or awareness are diminished through the activation of ENDORPHINS. Twitching significantly increases

plasma levels of beta-endorphin, which returns to normal 30 minutes or so after the twitch is removed. Twitching could therefore be said to be analogous to ACUPUNCTURE.

'Tying-Up Syndrome'

Also known as set-fast, this condition in race-horses appears to be identical with azoturia. Symptoms include stiffness, a rolling gait, blowing and sweating and, if exercise continues, the adoption of a crouching attitude. Pain is evident. The animal may lie down and be unable to rise. (See azoturia, under BOVINE MYOGLOBINURIA.)

Tylan

The proprietary name of a preparation of tylosin.

Tylosin

A macrolide antibiotic effective against Gram-positive organisms; it concentrates in acidic conditions, as in the udder and the lung. It is used as a growth promoter in pigs. (See ADDITIVES.)

Tympanites

The drum-like condition of the abdomen, which results from distension of the stomach or bowels with gas, as the result of fermentation, constipation, or of simple obstruction. (See under STOMACH, DISEASES OF; INTESTINES, DISEASES OF; BLOAT; TYMPANY; TYMPANITIC.)

Tympanitic Resonance in Cattle

Right-side tympanitic resonance (ping) caused by gas distention of intra-abdominal structures was diagnosed in 366 adult cattle, in a USA study. The source of the ping was identified as the abomasum in 137 animals, various segments of the intestinal tract in 157 and peritoneal gas in two. The source of the noise was not identified in 70. The principal final diagnoses were: left displacement of the abomasum (116), right displacement of the abomasum (77), abomasal (and omasal) volvulus (60), other gastro-intestinal conditions (73) and non-gastrointestinal conditions (40).

Tympany

Tympany is distension of a hollow organ with gas. (See TYMPANITES; BLOAT.)

Typhilitis

Inflammation of the caecum or 1st part of the large intestine, into which the termination of the small intestine opens.

Typhus of Rats and Mice

Typhus of rats and mice, caused by *Rickettsia mooseri*, may kill about 5 per cent of people infected by it.

Tyzzer's Disease

This was first described in mice in 1917, and has since been reported in horses, cats, and laboratory animals including rats, rabbits, gerbils, and rhesus monkeys.

Cause The spore-forming, Gram-negative, motile *Bacillus piliformis*.

Signs The disease is characterised as a rule by severe diarrhoea, debility, and death; though sudden death in foals without preliminary symptoms has been reported in the USA. Jaundice, slight or marked, was a post-mortem finding, together with some liver necrosis and enteritis.

In the cat, the infection gives rise to symptoms of loss of appetite, depression, diarrhoea, collapse and death. Necrosis of the ileum and hepatitis are among post-mortem findings.

Tzaneen Disease

This is a tick-borne infection with *Theileria mutans* in cattle, the African buffalo, and the Indian water buffalo, and often occurs simultaneously with other infections. There may be only a mild fever or, less commonly, serious illness, and death. Anti-malarial drugs are of use.

Udder
(see MAMMARY GLAND)

Uitpeuloog
'Bulging eye disease'– an oculovascular myiasis of domestic animals in South Africa.

Ulcer
A break on the surface of the skin, or of any mucous membrane of a cavity of the body, which does not tend to heal. The process by which an ulcer spreads, which involves necrosis (death) of minute portions of the healthy tissues around its edges, is known as ulceration. Most ulcers are suppurative; bacteria prevent healing and often extend the lesion.

An ulcer consists of a 'floor' or surface which, in consequence of the loss or destruction of tissue, is usually depressed below the level of the surrounding healthy structures; and an 'edge' around it where the healthy tissues end.

Callous ulcer is a type of chronic ulcer often encountered in horses and dogs, when there is any pressure or irritation that interferes with the blood supply but does not necessarily cause immediate destruction of the skin. In most cases it is covered by a hard, leathery piece of dead skin from under which escapes a purulent fluid. 'Bedsores' in all animals may be of this nature.

'Rodent ulcer' is a term reserved in human medicine for an ulcerating carcinoma of the skin, but it is often colloquially used by dog- and cat-owners for an EOSINOPHILIC GRANULO-MA. Skin cancer occurs in domestic animals, and such malignant tumours may ulcerate.

Tubercular ulcers may occur in dogs' and cats' skin in the form of raised plaques which ulcerate.

Internal ulcers may occur in the mouth (see MOUTH, DISEASES OF), in the stomach (see GASTRIC ULCERS), in the bowels (see INTESTINES, DISEASES OF), and in other parts.

Glanders ulcers are typically encountered in the mucous membrane of the nostrils, and have a 'punched-out' appearance.

Lip-and-leg ulcers occur in sheep with ORF.

Causes Any condition that lowers the general vitality of the animal, such as old age, chronic disease, malnutrition, and defective circulation, will act as a predisposing cause. Among direct causes may be bacteria gaining access to wounds; irritation from badly fitting harness, pressure of bony prominences upon hard floors insufficiently provided with bedding, and application of too strong antiseptics to wounds.

Treatment In the smaller animals a vitamin supplement may be indicated. An antibiotic or one of the sulfa drugs may be used.

Local treatment aims at converting the ulcer into what virtually becomes an ordinary open wound. The surface is treated with some suitable antiseptic, such as cetrimide, gentian violet, dilute hydrogen peroxide, etc. If one or two days of such treatment does not result in a clean, bright-red, odourless wound, or where there are shreds of dead tissue adherent to the surface, it may be necessary to curette the surface so that the dead cells may be separated from the healthy ones below them.

Animal-owners should note that after the surface of the ulcer has been rendered as healthy as possible, use of strong antiseptics or (worse still) disinfectants should cease, as these retard healing by the destruction of surface tissues.

Corneal ulcers are referred to under EYE, DISEASES OF – Keratitis. (See also CRYOSURGERY.)

Ulcerative Dermatosis of Sheep
A viral infection, which has to be differentiated from ORF, and is characterised by ulcers on the face, feet, legs, and external genitalia. It also in Europe and Africa.

Ulcerative Dermal Necrosis
A disease of adult salmon which occurs when they enter fresh water on their way to spawning grounds. Grey lesions are seen above the eyes, on the snout and on the side of the opercula (gill coverings). If they do not heal, the lesions spread to the skin of the head, ulcerate, and become prone to infection by *Saprolegnia* fungus. The fungal infection may be treated with zinc-free malachite green. The cause is unknown.

Ulcerative Enteritis of Chickens, Pheasants and Quails
Ulcerative enteritis is seen in chickens between 4 and 7 weeks, and in quail, turkeys, partridge and grouse at any age. Birds are depressed, with watery droppings; mortality can be very high, reaching 70 to 100 per cent. The cause is a virus.

Ulcerative Lymphangitis
Ulcerative lymphangitis, also called ulcerative cellulitis, is a contagious chronic disease of horses, characterised by inflammation of the

lymph vessels and a tendency towards ulceration of the skin over the parts affected.

Cause *Corynebacterium bovis (pseudotuberculosis)*. It gains access through abrasions. Infection may be carried by grooming tools, harness, utensils, etc., from one horse to another.

Signs The commonest seat of the disease is the fetlock of a hind-leg. This part becomes swollen and slightly painful. Small abscesses appear; ulcers follow. The condition gradually spreads up the leg.

Treatment Antibiotics.

Ulcerative Spirochaetosis of Pigs

This has been reported in the UK, Australia, New Zealand, South Africa, and the USA. It may give rise to foot-rot in pigs, ulceration of the skin, and scirrhous cord.

Ulna

This is the inner of the 2 bones of the fore-arm. The shaft has gradually reduced in size as the number of digits has decreased, so that while the ulna is a perfect bone in the dog and cat, in the horse its shaft has almost completely disappeared and the bone is only represented by the olecranon process which forms the 'point of the elbow'. The shaft of the ulna is liable to become fractured from violence to the fore-limb, but the commonest seat of an ulnar fracture is the olecranon process. This occurs from a fall in which the fore-limbs slip out in front of the animal, and the weight of the body comes down suddenly on to the point of the elbow. (See FRACTURES.)

Ultra-High-Temperature Treatment of Milk (UHT)

Ultra-high-temperature treatment of milk (UHT) involves heating it to between 135° and 149°C (275° and 300°F) for a few seconds. Suggested in 1913, UHT is used to produce long-life milk, on sale in Britain from 1965 onwards. This process does not affect the calcium nor the casein, but destroys some vitamins and probably some serum proteins (immune globulins). Calves grow less well on it than on raw or pasteurised milk.

Ultrasound

Sound at a frequency above 20,000 cycles per second. Propagated by applying an electric current to one side of a piezoelectric crystal, which deforms and produces a sound wave.

Ultrasound is generally defined as an auditory frequency beyond that perceived by the human ear. Most humans hear and emit sound in the frequency range 2 to 20 kHz, while in some animals ranges are much greater. Bats, dolphins, many rodents and some insects have ranges that extend as high as 120 kHz – well beyond the limit of human detection. Pigs and poultry can detect higher ultrasound frequencies and may be disturbed by the noise given off by, for example, certain electronic equipment and dripping nipple-drinkers. Female rabbits communicate with their litters in ultrasound.

Ultrasound, in the range of 1 million to 10 million hertz, is used in non-invasive diagnostic imaging of internal body structures. It is widely used in pregnancy diagnosis of animals. (See also PREGNANCY DIAGNOSIS.)

In human medicine, ultrasound has been shown to be beneficial for wound healing, both in the treatment of pressure sores and in the preparation of trophic ulcers for skin grafting. Studies have shown that it influences the activity of fibroblasts.

Ultra-Violet Rays

Ultra-violet rays are used in the treatment of various skin diseases, etc., and in the diagnosis of ringworm and porphyria; also in the fluorescent-antibody test for various infections including rabies.

Ultra-violet rays and eye cancer

Analysis of data from 14 veterinary colleges in the USA, where 147 cases of eye cancer in horses were studied, led to the conclusion that ultra-violet radiation may be of primary importance in triggering cancer.

Umbilical Cord, Cutting The

(see under PARTURITION)

Umbilicus

Umbilicus is another name for the navel.

Umgana Tree

Elephants seek out and gorge themselves on the fruits of this tree, leading to in sexual excitement. Ostriches may behave similarly.

Uncinariasis

Infection with *Uncinaria stenocephala*, one of the hookworms of the dog.

Unconsciousness

(see under COMA; FITS; SYNCOPE; EPILEPSY; NARCOLEPSY)

Undecylenate Ointment

A fungicide, used in the treatment of ringworm, etc.

Undulant Fever in Man

Undulant fever in Man is caused by *Brucella melitensis*, *B. abortus suis*, or *B. abortus*. The latter organism is responsible for 'contagious abortion' (brucellosis) of cattle, and it is probable that most cases of undulant fever in man caused by *B. abortus* arise through handling infected cows or from drinking their milk. Infection can readily occur through the skin. Numerous cases have occurred in veterinarians, following mishaps with Strain 19 vaccine, e.g. accidental spraying into the eyes or injection into the hand. In America, *B. abortus suis* is an important cause of undulant fever in man; *B. canis* likewise.

Signs are vague and simulate those of influenza except that undulant fever lasts for a much longer time, even many months. Temperature is generally raised but fluctuates greatly; there are muscle pains, headache, tiredness and inability to concentrate. One or more joints may swell. There may be constipation. The organisms are present in the bloodstream and in the spleen.

The disease is serious, not so much because of its mortality (1 to 2 per cent), but because of incapacity occasioned by its long duration. (See BRUCELLOSIS and CHEESE.)

Prevention Anyone handling aborting cows, or their fetal membranes, or even calving an apparently normal cow, should wear protective gloves or sleeves (which nevertheless sometimes tear), and wash arms and hands in a disinfectant solution afterwards. Avoid drinking any cold milk that has not been pasteurised.

Unsaturated Fatty Acids

(see under LIPIDS; VITAMINS – Vitamin E)

Unstable Substances

(see under INJECTIONS)

Uraemia

Uraemia results when the waste materials that should be excreted into the urine are retained in the body, through some disease of the kidneys, and are circulated in the bloodstream. Blood urea is in excess. Death may be preceded by convulsions and unconsciousness. In the slower types there is usually a strong urinous odour from all the body secretions. In acute cases the administration of glucose saline subcutaneously may help; likewise, withdrawal of a quantity of blood (provided that saline is given). (See URINE – Abnormal constituents; LEPTOSPIROSIS; KIDNEYS, DISEASES OF.)

Urates

(see URIC ACID)

Urea (Carbamide)

Urea (carbamide) is a crystalline substance of the chemical formula $CO(NH_2)_2$, which is very soluble in water and alcohol. It is the chief waste product discharged from the body in the urine, being formed in the liver and carried by the blood to the kidneys. The amount excreted varies with the nature and the amount of the food taken, being greater in the carnivora, and when large amounts of protein are present in the food. It is also increased in quantity during the course of fevers. Urea is rapidly changed into ammonium carbonate after excretion and when in contact with the air, owing to the action of certain micro-organisms.

Determination of the blood urea level is an important aid to the diagnosis of kidney failure.

Urea As a Ruminant Feed

Some of the micro-organisms which inhabit the rumen can synthesise protein from urea. It was accordingly suggested that urea might be substituted for protein in concentrates fed to cattle. This has been called the protein-sparing effect of urea, which is a non-protein source of nitrogen.

The emphasis has now shifted more to the value of urea in increasing the intake and aiding the digestion of low-quality roughages, and it has been widely used as a dietary supplement for cattle and sheep on poor pasture in many parts of the world. Where extra energy, in the form of readily digestible carbohydrate, is provided in addition to the urea, both roughage digestibility and feed intake improve. In these circumstances the urea stimulates multiplication of cellulose-digesting organisms, so that the urea-fed animal may be able to make more effective use of roughage than the one receiving no urea.

In the ruminant animal, any injudicious feeding of urea can give rise to poisoning by ammonia, since it is this which is released in the rumen and then converted into microbial protein. Excess ammonia can cause the animal's death. It is essential, therefore, that urea is taken in small quantities over a period, and not fed a large amount at a time.

Urea is often added to molasses and fed via ball feeders which prevent rapid and excessive uptake of the liquid and ensure maximum utilisation of urea. Under optimum farm conditions only 15 to 30 per cent of the dietary protein can be replaced by urea. As a rule of thumb, urea, if

U

incorporated uniformly within the dairy ration, has been shown to be safe at a level of 1 per cent. Combined with 5 per cent barley, that mix can replace 5 per cent ground-nut meal in the ration. In the diets of finishing beef cattle, the animals can gradually have the proportion of urea increased.

Some guidelines for urea feeding

1. Introduce urea feeding gradually, i.e. at a slowly increasing level over a period of 3 to 4 weeks, with adequate minerals and vitamins provided.

2. Avoid starting newly calved cows on it (but it may be included in the steaming-up ration), or giving it to calves under 3 months of age.

3. Ensure that urea is fed with adequate readily digestible carbohydrate, as is contained in cereals, molasses, sugar-beet pulp, maize silage, etc.

4. Do not exceed levels of urea recommended by the supplier.

5. Ensure that urea is fed little and often, and not irregularly or at long intervals.

Urea poisoning Symptoms include salivation, excitement, running and staggering, jerking of the eyeballs, and scouring.

Acute urea poisoning killed 17 beef cows in a group of 29 in the south of Scotland. The animals died over an 8-hour period as a result of drinking water which had been carried to a trough in a tanker previously used for transporting urea fertiliser. It was calculated that as little as 10 litres of the water would have provided a fatal dose of urea to a 500 kg cow.

Ureaplasmas

Formerly known as T-mycoplasmas, these have been isolated from the lungs, and also the urogenital tract of several species of animals. They are a likely cause of pneumonia and infertility.

Ureter

The ureter is the tube which carries the urine excreted by a kidney down to the urinary bladder. Each ureter begins at the pelvis (main cavity) of the corresponding kidney, passes backwards and downwards along the roof and walls of the pelvis, and finally ends by opening into the neck of the bladder. The wall of the ureter is composed of a fibrous coat on the outside, a muscular coat in the middle, and this is lined by a mucous membrane consisting of cubical epithelium.

Urethra

The urethra is the tube which leads from the neck of the bladder to the outside, opening at the extremity of the penis in the male, and into the posterior part of the urino-genital passage in the female. It serves to conduct the urine from the bladder to the outside; also the semen.

Urethra, Diseases of

Owing to its extreme shortness in the female, the urethra is not subject to the same disease conditions as in the male, where the tube is considerably longer. In fact, disease of the urethra in the female hardly ever arises except as a complication of either disease of the bladder, on the one hand, or of the vagina on the other.

Urethritis Inflammation of the urethra is usually associated with cystitis, and may be the result of an infection, or of some irritant poison (such as CANTHARIDES) present in the urine. The lining mucous membrane may also be inflamed by crystalline deposits. (See FELINE UROLOGICAL SYNDROME; UROLITHIASIS; URETHRAL OBSTRUCTION.)

In most cases of urethritis there are signs of pain and distress whenever urine is passed or when the parts are handled. A little blood may be seen.

Stricture is an abrupt narrowing of the calibre of the tube at one or more places. In almost all cases of true stricture there has been some injury to the urethra or penis, resulting in the formation of scar tissue, which eventually contracts and decreases the lumen of the tube. A few cases, however, are caused by a rapidly growing tumour.

Injuries to the urethra may follow a severe crush or blow which causes fracture of the pelvis or of the os penis in the dog. They are usually obvious when the injury has involved the surface of the body, and may be suspected if there is an inability to pass urine, or if the urine contains blood or pus following upon a severe injury to the hindquarters of the body. A complication of urethral injuries is abscess formation around the urethra and consequent stricture at a later period.

Urethral Obstruction

In sheep, the injudicious use of hormones to increase liveweight gain has killed lambs, apparently as the result of urethral obstruction. In one incident in the USA, 200 out of 9000 lambs died after receiving 12 mg stilboestrol by injection.

In the UK, an increased incidence of urethral obstruction in male calves and lambs followed the incorporation of too high a level of magnesium in the concentrates fed.

Analysis of the calculi (stones) causing the obstruction showed them to be crystals of magnesium ammonium phosphate. After reducing the level of magnesium supplementation to 200 mg MgO per tonne of feed, there were no cases of urolithiasis in intensively fattened male lambs offered a cereal-based diet ad lib. (See also under URINARY BLADDER, DISEASES OF – Urinary calculi.)

Five outbreaks in male calves of various ages investigated by the Veterinary Research Laboratory, Stormont, showed a magnesium content of the concentrates (fed from the first week of life) to range from 4.9 to 9.2 g/kg dry matter. (The AFRC recommendation is not more than 1.4 g/kg dry matter.)

Obstruction of the male urethra is a common condition in cats, and fairly common in the dog. (See FELINE UROLOGICAL SYNDROME.)

Unless relieved, urethral obstruction can lead to rupture of the bladder and death.

Urethrostomy

Perineal urethrostomy is a surgical operation for the treatment of urethral obstruction; it consists of making a permanent opening in the urethra, the lining mucous membrane and the skin being joined by sutures. (Urethrostomy differs in this respect from urethrotomy, in which the urethra is incised – to remove a wedged calculus, for example – but immediately closed.)

Urethrostomy is performed mainly in cats suffering from feline urological syndrome. It is not in itself a cure for this, but rather for the often-associated urethral obstruction. The operation is an alternative to euthanasia when the cat cannot be catheterised, or has already been subjected to this on 2 or more occasions, when repetition could be regarded as inhumane.

Urethrostomy, skilfully performed, can be successful, in both the short and the long term.

Complications can arise, however, after both urethrotomies and urethrostomies, and include: extravasation of urine into surrounding tissues; haemorrhage; and stricture, as the result of scar formation. Should the latter occur, it leaves the cat in the same state as it was before the operation, so that nothing has been gained.

Urethrostomy makes the male cat anatomically similar to the female, so that ascending infections may occur.

Uric Acid

Uric acid is a crystalline substance, very slightly soluble in water, white in the pure state, and found in the urine of flesh-eating animals in normal conditions. It is also found in some kidney stones and urinary calculi, and may be present in joints affected with GOUT.

Urinary Antiseptics

Urinary antiseptics include hexylresorcinol, mandelic acid, hexamine (for acid urine; not effective in alkaline urine), buchu.

Urinary Bladder

In some animals the bladder is situated in the pelvis, but in the dog and cat it is placed further forward in the abdomen, while in the pig and ox it may be almost entirely abdominal when distended. The size of the organ varies with the breed and sex of the animal, and its capacity depends upon the individual. Two small tubes – called ureters – lead into the bladder, one from each kidney, and the larger, thicker urethra conveys urine from it to the exterior. The constricted portion from which the urethra takes origin is called the neck of the bladder, and is guarded by a ring of muscular tissue – the sphincter.

Structure The wall of the bladder is somewhat similar to that of the intestine, and consists of a mucous lining on the inside, possessing flat, pavement-like epithelial cells; a loose submucous layer of fibrous tissue very rich in blood vessels; a strong, complicated muscular coat in which the fibres are arranged in many directions; and on the surface an incomplete peritoneal coat covering the organ. In places this peritoneal covering is folded across to parts of the abdominal or pelvic wall in the form of ligaments which retain the bladder in its position.

In young animals the bladder is elongated and narrow, and reaches much further forward than it does in the adult. In the unborn fetus its forward extremity communicates with the outside of the body until just before birth, when the passage becomes closed at the umbilicus, or navel, and the bladder shrinks backwards.

Urinary Bladder, Diseases of

Cystitis Inflammation of the bladder is often infective in origin, with micro-organisms coming either from the kidneys via the ureters, or, in the female, in the reverse direction – i.e. via the urethra from an infected vagina.

Leptospirosis is a common cause of nephritis and cystitis in farm animals and in dogs. *E. coli* is another common pathogen in dogs; and *Corynebacterium suis* in pigs.

In dogs, cystitis is occasionally found to be due to the bladder worm *Capillaria plica*; and in cats to *C. feliscati*. The parasites' eggs may be found in the urinary sediment. Anthelmintics may be used for treatment.

Inflammation of the bladder may be caused by the abrasive action of a sand-like crystalline deposit as in the FELINE UROLOGICAL SYNDROME or, to a lesser extent, by sizeable urinary calculi.

Signs In acute cystitis, small quantities of urine may be passed frequently, with signs of pain and/or straining on each occasion. Blood may be seen in the urine. The larger animals may walk with their hind legs slightly abducted, and the back is often arched in all animals.

Treatment This will naturally vary according to the cause. An appropriate antibiotic may be used to overcome infection, along perhaps with a urinary antiseptic. Urine acidifiers, such as ascorbic acid or ammonium chloride, or alkalisers, such as potassium citrate or sodium bicarbonate, may also be used to adjust the pH of the urine. Pain-relievers may be needed.

Urinary calculi These, associated with high grain rations and the use of oestrogen, produce heavy losses among fattening cattle and sheep in the feed-lots of the USA and Canada. However, this condition does not seem to present the same problem in the barley beef units in this country, although outbreaks do occur in sheep fed high grain rations. The inclusion of 4 per cent NaCl in the diet decreased the incidence of urinary calculi.

In male calves and lambs, crystalline deposits of magnesium ammonium phosphate cause urethral obstruction if the animals are receiving too high a level of magnesium supplement in their concentrate feed. (See URETHRAL OBSTRUCTION.)

Urinary calculi may occur in an individual animal irrespective of its diet, or of hormone implants. There may be one large calculus present in the bladder, or several small ones, or the crystalline sand-like deposit already mentioned. In such cases, although hyaluronidase might be tried, treatment usually has to be surgical, i.e. cystotomy.

Rupture of the bladder This condition is usually quickly fatal, and is brought about by a painful over-distension of the bladder due to urethral obstruction.

Tumours These may cause difficulty in passing urine, and sometimes the presence of blood in the urine.

In a study of 70 cases in the dog, no urinary signs were found in 9. In the other 61, signs included haematuria, dysuria, tenesmus, incontinence, and polyuria. Sixty-two dogs had primary tumours; 44 of these were carcinomas. Several papillomas were found during cystotomy for urinary calculi.

Urinary Calculi
(see above, and under URINARY BLADDER, DISEASES OF)

Urinary Incontinence in Dogs and Cats
(see INCONTINENCE)

Urinary Organs
(see KIDNEYS; URETER; BLADDER; URETHRA)

Urine
A brief outline of the formation of urine is given under KIDNEYS – Function. (See also HOMEOSTASIS.)

Not only are waste products removed from the bloodstream by the kidneys, but most poisons taken into the body are eliminated from the system by way of the urine; thus, quinine, morphine, chloroform, carbolic acid, iodides, and strychnine can be recognised in the urine by means of appropriate tests, while there is abundant evidence to show that during bacterial diseases, the kidneys eliminate toxins.

Specific gravity The specific gravity of the urine of animals varies between wide limits; for average purposes the following figures are given:

	Lowest	Average	Highest
Horse	1014	1036	1050
Cow	1006	1020	1030
Sheep	1006	1010	1015
Pig	1003	1015	1025
Dog and cat	1016	—	1060

Reaction The urine of the herbivorous animals is usually alkaline, and that of the flesh-eating animals, acid. The alkalinity in herbivores is due to the salts of the organic acids that are taken in with the vegetable diet, such as malic, citric, tartaric, and succinic; these acids are converted into carbonates in the body, and these latter are excreted in solution. In the case of some foods, such as hay and oats, an acid urine may be produced when they are fed to the horse. In the carnivorous animals the acidity is due to sodium acid phosphate. The pig's urine may be acid or alkaline according to the nature of its food.

Amount The quantities of urine excreted depend upon many factors, among which may be noted: season, diet, amount of water consumed, condition of the animal, secretion of milk, pregnancy, age, and size of the animal. (See also PREGNANCY DIAGNOSIS.)

The following are average figures of the amounts excreted during 24 hours:

Horse: 3 to 11 litres (5 to 20 pints), average 5 litres (9 pints).

Cow: 5.7 to 22 litres (10 to 40 pints), average 12.5 litres (22 pints).

Sheep: 285 to 855 ml (0.5 to 1.5 pints), average 570 ml (1 pint).

Pig: 1.4 to 8 litres (2.5 to 14 pints), average 4.5 litres (8 pints).

Dog: 440 to 995 ml (0.75 to 1.75 pints), average 680 ml (1.25 pints).

Abnormal constituents of urine

Albumin may be excreted when there is some disease of the kidneys. Sugar is found in diabetes and it is also found in smaller amounts after an animal has been fed on a diet that is too rich in sugar. In this latter case – known as glycosuria – the sugar disappears when the feeding is corrected. Pus and tube-casts are the signs of inflammation or ulceration in some part of the urinary system. Bile in the urine is a sign that there is some obstruction to the outflow of bile into the intestines, and that the bile is being reabsorbed into the bloodstream and excreted by the kidneys.

Urine-Drinking, or Licking

Urine-drinking, or licking, by cattle may be a symptom of sodium deficiency. (See 'LICKING SYNDROME'.)

Urine Scald

Loss of hair and inflammation of the skin caused by persistent wetting with urine.

Urine-Spraying by Cats

This is the normal method used by the male cat to mark out his territory. Under natural conditions this may be some 2 km² (5 acres) or so in extent. The territory-marking serves as a warning to other males to keep out, and perhaps also as an invitation to females in oestrus to enter.

Urine-spraying is not confined to the entire male, but may also be indulged in by the entire female, and even by neuters of either sex. It may also be an expression of sexual excitement.

Spraying indoors is often the result of the invasion of a cat's territory by an intruder such as a new person (if the owner marries, for example), the arrival of a baby or another pet. The appearance of a cat at the window of a house or in the garden may trigger spraying. Another cause is the installation of a cat flap, if the flap does not keep other cats out of the house. A move to a new home, or even the rearrangement of furniture, may initiate urine-spraying indoors. Spraying is common in households where several cats are kept.

Hormonal drugs such as progestins, which block the effects of male hormones, can be used in male cats. Tranquillisers may be of benefit in more intractable cases. If a particular area is targeted, the cat's food bowl can be placed there, as cats will not spray close to where they eat. Feline pheromone, in an aerosol, is said to inhibit the cat's desire to spray.

Urinometer

An instrument designed for the estimation of the specific gravity of urine.

Urogenital Papilla

A small projection at the urogenital opening of fish. Damage or infection at this area can lead to problems in shedding eggs or semen ('milt').

Urolithiasis

The formation of calculi (stones), or of a crystalline sand-like deposit, in the urinary system. A bacterial or viral infection may precede or follow the condition. (See URETHRAL OBSTRUCTION; URINARY BLADDER, DISEASES OF; FELINE URINARY SYNDROME; and URETHRA, DISEASES OF.)

Uroliths

The mineral composition of 2700 of these were studied, after their removal from dogs. Their composition was struvite in nearly 60 per cent of those tested. In horses the most common mineral was calcium carbonate.

Urotropine

(see HEXAMINE)

Urticaria (Nettle Rash)

Urticaria (nettle rash) is a disease of the skin in which small areas of the surface become raised in weals of varying sizes. It occurs in horses, cattle (when it is often called blaines), pigs, and dogs.

Causes The condition is not necessarily specific. It may follow exposure to the leaves of the stinging nettle (hence one of its names); insect bites may produce it; it may be associated with diet; it may occur during the course of certain specific conditions, such as purpura, dourine, influenza, etc. Urticaria is usually, if not always, of an allergic nature.

Factitious urticaria, common in the dog but not recorded in the cat, is a term for an abnormal tendency for the skin to weal when rubbed or scratched.

Signs As a rule there is little to be seen beyond the local swellings of the skin. These may vary in size from a pea to a walnut, and are generally more or less almond-shaped. They are painless to the touch, show no oozing discharge, are scattered irregularly over the whole body, and sometimes involve the skin of the eyelids, nostrils, and perineum. In cattle especially they may attain a great size in the throat region and produce difficulty in breathing.

Treatment Consists of the use of ANTIHISTA-MINES, a light diet, and calamine lotion. An antibiotic may be used to prevent infection from occurring.

Ustu Virus

Ustu virus is closely related to WEST NILE VIRUS. An outbreak in Vienna in 2000 is thought to have been carried by swallows migrating from Africa. The disease is transmitted by mosquitoes, In humans, the signs are fever and a rash, but serious illness has not been reported. Humans and primates are terminal hosts for the virus and so are not a source of infection for other animals.

Uterine Infections

These are discussed under UTERUS, DISEASES OF and INFERTILITY. A list of the principal organisms which infect the uterus in the various species is given under ABORTION; but for the mare, see EQUINE GENITAL INFECTIONS.

Uterus

The uterus is a Y-shaped organ consisting of a body and two horns, or cornua; it is lined by an elaborate mucous membrane which presents special features in different species of animals. The uterus lies in the abdomen below the rectum and at a higher level than the bladder. It becomes continuous with the vagina posteriorly. Its most posterior portion, known as the cervix, usually lies partly in the pelvis. From the tip of each horn to the ovary on the corresponding side runs the Fallopian tube or oviduct, which conducts the ova from the ovary into the uterus.

In the human female the body is large and horns, for practical purposes, do not exist. In rabbits the 2 horns open into the vagina separately. The uteri of domesticated animals are intermediate between these types.

The walls consist of 3 coats: a peritoneal covering on the outside continuous with the rest of the peritoneum; a thick muscular wall arranged in 2 layers, the fibres on the outside being longitudinal and those on the inside circular; an innermost coat, which is mucous membrane. This latter is very important, since it is by its agency that the ovum and the sperms are nourished before they fuse; it is through the mucous membrane that nutrients and oxygen are conveyed from dam to fetus, and that much of the waste products leave the fetal circulation to pass into the maternal bloodstream. It consists of epithelial cells, amongst which lie the uterine glands which secrete the so-called 'uterine milk' serving to nourish the newly fertilised ovum.

The most posterior extremity of the uterus is called the os uteri, and this forms the opening into the cervix uteri, which is a thick-walled canal guarding entrance into the cavity of the body of the uterus. Normally this is almost or completely shut, but during oestrus it slackens, and during parturition it becomes fully opened to allow exit of the fetus. The uterus is held in position by means of a fold of peritoneum attached to the roof of the abdomen, which carries blood vessels, nerves, etc. This is known as the 'broad ligament'; it is capable of a considerable amount of stretching.

The mare The shape of the uterus of the mare most nearly approaches that of the human being. It possesses a large body and comparably small horns. During pregnancy the fetus generally lies in horn and body. The mucous membrane is corrugated into folds.

The cow The body is less in size than the horns, which are long, tapering, and curved downwards, outwards, backwards, and upwards to end within the pelvis at about the level of the cervix. The fetus lies in the body and one horn in single pregnancy, and when twins are present each usually occupies one horn and a part of the body. The mucous membrane presents upon its inner surface a large number (100 upwards) of mushroom-shaped projections – cotyledons. The fetal membranes are attached to the domelike free surface of the cotyledons, in which are a large number of crypts, which receive projections called villi from the outer surface of the chorion.

The ewe has a uterus similar to that of the cow except that it is smaller and that the cotyledons are cup-shaped.

The sow has a small uterine body and a pair of long convoluted horns that resemble pieces of intestine. The mucous membrane is ridged but has no cotyledons. The young lie in the horns only.

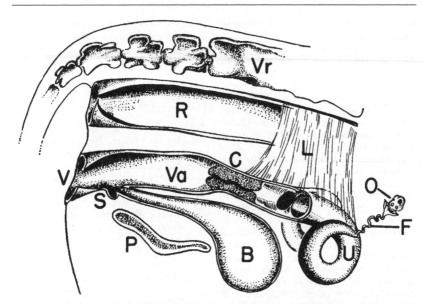

The reproductive tract of the cow (side view). *B*, Urinary bladder; *C*, cervix; *F*, Fallopian tube; *L*, broad ligament; *O*, ovary; *P*, pelvic bone (*os coxae*); *R*, rectum; *S*, suburethral diverticulum; *U*, uterine horn; *V*, vestibule; *Va*, vagina; *Vr*, vertebral column. (Hafez, *Reproduction in Farm Animals*, Lea & Febiger as reproduced in R. D. Frandson, *Anatomy and Physiology of Farm Animals*, Baillière, Tindall.)

The bitch and cat have uteri with comparatively short bodies and long, straight, divergent horns that run towards the kidneys of the corresponding sides.

(See PREGNANCY; PARTURITION.)

Uterus, Diseases of

Inflammation of the uterus (metritis) may be acute or chronic, localised (e.g. confined to the cervix), or involving more than one uterine tissue.

A list of uterine infections giving rise to infertility and abortion in the various species will be found under ABORTION, but for the mare, see under EQUINE GENITAL INFECTIONS.

The mare

Acute Metritis This may occur either before or after foaling. When it takes place prior to the act it is usually associated with the death of the foal and its subsequent abortion, with or without discharge of the whole or a part of the membranes. In such cases the inflammatory condition may persist in an acute form and cause the death of the mare, or it may assume a chronic form after the abortion and render the mare incapable of further breeding; other cases are followed by recovery. Acute metritis occurring after normal foaling may arise through the conveyance of infection into the uterus by the arms or hands

of the attendants, or by the ropes, instruments, or other appliances that are used to assist the birth of the foal; or it may be the direct result of retained membranes that undergo bacterial decomposition. (This may happen after a large part, but not all, of the fetal membranes have come away.)

Signs Acute metritis is a severe and often fatal condition. Within 24 to 48 hours, the mare becomes greatly distressed and loses all interest in the foal. She lies most of the time and refuses food; her temperature is usually high. Greyish blood-flecked discharge escapes from the vagina and soils the tail and hindquarters. The mare may become tucked up in her abdomen and stands with her back arched.

LAMINITIS may develop.

Prevention During foaling and after the act the greatest attention should be paid to the cleanliness of everything that is to come into contact with the genital tract of the mare. The attendant's fingernails should be trimmed short, and the hands and arms should be well scrubbed with soap and water containing some antiseptic, such as Dettol. Finally the hand and arm should be lubricated with a suitable preparation marketed for this purpose. All appliances that are to be used should be boiled and kept in a pail of hot water when not actually in use.

One other factor is of the greatest importance: after a mare foals, the fetal membranes should be given attention. Normally they are discharged by means of a few comparatively mild labour pains within an hour of the birth of the foal. If however they are retained for longer than this period, the person in attendance should suspect that something may be wrong and seek veterinary advice.

In other cases a series of violent pains may commence, when the bulk of the membranes are passed to the outside, where they hang suspended. Should this happen a sack or sheet should be placed under the dependent mass, and held so as to support the weight and relieve the tension on that portion that is still retained in the uterus. This is necessary lest the weight of the external membranes causes a tearing away from the non-separated part. **Gentle** traction should then be exerted upon the imprisoned portion; as a rule it will gradually detach itself and come to the outside. If no progress is made, veterinary assistance should be sought promptly.

Injections of PITUITRIN may obviate manual removal of the fetal membranes. A synthetic oestrogen may be preferred. (See HORMONE THERAPY.)

Regarding complete retention of the fetal membranes – when only a very small portion is seen hanging from the vagina – professional help should be obtained if there is no sign of any attempt at expulsion within 4 to 6 hours after foaling.

Generally speaking, membranes that have remained in position for 8 to 12 hours are starting to decompose, and decomposition means bacterial infection of the uterus (i.e. metritis) in almost every case.

Treatment The case must be considered most serious. The use of antibiotics or one of the sulfa drugs is indicated. (See also under NURSING.) Any retained fetal membrane must be removed from the uterus by hand and as much discharge as possible cleared out. A solution of acriflavine, proflavine, or brilliant green, 1 part in 1000 of boiled water, or some other suitable non-irritant antiseptic solution at blood heat, is douched into the cavity of the uterus by a length of rubber tubing, and, after allowing it to act for 2 to 5 minutes, is syphoned off. A special 2-way tube is sometimes used for this purpose – the solution entering by one channel and leaving by the other. When all the fluid has been removed, an antiseptic pessary may be inserted. When complications such as LAMINITIS or PNEUMONIA co-exist, they must receive separate attention.

Chronic Metritis This may originate as a sequel to an acute attack in some cases, but more commonly it is directly due to an injury or infection which is not sufficiently severe to produce an acute attack.

Signs There may be a general unthriftiness following upon foaling. The mare's appetite is capricious, but her thirst is unimpaired. The temperature fluctuates a degree or two above normal. There may or may not be a dirty, sticky, grey, or pus-like discharge from the vagina, which causes irritation and frequent erections of the clitoris. The mare resents handling of the genital organs, but if the lips of the vulva are gently separated the mucous membrane is seen to be inflamed and swollen.

In other cases the pus collects in the cavity of the uterus and is retained there through closure of the os. (See PYOMETRA.) It sometimes happens that after the pus has collected for a certain period the os suddenly opens and 4.5 litres (1 gallon) or more of pus is discharged. The os then closes once more. Intervals between these evacuations may vary from a few days to 3 or 4 weeks. The mare's general condition shows an improvement immediately following a sudden discharge of pus, but as it re-accumulates she relapses into her former chronic state. Chronic metritis may get gradually worse, and the mare dies. Cases taken in time usually recover with treatment, but further breeding is often impossible.

Treatment An early opportunity should be taken to evacuate the pus from the uterus, by douching and siphonage, or by irrigation as already described under 'Acute metritis'.

Sulfa drugs or antibiotics may be used.

It should be emphasised that expert advice should be sought at the earliest opportunity.

(See also CONTAGIOUS EQUINE METRITIS.)

The cow In the following brief account, much of what has been said in relation to the mare must be understood to apply to the cow as well, and only the main differences will be stated.

Acute Metritis In some cases where birth of the calf has taken place easily and naturally, metritis supervenes in the course of the first week or 10 days after calving, but in the majority of cases there has been some injury or infection at, or shortly after, parturition. Retention of the fetal membranes, which is so much more common in the cow than in other animals, is very often the contributory factor to an attack of acute metritis. The conveyance of infection by the hands and arms of the attendant, in his capacity of *accoucheur*, or insemination of a cow not in oestrus, are other causes.

Signs The cow generally becomes obviously affected between the 2nd and 8th day after calving. The vulval lips swell and are painful when touched; the lining membrane of the vagina is intensely reddened and swollen. There are frequent and painful attempts at the passage of urine, the temperature rises to 41.5° or 42°C (107° or 108°F), the appetite is lost and there is a gritting of the teeth. Rumination is suppressed, the pulse is hard and fast, the milk secretion falls off or stops altogether. A discharge appears at the vulva.

Treatment Acute metritis in the cow should be looked upon as a contagious disease and precautions taken to prevent infection being conveyed to other cows that are soon due to calve. Actual treatment is similar to that as applied to the mare.

Chronic Metritis very often follows an acute attack in the cow. The animal partially recovers, the more acute symptoms subside, and there is apparently little or no pain. Milk yield may be reasonable, and the animal may appear bright. The general health, however, remains indifferent and there may be either a constant or an intermittent discharge from the vulva, which soils the tail and hindquarters, and has in many cases a putrid smell.

Chronic metritis may be due to *Brucella abortus* (see BRUCELLOSIS), *Trichomonas fetus*, *Actinomyces pyogenes*, or *Campylobacter fetus*, among other organisms. Another form of chronic metritis that attacks cattle is seen in virgin heifers that have never bred.

Pyometra (a collection of pus in the uterus) may result from infection introduced during natural service, insemination, or at or after calving. Treatment with cloprestenol may be helpful.

Treatment of chronic metritis in the cow is much the same as that in the mare, but see also under HORMONE THERAPY.

The ewe, sow and goat What has been said in respect to the larger animals applies to these animals to a great extent. It should be remembered that flesh from an animal that is suffering from a severe inflammatory condition, such as metritis, is not fit for human food. (See also SOW'S MILK, ABSENCE OF.)

The bitch and cat In these carnivores, owing to the diffused placenta, and to the consequent sudden stripping bare of protective covering of a large surface, inflammation of the uterus is very prone to follow protracted or difficult parturition, especially when manual assistance from unskilled persons has been undertaken. As in other animals, an acute and a chronic form are recognised.

Acute Metritis may follow difficult whelpings, and retention of one or more fetal membranes. The membrane most commonly retained is that which belonged to the fetus that was born last and occupied the extremity of one of the horns of the uterus.

Signs The onset of inflammation of the uterus generally occurs within a week after whelping, but some cases are delayed a little longer than this, especially in cats. A rise in temperature, increased pulse and respiration rates, dullness, disinclination for movement, and an absence of appetite occur.

Cats and dogs seem to get ease from the pain by sitting crouched in an upright position on their hocks and elbows, and this posture is almost continually assumed. A discharge appears at the vulva. Vomiting may occur. The secretion of milk ceases and the puppies or kittens become clamorous for food. The sides of the abdomen are held tense and rigid, and any attempt at handling these parts is resisted. The animal may groan or grunt if the flanks are firmly pressed between the hands.

Treatment The use of antibiotics or sulfonamides is important. The uterus is syringed out with a non-irritant antiseptic such as dilute cetrimide solution; and pituitrin, ergometrine or dinoprost is given. Antiseptic pessaries may be introduced into the uterus. (See NURSING; NORMAL SALINE; ANTIBIOTICS.) The puppies or kittens should be removed from their mother, and may be reared either by hand or through the agency of a foster-mother.

Chronic Metritis is very common in the smaller animals, and is sometimes the sequel of an acute attack that has never completely cleared up. The cervix remains closed in most cases, so that the uterus becomes filled with pus (PYOMETRA) and the abdomen consequently enlarges. It is this increase in size that first draws attention to the condition, as a rule.

Treatment In cases of pyometra where some pus is coming away, a course of pituitrin injections may be useful (and it may be tried even where the cervix is closed). (See PITUITRIN.) Stilboestrol is no longer an alternative in EU countries. A 2-way catheter may be used to wash out the pus. Penicillin or acriflavine may be used for irrigation of the uterus, and antibiotics or sulfonamides systemically. Ovario-hysterectomy is indicated in a number of cases but should not be postponed until toxaemia is far advanced or the animal too weak to stand the operation. Shock is severe.

Stricture of the cervix is one of the results of an inflammatory condition of this part. When inflammation has been severe, a certain amount of fibrous tissue is laid down around the canal, contracts and causes a narrowing of the passage.

Treatment is described under 'RINGWOMB' – a term used only for stricture in ewes, in which it is most often seen.

Tumours Benign tumours include lipoma, fibroma, papilloma, myoma, and haemangioma (rare). Malignant tumours include lymphosarcoma, adenocarcinoma, and squamous cell carcinoma.

Prolapse A partial or complete turning-inside-out of the organ, in which the inside comes to the outside through the lips of the vulva and hangs down, sometimes as far as the hocks. When the displacement is only slight nothing may be seen at the outside – as, for example, when one horn only is inverted into the body of the uterus. It is most common in ruminants, less frequent in the mare.

Signs With an incomplete inversion, the uterine horn that carried the fetus becomes turned in upon itself like the finger of a glove, but it remains inside the passages, and nothing is seen to the outside. The animal is distressed for a time, paws the ground, stamps, lies and rises from the ground frequently, and a series of mild or violent labour pains occurs. She may settle down in a short while, but in a few hours she generally has a repeated attack, when the bulk of the uterus will be expelled to the outside of the body. In the early stages of such a case the real nature of the condition is seldom suspected unless a large pear-shaped mass is seen hanging from the vulva.

The state of the mucous membrane lining of the uterus, which in the prolapse is of course on the outside of the mass, serves as a rough guide to the length of time that has elapsed since the accident occurred. For the first 2 or 3 hours the mucous membrane appears moist and of a reddish or brownish colour over the whole surface in the mare and sow. In the cow, sheep, and goat, the general surface is red or pink, but the cotyledons show as deep-red mushroom-like eminences scattered over the outside of the tumour. In the bitch and cat there is a wide dark-brown zone. Later, the surface becomes dry – owing to its exposure to the air – and becomes deep reddish, violet, or purple, according to the amount of congestion and strangulation.

In the cow the whole of the outer upper surface may be covered with the faeces that are passed as the result of the severe straining. In all animals – but especially in ruminants – parts of the fetal membranes may be adherent to the outer surface of the mass, and can be easily recognised.

The surface is not sensitive to the touch, but any manipulation of the mass is provocative of further straining.

Various complications may occur. The vagina is always displaced when the prolapse is complete; this obstructs the urethra, and dams back the urine.

Treatment Prolapse of the uterus is always an extremely serious condition in any animal, and in the mare and sow very often proves fatal. A percentage of cows and ewes recover, when the prolapse is replaced without loss of time, and when there are no complications.

When treating a case – in whatever animal – it is absolutely necessary to comply with certain essentials as follows:

(1) The prolapsed uterus must be protected from further damage. To ensure this the animal must be secured at once, and a large sheet or blanket – which has been previously dipped in mild antiseptic solution – must be placed under the mass, and held by 2 men so that the tension is relieved from the neck, and so that it cannot be further contaminated or injured.

(2) The surface of the organ must be carefully cleansed. For this purpose a clean pail containing a warm solution of potassium permanganate and common salt (1 teaspoonful of the former and 100 g (4 oz) of the latter to 4.5 litres (1 gallon) of water) or diluted Dettol or cetrimide solution may be used. All the larger particles of straw, debris, etc., are picked off, and the smaller pieces removed by gentle washing. Care must be taken not to make the surface bleed.

(3) The prolapsed portion must be replaced. To effect this the larger animals may require epidural or general anaesthesia to prevent

the powerful expulsive pains that otherwise accompany the process, and make return difficult. When the animal has been anaesthetised the hindquarters are raised as high as possible by building up the floor with straw bales, by hoisting the hind-legs, or by other means. When the protruded mass is very large and has a distinct neck, the main bulk is raised to a slightly higher level than the external passage, and a process of 'tucking in' is begun near the vulva. This is carried out by the 2 hands – one at either side – using the hands half closed, so that the middle joints of the fingers come into contact with the uterus. The fingertips should not be employed owing to the danger of laceration or even puncture of the walls. The resistance is gradually overcome and the mass eased along the passages back into the pelvis – a labour that often makes great demands upon the strength and endurance of the operator, and frequently takes an hour or more to effect. Moreover, when once the organ has been returned, unless it is straightened out into its normal position, it may be reinverted a 2nd time.

(4) Measures must be taken to retain the uterus in position: the animal may be given an analgesic or a tranquilliser to lessen the chance of subsequent straining; and sutures may be inserted.

Bedding, etc. is arranged so that the animal is compelled to both stand and lie with the hindquarters raised above the level of the forequarters. This throws the abdominal contents forwards, and helps to maintain the uterus in place. It is, of course, mainly applicable to mares and cows. Bandages may prove helpful.

Amputation of the prolapsed uterus becomes necessary when all attempts at its reduction are futile; when the organ has received so much injury or has become so decomposed and gangrenous that it would be certainly fatal to return it to the abdomen; or when prolapse occurs time after time in spite of all attempts at retention.

In a survey of 103 cases of uterine prolapse, 19 cows died within 24 hours of replacement of the uterus.

Hydrops amnii A condition in which the quantity of amniotic (see AMNION) fluid is greatly in excess of normal. It is often associated with a similar condition of the ALLANTOIS, which is sometimes erroneously called hydrops amnii.

Occurring mainly in cattle, and only rarely in other farm/domestic animals, hydrops amnii is often associated with 'bulldog' calves and monsters. Sometimes a recessive gene is responsible. It may also occur when crossing an American bison on a cow, i.e. when producing hybrids.

Where oedema of the allantois alone occurs, the cause may be disease of the uterus, especially of the caruncles.

Sometimes oedema of both the fetal membranes and the fetus occurs. In mild cases the condition may not be suspected until calving, when an unusually large amount of fluid will be expelled. Retention of fetal membranes and subsequent metritis may follow.

In severe cases, the cow may lose appetite, appear distressed, be constipated, with rumination adversely affected or depressed. Abdominal swelling may suggest bloat. In extreme cases, the cow may be unable to get to her feet. Cases of dislocation of the hips or backward extension of the hind-legs have been seen in combined fetal and fetal membrane oedema involving amnion and allantois, and uterus (hydrops uteri).

Rupture, involving the uterine wall, may occur before or during parturition in any animal, during the reduction of a torsion or prolapse, or, in the bitch or cat, as the result of a car accident. (See ECTOPIC, PREGNANCY.)

Torsion, or twisting, of the uterus is commonest in the cow and other ruminants, and rare in other domestic animals. This accident consists of a partial or complete rotation of the uterus around its long axis, and usually involves the neck of the organ.

Signs As a rule there is no indication of the presence of the displacement until parturition is due to commence. The animal is then seen to prepare herself in the usual way, but the preliminary labour pains are exceptionally feeble and separated by long intervals. After the lapse of some hours – when the 'waterbag' and other signs of the approaching act should have become evident in an ordinary case – nothing happens. The animal is slightly disturbed, shows an occasional pain, walks round aimlessly, may feed spasmodically, but does not appear to be greatly distressed. This condition may persist for as long as 48 hours. In other cases the animal is very much distressed. It has spasms of violent and painful uterine contraction.

Treatment In the small animals laparotomy is performed, and the twisted organ untwisted. In the cow, it may be possible to rectify the twist by rolling the animal.

U

Congenital defects (see the diagram under INFERTILITY; also HYDROMETRA)

Uveitis

Inflammation of the uvea (iris, ciliary body and choroid coat of the eyeball).

Uvula

This is the small downward projection that is found on the free edge of the soft palate of the pig. It is not present in the other domesticated animals.

Vaccination

A method of producing active immunity against a specific infection by means of inoculation with a vaccine, i.e. a preparation of the necessary antigen(s). (See IMMUNITY; IMMUNISATION; IMMUNE RESPONSE; VACCINE.)

Vaccination in mammals is normally carried out by inoculating individual animals. The method of administration depends on the type of vaccine. Most inactivated vaccines are injected intramuscularly or subcutaneously; temperature-sensitive live vaccines may be administered as drops into the nasal passages; vaccines against husk are given orally.

Mass vaccination of poultry against Newcastle disease may be achieved by dispersing aerosols of vaccine over the heads of the birds with fine spray pumps or adding vaccine to the drinking water. Some fish are vaccinated by dipping the fish in a solution of the vaccine. Fox populations in Europe have been vaccinated against rabies by impregnating chicken heads or other baits and spreading them in known fox runs. Multiple-component vaccines containing antigens against a number of diseases are available. For example, sheep can be simultaneously immunised against pulpy kidney disease, lamb dysentery, braxy, blackleg, black disease, struck, *Clostridium oedematiens* infection and tetanus by a single 8-in-1 vaccine.

(In connection with foot-and-mouth disease, see also RING VACCINATION.)

Vaccine

When an animal is inoculated with a vaccine as protection against a specific disease, e.g. blackleg, this is carried out with the object of stimulating production of antibodies in its system, which will confer active immunity against blackleg organisms.

Vaccines may be prepared from live micro-organisms; from inactivated (killed) micro-organisms; from genetically engineered subunits of the pathogenic fraction of the organism; or from toxoids – heat- or chemically-treated micro-organisms that have lost their virulence but retain their antigenicity, i.e. ability to create resistance to disease.

Live vaccines are vaccines prepared from bacteria or viruses whose virulence is reduced by heat, chemicals or passage through an animal other than the normal host species. For example, cattle plague vaccine may be prepared from the virus *passaged* through (i.e. grown in) chick embryos. Occasionally the live viruses used are related but non-pathogenic strains, useful because they will stimulate antibody production but will not produce the disease.

Viruses may be inactivated by phenol or ultra-violet rays, for example; or they may be modified in some way, such as by artificially induced mutation, to produce a temperature-sensitive virus which will replicate in the nose but not in the lungs. Such a virus vaccine can be administered by nasal spray.

Tissue culture vaccines – live vaccines grown on cell cultures – are used in the prevention of canine distemper, rabies, etc., and in treatment of benign skin papillomata (warts) of cattle.

Vaccines are sometimes used for treatment as well as for prevention of a particular disease.

X-irradiated worm larvae vaccine is used in the prevention of PARASITIC BRONCHITIS.

It is important that, in the commercial production of live vaccines involving the use of chicken embryos (or of tissue cultures derived from them), contaminant viruses are eliminated. For example, the avian leukosis virus has contaminated distemper vaccine and would represent a risk to vaccinated poultry if contaminating vaccines for them. Scrapie was accidentally spread by an early louping-ill virus contaminated by the scrapie agent.

It is essential that vaccines are stored under suitable conditions of temperature, etc.; that they are not used after the expiry date shown on the package; that where 2 doses are stated to be necessary, both are given – and at the correct interval. Failure to observe these rules can mean that the vaccinated animal does not become an immunised animal; it has led to dogs presumed properly vaccinated against rabies becoming rabid after exposure to a natural infection. (See also INJECTIONS; GENETIC ENGINEERING.)

Inactivated vaccines are prepared from killed micro-organisms that retain sufficient antigenic activity to promote immunity. They are not as potent as live vaccines, and 2 doses at specified intervals are usually necessary to produce effective immunity. Inactivated vaccines often contain an adjuvant, usually an aluminium salt such as aluminium hydroxide, which enhances the immune reaction. Some are water-based, others formulated in an oily medium. Oil-based vaccines can cause serious reactions if accidentally self-injected into the operator. Leptospirosis vaccine is an example.

Subunit vaccines are genetically engineered so that only the antigenic fraction of a pathogen is utilised. The vaccine does not cause infection but does stimulate immunity. Feline leukaemia vaccine is an example; another is Aujeszky's disease vaccine. The virus component of the subunit vaccine has difficulty in penetrating the cells of the vaccinated animal; it does not multiply well within the cells and the animal does not shed the virus. By testing for the fraction missing from the vaccinial strain of virus, a vaccinated animal can be determined from one carrying the infection.

Toxoid vaccines are produced by treating toxins from micro-organisms so that their harmful effects are removed but the antigenic properties remain. Tetanus vaccine is an example.

Vaccinia Virus

This term may refer to the virus of naturally occurring cow-pox, or to a strain which has undergone mutation and was used for vaccination against smallpox. (See POX.)

Vacuole

A cavity within a cell.

Vacuum-Dipping of Eggs

A technique used in assisting the eradication of *Mycoplasma* spp. in poultry. Fertile eggs are dipped in a concentrated solutions of antibiotic (usually tylosin) and subjected to a negative pressure. Some of the air in the egg's air pocket is thus extracted and about 0.5 ml of antibiotic drawn through the shell into the egg and absorbed. This process is more effective in helping to eliminate *M. gallisepticum* than other mycoplasmas.

Vagina

The vagina extends from the cervix of the uterus to the vulva. Vaginal mucus is altered in character during pregnancy, a fact which can be made use of in pregnancy diagnosis. (For inflammation of the vagina, see VAGINITIS.)

An artificial vagina is used at AI centres for the collection of semen.

Vaginal prolapse in ewes This may precede lambing by up to 55 days, but most cases occur within the last 21 days of pregnancy.

Rupture of the vagina, with protrusion of the intestine and rapid death, occurs not uncommonly in ewes of a large breed, of mature age, carrying a twin – a week or two before lambing is due. Bulky foods – swedes, turnips, kale – are often involved.

Vaginoureteral fistula This has been recorded in dogs and cats, as a complication of ovariohysterectomy or a caesarean operation, and leads to urinary incontinence. It has been suggested that the fistula may occur following accidental ligation of the ureter during surgery, or because the ureter becomes involved in an inflammatory adhesion originating in the vaginal stump.

Intermittent haemorrhage occasionally occurs in mares having very prominent varicose veins at the dorsal aspect of the vulva-vaginal area; it does not appear to affect health or fertility. Persistent vulval haemorrhage from varicose veins of the dorsal wall of the vagina has also been described. It yields to local haemostatic treatment.

Vaginitis

Inflammation of the vagina. (See under INFERTILITY – Diseases of the genital organs in female; also 'WHITES'; EPIDIDYMITIS – Epivag; VULVO-VAGINITIS, GRANULAR; PROLAPSE.)

Vagotomy

Severing of the vagus nerve. (See HYPERTROPHIC OSTEOPATHY.)

Vagus (Pneumogastric Nerve)

The vagus (pneumogastric nerve) is the 10th cranial nerve. This nerve is remarkable for its great length, and for the attachments which it forms with other nerves and with the sympathetic trunks. It arises from the side of the medulla, passes out of the skull, and runs down to the jugular furrow of the neck, where, along with the sympathetic, it accompanies the carotid artery to the entrance to the chest. From this point the right and left vagi differ from each other in their course. They both pass through the chest cavity, giving branches to the pharynx (which run up the neck again), to the heart, bronchi, oesophagus, etc. Each nerve then splits into 2 parts and the 2 upper branches fuse with each other to form the dorsal trunk, the lower branches behaving similarly to form the ventral trunk. These 2 branches now pass through the diaphragm, with the oesophagus, into the abdominal cavity, and end by giving branches to the stomach, duodenum, liver, and various ganglia nearby. (See Parasympathetic system under CENTRAL NERVOUS SYSTEM – Autonomic; also BRAIN.) (See GUTTURAL POUCH DISEASE.)

Valgus

A bone growth-plate defect. (See under BONE, DISEASES OF.)

Valine

One of the essential amino acids.

V

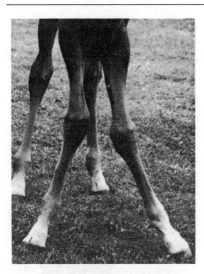

One-month-old foal with bilateral carpal valgus. (With acknowledgements to Professor L. C. Vaughan and the Royal Veterinary College.)

Valves

Valves are found in the heart, veins, lymph vessels, etc., and serve the purpose of ensuring that the fluids will only circulate in one direction. (See HEART; VEINS; ILEOCAECAL.)

Valvular Disease

(see HEART DISEASES)

Vampire Bats

Vampire bats are important transmitters of rabies in parts of South and Central America, the West Indies, etc. The bat laps blood from the wounds inflicted with its upper incisor teeth on cattle, horses, etc. In Mexico infected vampires have made necessary the preventive inoculation of 800,000 cattle a year. Trypanosomiasis can also be transmitted by vampire bats. Vampire bats imported into the UK remain in quarantine for the rest of their life.

Vanadium

A trace element essential in minute quantities for the growth of chicks; as little as 10 mg/kg of diet is an overdose that will suppress growth. It works with insulin to increase the amount of glucose and aminoacids taken up by muscle.

Varicose Veins

(see under VEINS)

Varied Diet, Need for

(see DIET AND DIETETICS; AMINO ACIDS; CAT FOODS; DOGS' DIET)

Variocele

Variocele is a condition in which the veins of one or both testicles are greatly distended.

Variola (Pox)

Variola (pox) is the inclusive term for fevers of animals and man, in which a skin eruption takes the form of a 'pock', caused by a POX virus.

Varroasis

Varroasis is a parasitic disease of honey bees, *Apis melifera,* caused by the mite *Varroa jacobsoni.* The mite feeds on the developing larvae and on the adult bees. The result is weak bees and sometimes the death of the queen. Whole hives can be wiped out, causing great economic loss not only to the apiculturalist but also to fruit and arable farmers; beekeepers often supply hives to fruit growers and to fields of rape and linseed. Varroasis is prevalent in the UK and is a NOTIFIABLE DISEASE.

As both parasite and host are arthropods, products used for control of the disease must have a fine division between toxicity to the mite and toxicity to the bee. Suspending strips impregnated with flumethrin or fluvalinate in the hive can be effective. Other treatments include tobacco smoke or a vapourising block containing thymol and aromatic oils. Eradication, however, is difficult. The disease came from Asia, where it does less harm because Asiatic bees groom each other, thus removing the mites. Long term, it has been suggested that European and Asian bees may be cross-bred to try to introduce the grooming habit into the European bee population. A leaflet available from DEFRA gives more details of the disease and its control.

Vas Deferens

(see under TESTICLE)

Vascular

Consisting of, or containing a high proportion of, blood vessels.

Vasculitis Inflammation of a blood vessel.

Vasectomised

A male animal in which the vas deferens has been cut. Such an animal is sterile though it retains its libido and may be used for the detection of oestrus (e.g. in cattle). In breeding catteries one or two toms are sometimes vasectomised for the sake of peace, quiet and contentment of queens not being bred from until a later oestrus.

Sterility does not immediately follow vasectomy (or castration), as some sperms will be in the seminal vesicles and can lead to conception

V

after mating. It may be 3 weeks or more before the animal is sterile.

Vasodilator

Anything which causes dilation of blood vessels. A drug used for this purpose is isoxuprine hydrochloride. (See NAVICULAR DISEASE.)

Vasomotor Nerves

Vasomotor nerves are the small nerve fibres that lie in or upon the walls of the blood vessels and connect the muscle fibres of the middle coat with the nervous system. By the continuous action of the nerves the muscular walls of the vessels are maintained in a moderate state of contraction. Any continuous and generalised increase in this action results in a raising of the blood pressure of the body, while a diminution produces a lowering of the pressure. Such vaso-motor nerves are called vaso-constrictors, but there are vaso-dilators as well. The latter are able to dilate the vessels, and cause either a general or a local fall in the blood pressure, along with an increased supply of blood to the part.

Vasopressin

A hormone secreted by the posterior lobe of the pituitary gland.It is also called ANTIDIURETIC HORMONE (ADH). (See PITUITARY.)

Vector

The carrier which transmits a disease from one animal to another. For example, the mosquito transmits malaria to man and a variety of diseases to animals.

Veins

With one or two exceptions, the veins lie along-side or near to the corresponding arteries – thus the renal vein brings back blood that has been carried to the kidney by the renal artery and lies alongside it. The veins are, however, more numerous and more irregular in their courses than are the arteries, especially on the surface of the body. In regions, such as the cheeks, brain meninges, and in the abdomen and thorax, there are veins arranged quite irrespective of the distribution of the arteries.

Structure A vein is a thin-walled tube which possesses a structure similar to that of an artery, and consists of 3 coats, viz. an outer fibrous, a middle composed of muscular and elastic fibres, and an inner coat composed of an elastic membrane and flattened epithelial cells. If an ordinary vein is split open along its length, there are seen to be a number of flap-like valves attached to its inner surface. These are like little

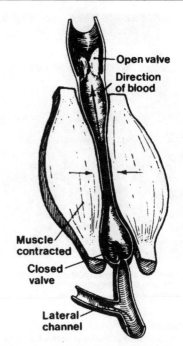

Valves of a vein showing pumping action of adjacent muscles. (Grollman, *The Human Body*, Macmillan Co., as used in R. D. Frandson, *Anatomy and Physiology of Farm Animals*, Baillière, Tindall.)

pockets, and are so arranged that they offer no resistance to the blood when it is flowing in the right direction, but prevent any back-flow. These valves are most numerous in the veins of the limbs, where gravity would naturally tend to produce a back-flow, and least numerous in the veins of the internal organs.

Chief veins The arrangement and relations of the veins are very different in animals of varying species, and even in different individuals, so that only a general description can be given here.

Pulmonary veins – as many as 8 or 9 in the horse and fewer in other animals – return the oxygenated blood from the lungs to the left auri-cle of the heart. They possess no valves. Opening into the right auricle are 4 veins: (1) coronary sinus; (2) anterior vena cava; (3) posterior vena cava; and (4) azygos vein. The coronary sinus is a short thick trunk that discharges the blood used by the heart walls back into the general circulation. The anterior vena cava drains the blood from the head, neck, 2 fore-limbs, and much of the chest wall. It is formed by the con-fluence of the jugulars and the brachial veins, and receives other branches from the neck, vertebral region, and the chest wall. The posterior vena cava drains all the remainder of the body except the region of the diaphragm, the posterior intercostal areas, the oesophagus, and the bronchial tubes, the blood from these parts being collected into the azygos vein which joins the right auricle separately in most animals. The posterior vena cava is formed under the lumbar region by the union of the right and left common iliac veins, which drain the blood from the pelvis and hind legs, and which are distributed in a more or less similar manner to the corresponding arteries of these parts. From here it passes forwards below the lumbar muscles in company with the abdominal aorta, until at the level of the last thoracic vertebra it passes downwards and forwards, past the pancreas, and reaches the liver.

Its further course is partly embedded in the liver substance until it arrives at a special opening in the diaphragm, called the foramen venae cavae, by which it gains the thoracic cavity. From here it passes along in a groove in the right lung to reach the right auricle. Its main tributaries are as follows: (1) lumbar veins, which empty blood from the lumbar muscles, etc.; (2) internal spermatics in the male, and utero-ovarian veins in the female, from the generative organs in either sex; (3) 2 renal veins, one from each kidney, satellites of the corresponding arteries; (4) several large hepatic veins, which return not only blood carried to the liver by the hepatic arteries, but also that which comes from the digestive organs by the portal vein to undergo a second capillary circulation in the liver (see PORTAL VEIN); and (5) phrenic veins returning blood from the diaphragm.

In the venous system, even more so than in the arterial system, there is an intricate arrangement of anastomoses by which, when one vein becomes damaged or diseased, lateral branches from it may enlarge and carry away the excess blood into other veins so that no great hindrance to the return flow of the blood to the heart may be occasioned. If this were not so, the circulation might be from impaired minor causes.

Veins, Diseases of

Those lying near to the surface are frequently injured along with other tissues when contusions or lacerations have been sustained, but so extensive is their communication with neighbouring veins that it is usually possible for these latter to enlarge and undertake the functions of the damaged vessels, and thereby prevent serious consequences. The deeper veins are protected from all but the most severe, and usually fatal, injuries.

Inflammation of a vein, or phlebitis, may follow the collection of blood samples when unclean instruments have been used, or when the resulting skin wound has not received attention. In other cases it follows THROMBOSIS and infection.

Varicose veins are those which have become stretched or dilated to an extent not justified by the blood flow. (See VARIOCELE and under VAGINA.)

Veld Sickness
(see HEARTWATER)

Vena Cava
Each of the 2 large veins that open direct into the right auricle of the heart. (For further details, see under VEINS.)

Thrombosis of the posterior vena cava, which may follow abscess formation in the liver or elsewhere, is in cattle not infrequently followed by the presence of clots in the pulmonary vessels, abscess formation and sometimes erosion of the pulmonary artery wall – giving rise to a fatal haemorrhage. Symptoms may include dullness, rapid breathing, a cough, chest pain, the presence of blood in material coughed up, anaemia, and widespread rhonchi. (See RECUMBENCY.)

Venereal Diseases
Animals, with the exception of the monkey, are not subject to infection by the 2 great human venereal diseases of syphilis and gonorrhoea, but there are several important contagious diseases that can be transmitted from animal to animal by coitus. These include brucellosis, trichomoniasis, *Campylobacter fetus* infection, and infectious vaginitis of cattle, venereal granuloma or venereal tumours of dogs, and dourine or mal du coit of horses. (See PROTOZOA; EPIDIDYMITIS; VULVO-VAGINITIS, GRANULAR; CONTAGIOUS EQUINE METRITIS.)

Venereal Tumours (Infective Granulomata)
Venereal tumours (infective granulomata) characterise a contagious disease of dogs.

Signs In the female the original tumour is a warty excrescence which soon grows and becomes cauliflower-like. In advanced stages there is a large mass of pinkish or greyish-red tissue, which easily bleeds when touched, occupying the greater part of the vaginal passage and

V

often causing a bulging and swelling of the perineal region. A dirty sticky blood-stained discharge accompanies the condition, and the animal's general health suffers. In the male the watery growths usually have a distinct stalk, and are attached to the skin or mucous membrane of the prepuce, or to the penis. (See also under WARTS.)

Venezuelan Equine Encephalomyelitis

A strain recognised in the 1930s. A severe outbreak occurred in Venezuela and Colombia in 1962–4, when thousands of horses died and about 30,000 people were infected. A later outbreak spread to Mexico in 1970 where 6000 or more horses died, and then to Texas, USA. (See also EQUINE ENCEPHALITIS.)

Venom

(see SNAKES; TOADS; BUFOTALIN; SPIDERS; SCORPIONS)

Vent Gleet

This condition in poultry is an inflammation of the cloaca, with which is associated a thin yellowish watery discharge which has a characteristic and particularly unpleasant odour. The cloaca and adjacent skin appear swollen and congested, and the bird exhibits signs of irritation. Other birds attracted by the reddening of the region may peck at vent; this leads on to cannibalism.

Egg production drops, and in some cases egg-binding and impaction of the oviduct result. Culling is advisable. There is a similar condition in ducks but the material round the vent is more solid. This must be removed and the affected area treated with antibiotic cream.

Cases of severe infection of the eyes of poultry-keepers treating this condition are not uncommon.

Ventilation

Ventilation may be summed up as 'the measures necessary to rectify the pollution of the air in a building – without the production of a draught'. Whenever animals are enclosed in a confined building they gradually use up the oxygen and discharge into the air quantities of carbon dioxide and water vapour, until, if no fresh air is supplied, the percentage of oxygen decreases below the amount required.

One of the problems in livestock buildings is condensation, which can lead to bronchitis and pneumonia. For buildings used for cattle and sheep, provision of Yorkshire boarding is one of the best and least expensive methods of avoiding or curing condensation.

Necessary air space

	m³	ft³
Cow, horse		
(Byre or stable)	5.6	200
(Loose box or yard)	16.8–33.6	600–1200
Bacon pig	1.7	60
Poultry		
(layers on slats)	0.17	6
(layers on deep litter)	0.34	12

The required amount of air for each animal must be continuously brought in from the outside, and an exit must be provided for an equal amount. This is arranged for by the provision of inlet and outlet ventilators.

Inlets These include windows, direct inlet pipes, perforated bricks and gratings, Yorkshire boarding, and electric fans.

Windows, of which the Sheringham Valve type is the most common and useful, serve the dual purpose of lighting and ventilation. Those on the lee side of a building serve as outlets when the wind is strong. In the Sheringham Valve windows, the incoming air is deflected upwards by the hopper-like flap that falls inwards, so that it is spread over a greater area than is the case with other openings. Inlet pipes are used, often in conjunction with windows, to ensure a supply of fresh air in the region of the animals' heads.

Ventilation rates – (maximum)

	Changes of air per hour	m³ per hour	ft³ per hour
Bacon pig	20	5.7–34	200–1200
Broiler chicken	40	6.8	240
Laying birds	30	10	360

Outlets These include an open ridge, louvre-board ventilators, outlet shafts, open eaves, exhaust fans, and other devices. The most satisfactory outlet is undoubtedly an open ridge along the whole length of the building. The heated impure air rises and is drawn through the open space by the suction of the wind. The disadvantages of this system are that the open space will allow entrance to a certain amount of rain or snow in bad weather; the system is also inapplicable to buildings possessing lofts.

Extraction area
(Necessary with natural ventilation)

Outlet per animal:	cm²	sq. ins
Cowhouse	930	144
Farrowing house	95	15
Fattening house	65	10
Calf house	65	10
Poultry (adult) house	13	2

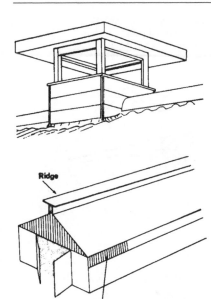

Ventilation methods for cattle houses: Top, Chimney; Bottom, Continuous ridge outlet. (With acknowledgements to *The UFAW Handbook on Care and Management of Farm Animals*, Churchill Livingstone.)

Mechanical ventilators may be either of the plenum or in-forcing type, or of the vacuum, exhaust, or outforcing variety. In the former a larger power-driven fan is enclosed in a chamber with communication to the outside of the building, and is connected by ducts or shafts with all parts that are to be ventilated. In the exhaust variety one or more electric fans are enclosed in turrets placed along the ridge of the roof.

Ventilation tunnel These have a fan to draw air into the building and force it out through vents over the stock.

The temperature in a livestock building is a result of the heat released from the stock (for example, a dairy cow gives off heat equivalent to 0.5 kW; and with a heavy milker the figure may be 1 kW) and the varying quantity of ventilating air drawn from outside. 'Because heating and refrigeration are only economic for young stock, the properties of the air entering the building are those of the outside air and vary considerably, depending on the weather. In hot weather a large amount of air is used, but in cold weather only a small amount is required and in many traditional systems this gives rise to different patterns of internal air flow. By studying the relevance of airflow patterns to the conditions near the stock and to the response of the ventilation system the Environment Department, NIAE, has designed a ventilation system which provides near uniform internal conditions as the outside temperature changes. The system ensures a desired airflow pattern by automatically adjusting the inlet gap to maintain an air speed of about 5 m/s. Calculations and experiments have shown that this system will maintain the required airflow pattern for outside temperatures down to 0°C (32°F).

'Another shortcoming of traditional systems is the influence of wind on ventilation rates, particularly in cold weather when fans are running slowly. For this reason the NIAE have discarded the method of varying fan speed to control rate of ventilation and recommends switching the fans on or off. When fans are off they are covered by simple backdraught shutters and when on they are at full speed and so are least affected by wind. The fans are switched on or off in predetermined steps and the inlet gap is adjusted automatically to match the steps in ventilation rate.

'The diagram [above] shows the essence of the system which has proved effective in fattening piggeries, broiler houses and turkey buildings and is fully described in the NIAE Report No. 28.' (See also HOUSING OF ANIMALS; CARBON MONOXIDE).

Fan failure (For this and the resulting mortality, see under CONTROLLED-ENVIRONMENT HOUSING.)

Ventral
Ventral in anatomy indicates that a particular organ or structure is situated towards the abdominal surface of the body, as distinct from the spinal or dorsal aspect.

Ventricle
A chamber of the heart, or a small cavity in the brain (see HEART; BRAIN).

Ventriculus
(see GIZZARD *and diagram for* PROVENTRICULUS)

'Verminous Aneurysm'
'Verminous aneurysm' is a misnomer for EQUINE VERMINOUS ARTERITIS.

Verminous Bronchitis
(see PARASITIC BRONCHITIS and GAPES)

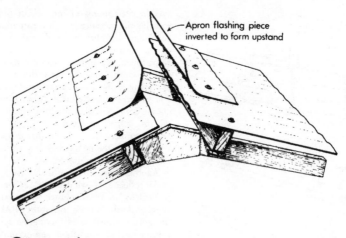

Open ridge

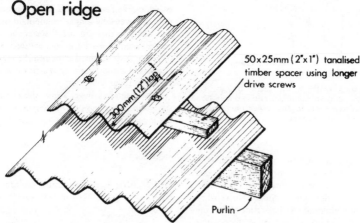

50 x 25mm (2" x 1") tanalised timber spacer using longer drive screws

300mm (12") lap

Purlin

Breathing roof

(With acknowledgements to the Scottish Farm Buildings Investigation Unit.)

Verminous Dermatitis
(see STEPHANOFILARIASIS; SUMMER SORES)

Verminous Ophthalmia
(see under EYE, DISEASES OF)

Vero Cells
A continuous heteroploid cell line derived from African green monkey (*Cercopithecus aethiops*) kidney tissue. These cells are approved as a substrate for the production of virus vaccines, including rabies. They are much easier to grow than human diploid cells, and provide a better yield; so that manufacturers are keen to use them for vaccine production. Latent virus in these cells is a potential danger.

Verotoxin
A total of 1012 milk filters were collected from 498 diary farms in south-west Ontario. The supernatants of 20 (2 per cent) of the milk filter cultures had verocytotoxic activity. Seven verotoxin-producing *E. coli* strains were isolated, 2 of which had been previously associated with disease in humans.

Verruca
(see PAPILLOMA)

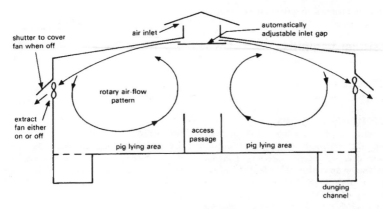

The NIAE ventilation system.

Verrucose

Covered with warts or vegetative growths. In pigs a verrucose endocarditis is recognised, the growth being found on the heart valves. The condition may be associated with swine erysipelas or be caused by staphylococci or streptococci.

Version (Turning)

Version (turning) means the changing of a presentation at parturition so that some other part of the fetus than that which was presented originally comes through the pelvic opening first.

Vertebra

(see SPINAL COLUMN)

Vesicle (Small Blister)

A vesicle (small blister) is a collection of fluid in the surface layers of the skin or of a mucous membrane. Vesicles are present in a number of diseases, and according to their location, some assistance is afforded for diagnostic purposes. For example, in foot-and-mouth disease the vesicles are present in the mouth and on the feet, while in cow-pox they are found on the teats, udder, and other parts.

Vesicles, Seminal

These secondary sex glands, like the prostate, have openings into the urethra and are situated close to the neck of the urinary bladder. (See also under SEMEN.)

Infected seminal vesicles can (rarely) cause problems. At a bull-rearing unit, 4 yearlings appeared fit and well. Their appetite was good and they showed no signs of pain or discomfort. When, however, samples of their semen were taken, clots of pus were noticed. This finding led to a careful examination of the bulls being

made, and it was then discovered that each had a hard, painful swelling of one of their seminal vesicles. Inflammation was found to be due to infection with *Actinobacillus actinoides*. Other organisms sometimes involved include tubercle bacilli, *Brucella abortus,* streptococci, *and Corynebactrerium pyogenes.*

Vesicular Disease of Pigs

Vesicular disease of pigs is described under SWINE VESICULAR DISEASE. (See also VESICULAR STOMATITIS.)

Vesicular Exanthema

A viral disease of pigs (and rarely of horses but not of cattle) which has to be distinguished from foot-and-mouth disease. It was eradicated from the USA in 1959 and has never been recorded elsewhere. It is thought that the vesicular exanthema virus may have been a 'land variant' of the San Miguel sea-lion virus, isolated from sea-lions off the coast of California.

Vesicular Stomatitis

Vesicular stomatitis is caused by a rhabdovirus transmitted by mosquitoes and biting flies, and may affect horses, cattle, pigs and, occasionally, sheep. The blisters seen on the tongue have occasionally caused confusion with foot-and-mouth disease, and vice versa – with serious consequences. Lesions can also occur on the udder or around the coronets. It is a disease of the summer, and mainly of the western hemisphere, especially in the Caribbean area.

In man the disease is influenza-like, with fever, sore throat, and several days' malaise.

Two strains of the virus are recognised – the New Jersey and the Indiana. Experimentally, numerous mammalian species can be infected – likewise ducks.

Vesicular Vaginitis
(see VULVOVAGINITIS, GRANULAR)

Vesiculitis
(see VESICLES, SEMINAL)

Veterinary Degrees

Veterinary degrees are conferred on graduates from the veterinary faculties of Bristol, Cambridge, Edinburgh, Glasgow, Liverpool and London universities. They lead to membership of the Royal College of Veterinary Surgeons (MRCVS) which allows the graduate to practise in the UK as a veterinary surgeon. Higher degrees (PhD, MSc, etc.) are available after postgraduate study, as well as certificates and diplomas in specialist areas of veterinary medicine and surgery. Graduates of veterinary schools in other EU countries may also become MRCVS. University degrees in veterinary nursing are also available.

Veterinary Facilities on the Farm

Every breeding cow and heifer in Britain has, during its lifetime, to be caught, ear-tag read, restrained and a blood sample taken from neck or tail vein. This will take place at least 2 or 3 times, quite apart from any herd or individual handlings necessary for clinical reasons or breeding management. Taking a blood sample can take as little as 30 to 45 seconds given efficient holding facilities; 200 cattle could be sampled in a morning's work. On most farms there is a lack of cattle-handling facilities of the right type, so that the catching of a single animal can and does take all the farm staff about 20 minutes with the very real possibility of broken gates and fences and varying degrees of personal injury, even before blood-sampling is attempted.

Experience in the design and erection of cattle handling units for dairy and beef cattle has shown the main points to be as follows:

Collecting pens should be large enough to hold all stock to be handled, or all the stock in units as they are housed, e.g. 50s or 100s. A post-and-rail pen 9 × 18 m (30 × 60 ft) or 12 × 13.5 m (40 × 45 ft) will hold 100 cows with calves at foot. A pen of 9 × 12 m (30 × 40 ft) will hold 60 adult cattle or 80 young cattle.

The forcing pen leads from the collecting pen to the race or chute, and should be funnel-shaped. It should hold no fewer than 12 cows plus calves, or 15 adult cattle – enough to provide a group for handling without having repetitive

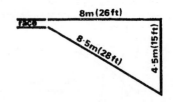

stops while 2s or 3s are run into the cow-race. The optimum dimensions are as shown in the diagram, and should not be made larger for large units. The dimensions are those within which cattle cannot evade pressure to go into the race by adopting a whirlpool movement.

Race An 18 m (60 ft) long race, 680 mm (2 ft 3 in) wide internally and 1.680 m (5 ft 6 in) to the top rail, will hold 10 to 12 cattle. It should be made up of verticals (sleepers) 2 m (6 ft 6 in) between centres sunk 900 mm (3 ft) into the ground, the bottom concreted with a brushed surface. There should be 4 horizontal rails. Height above ground of the 2nd and 3rd rails is specific in that it accommodates the large, fat or pregnant animal.

Catwalk and working space Catwalks should be provided on both sides of the cow race, 760 mm (2 ft 6 in) above ground level and not less than 300 mm (12 in) wide, in wood. Space should always be provided for 2 catwalks, even when building in close proximity to an existing wall – i.e. the face should be stood off from the wall, however tempting it may be to use an existing wall for one side. Cattle can then be run in either direction for procedures on either flank (vaccinations, branding, testing, etc.).

Crush and veterinary gates The crush should be stood off 1.079 m (3 ft 6 in) from the end of the cow race with the same internal width of 680 mm (2 ft 3 in), and suitable gates to hold animal No. 1 firmly, stop animal No. 1 from backing out of crush before being held and prevent animal No. 2 from pushing up. The materials and sizes are the same as for the race.

Yoke or headstock A device for restraining cattle by the neck, strongly made from wood or metal and designed so that the head cannot jerk about. While securing the animal firmly, it incorporates a quick-release frame to free it in an emergency.

Three-way cattle shedder If fat cattle are weighed, cows examined for breeding function or large stores sexed, then this at once dictates grouping by weight, pregnancy or other findings. A 3-way shedder immediately after the crush renders this separation an easy task.

Dispersal and recirculation Having dispersed any large group of cattle to their appropriate categories of in-calf, empty, etc., there should be a series of gates in the far end of all holding pens, allowing cattle to be recirculated, retained or individually extracted.

Suckler cows and calves Suckler cows are usually handled for clinical reasons (vaccinations, treatment, blood-sampling) or to find out breeding status at that time (in-calf, ovulating, empty). This usually means that calves are at foot. To simplify handling, calves can go with their dams right into the forcing pen without any attempted separation. If a calf race is then sited to run from near the mouth of the cow race, with a shedder gate, then calves of 1 to 7 months can be run off separately. This allows vaccination, castration, dehorning or weighing to be done very quickly with no time and energy dissipated on catching each calf individually. Critical dimensions for the calf race are 410 mm (1 ft 4 in) internal width and 1.040 m (3 ft 6 in) to top rail. The shedder gate should be close-boarded to prevent visual contact between calves and cows in cow race. Calves will run into the calf race quickly if the shedder is operated from an overhead platform, but they tend to flinch at an operator working through the rails at head or shoulder level.

In addition to the cattle-handling facilities described above, it is useful to have a footbath suitable for cattle (see FOOT-BATHS), and loose-boxes for calving or isolation purposes. With a very large herd of, say, 500 cows, 15 loose-boxes would not be too many.

Veterinary Investigation Centres (VICS)

Together with the Central Veterinary Laboratory, Weybridge, the VICs form the Veterinary Laboratories Agency. They provide laboratory facilities and a consultative service for veterinary surgeons in private practice, assisting with the diagnosis of disease and herd problems. Their work includes autopsies, serological tests, biochemistry and parasitology. VIC staff carry out research into disease problems of local importance, and also provide a surveillance function for DEFRA in warning of local disease which might become important nationally. In Scotland similar VICs operate but are affiliated to the Scottish agricultural colleges.

Veterinary Medicines Directorate (VMD)

The government agency with responsibility for overseeing the evaluation and licensing of animal medicines, protecting the consumer from unacceptable or hazardous residues, and advising the Veterinary Products Committee. Address: Veterinary Medicines Directorate, Woodham Lane, New Haw, Addlestone, Surrey KT15 3NB.

Veterinary Nurses

A title restricted to those who have completed the course of instruction and passed the examinations authorised by the Royal College of Veterinary Surgeons. People wishing to train as veterinary nurses must first find employment for not less than 35 hours per week in a veterinary practice or other veterinary centre approved by the RCVS. The greater part of the training is given while working; VN training is now part of the NVQ scheme

The practical training is supplemented by formal tuition to provide the necessary background knowledge. Residential courses are available.

All pre-enrolment queries about training are dealt with by the British Veterinary Nursing Association, Level 15, Terminus House, Terminus Street, Harlow, Essex CM20 1XA.

There are more than 80 training centres, approved by the RCVS, where student nurses can study for the 2 qualifying examinations.

A Diploma in Advanced Veterinary Nursing, and a university degree in veterinary nursing, can also be obtained.

Veterinary Poisons Information Service

Addresses are National Poisons Information Service, National Poisons Unit, Avonley Road, London SE14 5ER; and Leeds Poisons Information Service, The General Infirmary, Great George Street, Leeds LS1 3EX.

Veterinary Practitioner

Someone on the Supplementary Veterinary Register; not an MRCVS. The SVR was closed to new entrants in 1967.

Veterinary Products Committee (VPC)

This, under the Medicines Act 1968, advises the Medicines Commission, and ultimately, the Licensing Authority, on the marketing of medicines for animals. Its approval is needed before an animal medicine may be licensed for sale. It has to consider the safety, quality and efficacy of any veterinary medicine in relation to the treated animal, the safety of consumers of produce derived from treated animals, and the safety of farmer, pet-owner, and the environment. (See also SUSPECTED ADVERSE REACTION SURVEILLANCE SCHEME.)

Veterinary Profession

This comprises those engaged in private practice, in the Animal Health Division of the Ministry of Agriculture, the Royal Army Veterinary Corps, the overseas veterinary services, in research and teaching at the universities, and also at AFRC research establishments, and those of the Department of Environment, Food and Rural Affairs etc., in food inspection and other municipal services, in AI centres, in research and advisory appointments with, e.g. FAO, and in commercial undertakings. There are about 12,500 veterinary surgeons working in the UK and about 2,800 veterinary practices. Over the next few years the traditionally male-dominated profession will become about two-thirds female, as the majority of veterinary students are women.

Veterinary Surgeons Act 1966

This relates to veterinary education, the management of the profession, and the registration and professional conduct of veterinary surgeons and practitioners. The practice of veterinary surgery continues to be limited to veterinary surgeons and practitioners whose names appear on the registers maintained by the Royal College of Veterinary Surgeons. Unregistered persons may carry out only the very limited treatments, tests, or operations specified in section 19 of the Act, any exemption orders made thereunder, or schedule 3.

The Amendment Order to the Act permits a veterinary nurse to carry out any medical treatment or any minor surgery to a companion animal, provided that the latter is under the care of a registered veterinary surgeon who has authorised the treatment.

Veterinary Surgery (Epidural Anaesthesia) Order 1992

(see under LAW)

Vial

(see AMPOULE; GLASS EMBOLISM)

Vibices

Vibices are long tapering markings that sometimes occur on visible mucous membranes during certain diseases, such as purpura haemorrhagica and pernicious anaemia of horses.

Vibrio

Vibrio is a bacterium shaped like a boomerang. In stained smears they are often seen in pairs either in the form of an 'S' or of a flying seagull.

Vibrio fetus (see CAMPYLOBACTER INFECTIONS, FETUS)

'Vibrionic scours' in pigs (see SWINE DYSENTERY)

Vibriosis

Vibriosis caused by infection with *Vibrio anguillilarum* is a serious disease in marine fish farms. Affected fish suddenly lose appetite and turn dark in colour. Post-mortem examination reveals haemorrhagic internal organs; the kidney may be liquefied. Surviving fish may have ulcers that erode the back muscles and the base of the fins. Prompt treatment with antibiotics in the feed may save those still eating.. The infection has also been found in eels transported live in inadequate conditions.

Vibrissae

The thick, stiff hairs or whiskers which project from the faces of cats, dogs, and other animals. They are minor sense organs. (See SKIN.)

'Vices' and Viciousness

A definition comprehensive enough to include bad habits. (See TAIL-BITING (in pigs), SUCKING (in calves); and FEATHER-PICKING, CANNIBALISM (in poultry).) The following concern the horse.

Bad habits, mild vices, or whims

Horses which are shut in stables without exercise or work frequently learn vices and tricks which not only may be harmful to the animals themselves, but may be dangerous to persons who attend them. Perhaps the most objectionable is the habit of kicking when being approached. (See below, under 'Kicking'.)

Eating the bedding may be merely an endeavour on the part of the horse to acquire a sufficiency of coarse bulky food when the ration is too concentrated, or it may be a bad habit. It can be prevented by supplying sawdust instead of straw, or peat moss litter.

Refusing to lie is often due to fear, nervousness, or physical inability, such as ankylosis of the spinal column. Horses may lie when housed in a loose-box instead of a stall; a stout rope from one heel post across to the other may allow the horse to obtain some amount of rest. (See SLEEP, etc.). Gnawing the walls is usually a sign of the presence of worms, bots, a mineral or other deficiency, or indigestion, and appropriate measures should be taken to determine which condition is present, and to treat it accordingly.

Pawing in the stable may be a sign of impatience or loneliness; then it is not important, but sometimes it develops into a vice of such persistency that it entails great wear of the shoes, and may result in the production of holes in the stable floor. It should be remembered that pawing is sometimes a sign of abdominal pain (colic).

More serious vices (see CRIB-BITING AND WIND-SUCKING; WEAVING).

Aggressiveness may be due to pain (see HORSES, BACK TROUBLES); and, in countries where the disease is present, to RABIES. (See also BRAIN DISEASES.)

When an animal shows an ungovernable temper under the pressure of sexual disturbances, it is unfair to consider it vicious. Cruel treatment in the past may also be an underlying factor (and see also the effect of EQUINE VERMINOUS ARTERITIS).

Kicking (a) Rearing and striking with the fore-feet is a dangerous vice that is more common among the light horses than among the heavy draught. Sometimes the animal merely rears from a desire to get started with his work; sometimes he will not allow himself to be held by the head when in harness, but rears and strikes out at anyone approaching him; at other times he may strike out without rearing. A saddle horse, when rearing, may with his head strike the face or chest of his rider and unseat him, and may so lose his balance that he falls over backwards and perhaps crush the rider.

(b) Kicking with the hind-feet. 'With a kicking horse, pass in front' is a proverb that it is well to remember when dealing with the horse that uses his hind-feet for kicking. The hind-feet can be used to strike an object within a radius of from 1.2 to 1.8 metres (4 to 6 ft) all around them. It is a well-known fact that a mule can deliver a kick with his hind-feet to a person standing at its shoulder, and there are many horses able to do likewise. Two methods of kicking with the hind-limbs are commonly employed: in the first, which is the horse's natural method of defence and offence, the head is lowered, the body is lifted from the withers backwards, and both the hind-limbs are suddenly extended as far backwards as possible with tremendous force; in the second, the horse lifts one hind-foot and deals a short vicious backward or sideways kick without always fully extending the limb.

In addition to these there are 'cow kickers', which project one hind-limb forwards, outwards, and backwards, so that they may reach a person standing as far forward as the shoulder. These are especially dangerous.

Biting is commonest among stallions. It is well to take precautionary measures, such as muzzling while grooming, tying up short, using double head ropes, one to either side of the stall, etc.

Shying In many cases where horses suddenly stop, plunge to one side, snort, tremble, attempt to turn in the opposite direction and run away, when confronted by some unusual sight, sound, or smell, the same causes as occasion bolting are operative. The horse does not trust his eyesight, is unable to interpret an unusual sound or smell, and consequently takes fright. Among the many objects at which horses are liable to shy may be mentioned the following: pools of water shining in the sun-light, fluttering pieces of paper, clothes hung out to dry, dogs, cats, fowls, and other small animals darting into the roadway. The odour of wild beasts, and the smell of blood and offal, that an animal perceives when passing a menagerie or a knackery or abattoir, are also likely to frighten it and cause it to shy.

Aversion to special objects Occasionally a horse is encountered which has an absolute horror of some special, usually quite harmless, common object, e.g. pieces of white or coloured paper or rag, cock turkeys, pigs, goats, donkeys, small white inanimate objects of any nature, etc. Grey horses have been known to attack bay horses, and a brown-bay horse, light grey horses.

Villus

Villus is the name given to one of the millions of minute processes which are present on the inner surface of the small intestine. These are structures concerned in the taking up of fat. (See DIGESTION; INTESTINE.)

Viraemia

The presence of large amounts of infecting virus in the blood.

Viral

Relating to viruses.

Viral Haemorrhagic Disease of Rabbits

(see RABBIT HAEMORRHAGIC DISEASE)

Viral Hepatitis in Dogs

(see CANINE VIRAL HEPATITIS)

Viral Hepatitis of Ducklings

Viral hepatitis of ducklings is a disease which attacks ducklings under 3 weeks of age. There are usually no clinical signs before death except general malaise. On post-mortem examination, the liver shows enlargement and haemorrhaging. It can be prevented by vaccination at 1 day old.

Viral Infections of Cows' Teats

These include cowpox. Nowadays, true cowpox is (in the UK) considered to be a rare disease. Another infection common to man and cattle is pseudo-cowpox or milkers' nodules. The skin disease in herdsmen is indistinguishable from that in shepherds who have been handling sheep suffering from orf. It is now thought that the milkers' nodules virus very closely resembles the orf virus, but that they are 2 distinct entities.

Two doctors in Dorset who had 7 patients with milkers' nodules found, with the aid of a veterinary colleague, that the 6 dairy herds in which the men worked all had some cows with pseudo-cowpox (or milkers' nodules) lesions on the teats. There are 2 types of this infection: one is described as benign or chronic – this lasts for months, it is painless throughout, and starts with a mild redness of the teats, followed by the formation of many scabs which get rubbed off at milking. The second, or acute, form involves pain before scabbing begins, but not afterwards. First there is reddening, then blisters which burst, then very large scabs form. So-called proud flesh is formed beneath the scabs. When these drop off, a characteristic horseshoe-shaped ring of minute scabs at the circumference is left. All this takes 7 to 10 days. What looks like a wart remains for several months.

This pseudo-cowpox differs from true cowpox in that the latter infection is associated with more pain, fewer scabs, quicker development of them and recovery within 3 weeks.

The virus which causes pseudo-cowpox or milkers' nodules may be identical with, or closely related to, that of bovine papular stomatitis (BPS).

Raised, roughened, brownish plaques are seen on the muzzle, and lesions on the lips and inside the mouth.

An ulcerative infection of the teats of dairy cows has been described in Scotland, and given the name bovine ulcerative mammillitis. It is caused by a herpesvirus.

The disease has been seen only in early winter, and lasts for up to 15 weeks. In severe cases it is of sudden onset, often appearing between milkings; the whole teat being swollen and painful. Blue discoloration is common. The resultant ulcer covers most, if not all, the teat.

In a less severe form vivid red discoloration was noted.

On account of the impossibility of milking cows with badly ulcerated teats, and because mastitis often follows, several animals may have to be slaughtered.

The same disease has been seen in south-west England where the onset appeared to follow a prolonged period of wet weather. If the virus is of the herpes type, it may be that it is endemic in the cattle population and produces lesions only under conditions which result in devitalising of the tissues. Another possibility is that biting flies transmit the infection. (See also under FOOT-AND-MOUTH DISEASE.)

Viral Pneumonia of Cattle
(see infections listed under CALF PNEUMONIA)

Virginiamycin

An antibiotic used as a growth promoter which may be included in livestock rations.

Virino

A low-molecular-weight nucleic acid and a host-derived protein. (See SCRAPIE for a possible example.)

Virion

A mature virus; the ultimate phase in viral development.

Virology

The study of viruses.

Virus Diarrhoea of Cattle
(see BOVINE VIRAL DIARRHOEA)

Viruses

These are minute entities which carry their genetic information in one type of nucleic acid. They use the energy system of the host cell for their own biosynthetic needs, and can be differentiated from bacteria by their size and by their inability to multiply except in living cells.

Most viruses produce disease in man, animals and plants. They can be transmitted from one animal to another and stimulate the production of antibodies in infected animals.

Viruses are mostly invisible under the light microscope, although some of the larger examples (e.g. the pox viruses) can be seen readily under the light microscope. Most viruses can only be visualised in the electron microscope. There is considerable variation in size. Foot-and-mouth disease virus is about 25 nm in diameter, whereas African swine fever virus is about 10 times that size. (See NANOMETRE.)

Many pathogenic viruses are capable of altering their antigenic structure, or their pathogenicity, or both, in response to pressures put upon them by, for example, vaccination.

The classical example is provided by influenza viruses, which are able to change from harmless to extremely virulent forms very quickly within the same species.

The nomenclature and classification of viruses has in recent years undergone many changes, and further changes are likely as new viruses are discovered and new information on the properties of viruses accrues. (*See* table, page 762.)

Anti-viral agents Since viral infections are not controllable by antibiotics, there has been a long search for other compounds which might achieve anti-viral activity. Much hope was pinned on INTERFERON, but at present its use is very limited, and research has switched to attempts to stimulate natural production of interferon, or to find drugs effective against viruses.

Aciclovir may be used for ophthalmic infections by herpesviruses. Zidurodine alleviates clinical signs in cases of feline immunodeficiency virus (FIV). However, anti-viral drugs have to be used with great care as the margin between an effective dose and the toxic one (the therapeutic index) is narrow.

Vaccines are available against a number of viral infections, e.g. equine herpesvirus, canine distemper, and feline leukaemia.

(See also ROTAVIRUS; ASTROVIRUS; ONCOGENIC; DNA; RIBONUCLEIC ACID; CANCER.)

Viruses, Plant

Some of these can, by means of DNA technology, be adapted to produce 'potentially safe and inexpensive vaccines for use against disease in animals'. AFRC research workers have, for example, produced a harmless plant virus carrying a fragment of foot-and-mouth disease virus.

Viscera

Viscera is the name given to the larger organs lying within the chest and abdominal cavities. The term 'viscus' is applied to each of these individually.

'Visceral Gout'

A disease characterised by the deposit of urates over the internal organs; it is found in birds and reptiles.

Visceral Larva Migrans

A syndrome produced in man by the larvae of *Toxocara canis*. Occasionally it is the cause of death. (See TOXOCARA.)

Vision

(see also EYE) Rays of light pass, in the first place, through the cornea, then through the aqueous humour that fills the anterior chamber of the eye. The light then enters the hinder part of the eye, through the pupil – a round, slit-like, or elliptical hole in the iris, which can be automatically narrowed according to the strength of the light rays that are passing through it. Immediately behind the iris lies the crystalline lens, a clear structure arranged in layers somewhat like an onion, which also by automatic alterations in its curves, brings the rays to a focus upon the retina after they pass through a second clear jelly-like humour – the vitreous humour. The retina is the innermost of the 3 coats of the eyeball, and consists of the specialised terminations of the fibres of the optic nerve.

Monocular and binocular vision In animals whose eyes are laterally placed in the head it is impossible for both eyes to look at an object directly in front of them. One eye can be focused upon an object at any one time, while the other eye sees a completely different picture. This is called 'monocular vision'. When the eyes are placed towards the front of the head so that they can both be concentrated upon an object, as in man, horse, and dog, each eye sees a slightly different picture, but the 2 ranges of vision overlap. This is called 'binocular vision'. It is partly owing to the fact that in binocular vision each eye sees slightly 'round the corner' of the object, that a sense of depth and distance is conveyed to the higher brain centres. The 2 pictures are not quite superimposed, and the previous experience of the animal enables it to judge distance by this difference in superimposition. This is technically known as 'stereoscopic vision'.

A striking point in connection with the eyesight of animals is that, although many of them have their visual powers obviously very highly developed, they seldom trust their eyes in matters of emergency. The visual images alone do not convey to the mind the reality of the external world. It becomes necessary for the animal to verify its visual impression by tactile or olfactory impressions. In practically every case the fear of a harmless object may be immediately or shortly dispelled by allowing the animal to smell and examine it by touching it with the nose.

In birds, the central part of the lens has a magnifying power of up to 8x. As a result (stereoscopic) vision is very accurate, enabling birds to locate food easily. Birds, reptiles, amphibia and insects can 'see' ultraviolet light.

V

Some viruses of veterinary importance

Group	Diseases caused	Animals affected
Adenoviruses	Canine viral hepatitis	Dogs
	Fox encephalitis	Foxes
	(See also KENNEL COUGH.)	
Alphaviruses	Equine encephalitis	Horses, birds, man
Aphthoviruses	Foot-and-mouth disease	Cattle, sheep, goats, pigs, deer, hedgehogs; (very rarely) man
Arboviruses	(See Togaviruses *below*.)	
Arenaviruses	Lymphocytic choriomeningitis	Mice, hamsters, man
	(See also LASSA FEVER.)	(Man)
Bunyaviruses	Rift Valley fever	Sheep, cattle, goats, buffaloes, camels, man
	Nairobi sheep disease	Sheep, goats
	Gumboro disease	Poultry
Caliciviruses	Feline calicivirus disease	Cats
	Vesicular exanthema	Pigs; (rarely) horses
Circoviruses	Anaemia	Chickens
	Dermatitis and nephrosis syndrome	Pigs
	Post-weaning multisystemic wasting syndrome	Pigs
Coronaviruses	Transmissible gastroenteritis	Pigs
	Feline infectious peritonitis	Cats
	Infectious bronchitis	Chickens
	Enteritis	Calves, foals, dogs, cats
Enteroviruses	Swine vesicular disease	Pigs; (rarely) man
	Teschen/Talfan disease	Pigs
	Duck virus hepatitis	Ducklings
	Avian encephalomyelitis	Chickens
Flaviviruses	Louping-ill	Sheep, cattle, deer, dog, man
	Wesselbron disease	Sheep, man
	Japanese B encephalitis	Horses, man, pigs, birds
	Tick-borne encephalitis	Rodents, goats, cattle, man
	Kyasanur forest disease	Monkeys, rodents, man
	Omsk haemorrhagic fever	Rodents, man
	Murray Valley encephalitis	Wild birds, children
	St Louis encephalitis	Wild birds, bats, horses, man
Herpesviruses	(See table under HERPESVIRUSES.)	Horses, cattle, pigs, dogs, cats, man
Iridoviruses	African swine fever	Pigs, African warthog
Lentiviruses	Maedi/visna	Sheep
	Caprine arthritis-encephalitis	Goats
Morbilliviruses	Canine distemper	Dogs, ferrets, mink
	Cattle plague (rinderpest)	Cattle, sheep, goats
Oncoviruses	Leukaemia, leukosis, cancer	Mammals, birds
Orbiviruses	Bluetongue	Cattle, sheep
	African horse sickness	Horses (but not donkeys)
Orthomyxoviruses	Influenza	Horses, pigs, birds
Orthopoxviruses	Cowpox	Cattle, man
Papillomaviruses	Warts/papillomas/cancer/sarcoids	Cattle, horses, dogs, man
Paramyxoviruses	Newcastle disease	Poultry, pigeons
	Parainfluenza	Cattle, dogs (see KENNEL COUGH)
Parapoxviruses	Pseudo-cowpox	Cattle, man
	Orf	Sheep, cattle, goats, dogs
	Bovine papular stomatitis	Calves
Pestiviruses	Bovine virus diarrhoea	Cattle
	Border disease	Sheep
	Swine fever	Pigs
	Equine viral arteritis	Horses
Picornaviruses	(This group includes Aphthoviruses and Enteroviruses (see *above*) and Rhinoviruses.)	
Poxviruses	(See Orthopoxviruses *and* Parapoxviruses, *above*.)	
Reoviruses	Respiratory disease, enteritis	Calves, pigs, dogs, cats, rabbits, man
Retroviruses	(See Lentiviruses *and* Oncoviruses above.)	
Rhabdoviruses	Rabies (see LYSSA; DUVENHAGE; MOKOLA VIRUS; LAGOS BAT.)	
	Vesicular stomatitis	Horses
Togaviruses	(See Alphaviruses, Flaviviruses *and* Pestiviruses *above*.)	

Visna

A meningoencephalitis of sheep caused by a lentivirus. (See MAEDI/VISNA.)

Vitamins

Vitamins are substances present in natural foods, essential for health, and which exercise an influence in nutrition out of all proportion to the amounts consumed. Several vitamins are synthesised in the animal body, some being thus available independent of the diet, but it is important to note that a vitamin synthesised in the lower part of the alimentary canal may be available to an animal only if it eats its own droppings. (Nocturnal coprophagy is a regular practice in rabbits.)

Vitamin supplements now form an essential part of farm livestock feeding.

Animals, when feeding under natural conditions, with a free choice from a wide range of food-stuffs, consume, as a rule, all the vitamins they require. But under the influence of domestication, and especially of intensive rearing, animals often have no choice in the matter and suffer from vitamin deficiencies, either because their artificial diet is too restricted, or because vitamins naturally present have been destroyed in the preparation of the food.

Vitamin A is formed from yellow carotene found in carrots, green vegetables, egg-yolk, fish roe, liver, cod-liver oil, kidney and milk.

This vitamin is necessary for the growth and general well-being of the young animal in particular. Vitamin A is also necessary for healthy skin and teeth. Cats are unable to synthesise vitamin A and obtain it from fish and liver.

Too little or too much vitamin A can be harmful. In excess, it can adversely affect growth and bone development.

Vitamin B complex, water-soluble, includes riboflavin, nicotinic acid, pantothenic acid, choline, biotin, and thiamin. (See also CHOLINE; FOLIC ACID.) Most of these are present in yeast and liver. (For nicotinic acid, see NIACIN.)

Vitamin B_1 (thiamin, aneurine) is present in the husks of cereal grains, yolk of egg, yeast, and liver. A deficiency can be caused by overheating the food of pet animals, or by the enzyme present in some fish. Horse and cattle which eat bracken are affected by the thiaminase in that plant. (See BRACKEN POISONING.)

Vitamin B_2 (riboflavin) is present in milk (and is not destroyed by pasteurisation), as well as in foods mentioned under B_1.

Riboflavin is a constituent of the flavoproteins – hydrogen-transporting enzymes concerned with the animal's energy metabolism.

Biotin, formerly known as vitamin H, is another of the B group of vitamins. It is necessary for the health of skin and hoof. It is referred to below under 'Vitamin deficiencies'.

Vitamin B_3 (pantothenic acid). Necessary for skin health, and growth.

Vitamin B_6 (pyridoxine), present in liver, yeast and cereals, is important for growth and protein metabolism.

Vitamin B_{12} is the anti-pernicious anaemia factor of importance in human medicine, and contains cobalt. It is also known as cobalamin.

Vitamin C This is ascorbic acid; it is found in the juices of most fruits and vegetables. Most animals can produce sufficient vitamin C for their own requirements, with the exception of primates, guinea pigs and the bulbul family of birds. In hot weather and other stressful situations, additional vitamin C may be needed for all animals.

Vitamin D, or calciferol, is the anti-rachitic principle found in cod-liver oil, meat juice, cow's milk, and egg-yolk. The absence of this vitamin causes rickets. There is an intimate association between the presence of this vitamin, the action of sunlight or the artificial irradiation by ultraviolet rays, and the mineral balance in the body.

With its help, salts of calcium and phosphorus, instead of being eliminated from the intestinal canal, are absorbed into the system and made use of in the calcification of bone. (See COD-LIVER OIL.) Too much vitamin D is harmful. (See RODENTS – Rodenticides.)

Vitamin E (tocopherol) (fat-soluble). This vitamin is found in red meat, oil of seeds, milk, and egg-yolk. It is necessary for fertility, and its absence from a diet has been shown to cause sterility in rats by inducing firstly the death, and later the absorption, of the embryos.

Vitamin K complex – mostly fat-soluble vitamins concerned with the formation of PROTHROMBIN, and hence regarded as 'the anti-internal-haemorrhage factor'. Present in alfalfa. Synthetic preparations are available for therapy.

Vitamin excess (hypervitaminosis) may result in serious disease. (For an example, chronic hypervitaminosis A occurs in cats fed almost exclusively on liver.)

An excess of yeast, fed to pigs as a vitamin B supplement, has resulted in severe rickets.

Vitamin deficiencies These may occur as the result of a vitamin-deficient diet, or a failure

V

– in some instances – to synthesise a particular vitamin within the body. 'Secondary' or 'conditioned' deficiencies may also arise from any disease which impairs absorption from the alimentary tract, injuries to the liver, infections (which increase the consumption of vitamins), metallic poisoning, and as the result of some enzyme which destroys or inactivates a vitamin. (For examples of the last-mentioned cause, see 'CHASTEK PARALYSIS'.)

Biotin-producing bacteria live in intestines and contribute a variable amount. But biotin deficiency is not rare – except in adult ruminants. Signs of deficiency are: dermatitis on ears, neck, shoulder and tail of the pig, together with cracking of the walls and sole of the hoof; retarded growth and brittle feathering, foot dermatitis, swollen eyelids, eruptions on mouth and beak, perosis, leg weakness, poor hatchability and embryonic malformations in birds.

A report from Finland stated that bleeding from the navel, which was a serious problem in a breeding herd of 85 Finnish Landrace and 85 Large White sows, could be successfully controlled by vitamin C (not vitamin K as might have been expected). An ascorbic acid supplement was given to the sows for from 8 to 2 days before farrowing. Piglets from the treated sows were also 5.5 per cent heavier than those from untreated controls at 3 weeks of age.

Vitamin E (tocopherol) could with advantage be added to all compound feeds as a precautionary measure, particularly if the feed contains polyunsaturated fatty acids. Less vitamin E is absorbed from the intestine if the latter are present. Some feeds contain vitamin E antagonists – present in lucerne and beans. The activity of vitamin E may be reduced by a high nitrate content in feed or drinking water. Animals which do not receive an adequate supply of the trace element selenium need extra vitamin E, because selenium has a vitamin E sparing effect. Application of fertilisers rich in sulphates inhibits the absorption of selenium by plants from the soil, and in these circumstances grazing animals will require extra vitamin E.

Vitamin E contents of feeds as well as crops may be reduced to a dangerous level on storage. (See also Muscular dystrophy under MUSCLES, DISEASES OF.) Anti-vitamin E factor may be present in barley as well as fats of animal origin.

Despite a current tendency to increase vitamin levels in animal feeds, cases of vitamin E deficiency appear to be becoming more prevalent in all classes of farm livestock, resulting in mulberry heart in pigs, muscular dystrophy in calves, and 'crazy chick' disease in poultry. Perhaps this has something to do with the faster growth-rates expected of animals nowadays. Certainly the low vitamin E content of some cereals is important. This is especially the case with some samples of barley grown on selenium-deficient soil but fed on a farm where selenium is no problem, and where the possibility of such a deficiency might well be overlooked.

It is generally accepted that the daily requirement of vitamin E is, for cows, 1 g; for calves, 150 mg; for ewes, 7 mg; and for lambs, 25 mg.

Vitamin E deficiency leads to white muscle disease or muscular dystrophy; and a supplement of this vitamin has been shown to reduce the incidence of retained placenta, metritis, and cysts of the ovaries when given with SELENIUM.

Horses Vitamin A deficiency is unlikely to occur except in town horses denied adequate green food. Deficiency symptoms are stated to include night-blindness, hoof lesions, corneal lesions, respiratory symptoms, and reproductive difficulties. Some of the B vitamins are synthesised by adult horses, but backward foals may benefit from vitamin supplements. Infertility in the mare may sometimes be associated with a vitamin C deficiency. It has been suggested that splints, sidebones, ringbones, and spavins may be associated with a vitamin D deficiency.

Cattle Vitamin A deficiency in cattle denied adequate green food leads to abortion or the birth of weak, blind calves, or of those suffering from diarrhoea which die within a few days. Corneal lesions and blindness may also result in growing cattle. For example, Hereford bulls on a diet of beet-pulp nuts, high-protein nuts, and barley straw went blind owing to a lack of vitamin A. (See also HYPERKERATOSIS.) Vitamins of the B complex are mostly synthesised in the rumen, but in the newborn calf a deficiency may occur. (See THIAMIN.) Vitamin C is apparently synthesised by adult cattle, but some cases of infertility may, it is believed, be due to a deficiency, and some cases of navel-ill benefit, it is said, from vitamin C treatment. In some parts of Britain pasture or fodder crops contain too little vitamin D, while sunlight during the winter months is insufficient to enable the shortage to be made good within the animal's body; the result is rickets. Vitamin E deficiency is associated with muscular dystrophy.

Pigs Vitamin A deficiency results in failure to grow in piglets and infertility in adult pigs, as well as paralysis of the hindquarters. A nicotinic acid deficiency gives rise to a condition simulating necrotic enteritis and poor growth. Yeast supplements will correct deficiencies of the B complex, but excess may result in rickets.

A vitamin E deficiency in newborn piglets can result in their sudden death after being given iron injections to prevent anaemia. It is advisable to delay the injection until the piglet is a week old, when it is more tolerant of iron. Gilts' rations low in vitamin E or high in fatty acid predispose to this condition in the offspring.

Biotin deficiency in pigs gives rise to symptoms which include dermatitis. Lameness can affect a whole herd where there is a biotin deficiency causing cracks in the sole or wall of the hooves.

Dog and cat Vitamin A has been used with success in the treatment of diarrhoea in kittens. Corneal lesions, even blindness in extreme cases, and sometimes deafness, have also been attributed to a vitamin A deficiency. Vitamin B (thiamin) deficiency results in fatigue and loss of appetite, and may be associated with cramp. Yeast may prove effective in cases of depraved appetite and chorea. 'Black tongue' in the dog and an ulcerative stomatitis in the dog are seen in the USA in naturally occurring cases of nicotinic acid deficiency. Lack of riboflavin is associated with eye lesions and skin disease. Rickets results from lack of vitamin D, especially in the larger breeds, but overdosage is harmful and can lead to deposits of calcium salts in or between muscles.

Poultry Vitamin A deficiency will occur only in birds deprived of adequate green food. Maize and cod-liver oil (which must not be rancid) are alternative sources of this vitamin. Lack of it leads, in chickens, to drowsiness, weakness, staggering, stunted growth, and often a discharge from the eyes and nostrils. The presence of pustular lesions in the oesophagus is diagnostic. Adult birds become dishevelled looking, weak and emaciated, and show a watery or cheesy discharge from eyes and nostrils. Deficiency of riboflavin (vitamin B_2) in the diet is not uncommon, particularly in wire-floor battery brooders, in which the chicks have no access to droppings. (On solid floors chicks may correct the deficiency by eating their droppings, which contain riboflavin synthesised by organisms in the lower part of the gut, but not otherwise available to the body.) Symptoms are leg weakness and a curling inwards of the toes in chicks; also decreased egg production and poor hatchability. (*See also* biotin *under* 'Vitamin B', above.) Thin shells, reduced hatchability, and sometimes a temporary paralysis after laying, are indications of a vitamin D deficiency. Chicks are unthrifty, walk with difficulty, and later show typical symptoms of rickets. Bone deformity and softening of the beak occur in adult birds. Sunlight, green food, and the judicious use in winter of cod-liver oil overcome this deficiency. Vitamin E, necessary for hatchability, is present in whole grain and, to a lesser extent, in greenstuff. The latter also contains ample vitamin K, a deficiency of which leads to anaemia as a result of internal haemorrhage.

Voice

Voice is the sound produced as the result of the vibration of a column of air forced through the larynx by contraction of the respiratory muscles. The means by which this is produced are analogous to those by which sound is produced in a reed instrument, except that in the living animal the pitch of the voice can be altered at will. This is accomplished by the amount of tension exerted by muscular action upon the vocal cords; the more tense these are the higher is the pitch of the voice. In the majority of mammals the vibrations are produced when a blast of air is expelled from the chest, but in the donkey the higher notes of the bray result from inspiration of air, and the lower notes from expiration.

The character of the voice can be altered to some extent by changes in the resonating chambers of the nose, mouth, pharynx, etc.; thus, the false nostrils of the horse are used to produce the snort of fear or excitement, the nasal cavities transmit the whinny and neigh of pleasure, and the mouth and pharynx furnish the character of the neigh of impatience, loneliness, and sometimes the challenge of anger of the jealous stallion.

Neighing or whinnying in the horse is an expiratory act produced partly through the mouth and partly through the nose; the bray of the ass is expiratory for the low notes and inspiratory for the high; bellowing in the ox, bleating in the sheep, barking in the dog, and the mew of the cat are all produced by expiratory efforts.

Animals use their voices upon widely different occasions. It seems probable that they make the greatest use of this faculty for the purposes of enabling the young to recognise their dams from a distance, and to maintain cohesion of herds or flocks. Stragglers getting left behind, or separated from their special companions, can be heard calling for long distances. Male animals of many species will give a warning upon the approach of newcomers or danger. Females may produce little cries or screams when attended by males during periods of oestrus, or when making acquaintance with their newly born progeny. Almost all the domestic animals emit cries when

V

suffering pain. In the horse tribe the sounds are often merely grunts or groans, especially when the pain is abdominal. In other cases horses will scream when they are suddenly subjected to acute pain, or to very great fright. Cattle and sheep in agony behave similarly to horses; they usually groan, but cows, ewes, and heifers may issue a long drawn-out bellow or bleat during difficult parturition. The pig has a range of notes from the satisfied grunt of suckling a sow, to the frightened squeals and screams of those that are being handled by man. The dog has a note for all occasions; he generally expresses all the emotions of which he is capable by differences in his bark. (See also LARYNX and MUTING OF DOGS.)

In rabies the character of the voice may be changed. In the 'dumb' form, barking is suppressed.

Volar

Refers to the back of the fore-limb.

Volcanic Gases

Typically these comprise water vapour, carbon dioxide, sulphur dioxide, hydrogen sulphide, hydrochloric acid, hydrogen fluoride, and carbon monoxide.

Volvulus

An intestinal obstruction is produced by the twisting of a loop of bowel round itself. It is usually due to some spasmodic contraction of the muscular coat, or to the presence of gas, and is very dangerous owing to the great risk of strangulation of the blood supply and consequent necrosis. Excessive gas formation in the caecum and colon of whey-fed pigs may lead to volvulus. (See HAEMORRHAGIC GASTROENTERITIS OF PIGS and INTESTINES, DISEASES OF.)

Vomica

A cavity in the lung tissue produced by disease. Vomicae are most commonly met with in cattle suffering from either tuberculosis or contagious pleuro-pneumonia.

Vomiting

Vomiting involves not merely a contraction of the stomach walls and a dilatation of the gullet, but is a complex act in which the abdominal muscles, the diaphragm, the muscles of the chest and larynx, and those of the lower part of the neck all play a part.

Before the act there is usually a profuse secretion of watery saliva which serves to lubricate the passage of the stomach contents. The animal appears uneasy, and will usually seek a secluded spot. Soon rhythmic contractions of the abdominal muscles commence and culminate in the ejection of a quantity of frothy material. The diaphragm is generally fixed, and there is a powerful closing of the glottis to prevent any fluids from gaining access into the trachea.

The dog and cat vomit with relative ease. They are able to induce vomiting by eating portions of the green shoots of couch grass (*Triticum repens*), ingestion of which brings on vomiting within 5 to 10 minutes. In the pig, the process is more exacting than in the carnivores. Cattle and sheep may vomit occasionally, but it is not common and may be related to a serious stomach disorder or to rhododendron poisoning. Vomiting in the horse is rare, and often is associated with a rupture of the stomach; when it occurs it should be considered a very grave symptom indeed. The material always escapes through the nostrils in the horse.

Causes Vomiting can be considered under the following headings:

Travel sickness.

Stress.

Simple indigestion. When the stomach has received either a quality or a quantity of foodstuff with which it is unable to deal, the process of digestion does not proceed, or only proceeds up to a point. The material brought up is recognisable as food, but it is mixed with quantities of frothy mucus, water, and perhaps may be stained brownish from bile. It has a faintly sour smell which is greater the longer the process of digestion has been enabled to proceed. The ejecta is generally easily brought up, and the animal soon settles down and becomes normal.

Indigestion from foreign bodies. (See 'CHOKING'; IMPACTION; FOREIGN BODY.)

Gastritis. The walls of the stomach are inflamed and thickened, the mucous membrane is swollen and painful, and the nervous system is in an irritable state. Whenever food or water enters the organ, vomiting immediately takes place. The vomit consists of the solid material swallowed, coated on the outside with mucus and froth. If liquids have been taken they are returned almost unchanged. When the inflammatory condition is very severe there are quantities of blood that have undergone partial digestion and have an appearance not unlike coffee-grounds, seen in the vomit. In such animals there will be a very offensive smell both from the ejecta and from the mouth of the patient.

Pyloric stenosis, which may be congenital, is said to give rise to projectile vomiting.

Enteritis is associated with vomiting but there is diarrhoea as well.

Impaction of the rectum, whether from particles of undigested bone, or hair, hard faeces, etc., generally induces vomiting in which not only does the stomach expel its contents, but masses of bowel content as well.

Acute nephritis is an extremely common cause of thirst and vomiting in the dog.

Pyometra in the bitch, cat, and sow is frequently accompanied by vomiting.

Accidents. The shock of a severe burn or accident will cause vomiting, although the injuries have not been inflicted upon the stomach itself. In other cases, where the head has been injured, the area in the case of the brain which control the act of vomiting becomes disturbed and the animal evacuates its stomach.

Poisons. Many irritant substances will produce vomiting. Of the commonest may be mentioned tartar emetic, mustard, salt, carbolic acid, areca-nut, castor oil, etc.; and of substances less common, but more drastic, the following are examples: strychnine, arsenic, phosphorus, apomorphine, croton oil, zinc and copper sulphates, and many of the metallic salts. Some of these have special characteristics; for example, phosphorus vomit is luminous in the dark.

Diseases. The symptom of vomiting is common to many other diseases – meningitis, peritonitis, nephritis, leptospirosis, rabies, vomiting and wasting syndrome in pigs, etc.

Treatment In the dog and cat the use of normal saline or glucose saline by injection is frequently indicated as an alternative to giving food (liquid or otherwise) by mouth during an illness (such as nephritis, uraemia, and enteritis) in which vomiting is persistent.

Vomiting and Wasting Syndrome

This occurs in piglets 5 days old and upwards, and is characterised by vomiting, depression, loss of appetite, constipation, emaciation, and a hairy appearance. It is caused by a coronavirus, haemagglutinating encephalomyelitis virus (HEV). (See also 'ONTARIO ENCEPHALITIS'.)

Von Willebrand's Disease

An inherited bleeding disorder found in some 25 breeds of dogs, and associated with an autosomal trait causing a high morbidity but a low mortality. Signs may include epistaxis, haematuria, lameness, bleeding from genital mucosa, and prolonged bleeding from cut nails, etc.

Vultures

(see TROPICS; CARCASES, DISPOSAL OF)

Vulva

It has in domesticated animals only simple, single labia or lips.

Diseases of the vulva In Kenya, squamous cell carcinoma of the vulva is common in cattle of the Ayrshire breed. Cryosurgery has given good results when treatment has not been delayed until the tumour becomes too large. In 62 cases, 55 were successfully treated.

(For persistent bleeding from the vulva, see VAGINA.)

In the tropics, especially, a thick purulent discharge from the vagina may be a sign of tuberculosis involving the uterus/vagina.

Vulvovaginitis

(see under RHINOTRACHEITIS and VULVOVAGINITIS, GRANULAR)

Vulvovaginitis, Granular

A venereal disease of cattle caused by *Mycoplasma bovigenitalium*, affecting vulva and vagina or seminal vesicles and skin of the penis. The lesions are nodules.

V

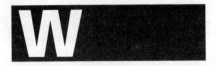

consequently unusual. It is not a serious defect except in tropical countries.

Wallabies

Smaller than kangaroos, these native Australian marsupials are a source of human HYDATID DISEASE in the southern tablelands of New South Wales. Lumpy jaw is a common finding. They may sometimes be found as feral animals in parts of England.

'Walkabout Disease'

(see KIMBERLEY HORSE DISEASE)

Wall Eye (Leukoma)

Wall eye (leukoma) is a condition in which the brown pigment of the iris is lacking, giving the iris a steely blue appearance. In dogs, it is usually unilateral and is not a problem. In the horse, wall eyes may occur when the greater part of the face, or that portion around the eyes, is white. The pupil of the eye appears to be encircled by a ring of bluish or greyish white, and the expression of the horse's face is

Warble Fly Order

The Warble Fly Order came into force in 1989. The presence of warble fly lesions in cattle is a NOTIFIABLE DISEASE in Britain. Where a blood test indicates that an infestation may be present, treatment under the supervision of an officer of the State Veterinary Service is required. Every herd and every bovine animal within 3 km of an infestation must be treated (the fly

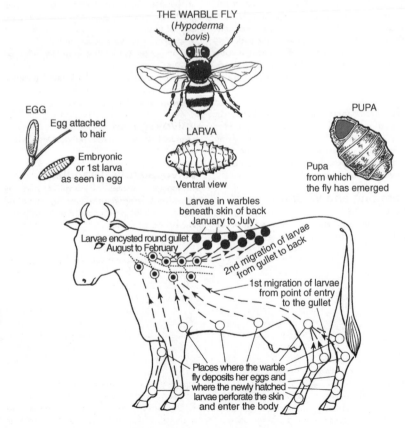

THE WARBLE FLY
(*Hypoderma bovis*)

EGG
Egg attached to hair
Embryonic or 1st larva as seen in egg

LARVA
Ventral view

PUPA
Pupa from which the fly has emerged

Larvae in warbles beneath skin of back January to July

Larvae encysted round gullet August to February

2nd migration of larvae from gullet to back

1st migration of larvae from point of entry to the gullet

Places where the warble fly deposits her eggs and where the newly hatched larvae perforate the skin and enter the body

The life-cycle of the warble fly.

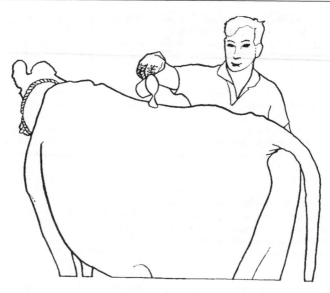

Dressing against warbles.

is able to travel only short distances). As warble flies are present in other countries, all cattle imported into Britain must be treated for possible infestation within 24 hours of arrival. The treatment must be supervised by a State Veterinary Service officer.

Warbles

Warbles are swellings about the size of a marble or small walnut occurring upon the backs of cattle in spring and early summer, caused by the presence in them of the larvae of one of the warble flies – *Hypoderma bovis* or *H. lineata*. These are of very great economic importance. The adults – especially *H. bovis* – cause great annoyance to stock during the period when eggs are being laid. Not only does this result in injuries, animals rushing around ('gadding') to avoid the attacks, but the milk yield is reduced, sometimes by as much as 25 per cent, and condition is impaired.

H. lineata in its migration through the body irritates the gullet; and both species may injure the spinal cord. The warbles on the back are really so many small abscesses which not only reduce condition very considerably but may, when many are present, result in the death of young animals. The accidental crushing of a number of the larvae in these cavities may cause the death of the animal from anaphylactic shock.

In the carcases there is considerable destruction of valuable meat around the warbles; 'butcher's

jelly' or 'licked beef' is an oedematous, straw-coloured, jelly-like substance, which infiltrates the tissue near the larvae. The holes which the larvae produce in the hides reduce their value; heavily infected hides are often useless for leather.

Warbles are most common in young animals, in which loss of condition is most serious; but they have been found in small numbers in animals up to 15 years old. They are sometimes found in young horses. The larvae occasionally enter the spinal canal and produce very serious lesions. Horses are attacked mostly by *H. bovis* larvae, which affect the area of the saddle chiefly; but brain involvement has been reported in the horse. In deer, larvae of the warble fly *H. diana* are often found.

Methods of control Satisfactory control depends upon artificial interference with the life-cycle. (See IVERMECTIN.) A systemic insecticide will kill a high percentage of larvae before they complete their migration and penetrate the back.

In Britain in 1978, 40 per cent of cattle in England and Wales, and 20 percent in Scotland, were affected with warbles. (See FLIES – FLY control measure.)

Autumn is the more effective time for treatment, even though infestation cannot be visually detected then, and cattle-owners in warble-affected areas are advised to treat their herds accordingly.

W

Pour-on warblecide compounds include phosmet and ivermectin. Parenteral preparations of abamectin, doramectin and moxidectin are also effective.

Reindeer In Canada they are attacked by the warble fly *Edoede magena tarandi*. Ivermectin has been used for control.

Goats Ivermectin has been used also against the goat warble *Przhevalskiana silenus*.
Following the introduction of the Warble Fly Order 1985, infestation by warbles was virtually eradicated by 1995.

The tropical warble fly of Central America is *Dermatobia hominis*, which lays its eggs on an intermediary vector – fly or mosquito – which it catches for the purpose. (See also under FLIES, and IVERMECTIN.)

Warfarin

An anticoagulant drug used in human medicine; its veterinary use is mainly as a rat poison. It causes death of rats and mice from internal haemorrhage. In the strengths used, 0.005 per cent and 0.025 per cent, it is considered that properly prepared baits will not prove dangerous to livestock if used with ordinary care. Cases of accidental poisoning have occurred, however, in domestic animals; and food contaminated by rodents' urine may be dangerous where warfarin is used.

Therapeutically, warfarin is used in the treatment of navicular disease.

Treatment of warfarin poisoning

Vitamin K_1 (phytomenadione) by intramuscular injection. Blood transfusion may be necessary.

Once symptoms have appeared, use of glucose saline, or blood transfusion, is indicated. The poisoned animal must be handled very gently, or further internal bleeding may occur. (See also NAVICULAR DISEASE.)

Warts (Papillomas)

Warts (papillomas) are small growths which appear on skin or mucous membrane, and occur in all farm and domestic animals. Papillomas are benign, but an individual wart can become malignant. (See PAPILLOMA.)

Around the mouth they may interfere with feeding, and when occurring about the nostrils they may obstruct the breathing. Soft warts in the oesophagus sometimes make swallowing difficult, and upon the penis or in the urethra they may hinder the passage of urine. (See also EYE.)

Horses The commonest situations are the skin of the udder or sheath, the lips and nostrils, the eyelids, outer and inner skin of the ears, the region of the breast, and the insides of the limbs.

Cattle The commonest seats of warts are the teats of cows. Young cows in winter are frequently affected about the skin of the eyelids and along the lower line of the abdomen, but the growths often drop off spontaneously from these positions when the young animals are turned out to grass in the early spring. Otherwise warty growths are found as in the horse.

Dogs and cats In the dog especially, less so in the cat, warts are common. Single small warts with a cauliflower-like extremity or with a rounded top are commonly found about the eyelids, lips, ears, paws, etc., as well as upon the general surface of the body. They usually grow very slowly and may be present for years without causing any pain or inconvenience. In other cases warts appear in connection with the gums, tongue, and insides of the cheeks; in these positions they arise in clusters and grow very rapidly. Cases such as these are usually accompanied by a great amount of salivation and a fetid discharge from the mouth.

Removal Of Warts Multiple warts in cattle have been treated by a variety of chemicals, including injections of lithium antimony tartrate, with varying degrees of success. Autogenous and other vaccines have also been used where there is a herd problem, and surgical removal may be resorted to.

Washing of Animals
(see BATHS)

Wasp Stings
(see under BITES)

Waste Food
(see BAKERY WASTE; SWILL; CHOCOLATE POISONING)

Wasting
(see ATROPHY)

Water and Watering of Animals

Amounts required The quantity of water needed per day by the various domestic animals depends upon the nature of the food, the climate, the temperature, and the size and the activity of the animals themselves. When very dry food is given, such as hay, bran, oats, etc., more water is required than when roots or growing grass is eaten.

Drinking water should be freely available to animals, so that they can drink as and when they choose. (*See below under* 'Water supply'.) Stress may occur in an animal deprived of the chance to drink sufficient water, and actual dehydration (which can lead to death) may be caused. Production of milk, etc., will obviously be adversely affected.

With an ad lib water supply, the amount of water required by various animals under various conditions is of mainly theoretical interest, apart from practical aspects of planning adequate supplies of piped water, trough space, etc. Water requirement figures can be taken only as approximate guidelines, and authorities differ to some extent.

Cattle Dry cows of the larger breeds require between 36.5 and 45 litres (8 to 10 gallons) per day. Those in milk need in addition about 5 times as much water as the volume of milk produced, while for the last 4 months of pregnancy, the daily consumption may rise to about 70 litres (approximately 15 gallons).

As the air temperature increases above 10°C (50°F), the water requirement rises rapidly.

Calves require much more water after they are weaned than before. A common mistake is to ignore this fact, with the result that the calves receive a check to their growth from which they may never fully recover.

Pigs are highly susceptible to water deprivation. (See SALT POISONING.) Approximate quantities required have been given as 4.5 litres (1 gallon) per day for a litter of 3-week-old piglets, and up to 22.5 litres (5 gallons) per day for a nursing sow. The benefits of creep feeding may be lost if the piglets are denied water.

Quality of water This is obviously of prime importance. Animals may suffer thirst and stress if the only drinking water available to them is disagreeable in taste. Where piped water is not available, and rainwater has to be stored in tanks, it is important to clean out gutters and the tanks themselves. Galvanised iron tanks should not be allowed to get rusty. Well-water may contain an excess of one or more minerals which may make it unpalatable or be harmful to the animal, so that sampling and analysis should be carried out.

Poisoning by water may result from the use of lead pipes or tanks. (See LEAD POISONING.)

The use of lead paints in storage tanks is also a danger. (See also ZINC POISONING.) Stored rain-water containing decaying organic matter (leaves, bird droppings, etc.) has led to the death of pigs from nitrite poisoning.

Diseases spread by water Apart from illness caused by some inorganic substance dissolved in the water, such as lead from lead pipes or tanks, or arsenic from contamination with sheep-dip, water-borne infection may cause disease.

Among diseases that can be distributed in this manner are the following: anthrax, from water used in tanneries or wool-washing premises, or when a carcase has been buried near a stream; Johne's disease, salmonellosis, and coccidiosis in cattle, from contamination of streams, ditches, and ponds. Liver fluke can be spread via infected mud snails, *Lymnaea truncatula*. *Leptospira hardjo* infection is 8 times more likely where cattle have access to a water course.

Washing water and water-tanks have been contaminated with, for example, *Bacillus subtilis*, leading to MASTITIS.

Water supply A good stockman will ensure that the animals in his care are never short of water; that all automatic drinking bowls or nipple drinkers are in working order; that frost has not cut off the supply of piped water (lagging of exposed pipes is obviously necessary in winter); and that the water has not been allowed to freeze in troughs, tanks, etc. It is also necessary to ensure that the levers of automatic drinking

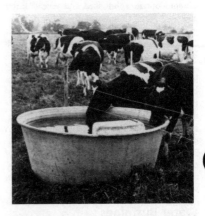

Designed for field use, this CemFil glass fibre-reinforced cement drinking trough is obtainable in sizes of up to 2000-litre capacity. The water supply is, of course, piped.

W

bowls are not too stiff for young animals to operate, and that young stock are shown working nipple drinkers – not left to find them for themselves. (See also ALGAE.)

In one incident, newly weaned pigs were put into a yard having automatic water-bowls fitted, but as the yard had been mucked out the bowls were out of reach of the young pigs.

Pigs deprived of water show nervous symptoms. They may walk in circles, or backwards, press their heads against a wall, champ their jaws, collapse and have convulsions. Of course, some pigs may be found dead without symptoms having been observed.

Sheep have shown symptoms suggestive of twin-lamb disease, and died, after being removed from a field where they had access to a stream and placed on pasture where the ball-valve of a drinking trough had been tied up. Sheep prefer to drink running water, and those of some breeds are so reluctant to drink anything else that, when housed, a running water supply must be arranged indoors.

A drop in milk yield may occur in dairy herds where the cows are moved periodically to a field too far from a water-trough; or where the water pressure is too low to ensure adequate supply.

Dogs, cats, and poultry should always be allowed an unlimited supply of water so arranged that they are unable to foul or upset the drinking vessels.

(See also DEHYDRATION.)

Horses Wherever possible, **water should be given before the food**, or not for 1 to 2 hours after feeding. The horse's stomach is small, and cannot contain a full feed and several litres/gallons of water simultaneously. Water in excess of requirements should be offered when horses are at rest, and they should be allowed to drink frequently when working.

Water intoxication This may occur in farm livestock when, as a result of bad management, they have been deprived of adequate drinking water and then suddenly find themselves in circumstances which enable them to drink as much as they want.

One symptom may be a red discoloration of the urine. Convulsions, recumbency, hyperaesthesia, aimless wandering, and death have been seen in calves.

Water Buffaloes

Water buffaloes are regarded by many as an under-utilised form of livestock. It is common practice in the tropics to immerse them in water

during the heat of the day as they have very few sweat glands and are prone to heatstroke. However, they can be reared away from water if shade is available. They are widely used as a draught animal in warmer countries, including the poorer parts of Italy. They are farmed in Britain to produce mozzarella cheese. Studies in the USA, Papua New Guinea, Trinidad and Australia have shown water buffalo perform well as regards growth rates, health and production of meat and milk. They are able to digest rougher material than cattle or sheep.

Water buffalo meat is similar in taste to beef; the milk is richer in butterfat and solids-not-fat than cows' milk. There is a general low incidence of mastitis, probably because on ceasing milking, the teat canal closes very rapidly. Water buffalo are generally quite docile unless severely stressed or in pain.

Some of the steps needed to permit greater exploitation of this valuable animal are:

1. Trials to compare growth rate, feeding, nutrition and other characteristics of water buffalo with those of cattle.

2. Selective breeding and protection of outstanding buffalo specimens, especially in Southeast Asia.

3. Replacement of the 1500-year-old inefficient wooden yoke (in rural Asia, where the water buffalo is the small farmer's 'tractor', improved harnesses could increase pulling power by up to 25 per cent. (See TRANSPORT OF ANIMALS.)

The limitation of water buffaloes must be taken into account. For instance, the animals suffer if forced to remain, even for a few hours, in direct sunlight. They cannot be worked for long periods during the heat of the day, and they are also susceptible to extreme cold. (*The Water Buffalo: New Prospects for an Underutilized Animal*, US National Academy of Sciences).

An important roundworm of the water buffalo (*Bubalus bubalis*) is *Paracooperia nodulosa*. This causes development of nodules in the intestine, and diarrhoea, anaemia, emaciation and sometimes death. (See LIVESTOCK PRODUCTION.)

Water-Dropwort

This is *Oenanthe fistulosa*, and while it and parsley water-dropwort (*O. lachenalii* and also *O. aquatica*) are all poisonous, they are less so than hemlock water-dropwort (*O. crocata*) – a weed of marshy places, ditches, and other wet locations. This is considered to be one of the most dangerous and poisonous of the commoner plants found in Britain, and many cases of

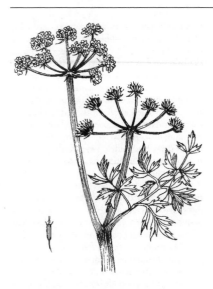

Water-dropwort (*Oenanthe crocata*). This should strictly be called hemlock water-dropwort. The roots are the most poisonous part of the plant, and are often dislodged during severe floods or ditching or drainage work. Height: about 1.3 m (4 ft).

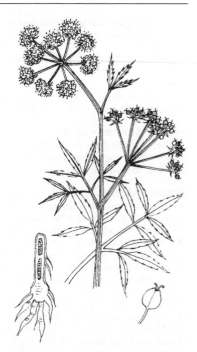

Water hemlock or cowbane (*Cicuta virosa*), showing the dahlia-like roots attached to the enlarged base of the stem, seed capsule, leaves and greenish-white inflorescence. The flowering stem may be 1.6 to 2.5 m (5 to 10 ft) tall.

poisoning, not only among animals but also among human beings, have been recorded. It is a member of the same botanical class as cowbane, hemlock, and fool's parsley, and like them the poisonous principle is found in all parts of the plant. In its leaves it has a great similarity to celery, and its rootstock has been mistaken for parsnip. The active toxic principle is called oenanthotoxin, and is most abundant in the root. Hemlock water-dropwort often causes problems when roots of the plant are exposed following hedging and ditching, and canal bank and stream clearances.

Signs The symptoms appear very quickly after the plant has been eaten, and death follows within 1 to 4 hours when large amounts have been taken. Cattle become very depressed in general appearance, and their respiration is fast and laboured. The mucous membranes become congested, the eye rolls, the pulse is weak and fast, and there is a certain amount of foaming at the mouth. Convulsions follow.

In some cases that are not fatal, one or more of the limbs may remain paralysed. In the horse the appearance of symptoms and the course of the illness are much more rapid and the nervous symptoms are exaggerated.

Treatment Barbiturates may save life.

Water-Fleas
Daphnia pulex, a brown water-flea found in British ponds, is the intermediate host of the roundworms of ducks, e.g. *Acuaria uncinata*.

Water Hemlock
Water hemlock, a common plant of damp marshy places in all parts of the Northern Hemisphere, has a short, stout hollow rootstock, and large much-divided leaves set on strong stems. Water hemlock (*Cicuta virosa*) is also known as cowbane.

The root in springtime contains the greatest amount of the poisonous principles, which are 3 in number, viz. an alkaloid, cicutine; an oil, oil of cicuta; and a bitter resinous substance, cicutoxin.

Signs Salivation, dullness, vomiting in pigs; colic in horses; bloat in cattle; together with diarrhoea, a staggering gait. Sudden death or a few hours' illness.

First Aid Owing to the rapidity of the appearance of symptoms it is not often that treatment

W

can be successfully carried out. Strong black coffee or tea may be given. Veterinary help should be sought.

Water, Loss of

Loss of water from the tissues – a serious condition – is referred to under DEHYDRATION. It occurs especially during the course of diarrhoea.

Waterhammer Pulse

The peculiarly sudden pulse that is associated with incompetence of the aortic valves of the left side of the heart.

Watery Mouth

An often fatal disease of newborn lambs in the UK. *E. coli* is commonly isolated but its involvement in the disease is unclear. The lambs appear strong and healthy but on taking milk from the ewe they soon show signs of abdominal pain, and a watery fluid drips from the mouth. There may be scouring. Death soon follows as a rule.

In a summary of the clinical features of 102 cases of watery mouth in lambs, the majority of cases were observed in ram lambs (73 per cent) and within the first 3 days of life (80 per cent). The results suggest that the incidence of watery mouth may be reduced by delaying castration until lambs are at least 3 days old. A similar condition occurs in calves, also due to *E. coli*.

WBC

White blood cells.

Weals

Weals are raised white areas of the skin which possess reddened margins. They may result from sharp blows or from continued pressure against some hard object. They are only visible upon the skins of pigs, as the hair of the other domestic animals hides the actual skin surface. (See URTICARIA.)

The term 'weal' is also used in surgery in connection with the use of local anaesthetic solution. A primary weal is made, and when the local anaesthetic has taken effect, the needle of the syringe may be reintroduced into the now insensitive area and further injections made painlessly in order to anaesthetise a given area.

Weaning

Weaning is a critical period in the life of the young animal unless carried out with care. Generally speaking, it is necessary to accustom the young growing animal to a diet in which its dam's milk takes a more and more secondary place for some weeks before actual separation occurs. In the case of dairy cattle there is an exception to this rule, in that newly born calves are often taken away from their mothers as soon as they have had some colostrum, and are then reared from a pail. Sudden changes in the diet are to be avoided at all times, and the changes from a milk to a herbivorous or omnivorous diet should be gradual, for obvious reasons. In modern pig husbandry, creep-feeding is practised before weaning. (See CREEP-FEEDING; COLOSTRUM.)

Early weaning of calves Most calves in the dairy herd are taken from their mothers within a day or two of birth, after they have received colostrum. They are then introduced to milk or milk-substitute feeding from a bucket, a teated container or an automatic machine feeder. The amount of liquid the calf receives with the first 2 methods is restricted, usually, to about 2 litres of milk or substitute containing 12.5 per cent solids. This does not completely satisfy the appetite of the growing calf, so it is introduced to roughage, in the form of creep feed and water. They continue on a fixed quantity of the liquid feed and gradually increase the amount of other feed consumed. This allows them to be completely weaned at a younger age than would otherwise be possible. Calves can be weaned when they are consuming 0.7 kg (1½ lb) daily if in single pens, or 1 kg (2 lb) on average if in group pens, for 3 consecutive days. It has, however, been suggested that calves should not be weaned until they double their birthweight or are at least 80 kg (175 lb), whichever is the heavier.

Early weaning of piglets Most piglets are weaned at 3 to 4 weeks. Earlier weaning is only permissible if the health and /or welfare of the sow or the litter would be adversely affected by the normal weaning age.

Piglets suckled to 8 weeks can cause marked loss of condition in the sow. Weaning at 4 weeks allows quicker turnround in the farrowing house, and consequently less accommodation is needed – as well as the attainment of more than 4 litters in 2 years. Food-costs per piglet are higher by this method, but weight at 8 weeks can be appreciably higher. The sow must be taken from the piglets, not vice versa, and housed out of earshot, as she will fret. (See also under SOW'S MILK.)

Early weaning of lambs (see SHEEP BREEDING)

Weatings

The particles finer than bran of the husk of wheat, containing not more than about 6 per cent crude fibre. They are also known as offals and middlings, and much confusion exists between these various terms.

Weaving

Weaving was thought to be a vice of horses and a form of stereotypical behaviour, but this is open to doubt. Affected animals swing the head and neck and the anterior parts of the body backwards and forwards; sometimes the affected animal appears not to be able to stand still on all 4 feet and lifts each foot in turn. The behaviour shown is thought to indicate pain. It has been postulated that the affected horse is suffering from trigeminal neuralgia, a recognised condition in man that causes excruciating pain. In some cases, a degree of relief has been obtained by tracheotomy; it appears that the mere passage of air through the nose is enough to cause the clinical signs.

Wedder (Wether)

A castrated male lamb, after weaning (see under SHEEP).

Wedge Osteotomy

An operation for treating an angular deformity of the horse's fetlock of 8° or more.

Weedkillers

Weedkillers used in agriculture include: DNOC, DNP, PARAQUAT, DIQUAT. Hormone weedkillers: MCPA, Agroxone 4, and 2, 4-D. MCPA, it is claimed, renders pasture more palatable and has no ill-effects upon cattle or their milk. Ragwort and buttercups also become more palatable, due to a temporary increase in their sugar content, and poisoning may consequently arise. (See also HERBICIDES.)

Weights of Cattle

At birth, calves of the larger breeds weigh 36 to 54 kg (80 to 120 lb) – 77 kg (170 lb) has been recorded. The averages for heifer calves are about: British Friesian, 39 kg (86 lb); Dairy Shorthorn, 36 kg (80 lb); Jersey, 25 kg (56 lb). Bull calves weigh about 2.25 kg (5 lb) more.

Weights of Horses

At birth, a Shire or Clydesdale foal averages 90 or 100 kg (1½ or 2 cwt).

Weights of Pigs

Averages in Britain are as follows: at birth, 0.9 or 1.4 kg (2 or 3 lb); at 3 weeks, 5.4 or 5.9 kg (12 or 13 lb); at 8 weeks, 16 or 16.6 kg (36 or 37 lb).

Weil's Disease

(see LEPTOSPIROSIS IN DOGS)

Weimaraner

A German breed of dog, medium to large, with long neck, pendulous ears and a smooth silvery coat. Originally used as a pointer and retriever. Close to extinction at the end of the 1939–45 war, it was saved by British troops. Distortion of the nictitating membrane may be found, as well as spinal dysraphism (an abnormal dilation of the central canal of the spinal cord). Cutaneous asthenia and ununited anconal process may be inherited, as may haemophilia A.

Welfare Codes for Animals

Welfare Codes for Animals produced under the Agriculture (Miscellaneous Provisions) Act 1968, make recommendations as to how animals should be kept. There are codes covering cattle, domestic fowl, ducks, farmed deer, goats, pigs, rabbits, sheep and turkeys. Anyone keeping any of those species must have, and have read, a copy of the appropriate code; staff looking after the animals must also have read it. While the codes are advisory only (but see below), if the recommendations are ignored and animals suffer in consequence, the code can be used in evidence in a court of law.

Regulations The regulations relating to cattle, poultry, pigs and rabbits (Welfare of Farmed Animal Regulations 2000) have converted some of the recommendations of the codes of practice into mandatory requirements (e.g. stocking densities for pigs). The regulations also prevent the routine tail-docking and tooth-clipping of pigs except where this is necessary (a case for performing such operations must be made). Tail-docking of cattle, surgical castration of poultry and interference with the vision of birds are also prohibited. (see also under FARM ANIMAL WELFARE COUNCIL; LAW).

Welfare of Animals at Slaughter Act

This amends the Acts of 1974 and 1980, and covers the formal training, examination, and licensing of slaughtermen, codes of practice relating to welfare, in both slaughterhouses and knackers' yards.

Welfare of Farmed Animal Regulations 2000

Welfare of Farmed Animal Regulations 2000 specify the minimum standards under which farmed animals are to be kept. There are special provisions for battery hens, calves, pigs and

W

rabbits. The regulations incorporate many of the guidelines in the WELFARE CODES FOR ANIMALS.

Wells (Well Water)
(see WATER AND WATERING OF ANIMALS)

Welfare of Animals (Slaughter or Killing) Regulations 1995
These cover the licensing of slaughtermen and knackermen, including the handling of animals at abattoirs. They detail the (only) methods by which animals may be slaughtered or killed.

Wesselsbron Disease

Cause A flavivirus. Transmitted by mosquitoes, and communicable to man, this infection was first reported in South Africa in 1955. It caused death of lambs, abortion, and some deaths of ewes; persistent muscular pain in man. It resembles Rift Valley fever.

West Highland White Terrier
A small, rough-haired breed, with pointed ears and black nose. The breed is prone to craniomandibular osteopathy, inguinal hernia, keratoconjunctivitis sicca and Perthe's disease.

West Nile Virus
Cause of an infection, mainly in wild birds; corvids (crows, magpies, jays) are particularly susceptible, with dead birds literally falling out of the sky. The disease was transported from Israel to the USA in 1998 and spread rapidly, reaching Canada. Virus is transmitted by mosquitoes; humans and other primates can be infected, but a mosquito biting an infected human is unable to transmit the disease to another person. There is evidence that the infection is present in British wild birds. The virus is related to yellow fever and Japanese encephalitis viruses.

Wether
A castrated male sheep after weaning (see under SHEEP).

Wetting Agents
Substances which lower the surface tension of water, so that the latter spreads out over the surface rather than remaining in the form of drops. Good wetting ability is a characteristic of detergents, which play an essential part in the disinfection of vessels, pipes, glassware used for milking equipment, etc.

Wharton's Duct
Wharton's duct is the name of the tube by which saliva secreted by the submaxillary gland reaches the cavity of the mouth. It opens in the floor of the mouth almost opposite to the canine tooth in the horse.

Wharton's Jelly
Wharton's jelly is the embryonic connective tissue that forms the basis of the umbilical cord in the fetus. In its substance are found the umbilical vessels and the other structures that constitute the umbilical cord.

Wheat Gluten
For the adverse effect of this in some instances in calves, see under SOYA BEANS.

Wheezing
(see BRONCHITIS; also 'BROKEN WIND')

Whelping
(see under PARTURITION, in the bitch)

Whey
Whey is the liquid residue left after the separation of the curds in cheesemaking. Used as a food, particularly for pigs. Can be a source of infection if made from unpasteurised milk.

Whippet
A medium-sized dog of the greyhound type. The breed is prone to alopecia.

Whipworm
Whipworm is the popular name for the Trichuris found in the caecum. (See ROUNDWORMS.)

Whirling Disease
A parasitic disease of fish caused by the protozoan *Myxosoma cerebralis*. The parasite spends part of its life-cycle in mud; after swallowing by the fish it migrates and penetrates the cartilage of the skull. Affected fish swim erratically. There is no treatment but the disease can be prevented by rearing young fish in plastic or concrete-lined ponds until the skull is ossified – the parasite cannot penetrate bone. It was formerly a notifiable disease.

Whistling
Whistling is a defect affecting the respiratory system of the horse. In many respects it is similar to 'ROARING', but the note emitted is higher pitched. It constitutes an unsoundness.

White Cells
(see under BLOOD. For white cells in milk, see under MASTITIS)

White Diarrhoea, Bacillary
(see under PULLORUM DISEASE)

'White Heifer Disease'
The name given to defects in the genitalia most commonly found in Shorthorn cattle. The defects can vary from the presence of fibrous tissue across the posterior part of the vagina ('persistent hymen') that may be corrected surgically, to the absence of all or part of the uterus.

White Line
White line is the margin of horn that runs round the outside of the sole, between it and the wall, in the horse's hoof. It acts as a slightly pliable cementing material between wall and sole. It is important as a guide to the shoeing smith, since it forms a line inside which it is unsafe to drive a nail without risk of pricking the sensitive parts of the foot.

White Muscle Disease
White muscle disease is another name for the result of vitamin E deficiency. (See MUSCLES, DISEASES OF – Nutritional myopathy.)

White Scour in Calves
White scour in calves is a disease affecting calves within the first 3 weeks of life. The disease is usually a rapid one. In the acute case the calf may be found dead or dying; in other cases death occurs within 3 to 10 days after symptoms are first noticed.

Cause is usually *E. coli,* but other organisms may be involved, including *Proteus vulgaris* and *Pseudomonas pyocyanea, Salmonella* spp.

Predisposing causes include: exposure to cold and damp; deprivation of colostrum; sudden

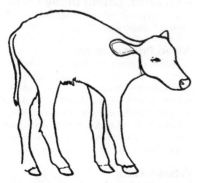

An arched back is characteristic of white scour; also a dejected appearance.

changes in diet; feeding with unsound milk or mouldy calf-meals from unclean utensils; overcrowding; and housing healthy calves in pens or boxes that have previously contained cases of the disease and have not been carefully disinfected afterwards.

White scour is very rare in beef cattle at pasture.

Calving-boxes should be disinfected and well littered before the pregnant cattle occupy them. A protective serum has been used with encouraging results. Where bucket-feeding is adopted, colostrum must not be withheld.

Treatment It is essential to overcome the dehydration resulting from the diarrhoea. (For details, see DEHYDRATION.)

Other treatment comprises the use of *E. coli* antiserum, sulfamezathine or one of the other sulfa drugs, and in some cases the inclusion of yeast in the diet. Serum from the dam has been given by subcutaneous injection in default of colostrum. (See also DIARRHOEA.)

White Spot
White spot is a parasitic disease in which white cysts are formed all over the surface of the fish, including the gills. It is more common in the carp family, including goldfish. The cause is *Icthyophthirius multifiliis.* Part of its life-cycle is spent at the bottom of ponds, from where the infective stage is released into the water and makes for the fish. It is only at this stage that the parasite can be treated. Zinc-free malachite green is used to create a very dilute solution in the pond (0.1 ppm), as the parasite will continue to be released until eradicated. Treatment instructions must be followed carefully if toxicity is to be avoided.

'Whites'
'Whites' is another name for leukorrhoea, and is a term popularly used in connection with *C. pyogenes* infection in cows. (See LEUKORRHOEA; UTERUS, DISEASES OF; VAGINITIS.)

Whiteside Test
This has been used for the detection of subclinical mastitis, by indicating an abnormally high white-cell count of the milk. A modified version consists of placing 1 drop of 4 per cent caustic soda (NaOH) and 5 drops of the milk on a glass plate, and stirring with a glass rod for 20 seconds or so. The presence of flakes indicates a positive result; a viscous mass at the end of the rod suggests a strong positive result. It is a laboratory version of the California Mastitis Test.

W

Whorls

These, as well as colour markings, assist in the identification of horses. A whorl is a pattern of hairs, often about 2.5 cm (1 in) across.

Wild Birds

For unintended poisoning of these, see under GAME BIRDS; also TEM.

Wild Dogs

Wild dogs are an important source of human hydatid infection in New South Wales, where a sylvatic strain of *Echinococcue granulosus* circulates predominantly between them and wallabies. The incidence of infection in domestic dogs, however, is much lower.

Wilting

Wilting of sugar-beet tops is highly desirable before feeding in order to avoid poisoning, and with a lush crop of grass on a new ley, cutting and allowing to wilt may obviate bloat.

Wind Puffs

A popular term for the rupture of one or more air sacs in birds, with escape of air under the skin. The birds appear very fat, until handled. The condition usually resolves without treatment.

Wind Galls

Distensions of the joint capsules, or of tendon sheaths, in the region of the fetlock. (See SYNOVITIS.)

Wind-Borne Infection

Under favourable conditions, viruses, including the virus of foot-and-mouth disease, may be carried from country to country, even where a long sea passage is involved.

Wind-Sucking

(see CRIB-BITING)

Windbreaks

(see under EXPOSURE)

Winter Diet

It is often wise to incorporate 5 per cent of animal protein in the winter rations of dairy cattle, which otherwise may be getting too little protein and give milk low in solids-not-fat. Succulent food such as silage or kale forms a high proportion of the winter diet for cattle, which may be receiving too little carbohydrate. On self-fed silage the NIRD have recorded a 33 per cent reduction in dry-matter intake, compared with a diet of hay and concentrates.

Winter Infertility

(see INFERTILITY)

Wire

(see STOMACH, DISEASES OF – Foreign bodies in reticulum) Barbed wire is responsible for many small wounds of the cow's udder which predispose to mastitis, and for accidents in the hunting field.

'Witch's Milk'

An old name for abnormal secretion, in rare instances, of milk by the newborn of either sex.

Withdrawal Period

The length of time that must elapse after treatment with a medicinal product before an animal can be slaughtered for food, or its milk or eggs used for human consumption.

'Wobbler'

A colloquialism for a horse which evinces a slight swaying action of its hindquarters and a tendency to stumble. The condition is likely to progress to a form of ataxia in which the horse cannot trot without swaying from side to side and falling.

Cause Pressure on the spinal cord in the neck region blocking nerve transmission to the hindlegs. The pressure may be caused by subluxation of the vertebrae of the neck, arthritis, or osteochondritis. Surgery to relieve the pressure may be a possibility.

The wobbler syndrome in the dog is referred to under SPINE AND SPINAL CORD, DISEASES AND INJURIES OF – Cervical spondulopathy.

Womb

(see UTERUS)

Wood-Ash, Eating of, by Cattle

This is suggestive of a diet deficient in salt, calcium or magnesium.

Wood Preservatives

Some of these are a source of arsenical poisoning; others, containing chlorinated naphthalene compounds, of hyperkeratosis. Creosote and pentachlorophenol are liable to cause poisoning in young pigs; the latter has caused fatal poisoning in cats bedded on sawdust from treated timber. Cats have been killed also by DIELDRIN used for treating floorboards, etc., against woodworm.

Wood's Lamp

A source of ultra-violet radiation, it is used in the diagnosis of ringworm – diseased hairs, etc., appearing fluorescent in the case of *Microsporum canis* infection, but only to the extent of 50 per cent or so. A useful screening method, nonetheless. The fluorescence is of an applegreen colour.

Wooden Tongue
(see ACTINOBACILLOSIS)

Wool Balls in Lambs
On opening a lamb's stomach after death from some unknown disease, if a mass of wool and greyish or greenish softer material is found in the 1st or 4th stomach and no other readily obvious symptoms are noticed, the shepherd or owner is prone to reach the conclusion that the cause of death was this mass of wool. In some districts, so-called 'wool balls' have in the past been held to account for a high mortality among lambs, when the real cause was often lamb dysentery.

There is no doubt, however, that wool balls do occasionally kill in dry seasons or when ewes have for some other reason a reduced flow of milk. The hungry lamb withdraws all the milk available, but when it reaches the age of 2 to 4 weeks or so, this proves insufficient to satisfy its needs. It empties first one teat, then the other, and finally, searching for a further supply it finds a small tag of wool on the udder or near to it and sucks at it. The somewhat salty taste of the contained wool grease may possibly be pleasing, and in time the lock of wool comes away and is chewed and swallowed. Another lock is found, sucked, and also swallowed.

The mass of wool may occasionally result in blockage of the outlet from stomach to small intestine (PYLORUS).

Prevention The removal of shed wool from the pastures, and 'udder-locking' (clipping all wool from the udder before or at lambing).

Wool-Eating by Cats
Wool-eating by cats may result from boredom (e.g. in Siamese) or from persistence of the sucking reflex, and cause an obstruction of pylorus or bowel.

Wool Rot
(see under LUMPY WOOL)

Wool Slip
Alopecia occurring in housed ewes shorn during the winter, reducing wool yield by up to 25 per cent.

In order to avoid this alopecia, it has been suggested that sheep should be sheared at the same time as [...] number of per[...] quality diet sho[...] The diet should [...]

Works Chim[...]
(see FACTORY CHIM[...])

Worm Egg Co[...]
The use of faecal e[...] ounts as a means of estimating the degree of infestation can be misleading. With *Ostertagia* worms in calves, for example, the pattern of faecal egg counts tends to be the same whether the worm burden is large or small, increasing or decreasing. Counts increase fairly rapidly to an early peak, from which they decrease according to a logarithmic curve. This means that the egg count at any one point in time bears a constant relation to the egg count a given number of days before. The limit to total egg output evidently depends on the host's degree of immunity.

Worms
(see ROUNDWORMS; TAPEWORMS; LIVER-FLUKES; RUMEN-FLUKES; SCHISTOSOMIASIS for 'blood flukes'; HEARTWORMS; also EARTHWORMS.)

In cattle and sheep, parasitic gastroenteritis and bronchitis (husk) are important diseases caused by worms. (See also LIVER-FLUKES; NEMATODIRUS, STEPHANOFILARIASIS; and WORMS, FARM TREATMENT AGAINST.)

In horses, strongyle worm larvae may cause a verminous arteritis with fatal results. (See HORSES, WORMS IN; EQUINE VERMINOUS ARTERITIS; DIARRHOEA; FOALS, DISEASES OF; HYDATID DISEASE.)

In dogs in Britain, the worms usually encountered comprise ascarids, hookworms, whipworms, and tapeworms. (See also ANTHELMINTICS; TOXOCARA; TRACHEAL WORMS; HEARTWORMS; KIDNEY WORM; FLUKES.)

In pigs *Ascaris* worms in the intestine reduce growth rate, while their larvae, migrating through the lungs, may give rise to pneumonia and the symptom known as 'thumps'. Metastrongylus lungworms cause bronchitis and sometimes pneumonia. (See also THIN SOW SYNDROME and WORMS, FARM TREATMENT AGAINST.)

Worms, Farm Treatment Against
Much effort has been concentrated on the development of effective and safe anthelmintic

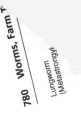

W

The principal parasitic worms of the pig, and their habitat.

drugs to control infestation of farm livestock by parasitic worms (endoparasites). There are many on the market, but often they derive from a relatively small group of chemical compounds. There is confusion among many users about which drugs to use in particular cases. A wide range of worms may be present in the gut (intestine), stomach or abomasum, lungs or liver; some endoparasites such as tapeworms and liver-flukes are found in other parts of the body during migratory stages of their development.

No wormer is completely effective against all worms, and one which may eradicate adult worms may not be effective against the larvae or eggs.

Thus the choice of which product to use depends both on knowing which worms are to be treated and the stage in their life-cycle at which they are to be destroyed.

Some anthelmintics act by killing the parasite, which may then be expelled in the faeces, broken down in the body or coughed up, depending on the site of infestation. Others work by immobilising the worm, thus allowing it to be expelled from the body.

Whatever worming procedures are used, they must be integrated with other animal-husbandry and grass-land-management procedures to prevent or reduce reinfection.

Wormers may be formulated to be given by mouth as a suspension, liquid, paste, in the feed or as a bolus; they may be given by injection; or as a 'pour-on' to be absorbed through the hide. Most have a wide margin of safety, but the effect of the medication on sick animals must always be considered. The effect of accidental contact, or ingestion, on the person administering the wormer must also be considered; the manufacturer's precautions and dosage instructions must be carefully read before use. Many products have a long duration of activity, and milk-withdrawal and meat-withholding times must be observed.

Administration The method of administering an anthelmintic is worth consideration. No method is perfect – each having some disadvantage. Drenching can, if not done with care, lead to 'drenching pneumonia', and the necessary restraint may be undesirable with yarded cattle or in-lamb ewes. The smaller dosages now required make drenching less hazardous, but see under DRENCHING.

Injection usually involves less restraint than drenching, but with any injection there is the slight risk of broken-off needles and an abscess at the site. Neither of these disadvantages applies to anthelmintics which can be given in the feed – a most convenient method which normally should not involve extra cost.

Long-acting boluses which lodge in the reticulorumen, and contain anthelmintics released over a period, are available for cattle. One containing morantel tartrate introduced by Pfizer provides several months' activity, depending on the type of roundworm present. The bolus is presented in the form of a cylinder made from a laminated sheet that unrolls to release the drug. Schering-Plough use a 'pulse' system which releases a dose of the anthelmintic oxfendazole at intervals of about three weeks. Other slow-release boluses contain fenbendazole and ivermectin. Such boluses are usually for use only in animals over a certain weight and age.

Husk – drugs or vaccine? Parasitic bronchitis or verminous pneumonia (known colloquially as husk or hoose) is mainly thought of as a disease of young stock in their first season at grass. Recovery from an attack can be expected to result in a useful degree of immunity to the lungworm.

While the disease is a virtually permanent problem on many farms, and a risk on most others except where zero-grazing is practised, some farms do escape it altogether – at any rate for a time; but then one day it may suddenly appear out of the blue with devastating results. When this happens it may be cows in milk which suffer, losses to the farmer arising mainly as a result of a lowered milk yield but also of the extra feed needed for recuperation. There may be deaths, too, following symptoms common to those of an allergic condition. Indeed one shocked farmer, in his first encounter with husk, lost several dairy cows from oedema of the lungs – and his bull as well!

Especially on farms where the disease is a perennial problem, the farmer's own veterinary surgeon should be consulted concerning the use of vaccine as a preventative.

The vaccine consists of 3rd-stage larvae of the lungworm *Dictyocaulus viviparus* treated by exposure to a specified level of radiation by X-rays. This type of vaccine, the first anti-worm vaccine commercially available, was developed at the University of Glasgow.

The irradiated larvae are left with the ability to stimulate antibody production in the host animal, but are deprived of their power to cause disease. The vaccine is administered in 2 doses (each containing 1000 irradiated larvae) with a 4-week interval.

Certain precautions are necessary in using this vaccine. For example, calves should not be less than 2 months old when vaccinated, and should be healthy. They should not be exposed to natural infestation with lungworms until 2 weeks after their 2nd dose; and should be introduced gradually to heavily infested pasture. Vaccinated and non-vaccinated calves should not be mixed.

Where the vaccine is not used, reliance must be placed on anthelmintics. It will be readily appreciated, however, that once severe symptoms of husk have appeared, the most that any drug can do is rid the animal of its lungworms. A drug cannot undo the lung damage, clear the blocked airways, or neutralise any subsequent infection; and the coughing will persist after the worms are gone. Vaccine can prevent such a situation from arising. Drugs, however, are a valuable means of lungworm control. If long-acting anthelmintics are to be used as well as vaccine, it is advisable to take veterinary advice.

Liver-flukes Years ago the problem with drugs intended to kill liver-flukes was their toxicity. The margin between an effective medicinal dose and a lethal dose was sometimes very small, especially in an already seriously ill sheep.

The introduction of safer drugs still left the problem of resistance to them shown by immature flukes which, by their massive invasion of the liver, cause 'liver rot' and a high mortality in affected flocks. Later developments brought drugs effective against both immature and mature stages of the fluke. Closantel (Flukiver; Janssen) has a claimed activity of over 97 per cent on adult flukes, 91 per cent of 5-week-old and up to 73 per cent on 3 to 4-week-old flukes. Triclabendazole (Fasinex; Novartis), at the appropriate dose level, is claimed effective against flukes from 2 weeks old. Nitroxynil (Trodax; Merial) is also claimed active against immature and mature flooks.

Other drugs with specific action on adult liver-flukes include oxyclozanide (Zanil) and albendazole.

Drugs in use include the following:

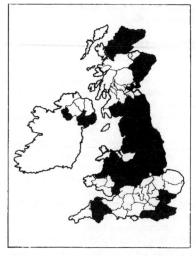

Areas where *Nematodirus* is more likely to be a problem.

Against PGE* worms in cattle and sheep	Against liver-flukes in cattle and sheep
albamectin	albendazole
albendazole	closantel
doramectin	clorsunol
febantel	oxyclonazide
fenbendazole	nitroxynil
ivermectin	triclabendazole
levamisole	
mebendazole	
moxidectin	
netobimin	
oxfendazole	
thiabenzadole	
thiophanate	
morantel tartrate†	

Against lungworms in cattle and sheep	Against worms in pigs‡
albamectin	flubendazole
albendazole	ivermectin
doramectin	levamisole
febantel	oxibendazole
fenbendazole	parbendazole
ivermectin (ivermectin only)	piperazine (ascarids
levamisole	tetramisole
mebendazole	thiophanate
moxidectin	thiabendazole
oxfendazole	
thiophanate	

*parasitic gastroenteritis
†a bolus, given by balling gun, for cattle only
‡given in the feed

(See also IVERMECTIN, for use against PGE worms and lungworms, in cattle and sheep; and against parasites of pigs.)

W

Dual-purpose and multi-purpose anthelmintics are available.

Parasitic Gastroenteritis For control of the parasites causing gastroenteritis, it is advised that calves should be dosed once with an efficient anthelmintic in mid-July and moved to pasture which has not been grazed that season by other cattle. The 1st pasture may then be grazed by animals not susceptible to parasitic gastroenteritis, such as adults.

The 2nd essential dose is in the autumn when cattle come in from grass. At housing, the wormer selected should be active against inhibited larvae, as well as maturing larvae.

Ostertagia worms, which are of considerable economic importance, are peculiar in that while most infective larvae living in the abomasum moult twice to become adults, some – especially perhaps those ingested by the calf during late summer and autumn – moult only once and remain as 4th-stage larvae in a dormant state. The larvae are resistant to many anthelmintics, but fenbendazole and albendazole are often effective. Later, they develop into adults causing a winter outbreak of gastroenteritis, with scouring and other digestive disturbance. Accordingly, it is usually recommended that calves be dosed in September and moved to 'clean' land.

Ivermectin (Ivomec) is effective against immature and even inhibited *Ostertagia* larvae; it can be given to both beef and dairy cattle, but not within 21 days of slaughter, or to dairy cows in milk, or within 28 days prior to calving. Three doses a year – in spring, summer, and autumn – are recommended to make the best use of this multi-purpose anthelmintic.

Ivermectin has no action against flukes or tapeworms, but is highly effective against all the important roundworms, both adult and larval forms.

Nematodirus in Lambs Lambs 4 to 6 weeks old and upwards may become severely ill as a result of infestation with *Nematodirus* worms. A well-recognised condition, it may show itself with dramatic suddenness in lowland flocks in spring, but – depending on locality and weather – the main period of incidence is probably the end of May until the 2nd week in July.

The worms, each about 1.70 cm (⅔ in) long, cause unthriftiness and poor liveweight gains; they may also cause a high mortality following 4 to 5 days' scouring resulting in a lethal loss of body fluids, i.e. dehydration. Where recovery

does take place, it is usually long-drawn-out and the animal may remain stunted.

These worms differ from others infesting the stomach/intestine of sheep in Britain in that their life-cycle takes about 12 months to complete, and the eggs require exposure to cold to initiate development; as infective larvae, they remain viable for only a few weeks. This fortunate fact offers an obvious method of control – the well-known rule, 'Never put lambs on the same pasture 2 years running.' On farms where it is impracticable to observe this rule, dosing 3 or 4 times with an appropriate anthelmintic is advisable. (See also 'CLEAN' PASTURE.)

Worms in Pigs Anthelmintics, complemented by good hygiene, play an essential part in maintaining health in the intensively managed pig unit. Pigs kept outdoors are vulnerable to worm infections.

Infestation by parasitic worms is best regarded as a herd problem, and the fact that anthelmintics are available in a palatable pellet form, or as a powder to mix in a meal, is a great help to the pig farmer. These are usually broad-spectrum drugs which will act against most of the species of worm normally found in the pig. Where a particular species has led to a severe health problem, an anthelmintic most effective against that species can be selected.

The main wormers used in pigs are febantel, fenbendazole, flubendazole, ivermectin, moxidectin and thiophanate.

Steering a middle course The farmer should, where necessary, seek veterinary advice on the spot, and aim to steer a middle course between inconveniently frequent dosing and high drug bills on the one hand, and tolerating poor liveweight gains, unthriftiness and even several deaths among his stock on the other hand. Internal parasites steal feed intended for their hosts, and often cause physical inury – sometimes very severe – as well.

Wounds

A wound may be defined as a breach of the continuity of the tissues of the body produced by violence. (See also under BRUISES.)

Varieties Wounds may be classified according to the nature of the effect produced, viz. incised, punctured, lacerated, and contused, and whether they are infected or contaminated.

Incised wounds are usually inflicted by some sharp instrument which leaves a clean cut; the tissues are simply divided without extensive damage to the surrounding parts. Bleeding from an incised wound is apt to be very profuse for a time, but it soon stops and is easily controlled.

Punctured wounds or stabs are inflicted with a pointed instrument or another animal's incisor or canine teeth. (A dose of tetanus antitoxin or toxoid is indicated in punctured wounds, especially in the horse, cow, and dog.)

Lacerated wounds are those in which great tearing takes place. They are usually very painful for a few days, and suppurate before they heal. They are usually followed by disfiguring scars when extensive.

Contused wounds are those accompanied by much bruising of the surrounding tissues, as in the case of blows from heavy sticks, kicks from shod horses, and from road accidents. There is usually little bleeding from the wound itself, but blood may be extravasated into the tissues. (See HAEMATOMA.)

Any one of these forms of wounds may become infected with pus-forming organisms, and develop into a suppurating, septic wound. (For other information, see under ACCIDENTS; FRACTURES; etc.)

First-aid treatment With a serious wound involving much haemorrhage, the first consideration must obviously be to stop the bleeding. (See BLEEDING – Bleeding, external; first aid for.)

With all wounds it is advisable to clip away the hair – preferably using blunt-pointed surgical scissors – first inserting a piece of cotton-wool moistened in antiseptic into the cavity of the wound (if large enough), so that the cut hair does not fall into the wound.

If the hair is not cut away, it is apt to become matted by blood or oozing serum, and the wound may later be found to be suppurating instead of healing. (What may look to the animal-owner like a normal healthy scab may be, in fact, a crust of blood, matted hair and dirt.)

The surface of the wound may be cleaned by gentle application of a piece of cotton-wool soaked in warm antiseptic such as diluted Dettol or Cetrimide, etc., or KY Jelly.

The wound may be covered in order to prevent contamination and infection by flies – in the case of farmyard animals – or to prevent excessive licking by dogs and cats. Before covering, a dry antiseptic dressing of sulfanilamide may be applied.

The covering of a wound cleaned and dressed as described should be removed daily so that the progress of healing can be observed, and cleaning repeated if necessary. An open, granulating wound should have a clean, pink appearance.

Large, gaping wounds may require suturing, which should be done by a veterinary surgeon, who should also always be consulted concerning the treatment of punctured and lacerated wounds.

Other points that should be noted are: (1) that stitches should be removed if they commence to suppurate, and in any case after being in position for a week, after which they serve no useful purpose; (2) that if pus burrows under the skin surrounding a wound, it must be given drainage by incision below the level of the most dependent burrowing or by drainage tubes; (3) that if the granulation tissue (i.e. 'proud flesh') rises to a higher level than the skin around, it may need professional treatment; and (4) that in cases of injury to parts such as the eyes, nostrils, lips, genital organs, feet, etc., it is essential to seek skilled advice rather than to persist in rule-of-thumb methods which often lead the enthusiastic amateur astray, and cause the animal unnecessary distress. (See also FRACTURES; GRANULATIONS; ULCER; ANTISEPTICS; ANTIBIOTICS; SULFONAMIDES; and under ACCIDENTS, INJURIES, and CORTISONE.)

Wounds, How They Heal

The blood forms clots; these consist of minute threads of fibrin, in which are enmeshed red blood cells and white blood cells. The threads of fibrin bridge the gap between the cut surfaces of the wound, at its base, forming a matrix, hardening into a scab under which tissue repair can take place. (See CLOTTING OF BLOOD.)

From the neighbouring blood capillaries come white cells (especially neutrophils) which engulf dirt, bacteria, etc. (See PHAGOCYTOSIS.) Monocytes arrive later, especially if the wound has become infected. They become macrophages which remove any disintegrated neutrophils and also bacteria. Meanwhile, the cells of the epidermis begin to multiply in order to restore the skin covering. (See LYMPHOCYTES.)

Healing of wounds may be delayed if the animal is being treated with corticosteroids.

Wry-Neck (Torticollis)

Wry-neck (torticollis), which occurs in foals, sheep and poultry particularly, is a lateral deviation of the head and neck to the right or left side of the body, usually so marked as to hinder or prevent foaling. The bones of the skull and neck are frequently distorted, and the ligaments, tendons, and muscles on the inside of the curve are shorter than those on the outside.

The condition may also be encountered in cattle.

When seen in rabbits, the cause may be middle ear infection.

W

X-Rays are high-energy radiation capable of passing through considerable thicknesses of many substances which are opaque to ordinary light, without undergoing material absorption, but other substances, even in very small thicknesses, are able to absorb the great majority of the rays: thus, flesh is very transparent; healthy bone is fairly opaque. Widely used for diagnostic imaging of internal body structures and (in human medicine) for radiotherapy.

Precautions Guard screens of lead glass, rubber impregnated with lead, or sheet lead, are used to protect the operators of radiographic apparatus, and precautions are necessary to shield the testes and ovaries of young persons and animals from the sterilising effects of the rays.

Detailed precautions are as follows:

1. Persons under 16 years must not take part in radiological procedures.

2. Fluoroscopy (imaging) or radiotherapy should not be carried out except under expert radiological guidance. Hand-held fluoroscopes must not be used in any circumstances.

3. Personnel radiation monitoring devices, such as film badges, must be worn by all persons who take part routinely in radiological procedures.

4. The animal should, if possible, be anaesthetised or tranquillised for radiography, and all persons should withdraw as far as practicable from the useful beam.

5. If it should be necessary to hold the animal for radiography, lead-protective gloves and aprons must be worn. Whenever possible, holding should be done by the owners, unless they are under 16 years or pregnant.

6. Persons should not expose any part of their bodies to the useful beam even when wearing protective clothing.

7. The useful beam should be restricted to the area being examined by means of a beam-limiting device.

Notes on protection against radiation will also be found in the British Veterinary Association's guide to the Health and Safety at Work Act.

Regulations In the UK, the Ionising Regulations 1985 require veterinary surgeons using X-ray equipment to notify their local Health and Safety Executive. Many veterinary practices now employ a radiation protection adviser to ensure compliance with the requirements of the regulations.

Radiography The production of a radiograph of the internal structure of a small animal is a comparatively simple matter once the difficulty of control is overcome. The animal is arranged upon the table in such a position as to allow the rays to pass down through the part and become registered upon a sensitive plate placed flat upon the table immediately below. The animal may lie upon its back, on one or the other side, or on its chest and abdomen with the legs pulled out from under it. To maintain this position it is always advisable to administer an anaesthetic. The discharge tube is best arranged immediately above the animal in such a position as to allow the rays to fall perpendicularly down through the body on to the plate. (For screening, the tube must be below the table, and the screen held or supported above the animal.) The period of exposure to the passage of the rays varies according to the tissues, to the type and power of the equipment, to the distance of the tube from the plate, and to whether or not an intensifying screen is used.

There are many conditions in which the actual extent of injury or disease can be accurately discovered by the use of X-rays, but the most important are diseases and injuries of bones. Fractures of the limb-bones are well shown, and their extent is better realised than is possible by palpation. Exostoses (overgrowths of bone) can also be clearly indicated, while tumour formation (usually sarcomatous) shows as a thinning and enlargement of the bone tissue. Where only one limb is affected it is advisable to arrange the animal so as to include a picture of the normal limb for comparison. Foreign bodies – especially needles, pins, nails, and other metallic substances – which have been swallowed are best shown by a profile view of the abdomen. Pieces of game bones (which are specially dense and show up well) can also be seen in the stomach or intestines, and are very often surrounded by gas, which, in the negative, appears as a dark shadow – the bone itself appearing light. Internal tumours can very often be diagnosed. They appear as more or less discrete pale areas in positions where a radiograph from a normal animal is denser under the same conditions of exposure, etc. Certain tumours can be made to show up well by giving the animal medicinal doses of a lead salt for a few days before taking the plate. Some of the

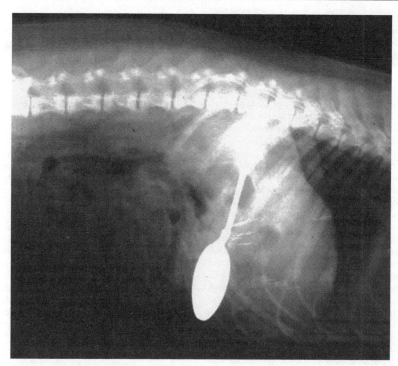

A teaspoon in the stomach of a cocker spaniel. The spoon was swallowed while the animal was being given cod-liver oil. (Reproduced by courtesy of Mr S. W. Douglas, University of Cambridge School of Veterinary Medicine.)

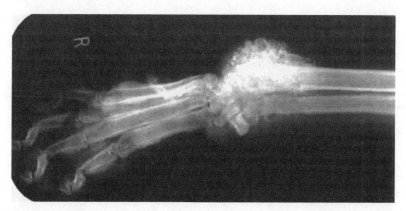

Radiography reveals that a painful swelling on the leg of a St Bernard is due to an osteosarcoma involving the radius. (Reproduced by courtesy of Mr S. W. Douglas, University of Cambridge School of Veterinary Medicine.)

lead becomes deposited in the tumour and intensifies the contrast. Where some displacement, stricture, or dilatation of the stomach or of part of the intestinal canal is suspected, the animal is given a feed or a draught containing an emulsion of bismuth or barium carbonate, or some other harmless metallic salt, or has some of the same material injected into the rectum. After waiting until the salt has become suitably distributed, a radiograph of the

X

abdomen is taken, and the outlines of those organs to which the salt has been carried by peristalsis, can be made out as pale areas in the negatives.

Other conditions in which X-rays are useful are as follows: stones in the kidney, urinary or gall-bladder; dilatation of a portion of a lung; and pleurisy.

Portable X-ray apparatus is available for use in, for example, examining the lower limbs of a horse at the stable.

Computed tomography A sophisticated and effective method of visualising the interior of the body, this has revolutionised radiography. A focused electronic imaging scanner is used to build up, by a series of consecutive exposures, a picture of an organ or specific area. The resulting image is enhanced by computer analysis and viewed on a visual display unit (VDU) which shows a clear picture without the the the superimposition of other body tissues which surround the targeted area. In the apparatus, whose British development was by Godfrey Hounsfield FRS, crystal detectors are used in place of the film in a normal X-ray system.

Radiotherapy X-ray therapy has been applied to a limited extent in the treatment of certain tumours in the dog.

Xanthosis
Xanthosis is a yellowish-brown pigmentation of meat, generally affecting the heart and the tongue. It gives the meat an objectionable colour, but is quite harmless.

Xenophthalmia
Inflammation of the eye caused by a foreign body.

Xerophthalmia
A disease of the eye associated with a vitamin A deficiency. There is thickening and cloudiness of the conjunctiva and cornea; blindness may result.

Xylazine
A sedative used to render animals easier to handle, it is widely used in dogs, cats, horses, farm livestock, and zoo animals. It is also used for pre-anaesthetic medication and for general anaesthesia in combination with ketamine.

Xylazine increases blood glucose levels and urine output. Side-effects may include bradycardia, slower breathing, and lowered blood pressure. In cattle tolazoline has been used as a xylazine antagonist.

X

Yarded Cattle

Before yarding cattle in the autumn, it is wise to make a gradual change from sugar-poor autumn pasture to things like roots; otherwise digestive upsets are likely to occur.

Similarly, in spring it is a mistake to turn calves straight out on to grass. This means a sudden change from protein-poor food to the rich protein of the early bite, and the resulting effect upon the rumen will set them back. It is best to get them out before there is much grass for a few hours each day; let them have hay and shelter at night to protect them from sudden changes of weather. Hypomagnesaemia, too, is far less likely under these circumstances. (See also HOUSING OF ANIMALS.)

Boss cows can be a nuisance in yards, but the provision of yokes for feeding overcomes the main diffculty.

When self-feeding of silage is practised, precautions are necessary in order to prevent foot troubles. (See SILAGE.)

Yarded animals fed on cereals, sugarbeet pulp, straw, and hay – but with little or no greenstuff – may suffer from xerophthalmia and go blind as a result of a vitamin A deficiency.

Yawning

Yawning is an important sign of KIMBERLEY HORSE DISEASE; it may also be seen in cases of LABURNUM POISONING and NARCOLEPSY.

Yeast

Yeast is a valuable source of vitamin B, but should not be fed in excessive amounts to pigs or it may give rise to rickets unless adequate vitamin D is simultaneously available. Yeast has proved successful in the treatment of tropical ulcers in humans, and success has been reported in a limited number of cases in horses in the tropics. The human patients were mostly those whose diet was deficient in vitamin B, a deficiency further increased by sweating. The yeast was applied directly to the ulcer, and a small quantity given internally also.

Yeasts

Yeasts sometimes cause enteritis, and are important in some cases of refractory otitis in the dog. (See FUNGAL DISEASES.)

Yellow Fat Disease of Cats

(see STEATITIS)

Yellow Fever

A viral disease affecting man and other vertebrates, principally monkeys, in large areas of tropical America and Africa. There are 2 known cycles of transmission, the urban and jungle cycles. In the urban cycle, man is the reservoir and *Aedes aegypti* probably the only vector. This cycle from man to *A. aegypti* to man is now virtually unknown in the Americas owing to efforts to eradicate the vector, but it is still common in Africa.

The jungle cycle has a primate reservoir maintained by various mosquitoes. Movement of virus from the monkey-mosquito-monkey cycle into man is accidental, and is the result of human penetration into jungle where the disease is endemic.

The causative organism is classified as a flavivirus.

Yelt

A female pig intended for breeding, up to the time that she has her 1st litter.

Yersiniosis

Infection with *Yersinia pseudotuberculosis* or with *Y. enterocolitica*.

Up to 1960, states WHO, only the former organism was regularly isolated in man and animals in Europe; but since then most of the isolations have been of *Y. enterocolitica*.

'Pseudotuberculosis' in the early 1990s was still occasionally found in rodents and birds, especially in France and the UK, and is a zoonosis. People may become infected through pets such as guinea pigs, hamsters, and cats, all of which may have a subclinical infection only but excrete *Y. pseudotuberculosis*.

An investigation in Invermay, New Zealand, resulted in *Y. pseudotuberculosis* being isolated from 675 apparently healthy small mammals and birds. In descending order of prevalence were feral cats (27.8 per cent), Norway rats (8.6 per cent), mice, hares, rabbits, ducks, sparrows, seagulls and starlings.

In New Zealand, yersiniosis has also emerged as a serious disease of farmed red deer. It appears to be triggered off by stress, and most cases occur during the winter.

Cats (which are liable to become infected by their prey) may also show clinical symptoms: loss of appetite, vomiting and diarrhoea. Also loss of weight.

Pheasants Yersiniosis is an important cause of death of these birds in the UK.

Yersinia enterocolitica **infection** in Europe was first found in hares, in outbreaks of disease on chinchilla farms, in monkeys in zoos, and in guinea pigs. There may be enteritis and other lesions, but symptomless carriers have been found among all the farmyard mammals and birds.

Occasionally *Y. enterocolitica* has been isolated from cases of mastitis in cows, endocarditis in bulls, and septicaemia in pigs. In cattle, the antibody produced may be difficult to differentiate from that produced by *Brucella abortus.*

Camels, foxes, and fleas may also carry the organism.

Public health *Yersinia enterocolitica* infection is not regarded as a genuine zoonosis by WHO. Person-to-person infection occurs, and also infection from soil-contaminated vegetables. The human illness is characterised by enteritis, and is a cause of diarrhoea, although less important than salmonella and campylobacter. Ileitis may be accompanied by acute pain, suggestive of appendicitis. A mesenteric adenitis is also seen, and sometimes polyarthritis, deep abscesses, eye lesions, and occasionally septicaemia.

In the UK in 1984, 250 cases were reported. Outbreaks in North America have been linked to raw milk. (For *Y. pestis see* BUBONIC PLAGUE, which can occur in cats and dogs in subclinical form.)

Yew Poisoning

All varieties of the British yew trees are poisonous, but owing to its more frequent cultivation, the common yew (*Taxus baccata*) is most often responsible for outbreaks of poisoning among animals. The Irish yew (*T. baccata* var.

fastigiata) and the yellow yew appear to contain less of the poisonous alkaloid, which is called taxine. The bark, leaves and seeds all contain it. The older dark leaves are more dangerous than the fresh green young shoots, which cattle have been known to eat in small amounts without harm. Cases of poisoning have been noted among horses, donkeys, mules, cattle, sheep, goats, pigs, deer, rabbits, and even pheasants, but the majority of cases occur in young store cattle and in dairy cows which have access to the shrubberies, graveyards, etc., where yew trees are most common.

Signs In many cases cattle drop dead without showing any preliminary symptoms at all. They may fall while cudding almost as suddenly as if shot. In other cases where less has been eaten, excitement and paresis may be seen.

Treatment Antidotes are as for alkaloids. If time allows, rumenotomy may be carried out.

Yolk Sac Infection
(see OMPHALITIS OF BIRDS)

Yorkshire Terrier
A long-haired, black-and-tan coloured toy dog. The breed is prone to tracheal collapse caused by a cartilage defect that may or may not be inherited. Patellar luxation is inherited as a recessive trait.

Yorkshire Boarding
Vertically arranged boards with a gap between each, used for partial cladding of a livestock building. It is a very useful means of improving ventilation and avoiding condensation, thereby reducing the risk or incidence of bronchitis and pneumonia in housed livestock.

Zearalenone

An oestrogenic toxin from the fungus *Fusarium graminearum* of standing corn. The toxin has caused abortion in sows, and possibly a splayleg condition in piglets.

Zebu

Bos indicus, the cattle of India, East and West Africa, and Southeast Asia. The American name is Brahman; in South Africa, the Afrikaner.

Zero-Grazing

Taking cut fodder to yarded cattle, or to cattle in exercise paddocks. Zero-grazing has a place on heavy land, with high stocking rates and large herds. It obviates poaching and the spoiling of grass, and a given acreage zero-grazed can provide more grass than if grazed. It means, however, cutting grass every day, and mechanical failures can upset the system. It is not yet considered economic for sheep.

Zinc (Zn)

Zinc (Zn) is a trace element, and a deficiency has occurred in pigs. (See PARAKERATOSIS.) A zinc supplement to prevent or correct this condition must be used with care, as 1000 parts per million can cause poisoning. It seems that a high calcium intake by pigs aggravates a zinc deficiency.

A zinc deficiency may also occur in dogs, especially in those fed largely on flaked maize or 'loose cereal-based diets'. Signs include a predisposition to skin infections, a poor coat, localised alopecia, and hardening of the skin in places. Response to a zinc supplement is usually quick. (See SHEEPDOGS.)

A zinc supplement has been used to protect sheep against facial eczema due to ingestion of the mycotoxin sporidesmin.

External uses Zinc oxide is an ingredient of ointments; the carbonate an ingredient of calamine lotion used for moist eczema, etc. The sulphate in weak solution has been used in wound treatment and in eye lotions; the chloride – a caustic – to repress granulations.

Zinc Bacitracin

An antibiotic formerly used as a feed additive to improve growth rate in most farm animals and egg production in poultry. (See ADDITIVES.)

Zinc Poisoning

Chronic zinc poisoning has been reported in a dairy herd as a result of contaminated drinking water – caused by interaction between copper pipes and newly galvanised tanks. The main symptom was chronic constipation throughout the herd, and a diminished yield from the cows in milk.

Fatal zinc poisoning has occurred in dairy cattle fed on dairy nuts to which zinc oxide has been added instead of magnesium oxide. The first death occurred after 3 weeks.

Zinc-responsive skin disease The most common cause of this is the feeding of soya or cereal-based diets – with little or no meat, which is rich in zinc. Some dogs may have an inherent defect which limits zinc absorption.

Signs A dull, harsh coat; sometimes with whitish crusts on the skin.

Zondek-Ascheim Test

(see PREGNANCY DIAGNOSIS)

Zoo Licensing Act 1981

The Zoo Licensing Act 1981 is intended to promote animal welfare and public safety at zoos. It covers any collection of wild animals (including mammals, birds, reptiles, fish, and insects) in Britain to which the public has access for more than 7 days in any 12-month period; but exempts pet shops and circuses, as these are covered by the Pet Animals Act 1951 and the Performing Animals (Registration) Act 1952.

Of 150 zoos inspected following the passing of the Act, only 5 were refused a licence; and in those cases it was public-safety considerations rather than the quality of animal care which brought about the refusal.

Zoonoses

Diseases communicable between animals and man. Information about them will be found under the following headings: ARIZONA INFECTION; BABESIA – Babesiosis; ANTHRAX; B VIRUS (from monkeys); BRUCELLOSIS; CAT-SCRATCH FEVER; CHAGAS DISEASE; EQUINE ENCEPHALITIS; EQUINE INFECTIOUS ANAEMIA; FOOT-AND-MOUTH DISEASE (very rare in human beings); GLANDERS; HYDATID DISEASE; LEPTOSPIROSIS; LISTERIOSIS; LIVER-FLUKES; LOUPING-ILL; LYME DISEASE; LYMPHOCYTIC CHORIOMENINGITIS (from mice); NEWCASTLE DISEASE; ORNITHOSIS; ORF; PASTEURELLOSIS; Q FEVER; RABIES; RATBITE FEVER; RIFT VALLEY FEVER; RINGWORM; ROCKY MOUNTAIN FEVER; RUSSIAN SPRING-SUMMER VIRUS; SALMONELLOSIS; SCABIES; SCHISTOSOMI-

ASIS; TAPEWORMS; TICK-BITE FEVER; TICK PARAL-
YSIS; TOXOCARA; TOXOPLASMOSIS; TRICHINOSIS;
TUBERCULOSIS; TULARAEMIA; VESICULAR STOM-
ATITIS; MARBURG DISEASE; WESSELBRON DIS-
EASE; YERSINIOSIS; YELLOW FEVER; SWINE VESIC-
ULAR DISEASE; PORCINE STREPTOCOCCAL
MENINGITIS; ROTAVIRUS; LASSA FEVER; BOVINE
ENCEPHALOMYELITIS; LEISHMANIASIS; BUBONIC
PLAGUE; ENCEPHALOMYOCARDITIS.)

It should be added that typhus and plague
may be transmitted, by flea-bite, from rats; and,
in jungle areas, yellow fever, by mosquito-
bite, from monkeys. (See also under RODENTS;
MONKEYS; INFLUENZA.)

Among skin diseases, the parasite of follicular mange may occasionally infest the human
eyelid. Among eye infections, INFECTIOUS
BOVINE KERATOCONJUNCTIVITIS should be
mentioned. Human enteritis has followed contact with sheep affected with campylobacter
abortion.

(See also BIRD-FANCIER'S LUNG; MELIOIDOSIS;
CAMPYLOBACTER INFECTIONS; CHLAMYDIA;
PSITTACOSIS; BOUTONNEUSE FEVER; LEISHMA-
NIA; HANTAVIRUS; TICK-BORNE ENCEPHALITIS;
EHRLICHIA CANIS; ABORTION, ENZOOTIC.)

Zoonoses in UK Veterinarians

A questionnaire was distributed to 1717 members of veterinary and support staff of the
Ministry of Agriculture and the Institute for
Research on Animal Diseases; 1625 (95 per
cent) responded, comprising 563 veterinary
surgeons, 690 scientific staff and 372 technical
support staff. A total of 1057 (61.5 per cent)
had apparently not suffered any zoonotic infection. Animal ringworm was the commonest
reported zoonosis. The incidences of ringworm,
brucellosis and Newcastle disease were higher
in the veterinary and support staff than in the
laboratory workers. In contrast, ornithosis,
salmonellosis and Q fever occurred at least as
often in the laboratory staff. Fourteen people
developed tuberculosis during their employment, although only 1 was caused by
Mycobacterium bovis. The veterinarians reported 441 injuries that resulted from accidents at
work; 397 (71 per cent) of these involved ani-
mal-handling. The comparable figures for laboratory workers and technical staff were 329 and
103 (15 per cent) and 198 and 179 (42 per
cent) respectively.

Zoonoses Orders 1988 & 1989

These include measures intended to reduce
the risk to humans of salmonella and brucella
infections of animal origin. The 1989 Order
recognises bovine spongiform encephalopathy
as a zoonotic disease.

Zootechny

Animal management.

Zygoma

Zygoma is the bridge of bone which runs from
near the base of the ear to the lower posterior
part of the eye-socket. It protects the side of
the bony orbit, forms part of the support of the
outside of the joint of the lower jaw with the
rest of the head, and serves as a base of attachment for part of the strong masseter muscle
which closes the mouth and is important in the
chewing of the food. The zygomatic arch
(another name for the zygoma) is formed by
projections from the temporal, zygomatic, and
maxillary bones.

Zygote

The body that results from the fertilisation of
an egg cell by a sperm.

Z